Essentials of
Basic Nursing Procedures

(As per the New Revised INC Syllabus for Nursing Students)

Second Edition

CP Thresyamma

(Ex Nursing Educator & Administrator)

Edited & Reviewed by
Vasantha Chitra PhD (MSN)

Foreword
BS Balachandran

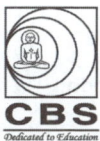

CBS
Dedicated to Education

CBS Publishers & Distributors Pvt Ltd

• New Delhi • Bengaluru • Chennai • Kochi • Kolkata • Mumbai
• Hyderabad • Nagpur • Patna • Pune • Vijayawada

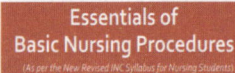

Essentials of Basic Nursing Procedures
(As per the New Revised INC Syllabus for Nursing Students)

ISBN: 978-81-945234-7-5

Second Edition: 2020-2021

Published by **Satish Kumar Jain** and produced by **Varun Jain** for

CBS Publishers & Distributors Pvt Ltd
4819/XI Prahlad Street, 24 Ansari Road, Daryaganj, New Delhi 110 002, India.
Ph: +91-11-23289259, 23266861, 23266867   Website: www.cbspd.com
Fax: 011-23243014
e-mail: delhi@cbspd.com; cbspubs@airtelmail.in.

Corporate Office: 204 FIE, Industrial Area, Patparganj, Delhi 110 092
Ph: +91-11-4934 4934   Fax: 4934 4935
e-mail: feedback@cbspd.com; bhupesharora@cbspd.com

Branches

- **Bengaluru:** Seema House 2975, 17th Cross, K.R. Road, Banasankari 2nd Stage, Bengaluru 560 070, Karnataka
  Ph: +91-80-26771678/79   Fax: +91-80-26771680   e-mail: bangalore@cbspd.com
- **Chennai:** 7, Subbaraya Street, Shenoy Nagar, Chennai 600 030, Tamil Nadu
  Ph: +91-44-26680620, 26681266   Fax: +91-44-42032115   e-mail: chennai@cbspd.com
- **Kochi:** 68/1534, 35, 36-Power House Road, Opp. KSEB, Cochin-682018, Kochi, Kerala
  Ph: +91-484-4059061-65   Fax: +91-484-4059065   e-mail: kochi@cbspd.com
- **Kolkata:** 6/B, Ground Floor, Rameswar Shaw Road, Kolkata-700 014, West Bengal
  Ph: +91-33-22891126, 22891127, 22891128   e-mail: kolkata@cbspd.com
- **Mumbai:** 83-C, Dr E Moses Road, Worli, Mumbai-400018, Maharashtra
  Ph: +91-22-24902340/41   Fax: +91-22-24902342   e-mail: mumbai@cbspd.com

Representatives

- **Hyderabad**   +91-9885175004
- **Pune**   +91-9623451994
- **Patna**   +91-9334159340
- **Vijayawada**   +91-9000660880

Printed at : Goyal Offset Works Pvt. Ltd. Haryana (INDIA)

Foreword

The book namely "Essentials of Basic Nursing Procedures" is a suitable and apt tool for professional and student nurses to keep abreast with new knowledge and techniques according to the continually advancing Preventive and Curative Aspects of Nursing.

Nursing is not an isolated or separate compartment of knowledge. It is an amalgamation of many subjects. As such, this comprehensive text covers almost all the subjects required to prepare an efficient nurse in our Indian culture to meet the basic needs of a patient in homes, small hospitals as well as in large hospitals.

The knowledge required from other medical subjects for performing proper healthcare is integrated in the book. This feature is an added credit. The excellent organization of the contents of the book gives an image of the ideas arising from the contemplation of the author.

The strenuous efforts of the author deserves real appreciation and I recommend that all the professional and student nurses should keep a copy of this book with them for their studies as well as for their future.

BS Balachandran
General Secretary
Bharat Sevak Samaj
Thiruvananthapuram

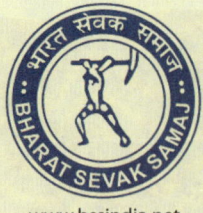

Founder President Pandit Jawaharlal Nehru

BHARAT SEVAK SAMAJ

National Development Agency, Promoted by Government of India
Founder Chairman: Bharat Ratna Gulzarilal Nanda
All India Chairman: M Swami Harinarayananand

Central Programme Office
Sadbhavana Bhavan, Brahmins Colony, PO, Kowdiar, Thiruvananthapuram,
Kerala 695003, India

www.bssindia.net

Phone: 0471 2433845, 0471 2434301, Fax: 0471 2431664
E-Mail: info@bharatsevaksamaj.org | bss.headoffice@gmail.com

TO WHOMSOEVER IT MAY CONCERN

This is to certify that the Book **"Essentials of Basic Nursing Procedures"** Written by Mrs CP Thresyamma is being recognized by Bharat Sevak Samaj as the study material for First Aid and Practical Nursing Course.

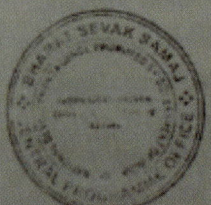

DIRECTOR

11/7/06

FLORENCE NIGHTINGALE PLEDGE

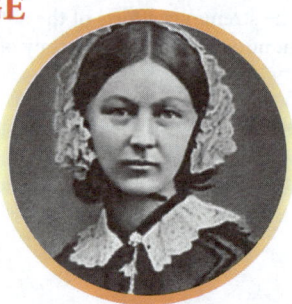

I solemnly pledge myself before God and this assembly to practise my profession faithfully. I will not take or knowingly administer any harmful drug. I will do all in my power to elevate the standard of my profession and will hold in confidence all personal matters committed to, my keeping and all family affairs, coming to my knowledge in the practice of my calling. With loyalty, I will devote myself to the welfare of those committed to my care.

Preface

Advancement in Science and Technology has placed more challenges and demands on nurses as guardian angels of health. In the present hospital settings, nurses need to play multiple roles and they have to deal with sophisticated modern technologies and equipment. Therefore, they need to develop adequate scientific knowledge, technical skill and positive attitude toward care giving, which are very essential for professional success and excellence.

Most of the available books, dealing with principles and practice of nursing are written by foreign authors and they suited for their culture and hospital settings. Moreover, these books are too costly and bulky. They are not simple enough to be effectively used in the present clinical settings of our country. Our country is in a progressive and hopeful stage of self-sufficiency now and trying its accomplishments in the near future. Therefore, a need was felt to present practical knowledge of nursing in easy language and that too in economical range.

During my very long service in medical department as Nursing Educator & Administrator, there were so many personal bitter experiences at the hospital wards in earlier periods, for practising and teaching nursing, due to the lack of proper books suited to our culture and environment. In this regard, an old saying that "Necessity is the mother of invention" is so meaningful. Hence, I felt the need of simple books on nursing for nurses of our hospitals. As per the philosophy, the OT functions are based on knowledge of all the subjects taught in nursing. This knowledge is integrated, reflected and effective in the scenario when the nurse interacts with the patients and doing the nursing procedures. With these facts in view and with the confidence that much of these troubles are surmountable, I was motivated to prepare a suitable book for the nursing procedures.

Under the valuable guidance of my respected teacher Miss Lucy Peters (Late) First Director of College of Nursing Thiruvananthapuram, the contents of this book were compiled from many other books and the procedures were experimented and arranged by trial and error in the Medical College Hospital, Kottayam with the generous help of the Nursing Leaders of that time. By the strenuous efforts over a long period, my first book namely "Fundamentals of Nursing Procedure Manual for General Nursing Course" was released in June 1990. It was approved and accepted by the Kerala Nurse's and Midwive's Council, Thiruvananthapuram and Registrar, for teaching in General Nursing Schools. Following this event, I prepared a few more books in other subjects on nursing, which are also widely used in the nursing field and my attempts became fruitful. I am sure that my books are suited to meet the challenging needs of the healthcare providers in the present clinical scene in India and I hope that the book *Essentials of Basic Nursing Procedures, 2nd Edition* will stimulate the learners, to refer more books too, to enrich and equip in the theme.

In 2003, I wrote a Malayalam Book in Nursing namely "Athurasusrusha" which is welcomed by all, especially by Practical Nursing Schools. As per the request of experts in this field, this book namely "Essentials of Basic Nursing Procedure" is prepared. This is exclusively for Student and Professional Nurses and almost a translation of "Athurasusrusha" with an addition of some extremely essential topics from Psychology, Sociology and First Aid as salient features.

The first edition of this book came in 2009. And now the second edition is before you with a lot of hard work put by Dr Vasantha Chitra, who has updated this book according to the new revised INC syllabus for nursing students.

Finally, I request the users of this book to inform me about their criticisms, suggestions and corrections, if any, for further improvements. Thanking the Almighty with great pleasure.

CP Thresyamma

Acknowledgments

It is my sincere hope that this textbook *Essentials of Basic Nursing Procedures, 2nd Edition* will be welcomed by Nursing Educators and Nursing Students, equally.

Before concluding my words, I remember with gratitude the Director, President and Committee Members of J.S.S. and B.S.S. for motivating and propelling me, accepting the course outline prepared by me, and recommending this book to their schools. Moreover, I express my sincere thanks to the leaders, experts, well-wishers and family, for their timely help and encouragements given to me directly and indirectly, during the strenuous work and accomplishing this venture. Although their names are not mentioned here, I am indebted to each and everyone of them.

I am thankful to Dr Vasantha Chitra for her contribution as a Reviewer & Editor of this book.

I would like to thank **Mr Satish Kumar Jain** (Chairman) and **Mr Varun Jain** (Managing Director), M/s CBS Publishers and Distributors Pvt Ltd for providing me the platform in bringing out the book. I have no words to describe the role, efforts, inputs and initiatives undertaken by **Mr Bhupesh Arora,** (Vice President – Publishing & Marketing, PGMEE and Nursing Division) for helping and motivating me.

I sincerely thank the entire CBS team for bringing out the book with utmost care and attractive presentation. I thank Ms Nitasha Arora (Production Head & Content Strategist), Dr Anju Dhir (Project Manager & Senior Scientific Coordinator), Mr Shivendu Bhushan Pandey (Senior Editor), Mr Ashutosh Pathak (Senior Proof Reader) and all the production team members Mr Prakash Gaur, Mr Phool Kumar, Mr Bunty Kashyap, Mr Chaman Lal, Mr Chander Mani, Ms Manorama Gupta, Ms Babita Verma, Mr Raju Sharma, Mr Manoj Chaudhary, Mr Vikram Chaudhary, Mr Arun Kumar and Mr Rahul Negi for devoting laborious hours in designing and typesetting of the book.

Finally, I request the users of this book to inform me their criticisms, suggestions and corrections, if any, for further improvements. Thanking the Almighty with great pleasure.

Special Features of the Book

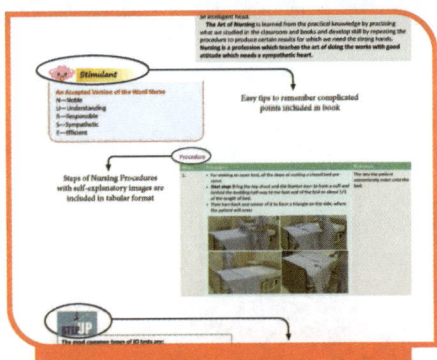

Includes up to 100 procedures of all 7 basic subjects/new procedures have been added in the 2nd edition as per the new revised INC syllabus.

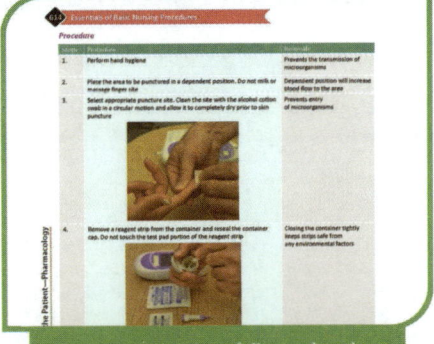

Step-wise presentation of all procedures have been given for easy implementation in clinical practices.

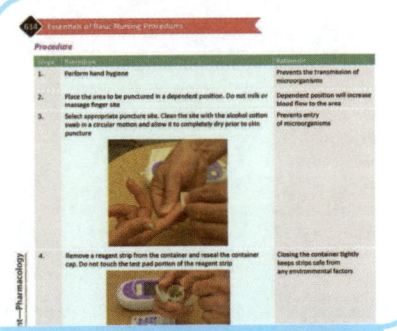

Rationale of all the procedural steps are given in separate column to correlate their importance with the relevant procedure.

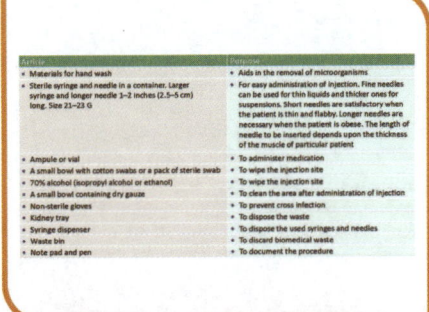

Article trays have been provided for all procedures to acquaint the young nurses with the equipments required for performing the procedure.

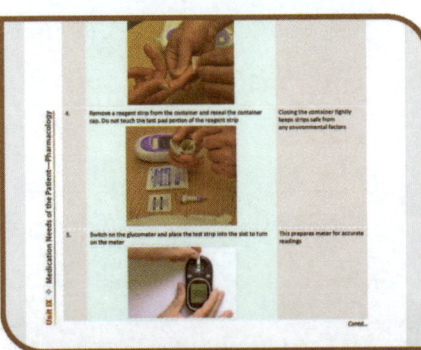

Fully colored diagrams and real-time photographs of performing procedures have been included wherever relevant.

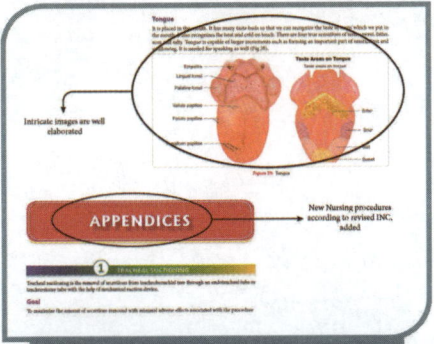

15 Appendices have been added covering all new basic procedures according to new revised INC syllabus.

Contents

PART 1   NURSING FOUNDATION

PART 2   ANATOMY AND PHYSIOLOGY

PART 3   MICROBIOLOGY

PART 4   PSYCHOLOGY

PART 5   SOCIOLOGY

PART 6   FIRST AID IN EMERGENCIES

PART 7   NUTRITION

APPENDICES

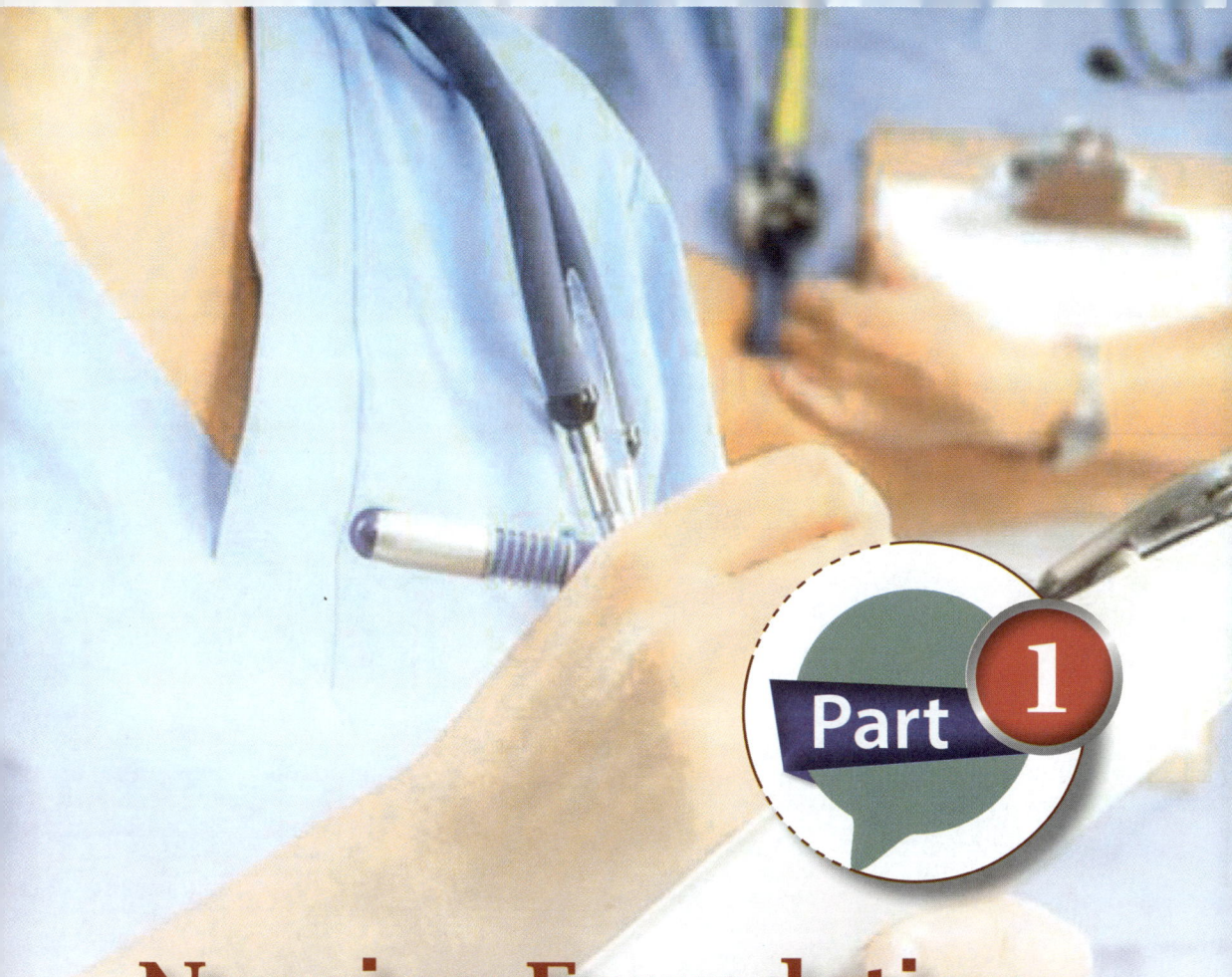

Nursing Foundation

Part Outline

Introduction to Nursing

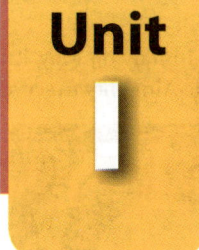

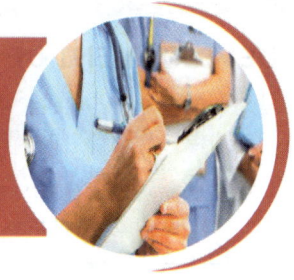

A GENERAL VIEW

As a first impression, the word nursing represents the care given to a patient or looking after sick person. But the real expectation of nursing is not only giving care to the patient for a temporary relief, cure or well-being, but also the restoration and improvement of health and prevention of disease. By doing such a service, the client gets physical and mental comfort along with the maximum effect of the treatment given by the physician. The patient should be considered as a valuable individual with body and mind and we should remember that the disease of the body will affect the mind and the illness of the mind will affect the body. It is because of this understanding, that any procedure being performed on/for the patient should be done only with his/her knowledge about the procedure, his/her consent and cooperation if patient is conscious, to achieve maximum effect and satisfaction. Therefore, a nurse should provide care of not only the mind but also the body of normal and abnormal/diseased human beings.

The word 'nurse' comes from the Latin word 'nutire' which means nursing mother 'that nourishes, fosters and protects'. We find in the dictionary that 'Nursing' has a wide range of meanings, like 'to nourish', 'to sustain' and 'to give curative care and treatment to sick and infirm'.

ORIGIN OF NURSING

Nursing in its simplest form has been practiced since the time immemorial. Mothers are the first practitioners of the art of nursing and women have always taken care of children, the aged and the sick. From old days to the modern times, we find women protecting children and caring for the sick and old members of the family. The impulse to serve is the basis on which the spirit of nursing has been fostered through the ages.

Throughout the history of civilization, it has been observed that the family is the smallest unit in the society or a living group. It became the duty of the women of the family to care for the young and helpless and to look after the sick. So, for many years the nursing was carried on only inside the family or a group. Women also offered their services to the neighbors during illness. Later, the meaning extended to cover the care of sick and suffering people of all ages and in helpless conditions of human beings. Simple procedures, like the application of cold compress to the forehead, applying pressure over a bleeding injury, etc. were adopted in olden times.

As society became highly organized and religious, the vocational groups shared this responsibility with the family members. With different times and conditions, the needs of the humanity changed. Nursing developed as broader interests and functions, out of the same impulse to serve. This development explained the need for nursing care of the patient's mind and body as a whole, and the care of the patient's environment—physical as well as social, health education and health services to the individual, family and society for the prevention of disease and promotion of health.

DEVELOPMENT OF MODERN NURSING

Miss Florence Nightingale is the founder of modern professional nursing. She was born in Italy on May 12, 1820. Right from her childhood she had a feeling of an inner call that she was created by the Almighty to serve humanity and she directed her life in such a way to fulfill the 'Mission of Mercy. From the period 1854–1856, during the Crimean war, she looked after the wounded soldiers at Crimea. Her services were accepted and appreciated by the people and rulers of that period. She proved the need of education, developed theories of nursing practice and hygienic techniques, and emphasized the preparation of nurses to care the sick and wounded to protect and promote the health of the individuals and families. Her performances demonstrated that leadership is needed to train the nurses to be efficient workers in the field of healthcare (Fig. 1).

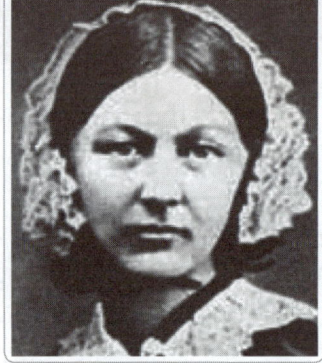

Figure 1: Miss Florence Nightingale

During her services in the Crimean War, she used to walk with a lamp in her hand, among the wounded soldiers at night and because of this, she is named as 'Lady with the Lamp'. She collected a number of educated ladies from Europe and started the first Nursing School at St Thomas Hospital, London in 1860, under the name as "The Nightingale School of Nursing, St Thomas Hospital London". She chalked out the rules and regulations, and the curriculum for the school. A good number of women were trained and they were sent to other countries to start nursing schools. In India, the first Schools for Midwives were started in 19th Century in Madras and Calcutta by Europeans and Anglo Indians, which later evolved as nursing schools and colleges. Thus nursing flourished as a profession of educated people, noble service and a career avenue having a global glitter.

On August 13, 1910, Florence Nightingale died peacefully in her sleep. In respect of her, May 12th, the birthday of Florence Nightingale, is celebrated as 'International Nurses Day' throughout the world. Her humanitarian services are followed and remembered by all.

In Kerala, the first Nursing School was started in 1942 with two-year training for general nursing at Thiruvananthapuram and in 1945 it was upgraded as four-year General Nursing and Midwifery course. Post-Basic BSc Nursing course was started at Thiruvananthapuram in 1963, later it was stopped and was restarted as Basic BSc Nursing Training, in college of nursing. The number of General Nursing Schools, Junior Public Health Nursing Training (JPHNT) Schools and Colleges increased in the State. Now, there are many JPHNT Schools, general nursing schools and colleges of nursing in Kerala.

In our country, especially in Kerala, opportunities are available for:
- General Nursing and Midwifery (GNM)
- Basic BSc in Nursing [BSc (N)]
- Post Basic BSc in Nursing [PBSc (N)]
- MSc in Nursing [MSc (N)]
- MPhil in Nursing [MPhil (N)]
- PhD in Nursing [PhD (N)]

CONCEPTS OF NURSING

The word, 'concept' means an 'idea or general notion'. Therefore, concept of nursing means the idea or mental image of nursing. Concept formation results out of better understanding or the knowledge of nursing. Everybody has his/her own concepts regarding nursing based upon his/her understanding of the profession.

It is important to have a clear concept of one's own profession to perform the duties and responsibilities efficiently because one's own concepts will control his/her action and attitude toward the profession. Concepts are stepping stones by which theories are made. According to some eminent experts, "Nursing is a science, an art and a vocation for caring the patient, which requires head, hand and heart."

Florence Nightingale, the founder of modern nursing had a clear concept of nursing. According to her opinion, "nursing is to bring the healthy and those who are suffering from disease, to a condition for nature to act for preserving health, preventing disease and injury, to cure disease and to restore health".

DEFINITIONS OF NURSING

■ Nursing has been defined in many ways. The expansion of scientific knowledge and the changes in the social customs alter definitions of nursing and these definitions designed for one age won't fit into another age. Considering many aspects of Modern Nursing, we can define nursing as follows:

● Nursing is a science, art and a profession by which we render service to human beings to help them regain or keep a normal state of body and mind and when it's not possible to accomplish this, we help humans in getting relief from physical pain, mental anxiety or spiritual discomfort, for a peaceful death.

● Another definition for nursing accepted by the International Council of Nurses (ICN) is that "Nursing encompasses autonomous and collaborative care of individuals of all ages, families, groups and communities, sick or well and in all settings. Nursing includes the promotion of health, prevention of illness, and the care of ill, disabled and dying people. Advocacy, promotion of a safe environment, research, participation in shaping health policy and in patient and health systems management, and education are also key nursing roles (ICN, 2002)."

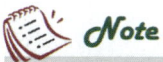 *Note*

3 H's in Nursing:
 i. H – Head
 ii. H – Hands
 iii. H – Heart

   The science of nursing is learned by the theory classes from the classroom and books and the student gets the knowledge of nursing for which we need an intelligent head.

   The Art of Nursing is learned from the practical knowledge by practicing what we studied in the classroom and books and develop skill by repeating the procedure to produce certain results for which we need the strong hands. **Nursing is a profession which teaches the art of doing the works with good attitude which needs a sympathetic heart.**

The Requirements to Become a Nurse

■ **Basic requirements:** Intelligent head, strong hands and a sympathetic heart.
■ **General education:** As prescribed by the governing board.
■ **Professional education:** This training is given in the nursing school.

A professional nurse is a graduate of a recognized nursing school, who has met the requirements for a Registered Nurse in a state in which he/she is licensed to practice.

Unit I ❖ Introduction to Nursing

NURSING—A PROFESSIONAL SERVICE

Nursing is a professional service (Fig. 2).

Goals of Nursing

The ultimate goals of nursing is **patient care** and it is achieved by:

- Alleviation of pain
- Curing of disease
- Restoration and promotion of health
- Prevention of disease
- Early detection and correction of defects

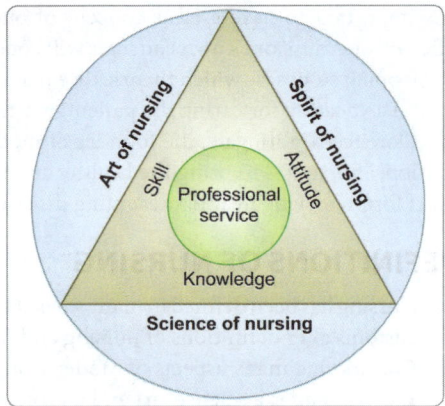

Figure 2: Nursing—A professional service

Scope of Nursing

By attaining the goals of nursing, a nurse renders service to individuals. Through individuals, his/her services reach families, society and ultimately to the country. Thus a nurse is an important member of the health team of a country (Fig. 3).

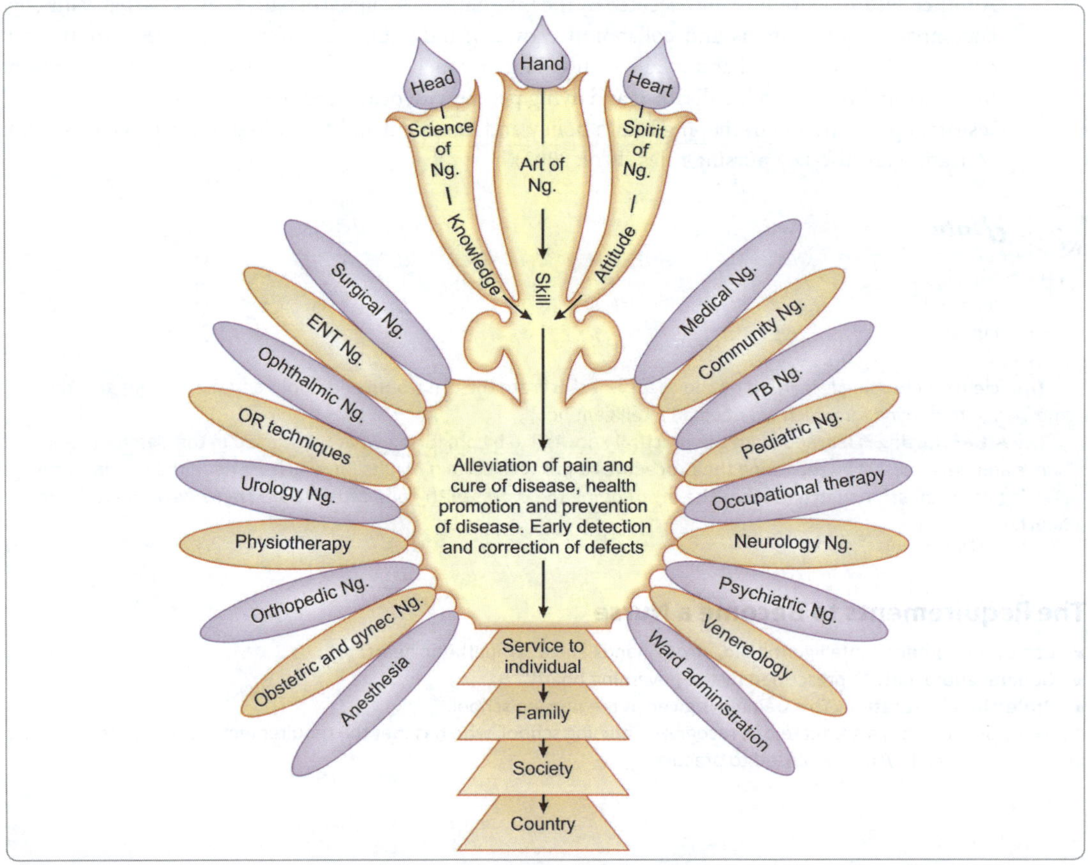

Figure 3: Diagrammatic representation of basic requirements, goals, branches and extent of service of nursing

Abbreviations: *ENT, ear, nose and throat; Ng., nursing; or, operation research; TB, tuberculosis*

REQUIREMENTS TO BECOME A NURSE

- **Basic Requirements:** Intelligent head, strong hands and a sympathetic heart.
- **General Education:** As prescribed by the governing board.
- **Professional Education:** This training is given in the Nursing School.

A professional nurse is a graduate of a recognized nursing school, who has met the requirements for a Registered Nurse in a state in which he/she is licensed to practice.

Qualities Required for a Nurse

Nursing is a career, which needs certain special qualities. In addition to the qualities of a good citizen he/she should not be a vain talker but should be a good listener. She should be a dedicated person, honest and must respect her vocation.

Some of the other essential qualities required for a nurse are:

- Honesty and loyalty
- Discipline and obedience
- Alertness and intelligent observation
- Technical competence
- Dependability and adjust ability
- Ability to inspire confidence
- Resourcefulness, economy of time, material and energy
- Courtesy and dignity
- Sympathy, empathy, tact and poise
- Intelligence and common sense
- Patience and sense of humor
- Good physical and mental health
- Generosity
- Gentleness and quietness

 Stimulant

An Accepted Version of the Word Nurse
N—Noble
U—Understanding
R—Responsible
S—Sympathetic
E—Efficient

Duties and Responsibilities of the Nurse

- Providing physical care and emotional support to the sick, injured and disabled.
- Helping in the diagnosis and carrying out the treatments prescribed by the physician.
- Observing, reporting and evaluating the response of the patient's illness, hospital treatment and care.
- Teaching patients and his/her family about good health habits and encouraging them to practice it in their life.
- Coordinating the services of all groups and departments of the hospital contributing to the care of patient and his/her family.
- Helping in the education of medical and paramedical students.

Unit I ❖ Introduction to Nursing

- Arranging and supervising the works of the auxiliary nursing personnel in the ward.
- Protecting and preventing the loss and damages of medicines and other articles in the hospital.
- Upholding and maintaining the dignity and status of the profession.
- Helping in the research works related to healthcare.
- Maintaining his/her own physical and mental health and planning a safe and happy future.
- Utilizing opportunities for continuing education to keep his/her knowledge up-to-date.

The nurse is a person who is directly or indirectly helping in the construction of the health of the nation. A nurse is directly helping the individuals for cure of disease, restoration of health and prevention of diseases. Indirectly, she is contributing services for the health of the nation, i.e., through the individual to the family and through the family to the society; and through the society to the nation.

By the intellectual capacity and technical competence and constant experience, a nurse has to realize and anticipate the needs of the individuals. In this way, he/she is conscious to unconsciousness, love of life to the desperate, crutches to the amputee, sight to the blind, walking stick to weak, mother to newborn, confidence to the young mother, knowledge to the illiterate and a real friend and support to the helpless.

His/her functions are directed toward herself also, by equipping physically and mentally and by renewing his/her professional weapon of knowledge, skill and attitude through further education and participating in the professional activities, and by enriching a happy personal life.

Some more responsibilities of the nurse are:

- A nurse should trustfully deal with the patient and relatives, and establish a desirable relationship with them. He/she should be polite while talking and behaving with a pleasing face, instead of always being highly official and such presentation will develop an unquestionable belief in others about him/her.
- When doing procedures, if at any time a nurse happened to touch the body of a patient, it should be soft and should not elicit any pain to him/her. If a nurse, while doing a procedure, makes unpleasant face, the patient would lose his/her confidence is that nurse and would not trust her.
- Do not disclose or share any unnecessary information about the patient, disease or treatment, to others
- Matters disclosed by the patient even in unconscious stage, should not be conveyed to others except to the doctor attending that patient.
- As if helping and trying to preserve the health of others, a nurse should take care of her own health and possess a good individuality.
- Considering the importance of risks in the service entrusted, the need of developing skill and attitude and the livelihood of the future, a nurse should give prime importance and seriousness to his/her own health and wellbeing.
- Nurse should try to improve himself/herself by reading, modeling the leaders of the profession and participating in the professional conferences to increase knowledge and skill.
- Nurse should not talk or whisper anything in front of the patient about disease or about his/her family. The unquestionable belief and affection entrusted upon the nurse by the patient and others, is the core of his/her success or work. In healthcare service caste, creed, wealth, status, beauty, age or sex should not be a bar to give care. We should respect and deal with the patient according to their personality and individuality.
- All must follow daily routines strictly and take the required amount of nutrients proper rest, sleep and exercise as is required to keep good health.

ETIQUETTES IN NURSING

Etiquette means the rules for the behavior or the good manners that the professional people should practice. A nurse is one of the important members of the health team and works in co-operation with others for the care of patients. People are of different kinds and cultures. For the smooth running and for good interpersonal relationship in the group, nurses should follow some rules for their good behavior.

Some of the common etiquettes to be followed by a nurse are:

- A nurse should be courteous, gentle and polite to all. He/she should be approachable and has a pleasing nature but it should not overcome his/her official status.
- Address the seniors appropriately as Sir, Madam, Miss, etc.
- Greet others according to the time of the day, e.g., good morning, good evening, etc.
- Stand up when senior members enter your room, if you are sitting there, or answering their questions.
- Open the door for seniors and stand aside for them to pass in or out.
- Say excuse me when overtaking seniors or passing between two persons.
- In staircases or corridors, stand aside and give way to the seniors.
- Maintain silence in group or whenever needed. Use neat and tidy dress to have a professional look such as combed hair and put up sarees/uniform well-arranged and fixed with pins.
- Do not use cutex/nail paint or jewellery during duty time as it may interfere in work.
- Obey seniors without arguing.
- Say 'Thank you' when someone do a favor to you or correct you.
- Give seats to seniors when traveling and help them to carry heavy loads if you find them on the way.
- Get permission from seniors if you need something from the department.
- Give proper answers in the proper time to others.
- Be punctual and honest in duty time and work.
- Follow mannerism while talking or listening to others like keep eye contact and sit face to face on such occasions.
- If you happened to hurt others accidently say 'excuse me'.
- Avoid talking about others unnecessarily, otherwise people will lose their confidence and trust in you.
- Always close the doors when you get into the room or when you get out of the room, if required.
- Knock at the door and wait for response before you enter in other's room.
- Cover the mouth when you cough or sneeze, but do not cover it when you talk to others.
- Say 'excuse me', when you interfere the talk or work of others.
- Do not receive gifts or presents from the patient or relatives of patient.
- If you happened to leave the patient alone or leave the ward, get the permission of the seniors or other responsible persons.

INTERPERSONAL RELATIONSHIP (IPR) IN NURSING

The smooth running of any work depends upon the proper relationship of the members of the team. A nurse being one of the important members of the health team, should establish a very good relationship with all the other members, for better cooperation and harmony in the working field. The principles of good interpersonal relationships are:

- Be familiar with the name of the patient and relations but do not use nick names
- Respect the individuals according to their status
- Do not impose any work upon others
- Always have good emotional control
- Willingly accept mistakes and ignorance
- Do not impose your mistakes on others
- Be calm in problems and focus attention to solve it
- Try to get the confidence of the patient, relatives and co-workers
- Be impartial to all
- Be honest and obedient to the seniors, doctors and all others
- Mingle with others as if you are one of the members of a family and always remember that the patient is the central figure of your work

- Behave nicely with all, as you expect from others
- Demonstrate responsibilities by your behavior and consider that the satisfaction of others is greater than yours
- Accept the work and problems of others, instead of projecting difficulties and works faced by you
- Include other people whenever possible to get the maximum effect of your work
- Do the procedures skillfully to get better cooperation and help of the patient and relatives
- Do not create situations for any arguments
- Consider the interests of others while talking to them
- Be a good listener than becoming a good speaker and answer in a soft voice while replying others
- Utilize the opportunities around, to enhance the knowledge
- When someone is angry unnecessarily or using foul language, do not try to defend yourself but approach and try to clear the misunderstanding when the person is calm
- Appreciate and encourage the goodness of others
- Always have a pleasant face
- Practice tolerance with others
- Avoid gossiping and try not to keep company with people who are in habit of gossiping
- Do not try to degrade any one as it may come back to you any time
- Show your interest in listening to the experience of the patients or elders
- Whenever possible, try to teach the healthy habits to patients and relatives and help them to practice these
- When work is finished or you get leisure time, try to help others to complete their work so that you may get from others more acceptance and help.
- You should not be selfish in dealing with others but should be dedicated for the welfare of the patient

People Interrelated with a Nurse

- **The persons related to nurses in the profession are:** Patients, relatives, physicians, nursing teachers, fellow nurses, nonprofessional hospital people, nursing administrators, senior nurses and ward sisters.
- **Members of the health team are:** Doctors, therapists, pharmacists, dietitians, technicians, medical representatives, social workers, chaplains and other nurses.

Central Figure and Triangular Connections

Wherever and whoever is the client, the most important aim of every treatment and care is the cure and welfare of the patient as an individual and not the name of the disease or 'case'. **Individual means a living mind in a living body**. The interconnected factors for the treatment and care of an individual are the relatives, doctors and the nurses (Fig. 4).

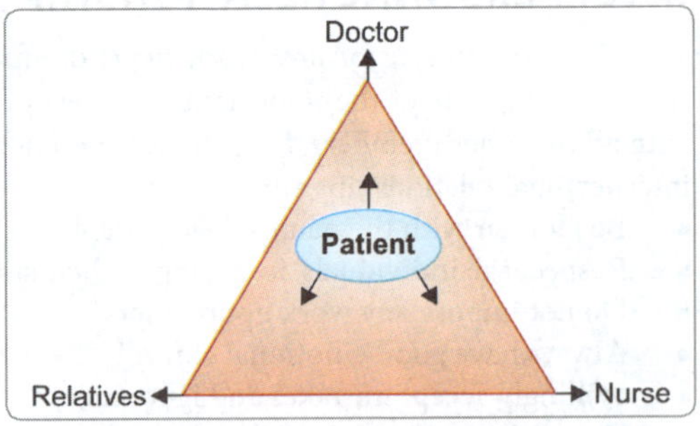

Figure 4: Triangular connection of patient care

- Relatives bring the patient to the doctor, disclose the required information about the patient and his/her illness and meet the expenses.
- A doctor examines the patient, does the investigations, diagnoses the condition and prescribes the expert treatment.
- A nurse carries out the instructions of the doctor and gives required efficient nursing care to the patients and deals with the relatives politely.

For the cure and wellbeing of the central figure, **the patient,** the three factors are connected with each other. Apart from this triangular connection, a nurse is a link between all the members and all departments of the hospital and the members of the health team in the healthcare system of the country.

Interaction with the Patient

The dealings of the nurse with the patient should be respectful and he/she should be considered as an important member of his/her family. More than a patient, he/she is an individual whose disease of the body will affect the mind and discomforts of the mind will affect the body too. When a person becomes a patient, he/she is more dependent, afraid, emotional and more anxious in that environment. He/she wishes to get love, sympathy and sincerity from the care givers as if he would have received from his/her family if he/she was at home. A patient expects expert treatment, efficient nursing care, perfect safety and full comfort when he/she is in the bed.

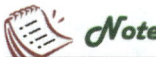 *Note*

> The nurse should not forget the fact that more than his/her own matters or mingling with the bystanders, the central point of attention is the patient, who is entrusted to care.

The patient is most valuable individual in the service field of a nurse. He/she should be alert to satisfy the basic needs of the patient such as rest and sleep, hygiene, food, elimination, diversion, etc. which are highly essential for healthcare and comfort.

Interaction with the Relatives

In connection with the treatment and care of the patient a nurse has to interact with the relatives or bystanders. Their fear and anxiety may be considered with sympathy and make situations favorable for them to talk with the doctor for clearing their doubts about the patient and diseases. A nurse should explain to them within limit. Out of ignorance, relatives may ask some flimsy or funny questions to the nurse about the patient or diagnosis and a nurse should console and comfort them with suitable answers. Visiting of close relatives may be soothing for the patient. But at times when the patient is extremely weak or expected to be tired because of visitors, the nurse should avoid such visitors tactfully. Talking for a long time or any other exertion is not desirable when one is sick or exhausted.

Interaction with Doctor

Instructions given by the doctor about the treatment should be carried out faithfully. If there is any doubt about any medicine or treatment, it should be cleared by asking the doctor without hesitation. Occurrence of any mistake in the treatment or care may result in a threat to the life of the patient. The reaction and the result of prescribed medicine or treatment should be observed and reported to the doctor during his/her next visit to the patient. Submission of a short report to doctor, about the patient and treatment given to the patient will increase the trust and faithfulness of the nurse. A written report should include the following points:

- Temperature, rate of pulse and respiration
- Details and frequency of urination and defecation
- Measurement of intake and output
- Type and time of sleep
- Details of appetite, food and eating
- Presence of pain and the given care or medication for it
- Vomiting, if any, and details

Unit I ❖ Introduction to Nursing

- Cough and details of sputum, if any
- Effects of given medicine and reactions, if any

BASIC NURSING PRINCIPLES

Schools of nursing prepares the nurses by instilling knowledge and skill in them so that they could do their work by fulfilling the basic nursing principles. In doing nursing procedures, the knowledge and skills are to be integrated to cover the following principles:

- **Safety:** It is the protection from hazards to patients and the members of the health team from the possible mechanical, chemical, thermal, bacteriological and psychological injuries.
- **Therapeutic effectiveness:** It is the result of the work, that is, whether the purpose of the procedure is fully achieved or not.
- **Comfort:** Every nursing procedure is aimed for the comfort of the patient. It should give the satisfaction to the patient, relatives and the nurse on completion of the work.
- **Use of resources:** The use of time, energy and material should be economic. A procedure should not be cancelled due to the shortage of one or two items required if they are not extremely essential. In such situations, adjustments can be done by improvising materials with the available resources.
- **Good workmanship:** It is the basic skill while doing procedures. There is great difference in doing things by a fresh hand and by an experienced hand. Such skill or the art of doing procedures is developed only by doing the same repeatedly. Nursing is learning by doing and not merely by reading.
- **Individuality:** The likes and dislikes are different in different persons. So when you are planning nursing care for a person, his/her needs are to be anticipated, problems are to be identified, and feelings are to be considered.

NURSING TECHNIQUES AND PROCEDURES

Nursing Techniques

The nursing techniques include the skillful handling of patient with the least discomfort, the skillful handling of sterile apparatus without contamination and the elimination of unnecessary movements so as to ensure the maximum speed with the highest efficiency.

Nursing Procedure

It means a method of carrying out a treatment. Details of procedure differs in various hospitals, although the underlying principles remain the same.

Important Factors of a Procedure

There are three factors involved in doing a procedure:

The Nurse

- Every nurse should have an interest in her work and should radiate joy while doing it.
- He/she should wash hands before and after every treatment.
- Have the correct equipment at hand before beginning, have it in good working condition and arranged conveniently.
- Always carry the equipment in a tray.
- Observe the condition of the patient while doing a treatment and report any unusual signs and symptoms to the supervisor. Note the effect of treatment and report it.
- Always chart procedure only **after** they have been done, not before. Otherwise, the charting may be dishonest.

The Patient

- The patient's mental and physical comfort should always be the first priority.
- A brief explanation about the procedure should always be made to all patients undergoing treatment for the first time in order to make him/her understand the purpose and be willing to cooperate.
- The patient should be placed in a comfortable position as far as possible before beginning a procedure and should be left in a comfortable position after treatment.
- The patient should never be exposed more than what is absolutely necessary and if any exposure is necessary screens should be used.

The Environment

- The room should be in the right temperature and there should be proper light.
- Draughts should be avoided.
- The ward or room should be left in order, after carrying out a procedure.
- All equipment for a procedure should be clean and in a good working condition and must be checked for their efficiency before beginning the procedure.
- After use, all equipment should be given appropriate care, that is, it should be scrubbed, washed, boiled, dried, aired, etc. as needed and put back in their proper places in good condition for future use.
- All broken equipment should be reported and replacement obtained.

STEPS OF PROCEDURE

The steps of procedure have been discussed here as follows:

- **Preliminary assessment of the patient and situation:**
  - The first step before starting a procedure is to identify the patient.
  - Then he/she will see the doctor's order to note any specific instructions in doing the procedure.
  - He/she will meet the Senior Sister of the ward to get the further instructions about the patient and procedure.
  - After this he/she will see the patient and note general condition, ability of self-help, his/her mood for acceptance, hygienic status, positions to be changed, need of the procedure and need of assistance required or not.
  - Then nurse has to find out the availability of articles required in the unit, alterations to be made or improvisation of articles.

- **Preparation and organization of articles (requisites):** In this step, the nurse has to remember three important points:
  i. Articles for the preparation of procedure
  ii. Articles for the actual performance of procedure
  iii. Articles for the termination of the procedure

To collect and organize the articles according to the order of use, the nurse must have a thorough knowledge about the details of the procedure. That is, nurse should judge him/herself what all things are required to prepare for the procedure, what are essentially required to perform the actual procedure and what will be required to terminate the procedure. On the basis of this judgment, a thoughtful nurse will collect and organize all the articles to meet the needs throughout the procedure, and concentrate in the performance. Carelessness in this regard may cause adverse results on patient as well as on the concerned nurse and doctor.

Unit I ❖ Introduction to Nursing

- **Preparation of the patient:** If the patient is not prepared well then there is no meaning of a skilled nurse or arranging the articles in order. Patient has to be prepared mentally and physically.
  - **As far as mental preparation** of the patient is concerned, nurse makes the patient understand politely about the procedure and need of doing the same and the good effect that is expected after doing it. Thus win the trust, cooperation and confidence of the patient.
  - With regard to **physical preparation**, the nurse should provide privacy to the patient. He/she should expose only that part of the body which is necessary for doing the procedure, make only the minimum disturbance to the patient by movement and change of position and so on.

- **Performance of the procedure:** Even though the materials of the procedure are arranged well, if the nurse is not thorough about actual procedure to be done, it will not be accepted by the patient and the desired effect will not be obtained. This knowledge is obtained from the classrooms, books and demonstration and by assisting the senior sisters in the ward in the beginning. The sincere effort on behalf of students and junior staff in learning, observing and practicing is the real method of developing knowledge and skill in doing procedures.

- **After-care of the patient and articles:** Once the procedure is completed, the patient is made comfortable. The effect of the treatment is observed, proper recording is made in the chart with signature of the nurse. All the articles are well cleaned and sterilized (if needed) and replaced at the proper place, so that they could be ready for the next use.

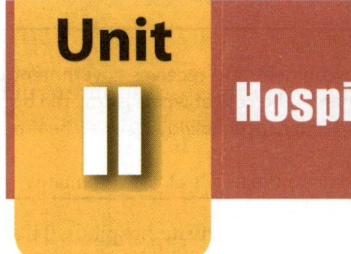

Unit II
Hospital

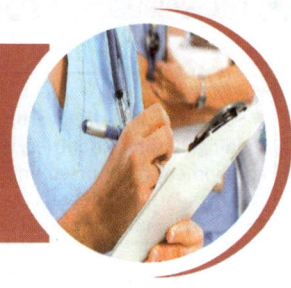

DEFINITIONS AND SET UP

A hospital is defined as an institution for providing medical and surgical treatment and nursing care for sick or injured people. It is a community health agency because a person comes to the hospital from a section of community and returns to it after the required hospital services.

An institution is composed of an established society or a group of people working together in a unit or group of units for a common goal, to meet any one of the basic needs of the man. Likewise, hospital is composed of patients, doctors, nurses and other members of the health team, functioning in a building or group of buildings and meet the needs of sick and injured. The student nurses should see it objectively the meaning of the hospital and not as a business center.

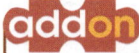

Definition of Hospital by WHO
WHO Expert Committee in 1963, defined hospital as: "A hospital is a residential establishment which provides short-term and long-term medical care consisting of observational, diagnostic, therapeutic and rehabilitative services for persons suffering or suspected to be suffering from a disease or injury and for parturitions. It may or may not also provide services for ambulatory patients on an out-patient basis".

CLASSIFICATION OF HOSPITAL

Hospitals can be classified in many ways:

- **Based on administration, ownership, control or financial income:**
  - **Governmental or public**
    - Medical college hospitals
    - District hospitals
    - City or town or headquarters hospitals
    - Primary health centers
    - Rural hospitals
    - Employees state insurance hospitals

    They are owned, administered and controlled by the government. They provide free care for patients.

    The governmental hospitals are owned by:
    - The Ministry of Health
    - The University
    - Others

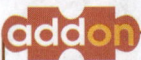

A public hospital or government hospital is a hospital which is owned by a government and receives government funding. In some countries, this type of hospital provides medical care, free of charge, the cost of which is covered by government reimbursement. In Australia, public hospitals are operated and funded by each individual state's health department. The federal government also contributes funding.

These government hospitals may be general hospitals or special hospitals according to the needs of the community.

- **Non-governmental or private hospitals:** These may be, nongovernment or private hospitals. They are privately owned or controlled by an individual or group of physicians or citizens or by private organization, e.g., Square Hospital. The purpose of these hospitals is to provide services for profit making.
- **Semi government hospital:** Hospitals run both by the government and private entity, e.g., Cantt Board Hospital
- **Voluntary agency hospitals: Not for profit hospitals. Such hospitals are run by the Voluntary Organizations,** e.g., HOPE Foundation Fistula Hospital

■ **Based on bed capacity (size):**
- Small hospital (up to 100 beds)
- Medium hospital (more than 100 to less than 300 beds)
- Large hospital (more than 300 beds)

■ **By teaching affiliation:**
- Teaching hospital
- Nonteaching hospital

■ **Based on system of medicine:**
- Allopathic hospital
- Ayurvedic hospital
- Homeopathic hospital
- Unani hospital
- Hospitals of other system of medicine

■ **Based on regionalism**
- Regional
- District
- Upazila health complex
- Union health and family welfare centers
- Community clinics

■ **As per WHO classification:**
- Regional hospital
- Intermediate/district hospital
- Rural hospital

■ **Based on the service offered, there are the following groups of hospitals:**
- **General hospitals:** In general hospital, care is given to many kinds of conditions such as medical, surgical, pediatrics and obstetrics. General hospitals are meant to provide a wide range of various types of healthcare, but with limited capacity. They care for patients with various-disease conditions for both sexes to all ages, medical, surgical, pediatrics, obstetrics, eye and ear, etc. Usually, general hospitals are devoid of super-specialist medical care.

Unit II ❖ Hospital

- **Special hospitals:** A special hospital limits its services to a particular condition or sex or age such as tuberculosis, maternity and pediatric hospital, respectively. They limit their services to a particular condition, orthopedics, maternity, pediatrics, geriatrics, oncology, etc.
- **Teaching-cum-research hospital:** College is attached for medical/nursing/dental/pharmacy education. Main objective is to provide medical care and teaching, research is secondary.

- **Based on the time of stay:**
  - **Short-term or short-stay hospitals:** These are hospitals where over 90% of patients stay for less than 30 days.
  - **Long-term or long-stay hospitals:** These are hospitals where over 90% of patients stay for 30 days or more, i.e. mental hospital.
- **The hospitals are also classified based on the type of staff they contain, like:**
  - **Closed-staff hospital:** In such types of hospitals, physicians are held responsible for all medical activities in the hospital including the diagnosis and treatment of patient; fee paying and emergency. In these hospital all doctors are on staff, and also doctors that are not on staff may not have access or privileges at said hospital.
  - **Open-staff hospital:** This type of hospital permits other physicians in the community to admit and treat patients. Open medical staff means any physicians can request to practice at the facility, regardless of their hospital affiliation.
- **Based on type of care:**
  - Primary care
  - Secondary care
  - Tertiary Car.

DIFFERENT DEPARTMENTS IN A HOSPITAL

- **Casualty:** This department, also known as the accident and emergency department, deals with patients who have been brought in by an ambulance in an emergency. Sometimes, patients find their own way to this department in case they have had an accident or they are in need of immediate treatment. This department works 24/7 and is equipped to deal with all sorts of emergencies. The patients are assessed according to the degree of injury or emergency and is then provided immediate treatment before being referred to a specialized department for further treatment.
- **Anesthetics:** Doctors in this department administer anesthesia on patients for various procedures and surgeries. They provide the following services:
  - Acute pain services post-surgery
  - Chronic pain services for patients suffering from bone-related illnesses like arthritis
  - Critical care services for those suffering from trauma
  - Obstetrics anesthesia and analgesia like epidurals during childbirth and anesthesia for C-sections.
- **Cardiology:** The department deals with problems of the human heart or circulation. It treats people on an inpatient and outpatient basis. Some of their procedures include:
  - Electrocardiogram (ECG) and exercise tests to measure the heart function
  - Ultrasound scan of the heart (echocardiogram)
  - Scans of the carotid artery in the neck to determine risks of stroke
  - 24-hour blood pressure tests
  - Insertion of pacemakers
  - Coronary angiography to see if there are any blocks in the arteries
  - Medical diagnosis and treatment of congenital heart defects, coronary artery disease, heart failure, valvular heart disease and electrophysiology
  - Cardiac surgery

- **Critical care:** This department also known as the intensive care unit (ICU) provides treatment for seriously ill patients. Certain patients need to be isolated and require close and individual medical attention. The ICU has very few beds and is usually managed by specialist doctors and nurses as well as consultant anesthetists, physiotherapists and dieticians. Patients can be transferred from any department to the ICU in case their condition gets worse.

- **Ears, nose and throat:** This department deals with ailments concerned with the ear, nose and throat and it includes treatment of a variety of ailments like:
  - General ear, nose and throat diseases
  - Neck lumps
  - Cancers of the head and neck area
  - Tear duct problems
  - Facial skin lesions
  - Balance and hearing disorders
  - Snoring and sleep apnea
  - ENT allergy problems
  - Salivary gland diseases
  - Voice disorders
  - ENT surgical procedures

- **Geriatrics:** This department is usually manned with doctors specialized in geriatric medicine.
  - The elderly suffers from a range of illnesses and seek treatment for stroke, gastroenterology, diabetes, locomotors problems, continence problems, syncope, bone disease, etc.
  - This department also provides a range of community services like home visits, mobile therapy units, palliative care, and this department is often linked to other community centers.

- **Gastroenterology:** This department deals with bowel related-medicine. Specialist consultants usually run it and they investigate and treat upper and lower gastrointestinal diseases, as well as diseases of the pancreas and bile duct system. It also involves endoscopy and nutritional services. Some sub specialties include:
  - Colorectal surgery
  - Inflammatory bowel disease
  - Swallowing problems

 *Note*

Special nurses are often appointed in this department and they are capable of performing a wide range of bowel investigations.

- **General surgery:** This department includes a wide variety of surgical procedures that include:
  - Thyroid surgery
  - Kidney transplants
  - Colon surgery
  - Laparoscopic cholecystectomy (gallbladder removal)
  - Endoscopy
  - Breast surgery
  - Minor surgeries such as hernia repairs, piles, etc.

These procedures are normally performed by general surgeons as these procedures do not normally require special surgeons.

- **Gynecology:** This department deals with the investigation and treatment of problems of the female urinary tract and reproductive system.
  - Infertility, incontinence and endometritis are some of the problems investigated in this department
  - Other services include cervical smear screen and postmenopausal bleeding checks

  This department usually has a special ward, day surgery unit, an emergency gynecology assessment unit and outpatient clinics.
- **Hematology:** This department can be part of the hospital laboratory or work closely with the hospital laboratory. Hematology includes the study of etiology, diagnosis, treatment, prognosis, and prevention of blood diseases that affect the production of blood and its components, such as blood cells, hemoglobin, blood proteins, and the mechanism of coagulation. A medical technologist carries the laboratory work. Hematologists also conduct studies in oncology—the medical treatment of cancer.
- **Maternity/neonatal/pediatrics:** All facilities concerning giving birth and childcare are provided in this department. In some hospitals, these facilities can be divided into different departments but most general hospitals provide this care under one department itself. Some of the facilities or treatments provided by this department include:
  - Childbirth
  - Midwifery
  - Antenatal and postnatal care
  - Pregnancy checkups
  - Surgical procedures on children or mothers
- **Neurology:** Neurology deals with the human nervous system. The doctors in this department investigate and treat patients for problems that affect their brain and spinal cord. Surgical procedures on the brain and spinal cord are extremely dangerous and require highly qualified and experienced doctors and nurses to provide such special care. Neurologists examine patients who have been referred to them by other physicians in both the inpatient and outpatient settings. A neurologist will begin his/her interaction with a patient by taking a comprehensive medical history. He/she then performs a physical examination focusing on evaluation of the nervous system. Components of the neurological examination include assessment of the patient's cognitive function, cranial nerves, motor strength, sensation, reflexes, coordination, and gait.
- **Oncology:** This department investigates and treats all kinds of cancers and provides a wide range of chemotherapy treatments and radiotherapy for cancerous tumors and blood disorders. This department is usually linked to all the other departments as referrals can be made when one department cannot diagnose the patient's problem. This department also requires highly qualified and experienced doctors and nurses. Doctors also carry out tumor-removal procedures, which are then sent for biopsy to confirm whether the tumor is malignant or not.
- **Ophthalmology:** This department deals with the investigation and treatment of eye problems of adults and children. Their services include:
  - General eye clinic appointments
  - Laser treatments
  - Optometry
  - Orthoptics
  - Prosthetic eye services
  - Ophthalmic imaging
- **Orthopedics:** This department deals with problems that affect the musculoskeletal system. Treating bones, muscles, tendons, ligaments, and nerves come under it. Services include bone setting, surgeries to repair damaged bones or ligaments or tendons, replacing bones like hip replacement, knee cap replacement, etc.

Unit II ❖ Hospital

Other outpatient services include treating fractures and dislocated joints, musculoskeletal injuries and soft tissue injuries.

- **Urology:** This department is usually a surgical department led by surgeons that perform certain specific services like:
  - Flexible cystoscopy bladder checks
  - Urodynamic research
  - Prostate assessments and biopsies
  - Shockwave lithotripsy to break up kidney stones
- **Psychiatry:** This department deals with investigating and treating patients with a wide range of mental illnesses and disorders. Some services include:
  - Providing psychosocial counselling
  - Investigating, diagnosing and treating psychiatric illnesses
  - Conducting IQ tests
  - Deaddiction services
- **Outpatient:** In this department, people come to the hospital only for consultation and not admission. The patients seek medical advice from a specific department depending on their problem and doctors provide a prescription of medication for them to take for a certain period. Patients are then asked to come back for a follow up. Patient's treatment within the boundaries of the hospital lasts only for a single day. Outpatient department runs for specific time during the day. Consultant doctors usually handle OPD.
- **Inpatient:** This department admits patients at least overnight for treatment. Here a case history of the patient is taken and the patients have a case sheet in which his/her progress is recorded. Nurses monitor patients throughout the day and doctors come on rounds to check on the patients conditions. The duration of stay will depend on severity of the patient's illness.

There are **supportive departments** in the hospital and they help in carrying out the functions of other departments in smooth way. These are:

- **Central sterilization unit:** This department is in charge of keeping all the instruments used in the hospital clean and sterilized to avoid spreading of infections throughout the hospital. They follow a strict procedure for sterilizing the medical and surgical instruments.
- **Housekeeping:** This department is in charge of keeping the hospital neat and clean. It involves doing the laundry and cleaning all the rooms of the hospital and effectively disposing of medical waste according to strict hospital disposal procedures.
- **Catering and food services:** This department provides food services to inpatients, their families and staff of the hospital based on a nutritional menu provided by the Nutrition Department.
- **Medical social work:** This department manned with medical social workers helps patients and their families dealing with a broad range of psychosocial issues and stresses related to coping with illness and maintaining health. This department addresses the challenges families face, increase accessibility to healthcare, and serves as a bridge between the doctors and the individual, family, and community.
- **Physiotherapy:** This department aims at rehabilitating patients. Mostly linked to the orthopedics department, this department offers a wide range of body-healing therapies that will help a patient resume normal functioning. This department offers outpatient as well as inpatient services.
- **Pharmacy:** Every hospital must be equipped with a pharmacy, which provides drugs for the entire hospital. It not only provides medication for patients but also ensures the supply of other drugs and instruments used by all the departments in the hospital for patient care or surgeries. The department is run by a pharmacist and provides the following services:
  - Purchase, supply and distribution of medication and pharmaceuticals
  - Inpatient and outpatient dispensing
  - Clinical and ward pharmacy

- **Nutrition and dietetics:** This department is manned with specialist in nutrition and dietetics. They are assigned to provide professional advice on diet for hospital inpatient wards as well as outpatient departments. Certain departments require that the patient be put on a diet and therefore the team works with many other departments that treat diabetes, cancer, kidney problems, pediatrics, elderly care, surgery and critical care, gastroenterology, etc. These specialists can also suggest a dietary chart to be followed by the hospital canteen to ensure that all patients get nutritious food during their stay at the hospital.
- **Microbiology:** This department deals with the microbial and viral aspects of medicine. This department is very important as the number of hospital-acquired infections is on the rise. These doctors usually carry out tests on samples from surgeries sent from various other departments and submit reports following biopsy.
- **Diagnostic imaging:** It is also known as the department of radiology, and provides the following services:
  - General radiology (X-rays)
  - Scans for accidents and emergency
  - Mammography (breast scans)
  - Ultrasound scans
  - Angiography (X-ray of blood vessels)
  - Interventional radiology (minimal invasive procedures)
  - CT scanning
  - MRI scanning (3D scans using magnetic and radio waves)

Patients are sent to this department for the above-mentioned services, as other departments do not have the required devices to perform diagnostic imaging. After the service is provided, reports are given about the imaging and all these reports will have to be handed over to the department from which the imaging was requested.

- **Medical records:** This department deals with recording, and maintains all the records/files of inpatients as well as outpatients. It is with these records that medical statistics can be formulated and later on used as a reference for future purposes.
- **Medical maintenance and engineering:** This department makes sure that the hospital is in operable condition. It makes plans and carries out various projects for the hospital. This department also makes sure that all electrical facilities are in perfect condition, carries out repair and replacement work for air-conditioning units, plumbing, steel works, and also takes care of the overall maintenance of the hospital.
- **Information technology and communication:** All hospitals today use computers to keep track of patient records and other medically-related affairs. Therefore, this department is in charge of providing technical support as and when needed, and keeping the systems updated and providing support when systems crash. They also aim to provide effective online services for patients and help to keep the entire hospital informed of certain events that take place within the hospital.
- **Human resources:** This department is given the objective of recruiting efficient human resources for the hospital. It also has the duty of creating policies and procedures that the staff members have to follow in the hospital. It aims at ensuring employee satisfaction, good working conditions and provision of monetary and non-monetary benefits for the employees. It is also responsible for providing compensation for the services rendered by the employees.
- **Finance:** This department looks after the financial aspects of the hospital. They make budgets, financial plans for the future and allocate financial resources to the various departments of the hospital for their upgradation. They also provide wage statements for the staff and oversee purchases of medical supplies and pharmaceuticals for the hospital.
- **Administration:** This department is in charge of looking after the day-to-day operations of the hospital. They look after all the paper work of hospital and ensure that every department follows administrative procedures of the hospital.

Unit II ❖ Hospital

FUNCTIONS OF A HOSPITAL

Now, we will focus on major functions of a hospital (Fig 1).

- **Investigations, diagnosis, and the care of the sick and injured:** The chief functions of the hospital are investigating the patient, making diagnosis and giving care to the sick and injured persons. They are examined according to the condition of the patient and the necessary investigations are done in the outpatient department for the diagnosis. The patients are treated either as an outpatient or inpatient. When the condition of the patient requires a detailed investigation or due to many other reasons, the doctor advises the patient to stay as inpatient in undiagnosed conditions, or the patient may be admitted only for observation.

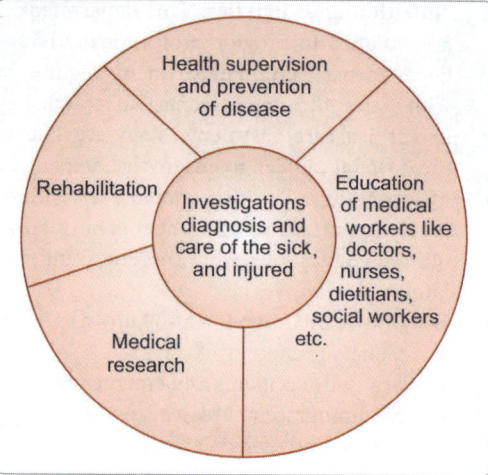

Figure 1: Functions of a hospital

For the care of the sick, the wards are of the following types:

- **According to the age of the patient**—General ward or pediatric ward
- **According to the type of disease**—Medical or surgical ward or in any special ward
- **According to the income and preference of the patient**—The patient may select a general ward or pay ward.

Several other departments as clinical laboratory, kitchen, X-ray, pharmacy, operation room, etc. work under the control of administrator for a common goal, i.e., taking utmost care of the sick. Therefore, several categories of personnel work together as doctors and nurses and other technical and non-technical persons in the hospital for achieving the common goal of taking maximum care of the sick.

- **Health supervision and prevention of disease:** The preventive aspects of medical work have been given so much emphasis in all aspects of medical practice at hospitals and health centers.
  - In the outpatient departments, provisions are available for the routine health examinations, supervision of antenatal and postnatal mothers, health supervision and immunization of sick and healthy children and other services to persons in normal conditions.
  - Hospitals prevent the spread of diseases by isolating the patients infected with communicable disease and also by raising the standard of health in the community by imparting health education.
  - Hospital staff and other medical social workers render great services while dealing with the social problems and recurrence of psychiatric conditions and the adjustments of such persons in the community.
  - Different types of home care are given to patients by community health programs.
  - Modern hospitals extend their services in the community by arranging camps and clinics by specialized doctors and other health supervisors for the health supervision. Eye camps, detection of cancer, diabetic clinics, immunization camps, family welfare program camps, etc. come under these services.

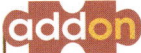

Preventive functions of hospital:
- It is an emerging secondary function for the hospital and concerned with health promotion.
- It is geared toward providing the preventive services through a community health center.
- It takes an active role to improve the health of the population.

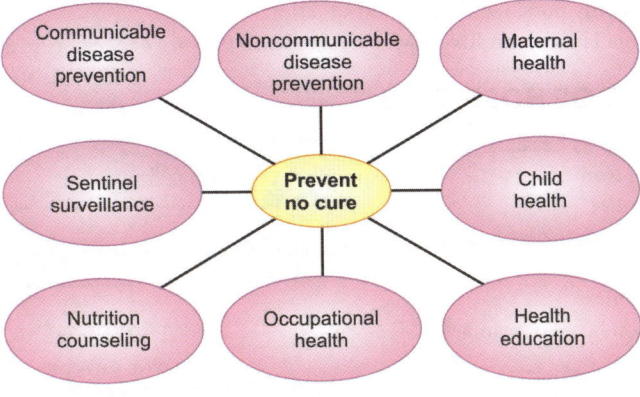

- **Education of medical workers:** Doctors, nurses, dietitians, social workers, physical therapists, technicians, hospital administrators and other medical and paramedical people are taught within the hospital in order to practice their profession efficiently. The theoretical part of their learning is conducted in an affiliated particular institution and they practice their knowledge in the actual situation of the hospital. Without hospitals or equivalent, it would be impossible to give an adequate preparation for almost any type of modern medical services, because such experiences are not available anywhere in the community other than a hospital or health clinic.
- **Medical research:** Hospitals offer medical workers opportunities for investigations in the form of laboratory facilities, trained personnel, patients and accumulation of records, which are not available elsewhere. This research is an important factor in the successful practice of medicine and the advancement of medical science. The modern trend is to establish a close association between the small rural hospitals and research centers and between all hospitals and other community health organizations so that their personnel may have provisions for an adequate research, diagnostic and therapeutic facilities. A large number of patients and workers in these research centers and District Hospitals should foster all kinds of medical research. The statistical side of the research works in the hospital helps to evaluate the occurrence and prevalence of a particular disease in locality or society and the health status of a country.
- **Rehabilitation:** Rehabilitation is an essential aspect of all health care facilities and it is one of the functions of hospital. Helping a person to regain independence or restoration of a person to normal or near normal function during and after hospitalization is considered as an integral part of nursing care. Rehabilitation involves the coordinated help of physicians, nurses, physical therapists, social workers, occupational counsellors and others. Such a comprehensive care restores each individual to his or her optimum physical, mental, social, vocational and economic usefulness. The modern concept of rehabilitation is stated clearly and accepted generally very recently.

  The Rehabilitation Services are dedicated to providing high quality, individualized, and effective interventions aimed at promoting both patient safety and a return to independent function. Services include Physical Therapy, Occupational Therapy, and Speech-Language therapy, etc. with compassion and empathy in a patient and family-centered care environment.

Unit II ❖ Hospital

Special units have been established in hospitals to help persons with physical disabilities that keep them moving freely in their environment. They admit both in-patients and out-patients in the unit. Furnishings and their arrangements are such that the independence of the individual is facilitated. Furnishings will vary depending on the type of service and economic status. Initially rehabilitation focuses on preventing complications and later, services begins toward maximizing the functioning and increasing the level of independence of the client. Such an effective rehabilitation involve the client, family and the whole health care team which is only possible in a hospital situation.

(Refer to Virginia Henderson RN. A.M. *Principles and Practice of Nursing*, p. 593 & 594)

CHANGING ROLE OF HOSPITALS

The role of hospitals (Fig. 2) has changed, with emphasis shifting from:

- Curative to preventive
- Inpatient care to outpatient and home care
- Acute to chronic illness
- Tertiary and secondary to primary health care

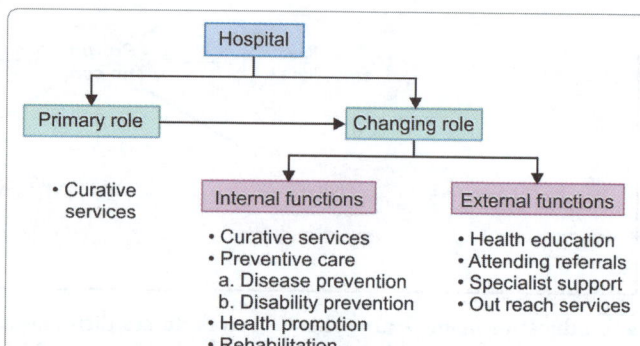

Figure 2: Changing role of hospital

The important factors that have led to the changing role and functions of the hospital are:

- Expansion of clientele from dying and destitute to all classes of people
- Improved socioeconomic status
- Increased health awareness
- Government's duty to provide comprehensive health
- Improved transportation and communication services
- Rapid advances in medical science and technology
- Increase in population leading to increase in demand for hospital beds
- Reorientation of health cum delivery system with an emphasis on primary health care

HOSPITAL—HOUSEKEEPING AND GENERAL CLEANLINESS

Housekeeping

- **Housekeeping:** It means the keeping up or managing of a house or the management of the domestic affairs of an institution.
- **Housekeeper:** The housekeeper is a person employed to take the utmost care of a house or to look after the domestic affairs of an institution. He/she spends maximum time there, as a dispenser of hospitality. He/she is responsible for the proper placements of furnitures and supplies, cleanliness, repairing, replacing and maintenance in the house or institution through the proper channel and also for entertaining the guests.
- **Hospital housekeeper:** This person manages the domestic affairs of the hospital under the supervision of the nursing superintendent and behaves generously to the guest (patients, relatives and co-workers).

General Cleanliness

- It refers to a place which is free from dirt, dust and stain and a stage of complete neatness of a house or institution. It also refers to cleanliness or purity. Cleanliness of a house or an institution includes the neatness of the total area such as rooms, walls, roof, fixtures, kitchen and other attachments, toilets, corridors and surroundings.
- Cleanliness is the key to the prevention of disease and promotion of health. It creates a dirt-free environment. Dirt may be organic or inorganic. Inorganic dirt is more dangerous. Dust is composed of sand, bacteria, lint from bedding, crumbs of food, scales from skin, dried secretion, etc. Therefore, to transfer dust from one place to another, that is from lockers and beds to the floor, is not cleanliness. It must be removed it harbors bacteria. For this reason, dusting must be done with a damp cloth and with firm even strokes.

Purposes of Cleaning

For the safety of the patients:
- To remove all dust and breeding places of germs with least disturbance to the patients
- To leave a clean, polished surface wherever possible so that dirt may not be accumulated
- To prolong the life of the articles
- To keep the articles in such a condition that they are ready for use at any time

Methods of Cleaning

Methods of cleaning are same in all cases. Dirt or stain is removed mechanically by brushes or mops, using water and soap, air and sunlight, by suction with a vacuum cleaner, or by use of an abrasive of some kind, a solvent or detergent or a chemical. Cleaning agents used in hospital may be acidic, alkaline or neutral.

 *Note*

Special Points in Cleaning
- For cleaning, choose the correct and simplest method for saving of time, material and energy.
- See that the ceiling and floor of the room have been cleaned before beginning to gather dust.
- Use clean water and clean dusters.
- Work should be done as quietly as possible. Dust with firm even strokes.
- Be economical in the use and care of materials.
- Use odorless cleaning agents. Use adequate room fresheners.
- Follow system to avoid waste of time and energy.
- Dust the corners well, use damp duster to collect dust.
- Always leave surfaces dry: clean from top to bottom; clean inside as well as out, back as well as front.
- After finishing the work, leave the place in order, everything neat and tidy and at its proper places.
- Clean the articles used in cleaning and put them away separately in a cup-board or room meant only for that purpose.

Materials used for Cleaning

- Mechanical agents: Brooms, mops, brushes, dusters, etc.
- Water and soap
- Absorbent agents
- Chemicals: solvents, detergent

Methods of Cleaning and Caring Equipment, Furniture, etc.

- **Polished surfaces:** Dust with soft cloth. The cloth may be little dampened. To remove greasy stains, wash with soap and warm water. Wipe with cloth wrung out of clean water. Dry well at once. Polished surface if left wet, becomes white. When necessary, polish with furniture polish. Use only a small amount of polish at a time, otherwise the surface will be sticky. Wipe off excess polish with a soft dry cloth (polish may be made from wax dissolved in turpentine).
- **Painted surface:** Wash with soap and warm water. A mild soap should be used. Strong soap takes off the paint. Do not use sodabicarb, sand or gritty cleaning powders as these take off the paint. Unpainted wooden surfaces can be washed with any soap and warm water. Cleaning powders may be used if needed.
- **Utensils: (sputum cups, receivers, basins, bedpans, urinals, etc.):** After use, clean re-usable bedpan holders/urinals/commode pans with hand hot water and general purpose detergent, rinse and dry. Or place disposables in a yellow plastic bag for incineration or registered landfill.
- **Enamel ware:** Wash in cold water first as hot water causes coagulation and sticking of albuminous material. Then wash with soap and hot water. Never heat or cool suddenly as it will cause cracks and chipping. Strong acids and alkalies destroy the polish. Kerosine or weak chlorine solution removes most stains. Sterilize by boiling for 10-15 minutes or by autoclaving.
- The spout of the feeding cup should be cleaned with a small bottle brush.
- If there is no bedpan washer, clean bedpans with a long-handled brush or mop.
- **Aluminum:** Wash with soap, cold water and then with hot water. Cleaning powders may be used. Frequent and excessive use of acids and alkalies ruins the metal. Aluminum vessels must be kept dry when not in use.
- **Porcelain:** Wash with soap and water. To remove stains, use lime juice, kerosine, vinegar or dilute hydrochloric acid. Cleaning powders can be used. To keep it free from grease, hot soda water should be poured into them frequently. Sand should not be used for cleaning porcelain.
- **Marble, tile, terrazzo:** Wash with soap and water; soda may be used to remove stains. Acids react with marble. Never use an abrasive on marble as it makes marks on surfaces.
- **Stainless steel:** Wash with soap and water and keep dry. To remove stain, use an abrasive.
- **Silver:** Wash with hot water and soap and polish with silver polish using a soft cloth.
- **Other metals like brass and copper:** May be washed with soap well. Cleaning powders may be used. Dry well and polish with metal polish. For brass, brasso may be used for polishing.
- **Glass and glasswares**
  - **Drinking glass:** Wash first in soap and warm water, rinse in clean water. Dry with soft cloth.
  - **Windows and mirrors:** Wash with soap and warm water. Use even strokes to avoid streaking. Rinse in clear water. A little ammonia or vinegar added to the water makes the glass shine.
    - Dry with soft cloth or crumpled newspapers. Wet newspaper cleans well.
    - Glassware when put to boil should be wrapped in clothes or cotton wool and should never be put directly in boiling water.
  - **Crockery:** Wash with soap and hot water, and dry. Use sodabicarb to remove stains.
- **Care of the environment:** It is the function of housekeeping department of the hospital to keep the hospital's environment clean.
- **Floors:** Depends upon the type of flooring. It should be made out of materials that will last long, fire resistant and easily maintained. It must be attractive and durable.
  - **Wooden floors:** These kept well-polished. They are mopped daily with clean mops. Vacuum cleaners if available may be used. Water or anything that sticks should be wiped off immediately.
  - **Mosaic floors:** These are washed with soap and water, and mopped. Occasional polishing is necessary.
  - **Cement floors:** These are washed with soap and water, and mopped.

- **Walls:** Hospital walls are usually washable, either paint, mosaic or tiles. A wall brush or a cloth tied to a light broom may be used for routine dusting. Periodic washing is done by male cleaners. Walls that can be whitewashed must be white-washed periodically, at least once in a year or whenever needed to do so.
- **Electric lights and fixtures:** These are dusted daily if they can be reached. If they are high, see that they are dusted at least once a week by male cleaners. Electric fittings should be cleaned only with dry clothes as water is a good conductor of electricity.
- **Diet kitchen:**
  - Cleanliness and order should prevail.
  - All appliances and equipment in the kitchen and dining room are kept scrupulously clean.
  - Dishes and serving utensils are kept in the cup-board.
  - After use, clean, dry and keep them in proper places, so that they could be easily found when needed.
  - The floor is cleaned and wiped after each meal.
  - The kitchen and pantry should be fly-proof.
  - The kitchen washbasin needs special attention.
  - Take care to prevent blockage of the drains.
  - Grease is removed by sodium bicarbonate solution or soap and warm water.

Care of Treatment or Utility Room

- Cleanliness and order should prevail. Everything should be in its proper place and ready for next use.
- All equipment such as basins, kidney trays, bowls and other utensils should be thoroughly cleaned as soon as they are used and should never be put away dirty.
- All soiled dressings are removed to a special receptacle from which they are later removed and burnt.
- Waste containers should be emptied and washed whenever necessary.
- The furniture, shelves and other wood work should be dusted daily with damp cloth.
- The wall should be cleaned and whitewashed as needed.
- The washbasin should be kept clean.
- Care must be taken to prevent blockage of the drain pipes.

Care of Bathrooms and Latrines

- Bathrooms should be kept free from unpleasant odors. Floor should be kept clean and dry.
- Waste containers should be emptied when necessary and cleaned daily.
- Toilets are cleaned with brush and cleaning powders.
- Bedpans and urinals are flushed well with cold water and then cleaned with mops. Bedpan washers are used wherever they are provided.
- **The commode:** The enamel or aluminum pail should be washed so that no stain or odor remains. Dish Wash powder may be used for cleaning. The outer seat should be washed with soap and water.

Care of Rubber Goods

All rubber goods must be cleaned, dried, powdered and put in as cool a place as possible. Do not put such goods under the sun to dry. Do not put rubber goods in boiling water, heat, sunlight, moisture, acids and grease as they will destroy rubber. Store them in airtight containers. Soap ruins rubber. Therefore, always rinse off soap thoroughly after cleaning with soap. Long boiling and sterilizing shorten the life of rubber goods. Folding cracks rubber, so roll them or hang on a wide rod.

- **Mackintoshes or rubber sheets:** Place on flat surface and wash well on both sides with soap and water. Rinse well and dry. Rubber sheets are dried either by hanging or by wiping with towel and never put them

Unit II ❖ Hospital

under strong sunlight. Put French chalk powder on both sides and roll in newspaper if they are to be stored. If used for an infectious patient disinfect before using it for another patient.

- **Rubber tubes:** After use, wash under running water, allowing water to run through, boil for three to five minutes. Dry it by hanging. Powder it in the outer surface of the tubes and store in a container lengthwise.
- **Catheters:** Clean the catheters with soap under running water. Use a stylette to clean the inside if needed. Hold the eye of the catheter upwards so that the water could run through the eye of the catheter. Dry it by hanging. Powder outside and store in a container, lengthwise.
- **Rectal tubes:** Remove Vaseline or lubricant well, using plenty of soap and water after wiping the Vaseline with dry cotton or rag pieces first. Rinse and soak in lysol 2% for 20 minutes. Allow water to run through. Then rinse off Lysol well or boil it for 5 minutes. Dry by hanging. Powder outside and store in containers lengthwise.
- **Rubber gloves:** Wash both inside and outside with soap and water. Boil for 3 minutes or soak in 2% lysol for 20 minutes. Then wash well, dry and put powder on both sides. Test for holes, fold back the cuff and keep in the glove bag in proper manner for ward use. A small packet of additional powder may be kept in the glove bag with each pair of gloves.
- **Rubber rings or air cushions:** Wash with soap and water, keep the valve closed to prevent water from getting inside. Dry well, paying special attention to the valves, to prevent them from getting rusty. Powder the outside part. Inflate with air and store.
- **Ice bags and hot water bags:** Wash with soap and water, dry well. Invert without closing so that water can drain out. Dry metal parts well to prevent rusting. Put in a layer of paper or cloth in the bag to keep the sides apart. Powder well only the outside part and store in proper place.

Care of Bedding

Mattresses

Mattresses should be protected by use of mackintoshes or large rubber sheets as needed. Change mattress cover as often as necessary. After use by one patient, air well and examine for tears and stains. If found wet, torn or stained, report to senior nurse. When a mattress is thin or lumpy, report to the senior nurse. Rubber loam mattresses should not be turned bent double or put in the sun. They may be washed and allow the water to drip off after wiping with a dry towel.

Pillows

If there is any danger of the pillow becoming soiled by blood, vomitus or any discharge, it should be covered by a rubber pillow case or a plastic case. Pillows used under the patients knees or crack also should be covered by rubber or plastic pillow case. After usage by one patient, pillows should be aired well in the sun. If it gets lumpy, thin, soiled or torn, report to head nurse. Air or foam pillows should not be put in the sun. They may be washed and hanged so that water may drip off and dry well.

Blankets

In ordinary cases, do not place blanket directly over patient's body. Place over a sheet and cover the blanket with a spread (counterpane). When it is necessary to place the blanket next to the patient's body, use old ones or cotton ones which can be washed easily. For seriously ill patients who may soil the blanket, use very old ones. Do not place or drag blankets on the floor at any time. Care must be taken to prevent staining of blankets. Small stains should be washed out at once. Sending blankets to washer-man frequently tears them, especially woolen ones. When the patient goes home, send the blanket to the washer-man only if it is too dirty or soiled, otherwise put in the sun and air it for 6 hours. Then shake off dust. Store in boxes preferably tin boxes. Put tobacco leaves or moth balls in the box to protect the blankets from insects. Do not put in the laundry box if damp. This will cause mildew.

Linen

Care of linen: To prevent staining on linen is a necessary economic measure. If drugs or other materials that produce stains or spoil the linen then proper measures should be taken immediately for the removal of the same.

Linen should be used only for the purpose for which it is intended. It should be kept as clean as possible. All articles should be separately marked and carefully checked before sending them to the laundry. Linen should be carefully checked when received from laundry. Check before putting them in cupboards for tears and send them for mending if needed so. Do not use torn linen on beds. Lending and borrowing from wards should be avoided. Do not put wet linen in the laundry box. For incontinent patients, save new sheets by using old ones folded up, as pads.

Linen cupboard: Have a definite place for each kind of linen. Place folded edge towards the front. Keep them neat and tidy always. Check them for wear and tear before arranging in the cupboard. Label the places for each articles of linen. Put moth balls in the cupboard. Inspect the cupboard frequently. Remove stains (blood, medicine, etc.) from linen immediately.

Removal of Stains from Linen

General instructions:
- Note the kind and color of material stained and the nature of the stain.
- Select the correct remover and follow an appropriate method.
- Remove stains as soon as possible.
- Try the simplest method first.
- See whether the stain can be removed by rinsing in cold water.
- For colored material, always test the remover first on a small part.
- Hot water and soap fix some stains.
- When using boiling water, stretch the stained part over a bowl and pour boiling water with force from a height until the stain disappears.
- When using an acid, stretch the part over a bowl of boiling water and apply the acid by means of medicine dropper, dipping the part occasionally in boiling water and again applying the acid.
- When bleaching by sunlight, wet the cloth or stain and lay it under the direct sunlight.
- Volatile liquids should never be used near a flame.
- Stains which contain proteins such as blood, excreta, milk, pus from wounds or body discharges are coagulated by application of heat therefore, clothes with such stains should be soaked in cold water for some time and washed in soap and cold water.
- Stains that contain fatty matter should be washed in hot water and soap.
- Use of absorptive materials such as salt, starch water, etc. will prevent the stains caused by liquids like Tincture of iodine, from spreading and damaging the linen.
- Bleaching agents like lemon juice, bleaching powder or hydrogen peroxide shall be used when simple methods fail to remove the stain in linen. But strong solution of bleaching agents will damage the linen very soon.
- Use equal parts of fresh peroxide of hydrogen and dilute ammonia (one teaspoon full of ammonia to one pint of water) and moisten the stain until it disappears. This is particularly useful in case of woolen articles.
- Strong chemicals are used only as a last resort because of their injurious effect.

Unit II ❖ Hospital

Removal of Specific Stains

Woolen articles: Strong chemicals are used only as a last resort because of their injurious effect on wool.

Stains due to	Removal of specific stains
Acids	Use water containing a little ammonia, or sodium bicarbonate or washing soda
Alkalies	Use warm water containing an acid such as vinegar or lime juice
Machine oils	Can be removed by using petrol or kerosene
Albumin	Wash in cold water
Argyrol	Soak in ammonia to fresh stains
Methylene blue	Use oxalic acid and wash thoroughly afterwards
Balsam of peru	Soak in alcohol or kerosene. Wash out grease stain in kerosene
Bichloride of mercury	Use oxalic acid and wash
Iodine	Apply ammonia or chloroform and wash in warm soapy water or apply alcohol and wash, or apply a starch paste, keep renewing until the stain is removed. Starch water is good to remove tincture of iodine (congee water)
Medicine	Use cold water for washing. If needed, use a little alcohol to soak the stained part
Silver nitrate	Ammonia or bichloride of mercury and wash
Blood	Wash in cold water using soap if fresh blood
If very dry	Apply hydrogen peroxide and wash with soap and cold water
If old	Soak in hydrogen peroxide or ammonia or milk for several hours (24 hours) and wash with soap and cold water
Tea, coffee, cocoa	First wash in cold water. Pour boiling water over stained part, If not successful apply lime juice or a little peroxide of hydrogen
Fruit stains	Rub with salt and pour boiling water over the stain, soak in alcohol. If unsuccessful, use oxalic acid or a bleaching agent in weak solution
Grease	Wash in warm water and soap. For materials harmed by water, use a grease solvent such as petrol and use an absorbent such as blotting paper or several folds of clean cloth under the stain
Paint or varnish	Shall be removed by turpentine, alcohol or ether

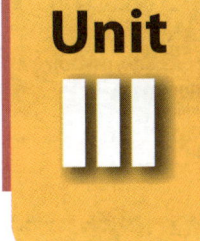

Unit III

Health and Illness

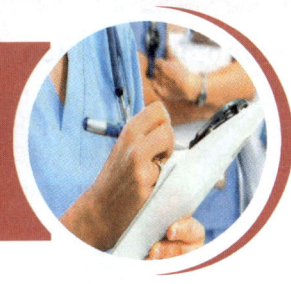

DEFINITION

The World Health Organization (WHO), has defined health in the following manner:

"Health is a state of complete physical, mental and social wellbeing and not merely an absence of disease or infirmity."

For a layman, health is a sound mind in a sound body. Physical, mental and social aspects of health are related to each other and cannot be separated. A person who is having these three aspects of health is said to be enjoying **optimum or positive health**. Achieving highest degree of health should be the aim of every individual.

FACTORS INFLUENCING HEALTH (FIG. 1)

Heredity

Height, weight, skin color, blood group, etc. are hereditary to certain extent. These factors cannot be changed completely. But due to the environmental changes of a living being these characteristics may change due to mutations in the genetic material. These changes are inherited through heredity and bring out the visible changes in the carriers. Still, hereditary characteristics are natural in people.

Environment

- **Physical environment:** Air, water, soil, house, atmosphere, food habits, etc. have good effect in the growth and development of the man.
- **Biological environment:** The living components such as plants, animals, insects, bacteria, viruses, etc. with which we are in constant relationship affect the growth and development of man.
- **Social environment:** This aspect is comprised of the customs, habits, income, occupation, religion, standard of living, etc. Social environment pertains to man by his relationship to others.

Mode of Life

Health cannot be transferred from one person to another. It depends upon one's education, hygiene and ways of living. People must assume the responsibility of their own health by observing the rules of hygiene, eating balanced diet, cultivating healthy habits, immunization and periodic medical check-up. Diseases like tuberculosis, leprosy, etc. can be eliminated by raising the standard of living. Cancer and heart diseases, etc. can be reduced by avoiding smoking. In short, health status can be improved by raising the standard of living of people.

Economic Condition

It has been observed that the people of developed countries are healthier than poor and undeveloped countries. This difference in status of health may be due to the difference in living standards of the people living in these countries.

Utilization of Health Services

In developed countries, people keep their health by the utilization of advanced medical facilities. Whereas in poor countries, the health status of the people is lower due to lack of advancement in medical facilities. Medical care, prevention of communicable diseases, family planning, maternal and child health care, environmental sanitation, health supervision of school children, collection and observation of health statistics and health education of the public are the basic health services (Fig. 1).

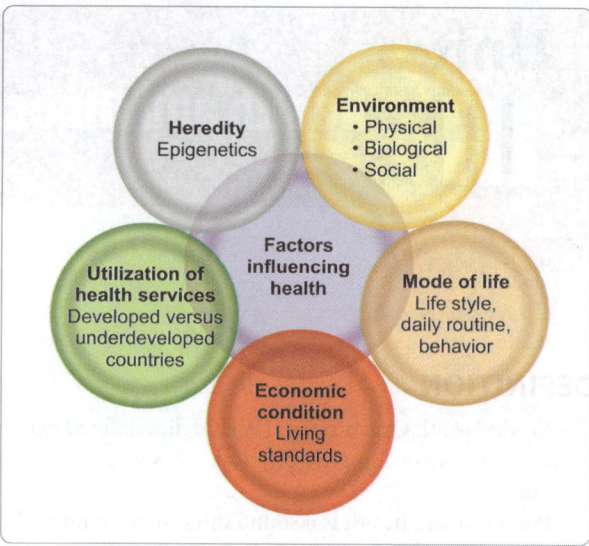

Figure 1: Factors influencing of health

CHANGING CONCEPTS OF HEALTH

Biomedical Concept

Health has been viewed as an 'absence of disease', and if one is free from disease, the person is considered healthy. This concept is known as biomedical concept, and it is based on the 'germ theory of the disease'. The medical profession viewed the human body as a machine and disease as an outcome of the breakdown of this machine, and one of the tasks of the doctor is to repair the machine.

Ecological Concept

Health implies the relative absence of pain and discomfort and a continuous adaptation and adjustment to the environment to ensure optimal function. Ecologists viewed health as a dynamic equilibrium between man and his environment, and the disease as a maladjustment of the human organism to environment.

Psychosocial Concept

Health is both a biological and social phenomenon. Advances in social sciences showed that health is not only a biomedical phenomenon, but one which is influenced by social, psychological, cultural, economic and political factors of the people concerned. These factors must be taken into consideration in defining and measuring health.

Holistic Concept

Holistic model is a synthesis of all the following concepts. A sound mind in a sound body, in a sound family, in a sound environment. Holistic concept recognizes the strength of social, economic, political and environmental influences on health (Fig. 2).

- The concept of holistic approach says that health is an ability to live to full potential and is a state of balance on seven levels—psychological, expression, connection, vocational, emotional, physical and spiritual.
- Every chronic disease is due to unresolved or incomplete healing. Physical, chemical and psychological disturbances create functional imbalances in body, which if not corrected will lead to diseases.
- The emerging science of psychoneuroimmunology (PNI) holds great promise in connecting immune system and mind, which results in incorporating methods to use the body's inherent abilities to live in state of balance on all above-mentioned seven levels. The holistic concept has been shown in Figure 2.

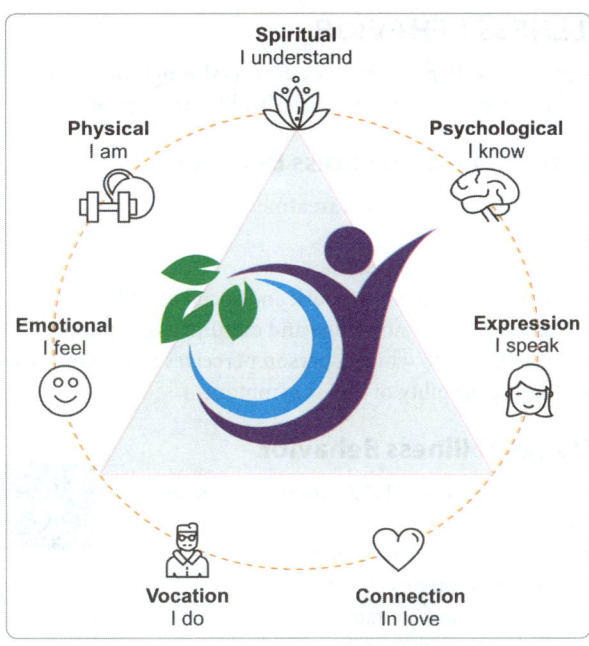

Figure 2: Holistic approach—seven levels of wellness

ILLNESS, SICKNESS AND DISEASE

The concept trilogy of 'illness', 'disease', and 'sickness', has been used to explain different aspects of ill health (Fig. 3).

- **Disease** is an objective term referring to diagnosable abnormalities in organs, body systems or physiology.
- **Illness** is a subjective term referring to an individual's experience of mental and physical sensations or states, and may not necessarily indicate the presence of disease.
- **Sickness** encompasses both disease and illness.

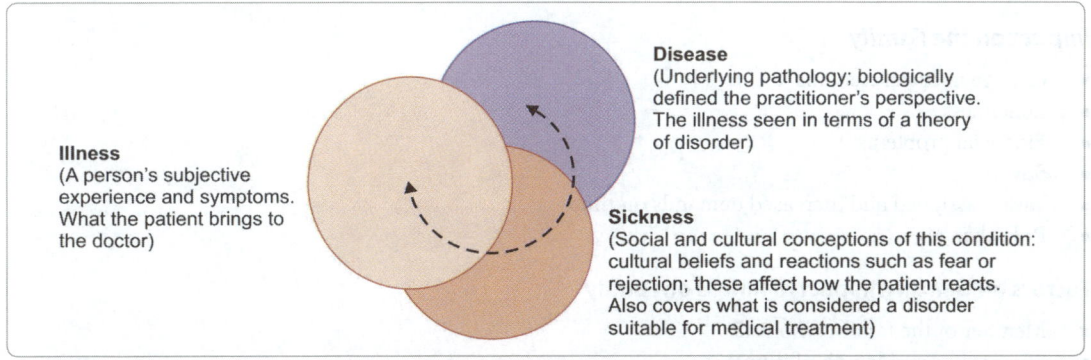

Figure 3: Three perspectives: disease, sickness and illness

Unit III ❖ Health and Illness

ILLNESS BEHAVIOR

A coping mechanism involves the way through which an individual describes, monitors, interprets symptoms, takes remedial actions, and uses health care system.

Determinants of Illness Behavior

- Physical proximity of treatment resources
- Toleration level
- Frequency of appearance
- Disruption in family work and social activity
- Information, knowledge and cultural assumption
- The extent to which a person perceives symptoms as serious
- Recognizability of illness symptoms

Stages of Illness Behavior

Edward Suchman (1972) identified stages of illness behavior (Fig. 4).
- Experience of symptoms
- Assumption of sick role
- Medical care contact
- Dependent client role
- Recovery and rehabilitation

Impact of Illness on Patient and Family

Impact on the Client

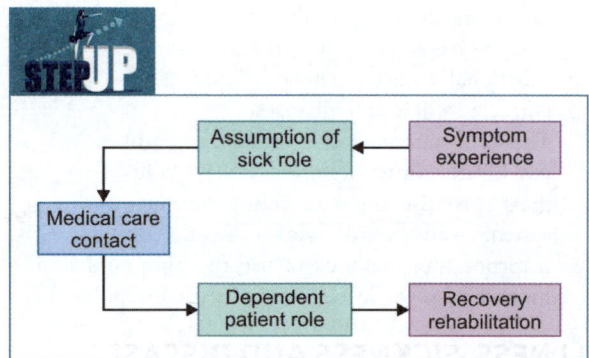

Figure 4: Suchman's stages of illness behavior

- Experience behavioral and emotional changes
- Changes in self-concept
- Loss of self-esteem
- Loss of self-concept
- Changes in lifestyle—diet, activity, exercise, rest and sleep.

Impact on the Family

- Change in social customs
- Loneliness
- Financial problems
- Stress
- Task reassigned and increased demands on time
- Role changes

Factors Influencing Impact of Illness on Family

- Member of the family, who is ill
- Seriousness and length of illness
- Cultural and social customs of the family

Unit IV

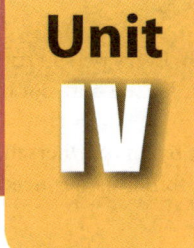

Basic Needs of the Patient

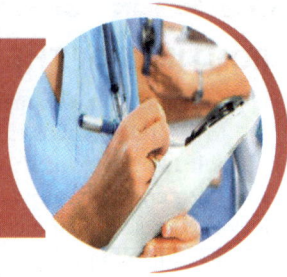

Psychological Needs of the Patient

DEFINITION

Psychology is the study of mind and mental processes. We should remember that the patient is an individual with mind and body. The disease of the body **will affect the mind and illness of the mind will affect the body.** Psychosocial care is part of a holistic patient perspective and allows patients to seek both informational and emotional support from care givers to help them manage their disease condition. The psychological needs of a patient are met by a nurse from the **time of admission of patient,** considering patient as an individual, satisfying the **routines of the day** and providing **safety in the hospital** during his/her stay. While giving care to a patient, his/her physical and mental conditions should be considered.

PATIENT AS AN INDIVIDUAL—THE REACTION OF THE PATIENT AND HIS/HER FAMILY TO ILLNESS

The position of the patient in the hospital is that of a paying guest. He/she has to pay certain medical fees for getting proper care and treatment in the hospital. However there are charity hospitals and government-aided hospitals where patients are given free treatment or are charged nominally. **The average person visiting the hospital expects adequate medical attention, expert and efficient nursing care, provision for his physical comfort and protection.** Sick persons are often dependent, sensitive, frightened and emotional. Therefore, they expect and need the kindness, consideration and support they would get from their family if they were at home. Every arrangement is made keeping in mind the patient care. If there is no patient there is no need of the existence of a hospital and no work for the people of the institution. Therefore, in every respect patient is the central figure in the hospital. In other words, a patient is the most important person in a hospital.

The patient and his/her family are unduly sensitive to all kinds of experiences in the hospital. When an individual is admitted in a hospital, the nurse is concerned primarily with his/her admission to the ward. Relatives accompanying the patient may be stressed and require help and understanding from nursing staff.

To a busy nurse, the relatives may seem selfish, but in fact their behavior is the result of preoccupation with their own family which gives them a different perception rather than selfishness.

Therefore, the relatives need reassurance that the patient will be taken a good care and will get better as early as possible. The nurse is not always able to reassure relatives on all points, particularly when diagnosis is in doubt. The nurse can give assurance to the relatives that **everything possible will be done for the benefit of patient** and that the nurse will be approachable and as helpful as possible.

ROUTINES OF THE DAY

- Individuals have to meet the basic needs of body daily, for healthy life and satisfaction. Every person tries to meet daily routines during his normal (healthy) life. But when one becomes sick, he/she may not be able to perform daily routines by himself/herself.
- The person may need help in some of the matters and he/she may do some activities by himself/herself.
- The nurse should recognize abilities and disabilities of patient and help him/her to fulfill his/her needs according to priority.
- Patient may be having several needs, at a time.
- The nurse should use intelligence to realize the importance and priority of the needs and act accordingly.
- By the sympathetic talk and tactful and intelligent behavior, the nurse should understand the reaction of the patient toward himself, toward disease, to the environment and treatment, to the family and to the nurse.
- The nurse should understand the position of the patient in his/her family and the society.
- The nurse should also understand the responsibilities of the patient in the family and compare the effect of his/her absence.
- A nurse should be interested to listen to the patient while talking to him/her.
- Try to retain the confidence and acquire patient's cooperation.

ADMISSION OF THE PATIENT

Admission of a patient means allowing a patient to stay in the hospital for investigation, diagnosis and treatment of the disease he/she is suffering from. The psychological aspects of admission of a patient to the hospital are quite valuable.

Purposes of Admission

- To receive the patient and to help in adjusting to the hospital environment and routines so that he/she may become the member of the hospital family
- To obtain the necessary identifying data concerning the patient
- To obtain his/her social and medical history for observation, investigation, diagnosis and treatment
- To secure safety of the patient and his/her belongings
- To institute immediate steps for the patient's diagnosis and treatment

Scientific Principles to be Observed on Admission

- Strange situation can cause fear, and changes in environment can cause anxiety
- Entering in a hospital for stay is threatening to one's personal identity
- Individual's response to situation is based on the previous experiences and the present response is expressed on the basis of that previous experiences.
- Individual's behavior depends upon the culture of the group from which one belongs and people have diversity of habits and mode of behavior.
- Illness can be a new experience for an individual and other's help may be required to understand and accept the condition.

Types of Admission

- **Emergency admission:** In this, patients are admitted in acute conditions requiring immediate treatment. They are taken utmost care in the emergency department. Examples of such disease are: Heart attack, patient with renal tubular acidosis (RTA), poisoning, burns and cardiac or respiratory emergencies, etc.
- **Routine admission or elective admission:** In this type of admission, patients are admitted for investigation and medical or surgical treatment. Treatment is given according to patient's requirements. Examples: patient with hypertension, diabetes mellitus, etc.
  - The admission itself may be delayed until a time is convenient for the patient and the doctor.
  - In most cases of elective admission, admission occurs at the hospital's admitting office.
    At the time of admission, hospital personnel must establish a desirable relationship with the patient to promote the feeling of confidence and security needed for recovery of patient. Hospital personnel must make special efforts to be friendly and courteous and make him/her feel that they are sincerely interested in welfare of patient. Since first impression is likely to be vivid and not easily erased, it is important that the patient and the family members should receive the most courteous attention and the patient himself should have the most effective service from the time of admission.
    The patient's first impression as received by the nurse when admitted to the ward, counts much toward the patient's future happiness and contentment. Remember that the hospital may be strange and even terrifying to the patients therefore, a nurse has to make all possible efforts to make him/her feel at ease and at home, as nurse is the host, welcoming these guests (patients) for a temporary stay in the house (hospital).

Admission Procedure

This can be divided into two areas, viz. outpatient department and inpatient department (Table 1).

Table 1: Types of admission procedure

Type	Explanation	Example
• Inpatient	Length of stay generally more than 24 hours	Acute appendicitis, acute pneumonia.
▪ Planned (nonurgent)	Is scheduled in advance	Elective surgery
▪ Emergency admission	Unplanned, stabilized in emergency department and transferred to nursing care unit	Unrelieved abdominal or chest pain
▪ Direct admission	Unplanned, emergency department bypassed	Acute condition as prolonged vomiting, and diarrhea
• Outpatient	Length of stay less than 24 hours	Minor surgery e.g., in case of 'warts'
▪ Observational	Monitoring required, need for inpatient admission determined within 23 hours	Head injury, RTA, FD

Outpatient Department (OPD)

Receiving the Client

- The admission procedure generally begins with the admitting department.
- The representative in admitting department should greet and make patient feel comfortable.
- The manner in which doctor or nurse receives the client is most important aspect of reception.

Recording of Social and Medical Data

- The representative in record section records data essential for identification of client.
- **Demographic data:** Including name, age, sex, education, address, occupation, religion, income, marital status, telephone number, etc.
- **Medical data:** Diagnosis, provisional diagnosis, duration of illness, name of the doctor, emergency contacts, etc. need to be registered.
- Privacy and confidentiality should be maintained while recording data.
- An interpreter should be available for translating the information if the patient does not speak the local languages.

ID (Identity) Band and Consent

- Once the necessary information is obtained, an ID band is placed on the patient's wrist.
- The patient signs a consent form that gives permission for general treatment.

The unit staff members are notified that a new patient is en route. They prepare the bed for admitting the client.

Inpatient Department (IPD)

Preparation of Records

Records such as general history sheet, doctors, orders, nurses' record, temperature, pulse, respiration chart (TPR), progress record, intake output record, investigation record, operation record, discharge sheet and other records as per patient's condition and institution's policy, should be kept ready.

Preparation of Equipment

Patient's bed, linen, sheets, patient locker, patient's chart, adequate light, clock, ventilation, wheelchair/ stretcher and other equipment such as oxygen, suction apparatus, etc. should be kept ready as per the need of the patient.

Transporting the Client from OPD to IPD

- Clients who are not very ill and are allowed to walk are escorted to ward by a nurse or attendant.
- Wheel chairs or stretchers should be available for those who are too sick, weak and unable to walk.

Reception of the Client by Ward Sister

- The ward sister or the nurse admitting the client should introduce herself and greet the client and his/her relatives with friendliness.
- Call the patient by his/her surname, unless otherwise directed by the patient.
- Introduce yourself with your name and designation.
- The ward sister or the nurse should gain the confidence and cooperation of the client.
- If the client is very sick, nurse should transfer the patient to the bed immediately.
- The client who is not very ill is allowed to move about and can be taken to a round.
- Introduce other clients to the patient and vice versa and also with nursing personnel in the ward.
- Orient the client to whole ward, duty room, toilet rooms and unit prepared for the client.
- Explain hospital policies, procedures, routines to the client and relatives.
- Explain to the client—the time for meal servings, doctor's visit, visiting time, prayer hours.

Patient's Room Orientation

Orientation should include the following:

- Explanation of policies applicable to the patient
- Adjustment of beds and lights
- Procedure to call the nurse from bed and bathroom and the operation of call bell
- Operation of the telephone and television
- Use of intercom
- Location of lounge areas
- Operation of bed
- Visitors timing
- Shift timing and changes

Preliminary Observation of Client

- Observe the first few moments with client. Assess immediate needs by patient's facial expressions like presence of pain, fatigue, shortness of breath or severe anxiety. Also note any discoloration of skin such as jaundice, cyanosis, facial paralysis, pallor, etc.
- Further observations can be made while giving care to the client.

Carrying Out the Routines

- A closed bed is converted to open bed on admission of client.
- The temperature, pulse and respirations of patient are recorded at the time of admission and later on at regular intervals.
- Check the doctor's orders that are to be carried out immediately.
- Document the date and time of admission, condition of patient and observations made on the client in the inpatient chart.
- Give time to patient to change his/her dress with hospital dress. Give assistance, if client is not accompanied by any relatives.
- Assist in bathing the client, if the client has to bath on admission.
- Bed bath should be given to a client who is not fit enough to use bathroom. Bed bath gives opportunity to the nurse to examine client carefully.
- Never leave a seriously ill client alone in the private room without any help.
- If any tests are ordered by the doctor, the nurse must make arrangements to carry out the test.
- Carry out other procedures prescribed by doctor, if any.

Care of Valuables and Clothing

- If patient is wearing hospital dress, patient's clothing should be handed over to relatives.
- In case of absence of relatives, clothing is numbered, labelled and kept in store until the time it is handed over to relatives.
- Encourage the client not to keep the jewellery, money and other valuables such as watch at hospital and send valuables to home. Make him/her understand that if he/she keeps something with him/herself, it is on his/her own risk.
- Get a written statement signed by the patient and relatives specifying the valuables handed over.

Unit IV ❖ Basic Needs of the Patient

Procedure

Steps	Procedure	Rationale
1.	Perform hand hygiene	Reduces spread of microorganisms
2.	Prepare the room before the patient arrives. • Keep the things in place. • Bed at proper height • Convert the closed bed into open bed • Lights on and well ventilated	Makes the patient feel expected and welcome
3.	Courteously greet the patient and family. Introduce yourself. Project interest and concern. If it is a general ward or sharing unit introduce the other patients.	Eases the patient and family if they know the people around them
4.	Check the ID band and verify its accuracy.	Ensures appropriate identification before every procedure and investigation
5.	Assess immediate needs and take appropriate actions to meet them.	Establishes trust
6.	Orient the patient to the: • Room • Unit • Nurses, station • Lounge • Policies and procedures • Facility routines, like meal time, visitors time, doctors rounds, etc.	Promotes safety and gives a feeling of security
7.	Instruct the patient to change to the hospital gown (as per the Institutions policy). Provide privacy if required.	Helps maintain dignity
8.	Follow Institutions policy in care of valuables, clothing and medications.	Helps to maintain legal proceedings with regard to valuables safety
9.	Perform initial nursing assessment within 30 minutes of routine admission or as early as possible.	Provides a basis for individualized care
10.	Take necessary safety measures such as: • Bed in low position • Raising the side rails • Call bell within easy reach	Promotes patient safety
11.	Monitor vital signs and record it. Perform care as per Doctor's order.	Develops positive attitude when care is started immediately
12.	Make the patient comfortable and tidy up the unit.	Decreases anxiety
13.	Perform hand hygiene.	Reduces spread of microorganisms
14.	Document the care given with date, time and signature.	Documentation fosters quality care

TRANSFERRING A PATIENT TO ANOTHER HEALTHCARE FACILITY

When a patient is admitted in a hospital, there are occasions when he/she must be transported to another healthcare facility to provide a continuation of care or within the hospital to another department. This transport is referred to as a 'patient transfer'.

Transfer combines admission and discharge. The patient is discharged from one unit and admitted in another unit.

Types

- **Intra-agency transfer:** Moving a patient from one unit to another
- **Interagency transfer:** Moving a patient from one healthcare facility to another.

Key Elements of Patient Transfer

- **Decision to transfer and communication:**
  - The decision to transfer the patient is important because of exposure of the patient and the staff to additional risk.
  - The decision to transfer the patient is taken by a senior consultant after thorough discussion with patient's relatives about the benefits and risks involved.
  - A written and informed consent of patient's relatives along with the reason to transfer is mandatory before the transfer.
  - A direct communication between the transferring and receiving facility should be undertaken with sharing of complete information on patient's clinical condition, reasons for transfer, treatment given, mode of transfer and time line of transfer in a written document.
- **Pretransfer stabilization and preparation:**
  - A proper and meticulous preparation and stabilization of patient should be done before transfer to prevent any adverse events or deterioration in patient's clinical condition.
  - The patient should be adequately resuscitated and stabilized to the maximum extent possible without wasting undue time.
- **Mode of transfer:** The two most commonly employed modes of transfer of patients are ground transport, with the inclusion of ambulances and mobile intensive care units (MICUs), and air transport which includes helicopter or aeroplane ambulances.
- **Accompanying the patient:**
  - It is usually recommended to have at least two competent personnel accompanying the patient to be transferred.
  - The accompanying person should be suitably trained, competent and experienced and preferably should have done training in patient transfer and should have sufficient training in advanced cardiac life support, airway management and critical care.
- **Equipment, drugs, and monitoring:**
  - A proper monitoring with the provision of all lifesaving drugs is mandatory for transfer of all patients.
  - The transfer ambulance must be equipped with all the drugs and instruments required for airway management, oxygenation, ventilation, hemodynamic monitoring and resuscitation.
  - The person in charge of patient transfer should ensure proper supplies of the emergency drugs.
  - The minimum standard of monitoring recommended for patient transfer includes continuous electrocardiogram monitoring, non-invasive blood pressure, oxygen saturation, and temperature monitoring.
- **Documentation:**
  - The documentation of patient transfer is most important at all stages of transfer.
  - A standardized document should be used and maintained both for intra- and inter-hospital transfer.
  - There should be a formal handing over at the receiving facility between the transferring team and the receiving team.

Unit IV ❖ Basic Needs of the Patient

The algorithm followed for transfer of a patient to other healthcare facility is as follows:

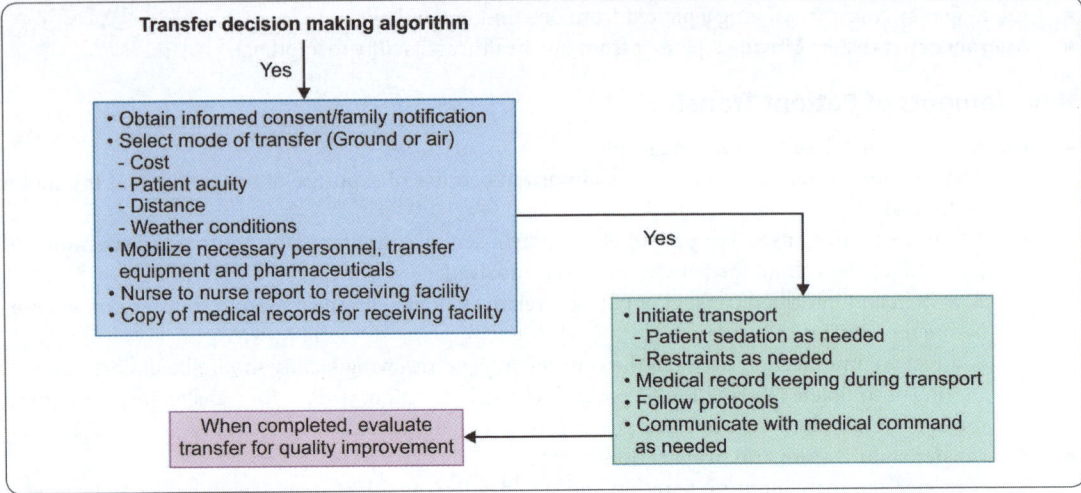

Steps of Transfer from One Unit to Another in Same Hospital

- Written order by physician
- Inform patient and family
- Inform ward incharge of another unit/ward
- Complete patient's documents and transfer summary
- Arrangement of transport
- Inform other departments
- Transportation of the patient
- Receiving of the patient in new ward
- Handing over and taking over of the personal belongings
- Documentation

Steps of Transfer from One Healthcare Facility to Another

- Be sure that patient and family are informed about the need for transfer.
- If the patient or family has some choice, encourage the family to investigate various facilities where patient can be transferred.
- Communicate with the agency or unit where the patient will be transferred.
- Make photocopy of medical records.
- Provide written transfer summary.
- Collect all the belongings of patient.
- Help in transportation of the patient.
- Give transfer personnel a copy of the medical records in a folder or envelop.
- Complete the medical records by adding transfer summary. All records should be kept for future reference.
- Notify other departments of hospital regarding patient's transfer. Each department has its own responsibility toward patient.

DISCHARGE PROCEDURE

It is the preparation of the patient and discharge records to leave the hospital. Discharge planning is the process of planning for patient care after discharge from a hospital or healthcare facility.

Purposes

- To ensure continuity of care to the patient after discharge.
- To assist the patient in discharge process.

Types of Discharge

- Cured and discharged
- Discharged against medical advice (DAMA)
- Discharged on request
- Absconded
- Death

Discharge Procedure

- No patient should be discharged without doctor's written orders.
- If there is no discharge order and the patient insists on leaving the hospital, have the patient signed the 'leaving against medical advice (LAMA) form'.
- Inform the hospital authorities about the discharge.
- See that the patient's personal hygiene is maintained and change the dress into his/her own clothing.
- Hand over the discharge slip to the patient or relatives.
- Provide discharge teaching including:
  - Medications
  - Diet
  - Exercise
  - Follow up care
- Ensure that the patient has taken all his/her belongings.
- Transfer the patient in a wheel chair or assist the patient to his/her vehicle.
- Use good communication skills and wish patient well as he/she leaves.
- Document entire discharge procedure including the teaching given, condition of the patient, time and method of discharge.
- Handover the case sheet and other records to the medical record department.

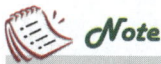 **Note**

Leaving Against Medical Advice (LAMA)

A client can decide to leave the hospital against medical advice. For this client must sign a form that releases the physician and the health care institution from any legal responsibility for his/her health status. The client is informed of any possible risks before signing the form.

Unit IV ❖ Basic Needs of the Patient

Role of the Nurse in Discharge Procedure

- Nurse must ensure that the patient leaves the unit with all belongings and personal effects, has the appropriate medications with him, and appointment for follow-up has been made and understood.
- All necessary instructions, especially regarding his/her medication regimen, side-effects etc. must be clearly given to the patient and his family members.
- Any paper work, signing of documents should be completed. The hospital file along with all charts and notes should be sent to the medical records section.

NEEDS OF HOSPITALIZED PATIENT

The needs of a patients vary according to the spiritual and cultural traditions of the patients. This is a dynamic concept that changes over time and the disease progression. The majority of studies showed that the main needs of hospitalized patients are information, communication, support and confidence. However, a nurse is also responsible for the following needs:

- **Safety needs:** The simplest definition of patient safety is the prevention of errors and adverse effects to patients associated with healthcare. Protect the patient from hazards like falling from the cot, slipping on the floor and damages due to electricity and safeguard from thermal, chemical and bacterial injuries.
- **Social needs:** Sociology is the scientific study of the development of man's social relationships and organizations. Humans live in groups. They need communication and interaction with people and organization in the society. The nurse has to help the patient in this matter as he/she is sick and dependent. If the patient is suffering from any communicable disease, dealing with others should be prevented, till the infection period is over.
- **Spiritual needs:** A patient's spiritual need is as important as his/her physical needs. It is the responsibility of the nurse to help the patient in this matter according to the caste and religion. Sustaining the spiritual needs of hospitalized patients requires building trust and having sympathy with patient, providing desirable environment, appropriate communication of medical team with patient, and respecting the patient's dignity and beliefs.

Physical Needs of the Patient

DEFINITIONS

- **Before discussing the physical needs of a patient, we must understand a few terms used here.**
- **Comfort** has been defined as 'a state of ease or well-being' when a person is comfortable, he is at ease with him/herself and with his/her environment.
- **Rest** is synonymous with repose of relaxation and implies freedom from emotional tension as well as physical discomfort.
- **Sleep** is a period of decreased mental alertness and lessened physical activity, which is a part of the rhythmical daily pattern of all living creatures.
- **Discomfort** is defined as want of comfort or ease due to pain or annoyance. Discomfort can result from stimuli of both psychological and physical origin. A person who is afraid or worried is uncomfortable, as he/she may be feeling cold or may be in pain or stressed due to some external stimuli.

IMPORTANCE OF PHYSICAL NEEDS IN HEALTH AND DISEASES

There are innumerable causes of emotional discomfort, for example, the newly-admitted patient is subjected to the stresses before going into strange environment. The ill person often fears pain, supposed death and disability and he worries about his ability to cope with forthcoming stresses. Neglect by the nursing staff or care by an unyielding, unconcerned nurse also contributes to a patient's discomfort. The patient looks toward the nurse for understanding and support in order to attain some degree of psychological comfort.

Physical discomforts can cause mental distress and interfere with a person's psychosocial equilibrium. Pain, nausea, heat and even an untidy environment are stimuli in which the patient feels uncomfortable and sometimes it becomes unbearable. By the selection of appropriate interventions, the nurse can prevent the development of many situations, which could be a source of discomfort. Many discomforts can be alleviated if they occur. The nurse should therefore be alert to the earliest signs of discomfort in a patient and be aware of interventions that can be used to relieve discomfort or prevent these from increasing.

The immediate source of providing physical comforts to a patient is to provide a healthy environment that is, patient's unit and suitable bed should be according to the condition.

PATIENT'S UNIT, REQUIREMENTS AND SET UP

Patient's Unit

It is the area furnished and equipped according to the necessity for the care of the patient. Unit may vary in size. It may be private unit or the immediate surroundings of patient in general ward. Whether the patient is in a single room or in a large general ward, there is definite unit of space and equipment assigned to a patient.

Variations in Units

Private room	Bed room with all other toilet facilities
Cubicles	Small or large, the partition may be of a wall or curtains
General ward	Where several patients are placed

Unit IV ❖ Basic Needs of the Patient

Furnishing and Supplies for the Patient's Unit

In the Private Rooms or Pay wards

- Bed and bedside table
- Cupboard or chest of drawers
- A sofa cum bed
- Chair and one table without drawers
- Wash basin
- A stool
- Kidney tray
- Other toilet facilities
- Bedpan and urinal
- Provision for drinking water and hot water

In a General Ward

- Bed
- Bedside locker
- Stool
- Some provision for drinking water and hot water
- All other things are used in common (bedpans, kidney trays, etc.). It is ideal to have individual equipment.

BED AND BED MAKING

Bed is an article or furniture to sleep or to take rest or to keep a patient for physical examination, or to do some procedures of treatment or for providing nursing care.

Selection of Beds and Beddings

As comfort, rest and sleep are important in maintaining health and promoting recovery from disease, special attention should be given in providing healthy beds and beddings both in the hospital and in homes. During the patient's stay in the hospital, he spends all or most of his/her time in bed. Since all of the patient's activities are carried on in the bed, it is of great importance as a comfort factor and in restoring his/her health.

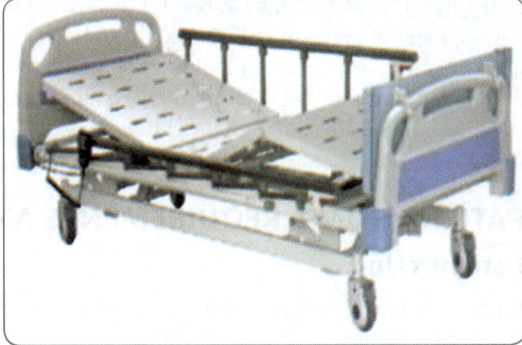

Figure 1: Hospital cot

- **Cot:** The hospital cot is adapted to the needs of the patient and to the needs of the doctors and nurses caring for them. Cots may be made of wooden or metal. It may be made-up of iron or steel tubing and painted. They are simple in design, light and easily movable, easy to handle, clean and disinfected, strong and durable. Modern hospital cots have hard rubber castors or tyres which make it possible to move the cot easily without jarring the patient. A standard hospital cot is 195 cm long, 95 cm wide and 65–70 cm high from the floor (Fig. 1).

■   **Mattresses**

- **Cotton mattress:** Hard and likely to lumpy

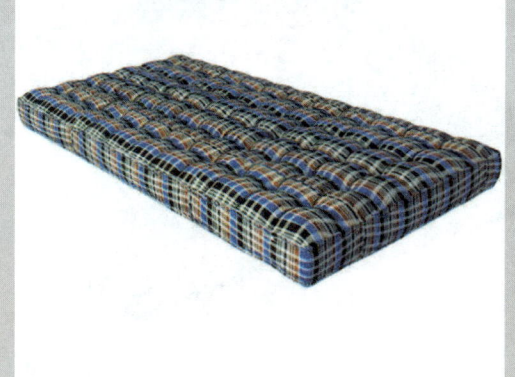

- **Horse hair mattress:** Firm, cool and light, nonabsorbent

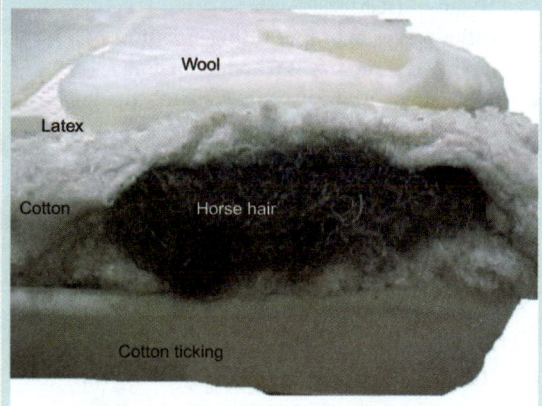

Wool

Latex

Cotton

Horse hair

Cotton ticking

- **Dunlop mattress**: Sponge rubber, useful for patients suffering from long-term illness. Disadvantage is that they are inflammable

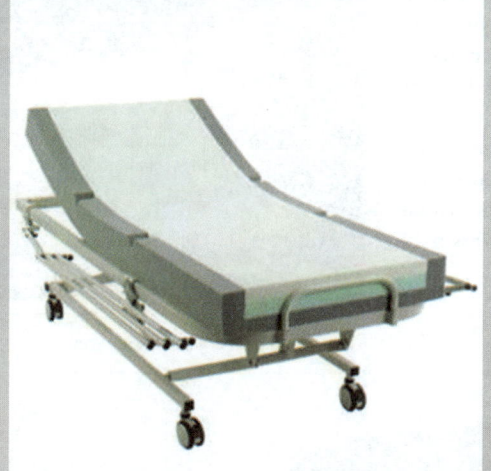

- **Coir mattress:** Common and cheap but hardly in use nowadays

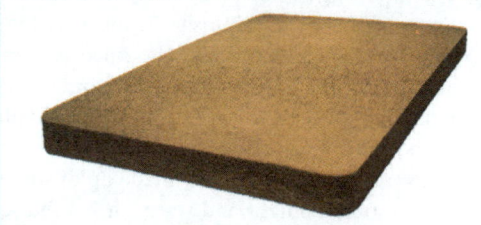

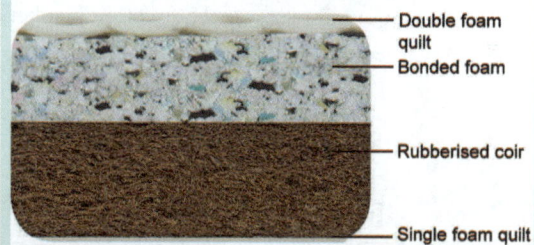

Double foam quilt

Bonded foam

Rubberised coir

Single foam quilt

- **Air mattress:** Inflated with air, rarely used in hospitals, should have washable covers

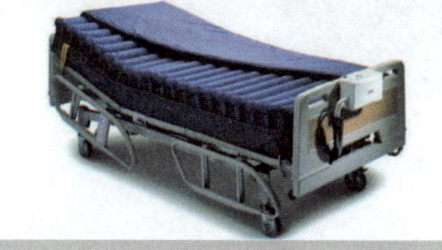

- **Water mattress:** Filled with warm water, blanket

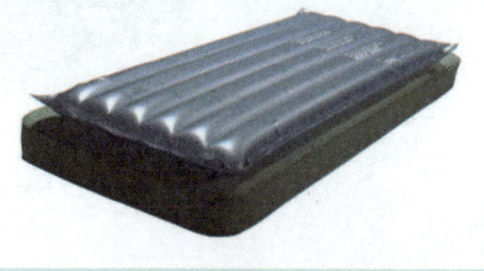

Unit IV ❖ Basic Needs of the Patient

- **Pillows:** These are usually made out of cotton. They are also stuffed with water or air. Dunlop pillows are available in 60 cm long, 45 cm width and 10 cm thick size.

  Pillow cases of proper fitting size must be taken. Average size is 65 cm × 50 cm.

- **Bed sheets:** Sheets are usually made out of cotton material. They are used to protect the mattress from soiling, to cover the patient and to protect the patient from irritation due to woolen blanket. These should be large enough to be tucked in all round the mattress and strong enough to withstand pulling. The ideal size should be 270 cm long and 190 cm wide.

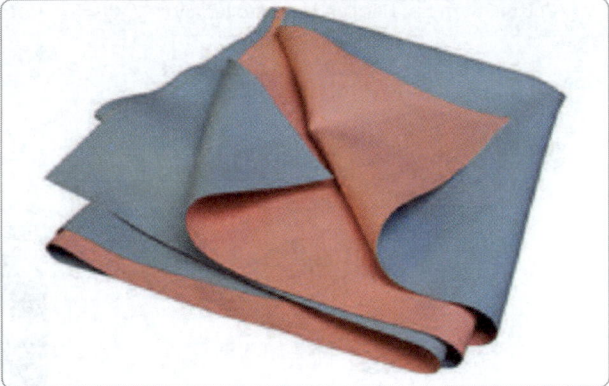

- **Rubber sheets or mackintosh:** Waterproof sheet or plastic sheet is used for protecting the mattress and bottom sheet (Fig. 2).

Figure 2: Water proof sheet or plastic sheet or Mackintosh

- **Draw sheets:** A draw sheet is made up of the same material and is as strong as the large sheet. It is used to cover the waterproof sheet (mackintosh). It must be long enough to extend from shoulders up to the knee and must be wide enough and strong to be pulled tightly and tucked well under the mattress on both sides. The ideal size should be 150 cm long and 110 cm wide (Fig. 3).

- **Blankets:** Blankets are usually made up of woollen material. Blanket should be light and warm. It is used for protecting the patient from draughts and chill. Woollen blankets irritate the skin. So use it over a sheet or cotton blanket covers may be used (Fig. 4).

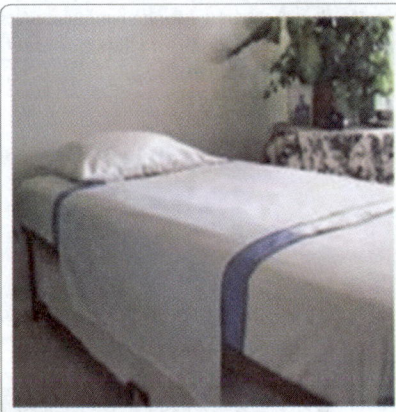

Figure 3: Draw sheets

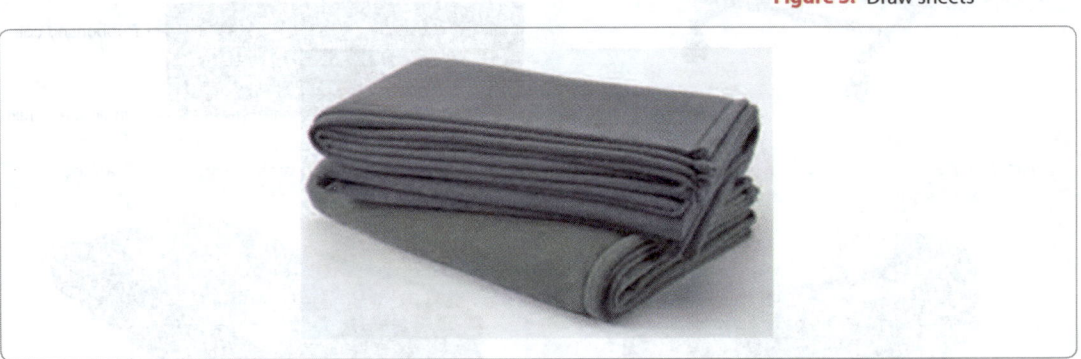

Figure 4: Blankets

■ **Bath blanket:** It is light in weight, narrow in width and about the same length as the blanket used for warmth. It is used to cover the patient during bed bath (Fig. 5).

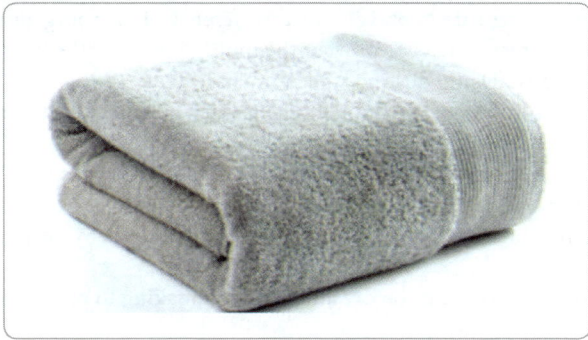

Figure 5: Bath blanket

■ **Bed spread or counterpane:** It is used for giving neat appearance (Fig. 6). It protects the blanket. It is usually made up of cotton which can be easily washed. The ideal size is 3 meters long and 2 meters wide (300 cm × 200 cm).

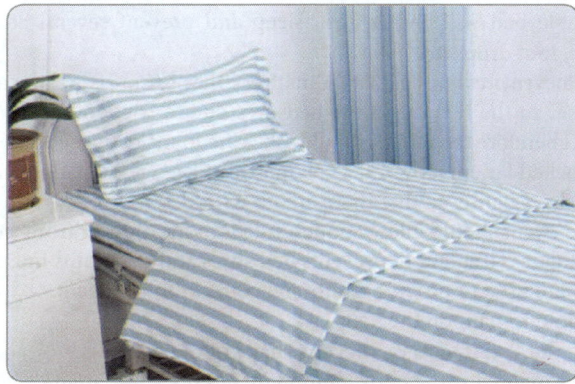

Figure 6: Bed spread

Objectives of Making Bed

■ To provide the patient with a comfortable and safe bed to take rest and sleep on arrival
■ To give the unit or ward a neat appearance
■ To give medical and nursing treatment to the patients
■ To prevent bed sore
■ To promote cleanliness
■ To provide active and passive movements to the patient
■ To create an effective nurse-patient relationship
■ To provide physical and psychological comfort and security to the patient
■ To promote fresh environment and cleanliness
■ To observe, identify and prevent patient's complications
■ To accommodate the patient's needs
■ To develop skill in the posture/body alignment of the nurse in bed-making

Unit IV ❖ Basic Needs of the Patient

Principles of Bed Making

- Microorganisms are found everywhere on the skin, on the articles used by the client and in the environment. The nurse takes care to prevent the transference of microorganisms from the source to the new host by direct or indirect contact or prevent the multiplication of the microorganisms.
  - Dry dusting raises dust. Damp dusting is recommended.
  - Do not place soiled linen on the floor. If clean linen touches the floor or any unclean surface, immediately place it in the dirty linen container.
  - Never shake the linen to avoid air currents that spread microorganisms.
  - Place soiled linen in special linen bags before placing in a hamper.
  - When changing bed linen, follow principles of medical asepsis by keeping soiled linen away from the uniform.
  - The nurse has to wash her hands before and after bed making to protect the client and herself from cross infection.
  - The linen removed from the isolation unit is disinfected first before they are sent to laundry.
  - Cleaning an area where there are less number of organisms before cleaning an area where there are numerous organisms minimizes the spread of organism to the clean area. For example, clean the bed first before cleaning the bedside locker.
  - The nurse keeps a reasonable distance from the client's face to prevent droplet infection.
- A safe and comfortable bed will ensure rest, sleep and prevent several complications in bedridden patients, e.g., bedsore, foot drop, etc.
  - The body exerts uneven pressure against the mattress, the pressure is greatest over the bony prominences. Lumps and creases in the bed can cause bedsores due to friction between the bed and mattress or wrinkled sheets. Therefore the nurses should take care to make the bed smooth and unwrinkled.
  - Keep the linen tucked far enough under the mattress, keep it fixed, tight and smooth.
  - Pull the bottom sheet tightly so that there are no wrinkles.
  - A bed made for a client should allow enough freedom for moving from side to side. The movement of the client stimulates circulation, prevents bed sores and maintains muscle tone.
  - Comfort devices are used to provide additional comfort to the client.
  - No wet linen should remain on the bed.
  - While tightening the sheets, do not alter the shape of the mattress.
- Good body mechanics maintains the body alignment and prevents fatigue.
  - During bed making use safe patient handling procedures and proper body mechanics.
  - Body mechanics and safe handling are very important while turning or repositioning the patient in bed.
  - Always raise the bed to the appropriate height before changing linen so you do not have to bend or stretch over the mattress. You move back and forth to opposite sides of the bed while applying new linen.
  - The nearer to center of gravity a weight is held, the less strain it produces. For example, when opening the linen it should be placed on the edge of the bed rather than holding it above the shoulder level.
  - The stability of the body is assured by keeping its centre of gravity over its base. When the base is wide it ensures that the center of gravity will fall through its base. In standing position the nurse can have a wide base by separating her feet.
  - When placing the linen on the bed and tucking them under the mattress face the direction of work and move with the work rather than twisting the body and over reaching.
  - When tucking the sheets under the mattress, flexing is done by knees and hips. This position shifts the work to the long and strong muscles of the thighs and keeps the back in good alignment. This reduces strain on the back.

- Systematic ways of functioning saves time, energy and materials.
  - The bed sheets are folded in such a way that it can be replaced easily.
  - When stripping the bed, remove the bed linen one by one holding the open end toward the floor, so that the client's belongings and the hospital articles are not sent to the laundry by mistake.
  - Finish on one side of the bed before going to the opposite side.
  - Arrange the linen in the reverse order of use.
  - Assemble all articles and arrange them conveniently before starting the bed making.
  - When patients are confined to bed, organize bed-making activities to conserve time and energy.
- General instructions of bed making:
  - Make all beds in a nursing unit alike for uniformity of appearance.
  - It is important to learn the skill of bed making in such a way where least amount of energy and time is required.
  - The patient's privacy, comfort, and safety are all important when making a bed. Using side rails to aid positioning and turning, keeping call lights within the patient's reach and maintaining the proper bed position help promote comfort and safety.
  - After making a bed, return it to the lowest horizontal position and verify that the wheels are locked to prevent accidental falls when the patient gets in and out alone.

Factors to be Considered while Bed-making

Factors to be considered in selecting and making bed are as follows:

- Have all equipment at hand before beginning and arrange conveniently to handle in the order of use.
- See that there is no draughts.
- Do not cover the patient's face while placing top linen on bed.
- Do not put linen on the floor at any time.
- Expose the patient only as much as necessary.
- Do not mix clean linen with that of soiled.
- When removing and replacing linen, make sure that it doesn't come into the contact of your uniform.
- To prevent wrinkles, pull linen tight as they are tucked.
  While tucking under the mattress the palm of the hand should be directed downwards in order to protect your nails.
- Never shake the blankets and sheets over the bed.
- Do not use torn linen or wet linen.
- Do not make a bed without mattress cover and rubber sheet.
- Use extra protection whenever necessary, for example, use a rubber pillow or pillow with plastic case when there is drainage from a wound on head.

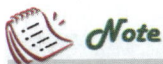 **Note**

Essentials of Basic Nursing Procedures
- The open end of the pillow should be placed away from the entrance of the ward.
- While preparing a bed, the crosswise free ends of the bottom sheet should be directed toward the head end of the bed and crosswise free ends of the top sheet should be directed towards the foot end of the bed before the sheets are unfolded to spread. This is applicable in the 1/4 size folding method. Three flaps folding also are practiced in some hospitals.
- Do not permit the patient to breathe, cough, or sneeze straight to the nurse's face.
- The time of bath and bed making is a good time to give instructions to patients on personal hygiene.

Unit IV ❖ Basic Needs of the Patient

Types of Beds

Simple beds	Special beds
• Closed bed or unoccupied bed	• Surgical operation bed
• Open bed	• Cardiac bed
• Occupied bed	• Blanket bed
	• Amputation or stump bed
	• Fracture bed
	• Burns bed

Simple Bed

- **Closed bed or unoccupied bed:** A closed bed is made when a patient has been discharged from the facility and no new patient is expected. An unoccupied bed is one that is made when not occupied by a patient.
- **Open bed:** An open bed is made when a patient is to be admitted in the unit.
- **Occupied bed:** An occupied bed is made when the patient is bedridden. An occupied bed is one that is made while occupied by a patient.

Special Bed

- **Surgical bed or postoperative bed or recovery bed or anesthetic bed:** A post-operative bed is used for a patient who had undergone surgery and who is recovering from the effects of anesthesia following a surgical operation.
- **Cardiac bed:** Cardiac bed is prepared for patients with cardiac diseases.
- **Blanket bed or rheumatism or renal bed:** Blanket bed is prepared for a patient with renal diseases or rheumatism.
- **Amputation bed or stump bed:** Amputation bed is prepared for a patient with amputation of the leg to take off the weight of the bed clothes off site of the operation. In this type of bed the top bed clothes are divided or split.
- **Fracture bed or plaster bed:** Fracture bed is prepared for the patient who is suffering from fracture of the trunk and extremities. A hard firm board is used to give support. It helps in immobilizing the part until the plaster dries.
- **Burns bed:** This is prepared for a patient with burns.

Let us discuss the simple bed and special beds in detail now.

Closed or Unoccupied Bed

It is an empty bed in which the top covers are so arranged that all linen beneath the spread is fully protected from dust and dirt.

Articles Required

Article	Purpose
Bed and mattress with mattress cover	For the patient to rest
Kinds of linens: Bed sheets–2 • 1 bottom sheet • 1 top sheet Mackintosh Draw sheet Blanket if necessary	For placing over the mattress

Contd...

Article	Purpose
Pillow one or more with cases	For patient's comfort
A chair or stool or trolley	For placing the linen and articles
A bowl with antiseptic lotion	To wet the duster for damp dusting
Dusters—2	One for dry dusting and one for damp dusting
Bucket or laundry bag	To put the soiled linen
Kidney tray	To put the dust particles from mattress, if any.

Prerequisites

- Raise the bed to a comfortable working height, if adjustable.
- Lower side rails, if present.
- Arrange all the equipment at the bedside.
- Wash the mattress, if necessary, turn the mattress to the opposite side, if necessary, and replace the mattress pad as needed. Observe the mattress for protruding springs.
- Collect all the supplies which are likely to be required, place on the stool or bedside table.
- Use a damp duster for enamel-painted iron bed and dry one for the varnished bed. Dust mattress and sheets with dry duster and furniture with damp duster.
- Remove your watch.

Procedure (By Single Person)

Steps	Procedure	Rationale
1.	Perform hand hygiene	Prevents the spread of infection
2.	Assemble the equipment at the bedside	Organization facilitates accurate skill performance

Contd...

Unit IV ❖ Basic Needs of the Patient

Steps	Procedure	Rationale
3.	Move the chair and bedside locker.	Facilitates adequate space for bed-making
4.	Adjust the height of the bed at comfortable position.	Prevents back strain
5.	Wear gloves.	Prevents the spread of infection
6.	Remove all soiled linen and pillow cases and place them in the laundry bag.	Prevents the spread of infection
7.	Fold the sheets and blankets as follows before arranging it on the chair or stool:	Systematic arrangement saves time, energy and material
7a	**Folding a Top Sheet**	
i	Take a top sheet and fold it once cross wise so that the folding is in the middle of the sheet	Systematic folding of the top sheet facilitates spreading of the top sheet toward the foot end first followed by the head end
ii.	Then fold it length wise with the folding in the middle. Ensure that the center point is on your left-hand side and fold it towards you	

Contd...

Steps	Procedure	Rationale
iii.	Now each layer of the sheet is ¼ of the total size with all free ends together length wise and cross wise and the foldings in the middle 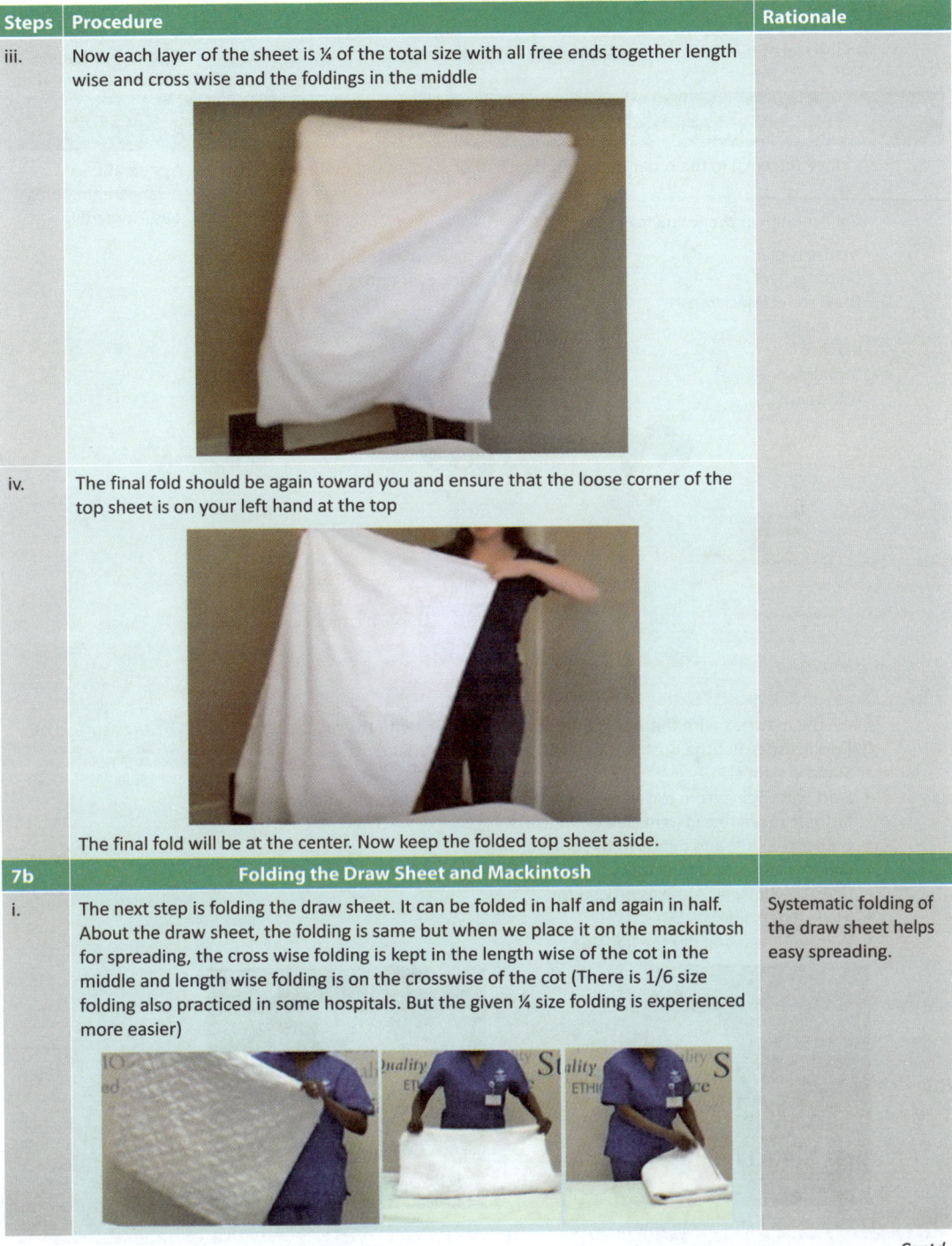	
iv.	The final fold should be again toward you and ensure that the loose corner of the top sheet is on your left hand at the top The final fold will be at the center. Now keep the folded top sheet aside.	
7b	**Folding the Draw Sheet and Mackintosh**	
i.	The next step is folding the draw sheet. It can be folded in half and again in half. About the draw sheet, the folding is same but when we place it on the mackintosh for spreading, the cross wise folding is kept in the length wise of the cot in the middle and length wise folding is on the crosswise of the cot (There is 1/6 size folding also practiced in some hospitals. But the given ¼ size folding is experienced more easier)	Systematic folding of the draw sheet helps easy spreading.

Contd...

Steps	Procedure	Rationale
ii.	On the top of the draw sheet place the rolled mackintosh.	Systematic folding helps easy spreading.
7c	**Folding a Bottom Sheet** **Whole procedure is same as followed for 'Folding a top sheet'.**	
8.	Arrange the linen in the order of use on the chair or stool at the foot end of the bed	Systematic arrangement helps easy spreading.

Collect linen in the following order:

Mattress pad Bottom sheet Draw sheet/Mackintosh Top sheet Blanket Bedspread Pillowcase	Once you have collected the linen, turn the stack over onto the other hand

Steps	Procedure	Rationale
9.	**Cleaning the Mattress**	
	Clean the mattress with the wet duster or a mitt and dry with the dry duster in the following order. Put the dust particles in the kidney tray, if any. • Stand in right side. • Start wet wiping from top to center and from center to bottom and from farthest to nearest in right side of mattress. • Gather the dust and debris to the bottom. • Collect them into kidney tray. • Give dry wiping as same as procedure. • Move to left side. • Wipe with wet and dry the left side.	Prevents spread of infection.

Steps	Procedure	Rationale
10.	Clean the cot in the same way.	

Contd...

Steps	Procedure	Rationale
11.	Turn mattress and pull the cover on. If loose, pull it on one side and tuck under the mattress. Pull the mattress to the top 	Prevents discomfort to the patient.
12.	There are two methods in performing bed making:	
12a	**Method 1:** Spreading each sheet one by one and tucking on both the sides simultaneously.	
	<div align="center">**Spreading the Bottom Sheet**</div>	
i.	Move to right side. Place and slide the bottom sheet upward over the top of the bed leaving the bottom edge of the sheet. Make sure that the central crease is in the middle and covering the right upper quadrant of the mattress. Open it lengthwise with the center fold along the center of the bed. 	Unfolding the sheet in this manner allows you to make the bed on one side.
ii.	Unfold it and spread it straight over the mattress allowing 30–37 cm to tuck under the top of the mattress and leaving just enough at the foot to tuck in figure 	Unfolding the sheet in this manner allows you to make the bed on one side.

Contd...

Steps	Procedure	Rationale
iii.	Tuck it securely just enough at the near side. Make a mitered corner • Pick up the selvage edge with your hand. • Lay a triangle over the side of the bed with 45°. • Tuck the hanging part of the sheet under the mattress by placing the hands on the top corner of the triangle. • Drop the triangle over the side of the bed. • Tuck the sheet under the side of bed.	A mitered corner gives a neat appearance to the bed and keeps the sheet securely under the mattress.
iv.	Spread the sheet to the foot end. Tuck at the foot end, secure the corner as before.	Unfolding the sheet in this manner allows you to make the bed on one side.
v.	Pull tight at the center and tuck in securely and then tuck sheet in, along the side. Tuck in with palms down and hands straight in front.	Unfolding the sheet in this manner allows you to make the bed on one side.

Spreading the Mackintosh and Draw Sheet

i.	Place the mackintosh or rubber sheet at the middle of the bed approximately 37 cm from the top and tuck in, along the side.	Mackintosh and draw sheet are additional protection for the bed and serve as a lifting or turning sheet for an immobile client.

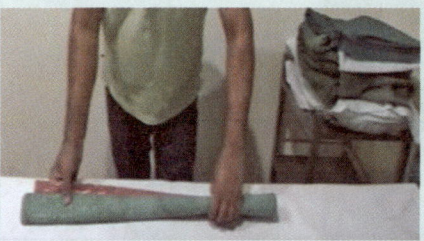
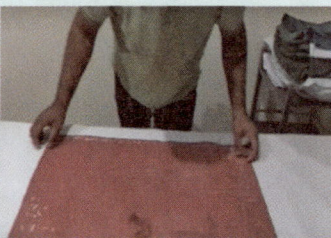

Contd...

Steps	Procedure	Rationale
ii.	Place the draw sheet over the rubber sheet 25 cm from the top of the mattress. Keep 7–12 cm above the rubber sheet. Tuck in well. (Rubber sheet and draw sheet can be tucked together too)	A draw sheet helps in lifting the patient easily.
iii.	Go to the opposite side; tuck in each article of linen separately as on the first side. Avoid folds and wrinkles before spreading top sheet	Securing the bottom sheet, mackintosh and draw sheet on the other side of the bed provides a wrinkle free bed and promotes comfort of the patient.

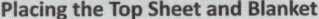

Placing the Top Sheet and Blanket

Steps	Procedure	Rationale
i.	Return to the right side of the bed and place the top sheet on the middle of the bed, making sure that the central crease is in the middle of the bed and covering the lower right quadrant of the mattress. Make the mitered corner and leave the edges hanging	Unfolding the sheet in this manner allows you to make the bed on one side.

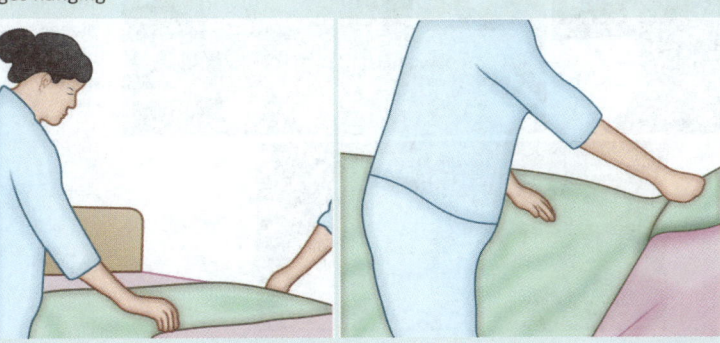

Contd...

Unit IV ❖ Basic Needs of the Patient

Steps	Procedure	Rationale
ii.	Unfold it and spread it so that the upper end is at the level of the top edge of the mattress. That means the upper end of the mattress and the upper edge of the top sheet must coincide. Move on to the other side and repeat the same procedure. 	Spreading the sheet in this manner allows you to make the bed on both the sides.
iii.	Tuck in at the foot end in both sides and make mitered corner allowing the side to hang free 	Tucking provides a neat appearance.
iv.	If blanket is used, spread it just like the top sheet. But the top edge of the blanket is covered with the top edge of the top sheet to prevent it rubbing on the chin of the patient while using. For this, fold the cuff (approximately 1 feet) in the neck part. Tuck all these together under the bottom of mattress Now the bed is ready to occupy.	Blanket provides warmth. Making the cuff at the neck part prevents irritation from blanket edge. Tucking all these pieces together saves time and provides a neat appearance.

Contd...

Unit IV ❖ Basic Needs of the Patient

Steps	Procedure	Rationale
12b	**Method 2:** Completing the procedure on one side of the bed and then moving on to the other side	
i.	The bed is made in the following manner, completing one side before going to the other. • Place the bottom sheet on the mattress. Center it lengthwise; fold at midline with the hem seam down and the bottom hem even with the foot edge. • Unfold the sheet across the bed. Tuck the surplus under the head of the mattress. • Pull the excess sheet taut and smooth over the top edge of the mattress, tightening it from the underside of the mattress. • Fanfold the bottom sheet to the center of the mattress. • To miter the corner, pick up a hanging side of the sheet edge about 12 inches from the head of the mattress. Lay it back on the mattress in a triangle fold. • Tuck the hanging corner of the sheet under the mattress, holding your hands palm down to protect your knuckles from the bedspring. • Place your hand at the side of the mattress and even with the top edge. Bring the triangle fold down over your hand to ensure a firm, smooth mitered corner. • Tuck the sheet under the mattress working from top to bottom. 	Unfolding the sheet in this manner allows you to make the bed on one side.
ii.	• Place a mackintosh at the middle of the bed. Spread it forward. • Fanfold the mackintosh toward the centre and keep it under the fan folded bottom sheet. • Tuck the near end of the Mackintosh under the mattress 	Systematic spreading promotes comfort and saves time, energy and material.

Contd...

Unit IV ❖ Basic Needs of the Patient

Steps	Procedure	Rationale
iii.	• Place the draw sheet on the mackintosh. Spread and tuck as same as above. • Fanfold the draw sheet to the middle and place it under the bottom sheet and mackintosh 	Systematic spreading promotes comfort and saves time, energy and material
iv.	• Center the top sheet on the top of the other sheets with the hem seam up and even with the head edge of the mattress. Permit the surplus to extend at the foot. • Center the blanket with the edge approximately 8 inches (about one hand span) from the head edge of the mattress and the surplus at the foot. • Fanfold the top sheet and blanket at the center and place in under all the sheets. • Place your hand under the foot end of the side of the mattress to hold the foundation sheet taut while raising the mattress slightly. Smooth and tuck the top sheet, blanket, and spread under the foot of the mattress. Miter the corner. Leave the side of the top covers hanging free 	Systematic spreading promotes comfort and saves time, energy and material

Contd...

Steps	Procedure	Rationale
v.	• Go to the opposite side of the bed and complete the making of the bed as follows 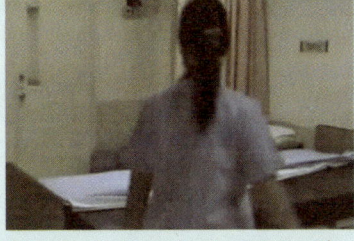 • Smoothen and straighten the bottom sheet, maturing the top corner and pulling the sheet taut while tucking the side under the mattress from head to foot. 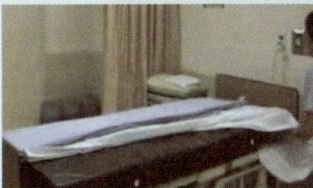 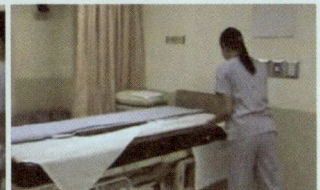 • Pull the mackintosh and draw sheets taut and tuck them under the mattress. 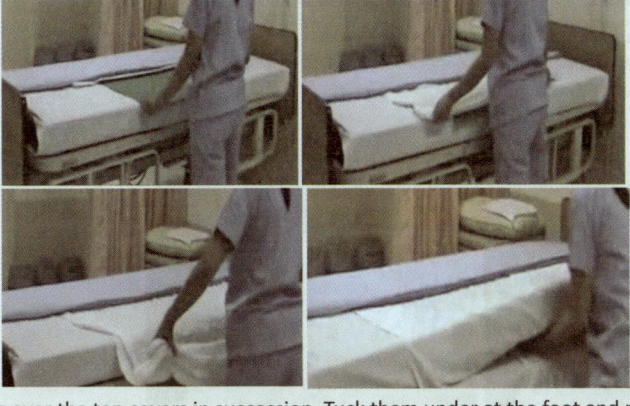 • Bring over the top covers in succession. Tuck them under at the foot and miter the corner. • Fold the top edge of the spread under the blanket edge. **Note:** Do not form a cuff when preparing a closed bed. 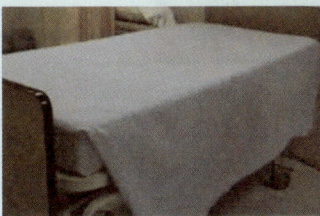 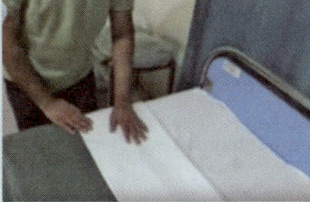 Now the bed is ready to occupy.	Systematic spreading promotes comfort and saves time, energy and material.

Contd...

Unit IV ❖ Basic Needs of the Patient

Steps	Procedure	Rationale
13.	**Replace the pillowcase and pillow** • Gather the open-end portion of the pillowcase to about midway of the pillowcase length. • Fit the pillow in the case with one hand while continuing to hold the gathered edges with the other. • Move one hand to the closed-end grasping the pillowcase and the pillow within. With the other hand, extend the pillowcase so that it covers the pillow. • Fit the pillow into the corner on one side of the pillowcase and pleat the excess under at the opposite side. • Place the pillow neatly at the head of the bed with the open end of the case away from the door. • Cover with the bed spread. 	Pillow cover keeps the pillow neat and clean. The open end may collect dust or micro organisms. The open end away from the door also makes bed look neat.
14.	• Damp-dust bedside cabinet, bed frame and chair. • Straighten the unit, adjust the bedside locker and stool. • Turn inward the bed wheels and crank handles. Lock the wheels and leave the unit in order. 	Prevents the spread of infection. Bedside necessities will be within easy reach for the client
15.	Clean the articles and replace in proper place. Discard lines appropriately. Perform hand hygiene.	Prevents the spread of infection.
16.	Document and report to the senior sister if there is any abnormality noted.	Documentation fosters quality care.

Open Bed

The term open bed is used to designate the hospital bed when it is about to be occupied by a patient either for a new patient or for an ambulatory patient. When a new patient is allowed to occupy the bed after changing to hospital dress or sponge bath on admission (whichever is the custom of the hospital) it is called an **Admission Bed.**

Procedure

Steps	Procedure	Rationale
1.	• For making an open bed, all the steps of making a closed bed are same. • **Next step:** Bring the top sheet and the blanket over to form a cuff and fanfold the bedding half-way to the foot end of the bed or about 1/3 of the length of bed. • Then turn back one corner of it to form a triangle on the side, where the patient will enter 	This lets the patient conveniently enter onto the bed.

Stimulant

Rules for Bed-making
- Use good body mechanics at all times.
- Follow the rules of medical asepsis and standard precautions.
- Practice hand hygiene before handling clean linens.
- Bring enough linens to the person's room. Do not bring extra linens.
- Place clean linens on a clean surface. Use the bedside chair, over-bed table, or bedside stand. Place a barrier (towel, paper towel) between the clean surface and the linens if required by agency policy.
- Do not use torn or frayed linens.
- Never shake linens. Shaking spreads microbes.
- Hold linens away from your body and uniform. Do not let used or clean linens touch your uniform.
- Never put used linens on the floor or on clean linens. Follow agency policy for used linens.
- Bag used linens in the room where they are used. Do not carry used linens un-bagged outside of the person's room.
- Keep bottom linens tucked in and wrinkle-free.
- Straighten and tighten loose sheets, blankets and bedspreads as needed.
- Make as much of 1 side of the bed as possible before going to the other side. This saves time and energy.
- Change wet, damp, or soiled linens right away.

Unit IV ❖ Basic Needs of the Patient

Stripping and Re-Making a Bed

It is the removal of used linen and airing the mattress.

Objectives

- To air the bed and beddings.
- To refresh the patient.

Prerequisites

- One chair or stool
- Dusters 2: One for dry dusting and one for wet dusting
- A bowl with antiseptic lotion
- Kidney tray 1: To put the dust particles, if any, picked from the mattress

Procedure

Steps	Procedure	Rationale
1.	Place a chair or trolley at the foot of the bed and lock the bed.	Stripping the bed in a systematic order prevents transfer of microorganisms.
2.	Remove pillow case from pillow and place the pillow on the chair.	
3.	Wipe off dust and food crumbs from the bed gently into the kidney tray using the duster.	
4.	Loosen all bedding starting from the head end 	
5.	Fold and set the blankets and spreads aside (to be reused) 	

Contd...

Steps	Procedure	Rationale
6.	Fold each linen with soiled part inside. Remove each linen separately 	To prevent spreading of microorganisms
7.	Fold the draw sheet. (Bring the end towards you from the opposite end and fold at the center) Strip the rubber sheet by rolling and place on the chair or stool. Roll rubber sheet and place on the chair 	
8.	Remove the spread, blanket and top sheet by folding into four as described in 1/4 size folding and place them on the chair or stool. The mode of 1/3 size folding is as follows. (Bring the lower third of the sheet or blanket over the middle third and fold the upper third over the lower third. Fold at the center toward you) 	

Contd...

Steps	Procedure	Rationale
9.	Wrap them all and place in a laundry bag	Prevents spread of infection
10.	Remove mattress cover. Wash the mattress, if necessary. Turn the mattress to the opposite side, if necessary, and replace the mattress pad as needed.	
11.	Replace the chair or stool and leave the unit neat and tidy. Wash the dusters, dry and replace in proper place. Change the gloves. Perform hand hygiene.	

Occupied Bed

It means making a bed with patient in bed.

Objectives

- To provide a comfortable bed for the patient.
- To change the soiled bed linen.

Preliminary Assessment of the Patient and Unit

- See the patient and assess the general condition.
- Identify the diagnosis and the extent of self-help.
- See the Doctor's order to note the restrictions in movement of patient or any part, if any.
- Get the instructions from the ward sister.
- Arrange help from others, if necessary.
- Collect the required clean linen to change.

Prerequisites

Same as for open bed.

Procedure (By One Nurse)

Steps	Procedure	Rationale
1.	Explain the purpose and procedure to the patient.	Providing information fosters cooperation
2.	Perform hand hygiene.	Prevents the spread of microorganisms.

Contd...

Steps	Procedure	Rationale
3.	Close the curtain or door to the room. Put screen.	Maintain the client's privacy.
4.	Assemble articles to bedside and arrange them in the order of use	Organization facilitates accurate skill performance.
5.	Straighten the bed. Adjust the height of the bed at comfortable position	Ensures proper body mechanics.
6.	Remove the client's personal belongings from bed-side and put them into the bed-side locker or safe place.	Prevents personal belongings from damage and loss.
7.	Remove all pillows except one (if necessary).	Extra pillows prevents undue disturbance during the procedure.
8.	Assist the client to turn toward left side of the bed away from you. If the patient is very ill, assistance may be needed to turn the patient. If the patient cannot be turned, lift him/her to the farther side of the bed. Raise the side rails if there are no assistants. Adjust the pillow.	Moving the client as close to the other side of the bed as possible gives you more room to make the bed.

Contd...

Steps	Procedure	Rationale
9.	Lower the side rails on one side. Loosen the bedding.	Facilitates easy removal.
10.	Fold the spread and blanket, if any, leaving the top sheet over the patient and place on the chair or stool	Top sheet keeps the client warm and protects his/her privacy.
11.	Fan fold the draw sheet toward the patient and push as close to the patient as possible	Placing folded (or rolled) soiled linen close to the client allows more space to place the clean bottom sheets.
12.	Dust the rubber sheet and roll it under the draw sheet	Placing rubber sheet protects the sheet.
13.	Fanfold the bottom sheet to the patient carefully under the rubber sheet	To place the clean bottom sheets.

Contd...

Steps	Procedure	Rationale
14.	Wipe the surface of mattress by sponge cloth with wet and dry cloth starting from head to foot end	Prevents the spread of infection.
15.	Place the clean folded bottom sheet in position on the mattress lengthwise and unfold the sheet making sure that the central fold lies in the middle of the bed leaving rest of the fold against the patient. 1/4 size folding is particularly convenient in this type of preparation of bed. But the first folding should be lengthwise and the second folding should be crosswise. Fanfold the bottom sheet to the middle of the bed. Tuck the head end. Make mitred corner at the top and bottom. Then tuck the sides as in the closed bed	This facilitates easy spreading of sheet on the opposite side.
16.	Bring the rubber sheet back into place over the newly-spread bottom sheet and tuck it tightly under the mattress or a new rubber sheet is used. Fanfold the mackintosh and place it in the middle down the bottom sheet.	Systematic spreading saves time, energy and material.

Contd...

Unit IV ❖ Basic Needs of the Patient

Steps	Procedure	Rationale
17.	Place the clean draw sheet in position. Fan fold it and place it in the middle under the mackintosh and tuck in together	Systematic spreading saves time, energy and material.
18.	Turn the patient back over folded linen	Moving the client to the bed's other side allows you to make the bed on the other side.
19.	Change the soiled pillow case which is kept on the head of the patient. Change pillow case, if necessary, and place pillow in position in the clean side. (Note: This step can also be done at the end)	Changing the pillow case and keeping it on the clean bed sheets promote comfort to the patient.
20.	Assist the client to roll over the folded (rolled) linen to right side of the bed toward you which is toward the clean side

Raise the side rails. | Moving the client to the other side of the bed allows you to make the bed on that side.

Raising the side rails ensures safety of the patient. |

Contd...

Steps	Procedure	Rationale
21.	Go to the opposite side, if there is no one to assist and lower the side rails 	This facilitates easy spreading of sheet on the other side.
22.	Loosen the bed sheets. Fold the sheets one by one in the same order. Remove dirty linen, hold them away from your uniform and put them in linen hamper or laundry bag or bucket 	Soiled linens can contaminate your uniform, which may come into contact with other clients.
23.	Wipe the surface of the mattress by sponge cloth with wet and dry cloth.	Prevents the spread of infection.
24.	Straighten the bottom sheet and tuck firmly as on the other side. Grasp clean linens and gently pull them out from under the client. Spread them over the unmade side of the bed. Pull the linens taut. Tuck the bottom sheet tightly under the head of the mattress and miter the corner. Tighten the sheet under the end of the mattress and make mitered the lower corner. Tuck in along the sides 	Wrinkled linens can cause skin irritation.
25.	Straighten the rubber sheet and draw sheet and tuck each separately and firmly as on the other side. Pull the linens taut.	Wrinkled linens can cause skin irritation.

Contd...

Steps	Procedure	Rationale
26.	Assist the client to the center of the bed	Promotes comfort.
27.	Replace the top sheet as in closed bed, providing privacy for the patient. Stand on one side. Place the clean top sheet over the patient. Hold the top of the clean sheet with one hand and with the other, draw the soiled top sheet from underneath toward the foot of the bed and take away. Then tuck in the bottom of the new one and make corners after removing the soiled one from the bed. After finishing the right side, repeat the procedure on left side.	Tucking these pieces together saves time and provides neat, tight corners.
28.	Place the blanket over the top sheet. Place the bed spread over the blanket. Tuck the foot end. Complete the bed by folding the top end of the bed spread under blanket by making a cuff and top sheet over spread if a bed spread is used	Making the cuff at the neck part prevents irritation from blanket edge.
29.	Place the side rails. Replace personal belongings back. Return the bed-side locker and the bed as usual.	Prevents personal belongings from loss and provides safe surroundings
30.	Leave the patient comfortable. Leave the unit in order.	Promotes comfort and well-being of the patient.

Contd...

Unit IV ❖ Basic Needs of the Patient

Steps	Procedure	Rationale
31.	Remove dirty linen and other articles. Send the dirty linen to the laundry. Clean and replace articles in their proper places.	Prepares for the next procedure.
32.	Then perform hand hygiene.	Prevents the spread of infection.

Surgical or Operation Bed or Postanesthetic or Recovery Bed

It is a bed, which is prepared for a patient who is recovering from the effect of anesthesia following an operation. It is prepared for all patients who had undergone a major or minor operation under general or spinal anesthesia.

Objectives

- To make a bed that will be comfortable and safe for the patient under anesthesia and that will provide the warmth necessary to maintain body heat.
- To secure a bed in which the mattress and pillows are protected and that will facilitate remaking parts as necessary.
- To have bed on which the patient may be placed quickly without unnecessary delay and movement.
- To observe the operated area easily and stay prepared to meet any emergency.

Prerequisites

Article	Quantity	Purpose
Mattress	1	For the patient to rest
Mattress cover	1	For placing over the mattress
Sheets	2	For placing over the mattress
Mackintosh	2	One small to protect the head end of the bed and the other is for draw sheet.
Draw sheet	1	For placing over the bottom sheet
Blanket	1	For providing warmth
Towel	1	To put over the small mackintosh
Pillow with case	1 or more as needed	As a comfort device
Kidney tray		For collecting secretions to maintain airway
Hot water bags as needed with hot water (104°–140°F)		To prevent hypothermia by warming the bed
Saline stand and other requisites for IV infusions depending on the patient's condition.		For administering IV fluids
Bed blocks	2	To raise the foot end or head end of the bed
Chart holder, pulse and BP Chart		For documenting vital signs
Vital signs tray with BP apparatus		For measuring vital signs
Duster or sponge cloth	2	To wipe the bed and mattress
Cotton swabs or clean rag pieces in a small bowl, gauze pieces		For wiping the secretions

Contd...

Article	Quantity	Purpose
• Oxygen cylinder with flow meter • O$_2$ cannula or simple mask • Suction machine with suction tube • Airway • Tongue depressor • SpO$_2$ monitor • ECG • Infusion pump • Syringe pump	As required	To use as required
Artery forceps, Tongue forceps, Tongue depressor, Mouth gag	1 each	For providing care as required
Paper bag	1	
Trolley	1	To place articles which can be used during recovery phase

Procedure (By One Nurse)

Steps	Procedure	Rationale
1.	Foundation bed is the same except for an additional rubber sheet and towel which is placed across the upper end of the mattress. Place the top sheet over the bed, top edge of the sheet beyond the top of the mattress and lower end hanging over the foot of the bed 	Tuck at foot may hamper the client to enter the bed from a stretcher.
2.	Place the blanket over the sheet, a hand's breadth below the top of the mattress and fold it as in closed bed. Fold back the blanket and top sheet over it at the level of the mattress at the bottom covering the edge of the blanket with the sheet 	Makes the client's transfer smooth.

Contd...

Steps	Procedure	Rationale
3.	Do not tuck along the sides. Bring the hanging ends of the top sheet and blanket on the side nearest to the door at the level of the bed. • Bring both head and foot corners to the center and form right angles. • Fold 1/3 side of top bedding to the opposite side • Roll the top bedding again. Tuck opposite side. Alternatively, form a triangle with the linen. Fanfold the linen triangle into pleated layers several times. After fan folding, form a tiny tip with the end so that it can be grasped quickly and pulled over the patient. This fan-folded triangle linen is kept in position opposite to the stretcher side of the bed	Tucking the top bedding on one side stops the bed linens from slipping out of place.

Contd...

Steps	Procedure	Rationale
4.	Keep the bed warm, if necessary, by means of filled hot water bags and additional blankets. Remove hot water bags before shifting the patient.	Hot water bags (or hot bottles) prevent the client from hypothermia.
5.	Place the pillow on a chair near or in an upright position at the head of the bed	Protects the patient's head from hitting against the beam. This helps to maintain airway.
	Ensure that the patients, head is not placed on the pillows. Keep the bed blocks ready, if necessary, use them	
6.	Keep the tray with the necessary articles already as mentioned, conveniently at the bedside on a stool or over the bedside locker • Place a kidney-tray on bed-side • Place IV stand near the bed • Lock the wheel of the bed	Kidney tray helps to receive secretions. IV stand facilitates to hang the IV soon. Prevents moving the bed accidentally when the client is shifted from a stretcher to the bed.

Contd...

Steps	Procedure	Rationale
7.	Fan fold top clothes length wise, toward the opposite side to the maximum, when the patient is brought back from the operating room. Keep him/her in bed, cover immediately by unfolding the top linen. Use hot water bags if needed. Observe the general condition of the patient, watch the BP, pulse, respiration, color and record it. Tidy up the unit. 	
8.	Perform hand hygiene	Prevents infection.

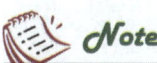 Note

Additional Mackintosh and draw sheet may be used according to the site of the operation to protect the bed.
If pillows are used to support the operated part, they should be protected with rubber sheets and towel or rubber pillow can also be used.

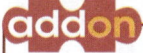

- For most of the abdominal operations, patient is kept in supine position in the operation bed for at least 12 to 24 hours. But for operations of the back and some other particular operations, like tonsillectomy, patient is kept either in prone position or lateral position.
- After tonsillectomy, many doctors prefer to keep the patient in prone position with one pillow under the chest. Three quarter prone position also is used to keep the patient after tonsillectomy.

The purposes of keeping the pillow under the chest in prone position are:
- To keep the head low turned to one side for the free flow of secretions from the mouth.
- To prevent the pressure on the soft abdominal organs and providing free movement of the diaphragm for easy breathing.
  - To attain these purposes the size of the pillow should be selected intelligently according to the age and size of the patient and it should be kept in the proper place.
    - Hands are extended and flexed at the elbow to keep on both sides of head extended and kept on both sides of the body with palms pronated.
    - A small roller pillow or sand bags should be kept under the ankle joints of the legs for support and comfort.

Another method is to keep the patient in lateral position. Here one pillow is kept at the back lengthwise to prevent the patient from falling flat and a spare small pillow is kept under the knee joint of the slightly flexed upper leg. Hands are kept conveniently without causing pressure on it.
(Prone position as described is used in the Medical College Hospital Kottayam after tonsillectomy)

Unit IV ❖ Basic Needs of the Patient

Fracture Bed or Traction Bed

It is a bed, which is prepared for patients with fracture, bone diseases and deformity (Fig. 7).

Purposes

- To keep the traction in position
- To restrict sudden jerky movements
- To immobilize the fractured part

Prerequisites

- Supplies as in open bed.
- Extra supplies:
  - Fracture boards
  - Bed cradle
  - Sand bags
  - Cover sheet
  - Hot water bottles with covers, if required
  - Extra pillows as required

Procedure

For making a traction bed, an assistant is required to minimize the risk of traction misalignment.

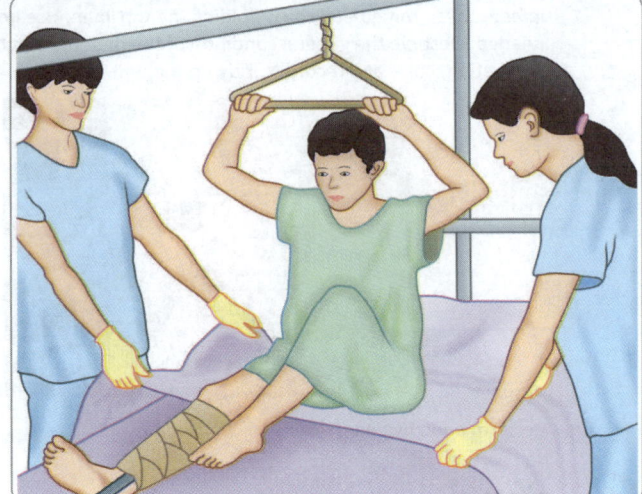

Figure 7: Traction bed

- Explain the procedure to the patient.
- Arrange the equipment at the bedside of the patient.
- Provide privacy
- Adjust the height of the bed to maintain body mechanics.
- Lower the side rails of both the sides.
- Perform hand hygiene.
- Don gloves.
- Stand near the headboard. Remove the pillows. Change the pillow case.
- Loosen the bed linens and roll them from the headboard toward the patients head.
- Place a clean bottom sheet across the head of the bed. Instruct the patient to raise the head and upper shoulders by grasping the trapeze. Quickly fanfold the bottom sheet from the head of the bed under the patients shoulders. Tuck at least 30 cm of the bottom sheet under the head of the mattress. Miter the corners and tuck in the sides.
- Instruct the patient to raise the buttocks by grasping the trapeze (as shown in figure). Quickly and safely remove the soiled linens through the buttocks and place the clean linens. Place the mackintosh and draw sheet simultaneously. Tuck in the foot end.
- Instruct the patient to release the trapeze and rest in a comfortable position. Replace the pillows under the head.
- Ensure that the traction apparatus is not disturbed. Place the top sheet over both the legs and above the traction apparatus. Don't press on the traction ropes.
- Tuck the sheet in the corner opposite the traction side under the foot of the bed taking mitered corners.
- Lower the height of the bed but ensure that the traction weight does not touch the ground. Raise side rails.
- Replace the soiled linens and wash hands.

Cardiac Bed

- Cardiac bed is prepared for patients who are suffering from cardiac diseases.
- Cardiac bed is made with special arrangements, which are required by a cardiac patient. The bed is provided with extra pillows to be kept on head side of patient to keep the patient in prop up position for better airflow. There is special cardiac table provided with the patient's bed with all equipment available for emergency cardiovascular support, like oxygen masks, nasogastric tubes, etc.

Purposes

- To relieve dyspnea
- To prepare the bed for the cardiac patients

Additional Requirements

- Additional pillows for back
- Air cushion
- Cardiac table
- Back rest where Fowler's bed is not available.
- Foot rest

Procedure

- Prepare the bed as open bed.
- Place back rest at the patient's back making it comfortable with pillows and adjust according to the need of the patient. Keep one or two pillows for extra comfort.
- Keep air cushion under the buttocks, a pillow under the knees and support the feet with foot rest board.
- Place the cardiac table in front of the patient with a pillow on it so that he or she can lean forward to rest his or her head and arms on it when gets tired in upright position (Figs 8A and B).

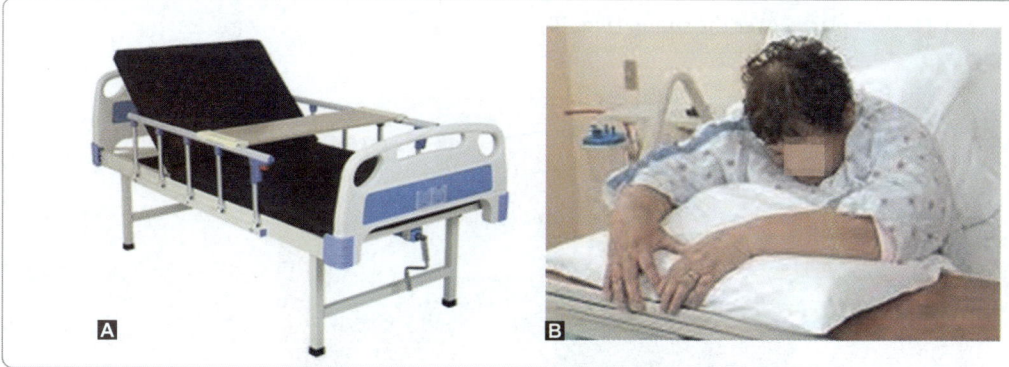

Figures 8A and B: Cardiac bed

Amputation or Stump Bed or Divided Bed or Cradle Bed

It is a bed in which the top linen is divided into two parts to visualize the amputated part of the lower limbs without disturbing the patient.

Unit IV ❖ Basic Needs of the Patient

Purposes

- To keep the stump in position
- To take the weight of the bed clothes off the patient
- To watch the stump for hemorrhage and apply tourniquet instantly.

Additional Requirement

- Waterproof/dressing mackintosh and dressing towels
- 2 sand bags in covers
- An extra dressing towel
- A cradle
- Bed sheets–2 or 3 as required.
- A tray with a tourniquet and dressing towel

Procedure

- The bed is modified depending upon where the amputation has occurred. The bed is made up to the level of a simple bed.

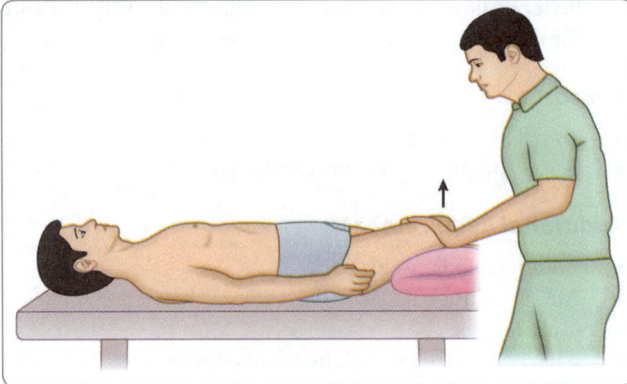

Figure 9: Place a pillow below stump

- A top sheet is placed over the patient's chest, trunk and the good leg.
- Place a pillow covered with protective cover and cotton cover under the stump for support (Fig. 9).
- The dressing mackintosh and dressing towel are placed where the stump lies. This prevents quivering of the stump.
- The second dressing towel is placed over the thigh and held firmly by placing the sandbags covered in a draw sheet over it at either side of the thigh to support the limb in order to keep the stump in good position.
- The cradle is then placed over the stump (Fig. 10).

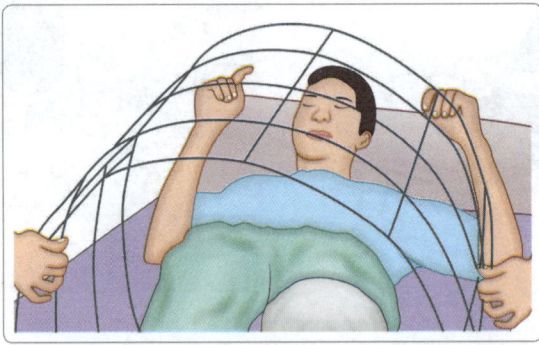

Figure 10: Place a cradle

- The bed is made up to the level of simple bed until the sheet and the bed cradle is in position but the top bed clothes at the stump side are turned back over the cradle. Arrange two sets of top clothes in such a fashion that they are divided into the middle so that there is a gap to visualize the stump. The foot end side of the top linen is folded back to the head end at the level of the part to be observed. Spread the second set of linen starting from the level of stump. The second set of top linen should overlap the first by 8–12 inches. The lower end is tucked in at the bottom on the foot end (Fig. 11).

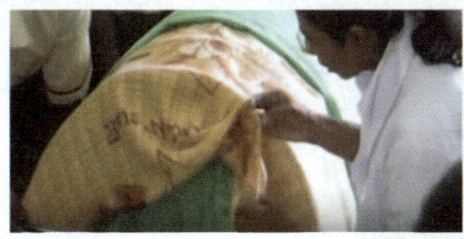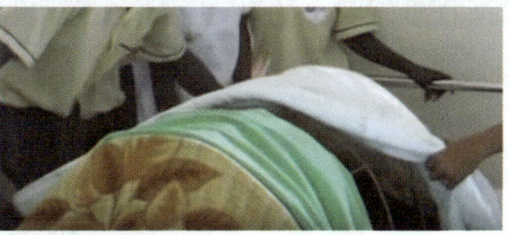

Figure 11: Amputation bed

■ Tie the tourniquet to the bed loosely to apply instantly when hemorrhage is detected (Fig. 12).

■ Keep shock blocks near the foot end of the bed ready in case of necessity.

■ When the patient is received in bed, cover with cover sheet except at the site where it must be folded back. Place a bed cradle over the stump to relieve the pressure of top clothes. Use hot water bottles or radiant heat (heat cradle) to supply warmth to the limb.

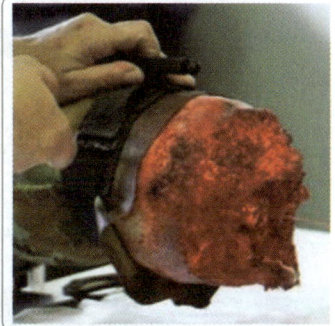

Figure 12: Tie tourniquet in hemorrhage

AMBULATION

Ambulation is defined as moving a patient from one place to another.

Benefits of Ambulation

■ Ambulation promotes oxygen rich blood flow throughout the body

■ It maintains normal breathing functions.

■ It stimulates circulation which can help stopping the development of stroke-causing blood clots.

■ It improves blood flow which aids in quicker wound healing.

Procedure

Steps	Procedure	Rationale
1.	Check physician's orders for any activity restrictions related to treatment or surgical procedures.	Helps to know the limitations.
2.	Explain the procedure to the patient	Allays anxiety and fosters cooperation
3.	Perform hand hygiene	Prevents spread of microorganisms.

Contd...

Unit IV ❖ Basic Needs of the Patient

Steps	Procedure	Rationale
4.	Ensure patient does not feel dizzy or lightheaded and is tolerating the upright position. Instruct the patient to sit on the side of the bed first, prior to ambulation 	Proper footwear is essential to prevent accidental falls.
5.	Apply gait belt snugly around the patient's waist if required. Gait belt should be snug, not tight 	Gait belt acts as a good support to hold the patient.
6.	Assist patient by standing in front of the patient, grasping each side of the gait belt, keeping back straight and knees bent.	Helps to maintain stability.
7.	While holding the belt, gently rock back and forth three times. On the third time, pull patient into a standing position 	Provides momentum to help patient into a standing position.

Contd...

Steps	Procedure	Rationale
8.	Once patient is standing and feels stable, move to the unaffected side and grasp the gait belt in the middle of the back. With the other hand, hold the patient's hand closest to you. If the patient does not require a gait belt, place hand closest to the patient around the upper arm and hold the patient's hand with your other hand 	Standing to the side of the patient provides assistance without blocking the patient.
9.	Before stepping away from the bed, ask the patient if they feel dizzy or lightheaded. If they do, sit patient back down on the bed. If patient feels stable, begin walking, matching your steps to the patient's. Instruct patient to look ahead and lift each foot off the ground. Walk only as far as the patient can tolerate without feeling dizzy or weak.	Always perform a risk assessment prior to ambulation.
10.	To help a patient back to bed, have patient stand with back of knees touching the bed. Grasp the gait belt and help patient into a sitting position, keeping your back straight and knees bent 	Allowing a patient to rest after ambulation helps prevent fatigue.

Contd...

Unit IV ❖ Basic Needs of the Patient

Steps	Procedure	Rationale
11.	When patient is finished ambulating, remove gait belt and settle patient into bed or a chair. When patient returns to bed, place the bed in lowest position, raise side rails as required, and ensure call bell is within reach	This provides a safe place for the patient to rest. Placing bed and side rails in a safe position reduces the likelihood of injury to patient. Proper placement of call bell facilitates patient's ability to ask for assistance.
12.	Perform hand hygiene.	Hand hygiene reduces the spread of microorganisms.
13.	Document patient's ability to tolerate ambulation and type of assistance required.	Documentation fosters quality care.

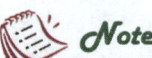 **Note**

Early ambulation after surgery is demonstrated to reduce complications and decreases patient length of stay (LOS) in hospital.

Assistive Devices for Ambulation

Ambulation device is a device designed to assist walking and improve the mobility of people who have difficulty in walking or people who cannot walk independently.

Purpose of Ambulation Devices

- Increase area of support or base of support
- Improve balance
- Maintain center of gravity over supported area
- Redistribute weight-bearing area by decreasing force on injured or inflamed part
- Helps to compensate for weak muscles
- Decrease pain

Types of Assistive Devices

- Cane
- Walker
- Crutches

Assisting with Cane

A cane is an ambulatory assistive device generally prescribed for people with moderate levels of mobility impairment

Purpose

To ensure safe ambulation with a cane

Types of Canes

- Standard cane
- Offset cane
- Offset 4-legged quad cane

Procedure

Steps	Procedure	Rationale
1.	Explain the procedure to the patient.	Allays anxiety and fosters cooperation.
2.	Perform hand hygiene	Prevents transmission of micro organisms
3.	Check the cane for presence of rubber tip(s).	Presence of intact rubber tips decreases the risk of falls by improving traction and preventing slipping.
4.	Assist patient to sit on edge of bed or chair and stand on count of three. Allow patient to gain balance with cane in one hand. Check for any discomfort and dizziness.	Allows patient to adjust position change. Change in position may cause dizziness due to a drop in blood pressure.

Contd...

Unit IV ❖ **Basic Needs of the Patient**

Steps	Procedure	Rationale
5.	Have patient place cane approximately 4 inches to the side of his/her stronger/unaffected foot. The height of the cane should be level with patient's hip 	Provides stability.
6.	Stand to the affected side and slightly behind patient 	Allows clear path for the patient and puts you in a position to assist patient if needed.
7.	Have patient move cane forward about 4–6 inches, step forward with weak (affected) leg to a position even with the cane. Then have patient move strong leg forward and beyond the weak leg and cane Take a step with the 'bad' leg and bring the cane forward at the same time. Move the cane and affected leg forward together.	Reduces risk of patient fall

Contd...

Steps	Procedure	Rationale
8.	Lean the weight through the arm holding the cane as needed. Repeat the sequence 	Maintains stability.
9.	Replace equipment and make sure the patient is comfortable.	Ensures comfort and wellbeing.
10.	Perform hand hygiene.	Prevents transmission of micro organisms
11.	Document the procedure with date, time, duration of ambulation, type of cane used and the patient response along with the signature of the nurse.	Documentation fosters quality care.

Note

- When standing up straight, the top of the cane should reach to the crease in the wrist.
- Elbow should be slightly bent when holding the cane.
- Hold the cane in the hand opposite the side that needs support. For example, if right leg is injured, hold the cane in the left hand.

Assisting With Walker

A walker is a walking aid that has four points of contact with the ground and usually has three sides with the side closest to the patient being open. It is a tool for disabled people, who need additional support to maintain balance or stability while walking.

Purposes

- To help increase the ability to walk independently and safely
- To increase the amount and distance of walk
- To decrease pain and discomfort while walking
- To increase endurance postural stability, control during transitional movements, and dynamic balance

Types

- Standard walkers
- Two-wheeled walkers
- 4 wheeled walker

Unit IV ❖ Basic Needs of the Patient

Procedure

Steps	Procedure	Rationale
1.	Explain the procedure to the patient.	Allays anxiety and fosters cooperation.
2.	Perform hand hygiene.	Prevents transmission of micro- organisms
3.	Assist patient to sit on edge of bed	Allows patient to adjust to position change.
4	Place walker in front of patient as close to the bed as possible. Instruct the patient to position his/her body within the frame of the walker and ask the patient to grasp the hand rests securely. Have patient grasp both arms of walker.	Helps steady patient.

Contd...

Steps	Procedure	Rationale
5.	Brace leg of walker with the foot and place the hand on top of walker. Check height of walker to ensure hand rests are at the level of the top of the femur and that elbows are flexed at a 250–300 degree angle	Prevents walker from moving.
6.	Assist patient to stand on count of three, check for balance and dizziness.	Allows coordination.
7.	Stand to side and slightly behind patient	Puts you in a position to assist patient if needed.
8.	Have patient move walker ahead 6 to 10 inches, then step up to walker moving the weak or injured leg forward to the middle of the walker while pushing down on the handles of the walker, and then bringing the unaffected leg forward even with the weak/injured leg. Instruct the patient to take a step forward with the weak leg. Instruct the patient to move his/her strong leg forward	Patient may fall forward if he steps too far into walker.

Contd...

Steps	Procedure	Rationale
9.	Instruct the patient to take short steps and keep his/her head up and eyes looking forward 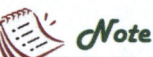	Helps to maintain stability
10.	Replace equipment and make sure the patient is comfortable.	Ensures comfort and wellbeing.
11.	Perform hand hygiene.	Prevents transmission of micro organisms
12.	Document the procedure with date, time, and duration of ambulation, type of walker used and the patient response along with the signature of the nurse.	Documentation fosters quality care.

Note

- Instruct the patient to move the walker forward by lifting it up, moving it forward and setting it down.
- Instruct the patient to position the walker so the back legs of the walker are even with the patient's toes.
- The patient should avoid sliding the walker.

Assisting with Crutches

Crutches are devices which are used to reduce weight bearing on one or both legs and also give support where balance is impaired and strength is inadequate.

Purposes

- To increase the size of an individual's base of support.
- To take some weight off one or both lower limbs resulting in more weight going through the arms.

Prerequisites for Crutches

- Good strength of upper limb muscles is required.
- Range of motion of upper limb should be good.
- Shoulder adductors, Elbow and wrist extensors and Finger flexors should be strong to support the weight.

Types of Crutches (Figs 13A to C)

- Axillary/Under arm crutches
- Elbow crutches/Lofstrand crutches
- Elbow extension crutches or Gutter crutches

Types of Gaits Using Crutches

When a patient is ready to start ambulating with crutches, they will start in the tripod position.

Four-point gait

- This type of gait is similar to the two-point gait but the crutch and leg move separately rather than at the same time.
- For example, the patient will move the injured side's crutch (example right crutch), then move the non-injured leg (example left leg), then move the non-injured side's crutch (example left crutch), and then move injured leg (example right leg).
- Move right crutch, then move left leg, then move left crutch, and then move the right leg.

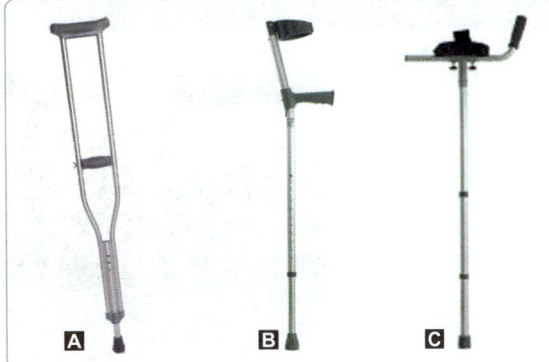

Figures 13A to C: Types of crutches. (A) Axillary crutches; (B) Elbow crutches; (C) Gutter crutches

Three-point gait

- The patient will not let the injured leg touch the ground.
- Therefore, the patient will move both crutches and the injured leg forward together and then move the non-injured leg.
- Move both crutches and injured leg forward together and then move the non-injured leg.

Two-point gait

- the patient will move the injured side's crutch (example right crutch) at the same time as the non-injured leg (example left leg) and then the patient will move the noninjured side's crutch (example left crutch) at the same time as the injured leg (example right leg).
- Move right crutch along with the left leg and then move the left crutch along with the right leg.

Swing-to-gait

- The patient will move both crutches forward and then swing both legs forward to the same point as the crutches.

Swing-through-gait

- The patient will move both crutches forward and then swing both legs forward, past the crutches.

Procedure

Steps	Procedure	Rationale
1.	Explain the procedure to the patient.	Allays anxiety and fosters cooperation.
2.	Perform hand hygiene.	Prevents transmission of micro organisms

Contd...

Unit IV ❖ Basic Needs of the Patient

Steps	Procedure	Rationale
3.	Assist patient to sit on edge of bed	Allows patient to adjust to position change.
4.	Place the crutches in front of patient as close to the bed as possible. Ensure that the crutches have rubber tips	Prevents device from slipping
5.	Ensure that the surface that patient walks on is clean and dry. Have patient grasp the crutches and choose appropriate crutch gait as described below.	Prevents injuries
	Four point gait	
6.	Begin in tripod position. Place crutches 15 cm (6 inches) in front and 15 cm to side of each foot. Instruct the patient to place weight on the handgrips and not on the underarms	Improve patient balance by providing wide base of support.

Contd...

Steps	Procedure	Rationale
7.	Move right crutch forward 0–5 cm (4–6 inches). Move left foot forward to level of left crutch. Move left crutch forward 10–15 cm (4–6 inches). Move right foot forward to level of right crutch. Repeat the above sequence	Requires bearing weight on both legs.

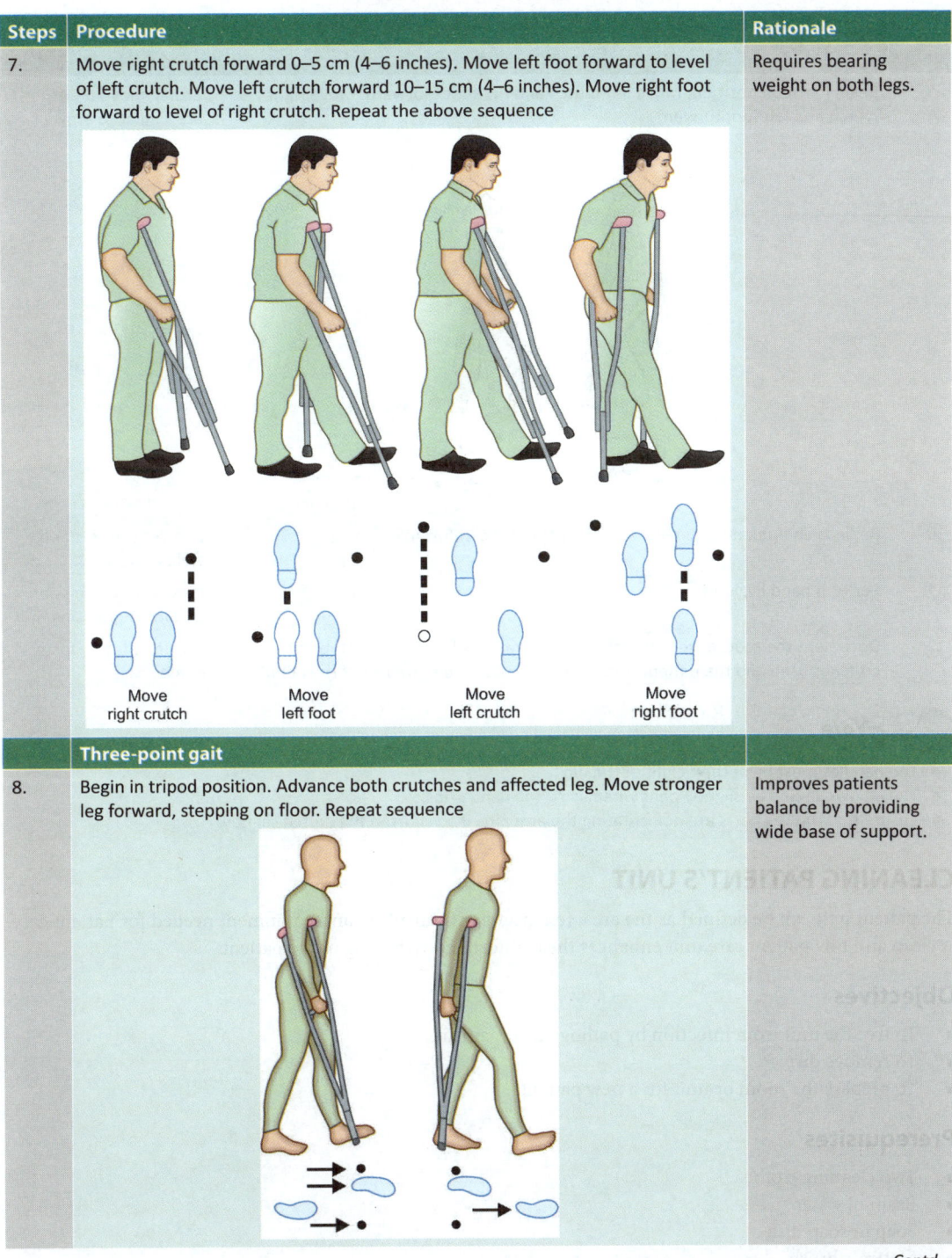

| Move right crutch | Move left foot | Move left crutch | Move right foot |

Three-point gait		
8.	Begin in tripod position. Advance both crutches and affected leg. Move stronger leg forward, stepping on floor. Repeat sequence	Improves patients balance by providing wide base of support.

Contd...

Steps	Procedure	Rationale
	Two-point gait	
9.	Begin in tripod position. Move left crutch and right foot forward. Move right crutch and left foot forward 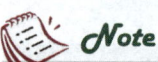	Crutch movements are similar to arm movements
10.	Replace equipment and make sure the patient is comfortable.	Ensures comfort and wellbeing.
11.	Perform hand hygiene.	Prevents transmission of micro organisms
12.	Document the procedure with date, time, duration of ambulation, type of crutches used and the patient response along with the signature of the nurse.	Documentation fosters quality care.

Note

- The handles must be at the height of the hip.
- The elbows should be slightly bent when using the hand grips.
- Ensure that the top parts are not irritating the arm pits, if so shorten the crutch slightly.

CLEANING PATIENT'S UNIT

The patient unit can be defined as the area, (environment) furniture and equipment needed for patient care. A clean and tidy patient care unit enhances the comfort and wellbeing of the patient.

Objectives

- To free the unit from infection by pathogenic organisms
- To remove dirt
- To prepare the room or unit for a new patient

Prerequisites

- Two cleaning clothes
- Basin of water
- Soap in soap dish
- Mattress brush

Procedure in Ward

- Wear appropriate PPE.
- Strip the bed.
- Ensure that the mattress is brushed (Do it outside if possible).
- The mattress, pillows and blankets are placed out in the sun to air.
- Rubber sheets are cleaned and dried.
- The bed is washed, paying special attention to the corners.
- The locker is cleaned inside and outside (Clean the painted surface with soap and water and polished surface with a damp duster).

 *Note*

When cleaning or carrying a mattress, avoid bending them in half as this breaks the fibers and the mattress soon becomes lumpy.

Procedure in a Room

- Wear appropriate PPE.
- Strip the bed as above.
- Ensure that the mattress is brushed.
- The mattress, pillows and blanket are placed in the sun (Strong sunlight will damage rubber mattress and pillows).
- Ensure that the walls have been swept down, bed is washed and all the furniture are clean (The walls are swept with a broom attached to a long pole or cobweb stick).
- All shelves and drawers are cleaned, all pictures and electric light fixtures are wiped with a duster.
- Check if the windows and doors are washed.
- Ensure that all the other equipment that are kept in the room are clean, e.g. Bed pan, Urinal, Kidney tray, Wash basin, etc.
- Ensure that the floor is clean and dry.
- See that the bathroom is clean and in order.
- Return cleaning articles to utility room and put them away in their proper places.
- Before going off duty, see that the bed or room is made ready to receive a new patient.

FACTORS PROMOTING PHYSICAL COMFORTS

Factors promoting physical comforts are as follows:
- Attending the immediate needs of the patient.
- Use of mechanical devices which will promote comfort of the patient.

Attending the Immediate Needs of the Patient

Morning Care

Care given to the patient in the early morning just prior to serving breakfast includes:
- Offering bedpan or urinal
- Attending to oral hygiene
- Washing face and hands (partial bath)
- Combing hair

- Remaking the bed
- Placing the patient in comfortable position in bed, etc.

Evening Care

Care given to the patient in the evening includes:

- Giving bedpan and urinal.
- Attending to oral hygiene.
- Washing the patient's back and rubbing with alcohol (partial bath).
- Remaking the bed and providing additional sheets or blankets if needed for the night according to the weather.
- See that all the treatments and medication are carried out and recorded before the nurse leaving the patient's unit.
- See that the food is served.
- Assist him/her, if necessary, to eat food. Leave the patient's unit in order.

Bed Time care

It is the care given in the evening prior to sleep. It includes:

- Offering bedpan or urinal and adjusting the bed clothes so that the patient is in a comfortable position for the night.
- The blanket should be kept folded across the foot end of the bed so that it will be ready for use if needed at night.
- The room should be adequately ventilated.
- All unnecessary lights disturbing the patient's sleep should be turned off.
- Shadow the light, if necessary.
- Silence should be maintained in the ward including the corridor, so that the patient's sleep will not be disturbed.
- Leave a glass of water or warm drink within reach of the patient.
- Whenever calling bells are provided, instruction should be given to the patient regarding the use of the same.
- Plants or flower pot, if any, should be removed from the room as plants produce carbon dioxide at night.

COMFORT DEVICES

Comfort devices are invented articles which would add to the comfort of the patient when used in the appropriate manner, by relieving the discomfort and helping to maintain correct posture.

Purposes

- To relieve discomfort
- To immobilize body part
- To relieve pressure on parts of body
- To prevent falls and accidents

The names and uses of common comfort devices are mentioned as follows:

Pillows

The use of pillows to support the parts of the body as head and neck, arms, legs and part of the back adds to the physical comfort of the patient. The comfort of the patient depends on the skillful arrangement of pillows according to the needs of the patient preventing strain and fatigue. It is used as a support to maintain correct body alignment.

Purposes

- Helps to maintain proper body alignment
- Helps to support body parts in good alignment
- Helps to reduce pressure
- Used to support head, neck arms legs and parts of the back

Back Rest

It is a mechanical device which provides a suitable support and rest for the back of the patient in sitting position. In the home, back rest may have to be improvised with canvas-covered adjustable back rests. A chair may be substituted. It can be adjusted to desired angle. Arms of patient are well supported. Extra pillows are needed. These are used for the patients who are suffering from cardiac and pulmonary distress (Fig. 14).

Purposes

- Helps to support back
- Helps to facilitate easy breathing
- It is used especially for heart patients and asthma patients
- Used even in postoperative patients
- Promotes drainage from abdominal cavity

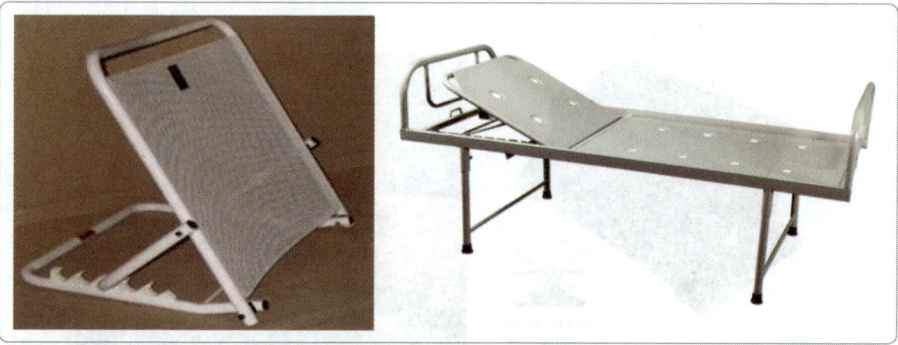

Figure 14: Back rest

Knee Rest

It is required to relieve pain on abdominal muscles and on tendons beneath the knees. A pillow may be used for this purpose. Change of position at frequent intervals is necessary so that the legs are not kept in a flexed position for a long period. Keeping the knees flexed, without movement for a long time will cause venous stasis which tends to produce thrombophlebitis in legs which is an inflammatory disease of the vein wall and may be accompanied by thrombosis (Figs 15A and B).

Unit IV ❖ Basic Needs of the Patient

Purpose

- Gives relaxation and thus relieves pain on tendons beneath the knees.

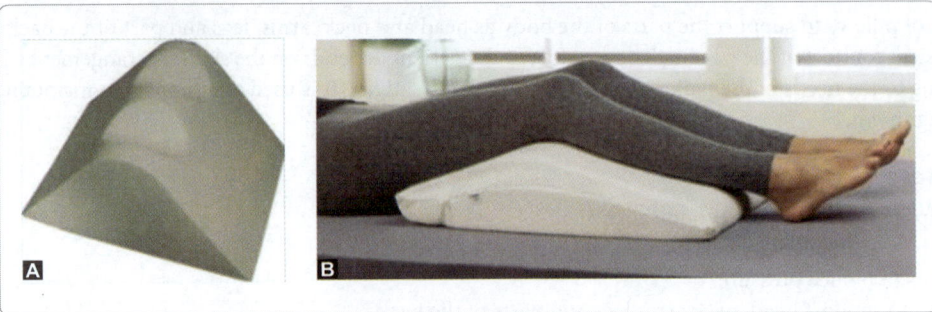

Figures 15A and B: Knee rest

Foot Rest or Foot Board

It is a device so placed that the feet rest firmly against it. It is used for comfort and to provide protection from foot drop. It is placed between the mattress and bed to keep the feet at right angles to the legs. A foot board is always padded. Hard pillows or sand bags or a board may be substituted. Foot rests are also provided for people engaged in office work to support the lower extremities and to prevent fatigue to the parts (Figs 16A and B). (Foot drop is a preventable condition that occurs in most cases due to inability to keep the foot in the correct angle due to lack of support or paralysis of the flexors of the ankle.)

Purposes

- Maintains the normal position of feet
- Promotes comfort
- Prevents foot drop

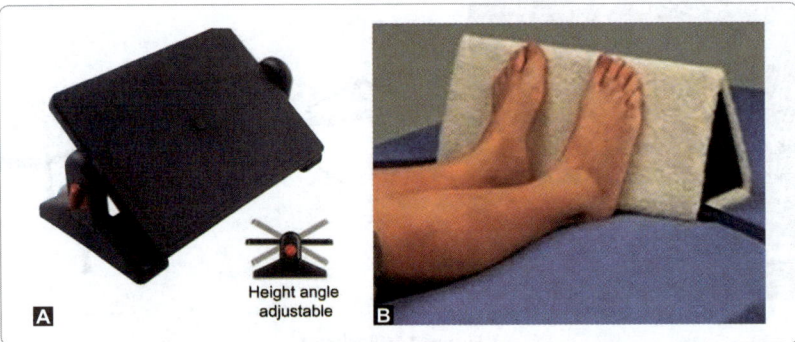

Height angle
adjustable

Figures 16A and B: Foot rest

Sand Bags

These are canvas rubber or plastic bags filled with sand. They are used to immobilize a part as in fractures and relieve discomfort. It may also be used to provide—needed support and to prevent foot or waist drop. They are made up of sand and are available in various sizes (Fig. 17).

Purposes

- Used to immobilize the body part
- Used to support fracture bone
- Helps to relieve discomfort
- Used to support body part
- Helps to prevent foot or wrist drop

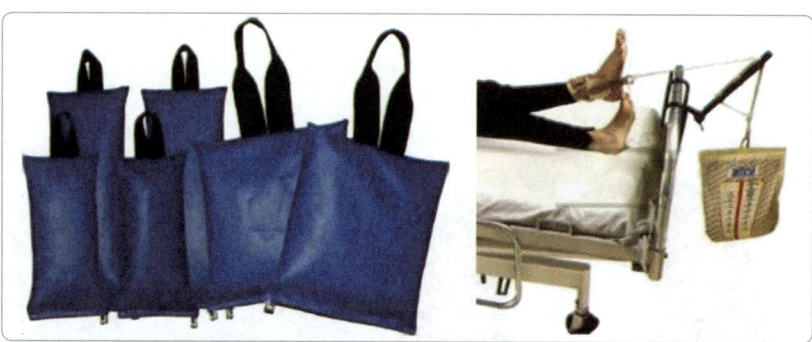

Figure 17: Sand bag

Bed Cradle

Bed cradles vary widely in size and in materials. These are semicircular or rectangular in shape made of wood and metal. Their purpose is usually that of supporting the weight of the top bed clothing, to prevent them from coming in contact with the patient as in case of patients with burns or when the plaster cast is to be dried. Small cradles are used for one or both extremities. Large cradles are available for use over the entire body. Cradles equipped with electric bulbs are used to supply the desired warmth. Coverings that maintain some degree of warmth within the cradle may be needed. Pad the cradle edges if necessary to prevent injury (Figs 18A and B).

Purposes

- Prevents the top cloth coming in contact with the patients especially burn patients. Helps to apply head in case of drying plaster casts.
- Electronic bed cradles are used to supply the desired warm in case of shock.

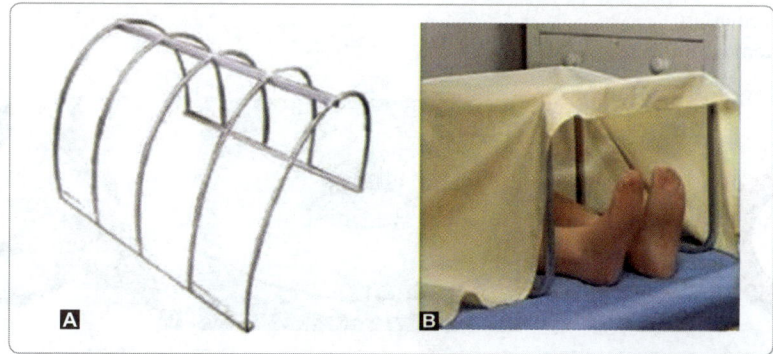

Figures 18A and B: Bed cradle

Unit IV ❖ **Basic Needs of the Patient**

Air Cushion

They are round in shape and can be inflated to any desired degree of firmness. It provides relaxation as it yields to shift off body weight and it relieves pressure on certain part of the body like coccyx. Air cushions should not be placed directly in contact with the skin as it is a rubber article and should have cover (Figs 19A and B).

Purposes

- Relieves pressure on certain part of body.
- Promotes comfort of client.

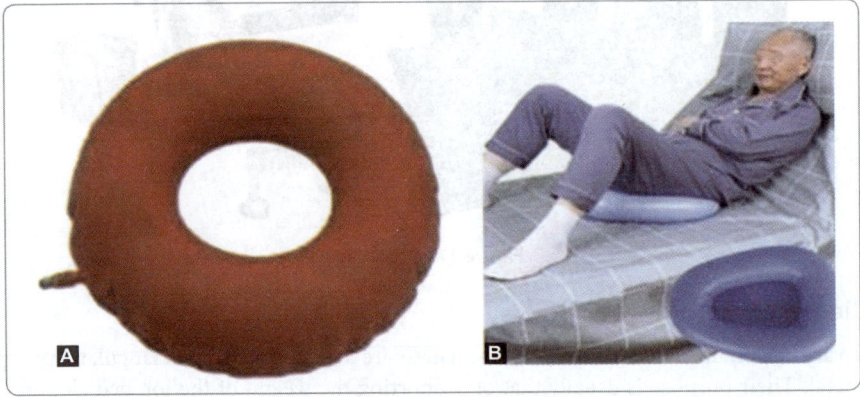

Figures 19A and B: Air cushion

Rubber and Cotton Rings

They are used to relieve pressure on certain parts of the body like elbows and heels. Cotton rings are made to fit the part to which they are to be applied. Cotton are wrapped with bandage. These are placed under bony prominence such as heels and fastened in place, if necessary (Figs 20A to C).

Purposes

- Helps to lift the hip from bed to prevent bed sores.
- Helps to prevent direct pressure on bony prominence.
- Improves circulation.
- Used after hemorrhoidectomy.

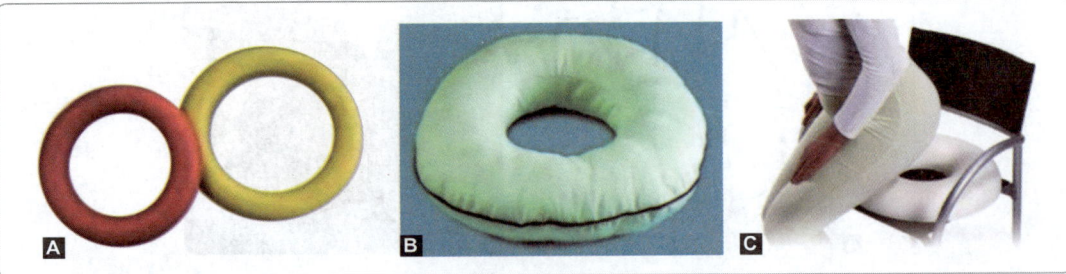

Figures 20A to C: Rubber and cotton rings

Air and Water Mattresses

They are used for very thin or very obese patients and those who must remain in bed for too long a time. The principle on which the use of such mattresses is based on that, pressure of air within closed or confined space is exerted equally in all directions. Thus pressure against bony prominences or areas subject to the development of pressure sores would be reduced. Air spaces between the honey comb structures of rubber foam mattress also equalizes the pressure in it to a certain extent when one is lying on it (Figs 21A and B).

Purposes

- Improves circulation
- Provides comfort
- Prevents pressure sores
- Used in very thin or very obese patients and chronic bed-ridden patients

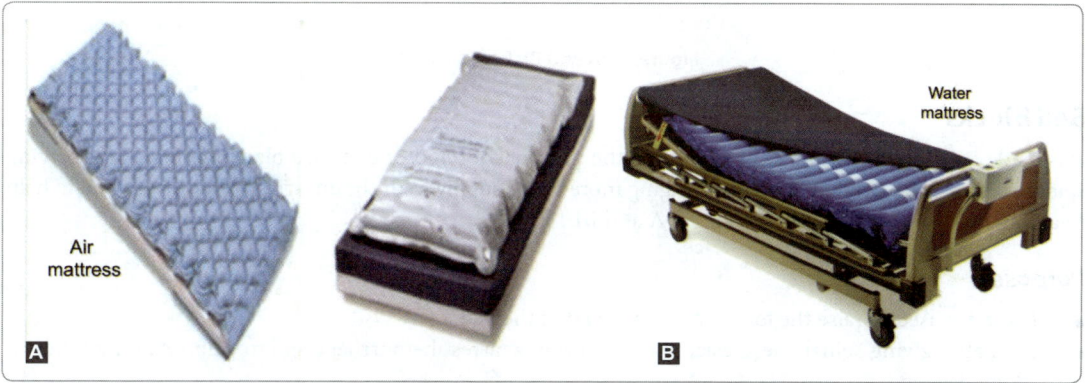

Figures 21A and B: Air and water mattresses

Cardiac Table

It is made up of wood or metal. Pillows should be arranged over the table for the comfort of the patient. This is used for the patient to lean forward, especially when he has been in the sitting position for a long time. This may also be used as a book support if the patient wishes to read or write and also to take food in bed itself. Generally, this is used by patients suffering from cardiac diseases (Figs 22A and B).

Purposes

- Used by cardiac patients who can lean forward with a pillow
- Used for writing purpose
- Used for serving food and other self-care activities

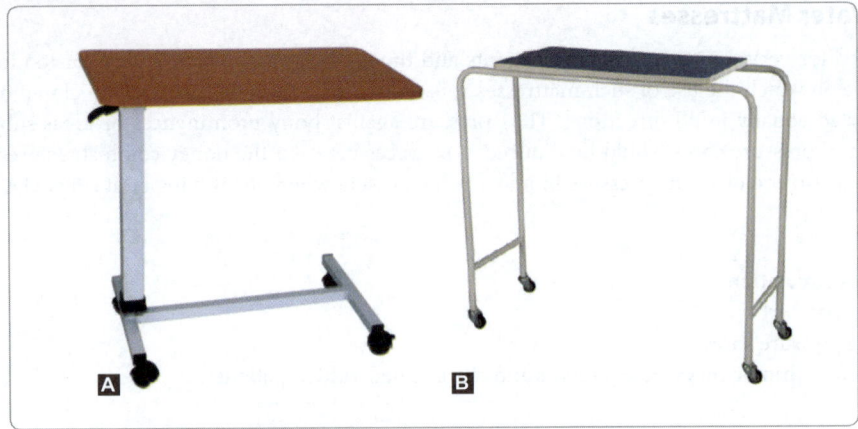

Figures 22A and B: Cardiac table

Bed Blocks

It is made up of wood or metal, used to raise the head or foot end of bed. Bed blocks are used after giving spinal anesthesia, to prevent shock by bringing more blood supply to the brain, arrest hemorrhage and to help retaining fluids in retained enema (Figs 23A and B).

Purposes

- These are used to raise the foot end or head end of the bed.
- Used after giving spinal anesthesia, to prevent shock, arrest hemorrhage and to help retaining fluids in retained enema.

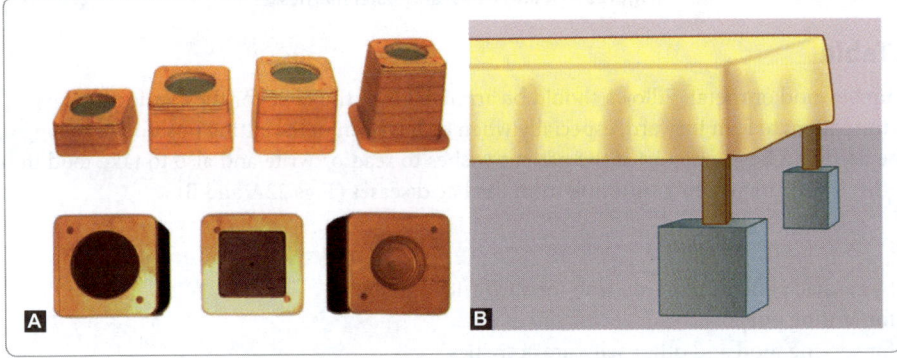

Figures 23A and B: Bed blocks

Hand Rolls

Hand rolls are made up of cloth that are rolled into a cylinder about 4–5 inches long and 2–3 inches in diameter and stiffed firmly securing roll with tape. Roll is placed against palmar surface of hand (Figs 24A and B).

Purposes

- Maintain thumb in slightly adducted and in opposition to fingers.
- Maintain fingers in slightly flexed position.
- Prevent contractures.
- Help client to improve functional mobility to grasp objects.
- Help to keep the fingers free being held in a tight fist.

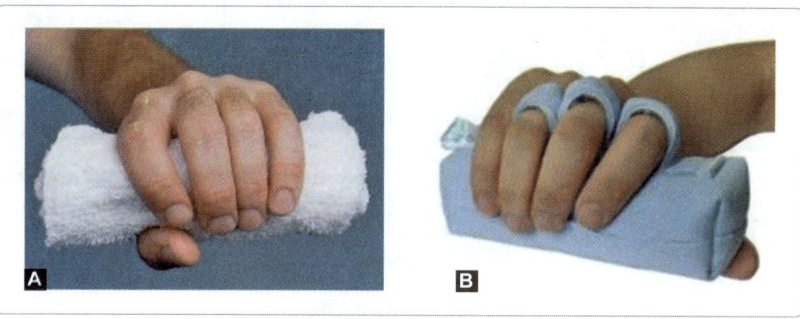

Figures 24A and B: Hand rolls

Foot End Elevator

A platform or an enclosure raised and lowered in a vertical shaft to transport people (Figs 25A and B).

Purposes

- It provides elevated support for feet and ankles.
- It is ideal for postoperative patients and for rehabilitation.

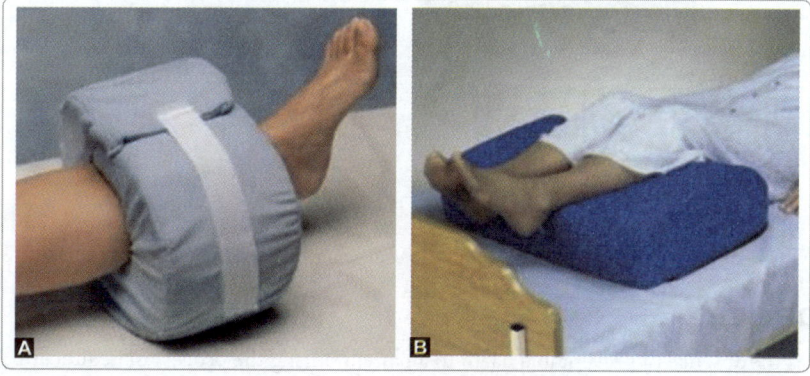

Figures 25A and B: Foot end elevator

Trochanter Rolls

This device is used to prevent the external rotation of the legs when the client is in supine position. To make a trochanter, take a cotton bath blanket /sheet. Fold it lengthwise to a width extending from greater trochanter of femur to the lower border of the popliteal space (Figs 26A and B).

Unit IV ❖ **Basic Needs of the Patient**

Purposes

- Prevents external rotation of legs when patient is in supine position.
- Used to prevent deformities in bedfast patients.

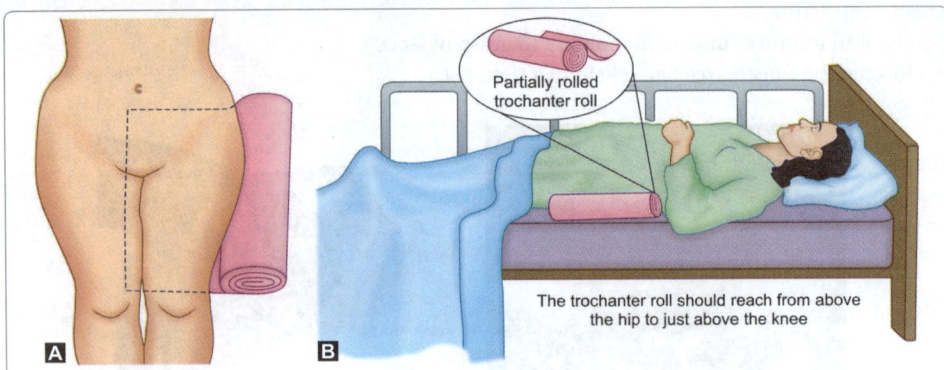

Figures 26A and B: Trochanter rolls

Wedge/Abductor Pillow

It is a triangular-shaped pillow made of heavy foam (Figs 27A and B).

Purpose

- Used to maintain legs in abduction following total hip replacement surgery.

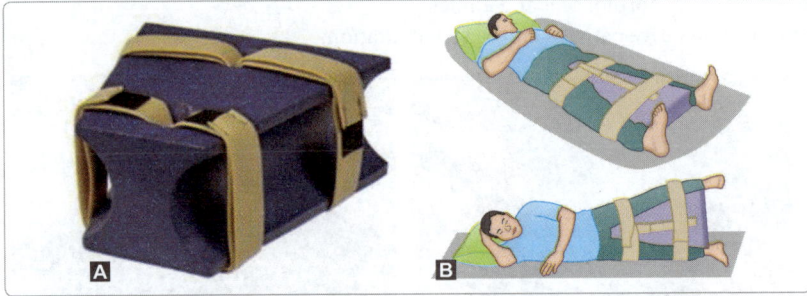

Figures 27A and B: Wedge/abductor pillow

SAFETY DEVICES

Patient safety is the absence of preventable harm to a patient during the process of healthcare. A safety device is one that is used to achieve proper body position, balance, or alignment to allow greater freedom of mobility in order to protect patients.

Side Rails

Side rails (also commonly known as cot-sides, safety rails and Bed rails) can be used as safety devices intended to reduce the risk of patients accidentally slipping, sliding, rolling or falling from bed. Bedrails may also be used as reassurance for patients who are anxious about falling from bed.

Purposes

- Aid in turning and repositioning within the bed
- Provide a hand hold for getting into or out of bed
- Provide a feeling of comfort and security
- Reduce the risk of patients falling out of bed
- Provide easy access to bed controls and personal care items

Uses

- If the patients are being transported on their bed
- In areas where patients are recovering from anesthetic or sedation and are under constant supervision

Grab Bars

Grab bars are safety devices designed to enable a person to maintain balance, lessen fatigue while standing, hold some of their weight while maneuvering, or have something to grab onto in case of a slip or fall.

Grab bars increase accessibility and safety for people with a variety of disabilities or mobility difficulties. Grab bars are most commonly installed next to a toilet or in a shower or bath enclosure (Fig. 28).

Uses

- Grab bars next to a toilet help people using a wheelchair transfer to the toilet seat and back to the wheelchair.
- They also assist people who have difficulty sitting down, have balance problems while seated or need help rising from a seated position.
- Vertical grab bars may help with balance while standing.
- Horizontal grab bars provide assistance when sitting or rising, or to grab onto in case of a slip or fall.

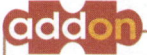

Grab Bar Guidelines

According to Americans with Disabilities Act of 1990

- The diameter of grab bars should be 1¼—1½ inch (32–38 mm) (or the shape shall provide an equivalent gripping surface)
- There shall be a 1½ inch (38 mm) clearance from the wall.
- Grab bars should not rotate in their fittings.
- The required mounting height is universally 33—36 inches (840–910 mm) from top of gripping surface of the grab bar to the finish floor.
- In a toilet, side grab bars must be a minimum of 42 inches long and mounted 12 inches from the rear wall and rear grab bars must be minimum of 36 inches long and mounted a maximum of inches from the side wall.

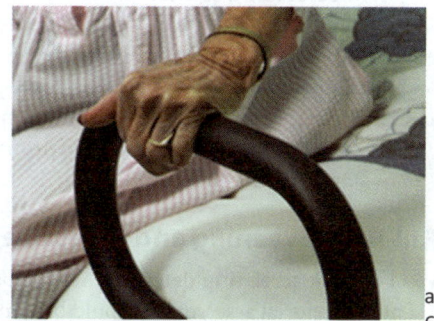

Figure 28: Grab bar

Ambu Alarm

A bag valve mask (BVM) known by the proprietary name **Ambu bag** (Air Mask **Bag** Unit) or generically as a manual resuscitator or 'self-inflating **bag**', **is** a hand-held device commonly used to provide positive pressure ventilation to patients who **are** not breathing or not breathing adequately. The alarm is used if the breathing system pressure fails to exceed a minimum threshold pressure within a fixed time. This low pressure alarm is used when there are:

Unit IV ❖ **Basic Needs of the Patient**

- Disconnections
- Leaks
- Accidental tracheal extubation
- Failures in the fresh gas flow system

Non-Skid Slippers

Non-skid slippers are commonly used for elderly patients, those with gait problems, problems with coordination, etc.

These slippers are light, very tender on the feet, low cut, easy to wear and crucially, must have a non-skid sole. It should be a pair they can wear the whole day and run their typical errands without slipping, falling, or feeling pain.

These slippers can assist patients on wet or slippery surfaces.

FALL RISK ASSESSMENT

Definition: Fall is "an unplanned descent to the floor with or without injury to the patient."

According to MDS, "**A fall** is unintentionally coming to rest on the ground, floor, or other lower level but not as a result of an overwhelming external force (e.g., resident pushes another resident)."

'**Risk**' refers to any external factor or characteristic of an individual resident that influences the likelihood of an accident.

Risk Factors for a Fall

Risk factors for falls can be classified as intrinsic or extrinsic.

- **Intrinsic risk factors for falls**: These are the factors, originating within the individual. These include:
  - Low blood pressure or orthostatic hypotension caused by standing, dehydration, or muscle weakness (most notable in the lower extremities)
  - Impaired mobility, unstable gait, and poor balance due to pain, musculoskeletal deformities, or neurologic disorders
  - Limited physical-activity endurance
  - Foot problems that cause pain or paraesthesia (such as peripheral neuropathy)
  - Impaired vision due to poor depth perception, glaucoma, or cataracts.
- **Extrinsic risk factors:** These originate outside the individual. They include:
  - Conditions in the physical environment, such as poor lighting, clutter, a slippery floor due to a spill and an uneven threshold.

Fall-Risk Screening and Assessment

- **Fall-risk screening** determines if the patient is at risk for falls and indicates whether a more in-depth multifactorial assessment should be done.
- **Fall-risk assessment** provides a systematic way to check for valid and reliable causes of falls in a particular patient and identify factors for which interventions are known to reduce the fall risk.

Fall-Risk Screening

When screening patients for fall risk, check for:

- History of falling within the past year
- Orthostatic hypotension
- Impaired mobility or gait

- Altered mental status
- Incontinence
- Medications associated with falls, such as sedative-hypnotics and blood pressure drugs
- Use of assistive devices
- Patients tethered to IV lines or other equipment are at increased risk for falls

Fall-Risk Assessment

There are currently approximately 50 instruments to assess fall risk. Typically, these tools use a scoring system that measures the cumulative effect of known risk factors. Few of them are discussed here:

1. **Morse Fall Scale**

    - The Morse Fall Scale (MFS) is a rapid and simple method of assessing a patient's likelihood of falling.
    - It consists of six variables that are quick and easy to score.

Item	Scale		Scoring
1. History of falling; immediate or within 3 months	No	0	
	Yes	25	_____
2. Secondary diagnosis	No	0	
	Yes	15	_____
3. Ambulatory aid			
Bed rest/nurse assist		0	
Crutches/cane/walker		15	
Furniture		30	_____
4. IV/Heparin Lock	No	0	
	Yes	20	_____
5. Gait/Transferring			
Normal/bed rest/immobile		0	
Weak		10	
Impaired		20	_____
6. Mental status			
Oriented to own ability		0	
Forgets limitations		15	_____

Items in the Scale

- **History of falling:**
    - This is scored as 25 if the patient has fallen during the present hospital admission or if there was an immediate history of physiological falls, such as from seizures or an impaired gait prior to admission.
    - If the patient has not fallen, this is scored 0.
    - Note: If a patient falls for the first time, then his or her score immediately increases by 25.
- **Secondary diagnosis:**
    - This is scored as 15 if more than one medical diagnosis is listed on the patient's chart.
    - If not, score 0.
- **Ambulatory aids:**
    - This is scored as 0 if the patient walks without a walking aid (even if assisted by a nurse), uses a wheelchair, or is on a bed rest and does not get out of bed at all.
    - If the patient uses crutches, a cane, or a walker, this item scores 15.
    - If the patient ambulates clutching onto the furniture for support, score this item as 30.

Unit IV ❖ Basic Needs of the Patient

- **Intravenous therapy:**
    - This is scored as 20 if the patient has an intravenous apparatus or a heparin lock inserted.
    - If not, score 0.
- **Gait:**
    - A normal gait is characterized by the patient walking with head erect, arms swinging freely at the side, and striding without hesitant. This gait scores 0.
    - With a weak gait (score as 10), the patient is stooped but is able to lift the head while walking without losing balance. Steps are short and the patient may shuffle.
    - With an impaired gait (score 20), the patient may have difficulty rising from the chair, attempting to get up by pushing on the arms of the chair/or by bouncing (i.e., by using several attempts to rise). The patient's head is down, and he or she watches the ground. Because the patient's balance is poor, the patient grasps onto the furniture, a support person, or a walking aid for support and cannot walk without this assistance.
- **Mental status:**
    - When using this Scale, mental status is measured by checking the patient's own self-assessment of his or her own ability to ambulate. Ask the patient, "Are you able to go the bathroom alone or do you need assistance?" If the patient's reply judging his or her own ability is consistent, the patient is rated as "normal" and scored 0.
    - If the patient's response is not consistent with the nursing orders or if the patient's response is unrealistic, then the patient is considered to overestimate his or her own abilities and to be forgetful of limitations and scored as 15.

Scoring and Interpretation

- The score is then tallied and recorded on the patient's chart.
- Risk level and recommended actions (e.g. no interventions needed, standard fall prevention interventions, high risk prevention interventions) are then identified.

Risk level	MFS score	Action
No risk	0–24	Good basic nursing care
Low risk	25–50	Implement standard fall Prevention interventions
High risk	≥51	Implement high risk fall Prevention interventions

2. The John Hopkins Fall Risk Assessment Tool (JHFRAT)

- It is an evidence-based fall safety initiative.
- This risk stratification tool is valid and reliable and highly effective when combined with a comprehensive protocol, and fall-prevention products and technologies.

Items and Scoring

If patient has any of the following conditions, check the box and apply Fall Risk interventions as indicated. **High fall risk:** Implement High Fall Risk interventions per protocol • History of more than one fall within 6 months before admission • Patient is deemed high fall-risk per protocol (e.g., seizure precautions) **Low fall risk -** Implement low fall risk interventions per protocol • Complete paralysis or completely immobilized **Do not continue with fall risk score calculation if any of the above conditions are checked**	
Fall risk score calculation: Select the appropriate option in each category. Add all points to calculate fall risk score (If no option is selected, score for category is 0)	Points
Age (Single-select) • 60–69 years (1 point) • 70–79 years (2 points) • Greater than or equal to 80 years (3 points)	
Fall history (Single-select) • One fall within 6 months before admission (5 points)	
Elimination, bowel and urine (Single-select) • Incontinence (2 points) • Urgency or frequency (2 points) • Urgency frequency and incontinence (4 points)	
Medications: Include PCA/opiates, anticonvulsants, antihypertensives, diuretics, hypnotics, laxatives, sedative, and psychotropics (single-select) • On 1 high fall risk drug (3 points) • On 2 or more high fall risk drugs (5 points) • Sedated procedure within past 24 hours (7 points)	
Patient care equipment: Any equipment that tethers patient (e.g., IV infusion, chest tube, indwelling catheter, SCDs, etc.) (Single-select) • One present (1 point) • Two present (2 points) • 3 or more present (3 points)	
• **Mobility** (Multi-select, choose all that apply and add points together) • Requires assistance or supervision for mobility, transfer, or ambulation (2 points) • Unsteady gait (2 points) • Visual or auditory impairment affecting mobility (2 points)	
Cognition (Multi-select, choose all that apply and add points together) • Altered awareness of immediate physical environment (1 point) • Impulsive (2 [points) • Lack of understanding of one's physical and cognitive limitations (4 points)	
Total fall risk score (Sum of all points per category)	
Scoring: 6–13 Total points = Moderate fall risk, >13 Total points = High fall risk	

 *Note*

For using these tools in the hospital, due permission has to be obtained from the concerned authority.

3. Fall Risk Assessment Scoring System (FRASS)

- The FRASS was originally developed by Suzanne Mac Avoy, Teresa Skinner & Maria Hines.
- This tool aims to identify patients at high risk of falling.

Unit IV ❖ Basic Needs of the Patient

This tool aims to identify patients at high risk of falling.
Instructions:
Assess patient's current status for each risk factor and record the relevant
rating in the scoring system. Add up total scores and record in space provided.

COMPLETED BY: _____

DATE: _____

Name:	
UR/MR number:	
Ward/Unit:	
DOB:	Gender:
Admission Date:	
Place UR sticker here or add patient details:	

Risk Factor	Rating	/ / 04 Score	/ / 04 Score	/ / 04 Score
AGE 65 – 79 years 80 and above	(1) (2)			
MENTAL STATUS Oriented at all times or Comatose Confused at all times – poor cognition, STM, lack of insight into own safety, impulsive Intermittent confusion – as above	(0) (4) (8)			
EMOTIONAL STATUS Moderately agitated/uncooperative/anxious Severely agitated/uncooperative/anxious	(2) (4)			
TOILETING Independent and continent Catheter and/or ostomy Needs assistance with toileting Ambulatory with urge incontinence or episodes of incontinence	(0) (1) (3) (5)			
HISTORY OF FALLING WITHIN 6 MONTHS No Has fallen one or two times Multiple history of falling	(0) (2) (5)			
SENSORY IMPAIRMENT Blind/Deaf/Cataracts/Not using corrective device	(1)			
ACTIVITY Ambulates/Transfers without assistance Ambulates/Transfers with assist of one or assistive device Ambulates/Transfers with assist of two Unsteady gait/mobility affected by pain/deconditioned	(0) (2) (1) (2)			
MEDICATIONS (MEDICATION REFERENCE TABLE OVER PAGE) □ Cardiovascular/Antihypertensives □ Antidepressants □ Psychotropics □ Tranquillisers/Sedatives □ Anti-Parkinson's/Anti-Convulsives □ Opioids □ Diuretics None of the above listed medications One of the above listed medication Two or more of the above listed medications Add one more point if there has been a change in these medications or dosages in the past five days.	(0) (1) (2) (1)			
TOTAL SCORE				

Level of Risk: *Score of 8 - 14 patient is at high risk for falls*
          Score of 15 + patient is at SUPER HIGH risk for falls
Document each patient's falls risk status in the medical history. Implement
appropriate fall prevention strategies (over page)

Unit IV ❖ **Basic Needs of the Patient**

4. Falls Risk Assessment Tool (FRAT)

- The Falls Risk Assessment Tool (FRAT) was developed by the Peninsula Health Falls Prevention Service.
- The FRAT has three sections: Part 1 - falls risk status; Part 2 – risk factor checklist; and Part 3 – action plan.

Part 1: Fall risk status

Risk Factor	Level	Risk Score
Recent Falls (To score this, complete history of falls, overleaf)	None in last 12 months............ One or more between 3 and 12 months ago.................... One or more in last 3 months....................... One or more in last 3 months whilst inpatient/resident	2 4 6 8
Medications (Sedative, Anti-depressants, Anti-Parkinson's, Diuretics, Antihypertensives, hypnotics)	Not taking any of these....................... Taking one.................................... Taking two................................ taking more than two........................	1 2 3 4
Psychological (Anxiety, Depression, ↓Cooperation, ↓Insight or ↓Judgement **Especially relational mobility**	Does not appear to have any of these............... Appears mildly affected by one or more........... Appears moderately affected by one or more................. Appears severely affected by one or more..............	1 2 3 4
Cognitive Status (AMTS: Hodkinson Abbreviated Mental Test Score)	AMTS 9 or 10/10 or Intact............ AMTS 7-8 Mildly impaired............ AMTS 5-6 Mod impaired............ AMTS 4 or less Severely impaired...........	
(Low Risk: 5-11 Medium Risk: 12-15 High Risk: 16-20)	Risk Score	/20

Part 2: Risk factor checklist

Vision	Reports/observed	Y/N
Vision	Reports/observed difficulty seeing - objects/signs/finding way around	
Mobility	Mobility status unknown or appears unsafe/impulsive/forgets gait aid	
Transfers	Transfer status unknown or appears unsafe i.e. over-reaches, impulsive	
Behaviors	Observed or reported agitation, confusion, disorientation Difficulty following instructions or non-compliant (observed or known)	
Activities of Daily Living (ADLs)	Observed risk-taking behaviours, or reported from referrer/previous facility	
	Observed unsafe use of equipment	
	Unsafe footwear/inappropriate clothing	
Environment	Difficulties with orientation to environment, i.e., areas between bed/bathroom/dining room	
Nutrition	Underweight/low appetite	
Continence	Reported or known urgency/nocturia/accidents	
Other		

Unit IV ❖ Basic Needs of the Patient

RESTRAINTS

Restraints are methods used by trained healthcare providers to stop or limit a patient's movement.

Definition: A "restraint" is defined as any physical, manual, chemical, mechanical means or device or material or equipment that restricts client's freedom and ability to move his/her arms, legs, body or head freely and cannot be easily removed or eliminated by the client.

Restraint is defined as 'the intentional restriction of a person's voluntary movement or behavior (Counsel and Care UK, 2002).

Purposes

- To carry out the physical examination
- To provide safety to child
- To protect from injury
- To complete the diagnostic and therapeutic procedures
- To maintain the patient in particular position
- To reduce the discomfort of patient during some tests and procedures like specimen collection
- To safely provide immediate and necessary care
- To prevent harm to himself or others
- To prevent the patient from removing lifesaving equipment, such as IVs or breathing tubes

Indications

- Displaying behavior that is putting themselves at risk of harm
- Displaying behavior that is putting others at risk of harm
- Requiring treatment by a legal order, for example, under the Mental Health Act 2007
- Requiring urgent life-saving treatment
- Need to be maintained in secure settings
- Restraints may be used to keep a person in proper position and prevent movement or falling during surgery or while on a stretcher.
- Sometimes hospital patients who are confused need restraints so that they do not:
  - Scratch their skin
  - Remove catheters and tubes that administers medicine and fluids
  - Get out of bed, fall and hurt themselves

Articles Needed

- Blanket or draw sheet
- Bandages for clove hitch knot
- Cotton pads
- Restraint clothes
- Wooden plastic sticks (Spatula) to restrain elbows
- Scissors for cutting the bandages
- Jacket for jacket restraint
- Adhesive tape for securing the restraints

Types of Restraints

- **Physical restraints:** Physical restraints limit a client's movement. For example, table fixed to a chair or a bed rail that cannot be opened by the client.

- **Environmental restraints:** Environmental restraints are the ones that change or modify a person's surroundings to restrict or control a client's mobility. For example, a secure unit or garden, seclusion etc.
- **Chemical restraints:** Chemical restraints are any form of psychoactive medication used not to treat illness, but to intentionally inhibit a particular behavior or movement.

Physical Restraints

Physical restraint is anything near or on the body which limit a client's movement. This may be attached to a person's body or create physical barriers.

Types of Physical Restraints

- Mummy restraint
- Elbow and knee restraint
- Extremity restraint
- Abdominal restraint
- Jacket restraint
- Mitten or finger restraint
- Crib net restraint
- Safety belt
- Side rails and splints

- **Mummy restraint:** It is a short-term type of restraint used on infants and small children (Figs 29A to F).

    Purposes
    - It is the safe temporary method for restraining young children for treatment or examination
    - Allows for unimpeded access to head and scalp
    - Individual extremities can be released to have access for examination or treatment
    - It is used during examinations, procedure and treatment of head, neck and face
    - It is used to immobilize the arms and legs of the child for a brief period of time. For example, scalp vein puncture, ear examination and eye irrigation, gastric lavage, etc.

    Articles required
    - Commercially available restraint ('papoose board') for larger infants
    - Clean blanket or small sheet
    - Safety pins or other device for securing final blanket fold

    Procedure
    1. Explain the reason for restraining.
    2. Place a small blanket on the examination table or bed on a diagonal, then fold down one corner.
    3. Put the child on the blanket, with his shoulders along the folded edge and his head and neck above the edge of the fold.
    4. Keep one hand of the baby near the body.
    5. Firmly pull one corner of the blanket across his body and secure it beneath his opposite shoulder or beneath the opposite side of his body if you need to keep his arm free.
    6. Bring the bottom up and secure the ends of the blanket with tape if needed to keep it in place.
    7. Bring the second corner across his body, tucking it into place under his back.
    8. Now take the rounded sheet at bottom near the leg and fold it towards the chest and tuck it.
    9. Continuously monitor the child's airway and circulation.

Unit IV ❖ Basic Needs of the Patient

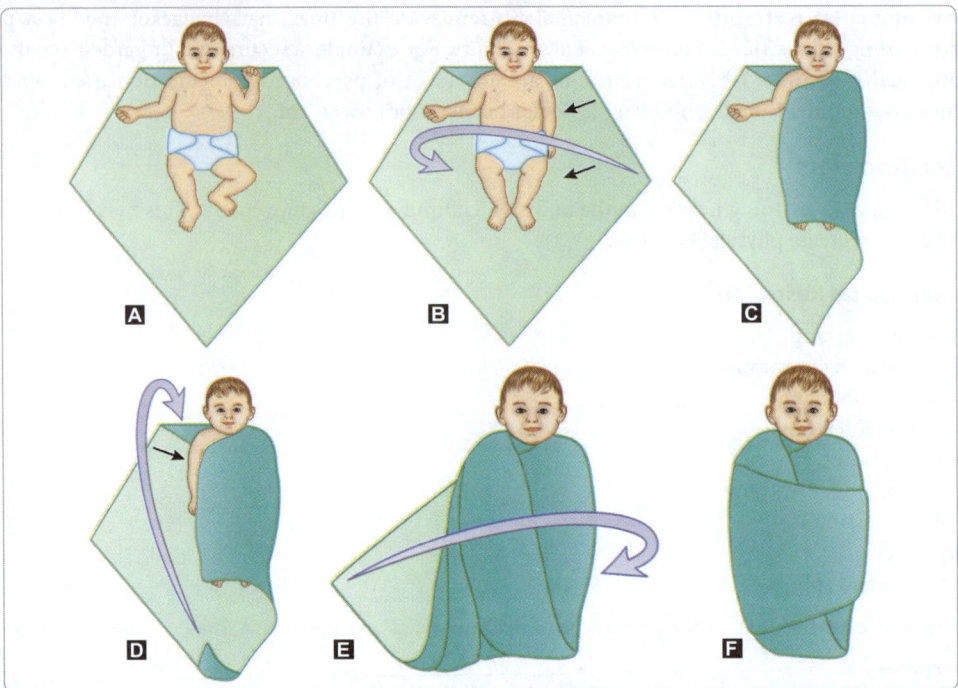

Figures 29A to F: Steps of mummy restraint

■ **Elbow and knee restraint (freedom splint):** This restraint is used to prevent flexion of the elbow and knee and to hold the elbow in an extended position so that the infant cannot reach the head and face. Knee joint also can be restraint like this so as to control the flexion of knee (Figs 30A to C).

Purpose

- Reduces ability of infant to flex elbow.
- This restraint is used in case of face and head surgeries.
- Cleft lip and cleft palate, scalp vein infusion, heart injuries and sutures are good examples of using this elbow restraint.

Articles required

- Commercially available restraints (sheepskin and/or foam padding) for larger infants OR
- Foam-padded arm board
- Adhesive tape
- Additional padding material, i.e., cotton balls, gauze pads
- Plastic elbow restraint, elbow cuff and well-padded wooden splint can also be used.

Procedure

1. In this a readymade cloth with 6-10 pockets is used
2. Cut four pieces of tape (appropriate size; tape should not completely encircle extremity).
3. Extend upper extremity.
4. Place armboard under elbow in order to eliminate ability to flex joint.
5. Tape extremity securely to armboard. Tape should be applied above and below elbow joint.
6. Pad bony prominences with cotton as needed.

7. Place the cotton on sides of elbow and knee and the wooden or plastic strips on pocket cloth.
8. These pockets are vertical.
9. Place the cloth on elbow and knee and adjust it with central location and tie the both side strips properly.

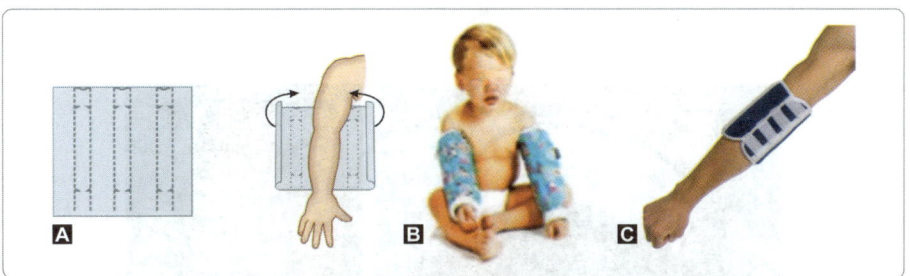

Figures 30A to C: Elbow and knee restraint

■ **Extremity restraint:** This restraint should be used with padding of wrist or ankle. It is used to immobilize one or more extremities (Figs 31A to C).

Purposes
- Immobilization of one or more extremities.
- Protects infant from interfering with or removing treatment regimens (IV access, feeding tube, mechanical ventilation, etc.)

Articles required
- Commercially available restraint (sheepskin and/or foam padding) for larger infants or
- Roll of gauze or gauze pads
- Adhesive tape
- Safety pins or other securing device

Procedure
1. Open gauze and fold in half lengthwise to reinforce material.
2. Wrap wrist or ankle with gauze at least three times to create secure restraint.
3. **Caution:** Do not wrap gauze too tight; this might interfere with distal circulation.
4. Use adhesive tape to ensure that gauze does not unravel.
5. Secure restraint to mattress, blanket, or light sandbag with safety pin.
6. One type of extremity restraint is clove-hitch restraint which is done with gauze bandage strip (2 inches wide) making figure-of-eight.
7. The end of the gauze to be tied to the frame of the crib/bed.

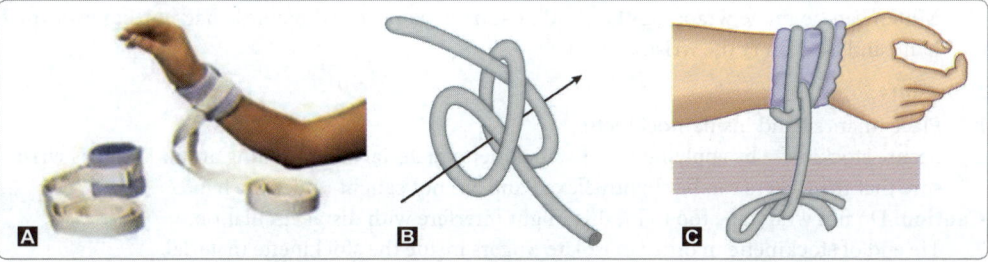

Figures 31A to C: Extremity restraint

Unit IV ❖ Basic Needs of the Patient

- **Abdominal restraint:** This restraint helps to hold the patient in a supine position on the bed (Figs 32A and B).
  - For this restraint, use wide size wooden strips.
  - Place the cotton pad appropriately to provide adequate comfort.
  - These restraints should not be too tight which may interfere with the respiration and bowel movement.

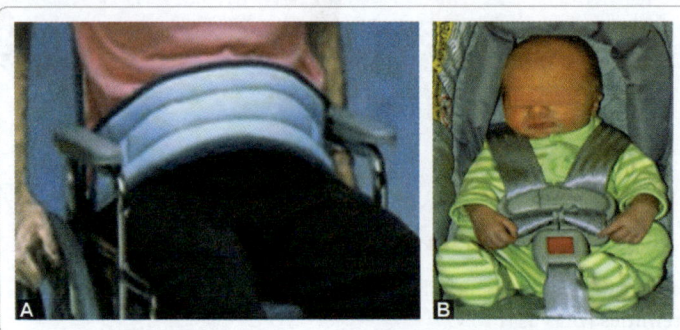

Figures 32A and B: Abdominal restraint in adult and infant

- **Mitten or finger restraint:** Mittens are thumb less device used to restrain or cover hand (Figs 33A and B).

  Purposes
  - Mittens are used for infants to prevent self-injury by hands in case of burns, facial injury or operations, eczema of the face or body.
  - Eliminates infant's ability to grasp and possibly dislodge necessary treatment regimens (IV access, feeding tube, mechanical ventilation, etc.).
  - It prevents infant from scratching self or removing dressings and activities that interfere with maintenance of skin integrity.
  - If the patient is confused and impulsive and doesn't follow directions but can be redirected, consider hand mitts to decrease grabbing ability. Or consider "freedom sleeves" (also called soft splints).
  - These are a good deterrent for patients who are trying to remove a medical device from the face or head (such as a nasogastric tube or drain).

  Articles required
  - Commercial mittens or
  - Stockinette material (cut to fit individual infant)
  - Adhesive tape
  - Safety pins or other securing device (optional)
  - Mitten can be made wrapping the child's hands in gauze or with a little bag putting over the baby's hand and tie it on at the wrist.

  Procedure
  1. Place infant's hand inside stockinette
  2. Secure stockinette by applying tape to stockinette material and fastening around infant's wrist. Make sure that the fingers can be slightly flexed and are not caught under the hand.

  Caution: Do not wrap tape too tight; this might interfere with distal circulation.
  3. Tie end of stockinette in order to isolate fingers inside the stockinette material.
  4. Secure restraint to mattress, blanket, or light sandbag with safety pin (optional).

5. With freedom sleeves, patients have difficulty bending their arms. Be aware, though, that the sleeves don't necessarily prevent them from removing IV lines.
6. Hand mitts and freedom sleeves let the patient move the arms up and down but limit the ability to bend and grab tubes or drains.
7. They can be removed by unstrapping the hook-and-loop closures and sliding them off the arms.
8. Mittens should be removed on a regular basis. This permits the client to wash and exercise the hands. It also helps in assessing the circulation of hands.

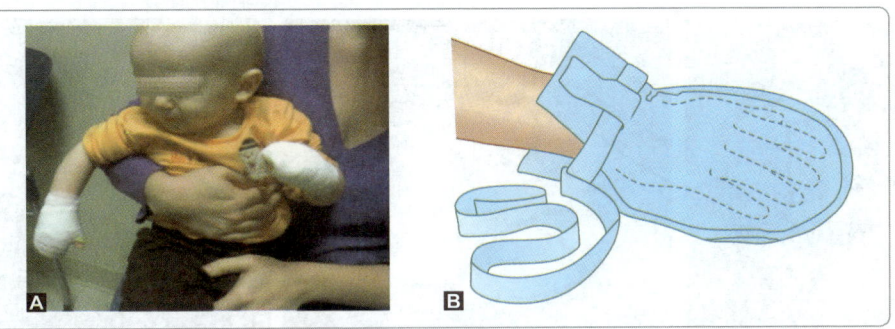

Figures 33A and B: Mitten or finger restraint

■ **Crib-net restraint:** A crib net is simply a device placed over the top of a crib to prevent active young children from climbing out of the crib (Fig. 34).

Purpose

• Crib restraints are used mainly to prevent children from falling out of the crib or climbing the crib rails.

Procedure

1. In this a net is used to cover the child cot.
2. Net is attached to the cot frame
3. The crib net or dome is not attached to the movable parts of the crib so that the caregiver can have access to the child without removing the dome or net.
4. Place the net over the sides and ends of the crib.
5. Secure the ties to the springs or frame of the crib.
6. Inside the crib net, the child is totally free to move, no movement is restricted

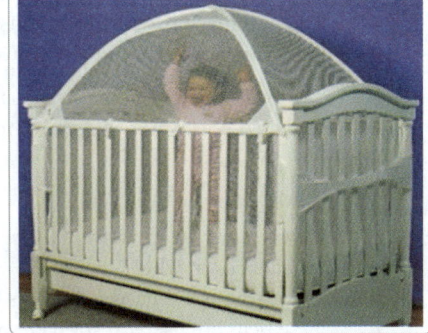

Figure 34: Crib net restraint

■ **Jacket restraint:** Jacket restraint is a device used to help immobilize the trunk of a patient (Figs 35A to C).

Purposes

• This restraint is used to avoid the child from climbing over the side rails, climbing out from chair, bed, cot, etc.
• It prevents the patient from fall and injury.

Procedure

1. In this method, a jacket made up of soft cloth and leather is used.
2. This jacket has laces at the back and two long strips.
3. Place vest on client with opening at the front or the back depending upon the type.

Unit IV ❖ Basic Needs of the Patient

4. Pull the tie on the end of the vest flap across the chest and place it through the slit in the opposite side of the chest.
5. The laces are tied at back and long strips tie at the side below the rails under the mattress.
6. Repeat for the other tie.
7. Use a half bow knot to secure each tie
8. Patient can sit and sleep in supine position while wearing jacket.
9. It can be used on chair also.

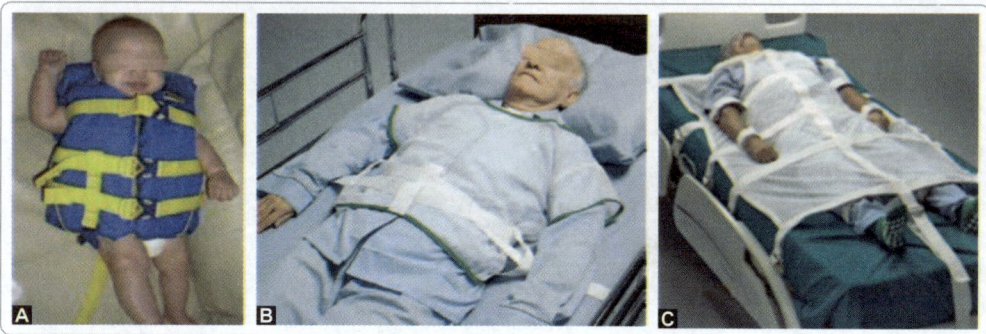

Figures 35A to C: Jacket restraint

- Safety vests and jackets can be placed on a patient like any other vest garment.
- They typically have a long strap at each end that can be tied behind a chair or to the sides of a bed to prevent injury or to settle patients for satisfying basic needs such as eating and sleeping.
- Posey vests are commonly used with elderly patients who are at risk of serious injury from falling.

■ **Belt restraint or safety belts:** Belt restraint is a common restraint that is designed to secure a patient to either a seated position, a bed, or simply to keep the arms secure to their torso, as with a straight jacket (Figs 36A to C).

Purposes

- Belt or safety strap restraints are used to ensure the safety of all clients who are being moved on stretchers or in wheel chairs.
- Belt restraints are used for clients who are confined to bed or chair.
- These belts are used on stretcher and operation tables to prevent the patients from falling.

Procedure

1. These are made up of electrically non-conductive material.
2. The belts go around the patients' waist and tied to the frame of bed under the mattress.
3. Place the patient in required position.
4. If the belt has a long portion and a shorter portion, place the long portion of the belt behind or under the client and secure it to the movable part of the bedframe.
5. Secure the belt to the frame of the bed.
6. To prevent the patient from slumping forward, attach a Y strap to the bar and over the clients' shoulders to the rear handles.
7. Some safety belt has three loop designs. One loop surrounds the patients' waist which is fastened to the back of the wheel chair.

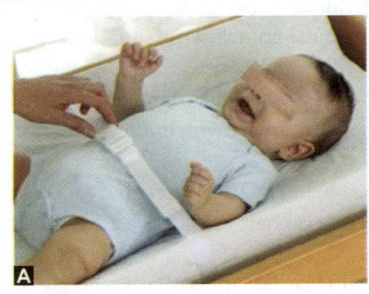 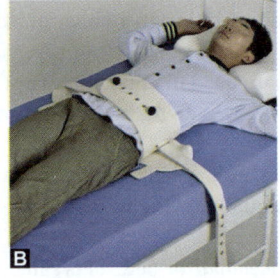 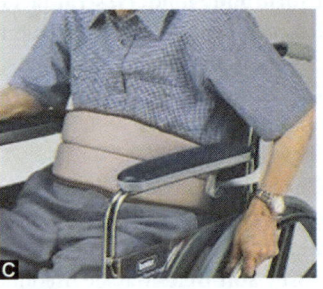

Figures 36A to C: Belt restraint

- **Side rails:** The rails are made up of iron or steel. These can be raised whenever need arises and can be decreased as per convenience (Fig. 37).
  - The main purpose of side rails is to prevent from fall and can be used along with other restraints.
  - These are used for patients with convulsive disorders also.

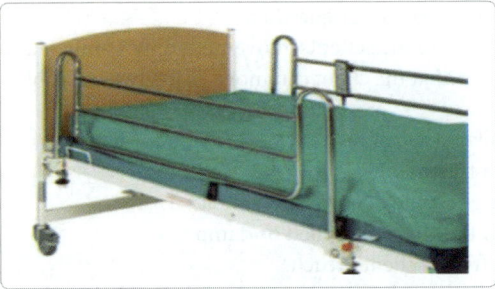

Figure 37: Side rails

- **Splints:** These are prepared devices which are used to restraint the movements of extremities (Figs 38A and B).
  - These are made up of plastic, card board, hard paper and cotton and gauze pieces.
  - These can be applied wherever needed.

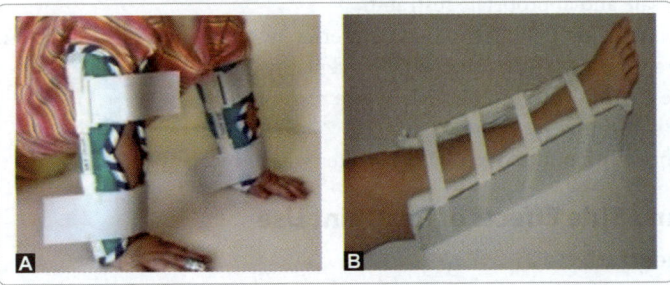

Figures 38A and B: Splints

Other Types of Restraints

- **Four-point restraints:** A four-point restraint restrains both arms and both legs. They are usually reserved for violent patients who pose a danger to themselves or others.

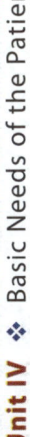
Unit IV ❖ Basic Needs of the Patient

- **Fabric body holders, straitjackets** are typically used temporarily during psychiatric emergencies.
- **Restraint masks** prevent patients from biting in retaliation to medical authority in situations where a patient is known to be violent.
- **Lap and wheelchair belts or trays** are used to clip across the front of a wheelchair so that the user can't fall out easily, may be used regularly by patients with neurological disorders which affect balance and movement.
- **Chest vests and lap belts:** Chest vests and lap belts (also called waist belts) may be warranted for confused or impulsive patients who are continually trying to get out of bed or a chair after repeated redirection, when it's unsafe for them to get up unaided.
- **Posey Soft Belt:** May be used in wheelchair or bed. This safety belt is perfect for patients who are at risk for forward sliding or require assistance with ambulation.
- **Enclosure bed:** An enclosure bed helps prevent patient injury by stopping the patient from getting out of bed unassisted. It may be a good option for patients who meet the criteria for this bed.

General Guidelines for use of Restraints

- Restraints should be applied only with the written order of the consulting physician.
- Obtain informed consent from patient or guardian.
- Restraints should be applied to reduce clients' movement only as much as necessary.
- Apply restraints in such a way that the client can move as freely as possible without defeating the purpose of the restraint.
- Nurse should carefully explain type of restraint and reason for its use.
- It should not interfere with treatment.
- Bony prominences should be padded before applying it.
- It should be changed when they become soiled or damp.
- It should be secured away from a client's reach.
- It should be secured in such a way that the device should quickly be released whenever necessary.
- Always tie a restraint with a knot that will not tighten when pulled.
- It should be attached to bed frame not to side rails.
- It should be removed a minimum of every 2 hours.
- When a restraint is temporarily removed, do not leave the client unattended.
- Frequent circulation checks should be performed when extremities are used.
- Always select the safe and appropriate restraint.
- Restraint should not be too tight; it should not interfere with the normal circulation.
- Monitor the restraint every 20–30 minutes to prevent any complications.
- All other possible alternatives must be tried before restraining.
- Offer bedpan or bathroom every 2 hours.
- Offer fluids and nourishment frequently, keep water within reach.

Potential Risks and Side Effects of Restraint Use

Psychological/Emotional effects:
- Increased agitation and fear
- Increased confusion
- Feelings of humiliation
- Loss of dignity
- Hostility

Physical effects:

- Contractures
- Loss of balance
- Decreased muscle mass, tone, strength, endurance
- Pressure ulcers
- Skin trauma
- Impaired circulation, obstructed and restricted circulation
- Physical discomfort, increased pain
- Dislocation/fracture

RESTRAINT ORDERS

- Initiation of restraints (try other alternatives always).
- May apply in emergency, but get physician order within 1 hour. The consulting physician must do face-to- face assessment within 1 hour of restraint initiation.
- Obtain written order within 12 hours of initiation.
- Renewing order—every 24 hours.
- Monitor a patient in restraint every 15 minutes for:
  - Signs of injury
  - Circulation and range of motion
  - Comfort
  - Readiness for discontinuation of restraint

Duration of Using Restraints

- Initial restraint orders are valid for three hours.
- After three hours, the nurse or physician assistant or authorized physician representative may continue the order if the rationale for the use of the restraints still exists.
- At six hours, the physician must examine the patient and determine if the order should be renewed.
- The maximum amount of time restraints or seclusion may be used is eight hours and a 24-hour period.
- If the physician determines that they should be used longer than that, a new order must be written every 24 hours.

Nurse's Responsibility while using Restraints

- Assess the client's behaviour and the need for restraint.
- Apply the least restrictive, reasonable and appropriate devices.
- Explain the client the reason for the restraint and cooperation.
- Comply with institutional policies and guidelines for restraint.
- Must communicate with the client and family members.
- Get written order and obtain informed consent as per Institution policy.
- Review the restraint regularly, or according to institutional policies.
- Institute a trial of restraint release.
- Ensure that particular attention is paid to the safety, comfort, dignity, privacy and physical and mental conditions.

Unit IV ❖ Basic Needs of the Patient

Monitoring the Client during Restraint

The scope of monitoring must include an evaluation or reassessment of the patient's physical condition, the patient's emotional state, and the patient's responses to the restraint or seclusion.

- Physical status, including vital signs, any injuries, nutrition, hydration, circulation, range of motion, hygiene, elimination and physical comfort
- Ongoing and frequent assessments called the **six P's** of the circulation checks - they're pulse, pallor, polar, paresthesia, paralysis, and pain.
- Psychological and emotional status, including psychological comfort and the maintaining of dignity, safety and patient rights
- Observe and monitor the following:
  - Is the patient safe?
  - Are the restraints still in place and safely applied?
  - Are the patient's vital signs normal?
  - Are the skin color, intactness of the skin, and circulation good?
  - Is the restraint too tight?
  - Is the patient comfortable and without any physical needs that you can attend to like toileting, food and/or fluids?
  - Is the person confused?
  - Is the patient or resident angry, upset or agitated?
  - Is the person afraid or fearful?
- After the restraint is applied, initial monitoring is done whenever necessary but at least every 15 minutes for the first hour by the qualified registered nurse.
- When the patient is stable and without significant changes, the monitoring and correlate documentation is then done at least every 4 hours for adults, every 2 hours for children from 9 to 17 years of age, and at least every hour for those less than 9 years of age.

Documentation

Document once in every 2 hours in restraint chart: (Sample enclosed) and it should include:

- The situation that initiated the use of the restraints.
- Who was contacted and what orders you received from that individual.
- The time when the restraints were initiated.
- How the nurse is maintaining safety for the restrained patient.
- Any other interventions the nurse is performing to calm the patient.

Acute Medical/Surgical Care (Restraint flow Chart)

| Restraint initiated | Date | Time |
| Order expires | Date | Time |

New verbal order required every 24 hours

Assessment should be based on individual needs. Patient must be assessed at least every 2 hours

		0700	0800	0900	1000	1100	1200	1300	1400	1500	1600	1700	1800	1900	2000	2100	2200	2300	2400	0100	0200	0000	0400	0600	0800
Restraints removed																									
Skin & Circulation Assessed																									
Toileting offered																									
Food/Fluids offered																									
Range of Motion & Patient Repositioned																									
Patient response	R - Restless C - Calm S - Sleeping U - Unaware																								
Effect of Restraint	A - Adequate I - Inadequate (explain)																								
Confined Need	Y- Yes N- No																								
Restraint Reapplied																									
Initials																									

Explain_____

T		SIGNATURE	TITLE

CARE OF CASTS AND SPLINTS

Definition: Casts are solid dressings applied to a limb or other body part.

Purposes

Casts are applied to:

- Immobilize a body part in a specific position
- Exert uniform compression to soft tissue
- Provide for early mobilization of unaffected body parts
- Correct or prevent deformities
- Stabilize and support unstable joints.

Types

- **Plaster casts:** Plaster casts mold very smoothly to the body's contours and are generally less expensive. The cast initially emits heat and takes about 15 minutes to cool and 24–72 hours to dry. It must be handled carefully until dry.
- **Fiberglass casts:** These plastic casts are typically lighter and more durable than plaster casts. Also, X-rays penetrate fiberglass casts better than plaster casts. They dry in 10–15 minutes and can bear weight 30 minutes after application.
- **Polyester-cotton knit casts:** Takes about 7–10 minutes to dry and can withstand weight bearing almost immediately.

Preparation of Client for Cast Application

- Explain the procedure and what to expect.
- Obtain informed consent if surgery is required.
- Clean the skin of the affected part thoroughly.

Care after the Cast Application

- Support an exposed cast, with the palms of the hands to prevent indentations.
- Ensure that the stockinet is pulled over rough edges of the cast.
- Elevate the casted extremity above the level of the heart using slings or pillows.
- Provide covering and warmth to uncasted areas.
- Expose the fresh plaster cast to circulating air, uncovered, until dry
- Instruct the client to avoid wetting the cast. Instruct him/her to dry a synthetic cast with a hair dryer on cool setting if it gets wet (Figs 39A and B).

Do's

- Do keep the cast clean and dry at all times.
- Do cover the cast with a plastic bag or cast cover for bathing or showering, but do not submerge the cast in the water. The bag or cover may leak and is only helpful to protect against splashes (Fig. 39).
- Do use a hair dryer on cool air setting to dry the cast if it gets wet by blowing air under the cast.
- Do cover any rough edges of the cast with tape to prevent skin irritation.
- Do elevate the cast above the heart if you have increased swelling, pain, numbness, tingling or change in color or circulation (Fig. 39B). If this does not relieve the symptoms, please contact the provider.

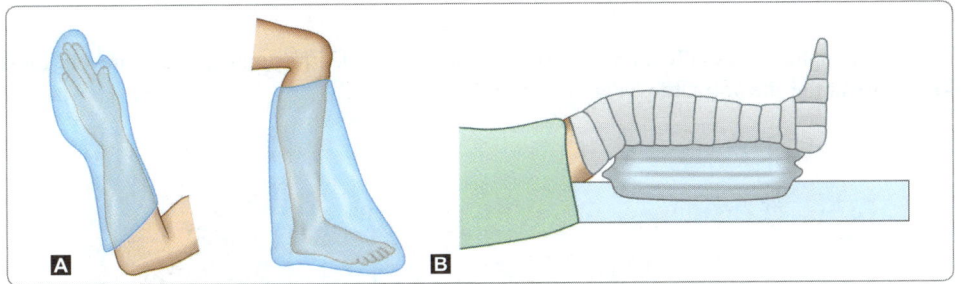

Figures 39A and B: (A) Cover the cast with plastic bag; (B) Elevate the affected body part

- Do contact the provider if the cast is damaged, cracked, or extremely wet. The cast will need to be changed.
- Do exercise the joints that are near to the casts (Fig. 40B).
- Do contact the provider if there is any red skin, irritation, blisters or sores around the edges of the cast or inside the cast.
- Use supportive tools such as crutches or slings (Fig. 40A).

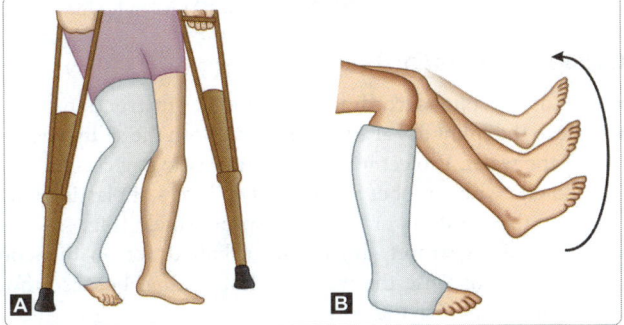

Figures 40A and B: (A) Use supportive tools; (B) Exercise

Don'ts

- Do not pull out any padding from under the cast.
- Do not get the cast wet.
- Do not stick anything into the cast to itch. Use a cool hairdryer to relieve any itching or irritation.
- Do not insert any object into the casts (Fig. 41A).
- Do not rest the heel of the leg cast on a pillow or bed. Keep the heel floating off the surface by elevating the leg with a pillow or blanket roll under the calf to prevent sores.
- Do not change or remove the cast without permission from the provider.
- Do not break off rough edges of the cast or trim the cast before asking the doctor.
- Inspect the skin around the cast. If the skin becomes red or raw around the cast, contact the doctor.
- Inspect the cast regularly. If it becomes cracked or develops soft spots, contact the doctor.
- Never attempt to remove the cast (Fig. 41B).

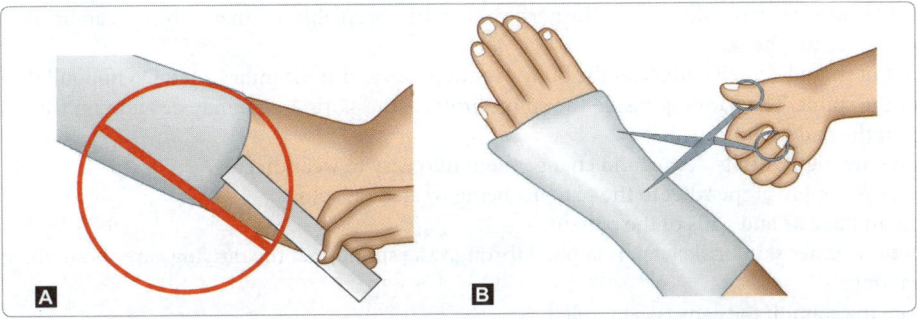

Figures 41A and B: (A) Do not insert anything in cast; (B) Do not remove cast by itself

Unit IV ❖ Basic Needs of the Patient

Splints

A splint is a rigid appliance, usually made of wood or metal, intended to support it and prevent movement from taking place at the site of fracture (Figs 42A and B).

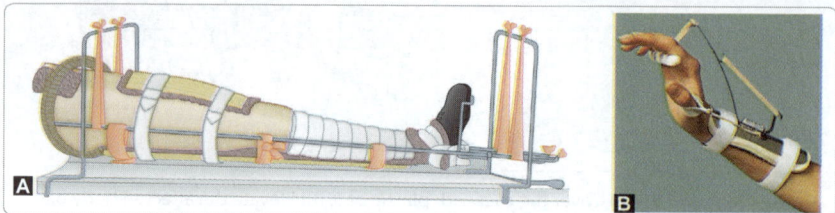

Figures 42A and B: (A) Splint for lower limb; (B) Splint for upper limb

Caring for the Splint

- Wear the splint according to the doctor's instructions.
- Keep the splint dry at all times. Bathe with the splint well out of the water. Protect it with a large plastic bag closed at the top end with a rubber band. Use two layers of plastic to help keep the splint dry or use a waterproof shield (Fig. 43).
- If a splint gets wet, dry it with a hair dryer on the 'cool' setting. Don't use the warm or hot setting, because those settings can burn the skin.
- Always keep the splint clean and away from dirt.
- Wash the Velcro straps and inner cloth sleeve (stockinet) with soapy water and air dry.
- Keep the splint away from open flames.
- Don't expose the splint to heat, space heaters, or prolonged sunlight. Excessive heat will cause the splint to change shape.
- Don't cut or tear the splint.

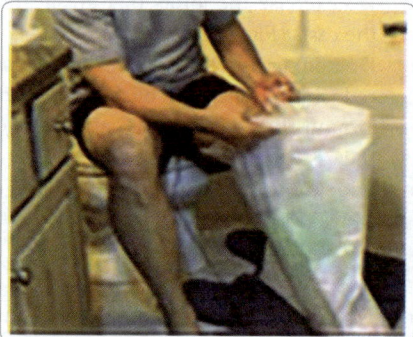

Figure 43: Cover the splint with waterproof material

- Exercise all the nearby joints not kept still by the splint. If you have a long leg splint, exercise the hip joint and the toes. If you have an arm splint, exercise the shoulder, elbow, thumb, and fingers.
- Elevate the part of the body that is in the splint. This helps reduce swelling.
- Check the splint and the skin around it each day. Check the splint for damage, such as cracks and breaks. Check the skin for redness, increased swelling, and sores.
- Loosen the elastic bandage around the splint if it feels too tight.
- Do not put powders or deodorants inside the splint. These can dry the skin and increase itching.
- Do not try to scratch the skin inside the hard splint with sharp objects. Sharp objects can break off inside the splint or hurt the skin.
- The splint should be well padded at the bony prominences and at the injury sites. Do not pull the padding out of the splint. The padding inside the splint protects the skin. A sore may develop on the skin if you take out the padding.
- Remove any tight fitting clothes and change them into easy to wear dresses.
- Arrange to supply proper diet to the patients being treated on splints.
- Attend to the hair and nails of the patient
- If traction, either skin or skeletal, is applied through the splint then the nursing care should include care on traction.
- Change the splint if the canvas gets soiled.

Activity, Exercise, Rest, Sleep and Positioning

DEFINITIONS

- **Activity:** It means exertion of energy or quality of being active or diligence or nimbleness.
- **Exercise:** It means exertion of muscles, limbs, etc. especially for the sake of health, bodily, mental or spiritual training or a task set for this purpose. Exercise is the performance of physical exertion for improvement of health or the correction of physical deformity.

IMPORTANCE OF ACTIVITY AND EXERCISE

All living creatures move. The cessation of all movement is the first observable sign of death. Movement is such a vital part of our lives that permanent loss of ability to move any part of the body is one of the major tragedies that can occur in a person's life.

All systems in the body function more efficiently when they are active. Disuse of the neuromuscular system quickly leads to degeneration and subsequent loss of functioning. If muscles are immobilized, the process of degeneration begins almost immediately. It has been estimated that the strength and tone of immobilized muscles may decrease by as much 5% per day in the absence of any contraction of the muscle.

The process of degeneration in muscles occurs very quickly. The restoration of muscle strength and tone, on the other hand, is a very slow process that may take months or years to accomplish.

In this case, prevention is the better part of cure. Nurses caring for patients during the acute stage of illness requiring more than a few days of bed rest, have a responsibility to do everything possible to prevent degeneration of unused muscles and the development of complications that will limit the person's mobility or prolong his recovery and restoration to health.

DANGERS OF PROLONGED BED REST

The dangers of prolonged bed rest have been well documented in numerous study reports, books and articles, in both the nursing and medical literature over the past 30 or 40 years. The custom of early ambulation of patients following surgery, child birth and acute illness was introduced just after the World War II. The results have been phenomenal in preventing complications and hastening patients' recovery.

Among the adverse effects of lengthy bed rest that have been noted are:

- A slowing down of the basal metabolic rate
- A decrease in muscle strength, tone and size
- Postural changes
- Constipation
- Increased vulnerability to pulmonary and urinary tract infection
- Circulatory problems such as thrombosis (the development of clot in the blood stream) and embolus. (Which occurs when the clot becomes detached and travels through the blood stream until it comes to a vessel too small for it to pass through, where it lodges).
- The degenerative process affects bone and skin tissue as well.
- The pulse rate increases as the heart works harder in an attempt to cope with the extra amount of blood 'dumped' into the general circulation from the legs when the body is lying down for long periods.
- There is increased excretion of calcium, nitrogen and phosphorus and the individual may suffer severe depletion of these elements.
- The person usually develops feelings of anxiety and frequent hostility as a result of disturbed functioning of physical and mental activities, as well as disruption of his sleep patterns.

Unit IV ❖ Basic Needs of the Patient

BENEFITS OF EXERCISES

Exercise in comparison increases the efficiency of performing all body processes. The physiological, psychological and social benefits of exercise have been receiving increasing attention in recent years. The predominantly sedentary way of life has been viewed as a major factor contributing to many of the illness with which we are plagued such as coronary heart disease, hypertension, diabetes and obesity.

The exact physiological changes that result from a regular exercise program are increased muscle strength, tone and size, increased efficiency of the heart; increased work tolerance, increased pulmonary efficiency, blood circulation, normal blood pressure, decreased deposits of fatty tissue; and decreased cholesterol

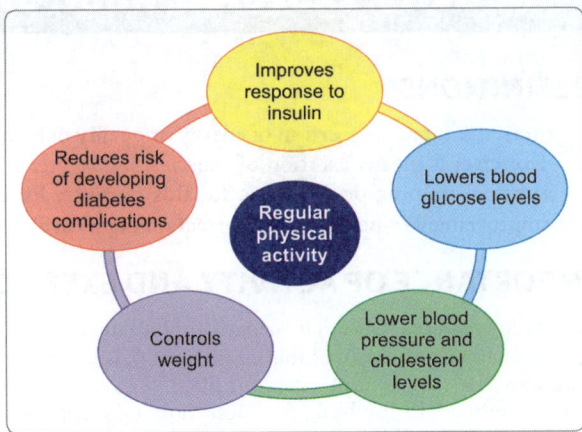

Figure 1: Benefits of exercise

levels in the blood. It has been demonstrated that the exercise following a fatty meal will help to clear the excess cholesterol level in the blood and thus it will increase the fat tolerance.

The benefits of exercise are shown in Figure 1.

CLASSIFICATION OF EXERCISE

Exercise is always required to make the sedentary muscles to become active. There are two types of exercises that are being done with patients: active and passive.

- **Active exercise** refers to the exercise, which the patient does for himself/herself by moving about in bed or by changing his/her position, reaching for objects that have been placed nearby or performing definite prescribed exercises, which can be done while remaining in bed. Simple exercises performed in bed will help the patient to overcome disabilities that may result from illness and prolonged rest in bed. Exercise during convalescence helps to maintain general muscle tone and strengthens the body (Fig. 2).

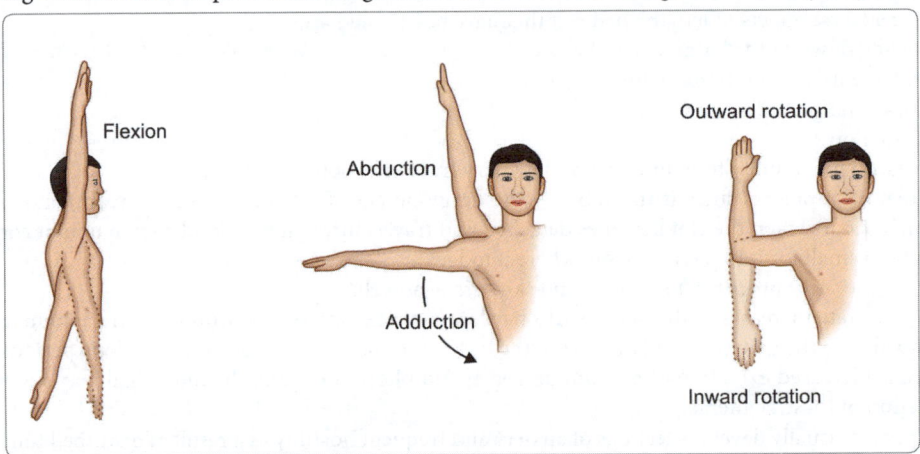

Figure 2: Active exercise

- **Passive exercise** refers to the exercise performed in the patient by another person. In passive exercise the movement or activity is carried out by another person (nurse or physiotherapist) and the patient makes no voluntary effort to assist or resist the action. Passive exercises are involved in such procedures as bed bath, turning the patient from side to side, moving arms and legs and application of alcohol massage (Fig. 3).

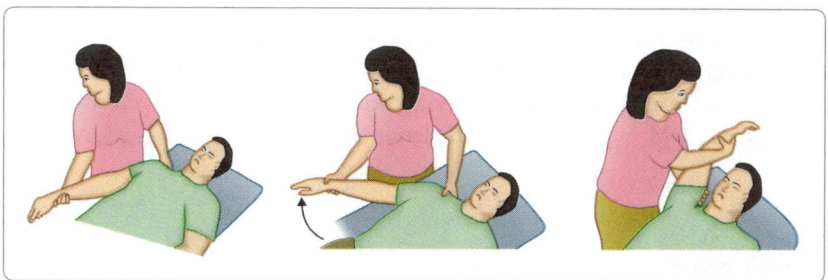

Figure 3: Passive exercise

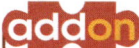

Foot Drop

Patients with prolonged rest and restricted movements develop a deformity called foot drop in which the foot is plantar flexed (The ankle bends in the direction of the sole of the foot). If the condition continues without correction, the patient will walk on toes without touching the heel of the foot in the ground.

This deformity is caused by the contraction of both gastrocnemius and soleus muscles. Prolonged bed rest, lack of exercise, incorrect positioning in bed and the weight of the bed clothes forcing the toes in the plantar flexion are some of the factors that contribute to this crippling deformity.

The foot drop can be prevented by the use of foot board (foot rest) to maintain the position of the feet at right angles to the legs, flexion and extension exercises to the feet and toes, frequently.

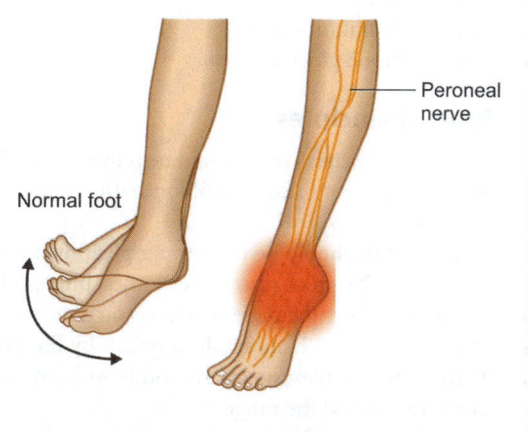

RANGE OF MOTION (ROM) EXERCISES

Exercise is physical activity for conditioning the body, improving health, and maintaining fitness.
- **Definition:** Range of motion exercise refers to activity aimed to improving movement of a specific joint.
- **Goal:** The goal of range of motion exercises is to keep movable joints flexible.

Purposes

- Promotes and maintains joint mobility
- Prevents contractures and shortening of muscles and tendons
- Increases circulation to extremities.
- Facilitates comfort for the patient

Unit IV ❖ Basic Needs of the Patient

Contraindications

- Any illness/disorder where increased use of energy or increased circulation is hazardous.

Example: Myocardial infarction, swollen, inflamed joints

Types of ROM Exercises

- **Active ROM exercises:** Exercises the client is able to perform independently.
- **Passive ROM exercises:** Exercises performed for the client by someone else.
- **Active assisted ROM exercises:** Performed by a client with some assistance. Client can move a limb partially through its ROM, but needs help completing the ROM.

Benefits

- Improves circulation
- Improves muscle strength
- Maintains flexibility
- Reduces pain
- Enhances physical performance
- Reduces stiffness
- Decrease injury potential.
- Better posture
- Improved joint function
- Reduces blood glucose levels

Technical Principles

The technical principles that should be remembered before performing ROM exercises are:

- Place the patient in comfortable position with proper body alignment and stabilization, to perform the exercise.
- The therapist should be in a proper position and effective stance.
- Free the region from restrictive clothes, linen, splints and dressings.
- Drape and cover the patient as necessary.
- Utilize the proper hand holds or grasps by the therapist.
- Perform the exercise slowly, smoothly with rhythm within the available pain free range of motion without any force behind the range.
- Do all ROM exercises smoothly and gently. Never force, jerk, or over stretch a muscle. This can hurt the muscle or joint instead of helping.
- Stop ROM exercises if the person feels pain. The exercises should never cause pain or go beyond the normal movement of that joint.
- Repeat the exercise 5–10 repetitions according to the patient condition and response.
- Do ROM exercises once or twice daily.
- Do each moves few times and build up to 12 times.
- Move until you feel a slight stretch but don't force a movement.

Patient Preparation

- Explain the steps and advantages of ROM exercises.
- Remove all restrictive clothing, linen, splint, and dressings.
- Position the patient comfortably—preferably supine position.

- Raise the bed to comfortable height.
- Drape appropriately

General Terminologies Used

- **Abduction:** Moving a body part away from the midline of the body
- **Adduction:** Moving a body part toward the midline of the body
- **Extension:** Straightening a body part
- **Flexion:** Bending a body part
- **Rotation:** Turning the joint
- **Internal rotation:** Turning the joint inward
- **External rotation:** Turning the joint outward
- **Plantar flexion:** Bending the foot down at the ankle
- **Pronation:** Turning the joint downward
- **Supination:** Turning the joint upward
- **Inversion:** Turning the sole of the foot towards the midline
- **Eversion:** Turning the sole of the foot away from the mid line

Procedure for ROM Exercises

Joint	Movements Possible	Procedure
• Neck	• Flexion	• Tuck chin in and bend head forward and chin towards the chest. Look at the toes.
	• Extension	• Look straight ahead

Contd...

Unit IV ❖ Basic Needs of the Patient

Joint	Movements Possible	Procedure
	• Hyperextension	• Look up at the ceiling
	• Lateral flexion	• Look straight ahead, tilt head to shoulder. Tilt left ear towards left shoulder, right ear towards right shoulder. Do not raise shoulder
	• Rotation	• Turn chin toward right shoulder, then towards left shoulder. Do not pull shoulder towards chin

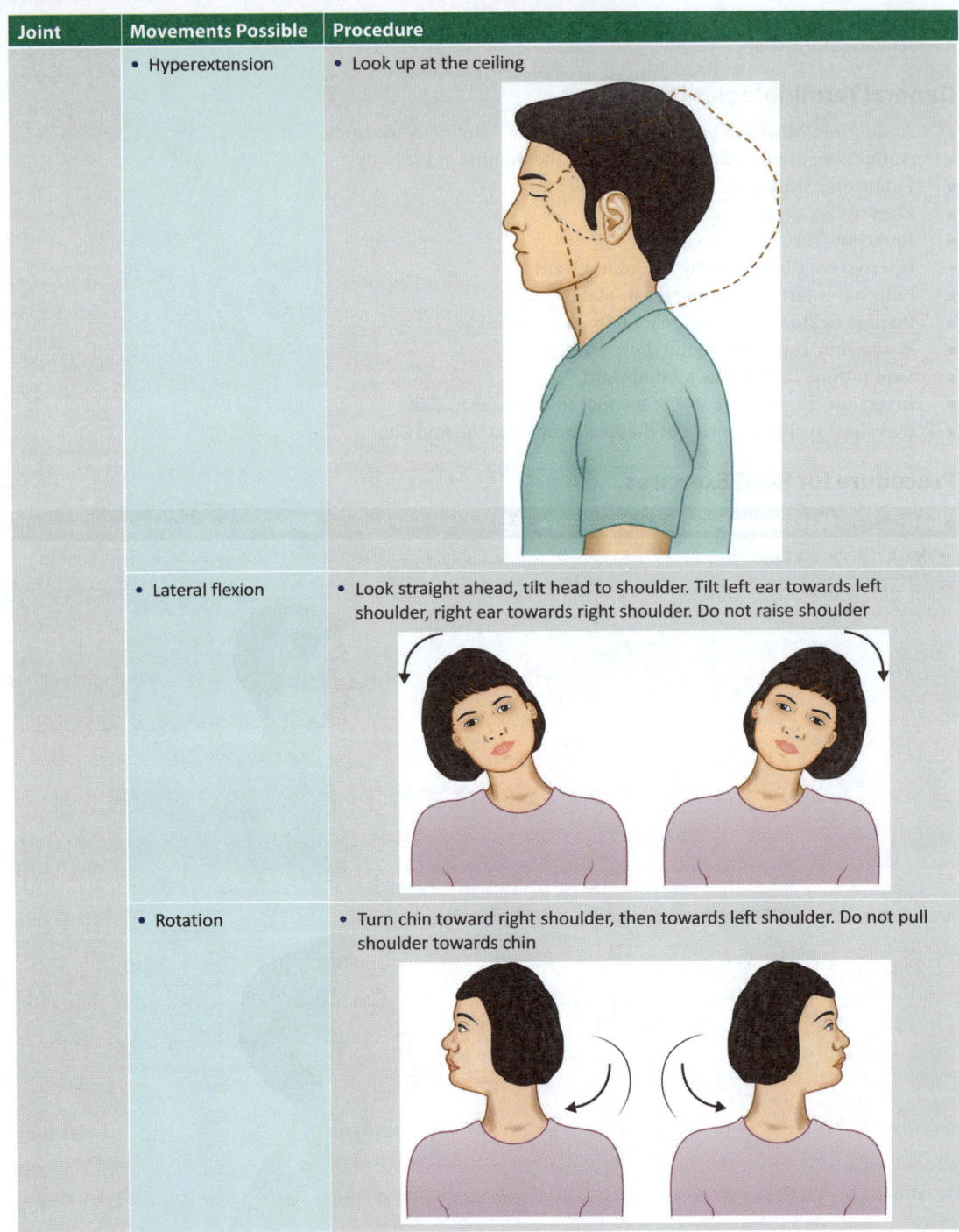

Contd...

Unit IV ❖ Basic Needs of the Patient

Joint	Movements Possible	Procedure
• Shoulder	• Flexion	• Lie on your back or stand straight. Raise your right arm over your head keeping your elbow straight. Try to flatten your arm slowly to your side. 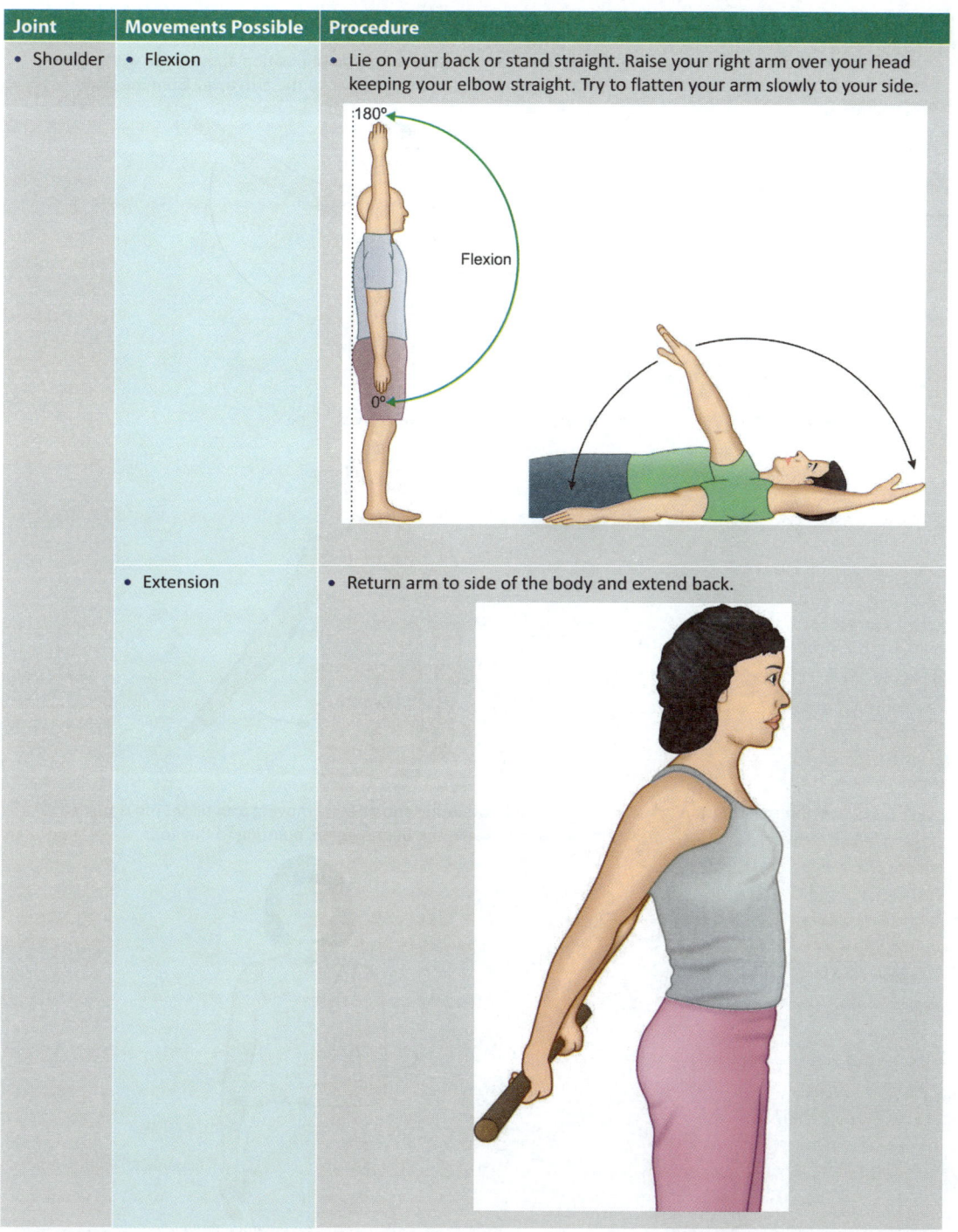
	• Extension	• Return arm to side of the body and extend back.

Contd...

Joint	Movements Possible	Procedure
	• Abduction	• Lie on your back. Raise arm to side to position above head with palm away from head toward ceiling. Move the arm away from the body.
	• Adduction	• Return arm and bring across chest
	• Internal rotation	• Elbow flexed, rotate the shoulder by moving arm till thumb is turned inward and towards the back. Fingers pointing to the floor

Contd...

Joint	Movements Possible	Procedure
	• External rotation	• Elbow flexed, move arm until thumb is lateral to head. Fingers pointing up
	• Circumduction	• Move arm in full circle.
• Elbow	• Flexion	• Bend elbow bringing forearm and hands towards shoulder.

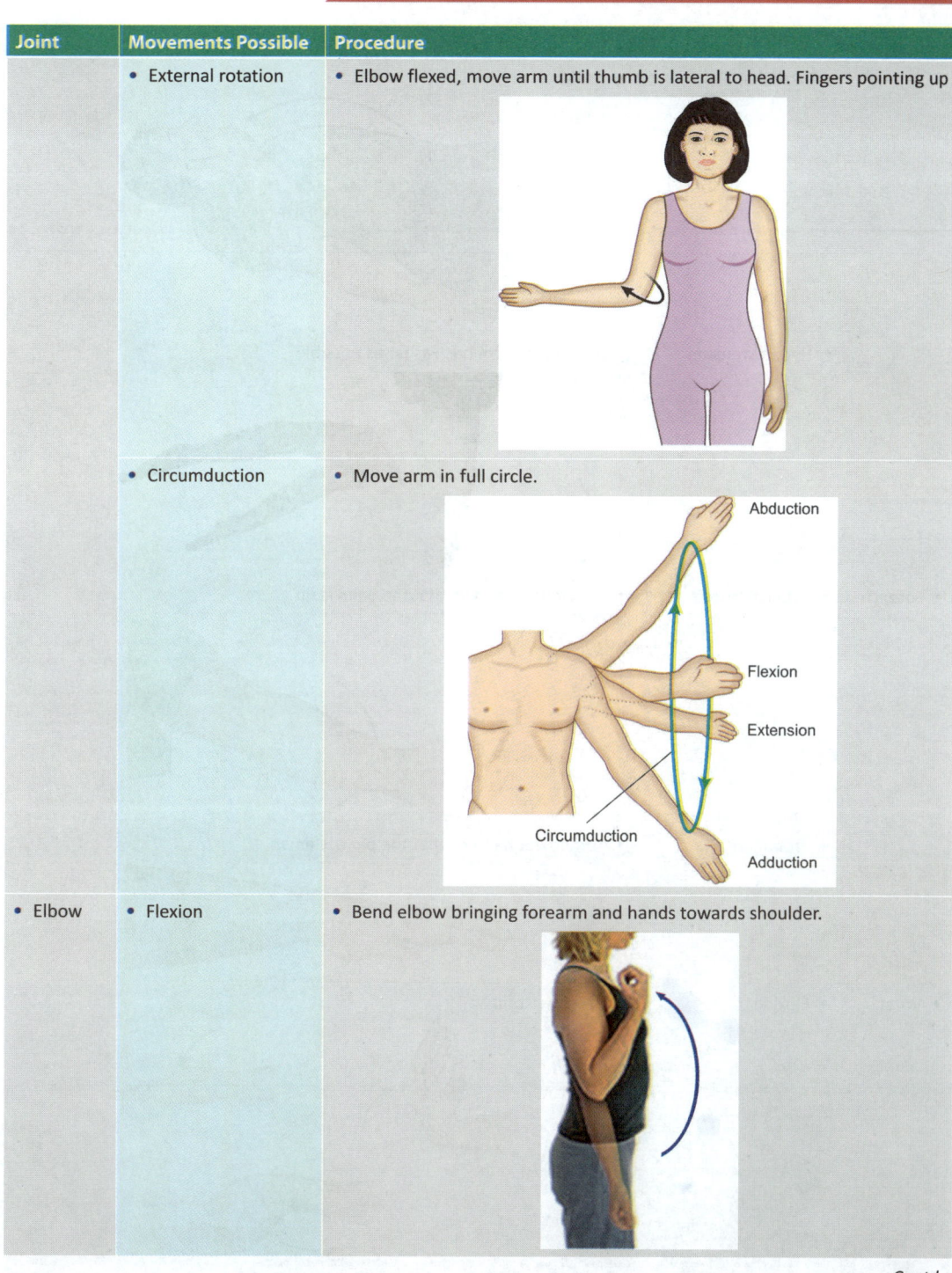

Joint	Movements Possible	Procedure
	• Extension	• Straighten elbow
	• Hyperextension	• Bend lower arm back as far as possible
• Forearm	• Supination	• Turn lower hand so that the palm is up
	• Pronation	• Turn lower hand so that the palm is down
• Wrist	• Flexion	• Bend wrist forward

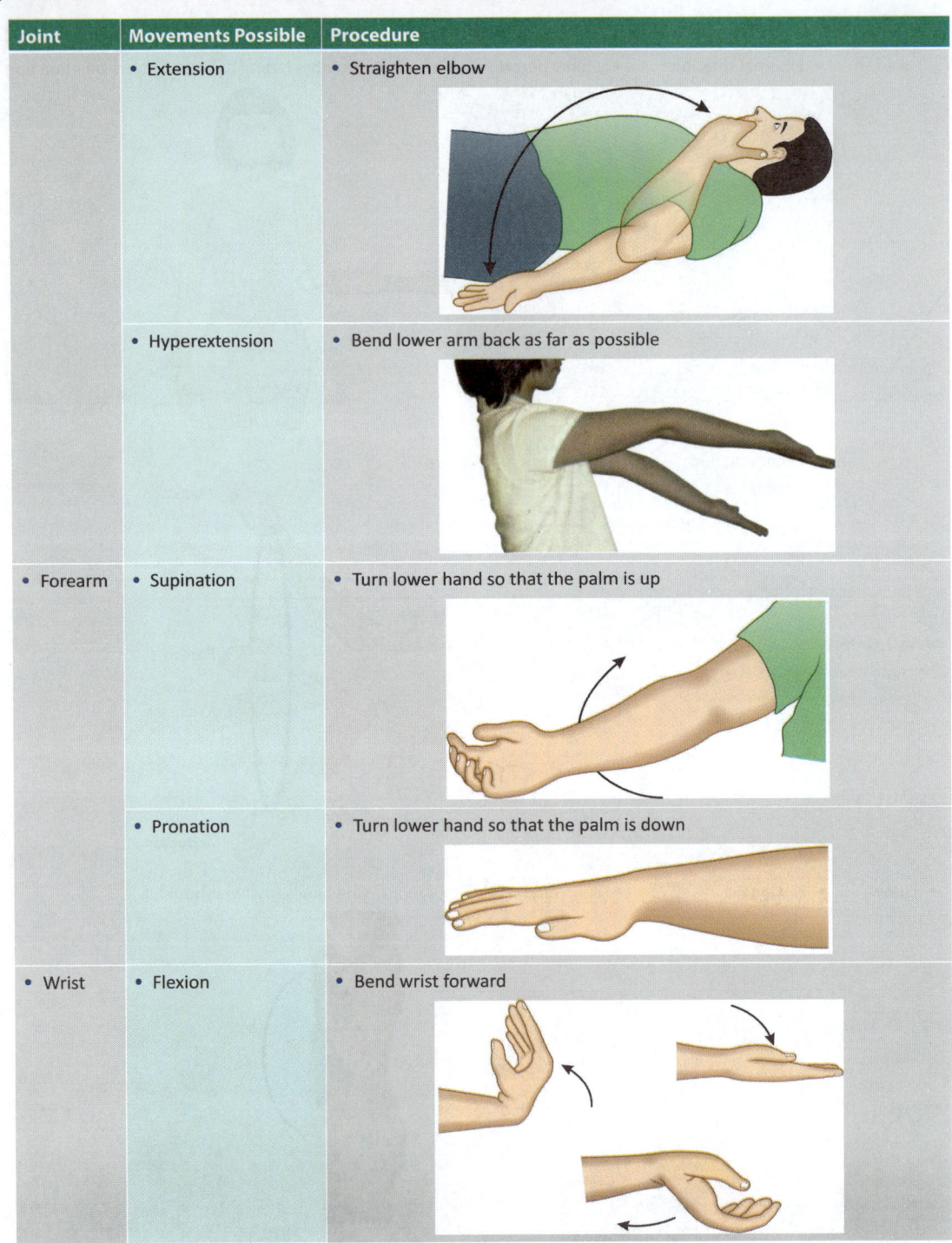

Contd...

Joint	Movements Possible	Procedure
	• Extension	• Straighten wrist so that the fingers, wrist and arm are in same plane
	• Hyperextension	• Bring dorsal surface of hand as far back as possible
	• Abduction	• Bring wrist medially towards the thumb
	• Adduction	• Bend wrist laterally towards 5th finger

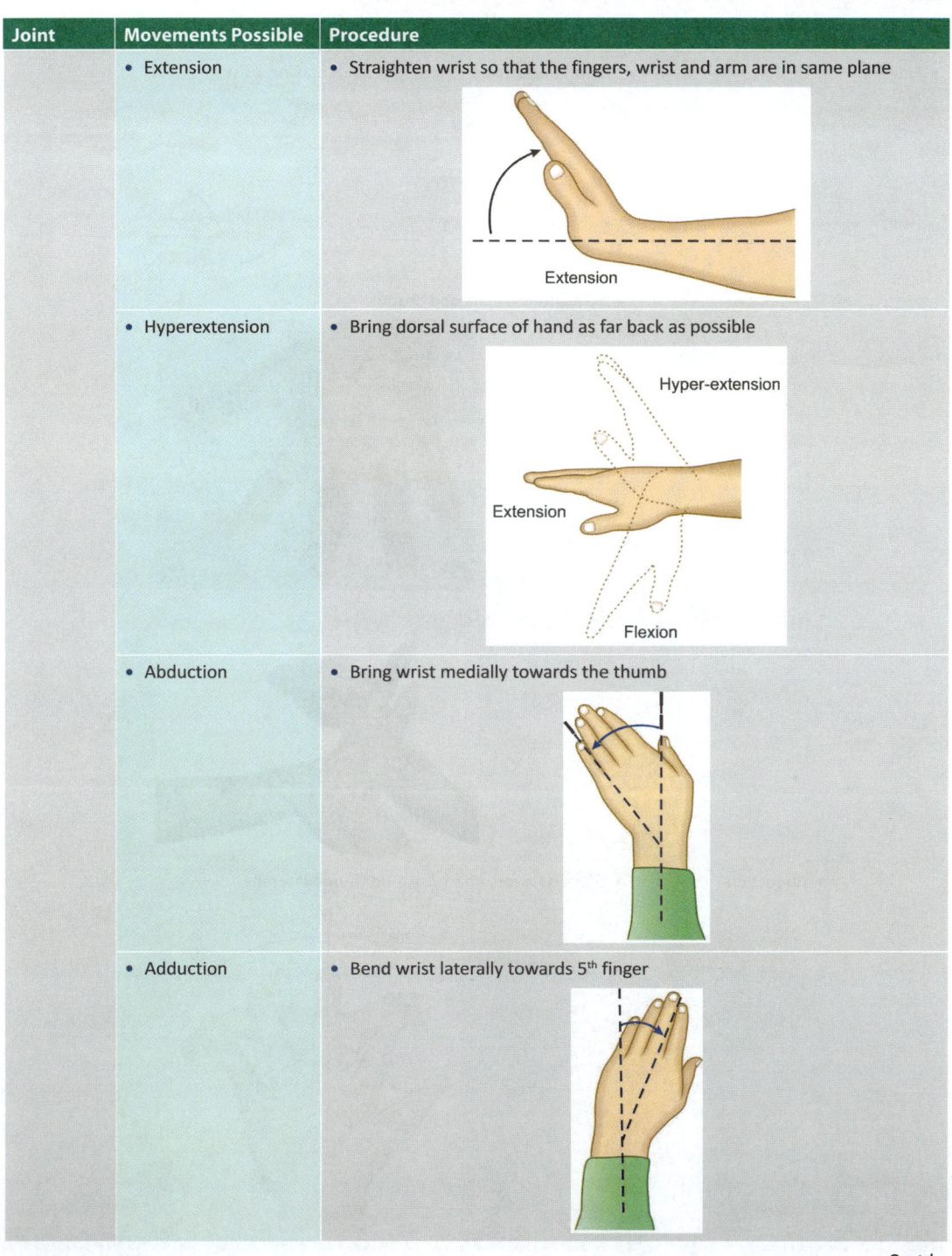

Contd...

Joint	Movements Possible	Procedure
• Fingers and Thumb	• Flexion	• Bend fingers and thumb into palm making a fist
	• Extension	• Straighten fingers and thumb
	• Hyperextension	• Bend fingers as far back as possible
	• Abduction	• Spread fingers apart / extend thumb laterally

Contd...

Joint	Movements Possible	Procedure
	• Adduction	• Bring fingers together/thumb back to hand
	• Circumduction	• Move finger/thumb in circular motion
	• Opposition	• Touch thumb to each finger of same hand
• hip	• Flexion	• Move leg forward

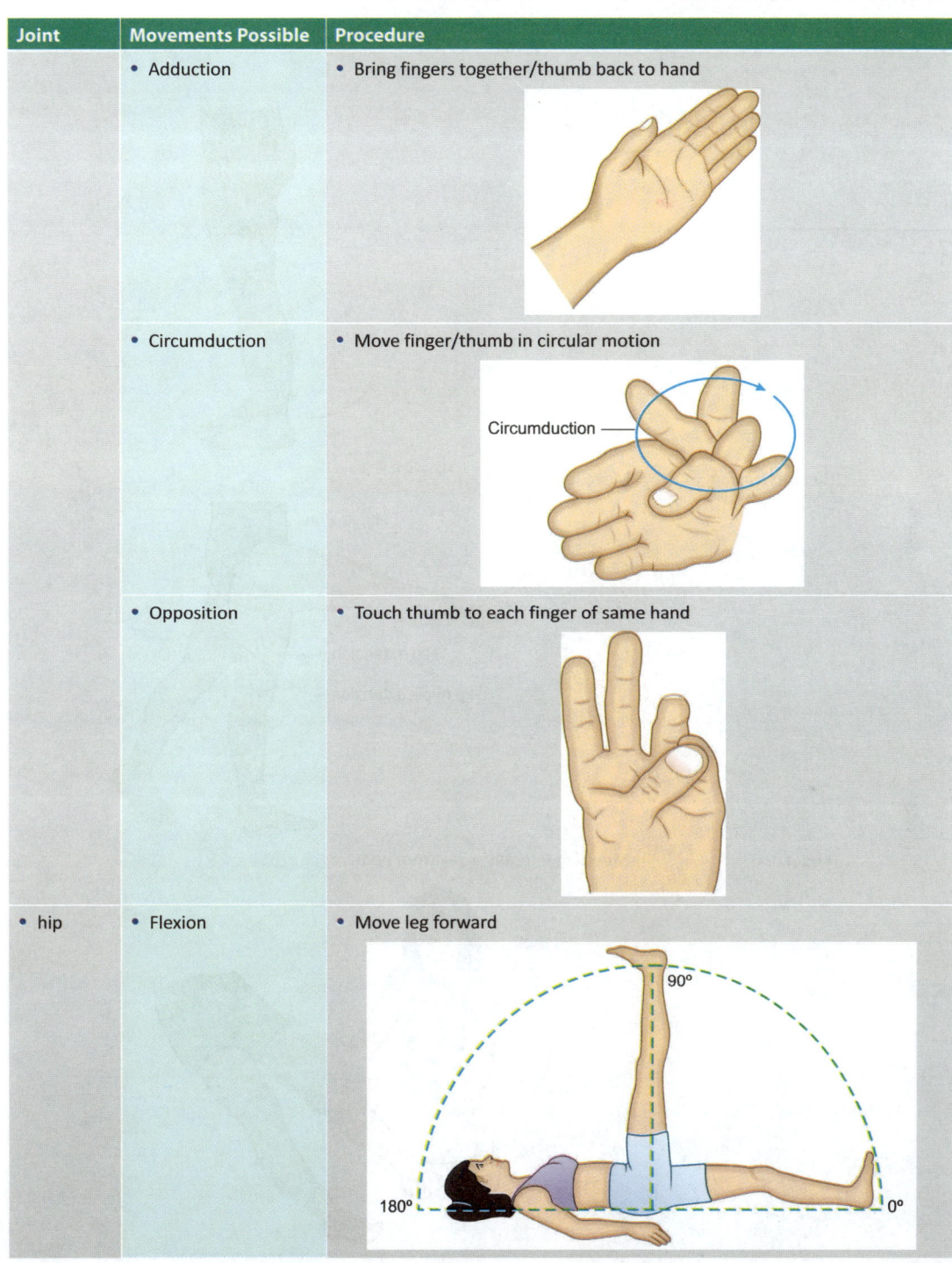

Contd...

Joint	Movements Possible	Procedure
	• Extension	• Move leg back beside other leg 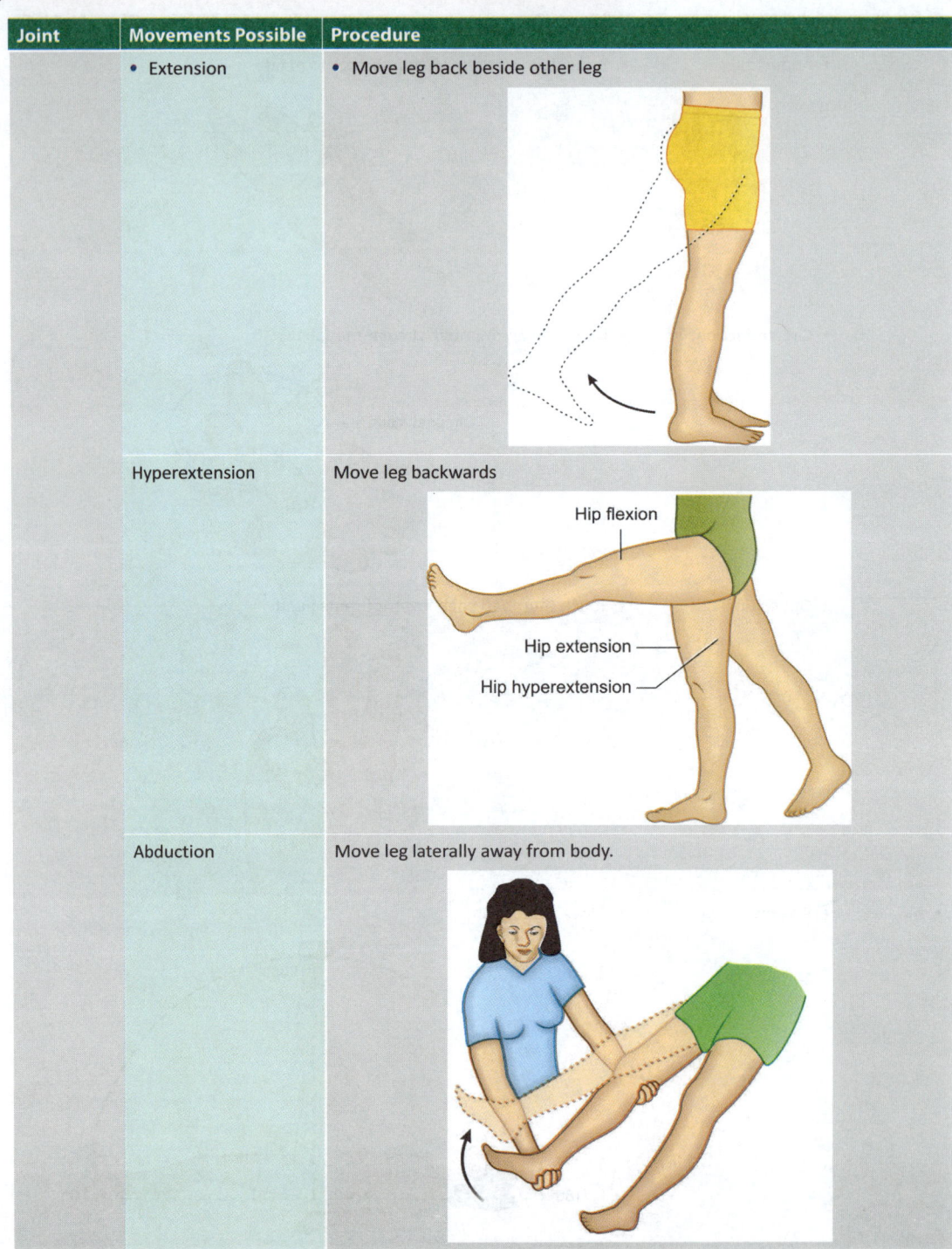
	Hyperextension	Move leg backwards
	Abduction	Move leg laterally away from body.

Contd...

Joint	Movements Possible	Procedure
		Hip abduction • Patient on back. Person assisting places one hand under patient's knee and other hand heel of feet. • Hold leg straight and lift slightly off the mattress. Take leg straight, keep knee pointing straight up. • Repeat
	Adduction	Move leg back to medial position and beyond if possible
Knee	Flexion	Bring heel toward back of thigh.
	Extension	Return leg to floor

Contd...

Unit IV ❖ Basic Needs of the Patient

Joint	Movements Possible	Procedure
• Ankle	Dorsiflexion	Move foot so that the toes are pointed upward Dorsiflexion
	Plantar flexion	Move foot so toes are pointed downward Plantar flexion Dorsiflexion Plantarflexion
• Foot	Inversion	Turn sole of foot medially
	Eversion	Turn sole of foot laterally Inversion Eversion

Contd...

Joint	Movements Possible	Procedure
	Abduction	Spread toes apart 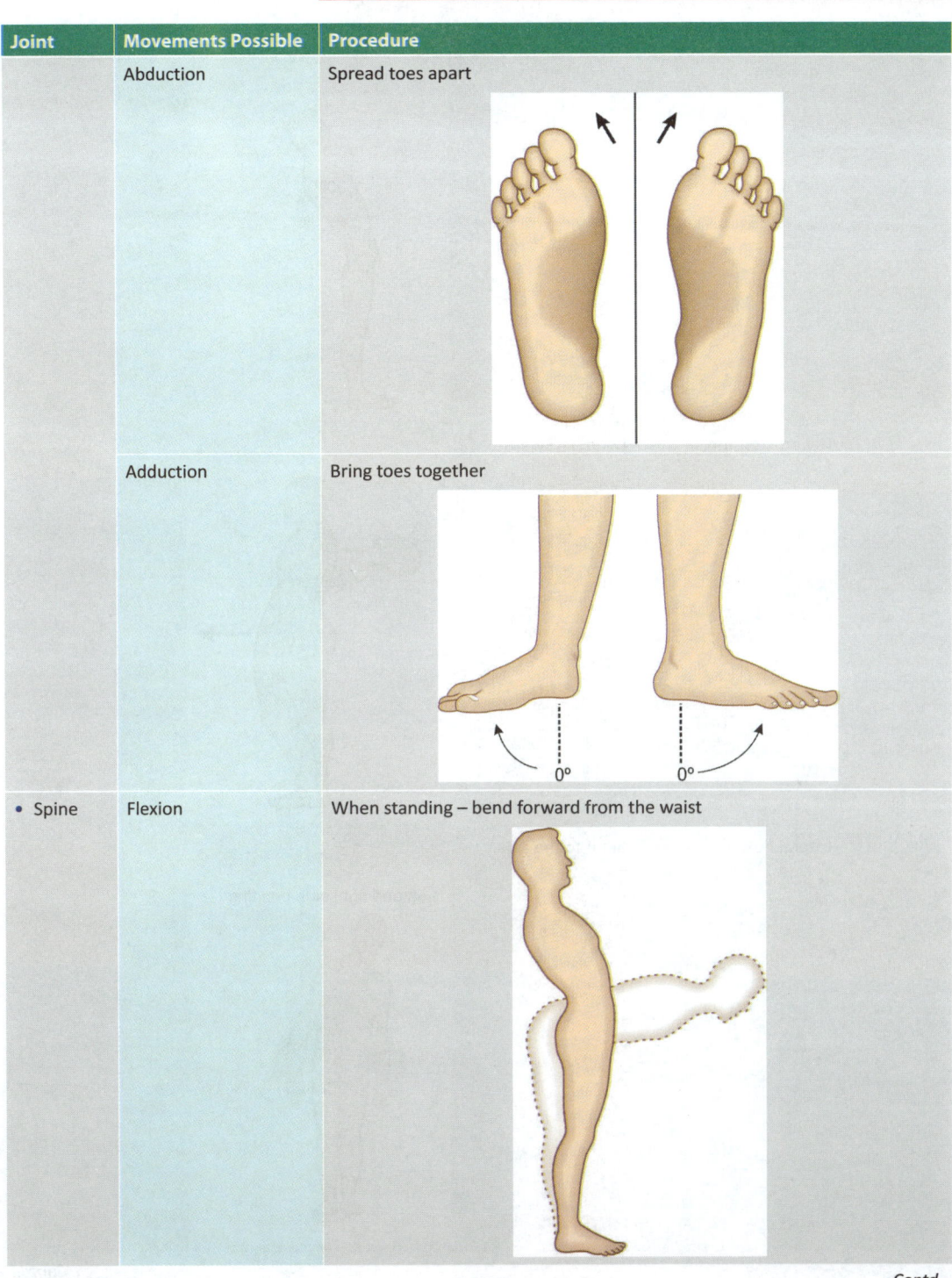
	Adduction	Bring toes together
• Spine	Flexion	When standing – bend forward from the waist

Contd...

Joint	Movements Possible	Procedure
	Extension	Straighten up 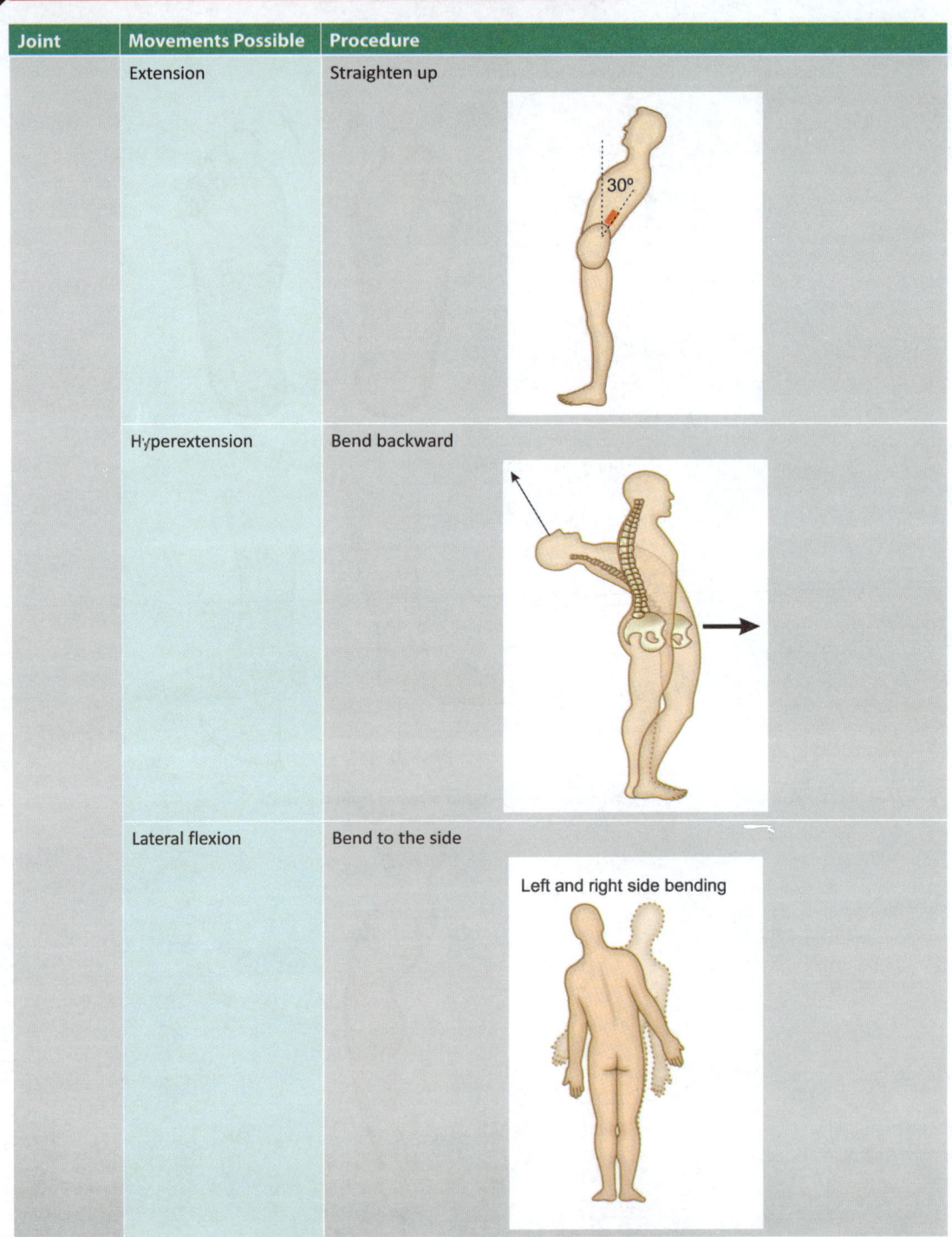
	Hyperextension	Bend backward
	Lateral flexion	Bend to the side Left and right side bending

Contd...

Joint	Movements Possible	Procedure
	Rotation	Twist from the waist 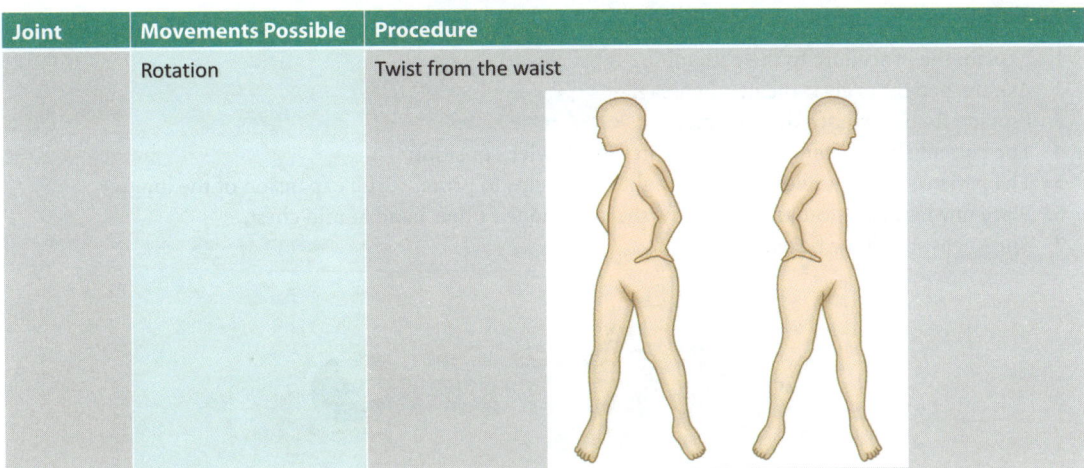

Documentation

Document the exercises given to patient, type and duration, patient's response along with date, time and signature of the nurse.

DEEP BREATHING AND COUGHING EXERCISES

Breathing exercises play an important role in overall pulmonary rehabilitation program of acute and chronic pulmonary disorders.

Purposes

- To retrain respiratory muscles
- To improve ventilation
- To make breathing easier
- Helps to expand the lungs; and forces an improved distribution of the air in all sections of the lungs.

Frequency of Performing Deep Breathing and Coughing Exercises

- Deep breathing exercises should be performed every hour while awake
- Patients who had undergone thoracic or abdominal surgeries need to perform these exercises at least 3 – 4 times a day.
- Each session should include at least 5 deep breaths

Common Types of Deep Breathing Exercises

- Diaphragmatic breathing
- Pursed lip breathing

Diaphragmatic Breathing Exercise

Diaphragmatic breathing strengthens the diaphragm, decreases the use of accessory muscles and allows for better emptying of the lungs. It helps the patient breath in a controlled manner during activities that produce dyspnea. Advice the patient to stop exercise if shortness of breath occurs.

Unit IV ❖ Basic Needs of the Patient

Procedure

1. Explain the procedure to the patient.
2. Ask the patient to clear the nasal passages.
3. Provide tissue paper to the patient.
4. The patient should stand firmly or sit in semi-fowler's position
5. The patient's back should be kept straight. This helps to promote full expansion of the lungs.
6. Place one hand on stomach just below the ribs and the other hand at mid chest.
7. The knees should be flexed.

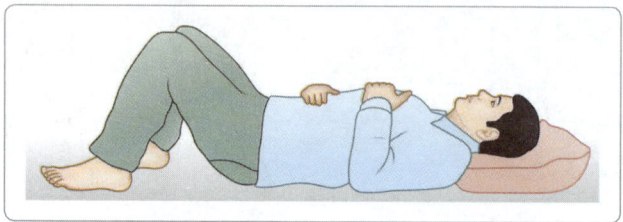

8. Instruct the patient to inhale slowly and deeply through the nose, letting the abdomen protrude as far as it could.

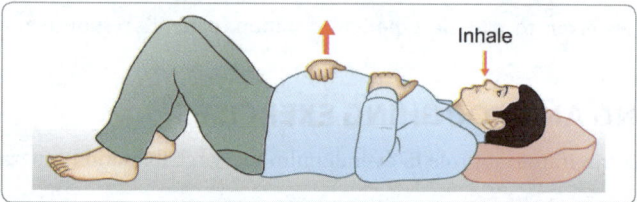

9. Instruct the patient to hold his breath for at least 3 seconds.
10. Instruct the patient to exhale slowly through pursed lips while tightening the abdominal muscles.
11. Press firmly inward and upward on the abdomen while breathing out. This facilitates slower and complete emptying of the lungs.

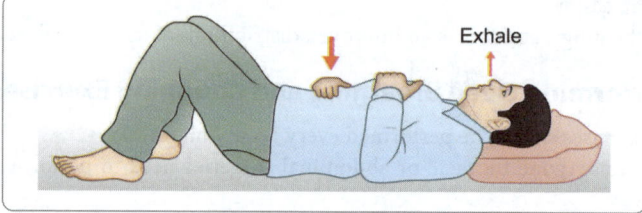

12. This procedure should be done for 1 minute followed by a rest period of 2 minute.
13. Work up to 10 minute, four times daily in different positions like supine, sitting, standing and walking.

Pursed-Lip Breathing

Pursed lip breathing slows the respiratory rate, decreases the dynamic compression of the airways and thus keeps the airways open longer.

Procedure

1. Explain the procedure to the patient.
2. Ask the patient to clear the nasal passages.
3. The patient should stand firmly or sit in semi-fowler's position
4. The patient's back should kept straight. This helps to promote full expansion of the lungs.
5. Have the patient inhale slowly through the nose to the count of 2.
6. Instruct the patient to exhale slowly and evenly against pursed lips to the count of 4 while contracting (tightening) the abdominal muscles.
7. Avoid exhaling forcefully.
8. Pursing the lips increases the intrabronchial, intra alveolar pressure (helps maintain them open)

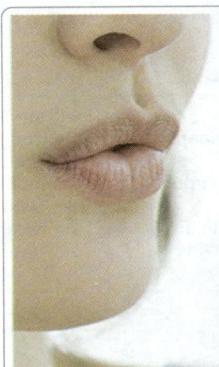

Pursed lip breathing:
1. Relax your neck and shoulder muscles
2. Breathe in for 2 seconds through your nose, keeping your mouth closed
3. Breathe out for 4 seconds through pursed lips. if this is too long for you, simply breathe out twice as long as you breathe in

Coughing

Airway clearance is an important part of management of all patients' especially patients with respiratory conditions. Coughing helps to break up secretions in the lungs so that the mucus can be expectorated or suctioned out, if necessary.

Purpose

Voluntary coughing in association with deep breathing facilitates movement and expectoration of secretion in the respiratory tract.

Procedure

1. Ask the patient to sit upright or in semi-fowler position. This facilitates deep inhalation.
2. Provide tissue paper to the patient.
3. Instruct the patient to place one hand on stomach just below the ribs and the other hand at mid chest with the knees flexed.
4. Instruct the patient to take slow inspiration deeply through the nose and watch for chest movement.
5. Instruct him to hold breath to count of 5.
6. Ask the patient to exhale forcefully and then release air while flexing forward and simultaneously having short puffs or coughs.
7. Repeat for 3 deep coughs or until mucus is expectorated.
8. This procedure is repeated several times a day.

Unit IV ❖ Basic Needs of the Patient

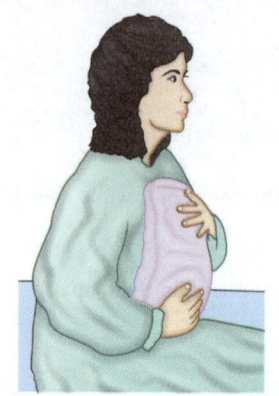

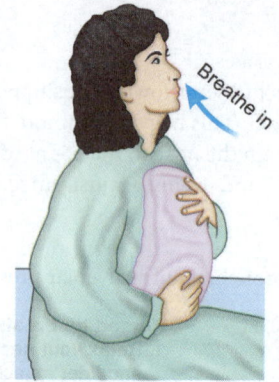

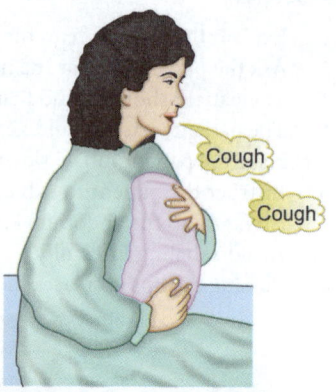

Step 1
- Sit on the edge of a bed or a chair. Or lie on your back with your knees slightly bent
- Lean forward slightly. Hold a pillow firmly against your incision with both hands
- Breathe out normally

Step 2
- Breathe in slowly and deeply through your nose
- Then breathe out fully through your mouth. Repeat
- Take a third deep breath. Fill your lungs as much as you can

Step 3
- Cough 2 or 3 times in a row
- Try to push all of the air out of your lungs as you cough
- Then relax and breathe normally
- Repeat as directed

Precautions While Effective Coughing

- Avoid uncontrolled coughing spasms
- Avoid forceful coughing instead advise patient to huff several times to clear the airways.
- Place the patient in a side-lying or erect position while performing coughing. This prevents aspiration of secretions.
- Manual pressure in the abdominal area while coughing helps in raising the abdominal pressure for a more forceful cough.
- Postoperative patients performing coughing exercises should guard the surgical site using a pillow.
- Frequent deep breathing exercises automatically triggers cough reflex.

REST AND SLEEP

Importance of Rest and Sleep

Rest and sleep are essential for health. Rest, both mental and physical, is essential to allow nature to rebuild and store energy. Even a few minutes of complete relaxation here and there throughout the day will go a long way toward conserving mental and physical energy, relieving tenseness and preventing fatigue. Sleep is recognized as one of the best means of securing rest.

Chief Methods of Ensuring Rest

- By meeting patient's need skillfully without delay.
- Use of comfort devices, by lessening discomfort or pain and to provide rest and relaxation.
- Protection from disturbing noises, unnecessary lights, bad odor and provision of adequate ventilation and a room free of dirt and dust.
- Procedures which make the patient feel refreshed and comfortable, increase physical comfort and rest. Besides, administration of drugs relieves pain.

- Ensuring mental relaxation by winning the patient's confidence through proper explanation of the nursing procedures, treatments and examination which the patient has to meet with.
- By helping the patient to solve his/her social or economic problems, if any.
- Giving all possible help to meet his/her spiritual need.

Sleep

Sleep is defined as a state of unconsciousness or of partial consciousness with the body and mind at rest. Approximately 1/3 of the normal life span of the individual is spent in sleeping. Fatigue is a normal process, ignoring it, usually results in nervousness and restlessness. Sleep is essential for the body to repair tissues worn out from activity and to rest the organs of the body. During sleep more energy is reserved. So children need more sleep than adults. The ability to fall asleep and stay asleep for an unbroken period is one of the measures of keeping mental and physical health. People feel very much refreshed after long hours of sleep.

The amount of sleep varies with individual's age, type of work, amount and kind of exercise, etc. An average healthy adult needs 8 hours of sleep to overcome fatigue.

Life stage	Daily sleep needs
• Newborns (0–3 months)	14–17 hours
• Infants (4–11 months)	12–15 hours
• Toddlers (1–2 years)	11–14 hours
• Preschoolers (3–5 years)	10–13 hours
• School age (6–13 years)	9–11 hours
• Teenagers (14–17 years)	8–10 hours
• Younger adults (18–25)	7–9 hours
• Adults (26–64)	7–9 hours
• Older adults (65+)	7–8 hours

Nursing Measures to Induce Sleep

The state of relaxation parallels the soundness of sleep. So sleep is promoted for relaxation.
- The patient should be prepared for sleep at a regular hour whenever possible. Habit formation plays an important part in inducing sleep. Nurses should explain the importance of sleep and encourage better practices.
- Prepare a conducive atmosphere for sleep. Avoid distractions caused by noise, light and improper ventilation or bad odor. Room should be clean, free from dust and dirt.
- Evening care induces physical relaxation by means of warm bath. If the weather is cool, additional sheet and blankets should be given, also hot water bags to feet and abdomen is often more conducive to relaxation and sleep.
- Give small warm pre-bed time drink to prevent hunger contractions of empty stomach.
- Make a comfortable position to sleep. He/she can use comfort devices also.
- Patients should not be disturbed at night or forced to awake from sleep to take temperature, pulse and respiration or to give a medicine or treatments unless specially ordered by the doctor.
- Ensure mental relaxation for the patient. Never try to solve a problem in the night or when one is sleeping.
- Excellent means of inducing sleep to children is by reading from a book which they like. Gentle massage on the back, neck and legs. Drugs are given to induce sleep when other measures fail. Avoid drugs to induce sleep, as it may become a habit. Serve a light meal in the evening. Bedpan and urinal should be supplied, if needed. Avoid insects, sounds, etc.

Unit IV ❖ Basic Needs of the Patient

POSITIONING

Putting a patient in proper body alignment to expose the operative site or area is known as positioning. Positioning is also defined as placing the person in a proper body alignment as needed therapeutically for the purpose of preventive, promotive, curative and rehabilitative aspects of health.

Purposes

- To promote comfort to the patient
- To relieve pressure on various parts
- To stimulate circulation
- To provide proper body alignment
- To promote normal physiological functions
- To prevent complications caused by immobility
- To perform surgical and medical interventions
- To carry out nursing intervention

Steps

Safe patient positioning involves several steps:

1. Assessing the patient's needs
2. Developing a plan of care
3. Assembling the necessary positioning devices
4. The actual positioning of the patient
5. Reevaluating body alignment and tissue integrity intermittently
6. Evaluating patient outcomes with respect to positioning-related complications

Positions

Gentle and skillful handling of the patient or the mattress and pillows as well as bed linen would prevent jerking and could reduce the pain to a minimum.

Supine Position

The patient lies on his/her back with one pillow under the head. Additional supportive devices may be added for comfort (Fig. 4).

Indications

- Post procedures to maintain hemostasis at insertion site
- Position for many surgeries
- Examination of the chest and abdomen

Procedure

1. Place the patient on back with one pillow under the head, arms and hands at the sides, knees flexed and separated.
2. Place the air ring under the hips and cotton or foam pads under the heels to reduce the pressure.
3. Place foot board under bottom of feet.
4. If the patient is paralyzed, place hand role in hand.
5. Align the patient's body in good position.

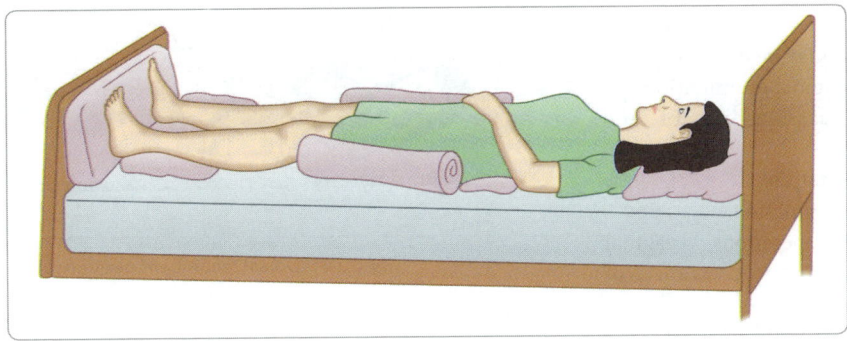

Figure 4: Supine position

Lateral Position

The client lies on the side with weight on hip and shoulder or the patient lies on his side with both arms forward and his knees and hips flexed. The upper leg is flexed more than the lower leg. The upper knee and hip should be at the same level. A pillow is given under the head, back and front to support the arms and abdomen. A small pillow is given in between the knees (Fig. 5).

Indications

- Patients who require periodic position changes
- In immediate postoperative patients
- Used for examination of perineum
- Inserting suppositories
- For taking rectal temperature
- For giving enema and colonic irrigation
- For giving back care

Procedure

1. Explain the procedure
2. Provide privacy
3. Lower the head of bed as low as patient can tolerate
4. Position the patient to side of bed
5. Turn the patient to one side
6. Place the air ring under the hips to reduce pressure in trochanters and at the hip joints
7. Position both arms in flexed position. Upper most arms are supported by pillow on level with shoulder.
8. Place pillow under back
9. Place pillow under semi-flexed upper leg at hip, from groin to foot
10. Place sand bag parallel to plantar surface of dependent foot

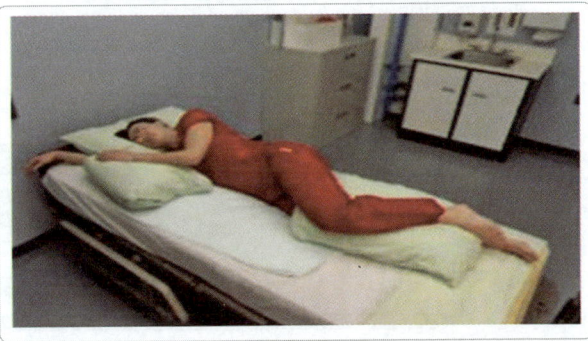

Figure 5: Lateral position

Dorsal Recumbent Position

Patient lies flat on back, knees bent, rotated outwards, feet flat on the bed (head/shoulders typically on a pillow). The legs are slightly separated and flexed so that the soles of the feet rest on the bed. In this position clients with painful disorders are more comfortable with knees flexed (Fig. 6).

Unit IV ❖ Basic Needs of the Patient

Indications

This position may be used for:

- Vulval, vaginal examination
- Digital examination of the rectum
- Catheterization
- Pelvic examination
- Vaginal operations, vaginal douche and insertion of tampons

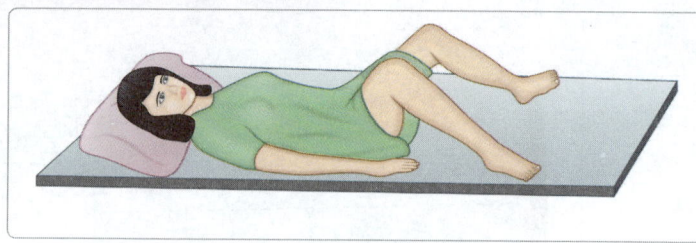

Figure 6: Dorsal recumbent position

Procedure

1. Place the patient on back in bed with two or more pillows under the head for patient's comfort.
2. Place the air ring under the hips and cotton rings or foam pads under the heels to reduce pressure.

Head-elevated Position

In a head-elevated position, the patient's head is elevated above the level of the heart to improve drainage of blood and cerebrospinal fluid away from the surgical site. Variations of the head-elevated position include the sitting position, the low sitting position and its variant, the reclining shoulder position, the head-elevated prone position and the head-elevated supine position (Fig. 7).

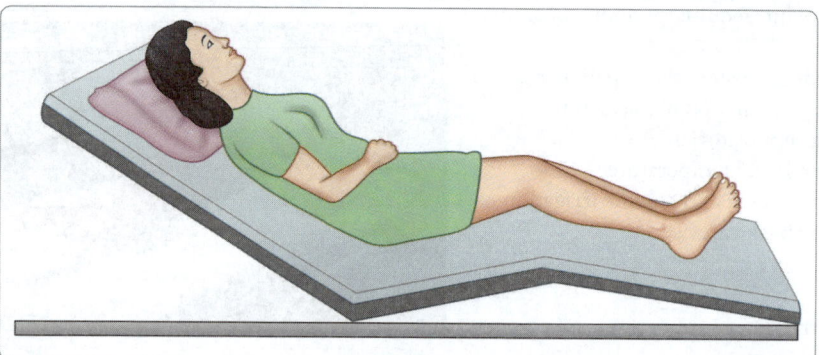

Figure 7: Head-elevated position

Sitting Position

Sitting in bed is sometimes referred to as orthopneic position. In this, the patient is made to sit at the side of the bed, leaning over a table. This position facilitates respiratory expansion, makes it easier to breathe in the patients with respiratory difficulty, and is used during thoracentesis (Fig. 8).

Indications

- Patients with severe dyspnea
- Patient with chest drainage tubes
- Cardiac patients
- Position for thoracentesis

Procedure

1. Explain the procedure
2. Provide privacy
3. Lower bed and ensure brakes are applied.
4. Have patient turn onto side, facing toward the caregiver. Assist patient to move close to the edge of the bed if the patient sits with dangling the legs. Or place the patient in High Fowler's position with over bed table to be placed across the front of the patient.
5. Assist the patient to sit.
6. Ask the patient to rest both hands on over bed table/on pillow placed in it and leans forward.

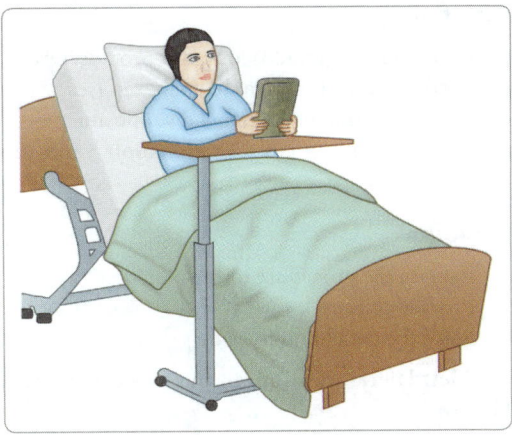

Figure 8: Sitting position

Lithotomy Position

The patient lies on his/her back with one pillow under the head. The legs are well separated and thighs are flexed on the abdomen and the legs on the thighs. Upright rod with stirrups attached are fastened on the sides of the table. The patient's buttocks are brought to the extreme edge of the table and the legs supported on the stirrups (Fig. 9).

Indications

This position is used for:

- Cystoscopic examination
- For rectal examination and surgeries
- For delivery of baby
- Operations on the perineum, vagina, cervix, bladder and rectum
- For vaginal examination and hysterectomy

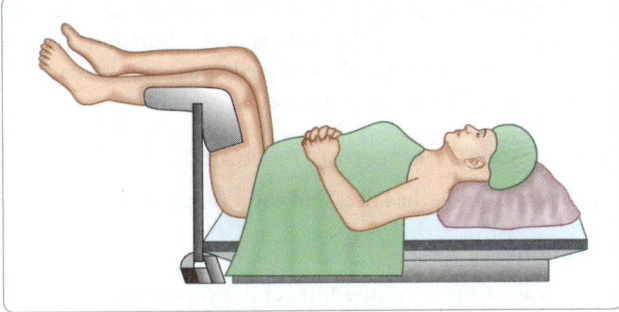

Figure 9: Lithotomy or dorsal sacral position

Procedure

1. Explain the procedure to the patient
2. Provide privacy
3. Position the patient to lie on his back with one pillow under the head
4. Keep the legs well separated from the midline into 30°–45° or unforced abduction and elevated in leg holders.
5. The hips are flexed until the thighs are angled between 80° and 100° on the trunk, with the knees being bent until the lower legs are roughly parallel to the frontal plane of the torso.
6. Buttocks are kept on the edge of the table and the legs are supported on stirrups
7. The draping is done by means of leggings, towel or sheets or by one fenestrated towel.

Sims' Lateral Position

In this position the client lies on either the right or left side. The lower arm behind the body and upper arm is bent at the shoulder and elbow. The knees are both bent, with the upper most leg more acutely bent. This position is similar to the lateral position except that the patient's weight is on the anterior aspect of the patient's shoulder girdle and hip.

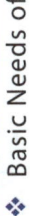

Unit IV ❖ Basic Needs of the Patient

Indications

- Position for sigmoidoscopy and proctoscopy
- Used for relaxation in antenatal exercises
- Administration of enema and suppository
- Vaginal and rectal examination and its treatments.

Procedure

1. Explain the procedure to the patient
2. Provide privacy
3. Place the patient on the side

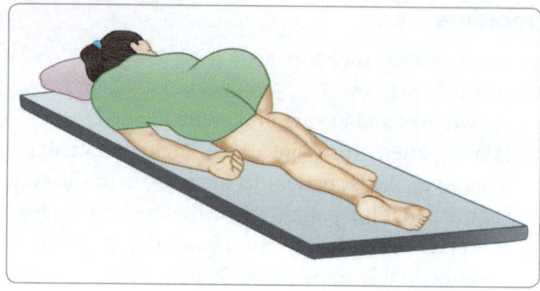

Figure 10: Sims' left lateral position

Sims' left lateral position: In this position a patient lies on the left side obliquely across the bed or table (Fig. 10).

4. Place small pillow under head and neck. One pillow is placed under the head with the left cheek resting on it.
5. Place pillow under flexed upper arm, supporting arm level with shoulder. The left arm is drawn behind the body and the right arm may be in any position comfortable for the patient.
6. Place pillow under flexed upper leg, supporting leg level with hip. The right thigh is flexed against the abdomen. Left thigh is extended well.
7. Place sand bags parallel to plantar surface of dependent foot.
8. Draping is practically the same as for the horizontal recumbent but exposing the area required.
9. This position without pillow is used for giving evacuant enema because the rectum and sigmoid colon are situated in the left side of the body.

Knee Chest or Genupectoral Position

The patient rests on the knees and chest (Fig. 11).

Indications

- As exercise for postpartum and gynecology patients.
- Used in first aid treatment in cord prolapse or retroverted uterus
- Used for vaginal and rectal examination
- This position is used for examinations of the rectum and vagina.

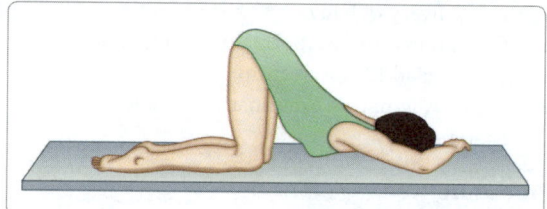

Figure 11: Knee chest or genupectoral position

Procedure

1. Explain the procedure to the patient.
2. Make the patient rest on the knees and chest.
3. The head is turned to one side with the cheek on a pillow.
4. The arm should be extended on the bed and flexed at the elbows to support the patient partially.
5. The body is at 90° to the hips with back straight, the arm above the head, and the head turned to one side.
6. The weight should rest on the chest and knees, which are flexed so that the thighs are at right angles to the legs.
7. A small pillow may be placed under the chest but the abdomen remains unsupported.
8. Draping may be done with two sheets one for the upper and one for the lower part of the body, or with a large sheet having an opening in the center (fenestrated towel).

Trendelenburg Position

Used during operations on the pelvic organs in order to displace the intestines from the pelvic cavity into the upper abdomen. In this the patient lies on the back with the head low. The foot of the bed is elevated at 45°. Entire frame of bed is tilted with head of bed down. A special table is required, one that can be adjusted so that the patient's head is low, the body is on inclined plane and the knees flexed over the adjustable lower section of the table which is lowered (Fig. 12).

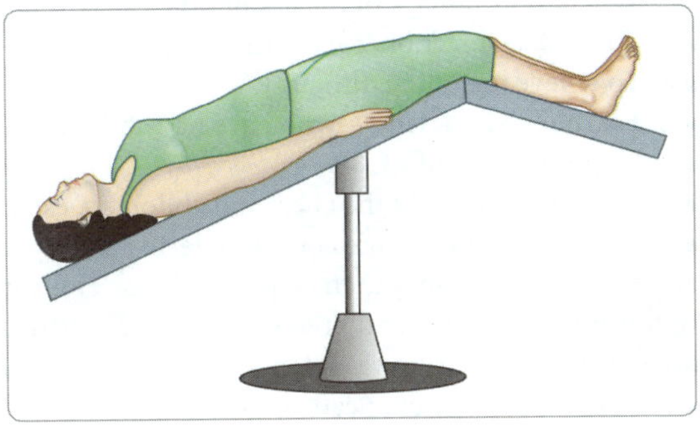

Indication

This position is used in:

- Emergency situations like shock, hemorrhage and hypotension
- Postural drainage
- Patients with deep vein thrombosis

Procedure

1. Explain the procedure to patient.
2. Place the patient in supine position.
3. Lower the head end of the bed.
4. If it is not adjustable type, use bed block at foot end and tilt entire frame of bed down. OR elevate the foot end at 45°.
5. The patient is carefully supported to prevent from slipping.
6. Draping depends upon the kind of operation to be performed.

Figure 12: Trendelenburg position

Fowler's Position

It is a sitting position in which the head is elevated at 45° to 60°, and the client's knees are slightly elevated, avoiding pressure on the popliteal vessels. Backrest and two pillows are used for the back and head. Pillows can be used to maintain natural alignment of the hands wrist and forearms. This is a more erect position in which an effort is made to maintain the patient in a sitting posture as nearly upright as possible. This position may be maintained by means of the watch frame attached to bed or by propping up the patient by means of backrest and pillows or by using only pillows. The arms should be supported on pillows so that the patient sits with his forearms supported as in an arm chair. An air cushion is frequently used to prevent pressure over the sacrum (Fig. 13).

Indications

- To relieve dyspnea
- To improve circulation
- To relax the muscles of the abdomen, back and thighs
- To relieve tension on abdominal stature

Procedure

1. Explain the procedure
2. Elevate the head of the bed
3. Rest the head against mattress or small pillow.
4. Use pillow to support arm
5. Place a small pillow at lower back

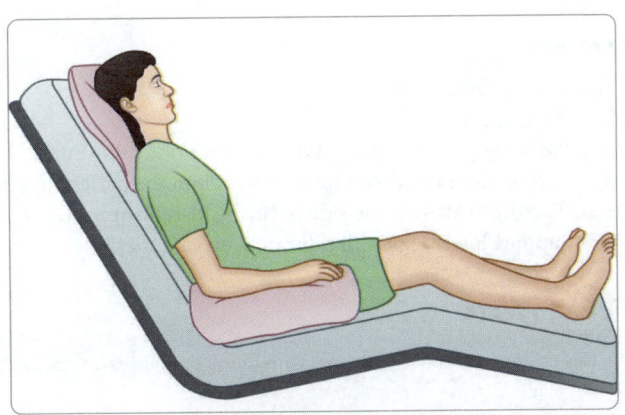

Figure 13: Fowler's position

Unit IV ❖ Basic Needs of the Patient

6. Place foot board at bottom of patient's feet
7. Place the patient in sitting position with arms at sides and knees raised with pillow

The knees may be raised over a knee pillow or a bolster to prevent the patient from slipping. But thrombophlebitis in leg should be prevented by frequent change of position of the knees and legs.

This position is used:

- Whenever drainage of the abdominal cavity is desired.
- To localize infection, e.g., peritonitis.
- To relieve breathing difficulty.
- For nursing patients—who have had abdominal operation, to relieve tension on sutures.
- To promote comfort.
- To relieve edema of the chest and abdomen, especially in cardiac diseases.
- To make a patient more comfortable, in an upright position, place one or two pillows on an over bed table. Several pillows may then be put at his back for support. He may lean forward to rest on the padded table.

In this position there is no pressure from the mattress against the back and the patient can breathe with less discomfort. This position is often used for cardiac patients with breathing difficulty.

- In Fowler's position, head and trunk are raised 40–90°.
- In low Fowler's position, head and trunk are raised to 15–45°.
- In high Fowler's position, again head and trunk are raised to 90°.

Prone Position

Patient lies on the abdomen with head turned to one side and the arms rest in a comfortable way with one pillow under the head and one under the ankles to support the feet (Fig. 14).

Indications

- Postoperatively
- To relieve abdomen distension
- Patient with pressure sores, burns, injuries and operations on the back
- For patients after 24 hours of amputation of lower limbs
- Examine the back
- Renal biopsy

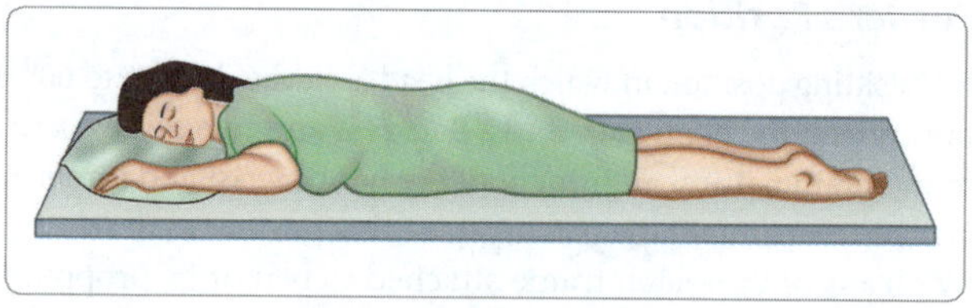

Figure 14: Prone position

Procedure

1. Explain the procedure
2. Provide privacy
3. Place the patient flat on abdomen with one pillow under the head
4. Turn patient's head to one side and align the patient in good position
5. Place both arms at the side of the head and support arm in flexed position at the level of shoulder
6. Support lower legs with pillows to elevate toes

 *Note*

This position is used for patients with burns or injuries on the back or tired back muscles.

Unit IV ❖ Basic Needs of the Patient

Horizontal Recumbent Position

The patient lies on his back with legs extended. One pillow is placed under the head (Fig. 15).

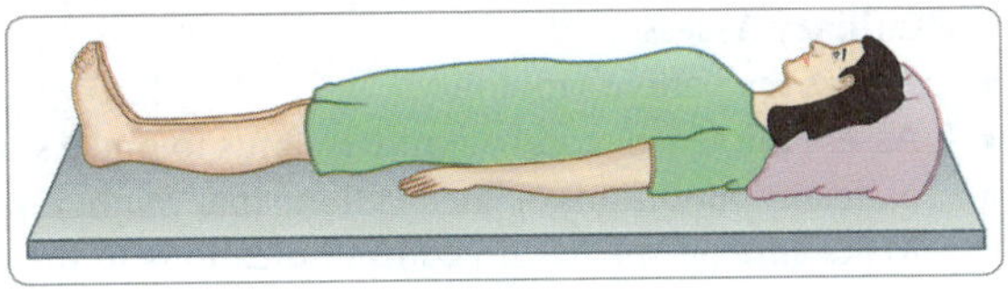

Standing or Erect Position

It the standing position, that is standing with both feet on the floor, the patient is examined for orthopedic and neurological conditions (Fig. 16).

Figure 15: Horizontal recumbent Position

Patient Position

- Patient stands with the back against the vertical Bucky.
- Patient's legs separated well apart to maintain a comfortable position.
- The median sagittal plane is adjusted at right angles and coincident with the midline of the table.
- The pelvis is adjusted so that the anterior superior iliac spines are equidistant.

MOVING, TURNING AND TRANSFERRING THE PATIENTS

Transferring refers to moving a patient from bed to a chair or to a stretcher, or to a wheelchair with maximum comfort and safety for patient and nurse.

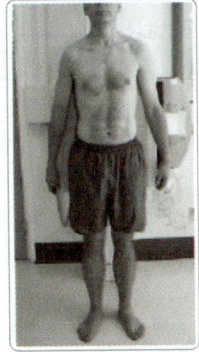

Figure 16: Standing erect position

Reasons for Moving

- Change position
- Repositioning the client
- Client's slid down in bed from Fowler's position
- Changing the bed linen

Reasons for Transferring

- Improvement of the patient's condition (from ICU to medicine unit)
- Worsens of patient's condition (to ICU)
- The need for surgery or X-ray
- Transfers at the patient's request
- For any other diagnostic tests.

Methods of Transferring

- By wheel chair
- By stretcher
- By a movable bed

Transferring the Patient from Bed to Chair

Transferring an individual from a bed to a chair needs skill. Being transferred on a chair enables the patient to execute some slight movements that is beneficial in improving circulation.

Purposes
- To strengthen the patient gradually
- To provide a change in position

Unit IV ❖ Basic Needs of the Patient

Preliminary Assessment

- Assess the patient's mobility.
- Assess the sensory and cognitive status to make sure he/she can assist with the transfer.
- Note any conditions or medications that might affect his/her alertness or balance.
- Make sure he/she has no contraindications to the use of a transfer belt, such as a spinal injury or recent abdominal surgery.
- Reduce the patient's anxiety by announcing each step of the transfer before it begins.

Articles Required

Articles	Purpose
• Chair	• For transferring the patient
• Patient's robe and slippers	• For covering the patient and prevent soiling of feet
• Pillows	• For supporting the back
• Blanket, sheet or draw sheet	• For draping the patient
• Safety belt	• For lifting the patient while transferring

Procedure

Steps	Procedure	Rationale
1.	**Bed to chair** Explain the procedure to the patient, how the maneuver will be done	Providing information fosters cooperation and wins confidence
2.	Close the door or draw the curtain for privacy	Maintains clients self-esteem
3.	Perform hand hygiene and maintain standard precautions	Prevents transfer of microorganisms
4.	See that the chair is in good condition. Bring the chair as close as possible to patient's bed	Prevents patients fall. This reduces the distance of the transfer
5.	Slide the patient's buttocks close to the edge of the bed by shifting his weight alternatively from right to left buttock till his/her feet are placed on the floor. Assist the patient to a sitting position on bed, i.e., put one arm under the head and shoulders and the other arm under his/her knees and pivot to a sitting position with the legs hanging over the side of the bed 	Rocking motion lifts weight on alternate buttocks and enhances forward movement

Contd...

Steps	Procedure		Rationale
6.	Lower the bed and ensure that brakes are applied Place the chair preferably at the right side of the bed conveniently at right angles to the bed. Place the chair against the wall or another person. Help the patient to sit on right side of the bed. 		Minimizes transfer distance and Helps to reduce energy expenditure by the patient Prevents falling of chair during transfer of the patient
7.	Place pillow on the seat of the chair. Stand in front of the patient, facing him/her.		To extend help to the patient, when needed.
8.	Apply proper robe and footwear prior to ambulation. Place the foot stool under the patient's feet.		Ensures patient dignity and prevents patients fall.
9.	Instruct the patient to stand on command by simultaneously leaning forward, pushing with the foot placed at the back as he straightens his legs. Balance the patient on the armchair/side rail or mattress.		Do not risk the danger of the patient falling to the floor. Observe for symptoms of orthostatic hypotension.
10.	Stand directly in front of the patient and with a hand under each axilla, assist the patient to stand, step down and turn around, with his/her back to the chair. Let patient flex his/her knees and lower body to seat him/her to the chair. Anchor chair with foot or have someone hold it on. (Or let patient place his/her arm over your shoulders while you put your arm around his/her waist. Turn patient around with his/her back to the chair and seat him/her gently). Help the patient to get comfortable in the chair. 		Provides stability by preventing slipping of the patients' foot.

Contd...

Steps	Procedure	Rationale
11.	Instruct the patient to step back to the chair/wheel chair until he/she touches the seat and grasps the other arm of the chair with his/her right hand. Instruct the patient to lean forward and lower his/her buttocks slowly to the seat by bending knees and elbows.	Facilitates sitting in the chair with ease.
12.	Help the patient in positioning him/herself properly when seated. Make sure that his/her buttocks are entirely rested on the seat and his/her back is firmly resting on the back support. Check for any discomfort. Adjust the pillows and wrap blanket over patient's lap.	Helps to check for orthostatic hypotension.
13.	**Back to bed** To put him/her back to bed, assist to stand, help to turn and stand on stool and back to bed. Support patient while he/she sits on the side of bed. Remove robe and slippers. Pivot to a sitting position in bed, supporting his/her head and shoulders with one arm and her knees with the other arm, and lower slowly to bed in lying position. Draw up bedding.	Ensures patient stability and prevents the risk of falling.

Contd...

Steps	Procedure	Rationale
	Help the patient into a comfortable position in bed.	Promotes comfort and well-being.
14.	Remove gloves and perform hand hygiene.	Prevents transfer of microorganisms.
15.	Document the transfer, including the patient's ability to bear weight and pivot, number of staff needed for transfer, and the patient's response to transfer and to being in a chair along with date, time and signature of the nurse.	Documentation fosters quality care.

Special Considerations

- Avoid lifting patients. Let them stand using their own strength.
- Stay close to your patient during the transfer to keep the patient's weight close to your centre of gravity
- If the patient has hemiplegia due to a **CVA**, place the chair on the strong side.
- Assess the patient for hypotension and fall risk before attempting a transfer.
- Don't let the patient put her **arms around** your neck or shoulders during the transfer; this could cause neck or back injuries.
- For maximum stability, keep the patient close to you during the transfer.
- Make sure the patient understands what's going to happen and when. Count "1, 2, 3" out loud and move on the count of 3.

Transferring Patient from Bed to Wheelchair

A wheelchair is a chair with wheels, used when walking is difficult or impossible due to illness, injury, or disability.

Transferring an individual from a bed to a wheelchair needs skill. Patients who are debilitated or overweight require more than minimal assistance to transfer between a bed and wheelchair.

Purposes

- To strengthen the patient gradually
- To provide a change in position

Preliminary Assessment

- Assess the patient's mobility.
- Assess the sensory and cognitive status to make sure he can assist with the transfer.
- Note any conditions or medications that might affect his alertness or balance.
- Make sure he has no contraindications to the use of a transfer belt, such as a spinal injury or recent abdominal surgery.

Unit IV ❖ Basic Needs of the Patient

- Know and follow the Institution's lifting policy, including how much weight an individual can lift.
- Call for assistance if indicated; use a hydraulic lifter to transfer a very heavy or weak patient.
- Reduce the patient's anxiety by announcing each step of the transfer before it begins.

Articles Required

Articles	Purpose
• Wheelchair	• For transferring the patient
• Patient's robe and slippers	• For covering the patient and preventing soiling of feet.
• Pillows	• For supporting the back
• Blanket, sheet or draw sheet	• For draping the patient
• Safety belt	• For lifting the patient while transferring

Procedure

Steps	Procedure	Rationale
1.	Explain the procedure to the patient.	Providing information fosters cooperation and wins confidence.
2.	Close the door or draw the curtain for privacy.	Maintains clients self-esteem
3.	Perform hand hygiene and maintain standard precautions.	Prevents transfer of micro organisms.
4.	Apply proper robe and footwear prior to ambulation.	Ensures patient dignity and prevents patients fall.
5.	Lower the bed and ensure that brakes are applied. Place the wheelchair next to the bed at a 45° and apply brakes. If a patient has weakness on one side, place the wheelchair on the strong side. Elevate the foot pedals. Line it with a blanket or sheet and arrange pillows on the seat and against the back.	Minimizes transfer distance. Ensure brakes are applied on the wheelchair.
6.	Make the patient sit on the side of the bed with his or her feet on the floor. Assess client for dizziness. Remain in front of the client until the client is stable.	Reduces possibility of orthostatic hypotension

Contd...

Steps	Procedure	Rationale
7.	• Apply the gait belt snugly around the waist (if required). • **Place the transfer belt around** the patient's waist over her clothing. (Never apply it on bare skin or over a woman's breasts.) • To apply the transfer belt, lift the buckle and feed the belt through the slot. • Tighten the belt and close the buckle to secure the belt. • It should fit snugly, but with enough slack for you to fit both hands underneath comfortably. 	Reduces risk of falling by maintaining stability during transfer.
8.	**Position yourself directly in front** of the patient, assuming a broad-based stance with your feet outside of her feet. • Flex your knees and hips but keep your back straight. • Grip the belt by sliding your hands upward under it, with your palms away from the patient. • Instruct the patient to put her arm on your shoulder, but never around your neck or shoulder. 	Maintains client stability
9.	As the patient leans forward, grasp the gait belt (if required) on the side of the patient, with your arms outside the patient's arms. Position your legs on the outside of the patient's legs. The patient's feet should be flat on the floor. 	Maintains client stability

Contd...

Unit IV ❖ Basic Needs of the Patient

Steps	Procedure	Rationale
10.	Place hands on waist to assist into a standing position. Count to three and, using a rocking motion, help the patient stand by shifting weight from the front foot to the back foot, keeping elbows in and back straight.	Shifting weight to back leg helps client to stand safely.
11.	Once standing, let the patient take a few steps back until they can feel the wheelchair on the back of their legs. Have patient grasp the arm of the wheelchair and lean forward slightly. **Instruct him/her to reach over** the wheelchair and grasp the handrail as you help him/her to pivot toward the seat.	Ensure the patient can feel the wheelchair on the back of the legs prior to sitting down. Allows client to judge distance to seat.
12.	• As the patient sits down, shift your weight from back to front with bent knees, with trunk straight and elbows slightly bent.	This allows the patient to be properly positioned in the chair and prevents back injury.

Keep your knees bent

Contd...

Steps	Procedure	Rationale
	• Allow patient to sit in wheelchair slowly, using armrests for support. • Make sure that patient is properly aligned and comfortable. • You can leave the transfer belt in place for the transfer of patient back to bed, later. Secure the safety belt on the wheel chair, place clients, feet on foot pedals and release brakes. 	Ensures client safety and prepares the client for movement.
13.	Shift the patient to the desired area for completing the appropriate tasks may be a diagnostic procedure.	Ensures safe transfer.
14.	**To transfer the patient back to bed**, make sure that the wheels on bed and wheelchair are locked and that the transfer belt is securely fastened as described previously. Assume a broad base of support. Instruct him/her to grasp the wheelchair's arms for leverage. 	Ensures safety of the client.

Contd...

Steps	Procedure	Rationale
15.	**Grasp the belt with both hands**, palms facing you. On the count of 3, flex your hips and knees and help the patient stand.	Ensures patient stability
16.	**Have the patient rest his/her hands** on your shoulders for balance.	Ensures patient stability
	Pivot with him/her toward the bed, shifting your weight to your back leg and keeping your knees flexed. Bed height set at lowest setting Patient's knee should be between your legs	

Contd...

Steps	Procedure	Rationale
17.	**Flexing your knees and shifting** your weight toward the leg nearer the bed, guide her to a sitting position on the side of the bed. Remove the belt and help her into a comfortable position in bed. 	Ensures patient stability and prevents the risk of falling.
18.	Remove gloves and perform hand hygiene.	Prevents transfer of microorganisms.
19.	Document the transfer, including the patient's ability to bear weight and pivot, number of staff needed for transfer, and the patient's response to transfer and to being in a wheelchair along with date, time and signature of the nurse.	Documentation fosters quality care.

Special Considerations

- Avoid lifting patients. Let them stand using their own strength.
- Stay close to your patient during the transfer to keep the patient's weight close to your centre of gravity.
- If the patient has hemiplegia due to a **CVA**, place the wheelchair on the strong side.
- Don't try to transfer a very heavy patient without a hydraulic lifter.
- Assess the patient for hypotension and fall risk before attempting a transfer. Make sure she can bear weight, has adequate upper body strength and coordination, and can cooperate and follow directions.
- Don't let the patient put her *arms around* your neck or shoulders during the transfer; this could cause neck or back injuries.
- For maximum stability, keep the patient close to you during the transfer.

Unit IV ❖ Basic Needs of the Patient

- Make sure the patient understands what's going to happen and when. Count "1, 2, 3" out loud and move on the count of 3.
- Don't twist at the waist at any point during the transfer. Keep your body in proper alignment with your back straight and hips and knees flexed.

LOG ROLLING

Logrolling is a technique used to turn a patient whose body must at all times be kept in a straight alignment (like a log). It is used to roll a patient onto their side without the patient helping and while keeping the patient's spine in a straight line (Fig. 17).

Definition: The log roll technique can be described as a maneuver used to roll a patient, from the supine position, onto the patient's side or completely over without flexing the spinal column.

Purpose of Logrolling

To maintain alignment of the spine while turning and moving the patient who has had spinal surgery or suspected or documented spinal injury.

Principles

The main principles underlying the log rolling procedure are the strict adherence to correct anatomical

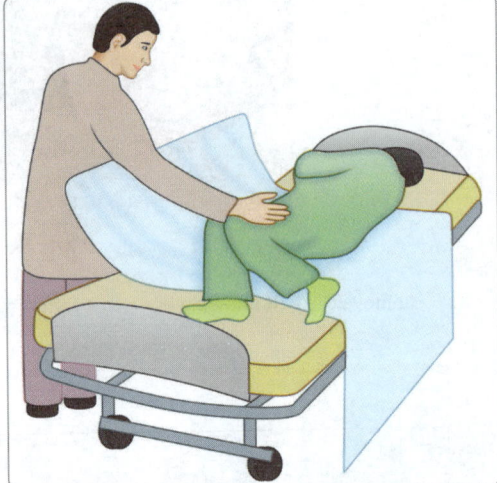

Figure 17: Log rolling

alignment in order to prevent the possibility of further, catastrophic neurologic injury, the prevention of pressure sores, and the safe performance of some medical interventions.

Indications

- For examining the patient's back.
- For providing cervical collar care
- For performing pressure care
- For facilitating chest physiotherapy

Members Required

A minimum of four to five members are required to assist in this procedure:

- 1 to hold the patient's head and direct the procedure called **the Roll Lead (RL).** The RL ensures that all of the team members are ready to turn in a coordinated manner (decide if rolling on three or after three).
- 2 or 3 to support the chest, abdomen and lower limbs.
- 1 to carry out the planned activity, i.e. pressure care, observation of back or any other interventions.

Preparation of Patient

- Explain the procedure to the patient.
- Ask the patient to lie still and to refrain from assisting.
- Ensure that the cervical collar is well fitting prior to commencement.
- Ensure that all patient assist devices such as indwelling catheters, intercostal catheters, ventilator tubing, etc. are repositioned to prevent overextension and possible dislodgement during repositioning.

Procedure

Steps	Procedure	Rationale
1.	Explain the procedure to the patient.	Allays anxiety and wins confidence and cooperation.
2.	Perform hand hygiene.	Prevents transfer of micro-organisms
3.	Provide privacy.	Reduces embarrassment
4.	• Position the bed. The bed should be in the flat position at a comfortable working height. • Lower the side rails on the side of the body at which you are working. 	Maintains body mechanics and ensures safety.
5.	Ensure that all the four members are ready. 	Ensures a coordinated effort in changing the patient's position.

	• The RL will be positioned at the head of the patient.
	  ▪ He/she is responsible for ensuring that the patient's head and neck are suitably immobilized and supported throughout the maneuver.
	
	  ▪ He/she is responsible for supporting the airway and any equipment involved in maintaining the airway and keeping the patient informed of all actions taking place.
	  ▪ The RL will ensures that the team involved in the move, fully understands their roles and asks the team to confirm this before the roll takes place.
	Assistant 1: The assistant supporting the patient's upper body, places one hand over the patient's shoulder to support the posterior chest area and the other hand around the patient's hips on the top.	

Contd...

Steps	Procedure	Rationale
	Assistant 2: The assistant supporting the patient's abdomen and lower limbs overlaps with assistant 1 to place one hand under hip level and second hand underneath furthest thigh. **Assistant 3:** Places the first hand under the knee of the furthest leg and second hand under the ankle of the same leg. 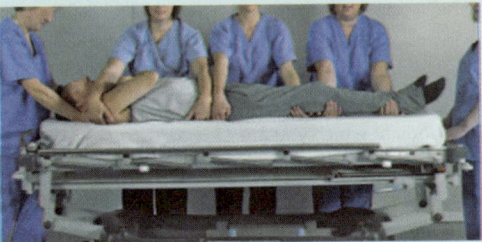 Ensure that the positioning of hands are in contact with the patient's natural skeletal landmarks. 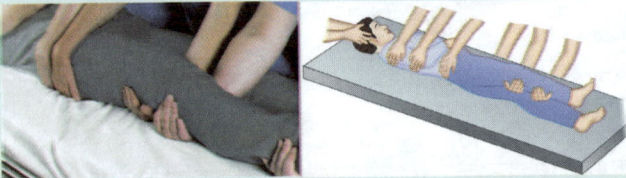 If the patient is on the floor, the following positioning is maintained. 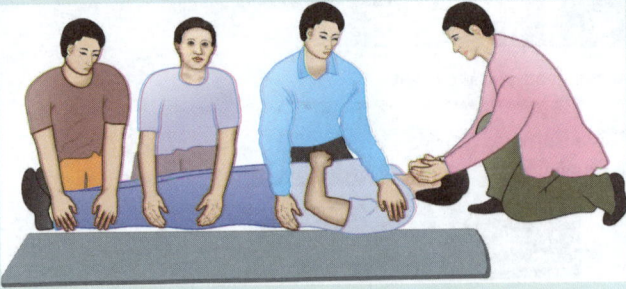	
6.	Position yourself with your feet apart and your knees flexed close to the side of the bed. 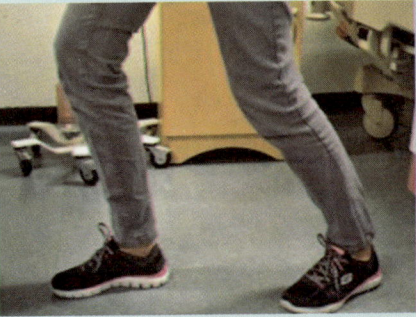	Flexing the knees ensures use of large muscle groups on the legs and lowers the centre of gravity

Contd...

Steps	Procedure	Rationale
7.	Fold the patient's arms across his chest. The patient's proximal arm must be adducted slightly to avoid rolling onto monitoring devices, e.g., arterial or peripheral intravenous lines. The patient's distal arm should be extended in alignment with the thorax and abdomen (see below), or bent over the patient's chest if appropriate, i.e. if the relevant arm is uninjured.	Protects the natural skeletal landmarks from injury.
8.	The RL will state in the following order: **1. 'READY':** This is a question. Everyone involved in the move is required to answer YES or NO. If anyone answers NO then the move is to be stopped immediately. If everyone answers YES the manoeuvre can continue to the next step. **2. 'BRACE':** The team involved in the manoeuvre PREPARES to roll the patient. All members have to ensure that they have a firm hold/ hand placement on the patient. They should also ensure that they have the correct posture, i.e. legs in correct position (lead leg slightly in front of the other) and their back straight. **3. 'ROLL':** All members have to roll the patient in one smooth controlled technique simultaneously. The persons responsible for the leg should ensure it is supported and kept straight in order to prevent any movement that could affect the spine. 4. Once the patient has been rolled onto their side the person examining the patient, who should be prepared to start as soon as the roll has been completed, can complete all relevant observations and tests. The steps of log rolling have been elaborated in Figures. 	Ensures uniform rolling of the patient and prevents back strain.

Contd...

Unit IV ❖ **Basic Needs of the Patient**

Steps	Procedure	Rationale
	5. On the count of three, move the patient to the side of the bed, rocking backward on your heels and keeping the patient's body in correct alignment. 	
9.	Place a pillow under the patient's head and another between his/her legs. Place pillows in front of and behind the patient's trunk to support his/her alignment in the lateral position. The patient must be left in correct anatomical alignment. 	Facilitates proper maintenance of body mechanics.
10.	If the patient is conscious, • Position the call bell. • Place personal items within reach. • Be sure the side rails are up and secure. • Place the side rails	Ensures patient's comfort and safety.
11.	Perform hand hygiene.	Prevents transfer of microorganisms.
12.	Document procedure including date and time, patient's response with signature.	Documentation fosters quality care.

TURNING A CLIENT TO THE LATERAL SIDE IN BED

Purpose

Movement to the lateral position may be necessary when placing a bedpan beneath the client. When changing the client's bed linen, or when repositioning the client.

Procedure

1. Pull or roll the client toward you to the lateral position.
2. Document all relevant information.
3. Wear PPE wherever required or as per the Institution's policy.

Patient Transfer

A transfer is the safe movement of a person from one surface to another.
Transfer is the activity of moving a person with limited function from one location to another.

Types of Patient Moves and Lifts

- **Lateral transfers:** Moving a patient sideways
- **Repositioning:** Moving a patient up and down or side to side in a bed or chair
- **Transfers involving sitting position:** bed to chair, bed to bed, chair to toilet, car to chair
- **Transfers involving lying down position:** Bed to stretcher
- **Floor:** Recovering a patient that has fallen on the floor

General Rules/Principles for Transferring

- Maintain a wide, stable base with your feet.
- Put the bed at the correct height (waist level when providing care; hip level when moving a patient.)
- Try to keep the work directly in front of you to avoid rotating the spine. Keep back straight.
- Keep the patient as close to your body as possible to minimize reaching.
- Proper attention to body mechanics and the relationship between center of mass and base of support allows to maintain the safest position while working with a patient.
- Position the patient close to your body to decrease stress on your back and arms.
- Ensure that stretcher and bed are locked.
- Always remember basic safe lifting techniques while performing duties.
- Get a good grip on the patient.
- Lift with legs when possible. Moving the client up in bed
- Review the medical record and nursing plan of care for conditions that may influence the patient's ability to move or to be positioned.
- Assess for tubes, IV lines, incisions, or equipment that may alter the positioning procedure. Identify any movement limitations.
- Consult patient-handling algorithm for moving the patient.
- Perform hand hygiene and put on PPE.
- Identify the patient. Explain the procedure to the patient.
- Close curtains around bed and close the door to the room, if possible.
- Adjust the head of the bed to a flat position.
- Remove all pillows from under the patient. Leave one at the head of the bed, leaning.
- Position at least one nurse on either side of the bed, and lower both side rails.
- Ask the patient (if able) to bend his/her legs and put his/her feet flat on the bed to assist with the movement.
- One nurse should be positioned on each side of the bed.
- Grasp the friction-reducing sheet securely, close to the patient's body moving the client up in bed.
- Flex your knees and hips. Tighten your abdominal and gluteal muscles and keep your back straight.
- On the count of three, move the patient up in bed.
- Assist the patient to a comfortable position and readjust the pillows and supports, as needed. Return bed surface to normal setting.

Unit IV ❖ Basic Needs of the Patient

MOVING A PATIENT FROM BED TO STRETCHER

Preliminary Assessment

- Assess the patient's mobility and sensory and cognitive status before transferring.
- Note any conditions or medications that might affect the patient's alertness or balance.
- Make sure that the patient has no contraindications to the use of a transfer belt, such as a spinal injury or recent abdominal surgery.
- Predetermine the number of staff required to safely transfer a patient horizontally.

Procedure

Steps	Procedure	Rationale
1.	Explain the procedure to the patient. Assess her level of consciousness, ability to understand and follow directions, and ability to assist with the transfer.	Allays anxiety and wins confidence and cooperation.
2.	Close the door or draw the curtain for privacy.	Helps to promote dignity.
3.	Arrange the articles at the bedside	Organization promotes skilled performance.
4.	Perform hand hygiene and wear required PPE.	Prevents the transmission of microorganisms.
5.	Ask the patient to tuck the chin in and keep his hands on chest.	This helps with the transfer.

Contd...

Steps	Procedure	Rationale
6.	Lower head of bed and side rails. Cover the patient with a sheet or blanket. Raise bed to safe working height so it's slightly higher than the stretcher. Make sure the brakes are locked on both the bed and stretcher. Position the patient closest to the side of the bed where the stretcher will be placed. 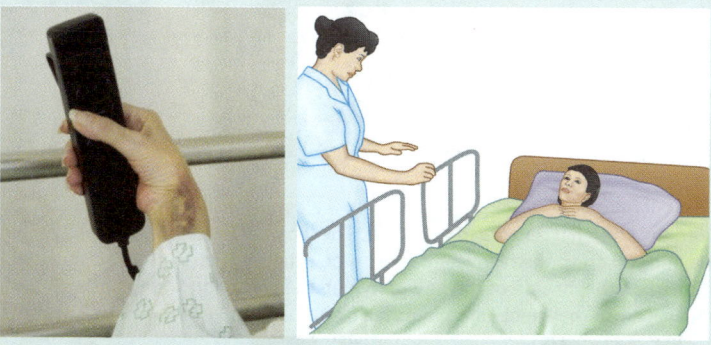	This maintains privacy and provides warmth. The patient must be positioned correctly prior to the transfer to avoid straining and reaching.
7.	Remove the pillow from the bed and place it on the stretcher. Roll patient over and place slider board halfway under the patient, over the gap between the bed and stretcher. 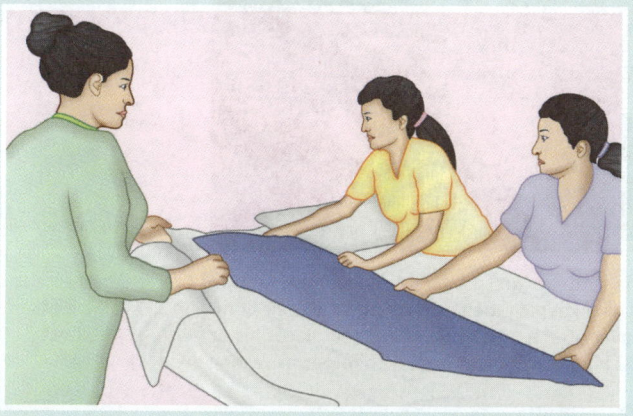	This forms a bridge between the bed and the stretcher.
8.	Place sheet on top of the slider board. 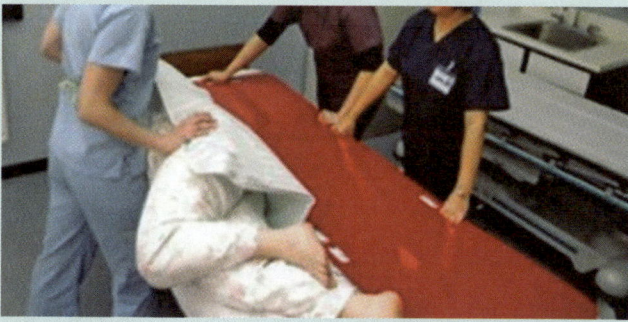	This decreases friction between patient and board.

Contd...

Steps	Procedure	Rationale
9.	Place the patient in supine position. Position stretcher beside the bed on the side closest to the patient, with stretcher slightly lower. Apply brakes. 	Positioning helps to maintain proper body mechanics
10.	Two persons climb onto the stretcher and grasp the sheet. The lead person is at the head of the bed and will grasp the pillow and sheet. The other health care provider is positioned on the far side of the bed, between the chest and hips of the patient and will grasp the sheet with palms facing up. 	This helps to maintain centre of gravity for stability.
11.	The two caregivers on the stretcher grasp the draw sheet using a palms up technique, sitting up tall, and keeping their elbows close to their body and backs straight. The caregiver on the other side of the bed places his or her hands under the patient's hip and shoulder area with forearms resting on bed. 	This helps to maintain centre of gravity for stability.

Contd...

Steps	Procedure	Rationale
12.	The designated leader will count 1, 2, 3, and start the move. The person on the far side of the bed will push patient just to arm's length using a back-to-front weight shift. 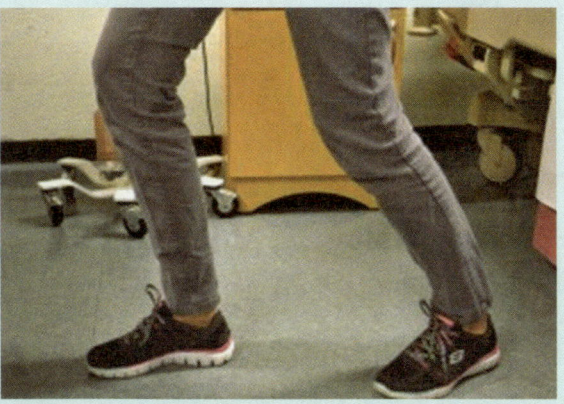 At the same time, the two caregivers on the stretcher will move from a sitting-up-tall position to sitting on their heels, shifting their weight from the front leg to the back, bringing the patient with them using the sheet and slide the patient into the middle of the bed. 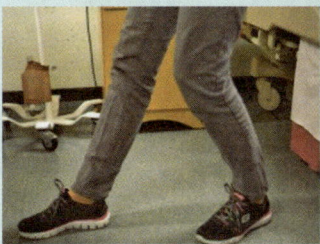 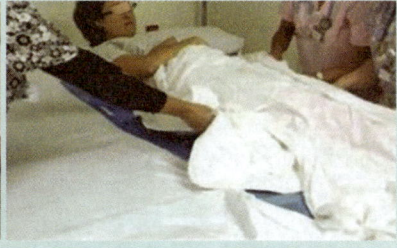	Coordinating the move between health care providers prevents injury while transferring patients. Using a weight shift from front to back uses the legs to minimize effort when moving a patient. This allows the patient to be properly positioned in the bed and prevents back injury to health care providers.
13.	At the same time, the caregiver on the other side slides the slider board out from the patient. 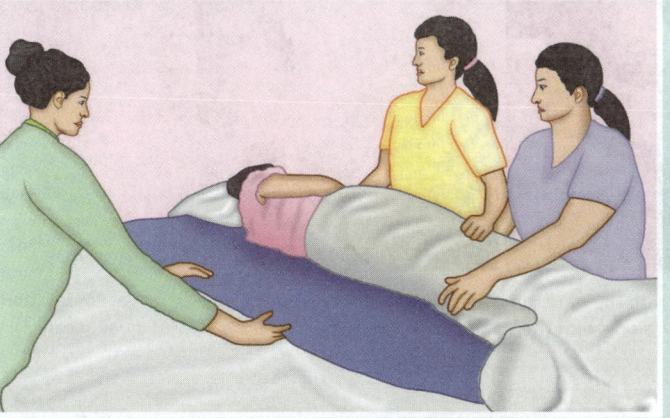	This step allows the patient to lie flat on the bed.

Contd...

Steps	Procedure	Rationale
14.	Replace pillow under head, ensure patient is comfortable and cover the patient with sheets. 	This promotes comfort and prevents harm to patient.
15.	Lower bed and lock brakes, raise side rails as required, and ensure call bell is within reach. 	Placing bed and side rails in a safe position reduces the likelihood of injury to patient. Proper placement of call bell facilitates patient's ability to ask for assistance.
16.	Remove PPE and Perform hand hygiene. 	This reduces the spread of microorganisms.
17.	Document procedure with the date, time including patient response, any untoward incidents etc along with the signature of the nurse.	Documentation fosters quality care.

TRANSFERRING THE PATIENT FROM BED TO STRETCHER AND FROM THE STRETCHER TO THE BED

It is done for patients who cannot help themselves and need help. The selection of transfer technique is individualized. The following methods can be used.

- Draw sheet method
- Patient lifted by three persons
- Mechanical devices like hydro-ureter lift

Precautions

- Lower the head of the bed until it is flat.
- Raise the bed so that it is slightly higher than the surface of the stretcher.
- Ensure that the wheels on the bed are locked.
- Pull the draw sheet out from both sides of the bed.

I. Draw Sheet Method

- **Requirements**

  Four nurses or helpers are required:
  - One stands at the opposite side of the bed.
  - Remaining three stand across the stretcher: one supporting the head and shoulders, second one supporting the hips and thighs.

  - **Procedure**
    1. Grasp the draw sheet tightly
    2. Coordinate lifting by counting the numbers of 1, 2, 3 and receive the patient in stretcher by pulling the draw sheet and the patient toward the stretcher, quickly and gently.
    3. The sheet can be removed by turning the patient from side to side.

II. Patient Lifted by Three Persons

1. Three people, all standing on the same side of the patient, slip their hands, palms facing up, beneath the patient.
2. First person holds the head, shoulder, second person holds the trunk up to thigh, and the third person holds the legs.
3. Cradle the patients in the arms so that the patient's weight rests against the nurses chests and the patient faces nurses.
4. Care must be taken so that the patient will not be dropped down suddenly.
5. The nurses should bend over and release the weight of the patient gradually and until it rests gently upon the bed or stretcher.

III. Mechanical Devices like Hydro Ureter Lift are also Used

Unit IV ❖ Basic Needs of the Patient

Hygienic Needs of the Patient

IMPORTANCE OF MAINTAINING GOOD PERSONAL HYGIENE IN HEALTH AND DISEASE

Hygiene is the science of health and its preservation; it also refers to practices that are conducive to good health. Good personal hygiene is important to a person's general health.

Good personal hygiene usually refer to those measures a person takes to keep his skin and its appendages (his hair, fingernails and toe nails) and his teeth and mouth clean and in good condition. The healthy unbroken skin is the body's first line of defense against infection and against injury to underlying tissues. The skin is also important for the regulation of body temperature. In addition, it serves as one of the means for the excretion of body wastes. Healthy teeth and gums are essential for maintaining nutritional status. Decayed teeth and poor condition of the oral cavity are potential sources of infection as well as sources of discomfort and pain for the individual.

NURSE'S ROLE IN MAINTAINING GOOD PERSONAL HYGIENE

The nurse must acquire a knowledge of health and hygiene—the science of health. She must accept responsibility for teaching good health practices to patients.

Personal hygiene for the patient is a continuous process of learning about and observing desirable health practices. Some patients come to the hospital with a good health practice already well-established and need only to continue those practices as much as is permitted by their physical conditions. Other patients will need instructions in the matters of hygiene and for them the nurse becomes a health teacher. In giving daily care to patients, nurse gets opportunity to demonstrate all the essential procedures for personal cleanliness and to set an example by observing good health practices herself.

Cleanliness of the body is essential for the comfort and welfare of the patient and is the basis for many nursing procedures performed in giving daily care. It is especially important that the patient's body be kept clean and the skin is in good condition. For a healthy person proper care of the skin is one of the major factors in maintaining good health. For a sick person skin care becomes even more important.

ORAL HYGIENE

Oral hygiene means the cleanliness of the mouth. Oral hygiene includes measures to prevent the spread of disease from the mouth and increase the comfort of the patient.

Objectives

- To keep the mouth and teeth in good condition.
- To prevent the mucous membrane from becoming dry and cracked.
- To prevent ordes which result in ulceration.
- To prevent bacteria in the mouth from causing local and general infections.

Complications Arising from a Neglected Mouth

It is divided into local complications and general complications

Local complications	General complications
Offensive breath	Loss of appetite
Parotitis	A general run down condition
Stomatitis	Joint diseases
Glossitis	Inhalation pneumonia
Pyorrhea	Rheumatism and heart disease from focus of infection of mouth and throat
Sordes and crust	Adenitis
Root abscess	Nephritis, gastritis
Tonsillitis	
Halitosis	
Otitis media	
Sinusitis	
Dental caries	
Decayed teeth	
Cracked lips	
Herpes	

Prevention of Complications

- The teeth of every patient needs thorough cleaning and brushing at least twice a day with reliable tooth paste and brush or salt, soda-bicarb or charcoal.
- Washing out the mouth before and after meals, thus eliminating the food particles immediately after the meal, keeps the mouth clean, prevents tooth decay, aids appetite and digestion.
- If the teeth or gums are in bad condition, they must be brushed and cleansed every four hours with salt, soda-bicarb or a reliable tooth paste, followed by mouth wash and gargle. When the mouth is dry, local treatments with fluorides and emollients give temporary relief.
- Patients who are very sick should have careful cleaning of mouth every four hours and before and after each meal.
- Dehydration of the tissue generally should be avoided by administration of fluids through routes prescribed by the physician.
- Patient's diet should be adequate in calories and high in vitamins, especially B and C. Citrous fruits if permitted should be given in plenty for their beneficial effects in building up resistance. Also it has an immediate effect of increasing salivary secretions in the mouth.

Essentials to Keep Good Oral Hygiene

- An optimum diet and general health are conducive to the development and maintenance of a normal condition of mouth and teeth
- It also depends upon favorable parental factors: such as the mother's diet during pregnancy and lactation. A balanced diet with enough calcium, phosphorus and vit-D are required during the antenatal period.
- By proper use of tooth brush and non-irritating dentifrice or cleansing agent.
- Periodic supervision of teeth by an expert dentist who will help for the correction of defects.

Unit IV ❖ Basic Needs of the Patient

MOUTH CARE (MOUTH CLEANING)

Objective

To keep the patient's mouth and teeth clean and healthy and thus prevent complications which may arise from a neglected mouth.

Importance of Mouth Care in Health

The mouth is one of the chief portals of entry of disease--causing bacteria and is an ideal incubator for germs. It is an entrance to both respiratory and alimentary tracts—A double gateway needing double guarding. Care of mouth and teeth helps to prevent tooth decay, gum disease, parotid gland infection and mouth sores. Mechanical cleansing and forceful rinsing is important to get rid of food particles from around teeth and gums. The remote damage from infected or diseased teeth and gums may be serious. Pus may be absorbed from such a place which forms a focus of infection, into the blood and lymph, be carried to joints, kidney and heart, causing the diseases. A clean mouth has a markedly good effect on appetite and digestion. Cleansing the mouth gives great relief from discomfort and frees the mouth from bad tastes and odours.

There is a social and psychological value in increasing one's sense of well being as well as economic value in saving his teeth.

Importance of Mouth Care during Illness

Mouth care is much more important during illness. High temperature, mouth breathing, malnutrition and other conditions accompanying illness cause drying and cracking of lips and predispose all mouth tissues to infection. The salivary secretion will be diminished during illness. The mouth and teeth may be kept clean by careful attention. The frequency of mouth care depends upon the condition of the patient.

Patients Who Need Special Care of Mouth

- Seriously ill patients
- Unconscious patients
- Patients with fever and patients breathing through the mouth
- Patients who are on liquid diet, or not taking oral feed
- Post-operative patients and paralyzed patients
- Patients on tube feeds, gastrostomy feeds, etc.
- Patients with infections and diseases of the mouth
- Dehydrated patients
- Patients with heavy sedation or under anesthesia for prolonged period

Solutions Commonly Used for Mouth Wash

- Potassium permanganate—1:5000 ($KMNO_4$) 1 crystal in a glass of water
- Sodium chloride 1 teaspoon to a pint of water (normal saline)
- Potassium chloride—4–6%
- Hydrogen peroxide (H_2O_2) 1:8 solution
  Many other commercial preparations are also available which shall be used according to the instructions of the dentists.

Dentifrices Used

- Glycerine with lime juice equal parts
- Sodium bicarbonate paste
- Reliable tooth paste or powder
- Hydrogen peroxide solution: Removes decaying food by its bubbling action and reduces bacterial activity from the cavities of the tooth.
- A homemade preparation of equal parts of sodium chloride, sodium bicarbonate with prepared charcoal seasoned with oil of peppermint is good for mouth cleaning. Charcoal powder alone is also good when one is able to do mouth cleaning by himself/herself.

Commonly Used Emollients

Cream or butter	White Vaseline	Liquid paraffin
Glycerine	Borax	Olive oil

Readymade preparation of emollients are also available.

Preliminary Assessment of the Patient and Environment

- Identify the patient and observe the general condition of the patient
- Check the condition of the mouth
- Find out the ability of the patient to cooperate for the procedure
- See the mood of the patient for acceptance
- Assess the status of health habits of the patient to give health education accordingly
- Decide the type of dentifrices and emollients to be used
- Assess the frequency of mouth care needed
- Note the precautions to be observed while moving the patient
- Make sure about any food or drink to be given after mouth care, if advisable

Requisites

A tray containing:

Articles	Purpose
Hand washing articles	For hand washing
Small mackintosh and towel	To protect the bed and dress of the patient
Small jug with warm water	For rinsing the mouth
Tooth brush/foam swabs/cotton ball/rag pieces	For cleaning the mouth
Gauze padded tongue depressor	To suppress tongue
Dentifrice to be used in a container—tooth paste or antiseptic solution	For mouth care
Gallipot—2	For preparation of oral care agents
Feeding cup	To pour water in the mouth in lying position
Two small cups—one for rag pieces or cotton, one for the paste	To clean the mouth
Artery forceps and dissecting forceps one each. Swab stick can be used if dissecting forceps is not available.	For cleansing mouth of unconscious patient

Contd...

Unit IV ❖ Basic Needs of the Patient

Articles	Purpose
Paper bag	To receive the soiled cotton balls and dirt
Kidney tray	To receive the waste water
Paper bag or any receptacle	To discard dirty swabs
Face towel	To wipe the face after mouth care
Warm water in a bowl	To wipe the face after mouth care
A bowl with gauze pieces/swab	To apply the lubricant
Lubricants—Vaseline/Glycerine/soft paraffin gel/lip cream	To apply in the lips
Disposable gloves and face mask	To prevent cross infection
Suction catheter with suction apparatus	To provide oral care in unconscious client

Procedure

Steps	Procedure	Rationale
1.	Explain the procedure to the patient including proper explanation of how and why it is done to win his confidence.	Ensures cooperation of the patient
2.	Bring the equipment to the bed side.	Proper organization facilitates skilled performance
3.	Provide privacy.	Reduces embarrassment
4.	Don disposable gloves and face mask.	Prevents transfer of microorganisms

Contd...

Steps	Procedure	Rationale
5.	Place the patient in sitting or semi-sitting position if possible; if not, the head is turned to one side with the face along the edge of the pillow at the near side of the nurse 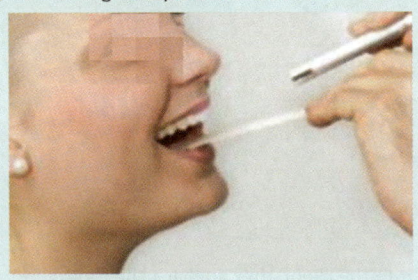	Promotes comfort and safety and effectiveness of the care including oral inspection and assessment
6.	Inspect whole of the oral cavity, such as teeth, gums, mucosa and tongue, with the aid of gauze-padded tongue depressor and torch. 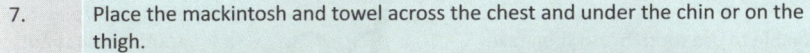	Comprehensive assessment is essential to determine individual needs
7.	Place the mackintosh and towel across the chest and under the chin or on the thigh. 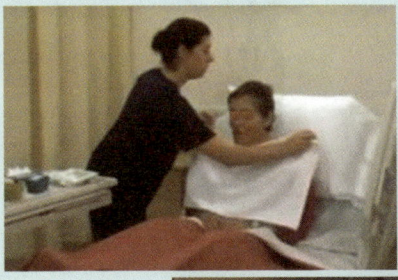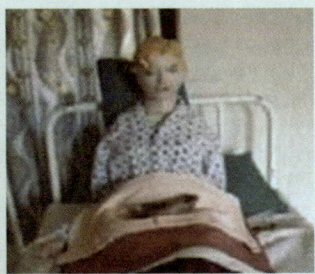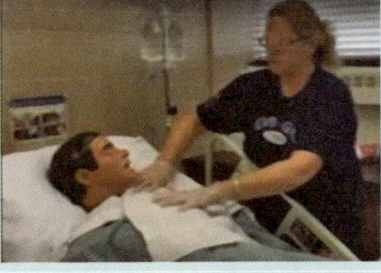	Prevents the clothing from wetting and to promote comfort.
8.	Fill the feeding cup half full of potassium permanganate solution 1:5000. Place it conveniently for use on the table.	Facilitates cleansing

Contd...

Unit IV ❖ Basic Needs of the Patient

Steps	Procedure	Rationale
9.	Make the paste with soda bicarb or salt or use the dentifrice used by the patient.	Solutions must be prepared each time before use for maximum efficiency
10.	Place the kidney tray close to the cheek with concave side towards the patient. Allow the patient to adjust the kidney tray if he is able; as it is convenient to him. Help the patient to turn his head to one side and support to rinse out his mouth, if he is able to do so. 	Proper positioning helps to receive disposal.
11.	Wash the soft tooth brush and give it to the client after applying the tooth paste on it. (Or) if the client is unable to use tooth brush then take the square gauze or rag or cotton and wrap it around the forceps covering the tips completely. Cotton when wet is slippery and does not thoroughly clean a coated tongue or teeth. Gauze or rag pieces are preferable. 	When the client is prone to bleeding and/or pain, tooth brush is not advisable
12.	Moisten the gauze or cotton after wrapping. Dip in cleansing agent, swab gently but firmly Use, up and down and circular strokes on both back and front of teeth..	Gentle and firm movement prevents injury to the oral mucosa and removes debris by friction.

Contd...

Steps	Procedure	Rationale
13 (a).	**Procedure steps for conscious patients:** • Instruct the client to brush teeth in the following manner • Place the soft toothbrush at a 45° on the teeth. • Brush under the gum line. Rotate the bristles using vibrating or jiggling motion until all outer and inner surfaces of the teeth and gums are cleaned. Brush biting surfaces of the teeth • Clean tongue from inner to outer and avoid posterior direction.	Ensures dislodging debris and dental plaque from teeth and gingival margin. Cleansing posterior direction of the tongue may cause the gag reflex

Procedure steps - for conscious

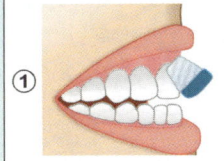 ① Place the brush at a 45° angel to the front tooth surface. Bristles must contact both lines of tooth and gum	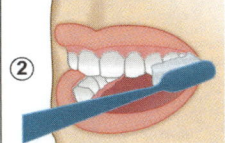 ② Move the brush in a small, jiggling, circular motion	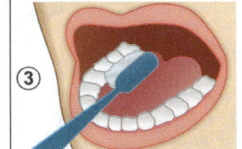 ③ Clean the inside surfaces of the back teeth by moving the brush in a small back and forth motion
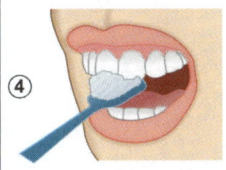 ④ Clean the inside surfaces of the front upper teeth by tilting the brush vertically using small up and down strokes	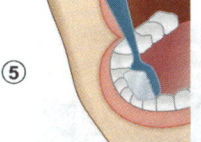 ⑤ Clean the inside surfaces of the front lower teeth by tilting the brush vertically using small up and down strokes	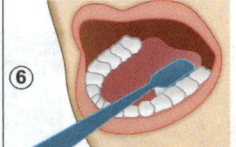 ⑥ Move the brush in a back and forth motion to clean the biting surfaces

	Mouth is cleansed in the following order: • Outer and inner surface of the upper teeth and gums-left, front and right • If brush is used, moisten the brush with solution and brush teeth thoroughly using the same movements. • Clean the client's teeth from incisors to molars using up and down movements from gums to crown. Clean oral cavity from proximal to distal, outer to inner parts, using cotton ball for each stroke.	Friction cleanses the teeth.

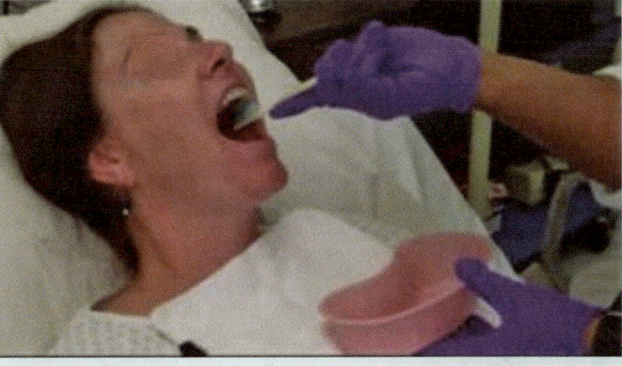

Contd...

Unit IV ❖ Basic Needs of the Patient

Steps	Procedure	Rationale
13 (b).	**Procedure steps in unconscious patient:** • Support the mouth with a gauze-padded tongue depressor in an unconscious patient. • Each part is cleansed gently and thoroughly using the forceps or swab sticks. Use fresh swab for each area and discard the used swab into the kidney tray or paper bag. 	Prevents cross contamination
	• Pour solution on brush, holding over the kidney tray when cleaning it in between brushing. A practical way to ensure an equal amount of brushing on every tooth is repeating each stroke a definite number of times, 3 or 5 preferably in each area, brushing one area at a time in proper sequences. All surfaces of the teeth and curves between the teeth and gums should receive attention. 	Repeated cleaning ensures complete removal of debris.

Contd...

Steps	Procedure	Rationale
	• Gentle brushing of gums and tongue is often desirable. • Rinse brush frequently. 	Microorganisms collect and grow on tongue surface and contribute to bad breath.
14.	Rinse the mouth with solution • Then rinse with clear water and gargle, letting the fluid run gently out through the corner of the mouth. Ask the client to rinse with fresh water and void contents into the kidney tray. Advise him/her not to swallow water. • If the client cannot gargle by himself rinse the areas using moistened cotton balls or insert the rubber tip of irrigating syringe into the client's mouth and rinse gently with a small amount of water. If needed, use suction apparatus to remove any excess. 	Ensures comfort and not to remain any fluid and debris and reduce potential for infection
15.	Ask the client to wipe mouth and around it. 	Ensures comfort and provides a sense of well-being.
16.	Wipe lips with the wet cotton. 	Ensures cleaning of lips

Contd...

Unit IV ❖ Basic Needs of the Patient

Steps	Procedure	Rationale
17.	Apply Glycerine with borax on the lips, gums and tongue with swab stick.	Moisturize lips and reduce risk for cracking
18.	Clean the eyes using separate cotton swabs for each eye with special care not to spread the discharges from the corner of the eye. Ask the patient to close the eyes when wiping corners. Inner corner of the eyes are wiped towards the nose to prevent the spreading of discharge to the total area and one swab is used only once.	Enhances comfort of the patient
19.	Wipe the face with a wet face towel.	Ensures more refreshing to a bed patient.
20.	Rinse the brush with running solution and water and dry tooth brush thoroughly. Return it to the proper place for personal belongings after drying up.	Prevents infection
21.	Make the patient comfortable and tidy up the unit.	Promotes comfort
22.	Remove the kidney tray, mackintosh and towel. Discard the waste, clean the articles used, boil the forceps and replace them in their proper place (artery forceps may be washed with plenty of water using soap and brush taking special care in its joints and teeth and boiled for 5—15 minutes before the next use)	Facilitates for next use

Contd...

Unit IV ❖ Basic Needs of the Patient

Steps	Procedure	Rationale
23.	Remove gloves and perform hand hygiene	Prevents infection transmission
24.	Record the time and nature of treatment and condition of the mouth along with the nurse's observations.	Documentation fosters quality care and ensures professional accountability
25.	Report any abnormal findings to the senior staff.	To provide continuity of care

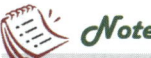 *Note*

An astringent mouth wash is used when excessive salivation is present. When mouth is dry, lubricate at night and 15 minutes before cleansing the mouth. Do not use astringent mouth wash, when the mouth is dry.

CARE OF DENTURES (ARTIFICIAL TEETH)

People having artificial teeth are sensitive about it. It is the responsibility of the nurse to guard against offending patients, by helping them to take care of their mouth. If the patient is too ill to exert himself, the nurse must clean the dentures and help the patient to rinse their mouth.

Requisites

- Mouth care tray
- A covered opaque container with cold water
- A mixture of 1 part of salt and 3 parts of washing soda in a paper
- Tissue paper
- Toothbrush or denture brush, dentifrice
- Denture container
- A basin for cleaning the dentures

Procedure

1. Explain and secure the cooperation of the patient.
2. Arrange the articles conveniently for use and screen the patient.
3. Place the tray either on the bed side table or on the over bed table as the patient prefers, If he/she can give the care himself.
4. Ask the patient to remove dentures and place them in the container, which may be a glass of water if no other container is available.
5. Help him to rinse the mouth. Give him tissues to wipe his mouth.
6. Take it to the utility room if you are giving the care.
7. Place the basin in the sink and brush the dentures over the basin under running water. In event the denture is dropped, it will be cushioned by the water in the basin.
8. Brush the denture with a mixture of dry ingredients.
9. Brush both surfaces of the denture and around the teeth.
10. Be sure that metal clasps and areas near them are cleaned, in partial dentures.
11. Rinse the denture and container under running water holding securely under moderate flow or use plenty of water and large kidney tray if washed at the bedside.

Unit IV ❖ Basic Needs of the Patient

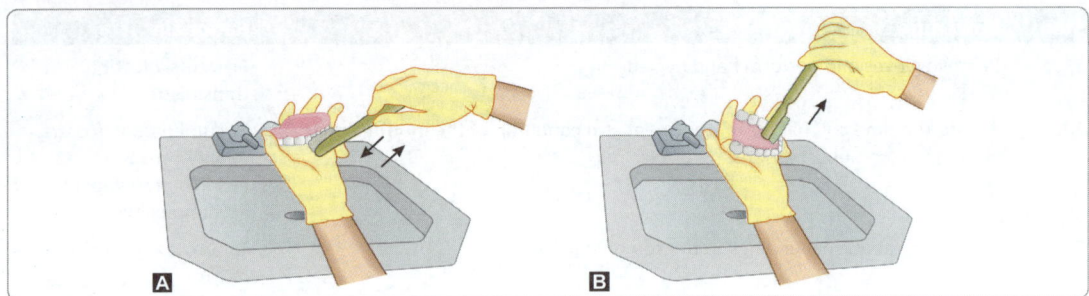

Figures 1A and B: Care of dentures

12. Have the dentures covered with cold water in the container when it is taken back to the patient.
13. Clean the mouth with solution, then with clear water, before replacing the denture. Massaging the gums stimulates circulation
14. Permit the patient who is able to replace his own denture (Figs 1A and B).
15. Keep dentures covered in cold water, in the container, if not in use, temporarily. A few drops of peppermint essence in the water give them a pleasant odor.
16. Tidy up the unit and make the patient comfortable.
17. Remove the articles to the utility room, clean them and replace them in their proper places. (Use only cold water to clean or keep the dentures).

Precautions

- In cleaning dentures, they should be held firmly as water reduces friction between the teeth and fingers. They are liable to slip and fall down.
- Dentures should be dipped in cold water to prevent friction with the mouth and make it slide easily into place.
- Hot water may destroy dentures. Dentures are expensive and not readily replaced if broken or lost.
- Privacy should be maintained.
- Dentures need to be kept moist when not being worn so they do not dry out or lose their shape. When not worn, dentures should be placed in a denture cleanser soaking solution or in water. However, if the denture has metal attachments, the attachments could tarnish if placed in a soaking solution.
- Remove and rinse dentures after eating. Run water over dentures to remove food debris and other loose particles.
- Handle dentures carefully. Be sure you don't bend or damage the plastic or the clasps when cleaning.
- Advise the patient to clean his mouth after removing the dentures. Instruct him to use a soft-bristled toothbrush on natural teeth and gauze or a soft toothbrush to clean the tongue, cheeks and roof of the mouth (palate).
- Brush the dentures once daily. Soak and brush them with a soft-bristled brush and nonabrasive denture cleanser, which helps to remove food, plaque and other deposits.
- If denture adhesive is used, it is essential to clean the grooves that fit against the gums to remove any remaining adhesive.
- Don't use denture cleansers inside the mouth.
- Soak dentures overnight.
- Most types of dentures need to stay moist to keep their shape. Place the dentures in water or a mild denture - soaking solution overnight. Follow the manufacturer's instructions on cleaning and soaking solutions that are used.

- Rinse dentures thoroughly before putting them back in mouth, especially if using a denture-soaking solution. These solutions can contain harmful chemicals that may cause vomiting, pain or burns if swallowed.
- When a denture is not in use, place it in a marked clean container filled with clean water. Patients should neither wrap a denture in tissue or other material nor store it in a pajama pocket, under the pillow, or in a drawer.

CARE OF HAIR

The care of the hair is a part of the daily hygiene. Some illness demands such complete rest that a certain amount of neglect of hair is inevitable, but in most cases it is possible to keep it in good condition. Generally, hair and scalp should receive the same treatment in sickness as in health.

Objectives

- To maintain cleanliness of the scalp and hair
- To prevent matting and tangles of hair
- To promote comfort and to stimulate circulation of the scalp
- To give an opportunity for observation of the scalp and hair
- To promote the growth of hair and prevent loss of hair
- To prevent itching and infection
- To get rid of dandruff and pediculi, which may be a factor in producing eruption of the face, neck, back and arms. Pediculi and nits lead to irritation and infection.
- To maintain a glossy and healthy appearance of hair and gives satisfaction to the patient.

General Instructions

- All the patients whether male or female should have their hair brushed or combed twice daily.
- Stiff brushes are most effective in caring for the hair.
- Teeth of the comb should be dull to prevent scratching of the scalp.
- Metal combs are injurious. Individual combs and brushes are advocated.
- If common comb is used, wash it with soap and water, disinfect it in carbolic acid 1:20 or Dettol 1:40 after every use.
- Tangles may be removed by application of oil.
- If tangles are difficult to remove, cut the tangles with the permission of the patient or his nearest relatives.
- Hair must be kept free from snarls, combed and brushed without hurting or irritating the patient and should be arranged in a comfortable manner.
- Appearance should always be considered.

Combing of Hair

Preliminary assessment of the patient and environment:

- Identify the patient and check the doctor's order for any restrictions for the movement and positioning of the patient.
- Get further instructions from the senior sister.
- See the general condition of the patient.
- Observe the condition of the hair and scalp.
- Assess the mood of the patient for acceptance, understanding and self-care.
- Check the articles available in the unit.

Unit IV ❖ Basic Needs of the Patient

- Provide privacy, light and win the confidence of the patient.
- If the client wears eyeglasses, remove them and put them in a safe place.
- Remove hairpins, combs, etc.

Preparation and Organization of Articles

A tray containing:

Articles	Purpose
Hand washing articles	For performing hand hygiene
Clean towels—2	One to place under the head to protect the bed and pillow and the other to protect the shoulders and garments.
Clean comb with coarse and fine teeth	Coarse one to remove tangles and fine one to remove nits if any, thus making the hair glossy.
Bath towel	For spreading under the shoulders
Paper bag—1	To collect the dropped hair
Carbolic: 1:20 or Dettol 1:40	To soak the used combs after use
Pair of scissors if necessary	To cut the tangles if needed
Kidney tray with lotion	To put the combs after use
A small bowl with rag pieces or cotton	To wipe the comb in between
Hair care articles like clips, rubber bands, oil	To provide hair care

Procedure

Steps	Procedure	Rationale
1.	Explain the procedure to the patient. Ask the client about personal hygiene preferences.	Proper explanation may allay patients anxiety, develops confidence and foster cooperation
2.	Assemble the equipment to the bed side. Place the kidney tray in a convenient place.	Organization facilitates accurate skill performance.
3.	Move the patient in a comfortable position close to the nurse and adjust the pillow for easy reach. Remove eye glasses if any.	Placing close to the nurse prevents back strain and helps the nurse to maintain body mechanics.
4.	Wash hands and don gloves if required.	Prevents the spread of microorganisms.
5.	Place a towel across the pillow if the client is in bed. For the sitting client, place a towel around shoulders.	Prevents soiling of linen.
6.	Inspect the hair and scalp for abrasions, lacerations, inflammation and infestations and determine whether patient needs any special treatments.	Observation facilitates planning of appropriate care.
7.	Loosen the hair and separate the hair in small strands.	Facilitates easy combing.
8.	Hold the strand above the part being combed so that pull comes on your hand, not on hair roots and comb the tangles out from the ends first and then go up gradually. Comb gently but remove all tangles. Application of oil may help to remove the tangles without injuring the patient.	Gentle stroke soothes the patient and promotes comfort and prevents pulling and further tangling.

Contd...

Steps	Procedure	Rationale
9.	If removal is very difficult, tangles may be cut off using scissors after getting due permission from the patient and the relatives.	Prevents unnecessary discomfort and pain while removing complicated tangles.
10.	Discard loose hair into the paper bag/kidney tray.	Safe disposal prevents cross contamination.
11.	After combing the hair thoroughly, braid the hair into two, one on each side of the head, so that the patient does not lie on them. Secure the ends with ribbon or tape. In braiding the hair straighted in front of the ears to make the patient more comfortable when lying on her back. Braids should not be too tight or too loose.	Promotes comfort and well-being of the client.
12.	Gather all used articles. Clean and disinfect brush and comb and return them into their proper places.	Ensures use for another patient.
13.	Replace eyeglasses if previously removed. Place the patient in comfortable position and tidy up the unit.	Ensures comfort and well-being.
14.	Perform hand hygiene.	Prevents transfer of microorganisms.
15.	Record the time and procedure into the nurse's record with signature on the chart. Report if any abnormalities were seen.	Documentation fosters quality care.

PEDICULOSIS AND ITS DANGERS

Pediculi or lice are blood suckers and parasites that live on the human body. They are found on the hair and hairy portions of the body.

Types of Pediculi

- Pediculus capitis—found in hair and scalp
- Pediculus corporis—the body louse that live on the body and clothing
- Pediculus pubis—found on the parts of the body covered with hair, especially pubic area

Pediculi are Harmful and Dangerous

- They are source of discomfort to patients, making them nervous and restless
- They cause itching and the patients scratches which may lead to infection and abscess formation
- They are blood suckers and cause anemia as well as infected glands
- They spread diseases such as typhus fever, relapsing fever and trench fever
- They spread rapidly on linen, blanket, beddings, towels, comb, brushes and other articles and may infect the whole ward in a short time if precautions are not taken.

Unit IV ❖ Basic Needs of the Patient

Treatment

Readymade parasiticide for removing pediculosis are available. It should be used according to the instructions of doctor and instructions given on the bottle.

Procedure

Steps	Procedure	Rationale
1.	Assess the scalp for nits and active lice. These are commonly found on the crown of the head, behind the ears, at the base of the neck.	Nits are small and firmly attached to the hair shaft. Shells of nits will still be present after they hatch. Adult lice may be more difficult to be seen as they are darker and move quickly.
2.	Use PPE for examining patient	As lice can be easily transmitted in clothing and on skin, use gloves to examine patient and change gloves between patients to prevent further transmission
3.	You can use Wood's lamp (black light) to see presence of lice or nits.	This method involves less chance of transmission of lice. It is done by shining the black light on the patients head. Lice and nits will glow as yellow or green dots.
4.	Apply pediculicide shampoo to patient's scalp and hair	Over the counter prescription, or strength shampoos are available. Hair should not be washed again for 1-2 days following treatment.
5.	Comb hair with nit comb	This is a long and tedious process, but it is required to remove lice and nits from the hair and prevent reinfestation. Some shampoos only kill adult lice and nymphs, so nits (eggs) must be manually removed.
6.	Administer oral medication as a last option (Ivermectin)	This medication is given orally when all other treatments have failed.
7.	Assess skin for signs of infection	Itching is the most annoying symptom, but it introduces bacteria into broken skin and can lead to skin infections.
8.	Ensure patient's nails are trimmed and clean	Scratching to relieve itching is a normal response, and is often done during sleep. Make sure nails are trimmed and clean to reduce likelihood of infection.
9.	Address patient or caregivers' emotional distress	People feel that lice is a reflection of poor hygiene therefore, reassure families that anyone can have lice and guide them on how to cope. It is only a medical condition and they avoid scolding or punishing the patient.

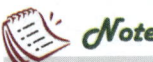 *Note*

There may be significant side effects to this medication, so monitor for signs of liver damage, joint or muscle pain, weakness, vision changes or rash.

- Provide education for patient and caregivers on ways to prevent further infestation
  - Treatment must be reapplied within 7–10 days to ensure that all newly-hatched lice and nymphs have been removed.
  - Wash all bed linens, towels and clothes belonging to the patient separately in hot water.
  - Make sure that the surrounding area of the patient is clean by vacuum cleaning the carpets, rugs, furniture and mattresses to remove lice that may be hiding there.

BED SHAMPOO (WASHING HAIR IN BED)

Special care of the hair may be required for patients who are in bed for a prolonged period of time, for those whose head is infected with lice and those who show evidence of neglect. If the patient is extremely weak or in a serious condition, he/she should avoid any form of exertion. With careful preparation, bed shampoo can be given in a very short time. Patient's hair can be thoroughly dried, combed and arranged in the usual manner.

Objectives

- To clean the hair
- To promote patient's physical and mental comfort
- To complete the treatment of pediculi

    (Preliminary assessment of patient and environment is same as that of combing of hair. In addition, get the help from assistants if needed).

Requisites

A tray consisting of:

Articles	Purpose
Articles for hand washing	For performing hand hygiene
Bath towel—2	One to cover the mackintosh One to wrap around the neck
Towels and safety pins or cloth pins or clips	To hold the towel in position
Shampoo solution or soap	For washing the hair
A small bowl containing cotton balls	To plug the ears.
Kelly pad or mackintoshes—2	One to prevent wet One to make Kelly pad
Basin and pitcher	For pouring water while giving hair wash
Buckets—2	One for collecting hair wash water One with hot water.
Jugs with hot and cold water	For hair wash
Small rubber sheet	To prevent soiling of linen
Wash cloth—1	For covering the eyes
A small tray or wooden board	For supporting the pillow
Comb and oil	For applying in hair after wash and combing
Kidney tray and paper bag	To dispose soiled waste
Newspaper	To make a trough

Procedure

Steps	Procedure	Rationale
1.	Explain the procedure to the patient including proper explanation of how and why hair shampooing is given at the bed side. Ask the client about personal hygiene preferences and ability to assist with the bath.	Proper explanation may allay patients anxiety, develops confidence and foster cooperation

Contd...

Unit IV ❖ Basic Needs of the Patient

Steps	Procedure	Rationale
2.	Assemble the articles on the bedside and arrange them conveniently for work.	Organization facilitates accurate skill performance
3.	Secure privacy by drawing curtains and by closing the doors. Close windows and doors.	Prevents embarrassment and draughts
4.	Place the bucket on the side of the bed where the nurse is to work. Remove all but one pillow unless contraindicated. Place chair or footstool at the side of the bed near the client's head and cover with a small towel. Set basin or bucket on chair.	Saves time and facilitates organized care.
5.	Perform hand hygiene. Don gloves and apron as per institution's policy.	Prevents transfer of micro-organisms.
6.	Inspect the hair and scalp for abrasions, lacerations, inflammation and infestations and determine whether patient needs any special treatments.	Helps to analyze the condition of the patient and decide care accordingly.
7.	Place the small tray or wooden board under the pillow on which head rests. Place the pillow or cushion or a rolled towel under the neck so that the head is slightly tilted back.	Prevents the head from sinking into the pillow. Putting a pillow or a cushion prevents discomfort during the procedure.
8.	Protect the bed with one mackintosh and towel or with the Kelly pad. If kelly pad is not available, roll one rubber sheet. Bend it as half circle and keep under the head a little beyond the occiput, directing the free ends towards the bucket on both sides to form a thorough flow for the water. The bucket on the floor receives the end of the second rubber sheet over the rolled one.	Prevents soiling of linen.
9.	Spread a towel over the rubber sheet or kelly pad. Place the basin on the bedside table.	Prevents soiling of linen.

Contd...

Steps	Procedure	Rationale
10.	Place the patient supine. Move the patient so that the head is as near to the edge of the bed as possible. 	Appropriate positioning helps in maintaining body mechanics.
11.	Protect the patient's shoulders with the small rubber sheet and towel and pin it in front. (If the patient is able to move, she may lie diagonally across the bed with her head hanging over the edge of the bed supported in nurse's hand. The rubber sheet is arranged in a similar fashion in the above method). 	Prevents soiling of linen.
12.	Fold and put wash cloth over the eyes for protection and put a piece of cotton on each ear.	Prevents water from entering into the ears.
13.	Loosen the hair and comb to remove all the tangles.	Facilitates easy washing without tangles.
14.	Mix hot and cold water and test the temperature of water. The water temperature should be 105°F. In addition, the room should be free of drafts, preferably 75°–80°F 	Correct temperature of water helps to prevent chills.
15.	Wet the hair with warm water. Apply shampoo solution and rub the scalp and hair with the balls of fingers.	Rubbing and massaging the scalp systematically adds to the comfort of the patient and effectiveness of the shampoo.

Contd...

Steps	Procedure	Rationale
16.	Rinse the hair well by pouring water with the pitcher protecting face, neck and ears while pouring.	Ensures thorough cleaning of hair.
17.	Repeat applying shampoo, rubbing and rinsing until the hair is thoroughly clean. Use plenty of water. Apply conditioner if requested or if the scalp appears dry. 	Increases circulation in the scalp.
18.	Squeeze off water from the hair. Remove the kelly pad or rubber sheet and towel holding the hair and head in the left hand of the nurse. Put the rubber sheet and towel into the second bucket and remove the bucket of dirty water. 	Prevents hair from wetting and soiling.
19.	Dry the hair by rubbing with the towel laid over the pillow. Drying is easy with bath towel.	Drying prevents chilling and promotes comfort.
20.	Wipe the face and neck if needed. Remove the wash cloth, cotton plugs, rubber sheet and towel from the patient's neck and place them into the bucket. 	Drying prevents chilling and promotes comfort.

Contd...

Steps	Procedure	Rationale
21.	Replace the wet towel with a fresh one and dry the hair thoroughly. Hot water bag may be used to dry the hair by placing it underneath the fresh towel and spread the hair over it. Hair dryers may be used instead, if available.	Prevents patient from becoming chilled.
22.	When dry, comb it.	Combing promotes comfort.
23.	Make the patient comfortable and tidy up the unit.	Ensures comfort and well-being.
24.	Remove all the articles. Clean and replace them in their proper places.	Prepares for the next procedure.
25.	Doff apron and gloves. Perform hand hygiene.	Prevents the spread of infection
26.	Document the condition of the scalp, hair and any abnormalities on the chart with date, time and signature. Report any abnormalities to the senior staff.	Documentation fosters quality care.

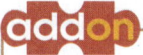

Kelly Pad

Kelly pad is a mechanical device used to protect the bed and bed linen from wetting while giving bed shampoo for a bed ridden patient.

- It is made up of water proof materials like rubber or plastic.
- It has a round double-layered head end with fittings and valve to inflate the round area with air while the article is in use like the air ring.
- The round double-layered head end is leading to a single layer of rubber sheet tapering down which leads to the bucket for the flow of water when hair wash is given.
- During bed shampoo the patient is kept diagonally on the bed and the Kelly pad is kept under the head after inflating the round head piece of it and the long tapering end leading to the bucket kept on the floor.

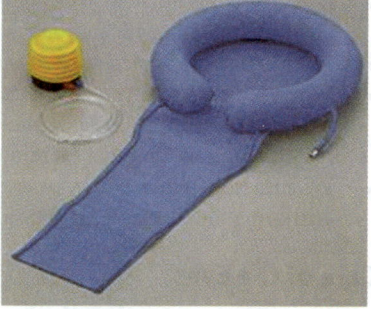

- The inflated end should be at the level of the shoulder of the patient and the head resting on the flat surface of the Kelly pad.
- A Kelly pad can be improvised by rolling one rubber sheet in the place of round inflated area and keeping another rubber sheet over the roll, leading one end to the bucket for the flow of water.
- The arrangements should be carefully made otherwise water may spread to the bed instead of flowing to the bucket.

Care of Kelly Pad after Use

Wash both sides with soap, brush and cold water after deflating the air in it. Dry by hanging. The metal piece should be dried carefully to prevent rusting. When all the parts are dry inflate air in the half circle ring to prevent sticking layers together. Put powder outside the inflated area and the flat surfaces. Roll the long tail toward the head end and keep with other rubber articles.

Unit IV ❖ Basic Needs of the Patient

CARE OF NOSE, EYES AND EARS

The eyes, ears, and nose require special attention for cleansing during the patient's bath. The nurse has the responsibility of assisting patients in the care of eyeglasses, contact lenses, or hearing aids.

When hygiene care is provided to the patient, the eyes, ears, and nose require careful attention. Assessments must be made of the patient's knowledge and methods used to care for the aids, as well as any problems he/she might be having with the aids. For example, patients with limited mobility cannot grasp small objects; patients who have reduced vision or are seriously fatigued require assistance from the specialist.

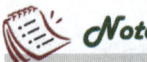 *Note*

- The eyes, ears, and nose are very sensitive areas and require extra care that should be taken to avoid injury to these sensory organs.
- Never use bobby pins, toothpicks, or cotton-tipped applicators to clean the external auditory canal. Such objects may damage the tympanic membrane (eardrum) or cause wax or cerumen to impact within the canal.

Care of the Nose

- The patient usually removes secretions from the nose by gently blowing into a soft tissue.
- If the patient is unable to remove nasal secretions, help him/her by using a wet washcloth or a cotton-tipped applicator moistened in water or saline. Never insert the applicator beyond the length of the cotton tip.
- The specialist must teach the patient that harsh blowing causes pressure that may injure the eardrum, nasal mucosa, and even sensitive eye structures.
- If the patient is not able to clean his/her nose, the specialist will assist using a saline-moistened washcloth or cotton tipped applicator. Do not insert the applicator beyond the cotton tip.
- Suctioning may be necessary if the secretions are in excess.
- When patients receive oxygen per nasal cannula, or have a nasogastric tube, nurse should cleanse the nares every 8 hours. Use a cotton-tipped applicator moistened with saline. Secretions are likely to collect and dry around the tube; therefore, it needs to be cleaned with soap and water.
- When nasogastric feeding, or endotracheal tubes are inserted through a patient's nose, change the tape anchoring the tube at least once a day.

Care of the Eyes

- Clean the sensitive sensory tissues in a way that prevents injury and discomfort to a patient, such as by taking care to not to get soap in his/her eyes.
- Cleaning the eyes involves simply washing with a clean washcloth moistened in water.
- Cleansing of the circular area around the eyes is usually performed during the bath, and involves washing with a clean washcloth moistened with clear water. Do not use soap because of the possibility of burning and irritation. The eyes are cleaned from the inner to outer canthus.
- A separate section of the washcloth is used each time. This is to prevent spread of infection. Place a damp cotton ball on lid margins to loosen secretions. Never apply direct pressure over the eyeball. Exudate from the eye should be removed carefully, and as often as necessary to keep the eyes clean.

- The eyelashes, tearing, and split-second blink reflex usually keeps the eyes well protected.
- An unconscious patient may need frequent special eye care. Secretions may collect along the margins of the lid and inner canthus when the blink reflex is absent or when the eyes do not completely close.
- The physician may order lubricating eye drops. In some cases, the eyes may be medicated and covered to prevent irritation and corneal drying.

CARE OF VISUAL AIDS

Eyeglasses

- Many patients wear eyeglasses. The specialist uses care when cleaning glasses, and protects them from breaking.
- Eyeglasses should be stored carefully. Glasses made of hardened glass or plastic can be easily scratched.
- Plastic glasses require special cleaning solutions and drying tissues. Warm water and a soft dry cloth may be used for cleansing glass lens.
- Wet lenses with warm water before wiping them with a microfiber cloth. For stubborn marks or dirt, use a cleanser available in the market for eyeglasses or a mild liquid soap.

 *Note*

- Avoid harsh products, like bleach, alcohol or ammonia as these can damage the anti-reflective coating on the eyeglasses.

Purposes

- To have a clear vision
- To prevent scratching of lens
- To prevent damage
- To facilitate proper fitting
- To prevent dryness of the lens

General Guidelines

Don'ts

- Don't clean your glasses with harsh chemicals or rough materials.
- Don't put your glasses lens-side down.
- Don't wear glasses with the wrong prescription.
- Don't wipe your glasses with your clothing.
- Don't clean your glasses with everyday cleaners.
- Don't set your frames/lenses down unprotected.
- Never use paper towels, tissue, or napkins to dry the lenses. All of these materials, regardless of how soft they are on the skin, have a textured surface and can easily scratch the lenses.
- Never leave them in places that get too hot—near a heater, fireplace, or in a hot car. Heat can warp lenses or cause them to peel.
- Avoid harsh products, such as window cleaner, bleach, alcohol, ammonia or even vinegar, which can damage the antireflective coating.

Unit IV ❖ Basic Needs of the Patient

Do's

- Eye glasses are costly. Protect them from loss or damage.
- Store glasses in a hard-shell protective case. Storing the glasses in their case will also prevent them from getting dusty or having anything spilled on them.
- Place the case in a safe place.
- Regularly clean the glasses.
- Always remove glasses from the face using two hands.
- Do use a gentle liquid soap.
- Do use lukewarm water to rinse them.
- When you want to push your glasses up on your nose, don't push on the nosepiece by one finger as well. It places pressure on the nose pads and weakens the whole frame. Use both hands again instead and move your specs back to the right position.
- Don't wear your glasses on the top of your head.
- Clean them daily and as needed.

Articles Required

Articles	Purpose
Eyeglasses in an eyeglass case	For storing the eye glasses
Cleaning solution or lukewarm water	For cleaning the glasses
Microfiber cloth or disposable lens cloth or cotton cloth	For wiping the glasses

Procedure

Steps	Procedure	Rationale
1.	Explain the procedure to the patient	Allays anxiety and fosters cooperation.
2.	Arrange the articles.	Organization facilitates accurate skill performance
3.	Wash hands.	Greasy or grimy fingers will make it harder to clean the glasses. Also, dirt on the fingers could scratch the delicate lenses.
4.	Remove the eye glasses by holding the frames in front of the ears. Lift the frames from the ears and bring the glasses down away from the face.	Prevents injury to the patient's face.

Contd...

Steps	Procedure	Rationale
5.	Inspect the glasses. Make sure that the screws are tight and the alignment is correct.	Ensures wearing appropriate glasses.
6.	Hold the frames by gripping the piece that crosses the bridge of the nose. The steps of cleaning glasses have been given in the Figures. Clean the lens with the cleaning solution or lukewarm water. Spray the lenses with an appropriate cleaner. Spray both sides of the glass lens one spray per side. Never attempt to clean the lenses dry. Rinse the glasses under a gentle stream of water. Rinse both sides of the lenses and the frame thoroughly. Clean in a circular motion. Do not use hot water Dry the lenses with the disposable lens cloth or a microfiber cotton cloth or allow the glasses to air dry. 	This will keep the frame from accidental bending while it is cleaned. Harsh cleaners on lenses can corrode the lens coating. Ensures your lenses are clean and there is no sticky residue left behind. Hot water may damage to the coatings
7.	If the patient is not going to wear the glasses: • Open the eyeglass case. • Fold the glasses and place the glasses in the case. • When you set down the glasses, make sure that you place them upside down with the bridge at the bottom. • Do not touch the lenses. 	Ensures that the eyeglasses are safe. This prevents scratching of lenses.
8.	• If the person wears the glasses: 　▪ Unfold the glasses. Hold the frames on either side and place them over the ears. 　▪ Adjust the eyeglasses so that the nosepiece rests on the nose. 　▪ Return the empty case to the top drawer of the bedside cupboard.	Ensures that the eyeglasses are safe.

Contd...

Steps	Procedure	Rationale
9.	Place the patient in comfortable position. Replace the cleaning solution and discard the disposable cloth.	Ensures comfort and well-being. Prepares for next procedure.
10.	Wash hands.	Prevents spread of infection transmission.
11.	Document the observations including the date, time, condition of glass and patient response along with the signature of the nurse.	Documentation fosters quality care.

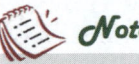 *Note*

- Plastic glasses require special cleaning solutions and drying tissues.

Contact Lenses

- Most patients prefer to care for their own contact lenses. A contact lens is a small, round transparent or colored disk that fits over the cornea.
- Care of contact lenses includes proper cleaning and disinfection, insertion and removal, and storage.
- It is very important that a nurse must take care of the patients who are unable to properly handle their lenses. Prolonged wearing of contact lens may cause serious damage to the cornea.

Remember 'Cradle'

- **Clean**
- **Rinse**
- **And**
- **Disinfect**
- **Lenses**
- **Every time**

When patients require help to clean their contact lenses, first perform hand hygiene, and then clean and disinfect the lenses with appropriate contact lens solution

Purposes

Helps to have:

- Safe lens wear
- Good vision
- Good comfort
- Clean lens

- Helps in preventing/minimizing deposits
- Maintaining wetness for comfort and clear vision
- Disinfecting lens to prevent ocular inflammation

Articles Required

Article	Purpose
Lens storage cases	For storing safely
Lubricating/Re-wetting solution	To wet the glasses
Disinfecting solution	To disinfect and reduce microorganisms
Rinsing solution	For cleaning chemicals off the glasses
Weekly/Protein cleaner/Daily cleaner	To keep the glasses under hygienic care

Procedure

Steps	Procedure	Rationale
1.	Explain the procedure to the patient	Allays anxiety and fosters cooperation
2.	Wash hands. Use soap that is free of oils, lotions, or perfumes. Dry hands with a lint-free towel.	Prevents transfer of microorganisms
3.	Place lens in palm of hand. Do not use fingernails and/or sharp objects like tweezers.	Using fingernails or sharp objects may damage the lens.
4.	Place 2-3 drop of cleaner on each lens.	Helps to clean the lens.
5.	Rub with forefinger for about 15 seconds per side using a to and fro action. Rolling the forefinger in both directions cleanse the lens periphery.	Facilitates thorough cleaning of lens.

Contd...

Steps	Procedure	Rationale
6.	Before replacing the lens into the lens case, empty, clean, rinse with solutions and allow to air dry. Rinse with hot water and rub thoroughly with a clean, dry tissue. Scrub with a toothbrush and oil free soaps or detergents weekly. Air dry by placing upside down.	Contact lens cases can be a source of bacterial growth.

Soak the lens overnight in fresh solution.

Steps	Procedure	Rationale
7.	Replace articles and wash hands.	Prevents spread of micro organisms
8.	Document the procedure with date and time along with signature of the nurse.	Documentation fosters quality care.

Special Considerations

- Before touching the contact lenses, wash the hands with soap and water and dry them with a lint-free towel.
- Avoid the use of soaps containing cold cream, lotion, or oily cosmetics before handling the lenses, as these substances may come into contact with the lenses and interfere with successful wearing.
- Never put contact lenses in the mouth to wet them. Saliva (spit) is not a sterile solution.
- Do not rinse or store contact in water (tap or sterile water).

- Never use a homemade saline solution.
- Do not use saline solution or rewetting drops to disinfect the lenses. They are not disinfectants.
- Use new solution each time you clean and disinfect the contact lenses.
- Never reuse or 'top off' with old solution.
- Do not pour contact lens solution into a different bottle. The solution will no longer be sterile.
- Make sure the tip of the solution bottle does not touch any surface. Keep the bottle tightly closed when you are not using it.
- Rinse the contact lens case with sterile contact lens solution (not tap water). Then leave the empty case open to air dry.
- Keep the contact lens case clean. Replace the case at least every 3 months or immediately if it gets cracked or damaged.
- Never wear the contact lenses if they have been stored for 30 days or longer without re-disinfecting.
- Handle the lenses with the fingertips and be careful to avoid contact with fingernails. It is helpful to keep the fingernails short and smooth.
- Stick strictly with the wearing schedule.
- If the eyes become red, or if you feel any irritation or changes in vision, remove the lens immediately and contact the doctor at the earliest.
  - The preservatives to store contact lenses are:
    - Thimerosal
    - Phenyl mercuric nitrate
    - Benzalkonium chloride
    - Chlorhexidine
    - Poly amino propyl biguanide
    - Polyquaternium-1

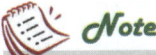 *Note*

- As RGP lenses are rigid and non-absorbent nature, they are easier to care for.
- Although, H_2O_2 is not normally used for rigid gas permeable lens (RGP lenses)

CARE OF THE EARS

- Routine ear care involves cleaning the ear with the end of a moistened washcloth rotated gently into the ear canal.
- The ears are cleaned during the bed bath. A clean corner of a moistened washcloth rotated gently into the ear, is used for cleaning.
- A cotton-tipped applicator is useful for cleansing the pinna.
- Gentle, downward retraction at the entrance of the ear canal usually causes visible cerumen to loosen and slip out. Nurse can usually remove excessive or impacted cerumen by irrigation with orders from healthcare specialist.

HEARING AID

A **hearing aid** is a small electronic medical device designed to improve hearing by making sound audible to a person with hearing loss. It makes some sounds louder so that a person with hearing loss can listen, communicate, and participate more effectively in daily activities. Hearing aids are delicate instruments that need attention to ensure good operation.

Unit IV ❖ **Basic Needs of the Patient**

Parts of Hearing Aids

A hearing aid has three basic parts: a microphone, amplifier, and speaker (Fig. 2).

- The hearing aid receives sound through a microphone, which converts the sound waves to electrical signals and sends them to an amplifier.
- The amplifier increases the power of the signals and then sends them to the ear through a speaker.

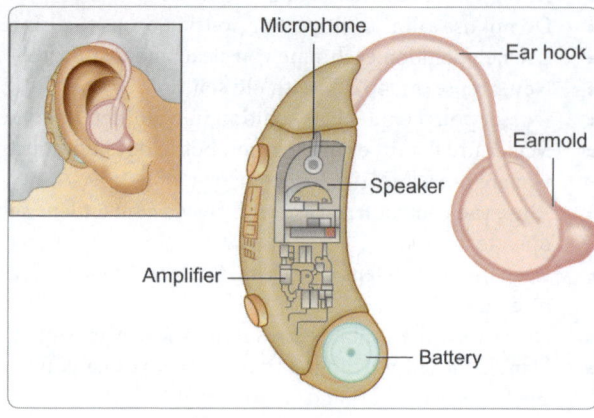

Figure 2: Parts of hearing aid

Types of Hearing Aids

- Body-worn
- Behind the ear (BTE) and in the ear (ITE)
- Invisible in-canal hearing aids
- Extended wear hearing aids
- CROS hearing aid
- Bone-anchored hearing aid (BAHA)
- Eyeglass aids
- Spectacle hearing aids
- Bone conduction spectacles
- Air conduction spectacles
- Directional spectacles

Caring of Hearing Aids

Hearing aids are delicate instruments that need attention to ensure good operation.

Purpose

- To maintain the proper hearing aid function

Inspection

- If the hearing aid has switches and/or volume controls, check them to be sure that they are working.
- Check the earmold tubing for cracks, holes or twists.
- Make sure the tubing fits snugly onto the hearing aid.
- Make sure the earmold opening is free of wax and moisture.
- Listen for static or crackling sounds.

General Guidelines

- It is important to keep the hearing aid, especially the earmold—clean, dry, and free of ear wax.
- Replace dead batteries in hearing aid with new ones of the same type, following the manufacturer's instructions.
- Before inserting the new batteries, make sure the hearing aid is turned off.
- Remember that moisture and excessive heat are enemies of hearing aid.
  - Don't store the hearing aid near a stove, a heater, in direct sunlight, or near any other heat source.

- Be careful wearing the hearing aid if it's raining or snowing, or when you are engaged in an activity that causes to perspire.
- Don't wear hearing aid in the bathtub or shower or while using a hair dryer, vaporizer, or hair spray.
  - Avoid dropping the hearing aid.
  - Clean hearing aids as instructed. Earwax and ear drainage can damage a hearing aid.
  - Avoid using hairspray or other hair care products while wearing hearing aids.
  - Turn off hearing aids when they are not in use.
  - Keep replacement batteries and small aids away from children and pets.

Articles Required

Articles	Purpose
Clients hearing aid	For cleaning
Soap and water	For washing the aid
Pipe cleaner or tooth pick	For cleaning the canal
New battery if required	For replacing the old battery
Towels or a damp cloth	For cleaning if can't be washed
Hearing aid brush	For cleaning the microphone and outside of the aid
Soft cloth	For drying
Wax cleaner	For removing the wax
Air blower	For drying and for removing the moisture
Kidney tray/paper bag	For disposing soiled waste

Procedure

Steps	Procedure	Rationale
1.	Explain the procedure to the patient.	Allays anxiety and fosters cooperation.
2.	Provide privacy by drawing the curtains or by closing the door.	Maintains clients self-esteem and dignity
3.	Arrange the articles.	Organization facilitates accurate skill performance
4.	Wash hands.	Prevents transfer of microorganisms.

Contd...

Unit IV ❖ **Basic Needs of the Patient**

Steps	Procedure	Rationale
5.	Remove the hearing aid. Remove the earmold by rotating it slightly forward and pulling it outward. Turn the hearing aid off and lower the volume.	Batteries continue to run if the hearing aid is not turned off.
6.	If the hearing aid is not to be used for several days, remove the battery.	Removal prevents the corrosion of the hearing aid from battery leakage
7.	Store the hearing aid in a safe place and label with client's name. Avoid exposure to heat and moisture. Store the hearing aid in a dry, cool place when not in use during the day and place it in a dry-aid or dehumidifier overnight.	Proper storage prevents loss or damage.
8.	Detach the earmold if possible. Disconnect the earmold from the receiver of a body - hearing aid or from the hearing aid case of behind the ear and eyeglass hearing aids where the tubing meets the hook of the case.	Facilitates easy cleaning
9.	Clean the microphone with the brush. Clean the entire hearing aid with brush. Then brush the ear mouth.	Removes the dirt and debris present externally.

Contd...

Unit IV ❖ Basic Needs of the Patient

Steps	Procedure	Rationale
10.	Clean the earmold. Wipe off the earmold with a soft tissue or cloth each time it is removed from the ear. 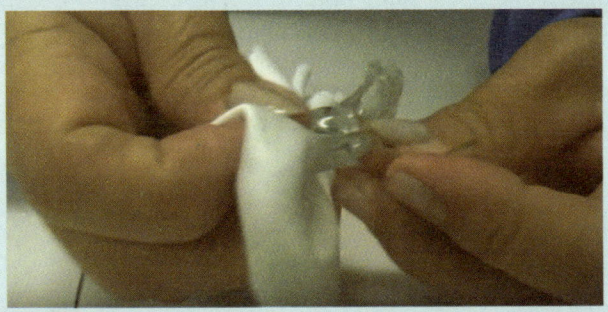 Use warm water and mild soap to wash the earmold. If the hearing aid doesn't detach, simply wipe the mold section with a damp cloth. Never immerse the hearing aid in water. 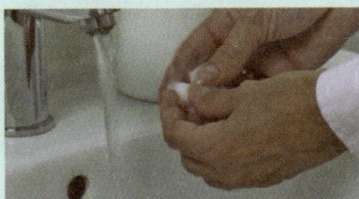 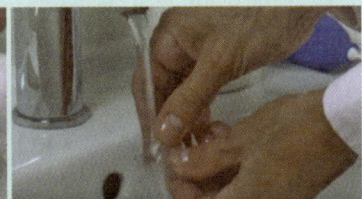 Carefully dry it and use an earmold air blower to remove moisture from the tubing. Allow it to dry overnight and reattach the earmold to the hearing aid the next morning. 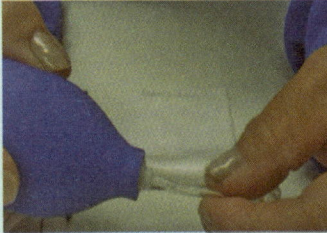 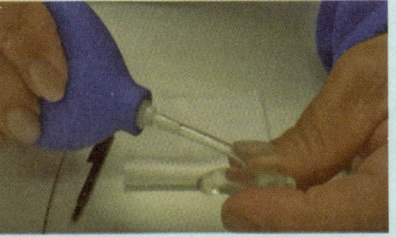	Helps in removing the dirt internally.
11.	Check the opening for earwax build-up. If wax is present, gently remove it with a pipe cleaner, tooth pick or wax tool. Do not poke the earmold with sharp objects. If the wax is deeper, use a vacuum. 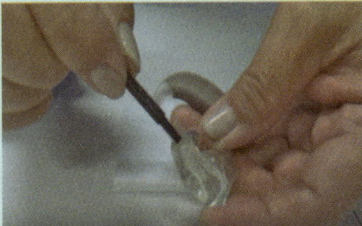 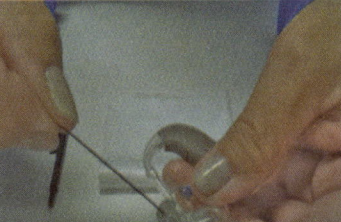	Keeping the earmold clean will usually prevent wax from building up.

Contd...

Steps	Procedure	Rationale
12.	Reattach the parts and fix it to the patient. Gently push the hearing aid into place while rotating it backward slightly to line up with your ear. The earmold should fit snugly and comfortably. Gently adjust the other pieces of the hearing aid. Place the behind-the-ear section carefully over the ear. Turn on the hearing aid and slowly raise the volume until it is placed at a comfortable level.	Promotes comfort of the patient.
13.	Replace the articles and wash hands.	Prevents spread of infection transmission.
14.	Document the procedure including the date, time, any presence of wax and patient response along with the signature of the nurse.	Documentation fosters quality care.

CARE OF SKIN

The chief method of caring the skin is bathing.

Objectives

- To clean the skin and promote elimination of waste products.
- To refresh and soothe the patient, to relieve fatigue and induce sleep.
- To stimulate circulation through slightly active and entirely passive movements.
- To promote comfort and relaxation by relieving fatigue and discomfort.
- To observe the condition of the skin of the patient.
- To provide the nurse an opportunity for health teaching.
- To regulate body temperature.
- To give care to pressure points.

Ideal Time for Bath

- Before breakfast
- One hour after the meal in order to avoid interference with the process of digestion.

Routine Cleansing Bath

- Bed bath
- Partial bath
- Self-administered bath
- Bath room bath
- Tub bath

Bed Bath (Sponge Bath)

Preliminary assessment of patient and environment:

- Identify the patient and see the order of the doctor and ascertain whether there are any restrictions in the movement of the patient or any part of the body.
- Get further instructions from the ward sister.
- Note the general condition of the patient.
- Assess the patient's need for bath and ability of self-help.
- Find out the mood of the patient for acceptance and the time the patient has taken meal or the time to take the meal.
- Assess the status of health habits of the patient to give the health education accordingly, during the procedure.
- Learn from the patient or relatives about his/her personal choice in using soap.
- Make ready the fresh linen and dress to use after bath.
- Find out the available articles in the unit.
- Provide privacy, avoid draught and maintain proper light.

Requisites

A tray consisting of:

Articles	Purpose
Articles for hand washing	For performing hand hygiene
Disposable gloves	For preventing cross infection
Soap dish with soap	For cleansing
Wash cloth one and a small towel or a readymade spongy cloth	For applying soap
Bath towels—2	One to spread underneath and one for drying the washed area
Basins—2	Big one for dipping wash cloth and other small one for dipping soap cloth. (Instead of small basin a small bowl can also be used)
Jugs—2	One with cold water and one with hot water
Bucket—1	For collecting soiled water.
Mackintosh	For protecting the linens from soiling
Lotion thermometer	For checking the temperature of water.
A bowl with cotton swabs	For cleaning the eyes and plugging the ears
Articles for mouth cleaning, if necessary	For performing oral care
Separate tray consists of articles for the care of hair and nail like comb, oil to attend hair, if necessary, nail scissors or nail file (if necessary)	For performing hair care and nail care along with bed bath.
Methylated spirit or back-rub-lotion	For providing back care
Dusting powder or talcum powder	For applying the body
Clean bed linen as necessary for changing	For performing comfortable bed
Clean dress for the patient.	To put after bathing
Kidney tray	To dispose the soiled things

Contd...

Unit IV ❖ Basic Needs of the Patient

Preparation of Patient

- Offer bedpan or urinal, if needed.
- Remove extra pillows or back rest if any. For cardiac patients arrange pillows according to their needs.
- Explain the procedure to the patient and win his/her confidence.

Preparation of Unit

- Arrange the articles near the bedside of the patient.
- Ensure that the room has proper lighting.
- Close the doors, windows and provide privacy.

Procedure

Steps	Procedure	Rationale
1.	Explain the procedure to the patient including proper explanation of how and why bath is given. Ask the client about personal hygiene preferences and ability to assist with the bath.	Secures cooperation of the patient and wins his confidence.
2	Secure privacy by drawing curtains and by closing the doors. Close windows and doors.	Prevents embarrassment and draughts
3.	Loosen the top bedding and remove the blanket leaving the patient with the top sheet. Remove personal clothing leaving the minimum dress at the waist as dhoti or skirt. Protect patient from exposure by draping the patient.	Ensures that the room is warm and the client's privacy is maintained.
4.	Arrange all articles in the order of use at a convenient place. (Tray and basin on the bed side locker and the clean linen on the stool or chair at the foot end of the bed).	Organization facilitates accurate skill performance
5.	Place client in supine position near the side of the bed close to you. Lower the side rails.	Placing close to the nurse prevents back strain and helps the nurse to maintain body mechanics.
6.	Perform hand hygiene.	Prevents the spread of microorganisms.

Contd...

Steps	Procedure	Rationale
7.	• Fill the basin with warm water. • Mix the cold and hot water and test the temperature of water and see that it is tolerated by the patient. Basin with less water is used for dipping cloth to apply soap and the other basin with plenty of water is used for dipping wash cloth. • Usually 110°–115°F (43.3°–46.1°C) temperature for the water is suitable for the ordinary bed bath. • Check the temperature of the water using a bath thermometer. • If you do not have a bath thermometer it should be comfortably warm to your elbow. Water will cool during the procedure. • Ask the client to verify the temperature of the water.	Water at proper temperature relaxes the patient and provides warmth.
8.	Don gloves.	Prevents the spread of organisms.
	Face, neck and ears:	
	Place the mackintosh and bath towel under the chin around the lower part of the neck, spreading to the chest. 	Prevents soiling of linen.
10.	Take two dry cotton balls and plug it in the ears.	Protects the ear from water entering into it.
11.	Take a cotton swab, wet with hot water and squeeze the water. Wash the client's eyes. Cleanse from inner to outer canthus. Use separate swabs for each stroke. Discard the used swab in the kidney tray. 	Washing from inner to outer canthus prevents sweeping of debris into the client's eyes. Using a separate portion of the swab for each eye prevents the spread of infection.

Contd...

Unit IV ❖ Basic Needs of the Patient

Steps	Procedure	Rationale
12.	• Take the cloth for soap and make a mitten to avoid dangling of the cloth. • Wet it and squeeze slightly so that water does not drip.	Making mitten prevents dangling of the cloth causing interference during the procedure.
13.	• Then wash his/her face, neck and ears with soap. Apply soap if the patient desires. • Leave the cloth on the brim of the basin. • Take the wash cloth and make mitten, dip in water and squeeze tightly and start wiping, rinse thoroughly several times. Use firm, gentle strokes. • Dry carefully with the other bath towel. • Note and report anything unusual such as rashes, cuts, bruises, reddened areas, swelling or vermin. • Dry the part with the bath towel and put powder on the face and neck.	Gentle stroke soothes the patient and promotes comfort.
	Hands & arms:	
14.	• Place the mackintosh and big towel lengthwise under the client's farther arm overlapping the abdomen. Uncover the far arm and then the other arm. 	Prevents soiling of the linen.
	• Wash the far arm with soap and rinse. Use long strokes: wrist to elbow→ elbow to shoulder→ axilla→ hand. Wash well, rinse well and dry thoroughly. 	Washing the far side first prevents dripping bath water onto a clean area. Long strokes improve circulation by facilitating venous return.

Contd...

Steps	Procedure	Rationale
	• Pay special attention to the axilla. • In between soaping and washing, the hand is kept resting comfortable over the abdomen on the towel or conveniently at the side according to the preference of the patient. Repeat the procedure on the other arm.	
	• Place the basin on the folded towel on the bed and let the patient place hands in the basin. Rinse and dry thoroughly, paying particular attention to skin in between fingers and nails using a nailbrush. Keep the washed hands up, resting on both sides of the head to prevent wetting again. 	Cleaning the nails using nailbrush facilitates removal of debris
15.	**Chest and abdomen:** • Fold the top sheet down to the abdomen. Move the mackintosh and bath towel under the upper trunk • Cover the chest with another towel. 	Additional towel provides warmth and privacy.

Contd...

Steps	Procedure	Rationale
	• Wash chest and dry without exposing, paying particular attention to the area under the breast of a female patient. Apply powder, keep the parts covered.	Keeping covered prevents chill.
	• Abdomen can be washed along with the chest or separately according to the condition of the patient. Wash abdomen with soap, rinse and dry giving special attention to the skin folds and umbilicus. Cover the trunk with top sheet and remove the bath towel from the abdomen.	Bacteria tend to get trapped in the skin folds and umbilicus.
	• Exchange the warm water. You may change water earlier, if necessary to maintain the proper temperature.	The water may probably be unclean. Cool water is uncomfortable.
	Legs:	
16.	• Place the mackintosh and bath towel under the far leg lengthwise. Expose one leg at a time; farther leg first, wash, rinse and dry the thigh and leg; from foot to knee→ from knee to hip.	Promotes comfort.

Contd...

Unit IV ❖ Basic Needs of the Patient

Steps	Procedure	Rationale
	• Pay particular attention to the skin between the toes while washing. Foot can be placed in the basin and cleansed. 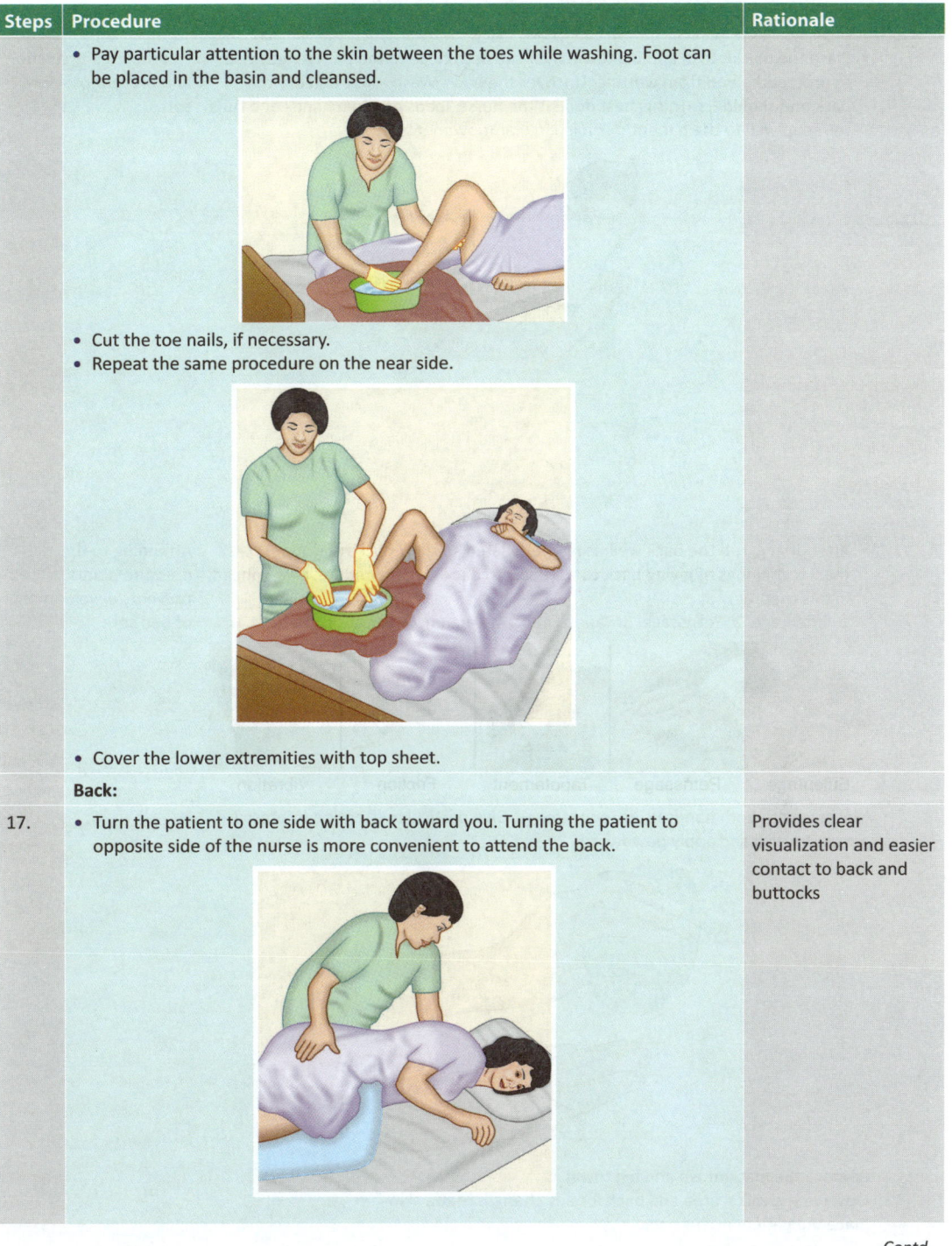 • Cut the toe nails, if necessary. • Repeat the same procedure on the near side. • Cover the lower extremities with top sheet. **Back:**	
17.	• Turn the patient to one side with back toward you. Turning the patient to opposite side of the nurse is more convenient to attend the back.	Provides clear visualization and easier contact to back and buttocks

Contd...

Steps	Procedure	Rationale
	• Place the mackintosh and big towel over the bed, close to the back lengthwise to protect the bed from wetting. Uncover the back. Wash, rinse and dry the back and shoulders. This is best done if the nurse soaps her own hands and rubs the soap well to the patient's skin in circular movements. 	It stimulates circulation and prevent pressure sores.
	• After drying, rub the back well using methylated spirit or back-rub-lotion. Use the 5 techniques of giving back care. (Refer to back care procedure, given ahead in this chapter.) 1. Effleurage, 2. Petrissage, 3. Tapotement, 4. Friction, 5. Vibration Effleurage Petrissage Tapotement Friction Vibration Massage with both hands using long strokes. Give particular attention to pressure areas. Dry well and apply powder. Remove the mackintosh and big towel. Observe the sacral area and back for any changes in the skin. Place the patient on his back.	Attending to the pressure points prevents development of bed sore.

Contd...

Steps	Procedure	Rationale
	Pubic region:	
18.	• Wash genital area. It is done by the patient if he or she is able to do so. If he/she is unable to do so the nurse should do it for her, making sure that the entire area is gently and thoroughly washed and dried.	Ensures cleaning from more clean to less clean area.
19.	Put the patient's personal clean clothing. Remove the plugged cotton swabs from the ear. Remove mackintosh and towel. Straighten bed linen and make the bed. Change linen, if necessary.	Provides warmth and comfort.
20.	Leave the patient comfortable and relaxed and the unit tidy.	Ensures comfort and well-being.
21.	Take the articles to the utility room. Disinfect, wash, dry and replace everything for the next use.	Ensures use for another patient.
22.	Doff gloves and perform hand hygiene.	Prevents transfer of microorganisms.
23.	Record the time and procedure into the nurse's record with signature on the chart. Report if any abnormalities are seen.	Documentation fosters quality care.

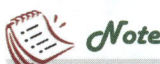 *Note*

- Change water as often as is necessary.
- Offer drink after the bath, if needed, comb hair in a female patient.
- Rinse and dry the areas of the body in the following order: face, neck, farthest arm, near arm, chest, abdomen, back, farthest leg, near leg and pubic region. In this order the upper trunk is fully bathed and lower extremities afterwards. In few books, e.g., 'Dugas' lower extremities and pubic area are cleaned; before back is bathed where back care is given last.

Tub Bath and Bathroom Bath

Objectives

- To encourage the patient and assist him/her to take bath himself/herself.
  Preliminary assessment of patient and environment is same as that of bed bath and in addition:
  - Have someone for help, if needed to take the patient to the tub or bathroom and bring back to the bed after procedure.
  - Tub bath or bathroom bath is allowed to the patient only if he/she has enough confidence for self-help and to withstand the procedure.

Unit IV ❖ Basic Needs of the Patient

Requisites

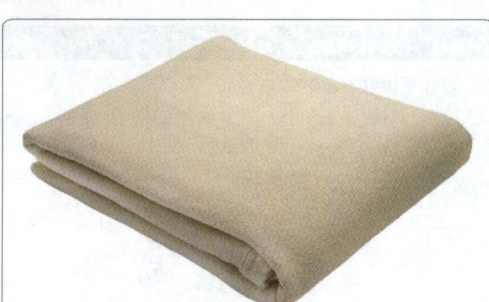

- Bath blanket, if needed
- Talcum powder
- Wash cloth
- Chair or stool
- Bath towel
- Patients clothing and slippers if he/she has
- Soap in soap dish

Procedure

1. Prepare the bath room for the patient, i.e., fill tub half full of water.
2. Instruct the patient to attend the oral hygiene if not done.
3. If the patient cannot walk, take him/her to bathroom in a wheel chair
4. Assist the patient to undress.
5. Pin the towel around his/her waist.
6. Hold the bath blanket around the patient until he/she is into the tub. This will prevent chilling and exposure.
7. Then, put it on the chair near the tub so that he/she can dry himself by sitting on the chair when he/she is out of the tub. Help him/her to be in the water in the tub in a comfortable position after removing the towel and blanket.
8. For tub bath or bathroom bath, the temperature of water should be 90–100°F (32.2–37.8°C)
9. Wash patient's back and assist the patient with complete bath, if necessary. Observe the patient for any unusual symptoms.
10. Dry the patient's back and chest before assisting him out of the tub. Allow the patient to sit on the chair where the bath blanket is spread. Dry the patient thoroughly, if patient needs assistance.
11. Apply powder according to the patient's wishes. Assist the patient to put on clothing and to go back to bed.
12. Clean the bath tub.
13. Remove the soiled linen after making the patient comfortable in bed.
14. Wash hands and record the time and procedure in the nurse's record. Leave bathroom ready for the next patient.

 Note

- Help the patient in coming out of the tub to chair if he/she becomes fatigued or dizzy. If no assistance around, let out the water in the tub, wrap the patient in bath blanket and call for assistance.
- Instruct the patient not to lock the door, if you are leaving the bathroom.
- Never leave the patient alone in the bathroom longer than 5 minutes. Call through the door after returning to make sure that the patient is alright and ask if he/she needs anything.
- Do not leave the patient in the tub longer than 10–15 minutes without doctor's order.
- There should not be any electric appliances near the tub. If electric appliances are there, caution the patient not to touch them when wet.
- Never leave a child, depressed person or unsteady person alone in the bathroom.

DECUBITUS ULCER/PRESSURE ULCER/BEDSORE

- **Definition:** Decubitus ulcer or bedsore or pressure ulcer is an ulcerated sloughed area of tissues resulting from pressure, slowing of circulation and causing death of cells. (also called decubitus)
- **Common sites:** This may happen more frequently over the bony prominences of the body where there is no rich supply of blood for nourishment and also where there is a thin layer of skin.

Unit IV ❖ Basic Needs of the Patient

- When the patient is in supine position, the pressure points are (Fig. 3):
  - Back of the head (occiput)
  - Scapula
  - Nape of the neck
  - Sacral region—most common area
  - Elbows and heels

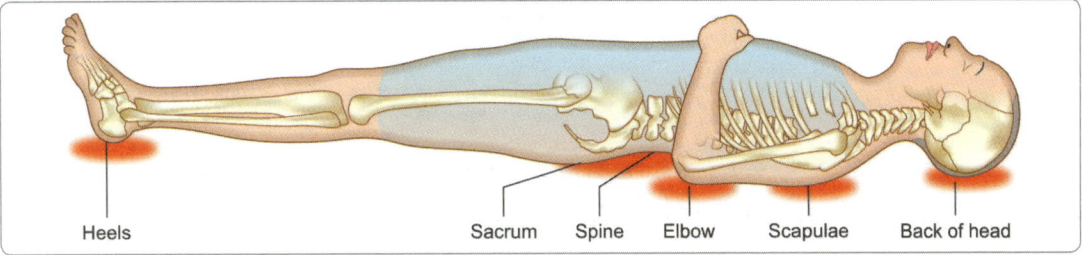

Heels   Sacrum   Spine   Elbow   Scapulae   Back of head

Figure 3: Pressure points in supine position

- In side lying position, pressure points are (Fig. 4):
  - Ears
  - Acromion process of the shoulder
  - Ribs, iliac crest
  - Greater trochanter of the hips
  - Medial and lateral condyles of the knee
  - Malleolus of the ankle joint

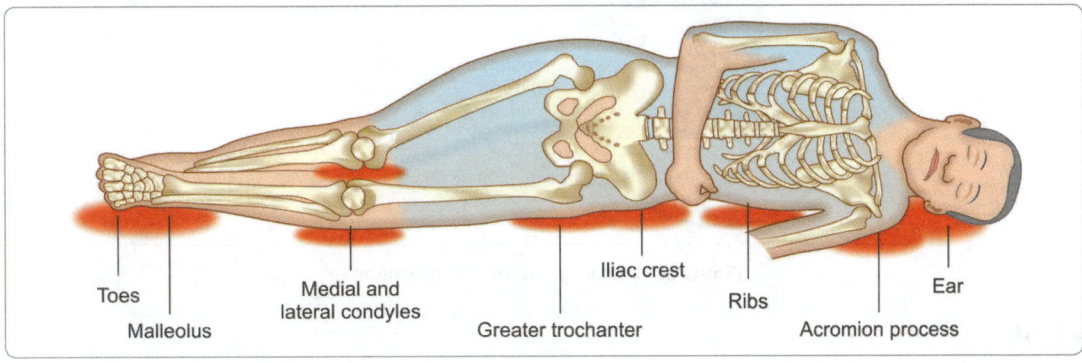

Toes   Medial and lateral condyles   Greater trochanter   Iliac crest   Ribs   Acromion process   Ear

Malleolus

Figure 4: Side-lying position

- In prone position, pressure points are (Fig. 5):
  - Back of the ears and cheek
  - Acromion process, knees and toes
  - Other areas that should be watched carefully are between the folds of flesh such as under the breasts in females and genitalia in males. The skin of patients, who are very thin or obese may break down quickly.

Unit IV ❖ **Basic Needs of the Patient**

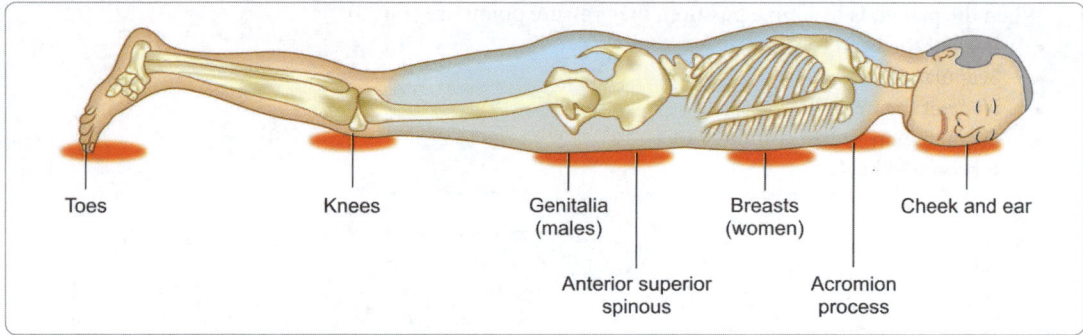

Figure 5: Pressure points in prone position

- In sitting position also the patients are at risk as shown here (Fig. 6):

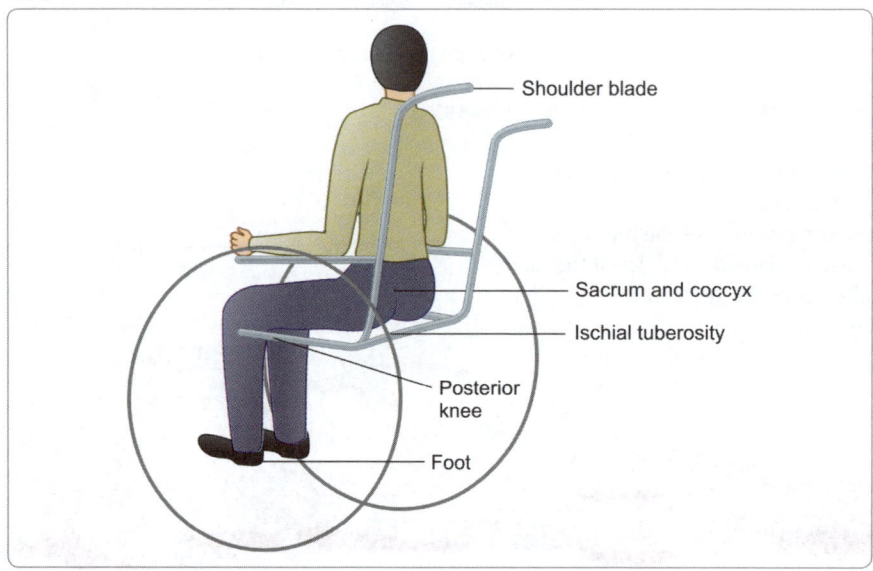

Figure 6: Pressure points in sitting position

Causes

Causes of bedsore may be predisposing or direct causes.

- Predisposing causes
  - Impaired circulation, which is the main cause due to interference in circulation, e.g., people with multiple fracture.
  - Lowered vitality due to disease, e.g., typhoid and due to old age and starvation
  - Emaciation
  - Edema
  - Obesity
  - Deficient nerve supply

- **Direct or immediate causes:**
  - **Pressure:** From lying in one position for a long time causing pressure because of the weight of the body. Splints, plaster casts and bandages may be sources of pressure when applied too tightly.
  - **Lack of cleanliness:** Directly act as an agent.
  - **Friction:** Rough surface, patches, seams or wrinkles on the bed linen or garments or other foreign bodies like orange peels, breadcrumbs, rice and food particles in bed, frictions with splints, plaster casts and chipped bedpan, restless movements of the patients, rubbing of two skin surfaces together, etc. can cause friction on skin.
  - **Moisture:** Resulting from perspiration, urine, feces and vaginal discharges that irritate the skin.
  - **Heat:** It is another cause for bed sore due to sameness of position or keeping the patient directly on rubber sheets.
  - **Presence of pathogenic organisms:** Lack of cleanliness accumulates pathogenic organisms and causes infection on the skin.

 Stimulant

Pressure ulcer or moisture lesion?		
Criteria	**Pressure ulcer**	**Moisture ulcer**
Causation	Usually pressure and/or shear are present	Usually moisture is present.
Location	More likely over bony prominences	Less likely over bony prominences
Shape and edge	Usually distinct edging and shape	Usually diffuse edging and shape
Depth	Pressure ulcers can be superficial or deep	Moisture lesions are rarely more than superficial
Necrosis	Necrosis may be present	Necrosis is never present

Types of Patients Most Susceptible to Bedsore

- Very thin, very fat and very old people.
- Person with long wasting diseases such as typhoid (because body tissues become poorly nourished).
- Persons for whom movement is difficult; as one with multiple fracture.
- Persons with paralysis.
- Patients who have incontinence of urine and motion.
- Unconscious patients.
- Patients with anemia, cancer and diabetes and others whose circulation is poor because of age, heart disease etc.
- Obese patients or edematous patients especially edema of the sacrum and buttocks.
- Severely ill patients whose general condition is very poor and rapidly deteriorating.
- Elderly patients who move very little in the bed.
- Sedated patients who do not move in bed frequently.
- Neurologic patients with lack of sensation in bony prominences.
- Surgical patients with limited movements in bed.
- Patients with hyperpyrexia who sweat profusely.
- Patients with excessive discharges and drainage from wounds.
- Chronic conditions, like diabetes who are in bed for a long time.
- Any bed patients who are neglected and getting poor nursing care.
- Malnourished patients or patients with deficiency diseases.

Unit IV ❖ Basic Needs of the Patient

Assessment of Pressure Ulcers

Pressure ulcer (PU) assessment requires quantification of multiple parameters of the ulcer and periulcer tissue. Ulcer assessment requires a systematic and objective approach.

Clinical Assessment

This should include:

- Ulcer history (including etiology, duration, and prior treatment)
- Anatomic location
- Stage
- Size (including length, width, and depth measured in centimeters)
- Sinus tracts, undermining, tunneling
- Exudate or drainage
- Necrotic tissue (slough and eschar)
- Presence or absence of granulation tissue
- Epithelialization
- Ulcer borders

Ulcer History

Focused history to assess ulcer history is as follows:

Adults	Geriatric	Pediatric
• Past skin diseases	• Dryness and itching	• Use/type of diaper cream or bathing products
• Sun exposure	• Bruising tendency	• Rashes or lesions
• Recent change in wart or mole	• Longer healing time	• Bruising
• Sore that has not healed	• Nail texture changes	• Allergy
• Signs of abuse	• Signs of abuse	• Signs of abuse
		• Injury history
		• Sun exposure

Anatomic Location

Correct terminology for location of pressure ulcers should be used at all times. This will assist in defining the etiology of the wound. For example, heel, sacrum, scapula, and so on....

Stages:

- Pressure ulcer assessment must include the stage of pressure ulcer: Stages 1, 2, 3, 4, unstageable, or suspected deep tissue injury.
- Pressure ulcers should never be reverse staged because once layers of tissue and supporting structures are gone they are not replaced. Instead, the wound is filled with granulation tissue. For example, once a pressure ulcer is at stage 4, it will become a healing stage 4 when it begins to granulate (Fig. 7).

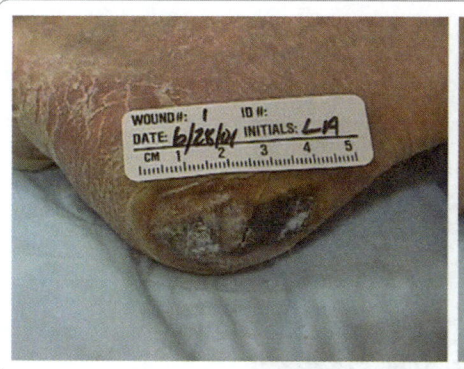 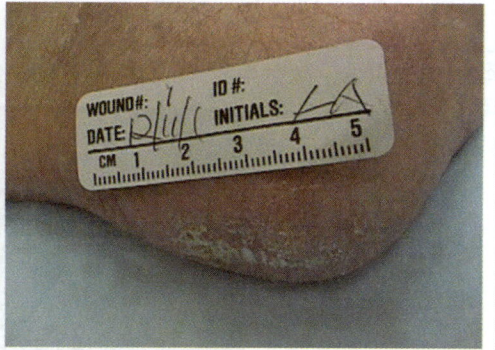

Figure 7: Pressure ulcer (left), healed ulcer (right)

Size:

Always use a single-use, metric tape for measurement.

- Length of a wound is measured by placing a ruler at the point of greatest length (head-to-toe).
- Width of a wound is measured by placing the ruler at the point of highest width (side to side; right to left) (Fig. 8).
- **Depth** is commonly obtained by placing a cotton-tipped applicator into the wound bed, at the deepest point and placing a mark on the applicator at skin level (or simply using the examiners thumb and index finger) and using a ruler to determine the depth of the wound at the skin level mark (Figs 9A and B).

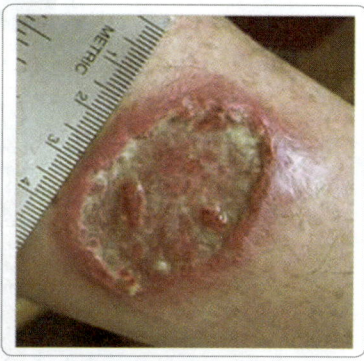

Figure 8: Measurement of pressure ulcer

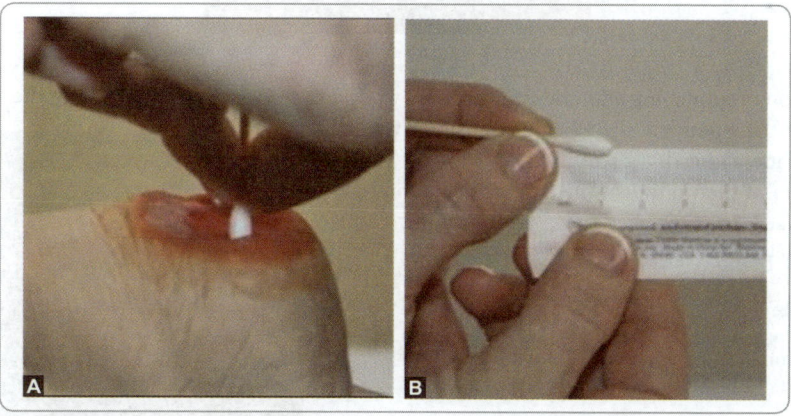

Figures 9A and B: Measurement of depth of ulcer

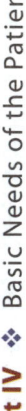

Unit IV ❖ **Basic Needs of the Patient**

Sinus Tracts, Undermining, Tunneling

- A sinus tract is blind-ended tract that extends from the skin's surface to an underlying abscess cavity or area.
- Tunnelling is a channel that extends from any part of the wound through subcutaneous tissue or muscle.

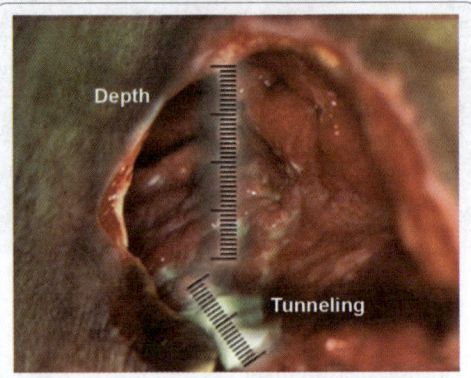

- Undermining is tissue destruction that occurs under intact skin around the wound perimeter.

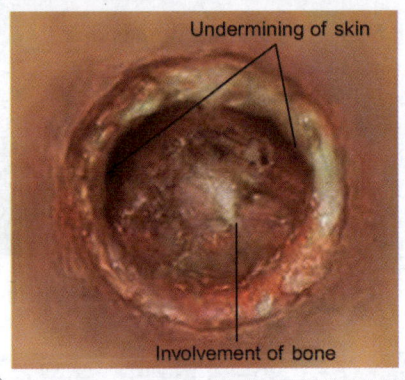

- The location of tunnelling and undermining in a wound can be determined by using the **clock method.**
- The top of the wound, at the 12 o'clock position would be at the patient's head.
- The bottom of the wound, at the 6 o'clock position will point toward patient's feet (e.g., undermining from 2 to 6 o'clock) (Fig. 10).

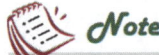 *Note*

Always remember that the patient's head represents 12 o'clock and the patient's feet represent 6 o'clock.

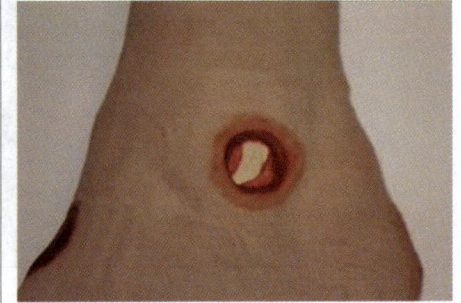

Figure 10: Location of tunneling and undermining

Exudate or Drainage

The amount, type and odor of wound drainage should always be assessed and documented.
- **Amount:** None, light, moderate, or heavy
- **Type:** Clear, serous sanguineous, sanguineous, purulent, tan, or bloody
- **Odor:** Absent, faint, moderate, or strong.

Tissue Type and Thickness

Necrotic tissue (slough and eschar)/presence or absence of granulation tissue/epithelialization. The wound bed tissue and its color, reveal the phase and progress of wound healing.

 Stimulant

- Epithelial tissue is 'pearly pink' in color.
- Granulation tissue is beefy red.
- Necrotic tissue is usually black, brown, or tan and known as eschar.
- Yellow necrotic tissue is known as slough (it can also be tan, gray, green, or brown).

Appearance of Wound Bed

Many pressure ulcers have a combination of different types of tissues in the wound bed.
- These combinations should be documented in percentages.
- Example: 80% of the wound bed contains yellow slough and 20% contains granulation tissue.

Condition of Periwound Skin

Periwound skin should be assessed for:
- Color (erythema or white)
- Temperature (cool or warm)
- Texture (moist, indurated, boggy or dry)
- Integrity (candidiasis, epidermal stripping, pustules)

Wound Margins

- Wound margins should be looking specifically for undermining or dead spaces.

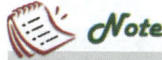 *Note*

Dead spaces are the areas where the wound edges have come away from the wound base. These areas may show signs of poor circulation such as gray or purple coloration.

Risk Assessment Tools to Assess Pressure Ulcers

Risk assessment tools are used to identify those patients who are at risk for developing pressure ulcers and are based on those factors, which have been identified as significant in the development of pressure sores.

Unit IV ❖ Basic Needs of the Patient

Purposes of Risk Factor Assessment

Risk factor assessment identifies:
- Patients, who are more likely to develop pressure ulcers
- Different components of risk for pressure ulcers
- Facilitates clinical decision making
- Helps selective targeting of preventive interventions

When to do Risk Assessment?

- On admission—within 8 hours
- Reassessment frequency—based on patient's acuity

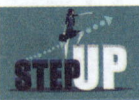

Comprehensive Pressure Ulcer Risk Assessment: Halt
- **H**istory—Collect history pertaining to formation of pressure ulcer
- **A**ssess comorbidities, medications, perfusion and oxygenation
  - Nutritional deficits
  - Higher rates of PU
  - Corticosteroid use
  - Disease conditions, like CHF, COPD, PVD, DM
  - Obesity
- **L**ook at the skin—Skin status, bony prominences, especially sacrum and heels, use of any medical devices that may precipitate formation of pressure ulcer. For example, oxygen face mask.
- **T**ouch the skin - Skin temperature may predict pressure ulcer risk.

Tools for Assessing Pressure Ulcer

There are three pressure ulcer (PU) risk scales:
1. The Norton scale
2. The Braden scale
3. The Waterlow scale

Norton Scale

This scale was created in England in 1962.
- This scale uses five criteria or parameters, relevant to skin condition. The criteria to score patients are as follows:
  - Physical condition
  - Mental condition
  - Activity
  - Mobility
  - Incontinence
- It makes deductions in the Norton score for associated conditions such as diabetes, hypertension, fever, low hematocrit, low hemoglobin and albumin, and changes in mental status and concurrent use of five or more medications (Table 1).

Table 1: **Norton scale**

Physical condition	Good	4
	Fair	3
	Poor	2
	Very bad	1
Mental condition	Alert	4
	Apathetic	3
	Confused	2
	Stuporous	1
Activity	Ambulant	4
	Walks with help	3
	Chair bound	2
	Bedfast	1
Mobility	Full	4
	Slightly Impaired	3
	Very Limited	2
	Immobile	1
Incontinence	None	4
	Occasional	3
	Usually urinary	2
	Urinary and fecal	1

Scoring in Norton score (Table 2)

- The five subscale scores of the Norton scale are added together for a total score that ranges from 5 to 20.
- A lower Norton score indicates higher levels of risk for pressure ulcer development.

Table 2: **Norton scores**

Greater than 18	Low risk
Between 18 and 14	Medium risk
Between 14 and 10	High risk
Lesser than 10	Very high risk

One of the benefits of Norton score is that this scale is quick to administer and straightforward, taking up to 10 minutes to complete.

Braden Scale

The Braden scale for predicting pressure ulcer risk is a tool that was developed in 1987 by Barbara Braden and Nancy Bergstrom (Table 3).

Purpose: The purpose of the scale is to help health professionals, especially nurses, assess a patient's risk of developing a pressure ulcer.

Categories: There are six categories under this scale that are as follows:

Unit IV ❖ Basic Needs of the Patient

Table 3: **Braden scale**

Braden Scale for Predicting Pressure Sore Risk						
Patient's Name_____ Evaluator's Name_____ Date of Assessment						
Sensory Perception ability to respond meaning-fully to pressure-related discomfort	**1. Completely Limited** Unresponsive (does not moan, flinch, or grasp) to Painful stimuli due to diminished level of consciousness or sedation. OR limited ability to feel pain over most of body	**2. Very Limited** Responds only to painful stimuli. Cannot communicate discomfort except by moaning or restlessness OR has a sensory impairment which limits the ability to feel Pain or discomfort over ½ of body.	**3. Slightly limited** Responds to verbal commands, but cannot always communicate discomfort or the need to be turned OR has some sensory impairment which limits ability to feel pain or discomfort in 1 or 2 extremities.	**4. No Impairment** Responds to verbal Commands. Has no sensory deficit which would limit ability to feel or voice pain or discomfort.		
Moisture degree to which skin is exposed to moisture	**1. Constantly Moist** Skin is kept moist almost constantly by perspiration, urine, etc. Dampness is detected every time patient is moved or turned.	**2. Very Moist** Skin is often, but not always moist. Linen must be changed at least Once a shift.	**3. Occasionally Moist:** Skin is occasionally moist, requiring an extra linen change approximately Once a day.	**4. Rarely Moist** Skin is usually try, linen only requires changing at routine intervals.		
Activity degree of physical activity	**1. Bedfast** Confined to bed.	**2. Chairfast** Ability to walk severely limited or non-existent Cannot bear own weight and/or must be assisted into chair or wheelchair.	**3. Walks Occasionally** Walks occasionally during day, but for very short distances, with or without assistance. Spends majority of each shift in bed or chair.	**4. Walks Frequently** Walks outside room at least twice a day and inside room at least once every two hours during walking hours		
Mobility ability 10 Change and Control body position	**1. Completely Immobile** Does not make even slight changes in body or extremity position without assistance.	**2. Very Limited** Makes occasional slight changes in body or extremity position but unable to make frequent or significant changes independently.	**3. Slightly Limited** Makes frequent though slight change in body or extremity position independently.	**4. No Limitation** Makes major and frequent changes in position without assistance		
Nutrition usual food intake pattern	**1. Very Poor** Never eats a complete meal. Rarely eats more than ⅓ of any food offered. Eats 2 servings or less of protein (meat or dairy products) per day. Takes fluids poorly. Does not take a liquid dietary supplement OR is NPO and/or maintained on Clear liquids or IV's for more than 5 days.	**2. Probably Inadequate** Rarely eats a complete meal and generally eats only about ½ of any food offered. Protein intake includes only 3 servings of meat or dairy products per day. Occasionally will take a dietary supplement OR receives less than optimum amount of liquid diet or tube feeding.	**3. Adequate** Eats over half of most meals. Eats a total of 4 servings of protein (meat, dairy products) per day occasionally will refuse a meal, but will usually take a supplement when offered OR is on a tube feeding or TPN regimen which probably meets most of nutritional needs	**4. Excellent** Eats most of every meal. Never refuses a meal. Usually eats a total of 4 or more servings of meat and dairy products. Occasionally eats between meals. Does not require supplementation.		

Contd...

Braden Scale for Predicting Pressure Sore Risk

Friction & Shear	1. Problem Requires moderate to maximum assistance in moving. Complete lifting without sliding against sheets is impossible. Frequently slides down in bed or chair, requiring frequent repositioning with maximum assistance. Spasticity, contractures or agitation leads to almost constant friction.	2. Potential Problem Moves feebly a requires minimum assistance. During a move skin probably slides to some extent against sheets, chair, restraints or Other devices. Maintains relatively good position in Chair or bed most of the tine but occasionally slides down.	3. No Apparent Problem Moves in bed and in Chair independently and has sufficient muscle strength to lift up completely during Maintains good position In bed or chair.			

Total Score

- **Sensory perception:** This parameter measures a patient's ability to detect and respond to discomfort or pain that is related to pressure on parts of his/her body.
  - Completely limited
  - Very limited
  - Slightly limited
  - No impairment

- **Moisture:** This parameter measures a patient's ability to detect and respond to discomfort or pain that is related to pressure on parts of his/her body.
  - Constantly moist
  - Very moist
  - Occasionally moist
  - Rarely moist

- **Activity:** This parameter measures a patient's ability to detect and respond to discomfort or pain that is related to pressure on parts of his/her body.
  - Bed fast
  - Chair fast
  - Walks occasionally
  - Walks frequently

- **Mobility:** This category looks at the capability of a patient to adjust his/her body position independently. This assesses the physical competency to move and can involve the client's willingness to move.
  - Completely immobile
  - Very limited
  - Slightly limited
  - No limitation

- **Nutrition:** The assessment of a client's nutritional status looks at his/her normal pattern of daily nutrition.
  - Very poor
  - Probably inadequate
  - Adequate
  - Excellent

- **Friction and Shear:** This category is assessed as the sliding motion can cause shear of tissues, which means the skin and bone are moving in opposite directions causing breakdown of cell membranes and capillaries.
  - Problem
  - Potential problem
  - No apparent problem

- **Scoring of Braden scale**
  - Score risk factors is from 1 to 4 except "Score friction/shear" from 1 to 3.
  - Total score ranges from 6 to 23 (Table 4)
  - Risk factor score of 1 is the lowest level of functioning
  - Do not rely on the total score alone
  - If a category falls between two numbers, choose the lower score

Table 4: Braden score

19–23	Not at risk	15–18	Preventive interventions
13–14	Moderate risk	10–12	High risk
6–9	Very high risk		

Unit IV ❖ Basic Needs of the Patient

Waterlow Score (or Waterlow Scale)

This scale was developed in 1985 by clinical nurse teacher Judy Waterlow.

Areas of assessment

The Waterlow scale consists of seven items:

1. Build/weight for height
2. Skin type/visual risk areas
3. Sex and age
4. Malnutrition screening tool
5. Continence
6. Mobility
7. The special risk factors are divided into tissue malnutrition, neurological deficit, major surgery/trauma, and medication.

Build/weight for height		Skin type visual risk area		Sex age		Malnutrition screening tool (MST) (Nutrition vol. 15, No. 6 1999 - Australia	
Average BMI = 20–24.9	0	Healthy Tissue Paper	0 1	Male	1	A - Has patient lost weight recently	B - Weight loss score
Above Average BMI = 25–29.9	1	Dry Oedematous	1 1	Female 14–19	2 1	Yes - Go to B No - Go to C	0.5–5 kg = 1 5–10 kg = 2
OBESE BMI > 30	2	Glammy, Pyrexia Discoloured	1	50–64 65–74	2 3	Unsure - Go to C And	10–15 kg = 3 > 15 kg = 4
BELOW AVERAGE BMI < 20	3	Grade 1 Broken/spots Grade 2–4	2 3	75–80 81+	4 5	Score 2	Unsure = 2
BMI = Wt (kg)/ Ht (m)^2						C- Patient eating poorly or Lack of appetite 'No' = 0; 'Yes score = 1	Nutrition score If > 2 refer for Nutrition assessment/ intervention

Continence		Mobility		Special risks			
Complete/ Catheterized	0	Fully Restless/fidgety	0 1	**Tissue malnutrition**		**Neurological deficit**	
Urine Incont.	1	Apathetic	2	Terminal cachexia	8	Diabetes, MS, CVA	4–6
Faecal Incont.	2	Restricted	3	Multiple organ failure	8	Motor/Sensory	4–6
Urinary + Faecal Incontinence	3	Bedbound e.g. Traction	4	Single organ failure (Resp, renal, cardiac)	5	Paraplegia (Max of 6)	4–6
		Chairbound e.g. Wheelchair	5	Peripheral vascular disease anemia (Hb < 8) Smoking	5 2 1		

SCORE
10+ At Risk
15+ High Risk
20+ Very High Risk

Major surgery or Trauma	
Orthopedic/Spinal	5
On table > 2 HR	5
On table > 6 HR	8

Revised Waterlow scale, 2005

Medication - Cytotoxics Long term/High dose steroids, anti-inflammatory   Max of 4
Scores can be discounted after 48 hours provided patient is recovering normally

Waterlow Scoring

Scores are totaled to produce a summary score from 3 (best prognosis) to 45 (worst prognosis).

- Potential scores range from 1 to 64.
- The tool identifies three 'at risk' categories:
  - A score of 10–14 indicates 'at risk'
  - A score of 15–19 indicates 'high risk'
  - A score of 20 and above indicates very high risk

BACK CARE

Back care means cleaning and massaging back, paying special attention to pressure points.

Purposes

- To improve circulation to the back
- To refresh the mode and feeling
- To relieve from fatigue, pain and stress
- To induce sleep
- To prevent bed sore

Steps in Performing Back Massage

Massage is an activity done by pressing the body/muscle gently to make someone more comfortable.

- **Effleurage or stroking**: It is a long sweeping movement with palm of hand conforming to the contour of the surface treated. Strokes should be slow, rhythmical and gentle with pressure constant and in the direction of venous stream. The thumb and fingers are used over small surface (on the neck). Using your palm, stroke from the buttocks up to the shoulders, over the upper arms and back to the buttocks (Fig. 11).

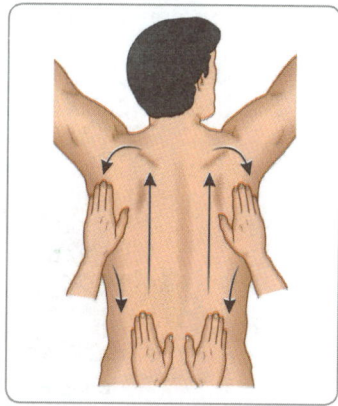

Figure 11: Effleurage or stroking

- **Petrissage or kneading**: It is performed with the clenched palm resting on the surface and the fingers, and thumble grasping the skin and subcutaneous tissues which move with the hand of the operator and by a squeezing movement by holding the tissue between the fingers. Using your thumb to oppose your fingers, kneed and stroke the back starting from the buttocks (Figs 12A and B).

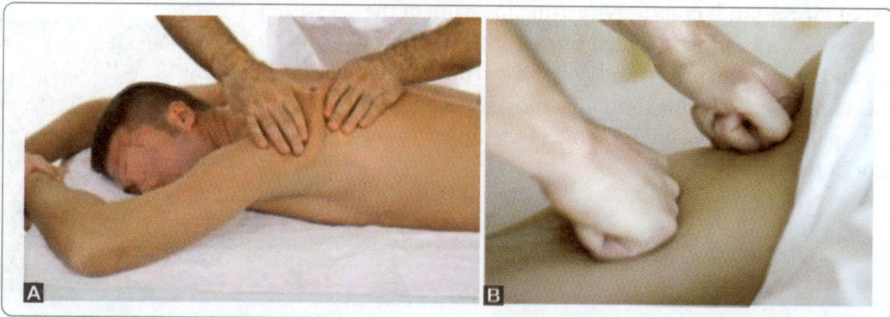

Figures 12A and B: Petrissage or kneading

Unit IV ❖ Basic Needs of the Patient

■ **Friction:** It is performed with the whole palmar surface of the hand or fingers and thumbs over limited areas. This movement is a circular form of kneading with pressure against the underlying part of tissue which cannot be grasped. Use circular thumb strokes to move from buttocks to shoulders; then using a smooth stroke, return to the buttocks (Figs 13A and B).

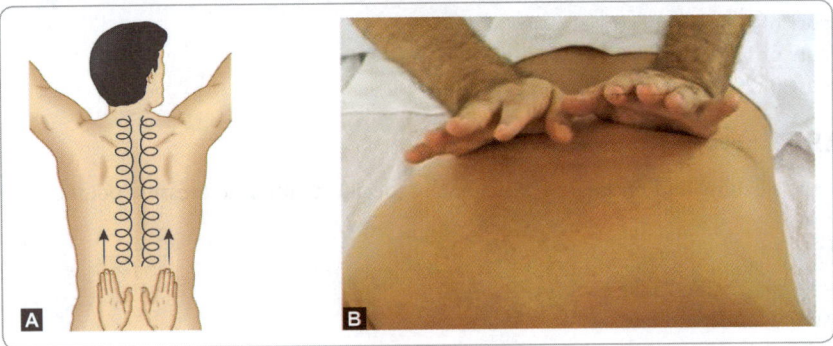

Figures 13A and B: Friction

■ **Tapotement or tapping:** It is movement produced by using the ulnar edge of the hand to stimulate circulation. It is a rhythmic percussion, most frequently administered with the edge of the hand, a cupped hand or the tips of the fingers. It includes hacking, cupping, pincement (pinching) and tapping and is performed with a light, fast tempo (Fig. 14).

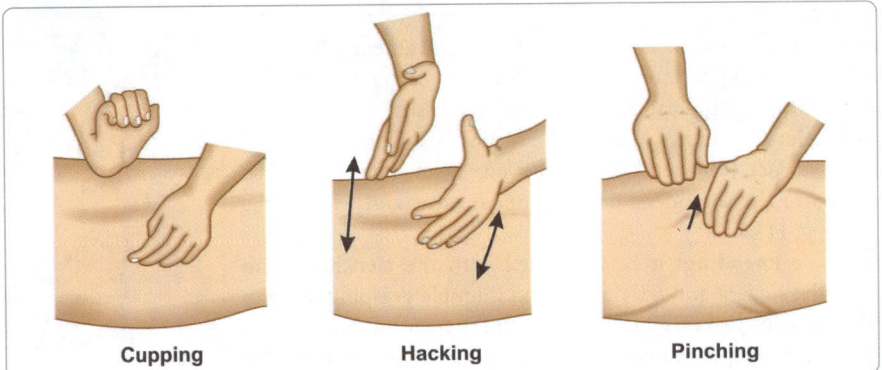

Cupping   Hacking   Pinching

Figure 14: Tapotement

■ **Vibrasi or vibration:** It is an activity using the palm of the hand to provide vibration in which tissues of the body are pressed and released in an 'up and down' movement. This often takes the form of a fine trembling movement applied using the palmar surfaces or just some of the fingertips of either or both hands (Fig. 15).

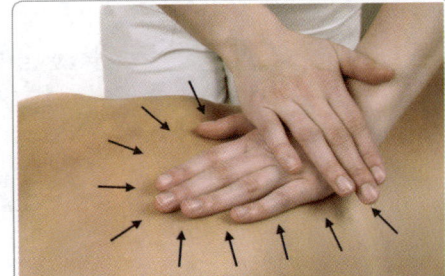

Figure 15: Vibrasi or vibration

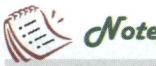

Note

- When performing effleurage and friction, keep your hands parallel to the vertebrae to avoid tickling the patient.
- For all the strokes, maintain a regular rhythm and steady contact with the patients back to help him relax.
- Perform each stroke at least six times before moving on to the next.
- Start with effleurage, go on to friction, then to petrissage and then to tapotement.

Requisites

A tray containing:

Articles	Purpose
Basin with warm water	For cleansing the back
Bucket	For receiving the waste water
Soap with soap dish	For cleansing the back
Face towel	For wiping the back
A bowl containing sponge cloth—2	1 for cleansing with soap and 1 for cleansing with warm water
Mackintosh	For spreading under the back to prevent soiling of linen
Big Towel	For covering the mackintosh
Oil/Lotion/Powder/other agents	For massaging the back
Gloves	To prevent cross infection
Kidney tray	To collect the soiled waste
Hand washing articles	For washing hands

Agents Used for Back Massage

- **Lotions or emollients:** Lotions and emollients reduce friction and lubricate the skin. They are appropriate for most patients, especially those with a tendency toward dry skin; that is, elderly patients.
- **Massage oil**
- **Rubbing alcohol:** Alcohol evaporates quickly, so it has a cooling but very drying effect. As certain amount of alcohol is absorbed by the skin, it should not be used on infants, elderly patients, or patients with liver disease.
- **Powder:** Powder reduces friction but also has a drying effect on the skin. It may be appropriate for those patients who perspire freely and/or are confined to bed.

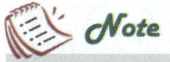

Note

General Guidelines
- A back massage should take about five to ten minutes.
- It can be given with the patient's bath, before bedtime, or at any other time during the day.
- Determine if any patient allergies or skin sensitivities exist before applying lotion to the patient's skin.
- The greatest relaxation effect of a massage occurs when the rhythm of the massage is coordinated with the patient's breathing.
- When massaging the patient's back, stand with one foot slightly forward and slightly bent the knees to allow effective use of the arm and shoulder muscles.

Unit IV ❖ **Basic Needs of the Patient**

Procedure

Steps	Procedure	Rationale
1.	Explain the procedure to the patient.	Helps to win confidence and cooperation of the patient.
2.	Perform hand hygiene	Hand washing deters the spread of microorganisms.
3.	Provide privacy. Close curtain or door.	Privacy increases relaxation
4.	Assist the patient to the prone position or side – lying position with the back exposed from the shoulders to the sacral area. Move the client near toward you.	This position exposes an adequate area for massage with privacy and warmth maintained.
5.	Untie the patients, gown and expose the patient's shoulders, back and the sacral region. Use the bath blanket to drape the patient. Raise the bed to the high position and lower the side rail closest to you. Put off the fan. 	Draping the patient prevents chills and minimizes exposure. Having the bed in the high position reduces back strain for the nurse. Putting off the fan prevents drought and chills.
6.	Assemble all the necessary equipment at the bed side of the patient. 	Organization facilitates accurate skill performance
7.	Don gloves.	Prevents cross contamination
8.	Place the mackintosh and a towel under the clients back.	Prevents wetting and soiling of linen.
9.	Warm the lubricant or lotion in the palm of your hand or place the container in warm water.	Cold lotion causes chilling and uncomfortable sensation.

Contd...

Steps	Procedure	Rationale
10.	Fold the wash cloth around your hand to form a mitten.	This prevents the loose ends of the cloth from dripping water onto the patient.
11.	Lather soap by sponge towel or the mitt. Wipe with soap and clean the back using gentle strokes. Use another sponge cloth and rinse the back with plain warm water until the soap is removed. Pat dry the back using a face towel. 	Facilitates cleaning the back before massaging with oil/ lotion/ powder.
12.	Put some lotion or oil into your palm. Apply the oil or the lotion and massage at least 3–5 minutes by placing the palms: • From sacral region to neck • From upper shoulder to the lowest parts of buttocks Don't apply oil or lotion directly to the back skin. Too much application of oil may bring irritation and discomfort. 	Lotion or oil reduces friction during back massaging.
13.	Apply lotion to patient's shoulders, back and sacral area using light gliding strokes (effleurage). 	Effleurage relaxes the patient and lessens tension.

Contd...

Unit IV ❖ **Basic Needs of the Patient**

Steps	Procedure	Rationale
14.	Place your hands beside each other at the base of the patient's spine and stroke upward to the shoulders and back downward to the buttocks in slow, continuous strokes. Continue for several minutes.	Continuous contact stimulates circulation and muscle relaxation. It also soothes.
15.	Massage the patient's shoulders, entire back, areas over iliac crests, and sacrum with circular stroking motion (Friction). Keep your hands in contact with the patient's skin. Continue for several minutes, applying additional lotion as necessary.	Continuous contact with a firmer stroke promotes relaxation.
16.	Gently knead the patient's skin by alternating grasping and compression motions (Petrissage).	Kneading increases blood circulation to areas.
17.	Continue rhythmic percussion with the edge of the hand, a cupped hand or the tips of the fingers (Tapotement).	Tapotement promotes muscular and systemic relaxation and desensitization of irritated nerve endings.

Contd...

Steps	Procedure	Rationale
18.	Complete the massage with additional long stroking movements. 	Long stroking motion is soothing and promotes relaxation.
19.	During massage, observe the patient's skin for reddened or open areas. Pay particular attention to the skin over bony prominences. 	Pressure may interfere with circulation and lead to development of decubitus ulcers. Back rub stimulates circulation to these areas.
20.	Use the towel to pat the patient dry and to remove excess lotion. Apply powder if the patient requests it.	This provides additional comfort for the patient
21.	Help the client to put on the clothes and return the client to comfortable position.	This provides warmth and comfort
22.	Replace all equipment in proper place.	Helps to prepare for the next procedure
23.	Remove gloves and discard. Perform hand hygiene.	To deter the spread of microorganisms.
24.	Document the patient's response and record your observations on the patient's chart including date, time and the skin condition. Record redness, abrasion or any change in the skin condition	Documentation provides coordination of care

NAIL CARE

Nail care is the care of the fingernails and toenails.

Purposes of Nail Care

Nail care is an important part of the client's personal care.

- It gives the client a neat appearance.
- It prevents scratches from long nails.
- Cleaning under the nails decreases bacterial growth that could cause infections.
- Good nail care plays an integral role in helping the client feel well groomed.
- It helps a nurse to use this time to talk with the client and meet the client's emotional needs as well.

Specific Measures Related to Nail Care

- The best time to perform nail care is after the client's bath.
- Nail care can also be given after soaking the hands or feet in a basin of warm water for 10-15 minutes to soften the nails.
- Ensure proper lighting when giving nail care.
- Fingernails should be cleaned every day.
- Fingernails are usually shaped with a slightly rounded edge.
- Trim toenails straight across.
- Do not trim the nails too close to the flesh.
- Use clippers rather than scissors.

Prerequisites

- Assess the patient's ability to self -care.
- Inspect all skin surfaces particularly between the toes for cleanliness, odor, dryness, inflammation, swelling, abrasions or other lesions.
- In case of unconscious or bed ridden patient, perform the procedure on the bed.
- Provide privacy if needed.

Requisites

Articles	Purpose
Basin or tub with warm water	For soaking the nails
Mackintosh	To prevent soiling of linen
Towel—2	One to spread on the mackintosh. Another to dry the hands or toes
Nail clippers or scissors (optional), nail file or orange wood stick	For nail care
Gloves	To prevent cross infection
Kidney tray	To collect the waste and nails
Bowl with cotton swabs	To clean the dirt after cutting the nails
Soap with soap dish (as required)	For cleansing the nails
Lotion or Vaseline	For lubrication.

Procedure

Steps	Procedure	Rationale
1.	Explain the procedure to the patient	Explanation fosters cooperation.
2.	Gather necessary equipment.	Organization facilitates accurate skill performance
3.	Perform hand hygiene. Don gloves.	Prevents spread of microorganisms
4.	If client is in bed, raise the backrest and assist the patient to sit in upright position. If the client is in a chair, place a table in front. 	Proper positioning promotes comfort.
5.	Place a Mackintosh and towel under the hand or toe.	Prevents soiling of linen
6.	Place a basin of warm, soapy water at 100°–110°F (38°–44°C) on the towel. Soak the fingers or toes in the warm, soapy water for 5–10 minutes. Soak one hand at a time or soak both at the same time. 	Makes nail soft.

Contd...

Unit IV ❖ Basic Needs of the Patient

Steps	Procedure	Rationale

1. Perform the beginning procedure actions. Soak each foot in a basin of warm water for 10 or 15 minutes.

2. Dry the foot well and look for any red or open areas. Use an orange-wood stick to clean under the toenails.

3. Apply lotion to the feet, especrfally the heels. Do not put lotion between the toes since it will be difficult to rub it in completely. Perform the ending procedure actions.

Steps	Procedure	Rationale
7.	Rinse hands with clear, warm water. Remove basin when finished soaking. Dry with the towel. If the client has just been bathed, the above step can be omitted.	Makes nails soft and prevents water causing interference during procedure.
8.	Place a kidney tray on the mackintosh and towel. Hold a cotton swab under the nails and place the patients hand over the kidney tray. Cut short the finger nails with nail clippers rounding the corners. Trim nails if needed. Ensure that the skin is not injured while trimming. Cut toe nails straight across and do not round off the corners.	Cutting the corners in toe nails causes growth of ingrown nails
9.	Gently remove dirt from around and under each fingernail. Wipe all nails side by side using a wet cotton ball. Use one cotton ball for one finger.	Prevents transmission of infection
10.	Rub lotion on hands and toes. Repeat the steps for the other hand and toe.	Promotes softening of foot and hands.
11.	Remove, clean, and store equipment. Place soiled linen in laundry bag. Place the patient in comfortable position.	Prepare equipment for the next procedure.
12.	Doff gloves and wash your hands.	Prevent spread of infection.
13.	Document in patient's record about the procedure and patient's response to procedure. Report anything unusual to nurse/supervisor like redness, swelling or other signs of infection around the nails.	Documentation fosters quality care.

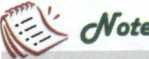 *Note*

- Patients with diabetes mellitus or peripheral vascular disease should be observed for adequate circulation of the feet.
- Care of hands and feet can be done along with the morning bath or at another convenient time.

Unit IV ❖ Basic Needs of the Patient

Nutritional Needs of the Patient

IMPORTANCE OF DIET

In Health

A person cannot exist for long without taking some form of nourishment. Food is the fuel with which we run our bodies. It is necessary for the growth and maintenance of bones and other tissues and for the regulations of all body processes. In order to function at optimal level, a person must consume adequate amounts of foods containing the nutrients considered essential for a human life. A nutrient is defined as any chemical substance found in foods that functions in one or more of the ways mentioned above. The amount considered adequate will of course vary from one individual to another, depending on age, sex, current physical status, lifestyle, physical environment and many other factors. The essential nutrients are carbohydrates, proteins, fats, vitamins, minerals and water.

In Diseases

Food as a source of nourishment is particularly important for those who are ill. Nearly all sick persons come across disturbances in gastrointestinal functioning. They may lose their appetite or be unable to tolerate food and fluids: there may be a problem in the digestion of food or in the absorption of nutrients from the gastrointestinal tract. Whatever the problem is, the sick person's nutritional needs are usually different from those of the healthy. Lack of exercise because of illness may decrease the body's need for energy giving foods but at the same time, there is a greater need for tissue-building nutrients.

 Stimulant

Benefits of Good Nutrition
The benefits of good nutrition go beyond weight. It can help:
- Reduces the risk of some diseases, including heart disease, diabetes, stroke, some cancers, and osteoporosis
- Reduces high blood pressure
- Lowers high cholesterol
- Improves well-being
- Improves ability to fight off illness
- Improves ability to recover from illness or injury
- Increases energy level

NURSE'S ROLE IN MAINTAINING GOOD NUTRITION

In hospital, usually dietician is responsible for planning meals for the patient. But on certain occasion, nurse may have to plan diet, as in a private nursing home. The nurse is responsible for observing and reporting the condition of appetite, patient's likes and dislikes for food, and can discuss it further with the doctor or dietician while planning the diet for patients. One of the other responsibilities of the nurse is to see that the patient gets the proper diet at the proper time and to note whether patient is taking the food and to give necessary help in feeding the helpless patients. He/she has to find out whether the patient is allergic to any food and should report to the person responsible for planning the diet.

Unit IV ❖ Basic Needs of the Patient

He/she can guide in planning diet on the basis of the general health needs of the patient and the family budget prior to his/her discharge from the hospital. The patient or the family member should be informed about the plan. It is the responsibility of the nurse to make the patient comfortable and surroundings pleasant at meal time.

The salient points to be observed by the nurse in maintaining good nutrition are depicted in Figure 1.

Preparation of the Environment

- The room or ward should be well ventilated, quiet and in order during meals.
- As far as possible all disturbing sights should be removed.
- Bed should be comfortable and in order.
- All unappetising objects like sputum cups and bedpans should be out of sight.
- The bedside locker and the food-serving tray should be set as attractive as possible.

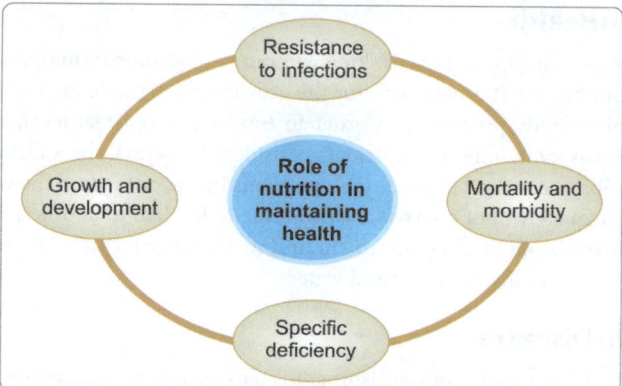

Figure 1: Role of nutrition in maintaining health

- Over bed tables whenever available should be used instead of bedside lockers.
- All equipment used for carrying out medical treatment or nursing procedure should be removed from the room or from the sight of the patient before serving meals.
- In every case, the food should be placed in front of the patient who is in a comfortable position.
- Ambulatory patients should be encouraged to eat in groups around a table (dining hall) where facilities are available.

Preparation of the Patient

- Make the patient as comfortable as possible in bed.
- Offer bedpan or urinal about half an hour before serving meals.
- Help him to feel fresh by washing hands, face and mouth.
- See that the patient is properly dressed up including hair.
- Bed linen should be straightened.
- If he/she is allowed to sit up, prop him/her up on a backrest and protect the chest with a towel.
- See that the dressings or painful treatments are finished at least an hour before meal is served.

Serving Diet

There is an old saying "that whoever is preparing the food, the one who serves it, should be a pleasing person."
- Meals should be served at regular time in order to make it more appetizing.
- If late, it may cause loss of appetite and lack of interest to eat food.
- The diet, which he/she likes best should be served as far as possible.
- The diet served must be suitable to the digestion of the individual and at the same time it should meet the requirements of the individual.
- Small servings are more appetizing than large servings.
- The tray should be large enough to hold the contents.
- It must be attractive.

- The food must be hot and tasty.
- Utensils used for serving meal must be scrupulously clean.
- Hot food should be served as hot and cold as cold.
- If the patient is able to sit up, help him/her to sit up in a convenient position.
- Keep the tray on the over bed table or on the bed side table.
- Remove the cover and hand it over to the patient or place everything in a convenient position.
- Complaint concerning food or food service should be given prompt attention.

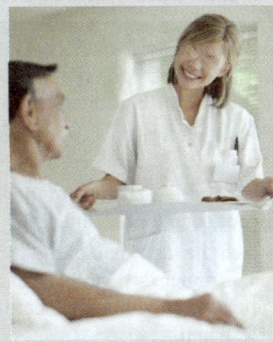

- Check the menu and patient's name on wrist band.
- Spread towel over patient's chest to catch food spills
- Help the patient to feed self by removing covers
- Do not accept any eatable from the patient and return unconsumed food to dietary department for disposal
- Remove the overbed table, collect the articles, raise the side-rails and make the patient comfortable
- Leave the unit tidy and clean

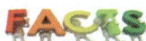

Conditions that Favor the Appetite and Digestion
- Sight and smell of food
- Food preference (likes and dislikes) of the individual
- Freedom from hurry, worry, pain, stress and fatigue
- Pleasant environment (attractive surroundings and a cheerful atmosphere) helps digestion and absorption
- Regularity in eating
- Spacing of meals (interval between feeds)
- Exercises

EXTRA ORAL/ARTIFICIAL FEEDING

Feeding given other than through mouth is called extra oral/artificial feeding.

General Rules in Artificial Feeding

- Make sure that there is Doctor's order for feeding.
- Explain the treatment to the patient if he is conscious and capable of understanding what is being carried out.
- Never apply undue pressure while passing the tube which can cause unnecessary pain to the patient.
- Temperature of the feed should be 90–100°F.
- Measure and strain the fluid to avoid blocking of the tube during the feeding.
- Special attention should be given to oral hygiene of the patient.
- Give well-balanced fluid food as far as possible, especially if the patient is on artificial feeding for a long period.
- Keep the patient either sitting or lying position conveniently while feeding.

Common fluids given: Milk and milk beverages, fruit juice, etc.

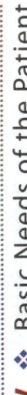

Unit IV ❖ Basic Needs of the Patient

Different Methods of Artificial Feeding

- Nasal feeding or nasal gavage.
- **Gastric gavage:** Feeding through orogastric tube.
- Gastrostomy and enterostomy feeding.
- Rectal feeding.
- IV Infusion (nutritive) or Total parenteral nutrition (TPN)

Differentiating the Placement of a Nasal Tube and Gastric Tube while Inserting

Digestive tract	Respiratory tract
During the insertion of the tube, the patient will experience no distress in breathing	The patient may experience dyspnea, violent cough and cyanosis if the tube is in the respiratory tract
The patient will have no difficulty in talking, if the tube is in the digestive tract	The patient will not be able to talk, if the tube has passed through the vocal cord
Listen to the distal end of the tube. No noise will be heard except a gurgling sound, if the tube has reached the stomach	A whistling sound is heard, if the tube is in the respiratory tract
Attach the distal end of the tube to a syringe barrel or a funnel and invert it into a glass of water. A few bubbles initially or no bubbles indicate that the tube is in the digestive tract	A steady stream of air bubbles indicate that the tube is in the respiratory tract
Attach a syringe to the distal end of the tube and aspirate. Some gastric fluid may be withdrawn	No fluid will be withdrawn if the tube is in the respiratory tract
Listen over the stomach with a stethoscope while injecting a small quantity (10 mL) of air into the tube. Sound of air entering in the stomach can be heard	No sound will be heard

Nasal Feeding or Nasal Gavage (NG)

The administration of liquid foods into stomach by a tube inserted through the nostril is called nasal feeding or nasal gavage.

Indications

- When patient refuses food, e.g., hysteria and mental conditions.
- When condition of the mouth or esophagus makes swallowing difficult or impossible, e.g., cleft palate, foreign body in throat, paralysis of pharynx.
- When operations in the mouth make it desirable to keep it clean, dry and as inactive as possible, e.g., mandibulectomy.
- When the patient is unconscious.
- Premature babies who may be weak and unable to suck.

Preliminary Assessment of Patient and Situation

- Recognize the patient by his/her identification band.
- Check the doctor's order to note the specific instructions about the tube feeding, precautions in the movement or positions of the patient, etc.
- Get the instructions from the senior sister and any help, if required.
- Check the consciousness and ability of the patient to understand and self-help.
- See that the required feed is ready.
- Check the articles available in the ward.
- Assess the reaction of the patient to tube feeding and his/her need for feeding according to the time of the day.

Requisites

A clean tray containing:

Article	Purposes
Nasal tube (catheter No. 7 or 8), funnel, glass connection and rubber tubing, Levin tube or *Ryle's tube* or Nasal tube (short) and clip for the tubing boiled and kept in a bowl of cold water	For nasogastric tube feeding To stiffen the tube
Required amount of feed in a graduated measure standing in a bowl of warm water	For feeding the patient
Lubricant such as water soluble jelly or glycerine or liquid paraffin	To prevent friction between mucous membrane and tube
Clean water in a container	To administer after introducing and after feeding
Mouth wash in a feeding cup	For providing mouth care after feeding
Clean water in a bowl, stethoscope, syringe	To test the location of the tube
Swab sticks	To clean the nostrils
Saline or soda bicarb solution 1% in a bowl	To clean the nose
Rag pieces or cotton swabs in bowl (wet swabs)	To wipe the secretions, if any
Kidney tray	For collecting waste and to give mouth wash before and after feed
Mackintosh and towel	To protect patient's cloths and linen
Adhesive plaster and scissors	To fix the tube in position
20 mL syringe	For feeding

Ryle's tube: A thin tube with a weighted end, introduced via the nose into the stomach. It may be used for the withdrawal of gastric contents or for the administration of the fluids (Fig. 2).

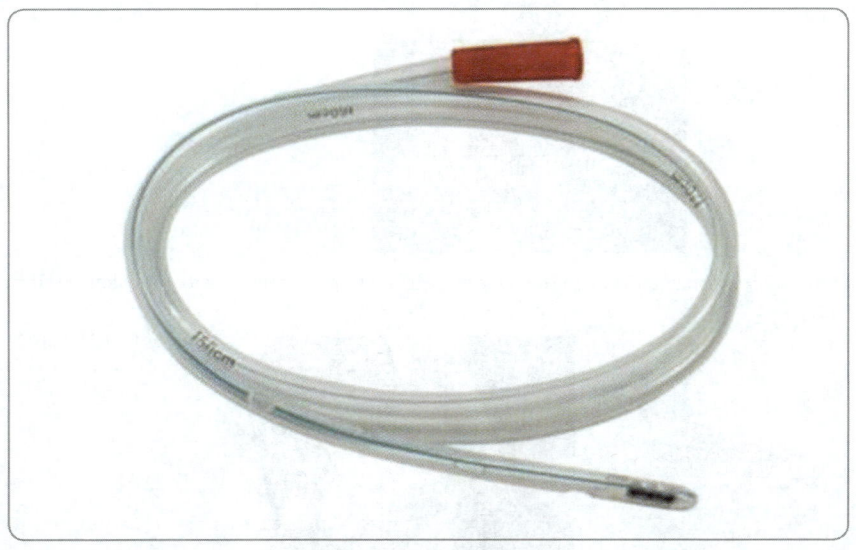

Figure 2: Ryle's tube

Unit IV ❖ Basic Needs of the Patient

Table 1: Size chart of Ryle's tube

CH/FR	6	8	10	12	14	16	18	20	22
Color name	LIght green	Blue	Black	White	Green	Orange	Red	Yellow	Purple
Connector color									
OD	2.0 mm	2.7 mm	3.3 mm	4.0 mm	4.7 mm	5.3 mm	6.0 mm	6.7 mm	7.3 mm

Abbreviations: CH, after the name of inventor, Cherriere; FR, French scale; OD, outside diameter

Levin tube: Levin tube is a single lumen, small bore NG tube used for the aspiration of gastric and intestinal contents and administration of tube feedings or medications (Fig. 3).

Preparation of Patient

- Explain the procedure to the patient and ask for patient's cooperation.
- Provide privacy.
- Place the patient in Fowler's position, make the patient comfortable.
- Clean the nostrils, if there is secretion or crust formation, using swab stick dipped in saline or soda bicarb solution.
- Give a mouth wash and help him/her to clean the teeth.

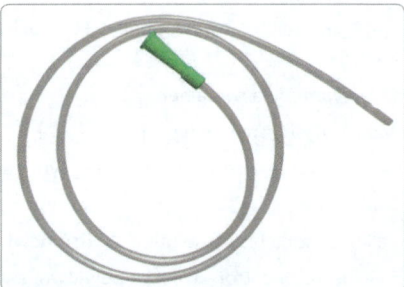

Figure 3: Levin tube

Procedure

Steps	Procedure	Rationale
1.	Explain the procedure to the patient if conscious. Adjust position (sitting or dorsal recumbent)	Proper explanation allays anxiety and ensures cooperation
2.	Screen the patient	Provides privacy and prevents embarrassment
3.	Assemble the equipment at the bedside	Organization facilitates skill performance
4.	Place the mackintosh and towel on the patient's chest. Place a kidney tray to the side	Prevents soiling of the patient's clothes and linen during the procedure by Nasal and oral secretions

Contd...

Steps	Procedure	Rationale
5.	Wash hands. Don gloves	Prevents the transmission of microorganisms.
6.	Elevate head end of the bed to 45°	Head elevation promotes safety during tube insertion
7.	Inspect the nasal and oral cavities for infection or skin breakdown. Assess the best nostril for insertion by occluding one side. If there is no blockage proceed	Assessment facilitates appropriate selection of the insertion site
8.	Measure the distance of the tube from the tip of the nose to the earlobe and from there to the tip of the Xiphoid process of the sternum and mark there. Mark this point	Determines the appropriate length of NG tube to be inserted

Tape masking tube length

Contd...

Unit IV ❖ Basic Needs of the Patient

Steps	Procedure	Rationale
9.	Clean the nostrils by using saline or soda bicarb solution with the swab stick	Prevents spread of infection
10.	Lubricate the tip of the tube using water-soluble lubricating jelly of about 6 to 8 inches with the lubricant using rag pieces. Or you can inject the jelly into the nose. Never use non-water-soluble lubricant (e.g., Vaseline), as it will not dissolve and may cause respiratory complications if it enters the lungs	Lubrication facilitates easy entry of the tube
11.	Pass the tube that is coiled around your hands through the nostril, gently but quickly in a backward and downward direction 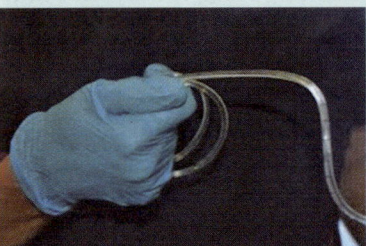 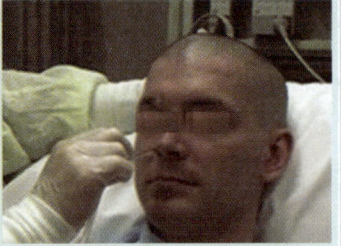 When it reaches the pharynx, some resistance may be felt. The patient's head may be slightly inclined forward and the tube passed gently till the mark When the tube is in the esophagus, irritation in the pharynx will cease. See that it has not come forward and curved up in the mouth. If it has gone into the trachea, patient may choke, cough and may become cyanosed. If the patient is conscious, advise him/her to swallow	Inclining the head forward closes the trachea and opens the esophagus, which allows the NG tube to pass more easily through the nasopharynx and into the stomach

Contd...

Steps	Procedure	Rationale
12.	Advance NG tube until you reach the mark/tape you had placed for measurement 	Ensures accurate placement
13.	**Verify tube placement** Make sure that it is in the right passage by: • Immersing the end of the tube in water for any air bubbles • Aspirate sample of gastric contents by attaching syringe to free end of the tube. Test the pH of the aspirated contents to ensure that the contents are acidic by a color-coded pH paper. The pH should be below 6 • **Auscultation:** Attach syringe to free end of the tube, place diaphragm of stethoscope over left hypochondrium. Inject 10 mL of air and auscultate abdomen for gushing sound. (But not used many times as it causes abdominal distention) • An X-ray is taken 	This aids in timely recognition and identification of tube displacement or migration

Contd...

Steps	Procedure	Rationale
14.	Close other end of tube with spigot. Secure tube on nose using adhesive in 'T' or butterfly	This keeps the NG tube in place

Step 1: Place the intact half of the tape strip over the bridge of the patient's nose

Step 2: Wrap one end of the split portion of the tape strip around the NGT

Step 3: Wrap the remaining end of the tape strip around the NGT in the opposite direction

Step 4: Place a tape strip over the bridge of the patient's nose horizontally

Steps	Procedure	Rationale
15.	Document the reason for the tube insertion, type and size of tube, the nature and amount of aspirate, the type of suction and pressure setting if for suction, the nature and amount of drainage and the effectiveness of the intervention	Documentation fosters quality care

Gastric Feeding (Gastric Gavage)

Gastric feeding or gastric gavage is the feeding with an orogastric tube passed through the mouth and esophagus into the stomach: (also called esophageal feeding).

(Preliminary assessment and situation is same as that of nasal feeding)

Requisites: As for nasal gavage plus sterile Levine tube or Ryle's tube instead of nasal tube in a bowl of ice water.

Procedure

Steps	Procedure	Rationale
1.	Explain the procedure to the patient if conscious. Adjust position (sitting or dorsal recumbent)	Proper explanation allays anxiety and ensures cooperation
2.	Screen the patient	Provides privacy and prevents embarrassment

Contd...

Steps	Procedure	Rationale
3.	Assemble the equipment at the bedside. Ensure that the feed kept in the container is warm	Organization facilitates skill performance
4.	Place the mackintosh and towel on the patient's chest. Place a kidney tray to the side 	Nasal and oral secretions may soil the patient's clothes and linen during the procedure
5.	Wash hands. Don gloves	Prevents the transmission of microorganisms
6.	Elevate head end of the bed to 45° 	Head elevation enhances gravitational flow of feed through tube and prevents risk of aspiration
7.	Attach syringe and aspirate stomach contents if there is doubt about tube placement 	Confirmation of tube placement promotes safety

Contd...

Unit IV ❖ Basic Needs of the Patient

Steps	Procedure	Rationale
8.	Pinch the feeding tube and attach barrel of feeding syringe to tube. Then connect the funnel and tubing, holding the funnel downwards to prevent the air from entering the stomach	Pinching of feeding tube prevents air from entering the stomach and causing distension
9.	Pinch the tube and hold the funnel upwards and pour some plain water into it and allow this to trickle down, checking the flow by constricting the tubing. The absence of distress will confirm the fact that the tube is not in the trachea. Pour the feed before the funnel is empty. **Keep on pouring feed/formula to barrel when it is three quarters empty, pinch tube whenever necessary**	Water clears the tube. The rate of flow is regulated by raising or lowering the syringe
10.	Document type and amount of feeding, amount of water given, reaction of the patient and tolerance of feed. Record with date, time with signature of the nurse. Record the intake and output chart	Documentation foster quality care
11.	When the feed is finished, pour little water to clear the tube. **Flush tube with at least 30 cc of plain water**	Water prevents clogging of feeding tube

Contd...

Steps	Procedure	Rationale
12.	Pinch the tube close up to the nostril and withdraw it gently and rapidly. Inspect the nostril, dry it and lubricate it, if necessary. When a patient is having nasal feeding at frequent intervals the tube may be left in position. It should be closed at the end of the tubing by a clamp or a knot and fastened to the side temple by means of a piece of adhesive plaster	Prevents leakage
13.	Remove the mackintosh and towel and leave the patient comfortable. **Keep head of bed elevated for 30–60 minutes after feeding.** Leave the patient comfortable Monitor for breath sounds, bowel sounds , gastric distension, diarrhea or constipation	Prevents aspiration Evaluates for aspiration effects on gastrointestinal (GI) system and therapeutic effect of feeding
14.	Wash the articles under cold running water first and then with warm water and soap. Rinse well, boil them and dry and keep in proper place	Prevents Bacterial Growth
15.	Doff gloves and wash hands	Prevents spread of infection

Nasogastric Tube Feeding in Kids has been Shown in Images as follows (Figs 4A to F). If the NG Tube is Connected to the Feeding Bag, Fill the Feeding Bag with the Liquid Food and Then Connect to the NG Tube

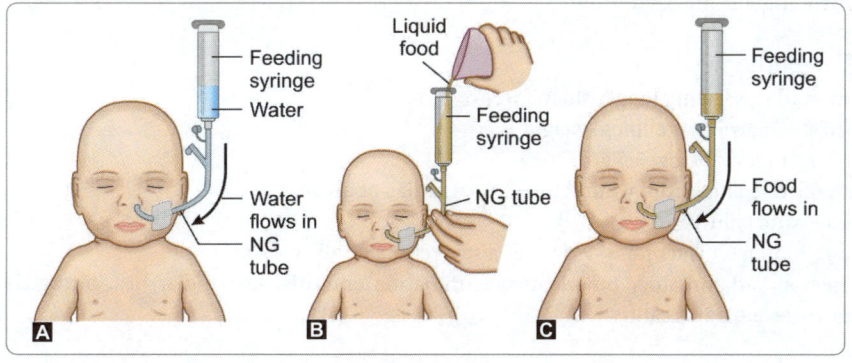

Figures 4A to C:

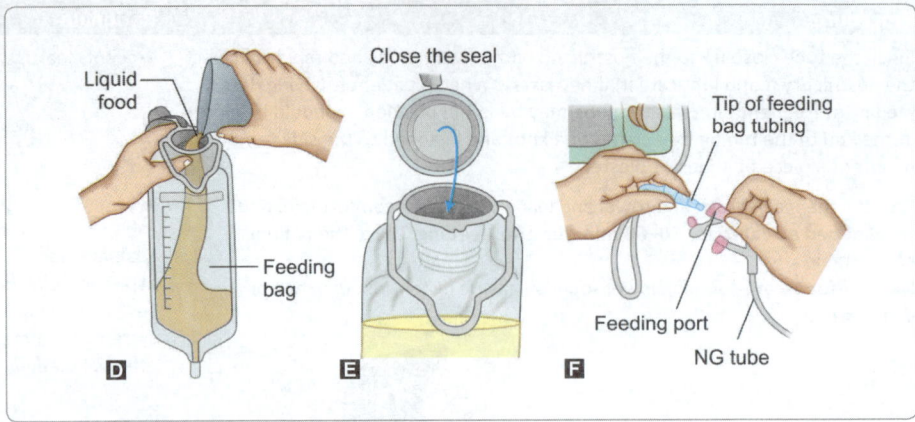

Figures 4A to F: NG procedure in kids

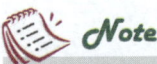

Note

- Avoid the entrance of air while feeding.
- Only strained fluids should be used.
- The feed should be warm.
- Be careful not to introduce the tube into the trachea.
- The nostrils should be cleaned before and after giving feed.

Total parenteral Nutrition (TPN)

When a patient can't meet his nutritional needs by oral or enteral feedings, he/she may require intravenous nutrition support or otherwise called as parenteral nutrition.

Total Parenteral Nutrition (TPN): Also known as parenteral nutrition (PN) is a form of nutritional support given completely via the bloodstream, intravenously with an IV pump.

Aims:

- To prevent and restore nutritional deficits, allowing bowel rest
- To supply adequate caloric intake and essential nutrients
- To remove antigenic mucosal stimuli

Indications:

- Debilitation illness lasting longer than 2 weeks
- Loss of 10% or more of preillness weight
- Serum albumin level below 3.5 g/dL
- Excessive nitrogen loss from wound infection, fistulas or abscess
- Renal or hepatic failure
- A nonfunctioning GI tract for 5–7 days in a severely catabolic patient
- Illness such as inflammatory bowel disease, radiation enteritis, severe diarrhea, intractable vomiting, moderate to severe pancreatitis

Unit IV ❖ Basic Needs of the Patient

- Major procedures like massive small bowel resection, bone marrow transplantation, high dose chemotherapy or radiation therapy, major surgery
  - Infants with congenital or acquired disorders like tracheoesophageal fistula, gastroschisis, duodenal atresia, cystic fibrosis, meconium ileus, diaphragmatic hernia, volvulus, malrotation of the gut, annular pancreas.

Candidates for TPN

- Patients with paralyzed or nonfunctional GI tract, or conditions that require bowel rest, such as small bowel obstruction, ulcerative colitis, or pancreatitis
- Patients who have had nothing by mouth (NPO) for 7 days or longer
- Critically ill patients
- Babies with an immature gastrointestinal system or congenital malformations
- Patients with chronic or extreme malnutrition, or chronic diarrhea or vomiting with a need for surgery or chemotherapy
- Patients in hyperbolic states, such as burns, sepsis, or trauma

Types of TPN

Parenteral nutrition has two types:

1. **Central parenteral nutrition** is the intravenous infusion of water, protein, carbohydrates, electrolytes, minerals and vitamins through a central vein.
2. **Peripheral parenteral nutrition** is the infusion of nutrients into the smaller peripheral veins.

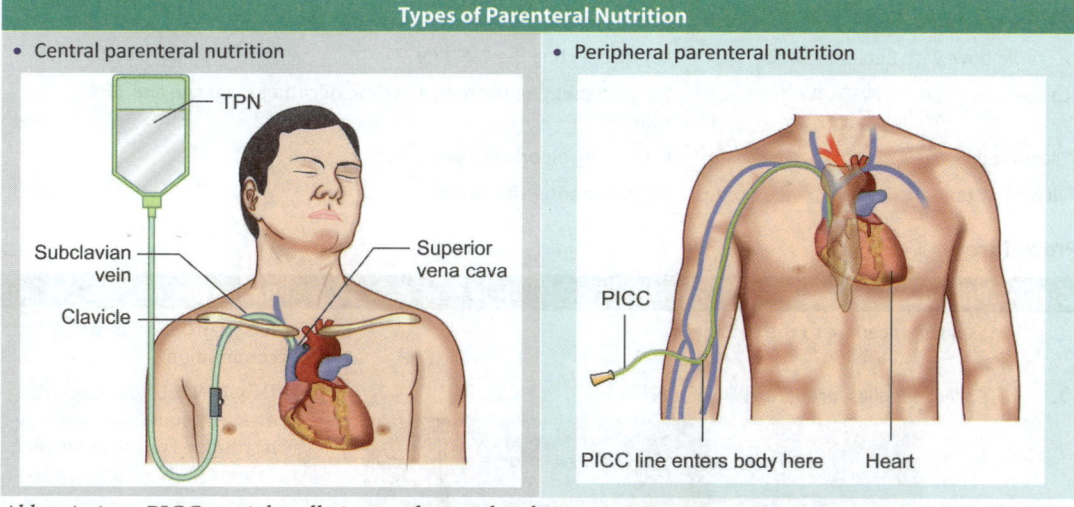

Types of Parenteral Nutrition

- Central parenteral nutrition
- Peripheral parenteral nutrition

Abbreviations: PICC, peripherally inserted central catheter

Types of TPN Solutions

- Dextrose water, electrolytes—D_5W, $D_{10}W$, $D_{25}W$
- Crystalline amino acids—2.5–8.5%
- Electrolytes, vitamins, trace elements, insulin
- Lipid emulsions 10%–20%

Unit IV ❖ Basic Needs of the Patient

Preliminary Assessment

- Review physician's orders and compare to medication administration record medication administration record (MAR) and content label on TPN solution bag and for rate of infusion. Each component of the TPN solution must be verified with the physician's orders.
- Check date and time of last TPN tubing change, lab values and expiry date of TPN to prevent medication error.
- Inspect the solution for cloudiness or presence of particles.
- Remove the ordered TPN solution from the refrigerator 1 hour before use, and check the proposed rate. (cold cause pain, hypothermia, and venous spasm and constriction)
- The solution must be used within 24 hours of preparation.

Articles Required

A tray containing:

Articles	Purpose
TPN solution	For administration of TPN
TPN tubing and set	For connecting the TPN solution with central venous catheter central venous catheter (CVC)
Infusion pump	For regulating the flow rate
Syringe and needle	For priming
Normal saline	For priming
Kidney tray/paper bag	For discarding the soiled waste
A sterile bowl with Betadine swab	For disinfecting the CVC line
Labels	For documenting the date and time of catheter change and TPN solution
Glucometer	For testing blood glucose
Vital signs tray	For monitoring vital signs

Procedure

Steps	Procedure	Rationale
1.	Explain procedure to the patient	Allays anxiety and wins cooperation
2.	Collect supplies, prepare TPN solution	New TPN tubing is required every 24 hours or as per Institutions policy to prevent catheter-related bacteremia

Contd...

Steps	Procedure	Rationale
	Change the solution container to the TPN solution ordered.	
3.	Provide privacy by closing the door and put on the screen	Maintains client's self-esteem
4.	Assist the client to a comfortable position	Ensures comfort
5.	Ensure that the tubing has an in-line filter connected at the end of the TPN tubing. Prime IV tubing with filter as per protocol	Ensure tubing is primed correctly to prevent air embolism
6.	Check the TPN solution before administering	Prevents medication errors
7.	Wash hands and wear appropriate PPE	Reduces transmission of microorganisms

Contd...

Unit IV ❖ Basic Needs of the Patient

Steps	Procedure	Rationale
8.	Complete all safety checks for CVC. Ensure that correct placement of the central line catheter by X-ray	This adheres to safety policies related to central line care
9.	If starting TPN for the first time, flush and disinfect CVC lumens as per agency policy. Use strict aseptic technique	Prevents transmission of microorganisms
10.	Ensure that the tubing has an in- line filter connected at the end of the TPN tubing	Infusion pumps must be used with all TPN administration to check air entry, regulate flow rate
	Attach the TPN solution to the IV administration tubing	

Contd...

Steps	Procedure	Rationale
	Insert new TPN solution and IV tubing into infusion pump	

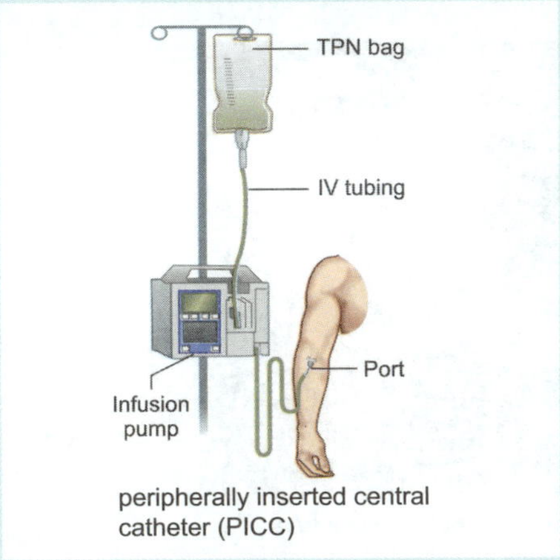

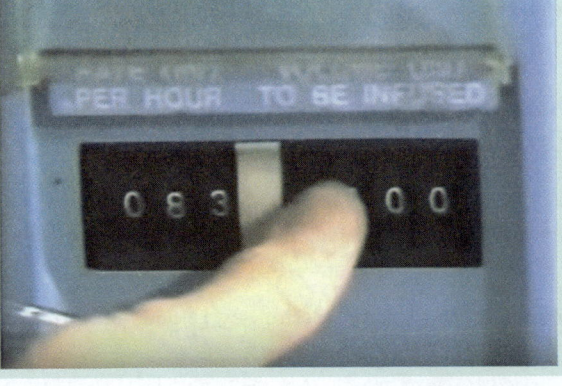

TPN bag

IV tubing

Infusion pump

Port

peripherally inserted central catheter (PICC)

| | Specify the date and time of opening the pack and catheter change | |

| 11. | Start TPN infusion rate as per physician's orders. Regulate and monitor flow rate | Prevents medication errors. Wide fluctuations in blood glucose can occur if the rate of TPN infusion is irregular |

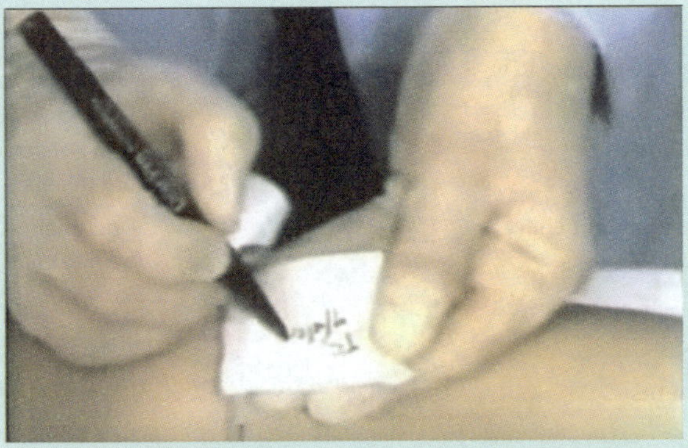

PER HOUR   TO BE INFUSED

0 8 3   0 0

Contd...

Steps	Procedure	Rationale
	Establish the prescribed rate of flow and monitor the infusion at least every 30 minutes Never accelerate an infusion that has fallen behind schedule	
12.	Monitor for signs and symptoms of complications related to TPN	Facilitates early identification of complications and take necessary steps
13.	Discard old supplies as per agency protocol	Ensures use for another patient
14.	Remove gloves and perform hand hygiene	Prevents transfer of micro-organisms
15.	Document the procedure in the patient chart • Type and amount of infusion • Date and time of infusion • Rate of infusion • Vital signs q4h • Anthropometric measurements • Client's weight daily • Fingerstick blood glucose levels • Complications, if any • Patient's response • Along with signature of the nurse	Documentation fosters quality care

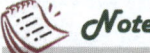 *Note*

Special Considerations
- Always infuse a TPN solution at a constant rate without interruption to avoid blood glucose fluctuations.
- Monitor the patients' vital signs every 4 hours or as often as necessary.
- Change the tubing and filters every 24 hours or as per Institution's policy.
- Closely monitor the catheter site for swelling, which may indicate infiltration.
- Check the patients' blood glucose every 6 hours.
- Record intake output chart daily.
- Monitor the values of laboratory tests, especially serum electrolytes, calcium, BUN, creatinine, albumin and blood glucose levels at least three times in a week.

Contd...

Unit IV ❖ Basic Needs of the Patient

- Weigh the patient at the same time every day preferably in the morning after he voids. Weight should be checked with similar clothing and on the same weighing scale. A gain of more than 0.5 kg/day indicates fluid excess and should be reported.
- Instruct the patient about the potential side effects of TPN. This includes:
  - Hepatic dysfunction
  - Hyperglycemia
  - Hypocalcemia
  - Hypokalemia
  - Hypophosphatemia
  - Hypercapnia
  - Hyperosmolarity
  - Hypoglycemia
  - Hypomagnesemia
  - Zinc deficiency
- Compare the patient's baseline vital signs; electrolyte, glucose and triglyceride levels, weight, and fluid intake and output with treatment values and investigate any rapid change in such values.
- To identify signs of infection early, be aware of the patient's recent temperature range.
- Use strict aseptic technique when caring for central venous catheters and PICC lines.
- Do not use TPN solution if it has coalesced, as evidenced by formation of a thick, dense layer of fat droplets on its surface. If the solution appears abnormal in any way, request a replacement from the pharmacy.
- Never try to catch up with a delayed infusion.
- Parenteral nutrition shouldn't be given to patients with normal functioning GI tract.

Gastrostomy Feeding

Gastrostomy feeding is the introduction of liquid food through a tube or catheter which the surgeon has introduced into the stomach through the abdominal wall (Fig. 5).

Indications

- Tumors or operation on the upper alimentary tract
- Cancer of the esophagus
- Stricture of esophagus caused by poisoning

Purpose

- To give nourishment to the patient
  (Preliminary assessment of patient and situation is same as that of nasal feeding)

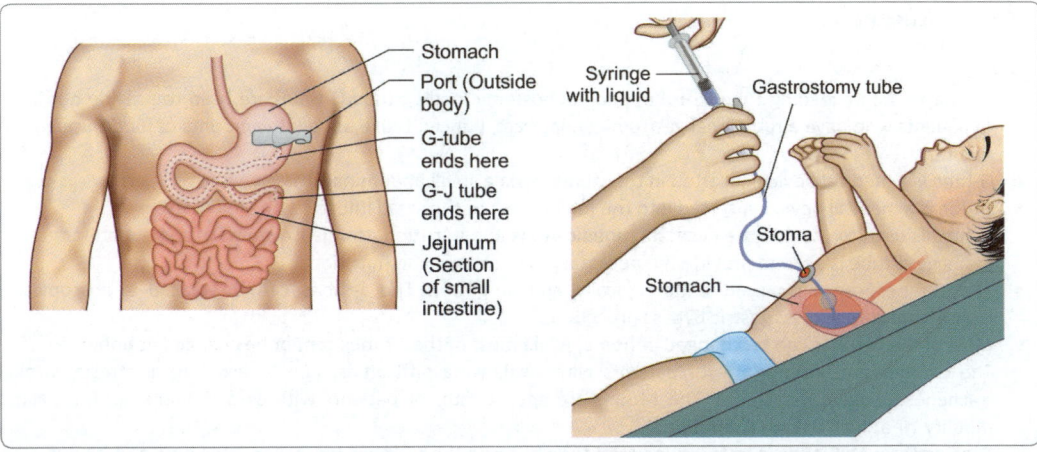

Figure 5: Gastrostomy feeding

Types of Feeding

There are 2 types of feeding with G or G-J tubes. They are:

The G tube or G-J tube is placed in such a way that liquid food or medicine is sent directly to child's stomach or small intestine.

- **Continuous feeding (Fig. 6A):**
    - Liquid food is dripped slowly through the tube for part or all of a day.
    - Continuous feeding can be done into either the stomach or the jejunum.
    - This type of feeding is only done using a pump.
    - The amount of food to be given and time frame are often set on the pump.
- **Bolus feeding (Fig. 6B):**
    - This is a meal-sized amount of liquid food given through the tube several times a day.
    - Bolus feeding is given using a syringe or a pump.
    - Bolus feeding is done into the stomach but not into the jejunum.

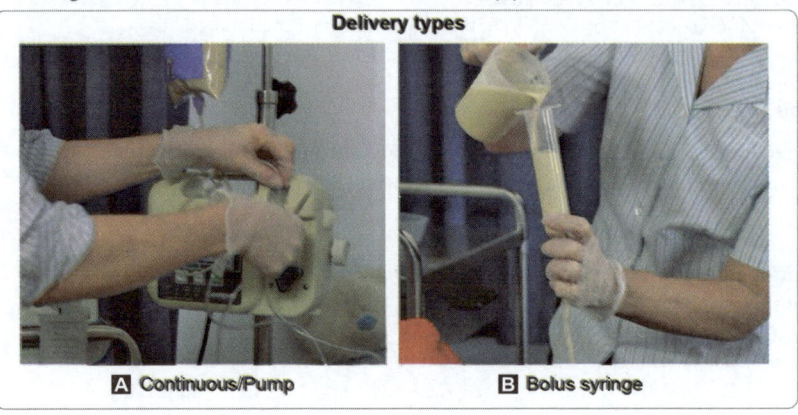

Delivery types

A Continuous/Pump   B Bolus syringe

Figures 6A and B: (A) Continuous feeding; (B) Bolus feeding

 Stimulant

G-tube versus J-tube
- The gastrostomy feeding tube (G-tube) and jejunostomy feeding tube (J-tube) are used to provide nutrients to patients who have a functional gastrointestinal tract, but can't take adequate amounts of food through the mouth.
- G-tube is a medical device, inserted in the stomach via a small abdominal cut.
- J-tube is a medical device, inserted into the middle part of the small intestine (the jejunum).
- G-tube is used to provide the necessary medications and nutrition, to release stomach gases, and for gastric drainage. J-tube is used to provide the necessary medications and nutrition.
- The G-tubes can be placed endoscopically and surgically. The J-tubes can be placed endoscopically, laparoscopically, and via gastric bypass procedure.
- Most of the G-tubes can be changed at home, while most of the J-tubes cannot be changed at home.
- The G-tubes are appropriate for patients with swallowing difficulties, due to esophageal atresia, stroke, tracheoesophageal fistula, etc. The J-tubes are appropriate for patients with chronic vomiting, low gastric motility, or at high risk for aspiration.
- Feeding through G-tube is faster than with J-tube because the stomach has expandable area and fundus.
- A complication of the presence of G-tube and J-tube can be the formation of granulation tissue, which can be irritating, painful and bleed easily. More complication can be expected to result due to the presence of a J-tube.

Requisites

A clean tray containing:

Articles	Purpose
A funnel, rubber tubing, glass connection and a screw clip boiled and kept in covered container	For connecting into the gastrostomy port
Feeding syringe: 20 mL or 50 mL	For administering tube feeding
Extension tubing	For connecting into the gastrostomy port
A cup of drinking water	For irrigating the tube
Required amount of feed in a jug kept in a bowl of warm water (100°F)	For nourishment
Sterile lubricant	To protect the surrounding area from the irritation produced by hydrochloric acid leaking from stomach
Sterile dressing, Many tailed binder and forceps in a sterile tray	For application of sterile dressing
Medicine ordered, if any	For administration along with feeding
Kidney tray	For disposing soiled waste
Small mackintosh and towel	To protect the dress of the patient

Procedure

Steps	Procedure	Rationale
1.	Explain the procedure to the patient	Reduces client's anxiety and increases cooperation
2.	Provide privacy by screening the bed either by putting the curtains or by closing the door	Places client at ease.
3.	Assemble the equipment at the bedside	Promotes efficiency during procedure
4.	Spread the small mackintosh and towel around the wound	Protect the dress and bed of the patient
5.	Observe for abdominal distension and auscultate for bowel sounds	Assessment ensures the clients ability to digest foods
6.	Perform hand hygiene and don gloves	Reduces transmission of pathogens
7.	Remove the dressing and clean the surrounding area and cover the wound with a sterile piece of gauze	Prevents wound infection

Contd...

Unit IV ❖ Basic Needs of the Patient

Steps	Procedure	Rationale
8.	Connect the extension tubing to the feeding port of the G or G-J tube. Make sure the clamp on the extension tubing is closed. Or Keep the tube pinched to prevent air from getting in Figure	Prevents air from entering the tubing
9.	Open the binder or the feeding port cap on the G or G-J tube	Prepares system for tube feeding
10.	Insert the syringe into the port and aspirate the stomach contents. Determine the amount of gastric residual. If the residual is more than 50–100 mL stop feeding until the residual diminishes. Instil the aspirated contents back into the feeding tube	Reduces the risk of regurgitation and pulmonary aspiration. Prevents electrolyte imbalances
11.	Pull the plunger out of the feeding syringe. Connect the feeding syringe to the other end of the extension tubing	Provides system to administer feeding
12.	Pour some clear water into the funnel and lower the funnel a little to let out the air. Hold it at the level of the stomach	Allows gravity to control flow rate

Contd...

Steps	Procedure	Rationale
13.	Open the clamp on the extension tubing 	Allows entry of feeding into the tubing
14.	Then pour the liquid food into the feeding syringe before the funnel is empty. If any medicine is ordered, add into it. Fill only to the amount that was prescribed 	Prevents entry of air thus reduces gaseous distension of stomach
15.	Hold the feeding syringe straight up. Adjust the angle of the feeding syringe to control the flow rate of the food 	Allows the food to run through the G or G-J tube by gravity
16.	If the food flows too slowly or doesn't flow at all, place the plunger in the syringe. Gently push the plunger a bit. Do not push the plunger all the way into the syringe or with force 	Helps remove anything that is blocking or clogging the tube

Contd...

Unit IV ❖ Basic Needs of the Patient

Steps	Procedure	Rationale
17.	After the feeding, flush the extension tubing with water 	Irrigates the tube and prevents the escape of gastric juice
18.	Clamp the tube. Disconnect the syringe from the extension tubing. Disconnect the extension tubing from the G or G-J tube 	Prevents air from entering the tube
19.	Close the feeding port cap on the G or G-J tube. After the feed, instruct the patient to remain quiet in the bed 	Prevents spread of infection
20.	Clean and apply sterile ointment; dress the wound, apply binder. (If required) 	Keeps the wound clean

Contd...

Steps	Procedure	Rationale
21.	Remove the equipment, clean, boil and replace them 	Keeps the articles ready for next procedure
22.	Doff gloves and perform hand hygiene	Prevents risk of transmission of microorganisms
23.	Record the time, kind and amount of feed, response to feeding and condition of the surrounding area. Record in Intake and output chart also	Documentation fosters quality care

Note

- The skin around the wound needs special care. Gastric juice which may leak is very irritating to the skin (because of the hydrochloric acid and enzymes in it) and it prevents the healing of the wound and will cause a very painful inflammation of the tissues. To prevent this condition, the area around the tube must be kept clean and protected by a sterile lubricant.
- The mouth also needs special attention.
- As this method of feeding must often be continued over a prolonged period, the patient should be taught how to insert and remove the tube, the proper care of the tube, care of skin, application of the dressing, the method of feeding and the variety, amount and most suitable food for feeds.
- Try to make the feed as natural as possible by giving the food to taste a little.
- The surroundings should be bright cheerful and pleasant and all efforts should be made to promote good appetite.

Elimination Needs of the Patient

Elimination in this context means the expulsion of waste products from the body by way of the lungs, the skin, the rectum and the urinary bladder.

HEALTH PROBLEMS IN SICKNESS

The problem of disturbed functioning of the gastrointestinal tract is an interference with the elimination of wastes from the tract. Elimination is of course, as vital to the healthy functioning of the human body as the intake of food and fluids.

The human body has the following mechanisms for the removal of waste products:

- From the gastrointestinal tract as feces
- From the urinary tract as urine
- Through the lungs as exhaled air
- Through the skin as perspiration

Each mechanism has its specific function in clearing the body wastes. Wastes eliminated from the gastrointestinal tract contain primarily the food residues and gases that result from the digestion of food.

Interference with the normal functioning of gastrointestinal elimination has serious repercussion on the body's total functioning. The patient is usually uncomfortable and often distressed. If normal functioning is not restored, all body systems will eventually be affected. Complete stoppage of bowel functioning is a medical emergency and surgical intervention is usually necessary to overcome the problem.

CONSTIPATION

Constipation is a very common problem among normal, otherwise, healthy people. Diarrhea is a frequent manifestation of stress and anxiety. Bacterial diarrhea is a part of the problem of gastroenteritis. The loss of essential nutrients and electrolytes by this route makes the problem one of the severe ones. It is particularly serious in infants and young children whose nutritional reserves can soon be depleted by excessive losses from the gastrointestinal tract.

Constipation is the passage of hard, dry stools due to undue delay in the evacuation of feces.

OR

Constipation is the infrequent or difficult evacuation of hard stool requiring much use of the supportive muscles.

Causes

- **Insufficient intake of roughage:** With very little roughage in the diet there is very little residue available to form the bulk of fecal material.
- **Insufficient fluid intake:** When fluids are restricted, the fecal material becomes hard causing difficulty in defecation.
- **Lack of exercise:** When exercise is restricted, normal peristaltic action may be decreased and the muscles of the digestive tract may lose their tone.
- Failure to establish a regular habit of defecation.
- Un-natural position for defecation when patients are confined to bed.
- **Surgery involving the intestines:** Trauma that results from handling of the intestines during the operation may interfere with elimination.

- Any obstruction in the lower bowel may lead to constipation.
- **Nervous tension and worry:** An undesirable mental state may distress vital physical functions so that digestion and elimination are affected.
- **The cathartic or enema habit:** For such people the bowels may not act without artificial stimulation.
- Malformations of the colon.
- Congenital weakness of the muscles of the abdominal wall.
- Pendulous abdominal wall.
- Use of certain drugs, e.g., sedatives.
- Excessive use of coffee or tea.
- Fecal impaction due to excessive absorption of fluid.
- Strange situations and unnatural positions.

Results of Constipation

May or may not give rise to symptoms of distension and local discomfort, headache and inertia; absorption of toxins possible with unhealthy membrane. Pressure on veins at anus and straining may cause hemorrhoids, varicose veins and menstrual pain.

Preventive Measures of Constipation

Removal of the cause is the main point of prevention. The following are some preventive measures of constipation:

- Diet containing foods that leave sufficient residue in the bowel.
- Sufficient amount of fluid intake every day.
- Reasonable freedom from stress and strain.
- Making an effort to empty the rectum at the same time or times every day.
- Sufficient exercise to maintain a normal tone of the muscles used in defecation.
- Squatting posture or the one that makes pressure on the bowel content as far as possible and provide privacy.
- Removal of the obstruction that prevents elimination.
- Use of laxatives or suppositories or enema according to the order of the doctor.

ENEMA

Enema is an injection of fluid into the lower bowel through the rectum for the purpose of cleaning or providing medication or nourishment. The types of enema have been given in Figure 1.

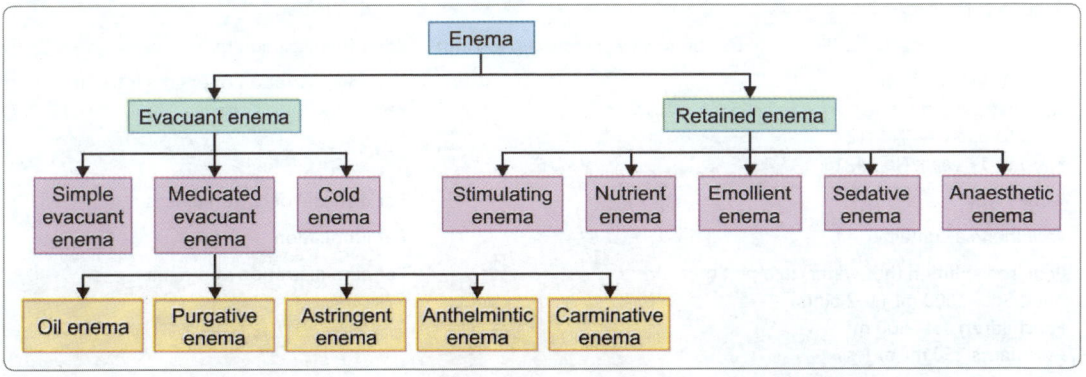

Figure 1: Types of enema

Unit IV ❖ Basic Needs of the Patient

Evacuant Enema or Cleansing Enema

Evacuant enema or cleansing enema is also called 'clyster' as it is derived from the Greek word, 'klysis', which means washing out of waste or stagnant material by means of injection of fluid.

Simple Evacuant Enema

Solutions used:

- Warm water
- **Soap and water:** Liquid soap 50 mL to 1 L of water or add soap in warm water till the color of solution resembles like diluted rice water.
- **Normal saline:** Sodium chloride 1 teaspoon to ½ L of water.

Purposes

- To remove waste products from the lower colon and rectum.
- To soften hard fecal matter or to relieve distension caused by gas.
- To relieve additional distension by stimulating peristaltic movement.
- To stimulate the bladder muscles and thereby relieving retention of urine.
- To cleanse the bowel prior to X-ray studies, surgery or sigmoidoscopy.

Preliminary Assessment of Patient and Environment

- Read the doctor's order and note the nature of enema, any precautions to be taken and any specimen to be collected.
- Get the instructions from the senior sister.
- Note the general condition of the patient and the diagnosis, operation, etc.
- Check the health status of the rectal and perineal area.
- Check the ability of the patient for self-help and the ability to understand and accept.
- Assess whether any assistance is needed to do the procedure or to maintain privacy of the room or unit.
- Note the availability of articles in the unit.

A tray containing:

Articles	Purpose
Screen	For providing privacy
Irrigation stand	For hanging the enema can
Bedpan with cover—2	For defecation
Enema can, tubing 3 feet (90 cm) glass connection, screw clip (clamp)	For administration of enema
Rectal tube or catheter Size No 22 for adults • Up to one year No. 12 • Up to 12 years No 14–18	For administration of enema into the rectum
Kidney tray	For disposal of cotton pieces
Vaseline in a container	For lubrication
Required solution (hot water) in a pint measure: Adult 500–1000 mL (1–2 pints) For children 250–500 mL For infants 250 mL or less	For administration of enema

Contd...

Articles	Purpose
Cotton swabs in a container	For wiping the perineal area
Mackintosh and towel or paper	For protecting the linen
Bath thermometer	For checking the temperature

Toilet Tray Containing

Articles	Purpose
Bowl with warm water (jug with warm water)	For washing the perineal area
Soap in a soap dish	For soap and water enema
Towel	For drying the anal area
Wash cloth	For draping the patient
Spirit and powder	For anal application to prevent bed sore
Rag pieces or cotton swabs in a container (wet swabs)	For wiping the anal area
Long artery forceps	For perineal care
Kidney tray	For waste disposal

Procedure

Steps	Procedure	Rationale
1.	Explain the procedure to the patient.	Fosters cooperation
2.	Close the door or put on the screen.	Secures privacy
3.	Wash hands. Wear required personal protective equipment (PPE).	Prevents spread of infection

Contd...

Unit IV ❖ Basic Needs of the Patient

Steps	Procedure	Rationale
4.	If using an enema bag, fill it with 750–1000 mL of warm tap water. Temperature: • **For adults:** 105°F–110°F (40.5°–43°C) • **For children:** 100°F (37.7°C) Close the screw clip and wind the tubing around the can. • Prepare the soap solution. Pour the solution into the can and remove the froth from the top. Rinse the pint measure and replace it. 	Cold water can cause abdominal cramps and hot water can burn the intestinal mucosa Keeps the solution intact
5.	Assemble the equipment to the bedside. 	Organization promotes skilled performance

Contd...

Steps	Procedure	Rationale
6.	Hang the can with the solution on the stand or IV pole. Height of the can must not exceed 18 inches (45 cm) from the level of the mattress for an adult patient. 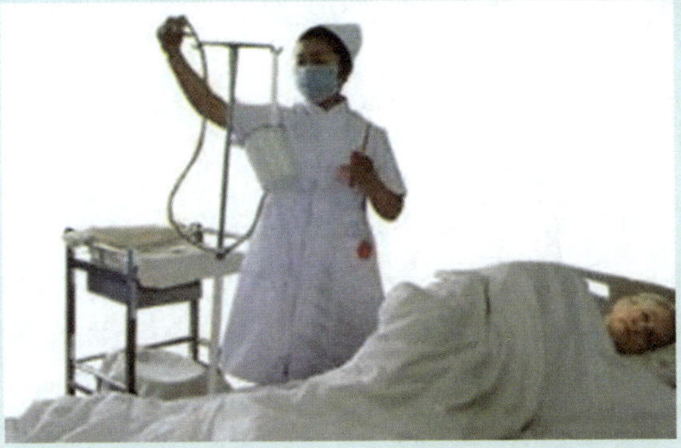	Raising the container too high causes rapid infusion and distension of colon
7.	Remove the top bedding leaving a sheet over the patient. Remove the pillows unless contraindicated. Fold back the patients, own clothes toward the waist. 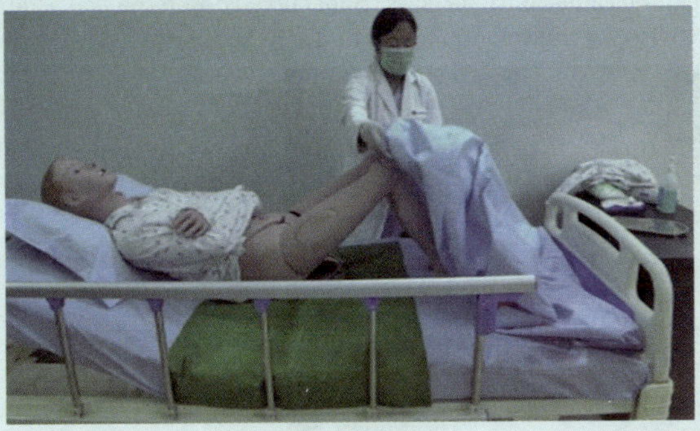	Prevents embarrassment and ensures privacy
8.	Place the mackintosh and towel under the hip.	Prevents soiling of linen.
9.	Turn the patient to the left side and put him/her in the left lateral position without pillow and with the buttocks resting on the edge of the bed. Cover the client with bath blanket and expose the rectal area. The positions of enema have been shown in the following figures. 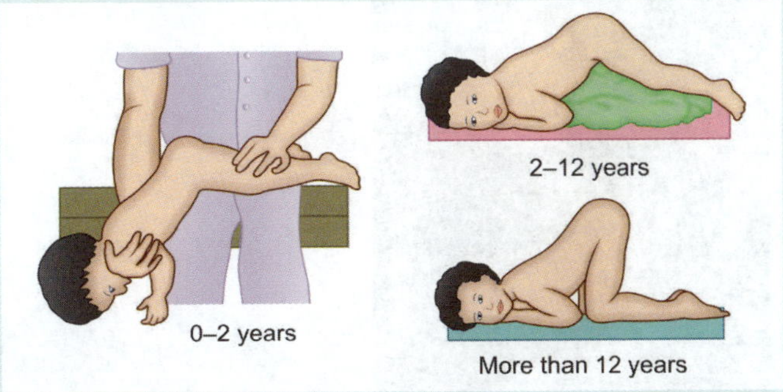	Positioning allows enema solution to flow by gravity. Covering provides warmth and promotes comfort

0–2 years

2–12 years

More than 12 years

Contd...

Unit IV ❖ Basic Needs of the Patient

Steps	Procedure	Rationale
	Left-side position: Lie on left aide with knee bent, and arms resting comfortably Knee–chest position: Kneel, then lower head and chest forward until left side of face is resting on surface with left arm folded comfortably	
10.	Unwind the tubing and connect the catheter to the glass connection. Loosen the screw clip and expel the air by allowing the solution to run through the tube.	Air entry may cause unnecessary discomfort by distending the abdomen
11.	Regulate the flow of solution by adjusting the screw clip. Pinch the tubing with the fingers.	Prevents air entry
12.	Lubricate the end of the catheter with Vaseline to a distance of 3–4 inches (7.5–10 cm).	Promotes smooth insertion without irritation and trauma to the mucosa

Contd...

Steps	Procedure	Rationale
13.	• Gently separate the buttocks with the thumb and forefinger of the left hand. • **Insert 3–4 inches (7.5–10 cm) of the catheter into the rectum gently and slowly.** • Instruct the client to relax and take deep breath. 	Ensures accurate exposure. Careful insertion prevents trauma to the mucosa. Relaxation and deep breathing relaxes the external anal sphincter
14.	Release the fingers and allow the fluid to run slowly. Instruct the patient to breathe through the mouth. Clamp tubing if client complains of abdominal cramping. 	Rapid infusion may stimulate abdominal cramping. Temporary cessation minimizes cramps
15.	When the level of fluid has come down to the level of the outlet in the can, clamp off flow. Inform the client that the procedure is completed and grasp the catheter near the anus and withdraw gently. Disconnect the catheter after pinching and place it in the kidney tray by wrapping the end in rag piece of paper.	Client may misinterpret the tube withdrawal as loss of control
16.	Wipe soiled end of the catheter with rag pieces or cotton and discard it. Place the tubing inside can and replace it in the tray.	Prevents cross contamination
17.	Encourage the patient to retain the solution for 5–10 minutes, if possible.	Longer retention promotes effective stimulation
18.	Turn the patient back on his back and place the bedpan with the head raised on pillows. Remove all the equipment and bring the toilet tray. 	Facilitates defecation

Contd...

Unit IV ❖ Basic Needs of the Patient

Steps	Procedure	Rationale
19.	When finished, remove the bedpan, cover and place it on the stool. Insert the second bedpan and finish the toilet hygiene. Assist the client to wash the anal area. 	Washing facilitates removal of fecal content
20.	Arrange the sheets and make the patient comfortable. 	Promotes comfort
21.	Take the bedpan to the bedpan room, inspect the same, if necessary, empty it, clean and keep it in the rack. (Take the specimen, if required, before emptying) Clean all other equipment and replace them. (Boil the catheter for 10 minutes)	Prevents spread of infection and prepares for next procedure
22.	Doff gloves and wash hands.	Prevents spread of infection
23.	Document the procedure with date, time, outcome and signature.	Documentation fosters quality care.

Medicated Evacuant Enema

Oil enema:

This enema is given to soften the fecal matter in case of severe constipation, also before the first bowl movement after operations on the rectum or perineum such as hemorrhoids and perineorrhaphy in order to avoid straining and injury to the sutures and wounds.

Amount and type of oil used:

- Olive oil 180 mL or olive oil and castor oil 1:2 strength
- Castor oil 2–4 ounces (60–120 mL)
- Gingelly oil 5–6 ounces (150–180 mL) Ref: Dugas

Temperature of the solution = 100°F (37.7°C)

Amount of solution = 150–180 mL

Oil enema is given by using a funnel and catheter. It should be retained for 1/2 to 1 hour to soften the feces. It may be followed by soap and water enema after 1 hour.

Equipment: Equipment will be the same as that of simple enema. Instead of can use funnel, tubing, glass connection and catheter placed in a bowl of warm water, oil is to be warmed at 100°F.

Procedure: Height of the funnel should not exceed 8 inches (20 cm) from the bed. Allow the patient to retain the solution by raising the foot end of the bed and pressing the buttocks. Give the fluid slowly at body temperature. Procedure is same as simple enema.

Retained Enema

Definition: Administration of a drug or liquid per rectum to be retained in order to treat mucus membrane, to quieten the patient, to stimulate or to supply fluids is called a retained enema.

Additional Principles for Retained Enema

- Effective absorption takes place when the solution comes directly in contact with the mucus lining of the colon.
- Reduced pressure and velocity of fluid favor retention of fluid.
- The atmospheric temperature, the length of the tube and rate of flow will influence the loss of heat from the fluid.

General Instructions

First of all, explain the purpose of treatment to the patient.
- The bowels must be cleared out by a simple enema before giving a retention enema.
- It should be given very slowly and at the body temperature.
- Use a fine catheter No. 8 or 10.
- Quantity used at a time should be about 180–240 mL so that the rectum will not be distended.
- Height of the can should not be more than 8 inches (20 cm) from the bed level.
- The foot end of the bed is raised to discourage the return flow.
- Instruct the patient to be in the same position for some time after the procedure.
- Encourage the patient to retain the fluid by pressing the buttocks together and discourage the use of bedpan immediately.
- If it is a continuous retention enema, maintain the temperature by applying hot water bag around container.
- The container should be refilled if it is a continuous retention enema, before it is completely empty.

INSERTION OF SUPPOSITORY

A suppository is a small, round or cone-shaped solid drug that is inserted into the rectum, vagina, or urethra, where it dissolves or melts and exerts local or systemic effects. Rectal suppositories are the most common type of suppository.

Unit IV ❖ Basic Needs of the Patient

Types of Suppositories and their Uses

There are three types of suppositories. They are:

1. **Rectal suppositories:** Rectal suppositories go in the rectum or anus. They are typically an inch long and have a rounded tip. They are used in conditions, such as constipation, fever, hemorrhoids, mental health issues such as anxiety, schizophrenia, or bipolar disorder, nausea, including motion sickness and pain.

2. **Vaginal suppositories:** Vaginal suppositories are typically oval and come with an applicator. They weigh about 3–5 g. People may insert vaginal suppositories into the vagina to treat bacterial or fungal infections, vaginal dryness.

3. **Urethral suppositories:** They are otherwise called bougies. They are pencil shaped and pointed at one extremity. A male urethral suppository weighs about 4 g each and are100–150 mm long and for females, they are 2 g each in weight and usually 60–75 mm in length. These suppositories are the size of a grain of rice. Men may use a type of urethral suppository to treat erection problems in rare cases.

Medicines that are Used as Suppository

- Emollients, astringents, antibacterial agents, steroids, and local anesthetics are dispensed in suppository for treating local conditions.
- Analgesics, antispasmodics, sedatives, tranquilizers, and antibacterial agents are dispensed in suppository for systemic action.

For examples:

- Glycerin—hyperosmotic laxatives
- Bisacodyl (dulcolax)—laxative
- Hydrocortisone acetate—Steroid
- Progesterone—vaginal suppository—hormonal
- Alprostadil—urethral suppository

Requisites

A tray containing:

Articles	Purpose
A bowl with suppository	For rectal insertion
Bowl with wet cotton swab	For cleaning the perineum
Kidney tray/paper bag	For disposing soiled waste
Bath blanket	For draping the patient
Mackintosh and towel	To prevent soiling of linen and clothes
Bedpan	For defecation and perineal care
Screen	For providing privacy
Lubricant	For applying in suppository

Insertion of Anal Suppository

Steps	Procedure	Rationale
1.	Explain the procedure to the patient.	Allays anxiety and wins confidence and cooperation.

Contd...

Steps	Procedure	Rationale
2.	Close the doors and windows. Screen the patient. 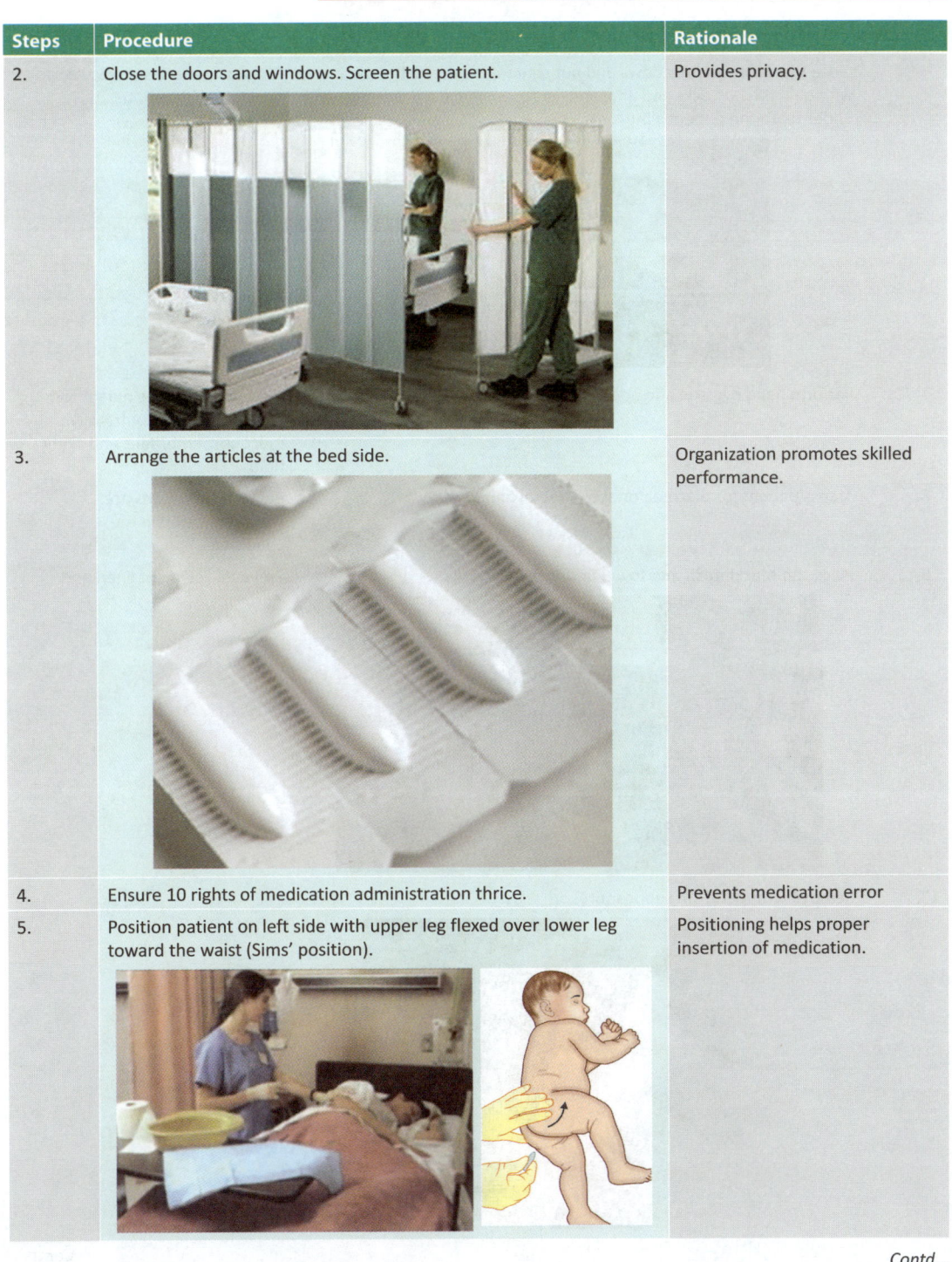	Provides privacy.
3.	Arrange the articles at the bed side.	Organization promotes skilled performance.
4.	Ensure 10 rights of medication administration thrice.	Prevents medication error
5.	Position patient on left side with upper leg flexed over lower leg toward the waist (Sims' position).	Positioning helps proper insertion of medication.

Contd...

Steps	Procedure	Rationale
6.	Close the doors and windows and put screen and drape the patient with only the buttocks and anal area exposed. Place a drape underneath the patient's buttocks.	Protects patient's privacy and facilitates relaxation.
7.	Perform hand hygiene and apply gloves	Gloves protect the nurse from coming into the contract with mucous membranes and body fluids.
8.	Assess patient for diarrhea or active rectal bleeding.	Rectal medications are contraindicated in these conditions.
9.	Place the Mackintosh and towel under the buttocks.	Prevents soiling of linen and clothes.
10.	Remove wrapper from suppository.	

Contd...

Steps	Procedure	Rationale
	Lubricate the rounded tip of suppository and index finger of dominant hand with a water-soluble lubricant such as K-Y Jelly, not petroleum jelly (Vaseline). 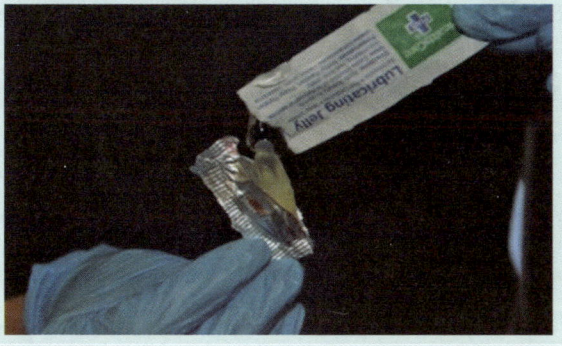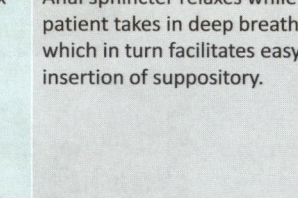	Lubricant reduces friction of anal mucosa.
11.	Separate buttocks with non-dominant hand and, using gloved index finger of dominant hand, insert suppository (rounded tip toward patient) into rectum toward umbilicus while having patient take a deep breath, exhale through the mouth. 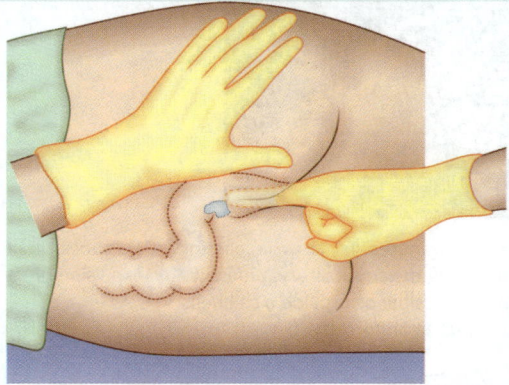 Push it in about 1 inch for adults, or half an inch for infants. 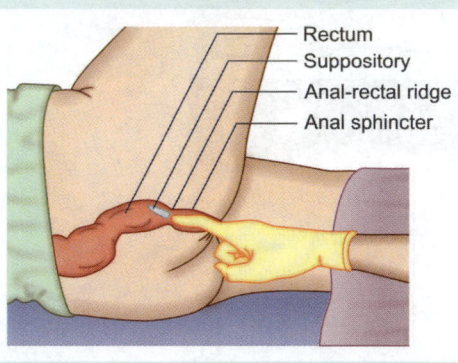 — Rectum — Suppository — Anal-rectal ridge — Anal sphincter	Anal sphincter relaxes while the patient takes in deep breath which in turn facilitates easy insertion of suppository.

Contd...

Unit IV ❖ Basic Needs of the Patient

Steps	Procedure	Rationale
	Alternatively, suppository can be inserted through a suppository inserter. The suppository inserter has a 5.1 cm long, hollow plastic tip that holds a standard suppository and spring-loaded design which pushes it out. Stimulator / Suppository inserter	
12.	Remove finger and wipe patient's anal area.	Wiping removes excess lubricant and provides comfort to the patient.
13.	Ask patient to remain on side for 5–10 minutes. Try to avoid passing stool for up to 60 minutes after inserting the suppository, unless it is a laxative. Ensure that bed pan is accessible or provide a call bell. Arrange the sheets and make the patient comfortable	This position helps prevent the expulsion of suppository.

Contd...

Steps	Procedure	Rationale
14.	Wash and replace the articles. Discard the soiled waste. Remove gloves and wash hands.	Prevents spread of infection
15.	Document procedure including date and time of administration, patient's response with signature	Documentation fosters quality care.

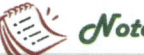 **Note**

If the suppository is soft, hold it under cool water or place it in a refrigerator for a few minutes to harden it before removing the wrapper.

Insertion of a Vaginal Suppository

- Unwrap the suppository and place it in the accompanying applicator.
- Either stand with the knees bent and feet apart or lie down with the knees bent toward the chest.
- Place the applicator into the vagina, as far as possible, without causing discomfort (Figs 2A to C).
- Press down on the plunger to push in the suppository.
- Remove the applicator from the vagina, and dispose it off.
- Lie down for 10 minutes to allow the medicine to enter the body (Figs 2A to E).

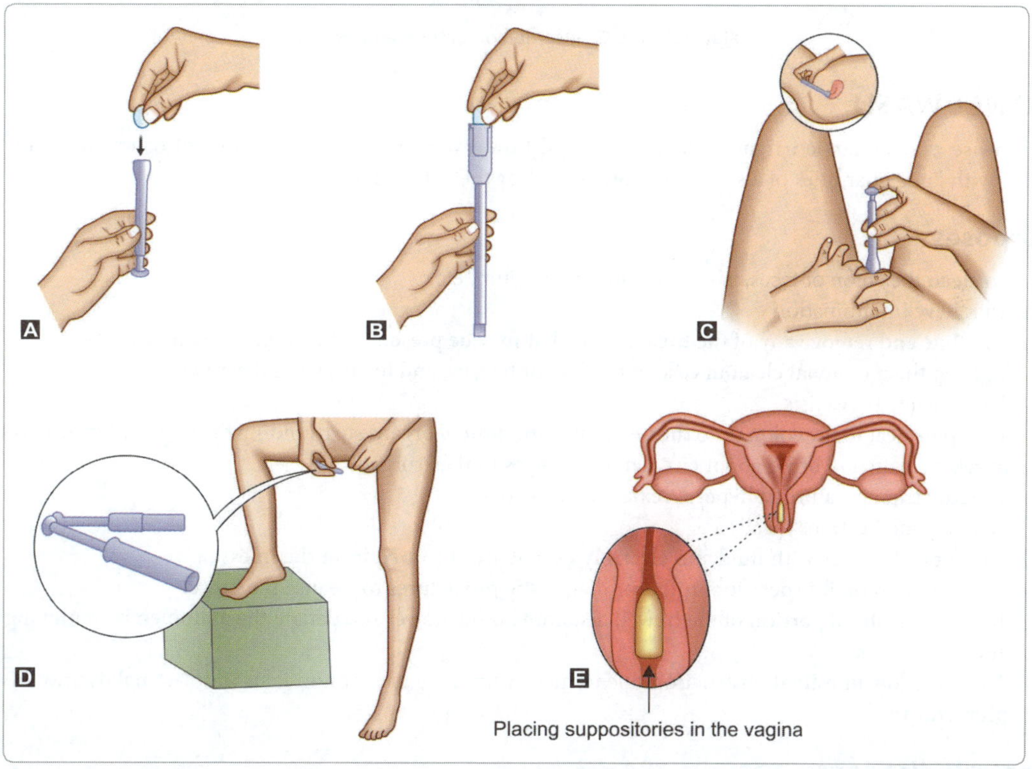

A

B

C

D

E

Placing suppositories in the vagina

Figures 2A to E: Procedure of inserting vaginal suppository

Unit IV ❖ Basic Needs of the Patient

Inserting a Urethral Suppository

- Empty the bladder.
- Stretch out the penis to open the urethra.
- Place the applicator into the hole at the tip.
- Push the button on the applicator and hold for 5 seconds.
- Gently move the applicator from side to side to ensure the suppository has entered the urethra.
- Massage the stretched penis firmly for 10–15 seconds to allow the medicine to be absorbed (Figs 3A to C).

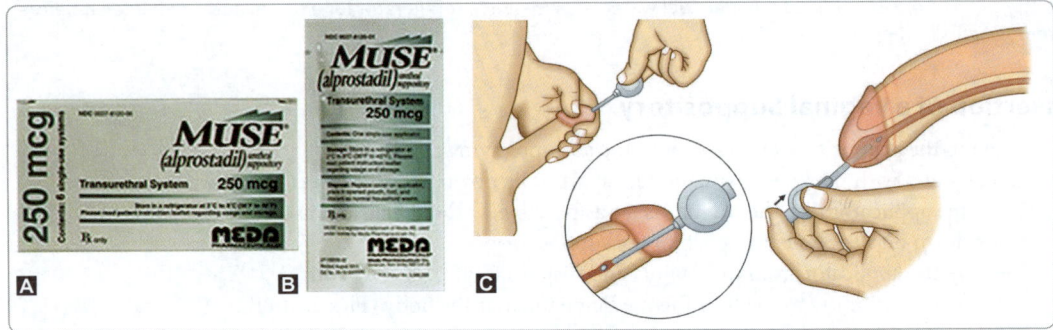

Figures 3A to C: Insertion of urethral suppository

BOWEL WASH

Otherwise called colonic irrigation or enteroclysis. Bowel wash refers to the treatment of washing out the colon with large quantities of a solution in order to clear the colon of feces.

Purposes

- To clean the colon of feces, gas, excess mucus, barium, etc.
- To relieve inflammation
- To dilute and remove any of the toxic agents that may be present in the large intestine
- To keep the individual clean in case of fecal incontinence and to check the diarrhea
- To stimulate peristalsis
- To supply heat to the colon or to the pelvic and abdominal organs surrounding the large intestine in order to relieve pain and bring about circulatory changes in these organs
- To reduce temperature in hyperpyrexia and heat stroke
- To apply medications locally
- To supply the body with fluid and electrolytes that are absorbed from the intestine
- To prepare colon for specific surgical or diagnostic procedures to cleanse the bowel
- To clean the distal portion of the bowel, decompress the bowel and deflate the abdomen by removing air and feces
- To relieve low intestinal obstruction due to meconium plug, meconium ileus or intestinal dysmotility of prematurity

Contraindications

- Loose sphincter
- Painful and bleeding hemorrhoids

- Fistula in anus
- Polyps and diverticulum of the intestines
- Rectal infections
- Painful skin lesions around the anus
- Massive carcinoma or tumors of the rectum
- Debilitation
- Rectal polyps
- Intestinal obstruction
- Rectal surgeries, infection
- Chronic diarrhea

Methods Used

- Funnel and catheter method
- 'Y' connector and rectal tube method
- 2 tube method

Solutions Used

- Plain water
- Cold water
- Normal saline
- Sodium bi-carbonate solution 1–2%
- Antiseptic solution such as:
  - Silver nitrate 1 : 5000
  - Potassium permanganate solutions 1 : 5000
  - Thymol 1 : 100
  - Alum 1 : 100
  - Boric solution 1–2%
  - Tannic acid 1 : 100 etc.

Amount of Solution Used

- 2–3 L or till the return flow is clear

Temperature of the Solution

- For cleansing purpose 104°F (40°C)
- For thermal effect 110–115°F (43.3–46°C)
- For reducing temperature 80–90°F (27–32°C)

General Instructions

- A cleansing enema should be given 1 hour before the bowel wash. This facilitates the rectum to be free from fecal matter.
- Ask the patient to empty the bladder before the bowel wash. This helps to reduce the intra-abdominal pressure.
- The temperature of the solution be kept constant throughout the procedure
- Do not allow air to enter into the intestine. This can be done by:
  - Expelling the air from the tube
  - Not letting the fluid to run in completely from the tube

- Make sure that the return flow is not blocked.
- Stop the procedure temporarily if the client complaints of pain or discomfort.
- Use a smooth and flexible rectal tube and lubricate it well to prevent damage to the rectal mucosa.
- Complaints of the client should not be ignored however small they may be.
- Stop the treatment if the client shows the signs of fatigue and collapse
- Allow only 200–300 mL of fluid to run into the rectum at a time. It should be drained out completely. Then the procedure may be repeated.
- Regulate the flow of fluid.
- Do not place the tube that is going inside the rectum higher than 45 to 60 cm above the bed level.
- Do not place the tube that is coming outside the rectum more than 30 cm below the bed.

Preliminary Assessment

- Check the diagnosis and general condition of the client.
- Check the abilities and limitations concerning movement.
- Check the consciousness and the ability of the patient to follow instructions.
- Check the doctor's orders and the specific precautions, if any, to be followed.
- Check for any lesions on the rectal or perineal area.
- Assess the need for extra help.
- Check the patient's chart for physician's order and any specific instructions

Articles Required

A tray containing:

Articles	Purpose
Colonic lavage set with tubing and glass connection • Funnel and catheter • Irrigation can, catheter with screw clamp • 'Y' connection	For colonic irrigation
Rectal tube placed in a kidney tray • **Children:** 12–18 Fr • **Adult:** 22–30 Fr	For irrigating the rectum
Required solutions	For irrigating the rectum
Mackintosh and towel	For protecting the bed and bed linen
Water soluble jelly or Vaseline	For lubricating the rectal tube
Rag pieces in a container and tissue papers	For applying the lubricant and for cleaning the perineum when necessary
Hot and cold water in jugs or any prescribed solution in jug	For irrigating the rectum
Paper bag	For discarding the soiled wastes
Kidney tray	For placing the rectal tube
Clean linen as needed	For changing after the irrigation
Bucket	For receiving the return flow
Perineal tray	For cleaning the perineum
Bedpan with lid/commode	For assisting in defecation
Duster/towel	For drying the perineum
PPE as required	For preventing transmission of microorganisms

Procedure

Steps	Procedure	Rationale
1.	Explain the procedure to the patient and how he/she has to cooperate	Allays anxiety and fosters cooperation.
2.	Arrange the articles at the bed side	Organization facilitates accurate skill performance.
3.	Close the door and put on the screen.	Maintains clients self-esteem and dignity.
4.	Place the patient in left lateral position with knees flexed toward the abdomen. • Bring close to the edge of bed. • Separate the patient's buttock's to visualize the anus clearly. • Drape the other parts exposing only the anal area. 	Minimum exposure lessens embarrassment and helps to provide warmth.
5.	Place mackintosh and towel under the buttocks. 	Prevents soiling of linen and garments.
6.	Keep the bucket on a low stool.	Helps to receive the outflow of fluid.
7.	Wash hands and don gloves.	Prevents transfer of microorganisms.

Contd...

Unit IV ❖ Basic Needs of the Patient

Steps	Procedure	Rationale
8.	Prepare the solution at the required temperature. Test the temperature of solution by pouring it at the inner aspect of the wrist. 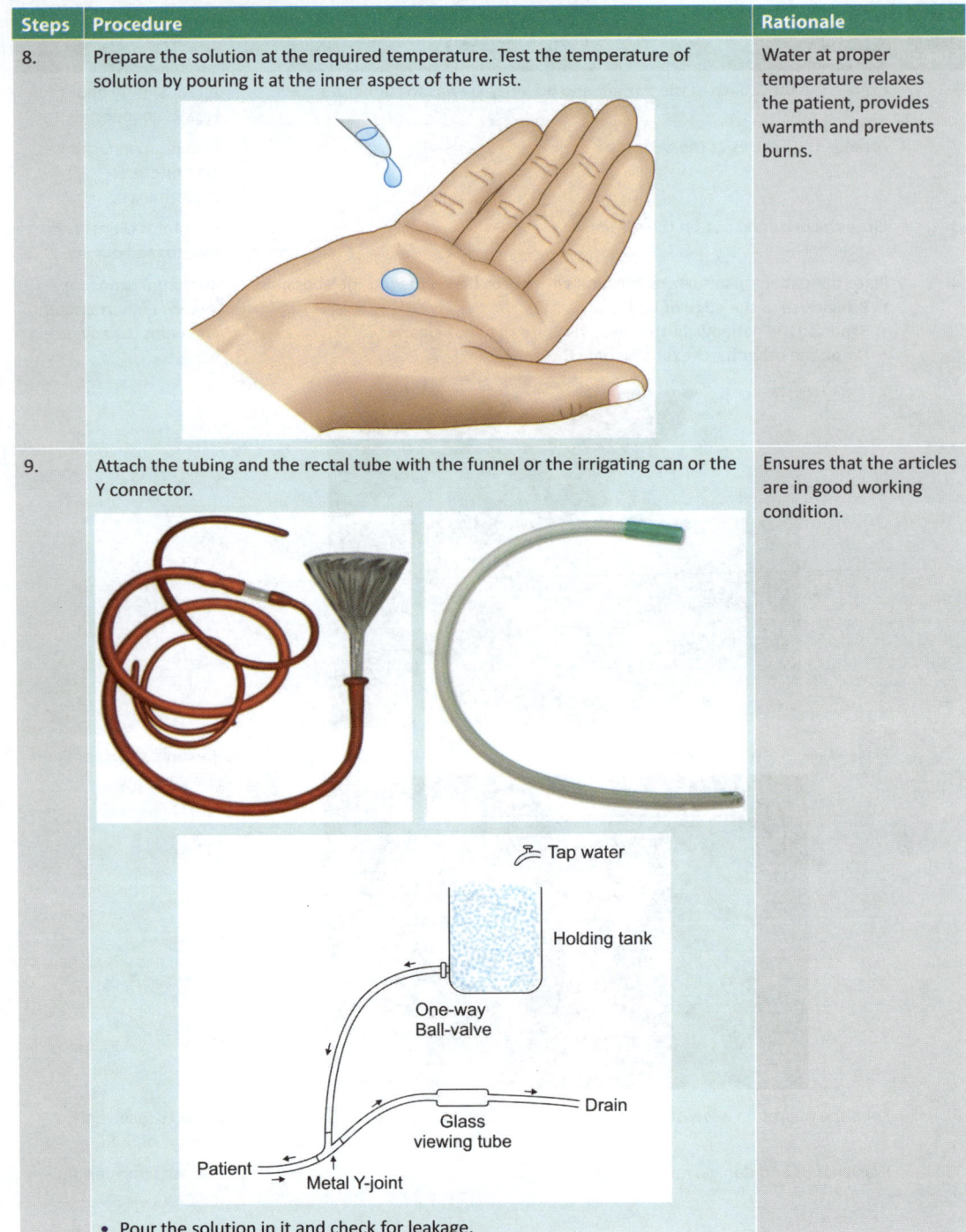	Water at proper temperature relaxes the patient, provides warmth and prevents burns.
9.	Attach the tubing and the rectal tube with the funnel or the irrigating can or the Y connector.	Ensures that the articles are in good working condition.

• Pour the solution in it and check for leakage.

Contd...

Unit IV ❖ Basic Needs of the Patient

Steps	Procedure	Rationale
10.	**By using funnel and catheter:** Fill the funnel with the solution and expel the air from tubing by allowing a small amount of fluid into kidney tray. Pinch the tube or close it with clamp. Lubricate the tip of the rectal tube about 4 inches. 	Expels the air and prevents air entry further.
	Using '2 tube' method: • Fill the can with solution and expel the air. • Mark the catheter about 6 inches from its tip and the rectal tube 4 inches from its tip. • Insert the tip of the catheter into the eye of the rectal tube and insert the tube together into the anal canal after lubricating them well. • When the tubes are in, pull the catheter slightly backward in order to dislodge it from the rectal tube. • Then insert the catheter alone until the marks on both tubes come together at the anus.	Lubrication facilitates passage of rectal tube through the anal sphincter and prevents injury. Catheter acts as the inflow tube and the rectal tube acts as the outflow tube.

Contd...

Unit IV ❖ Basic Needs of the Patient

Steps	Procedure	Rationale
	Using 'Y' Connection and Rectal Tube: • A 'Y' connection will permit the regulation of the inflow and outflow • The tube for inflow is attached to one prong of the Y connection and the outflow tube is attached to the other prong. • The stem of the Y connection is attached to the rectal tube. • Clamps on the inflow and outflow tubes make it possible to direct the flow of fluid into the rectum and then out of the rectum. • The solution flows from the inflow tube through the rectal tube into the rectum.	
11.	Gently separate the buttocks with the thumb and forefinger of the left hand. Insert the tip of tube about 4 inches while the patient exhales a deep breath. 	Careful insertion prevents trauma to the mucosa. Relaxation and deep breathing relax the external anal sphincter.
12.	Lower the funnel or the catheter or the tubing below the level of the rectum. 	Allows the flatus if any to escape from the rectum. It will be seen as bubbling through the fluid in the funnel.
13.	Raise the funnel or the irrigating can and allow the fluid to run in, continue to pour more fluid into funnel or the can before it is empty. 	Prevents entry of air into the bowel.

Contd...

Steps	Procedure	Rationale
14.	When 200–300 mL of fluid has gone inside, pinch the tube before the funnel or can is completely empty and invert it into the bucket and siphon off the fluid. Let the fluid drain. • In a 2 tube method, the fluid that flows from the irrigating can through the rectal catheter enters the rectum and return through the rectal tube which is situated 2 inches lower than the rectal catheter. • In a Y connector, when the clamp on the inflow tube is closed and the clamp on the outflow tube is opened, the fluid flows through the rectal tube to outflow tube and into the bucket. By opening and closing the clamps alternatively, the fluid enters the rectum and returns after washing out the rectum. 	Fluid drains by gravity. The fluid which has gone in should be drained out before introducing more fluid.
15.	When return flow ceases, turn the funnel upright and pour more solution, lower the funnel until air from the tube has been expelled. Then raise the funnel and repeat the procedure. Continue the procedure until all the fluid ordered has been given or until the return flow is clear. 	Ensures that the bowel is cleaned.

Contd...

Steps	Procedure	Rationale
16.	Temporarily stop the procedure (do not remove the rectal tube) if the client develops any discomfort and continue the procedure once the discomfort is relieved.	Entry of fluid into the rectum stimulates the peristalsis. Stopping the procedure for few moments will relax the bowels as the peristaltic movement is passed off.
17.	Gently remove the rectal tube by pulling it through 3–4 layers of rag pieces/tissue papers.	Gentle removal prevents mucosal injury and holding in tissue paper prevents soiling of hands and removes the feces from the tube.
18.	Discard the tissue papers or rag pieces in the paper bag. Place the funnel with tubing in the kidney tray. Assist patient to the toilet, commode or bed pan.	Safe disposal prevents transmission of microorganisms.
19.	Assist the client to wash the anal area or provide perineal care. Dry the area thoroughly.	Washing facilitates removal of fecal content.
20.	Put on garments and change the linen if needed and make the client in comfortable position.	Ensures comfort and well-being.

Contd...

Steps	Procedure	Rationale
21.	Take articles to utility room disinfect funnel, tubing, catheter and bucket. Clean, dry and replace. 	Prevents spread of infection and prepares for next procedure.
22.	Doff gloves and wash hands.	Prevents spread of infection transmission.
23.	Document the type of procedure, purpose, solution used, amount of solution, temperature of solution, nature of return fluid and the patient response along with date, time and signature of the nurse.	Documentation fosters quality care.

DIGITAL EVACUATION OF IMPACTED FECES

Digital removal of feces is an invasive procedure and should only be carried out when necessary.

Other names are:

■ Digital disimpaction
■ Digital removal of feces (DRF)
■ Disimpacting stool with digital maneuvers
■ Digital evacuation
■ Manual disimpaction
■ Manual elimination

Definition

Digital disimpaction is the insertion of one or two gloved fingers into the rectum to aid in the removal of stool from the rectum by manually breaking up the fecal impaction.

This technique is used for the treatment of acute fecal impaction or as a bowel management technique.

Indications

■ Fecal impaction/loading
■ Incomplete defecation
■ Inability to defecate
■ Patients in whom other bowel emptying techniques have failed
■ In patients with spinal injury as part of a bowel management program

Unit IV ❖ Basic Needs of the Patient

Complications

- Active inflammation of the bowel including Crohn's disease, ulcerative colitis and diverticulitis
- Recent radiotherapy to the pelvic area
- Rectal/anal pain
- Surgery/trauma to the anal/rectal area
- Tissue fragility due to age, radiation, loss of muscle tone in neurological diseases or malnourishment
- Obvious rectal bleeding
- Spinal injured patients (due to autonomic dysreflexia)
- Contraindicated in: Patient with known history of abuse
- Patient with known history of allergies (e.g., latex)

Preliminary Assessment

- Assess the date and quality of last bowel movement.
- Assess the client for signs of fecal impaction like nausea, anorexia, abdominal fullness, abdominal pain or cramps.
- Auscultate for bowel sounds.
- Obtain a baseline pulse and blood pressure whilst patient has rest prior to procedure.
- Observe for distress, pain, discomfort, rectal bleeding, collapse and stool consistency.

Articles Required

A tray containing:

Articles	Purpose
Required PPE—disposable apron, nonsterile disposable gloves	For preventing cross infection
Bowl with wet cotton swab	For cleaning the perineum
Kidney tray/paper bag	For disposing soiled waste
Bath blanket	For draping the patient
Mackintosh and towel	To prevent soiling of linen and clothes
Bedpan/commode/access to toilet	For defecation and perineal care
Screen	For providing privacy
Water soluble lubricant	For digital evacuation
Receptacle	For collecting faeces

Procedure for Digital Removal of Feces (DRF)

Steps	Procedure	Rationale
1.	Explain the procedure to the patient.	Allays anxiety and wins confidence and cooperation.
2.	Obtain informed consent and document.	Acts as a legal document
3.	Ask the patient to empty their bladder.	A full bladder may cause discomfort during the procedure.

Contd...

Steps	Procedure	Rationale
4.	Close the doors and windows. Screen the patient.	Provides privacy and ensures dignity of the patient.
5.	Arrange the articles at the bedside. Ensure that a bedpan, commode or access to the toilet should be readily available. 	Organization promotes skilled performance.
6.	Place the patient in the left lateral position with knees flexed with upper leg bent over lower leg (Sims' position) and expose the anal area. Drape the patient with only the buttocks and anal area exposed. 	Anal area can be easily visualized, facilitates easy access to anal canal and ensures privacy.
7.	Place a protective pad under the patient's hips and buttocks. Position a bedpan near to the client. 	Protects bed linen and clothing. Bedpan acts as a receptacle to receive stool once it is removed.

Contd...

Unit IV ❖ Basic Needs of the Patient

Steps	Procedure	Rationale
8.	Wash hands and wear necessary PPE.	Prevents transfer of micro-organisms.
9.	Apply local anesthetic gel into the rectum prior to the procedure or lubricate one gloved finger with plain lubricating gel.	Protects fragile mucosa from injury and may prevent local discomfort.
10.	Insert the lubricated gloved finger slowly into the patient's rectum.	Prevents possible injury to the bowel mucosa from a blind entry.
	Gently probe for stool by moving finger upwards towards the umbilicus and back and forth.	Stimulates peristalsis to facilitate removal of stool.

Contd...

Steps	Procedure		Rationale
11.	If stool is a solid mass, push finger into centre, split it and remove small sections until none remain. If stool is in small separate hard lumps remove a lump at a time.		Allows removal of stools without causing trauma to the anus.

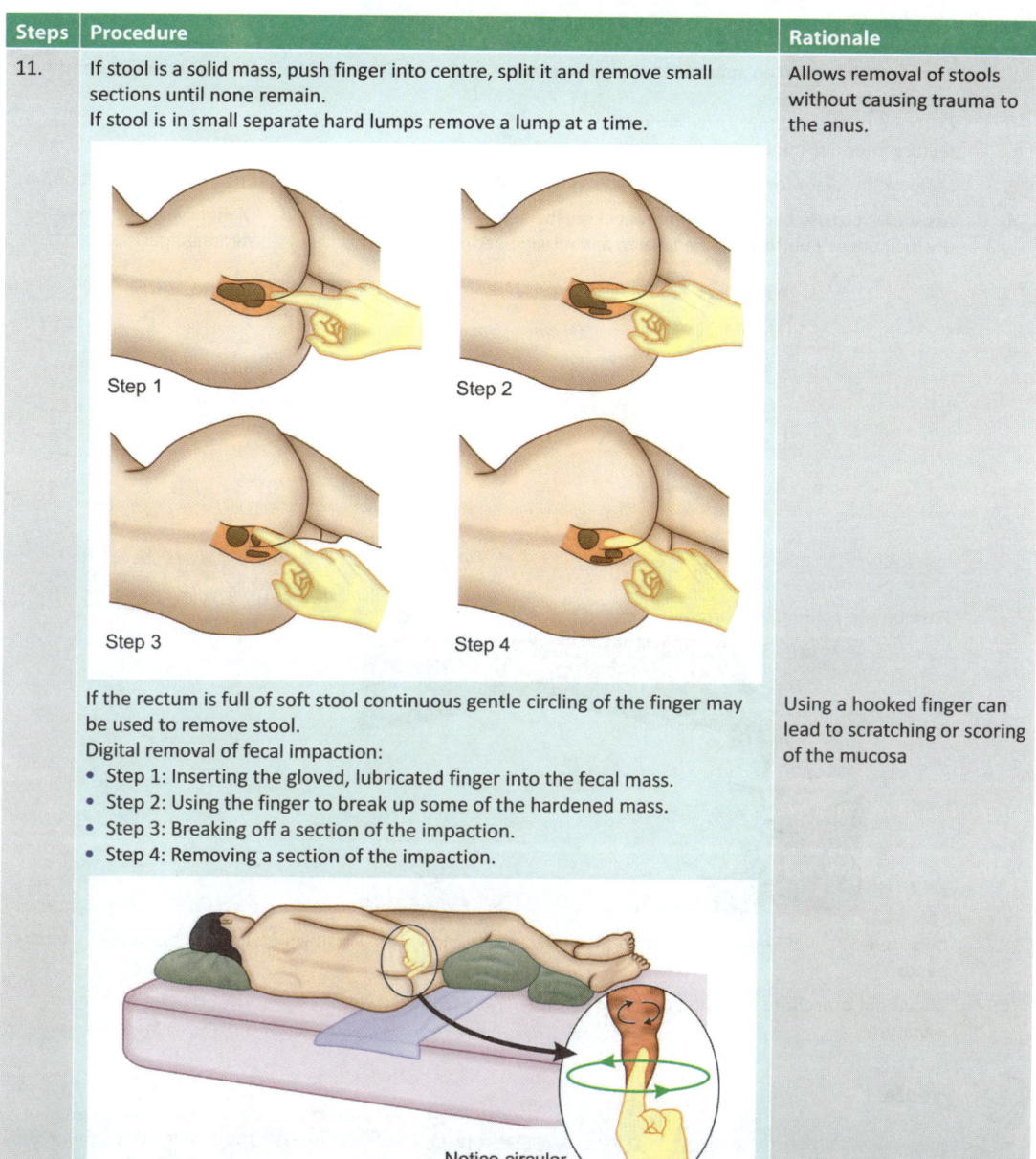

Step 1   Step 2

Step 3   Step 4

If the rectum is full of soft stool continuous gentle circling of the finger may be used to remove stool.

Digital removal of fecal impaction:
- Step 1: Inserting the gloved, lubricated finger into the fecal mass.
- Step 2: Using the finger to break up some of the hardened mass.
- Step 3: Breaking off a section of the impaction.
- Step 4: Removing a section of the impaction.

Using a hooked finger can lead to scratching or scoring of the mucosa

Notice circular motion of finger

Great care should be taken to remove stool in such a way so as to avoid damage to the rectal mucosa and anal sphincters.
Avoid using a hooked finger.
Move the stool pieces towards the anus and remove them.

Contd...

Steps	Procedure	Rationale
12.	Place fecal matter in an appropriate receptacle as it is removed. Dispose it appropriately. Once the rectum is empty on examination, conduct a final digital check of the rectum after five minutes to ensure that evacuation is complete.	Ensures infection control.
13.	Monitor the client for complications such as rectal bleeding or bradycardia.	Ensures early detection.
14.	Assist client to use bedpan or commode if he/she needs to defecate. Wash and dry the patient's buttocks and anal area and provide perineal care.	Digital evacuation may stimulate peristalsis.

Position the patient comfortably.

Steps	Procedure	Rationale
15.	Dispose waste and Replace articles. Remove the gloves and apron. Wash your hands.	Prevents spread of infection
16.	Document procedure including date and time, patient's response with signature.	Documentation fosters quality care.

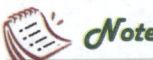 **Note**

- Take necessary caution for patients who have a spinal cord injury (SCI). Observe the patient throughout the procedure for signs of autonomic dysreflexia.
- During the procedure, the person delivering care may carry out abdominal massage to stimulate peristalsis.
- Where stool is hard, impacted and difficult to remove, other approaches should be employed in combination with digital removal of feces.

BOWEL DIVERSIONS OR OSTOMY

Bowel diversion refers to surgical procedures that reroutes the normal movement of intestinal contents out of the body when part of the bowel is diseased or removed.

Purpose of Bowel Ostomies

- To drain fecal material
- To divert the bowel to an opening in the abdomen

Types of Colostomy

Colostomy is a surgical procedure that brings one end of the large intestine out through an opening (stoma) made in the abdominal wall (Fig. 4).

According to stoma site:

- Transverse
- Ascending
- Descending
- Sigmoid

According to duration:

- Temporary
- Permanent

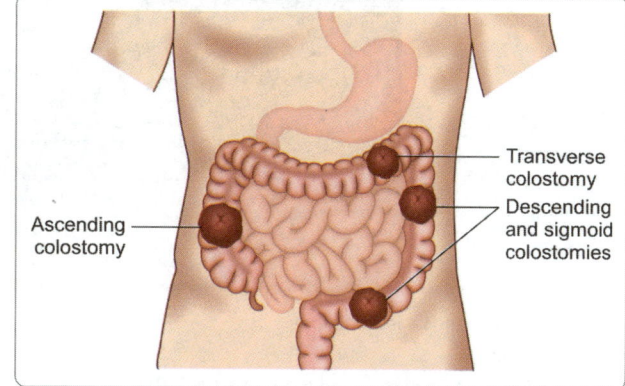

Figure 4: Types of colostomy

Articles Required

A tray containing:

Articles	Purpose
Colostomy bag or pouch	For changing
Mackintosh with draw sheet	For spreading under abdomen
Kidney tray/paper bag	For discarding the soiled waste
Basin with warm tap water	For cleaning the stoma
A bowl containing gauze pieces	For cleaning the stoma
Skin barrier	For sticking in the abdomen
Stoma measuring guide or sizing template	For measuring the stoma and size the opening
Pen or pencils	For tracing the size of the stoma
Bedpan	For discarding the fecal matter
Scissors	For cutting the stomatal opening

Procedure

Steps	Procedure	Rationale
1.	Explain the procedure to the patient.	Allays anxiety and fosters cooperation.
2.	Close the door and put on the screen.	Maintains clients self-esteem and dignity

Contd...

Unit IV ❖ **Basic Needs of the Patient**

Steps	Procedure	Rationale
3.	Assist client to a standing or sitting position.	Facilitates application of pouch by reducing wrinkles
4.	Gather equipment.	Organization facilitates accurate skill performance
5.	Wash hands and don gloves.	Reduces transmission of microorganisms.
6.	Spread Mackintosh and draw sheet.	Protects linen and garments
7.	Remove soiled pouch by gently pressing on the skin while pulling the pouch. Dispose the pouch.	Avoids trauma to the peristomal skin
8.	Remove clamp and empty the contents into the bed pan. Rinse the pouch with tepid water or normal saline.	Minimizes the odor and growth of microbes.

Contd...

Steps	Procedure	Rationale
9.	Cleanse the skin with soap and water using a gauze pad. Do not scrub the skin, dry completely by patting the skin with gauze.	Removes fecal material and prepare the skin for pouch reapplication
10.	Inspect the stoma and peristomal skin for redness, color, altered skin integrity or rashes.	Inspection helps to detect abnormalities at the earliest.
11.	Inspect the pouch opening and ensures that it fits the stoma. Trace same circle behind the skin barrier, using scissors, cut an opening 1/16th to 1/8th inch larger than stoma before removing the wrapper over adhesive part.	Ensures appropriate sized pouch and protects the peristomal skin.

Contd...

Unit IV ❖ Basic Needs of the Patient

Steps	Procedure	Rationale
12.	Remove excessive hair with a safety razor or electric razor. Apply a skin sealant and skin barrier as per indication.	Excessive hair is removed to promote the adhesives. Applying skin sealant protects the peristomal skin.
13.	Gently apply the pouch and press into place. Seal the inferior opening with the clip or a rubber band.	Prevents leakage of effluent from the pouch.
14.	Put on garments and change the linen if needed and make the client comfortable. Replace the articles after washing.	Ensures comfort and well-being. Prepares for next procedure.
15.	Remove gloves. Wash hands.	Reduces risk of transfer of microorganisms
16.	Document the type and size of pouch, condition of stoma and client response, amount, color, consistency of fecal matter with date, type.	Documentation fosters quality care.

INSERTION OF FLATUS TUBE

Insertion of flatus tube is defined as an introduction of a tube into the rectum for expulsion of gas to relieve flatulence and gaseous distension of the abdomen.

Flatus tube is a thick and stout tube usually made of Indian rubber and has a bulbous rod with two eyes at the tip.

Purposes

- To remove flatulence from the lower bowel.
- To relieve abdominal distension.
- It is used before giving a retention enema.
- To manage flatulence (gas) following abdominal surgery
- To alleviate dyspnea due to abdominal distension
- To control diarrhoea that cannot be controlled with medical management

Indications

- **Diagnostic:**
  - Diagnosis of volvulus
  - Diagnosis of intestinal obstruction
- **Therapeutic:**
  - To remove gaseous obstruction
  - In volvulus
  - In paralytic ileus
  - In typhoid lymphatics

Contraindications

- Recent rectal or prostatic surgery
- Diseases of the rectal mucosa
- Immunocompromised Patients

General Instructions

- Introduce the rectal tube 4–5 inches.
- Rectal tube should not be left in position more than 30 minutes.
- Longer periods of insertion can lead to permanent sphincter damage.
- The tube can be reinserted every 3–4 hours if necessary.

Requisites

A clean tray containing:

Articles	Purpose
Flatus tube/rectal tube or catheter, 22–30 French	For rectal insertion
Water-soluble lubricant, e.g., xylocaine jelly	For preventing friction
Wet swab in a bowl	For cleansing the perineum
Macintosh and towel	For preventing soiling of linen and clothes
Paper bag/kidney tray	To discard soiled waste
Kidney tray with water	For checking the passage of flatus
Screen	For providing privacy
Bedside drainage bag (optional)	If rectal tube used to manage diarrhoea

Procedure

Steps	Procedure	Rationale
1.	Explain the procedure to the patient.	Allays anxiety and wins confidence and cooperation.
2.	Arrange the articles near the bed side.	Organization promotes skilled performance.

Contd...

Unit IV ❖ Basic Needs of the Patient

Steps	Procedure	Rationale
3.	Close doors and windows and put curtain, so that the patient will not feel shy. 	Provides privacy
4.	Place the mackintosh and towel and draw sheet under his waist. 	Protects bed linen and clothes from soiling.
5.	Loose the garments of the waist and expose only the necessary portion. Drape the patient with a blanket. 	Prevents embarrassment
6.	Place the patient in left lateral position with right leg bent towards the abdomen and over the left leg. 	Facilitates easy access to anal canal.

Contd...

Steps	Procedure	Rationale
7.	Wash hands thoroughly and don gloves.	Prevents spread of microorganisms
8.	Lubricate the flatus tube at eye side, up to 3" to 4" with a water soluble lubricant.	Prevents friction, as the mucus membrane of the rectum is very delicate.
9.	Touch the tip of flatus tube to the anus so that the sphincter muscles of the anus constrict and immediately relax. Insert it in anal canal gently but quickly, keeping the free end of the flatus tube under the lotion in kidney tray.	Facilitates entry of the catheter into anal canal.
10.	Insert the tube 7 to 10 inches and observe the bubbles and liquid stools in the lotion. When the bubbles are stopped then move the tube little bit inside and outside and observe for the bubbles. If the patient has diarrhea, attach the other end to a drainage bag and secure with adhesives.	Ensures passage of flatus.

Contd...

Steps	Procedure	Rationale
11.	Remove the tube and keep it in other kidney tray. See that the tube does not touch the floor. Clean the area with wet cotton swabs. 	Promotes comfort.
12.	Remove the draw sheet and mackintosh. Make the patient comfortable. Wash and Replace the articles. 	Prepares the articles for next use.
13.	Doff gloves and wash hands.	Prevents spread of infection
14.	Document the date, time and result of flatus tube insertion, along with • Description of bowel sounds • Abdominal girth • Insertion and removal of rectal tube • Color and amount of diarrhea, if present • Presence of flatus release • Appearance of perianal skin and • Client tolerance to the procedure along with signature.	Documentation fosters quality care.

DIARRHEA

It is the discharge of loose watery stools due to excess rapidity in the passage of waste products of digestion through gastrointestinal tract. It is an abnormally frequent passage of fecal matter through the intestines resulting in loose stools.

Causes of Diarrhea

The causes of diarrhea are numerous and given as follows:

■ Direct stimulation or irritation of the central or autonomic nervous system. For example, tension diarrhea, pre-examination diarrhea.

- Use of certain drugs. For example, reserpine in the treatment of hypertension may cause hyper motility of the intestines resulting in diarrhea and cathartics cause irritation of the intestinal mucosa and produce diarrhea.

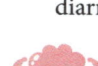 **Stimulant**

Some other drugs that may cause diarrhea are as follows:
- Magnesium containing antacids
- H_2-receptor antagonists, e.g., cimetidine, ranitidine
- Proton pump inhibitors, e.g., lansoprazole, omeprazole
- Misoprostol
- Aminosalicylates, e.g., mesalazine, olsalazine, sulfasalazine
- Digoxin
- Methyldopa
- Selective serotonin reuptake inhibitors (SSRIs), e.g., citalopram, fluoxetine
- **Antibiotics like:**
  - Sulfonylureas, e.g., gliclazide, glipizide
  - Metformin
  - Acarbose
  - Levothyroxine (usually at excessive dose)
  - Cytotoxic drugs, e.g., methotrexate
- Iron preparations:
  - Nonsteroidal anti-inflammatory drugs (NSAIDs), e.g., indomethacin, mefenamic acid, naproxen
  - Colchicine
  - Leflunomide

- **Reflex type of diarrhea** due to the irritation of the gastrointestinal tract. Irritation may be mechanical due to indiscretions of the food such as eating coarse foods or highly seasoned foods or the irritation may be chemical due to some drugs or it may be some allergic reaction of certain foods. For example, shellfish is a well-known allergen.
- **Infection of the gastrointestinal tract** may cause inflammation and produce loose motion.
- **Diarrhea due to defects in the anatomical processes** that are necessary for defecation. Some disease condition may increase the neuromuscular excitability of the intestine and cause diarrhea.
- **Malabsorption syndrome:** It is the failure on the part of the intestines to absorb water as the digestive product passes through and cause diarrhea.

Goals for Nursing Action in Diarrhea

- **Re-establishment of normal bowel action:** In establishment of normal bowel action, it is important to know the cause of diarrhea. If the cause is anxiety or tension the diarrhea will often disappear when the stressful situation is over. If the diarrhea is due to irritation of the gastrointestinal tract, the removal of the irritant will stop the symptoms. However, if it is a chronic symptom or due to any anatomical fault, medical intervention is necessary.
- **Relief of distressing symptoms:** Patients with diarrhea are uncomfortable due to distressing conditions like abdominal pain, dehydration, abdominal distension etc. Medications to coat the lining of the intestines or to reduce muscular spasm are often prescribed for patients with diarrhea. Some of these drugs are taken at regular intervals during the day and others are taken after each bowel movement. If the diarrhea is due to infection, appropriate therapy to combat the infection is prescribed by physician.

Unit IV ❖ Basic Needs of the Patient

- **Maintenance of fluid and electrolytic balance:** Adequate fluid and electrolyte balance is necessary for normal body functioning. Patients who have diarrhea, need extra fluid intake to compensate the fluid lost from the gastrointestinal tract. In diarrhea, fluid and electrolytes are lost because of hyper secretion of mucus from the membrane due to irritation and due to lack of reabsorption of fluid by the bowel. Normally 8 L of fluid is secreted into bowel in 24 hours period. Most of this fluid is reabsorbed. Due to severe diarrhea the level of the potassium and sodium chloride of the body is reduced resulting in an initial effect of acidosis due to the loss of base.
- **Maintenance of adequate nutritional state:** As the food moves quickly through the gastrointestinal tract, many food constituents are not absorbed in diarrhea patients. Taking of small amounts of nonirritating foods such as bland diets at frequent intervals is often helpful to prevent diarrhea and facilitate absorption.
- **Maintenance of comfort and hygiene:** Meeting the comfort and hygienic needs of the patients with elimination problem is valuable contribution to the sense of well-being.
  - Cleanliness is essential. The sight and smell of feces is distressing and the high bacterial count in feces is a source of contamination. Therefore, the patient is given opportunity to wash his/her hands after every defecation and if needed he/she is assisted to clean the rectal area and soiled linen should be removed immediately, if there is.
  - A bed patient with diarrhea should be provided with bed pan at hand and it should be emptied and cleaned after each use. The nurse should take initiative in ventilating and freshening the room after each defecation to eliminate unpleasant odors.
  - Many patients develop irritation of the skin and mucus membrane in the anal region due to constant diarrhea. Cleanliness is important to prevent infection and emollient creams help to keep the skin intact and to soothe irritated area.
  - Nurse's reaction to the patients with elimination problems is an important factor. He/she should show sympathy and accept his/her needs and extend the timely help to overcome the tension and anxiety.

(Ref: BW Dugas—Introduction to Patient Care)

Giving and Taking of Bedpan

Bedpan is a special container used to receive waste products such as urine and motion from the patient who is in bed.

Purposes of Giving Bedpan

- To give the patient necessary help and to ensure the correct and comfortable placement of the bedpan
- To receive the elimination of feces and urine
- To remove the bedpan correctly and to leave the patient and bed clean
- To measure and record the output accurately
- To collect the specimen for examination

Requisites

A toilet tray containing:

Article	Purpose
Warmed bedpan with cover	For the patient to defecate
Disposable gloves	To prevent cross contamination
Jug with warm water	For washing the perineum

Contd...

Article	Purpose
Soap in soap dish	For hand washing by the patient
Wash cloth and towel	For wiping
Small bowl with cotton or rag pieces	For cleaning the anus
Long artery forceps	For cleaning the perineum
Kidney tray	For disposing the soiled cotton pieces
Screen (if patient is in the private room there is no need of screen)	For providing privacy
Plastic apron	For protecting the dress of the nurse

Procedure

Steps	Procedure	Rationale
1.	Explain the procedure to the patient	Providing information fosters cooperation
2.	Screen the bed if it is in a common ward or close the door.	Minimizes embarrassment and ensure privacy
3.	Adjust the bed to appropriate height to prevent back strain. Elevate the side rail on the opposite side.	Ensures proper body mechanics. Elevating side rails prevent the client from falling out of bed
4.	Perform hand hygiene. Wear required PPE.	Prevents the spread of microorganisms
5.	A small Mackintosh may be placed over the draw sheet and under the buttocks to protect the bed before placing the bedpan under the buttocks. Keep the cloth away from the buttock.	Prevents soiling of the linen.
6.	Lower the top sheet to expose the area and loosen the pyjama. Ask the patient to flex the knees, resting the weight on the back heels, and raising the buttocks, or by using a trapeze bar, if present. Drape the patient	Provides privacy and facilitates easy defecation.
7.	Carry the bedpan to the bedside, cover it well and place it on a stool at the foot end of the bed. The bedpan should be clean and dry (Warm the bedpan either by washing it with warm water or by keeping it in the sun for a short time). Do not use chipped bedpan because it may injure the patient. So pad the seat of the bedpan if chipped. Remove the rubber ring or knee pillow if any and other articles that might interfere with the procedure.	Chilled bed pan may cause discomfort.

Contd...

Steps	Procedure	Rationale
8.	Keep the bedpan on the bed on your working side and keep the cover on the stool. If needed pour some water inside the bed pan.	Pouring water prevents sticking of feces in the bedpan.
9.	• With your left hand raise the patient's lower back and at the same time instruct him/her to lift himself/herself gently by pressing his/her heels against the mattress. • With your right hand, insert the bedpan under the patient's buttocks and lower the patient gently over the bedpan. Adjust comfortably for the patient. • Leave the patient alone unless he/she is too ill or weak and likely to faint or fatigued. Give the patient adequate time but do not leave the patient longer than the required time. • Raise the head end of the bed to 90°.	Allows space for bedpan between the individual and bed. Provides privacy and prevents embarrassment. Raising the head end facilitates easy defecation.
10.	Get the toilet tray ready to the bedside while the patient is on the bedpan. 	Organization facilitates accurate skill performance.

Contd...

Steps	Procedure	Rationale
11.	When removing the bedpan, return the bed to the position used when giving the bedpan, hold the bedpan steady to prevent spillage of its content, cover the bedpan, and place it on the adjacent chair.	Protects bedding and prevents odors.
12.	• In case of Indian patients supply a measure of water and let the patient wash himself/herself while he/she is on the bedpan if condition permits. Also, provide articles necessary for hand washing. In case of European patients supply with toilet paper and articles necessary for hand washing if condition permits. • In case of very ill patients, the nurse has to do it for the patient. Wash the part well with water while the patient is on the bedpan and remove the bedpan by supporting the hip as before and cover it immediately. Turn the patient to one side. Place the kidney tray near the buttocks. Use wet rag piece or cotton and clean the part using artery forceps. Clean it on above downward to prevent the entrance of bacteria into the urethra and vagina in case of a female patient. Discard the used swabs into the kidney tray. • Clean the perineal region and anus thoroughly and dry well. In case of bed patient, attend the back with spirit and powder after drying the area. 	Prevents excoriation and skin breakdown.
13.	Readjust pyjamas bedding, and patient's position. Remove the screen and leave the unit tidy. Make the patient comfortable.	Promotes comfort.
14.	Take the bedpan to the sluice room and inspect it for abnormalities before emptying the contents. If there is any doubt, keep the bedpan with its contents and call someone who knows about it. Empty the contents and clean the bedpan, rinse it with cold water. Then wash with hot soap water if available using a brush. Immerse it in (Lysol 2% for 2 hours and keep it ready for next use, on the bedpan rack)	Eliminates risk of cross contamination and spread of communicable disease.
15.	Remove all other articles from the bedside. Clean them and put them away in their proper places.	Prepares for the next procedure. Promotes comfort and well-being of the patient.
16.	Remove and discard your gloves. Wash your hands well.	Prevents the spread of infection.
17.	Air the area by opening a window, if possible. Spray the room with air freshener as needed unless contraindicated because of respiratory problems or allergies.	Controls odor
18.	Document color, odor, amount and consistency of urine and feces and the condition of the perineal area. Record the observations and time of elimination.	Documentation fosters quality care.

Unit IV ❖ Basic Needs of the Patient

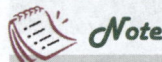

Note

- Never place a bedpan on the floor or on the bedside table.
- Cultivate observation regarding urine and stool and be careful in the selection of descriptive terms when charting or reporting.
- A routine stool and urine examination is done on every patient on the same day or the next morning of admission day.

Vital Points to be Observed

- The number of bowel movements in 24 hours
- Any accompanying pain or strain
- The consistency, shape, color and odor of the stool
- The presence of unusual matter like blood, worms etc.

RETENTION OF URINE

Retention of urine is a condition in which the urine is retained in the bladder and the patient is unable to expel the same. Urine production from the kidneys continues but the accumulated urine is not released from the bladder.

Symptoms of Retention

- Failure to void
- Feeling of fullness and discomfort on the lower abdomen
- Distended bladder

Possible Causes of Retention of Urine

- Temporary paralysis following anesthesia or any other cause. The abdominal muscles may not be able to contract sufficiently to produce contraction of the bladder to have micturition. In postpartum patients, atonic muscles of the bladder can lead to retention of urine. In patients with continuous catheter drainage, the tone of the bladder muscle will be lost temporarily and cause retention.
- Loss of tone due to debility or following over distension or paralysis following injury or disease of the spinal nerves.
- Dulled senses following shock or a dose of morphine or due to alcohol.
- Chill following pelvic operations. Surgery or trauma in urinary structures may interfere voiding. Edema or infection following operation on perineum or urethra can lead to retention due to pain.
- Nervous contraction of the urethral sphincters due to fear of pain.
- Obstruction due to stricture or enlarged prostate glands. This type of retention is not simple retention and therefore it should be treated by the doctor.
- Pressure on the bladder or urethra due to pelvic tumors or fetus in uterus or even a very hard fecal impaction.
- Use of certain drugs like analgesics and tranquilizers which suppress the nervous system and interfere with voiding, reducing the activity of the nerve reflexes of bladder.
- Lack of fluid intake may cause very slow urine production, which takes a lot of time to fill the bladder and accommodate an increased quantity of urine without causing the feeling for voiding as in normal case. Thus the contracting power of the bladder muscles is lessened due to over stretching and retention results.

Before resorting to catheterization or even reporting that the patient cannot pass urine, a good nurse, will use all knowledge and skill to aid the patient empty the bladder by natural means remembering that untold harm may follow frequent catheterization and that an attack of cystitis may occur following even one procedure of catheterization.

Nurse's Role to Relieve Retention of Urine

- Promote mental and physical relaxation through measures as the particular case demands. Provide enough privacy.
- Remove any distracting source of discomfort. See that the patient is not kept waiting for bedpan or urinal. Offer it soon, as they ask for it. Do not hurry the patients as this may cause further tension and contraction of the urethral muscles.
- Suggest the act by letting the patient hear the sound of running water by opening the tap or by pouring water from one jug to another.
- Relaxing the sphincter muscles of the urethra by pouring warm water over the vulva in female patients. Keep some hot water in the bedpan. The heat may relax the muscles. Apply a hot water bag over the bladder region.
- Let the patient splash her hands in cold water. Pour cold water over the vulva in female patients when pouring warm water is of no use.
- See that the patient is put as nearly as possible into the position in which she urinates normally.
- Give a warm drink and force fluids if allowed.
- Give a hot hip bath if not contraindicated.
- An enema may help.
- Stimulate bladder walls by gentle massage and pressure on the abdominal wall above the symphisis pubis.
- If voiding cannot be induced by nursing measures, catheterization will have to be done with the doctor's order.

INCONTINENCE OF URINE

Incontinence means uncontrolled urination: Urinary incontinence or involuntary voiding is a common urinary problem particularly among ill people. Sometimes there is complete inability to control the flow of urine and as a result a constant dribbling occurs. This is not only demoralizing and embarrassing to the individual, but urine can also be a source of irritation to the skin in the anogenital region. There are different types of incontinence, given as follows:

- **Sensory incontinence:** In very old people, the bladder loses sensitivity to fullness which may result in a lack of awareness of the need of micturition and hence the full bladder will dribble urine by itself. It is described as sensory incontinence.
- **Stress incontinence** is due to the weakness of the urethral sphincters by stretching of the pelvic floor during child birth. Urine is lost intermittently during coughing or sneezing but normally the patient remains dry.
- **Urge incontinence:** In severe inflammatory conditions of the bladder the desire to void is so urgent that the patient leaks urine before reaching toilet. This occurs usually rapidly after treatment of infection.

Possible Causes

- Urinary incontinence sometimes can occur temporarily after an operation on urinary tract
- Diseases of the nerves and muscles of the bladder

- Weakened or poor muscle control of the pelvic floor
- Weakness or damage to the sphincter muscles
- Any tumor or enlarged prostate or after prostatectomy
- Unconsciousness
- Old age (sensory incontinence)
- Extreme use of drugs like diuretics, sedatives, etc.
- Urinary infection
- Massive fecal impaction
- Neurological conditions like spinal fracture, paralysis, etc.
- Strictures of the urethra
- Hypertrophy of the tissues around the neck of the bladder
- Occasionally loss of bladder control can happen to anyone after drinking a lot of fluid and where a toilet is not immediately available specially in later life

Nurse's Role to Prevent Incontinence of Urine

- First, trace out the reason of the incontinence and try to correct it accordingly.
- Provide physical and psychological relaxation to the patient and make provision for voiding according to the condition and type of patient.
- Arrange for the toilet for walking patient. Provide bedpan for a conscious bed patient in his/her easy reach. This will improve the mental caliber of the patient to control voiding.
- Establish a regular voiding schedule frequently in the beginning and extend the interval gradually.
- Improve the muscle tone by perineal exercise which will strengthen the weak perineal muscles.
- Get medical aid for urinary infection and functional defects. Plenty of fluid may be administered in the treatment of infection if not contraindicated.
- The intake of fluids is limited before night so that urine production and overflow is reduced at night and the disturbances to patient are minimized.
- **Care of skin of patients with incontinence is of great importance:** Care should be taken regularly to clean and protect the patient's skin with barrier creams. Skin constantly moistened with urine will become irritated and macerated.
- Washing the perineal area and back of a bed patient and keeping the part dry will help to prevent complications. Not only will this reduce the possibility of pressure sores or infections occurring, but it will also reduce the offensive odor which arises from static urine.
- If the incontinence is not received by simple measures or by treatments such patients are advised to put an indwelling catheter in the bladder to keep them clean and dry.
- If it is a walking patient, the outer end of the catheter can be clamped and kept safely in position which can be released and the bladder is emptied when the patient feels a full bladder.
- If it is a bed patient, the indwelling catheter can be attached to a glass connection and rubber tube leading to a drainage bottle which can be emptied, cleaned and changed after clamping the tube when necessary.

Giving and Removing the Urinal

Urinal is a vase like container to receive urine.

Requisites

Articles	Purpose
Urinal	For meeting the urinary elimination needs of patient
Tissue paper or a basin with warm water or a wet wash cloth	For cleansing the perineal region
Mackintosh and towel	For spreading under the perineal area
Specimen collection container if required	For laboratory investigations
Kidney tray	To collect soiled waste

Procedure

Steps	Procedure	Rationale
1.	Explain the procedure to the patient and how he/she can cooperate	Reduces anxiety and promotes cooperation
2.	Screen the patient.	Minimizes embarrassment and ensure privacy
3.	Raise the level of the bed and position the patient comfortably.	Ensures proper body mechanics
4.	Perform hand hygiene and wear required PPE.	Prevents the spread of microorganisms
5.	Bring and place the urinal on the stool on the side of bed where the nurse is standing. Place a mackintosh and towel under the perineal region.	Prevents soiling of linen and clothes
6.	Make the patient to flex the knees slightly and keep the legs little apart so that the urinal can be placed on the bed in between the legs.	Proper positioning facilitates easy voiding

Contd...

Unit IV ❖ Basic Needs of the Patient

Steps	Procedure	Rationale
7.	Fold back the cloth and lift the top sheet and place the urinal in place. Do not expose the patient unnecessarily.	Provides privacy.
8.	The open end of the urinal should be directed to the patient. See that it is placed in the proper place and the penis is directed towards the opening of the urinal in case of male patient. The mouth of the urinal should be held higher than the lower portion so that the contents are not spilled when urinal is removed. Do not exert pressure against the patient's scrotum.	Proper positioning of the urinal prevents spillage of urine in the clothes and linen and prevents discomfort.
9.	Leave the patient for some time with the call bell within reach. Remove the urinal from the bedside as soon as he has finished using it. Measure the urine. Examine the urine for color, quantity and odor, etc., before emptying the urinal. Note whether specimen is to be saved or quantity is to be measured. Save specimen if anything seems abnormal.	Provides privacy. Assessment of urine facilitates in proper care.
10.	Empty the urinal, clean it and replace in its proper place.	Prepares for next use.
11.	Wipe the urethral orifice with a wet tissue. Make sure, the perineum is dry. Offer water, soap and towel to wash and dry the hands. Remove the mackintosh and towel. Make the patient and the unit tidy.	Promotes the hygienic care and patient's well-being.
12.	Remove gloves and wash hands.	Prevents transfer of microorganisms.
13.	Document the procedure with date, time, quantity of urine, color, odor with signature.	Documentation fosters quality care.

URINARY CATHETERIZATION

Catheter

A catheter is a hollow tube used to remove fluid from a body cavity like from the bladder or for distending a passage. Catheters are made from glass, rubber, metal, fibers and other similar materials and vary in size and in the shape of their tips. Depending upon the use of catheters, the tips may be flute type for urethral use, mushroom type for indwelling, filiform type for path finding and conical for dilatation.

Rubber and plastic catheters are flexible, whereas catheters made of metals and glasses are not.

Urethral metal and glass catheters are different in length for males and females depending upon the length of the urethra (Figs 5A to C).

Different Types of Urethral Catheters

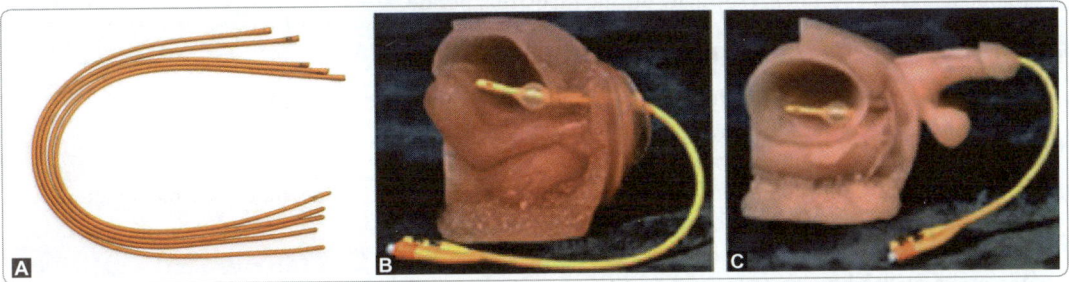

Figures 5A to C: (A) Different sizes of rubber catheters; (B) Female catheter; (C) Male catheter

- According to the use, the catheter can be classified into an **ordinary catheter** and **self-retaining catheter**.
- According to the part where a catheter is used, there are different types of catheters:
  - Urethral catheter used for drawing urine from the urinary bladder.
  - Self-retaining catheter used to retain in body cavities.

The size and length of catheter depends upon the type of it. A urethral catheter can be improvised for many other situations also in the common practice, such as fixing at the tip of the suction nozzle, aspiration syringe, oxygen cylinder to fix at the tip of mucus extractor to suck the mucus from the upper respiratory tract of the newborn babies, etc. It is more easy and safe to use an ordinary rubber catheter to catheterize the urinary bladder of the patients. The size of the catheter varies according to the age group of the patient.

Other types of catheters are:
- Nasal catheter for giving feeding or for gastric aspiration
- Tracheal catheter used for blowing air into the lungs
- Ureteric catheter used for drawing urine directly from ureters
- Eustachian catheter is one which is used for treating the middle ear
- Cardiac catheter to reach in the chambers of the heart through blood vessels

Catheterization of the Urinary Bladder

Catheterization is the introduction of a catheter into the urinary bladder through the external urethra for draining of urine.

It is a procedure to be done with the greatest care with strict aseptic precautions and it always involves the patient in considerable risk of developing cystitis. So this treatment is never carried out unless, especially ordered.

Therapeutic Uses

- To relieve distension of bladder caused by retention of urine
- To determine:
  - Whether inability to void is due to retention or suppression.
  - Amount of residual urine present in the bladder (in this case catheterization is done immediately after voiding).
- To ensure an empty bladder before certain pelvic operations, before bladder irrigation or before instillation of a drug.
- To avoid soiling and infection of the wound following operations on the genital region.
- To avoid scalding and the occurrence of possible bedsores in case of incontinence or retention with overflow

Unit IV ❖ Basic Needs of the Patient

- To secure a sterile specimen of urine when required for laboratory or culture examination.
- To obtain a clear specimen, especially during menstrual period.

Preliminary Assessment of the Patient and Situation

- Identify the patient, check the doctor's order and note any precautions to be taken.
- Verify physician's order for catheter insertion.
- Get the instructions from the ward sister.
- Note the general condition of the patient, his/her ability of understanding, mood and cooperation.
- Learn the purpose and reason for catheterization.
- See whether any specimen is to be preserved.
- Assess the availability of articles in the unit and assistance available.

Requisites

Sterile tray containing:

Articles	Purpose
Foleys catheter—2 with collecting chamber or urinary drainage bag	For urinary catheterization
Small bowl containing an antiseptic solution (Dettol—2%)	For cleaning the perineal area
Sterile cotton swabs or gauze pads	For cleaning the perineal area
Pair of gloves	To protect from contamination
Thumb forceps and artery forceps one each	For cleaning the perineal area
Sterile kidney tray—1	For collecting the urine
Sterile towel—1	For draping the patient
Test-tube or specimen bottle	For urine specimen collection
Small bowl containing lubricant	For lubricating the catheter facilitating easy insertion

Unsterile tray containing:

Articles	Purpose
Mackintosh or paper	To prevent soiling of linen
Flash light	For assessment of perineal area
Kidney tray	For discarding the wastes
Adhesive and scissors, if necessary	For securing the urinary bag
Screen	For providing privacy
Bedpan	To empty the urine from the kidney tray

Procedure

Steps	Procedure	Rationale
1.	Verify the physician's order. Explain the procedure to the patient.	Win the cooperation and confidence of the patient
2.	Provide privacy. Screen the patient.	Prevents embarrassment and promotes patient comfort.

Contd...

Steps	Procedure	Rationale
3.	Assemble the equipment to the bedside conveniently.	Organization facilitates skilled procedure.
4.	Check for size and type of catheter, and use smallest size of catheter possible. 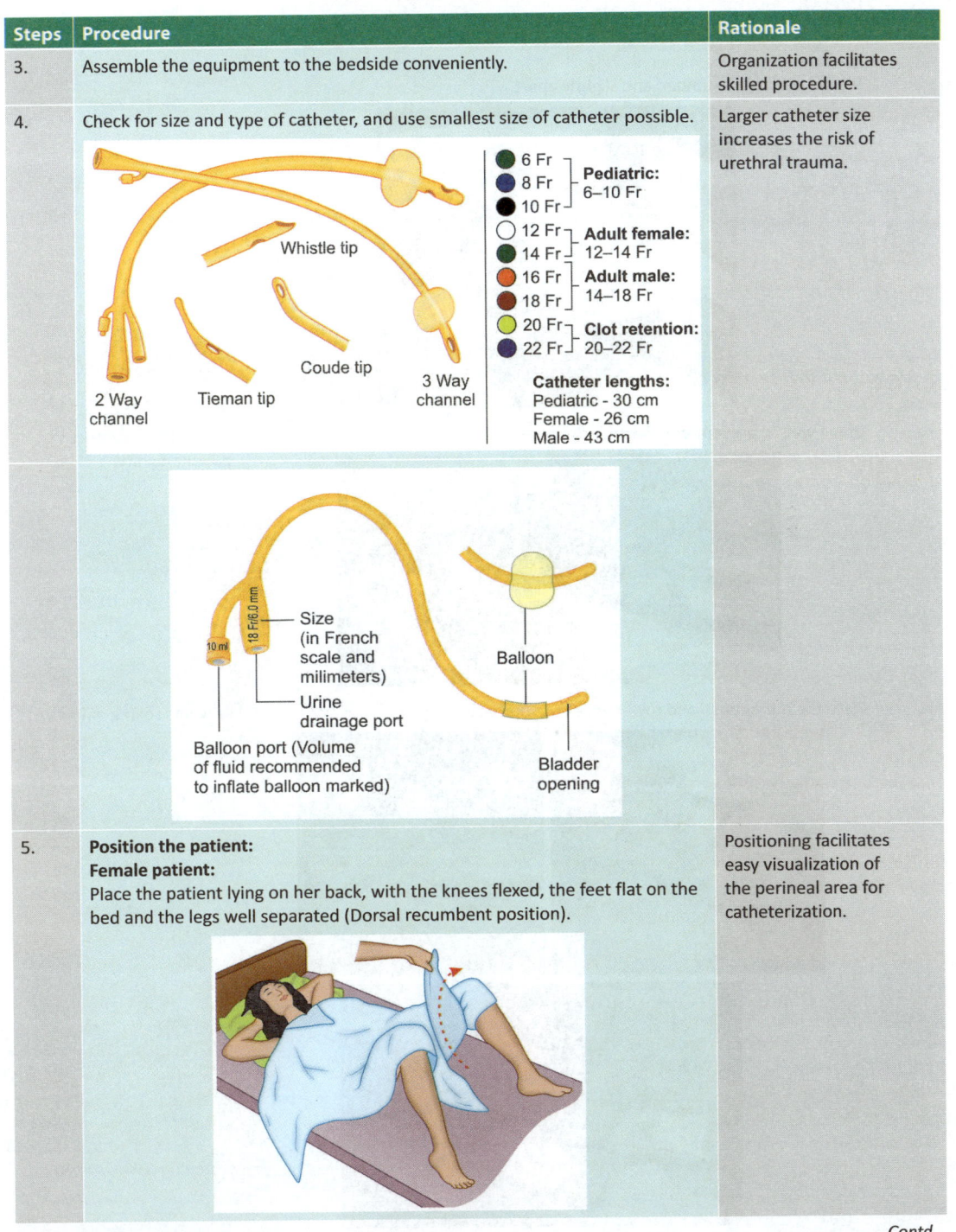	Larger catheter size increases the risk of urethral trauma.
5.	**Position the patient:** **Female patient:** Place the patient lying on her back, with the knees flexed, the feet flat on the bed and the legs well separated (Dorsal recumbent position).	Positioning facilitates easy visualization of the perineal area for catheterization.

Contd...

Steps	Procedure	Rationale
	Male patient: Supine with legs extended and slightly apart. 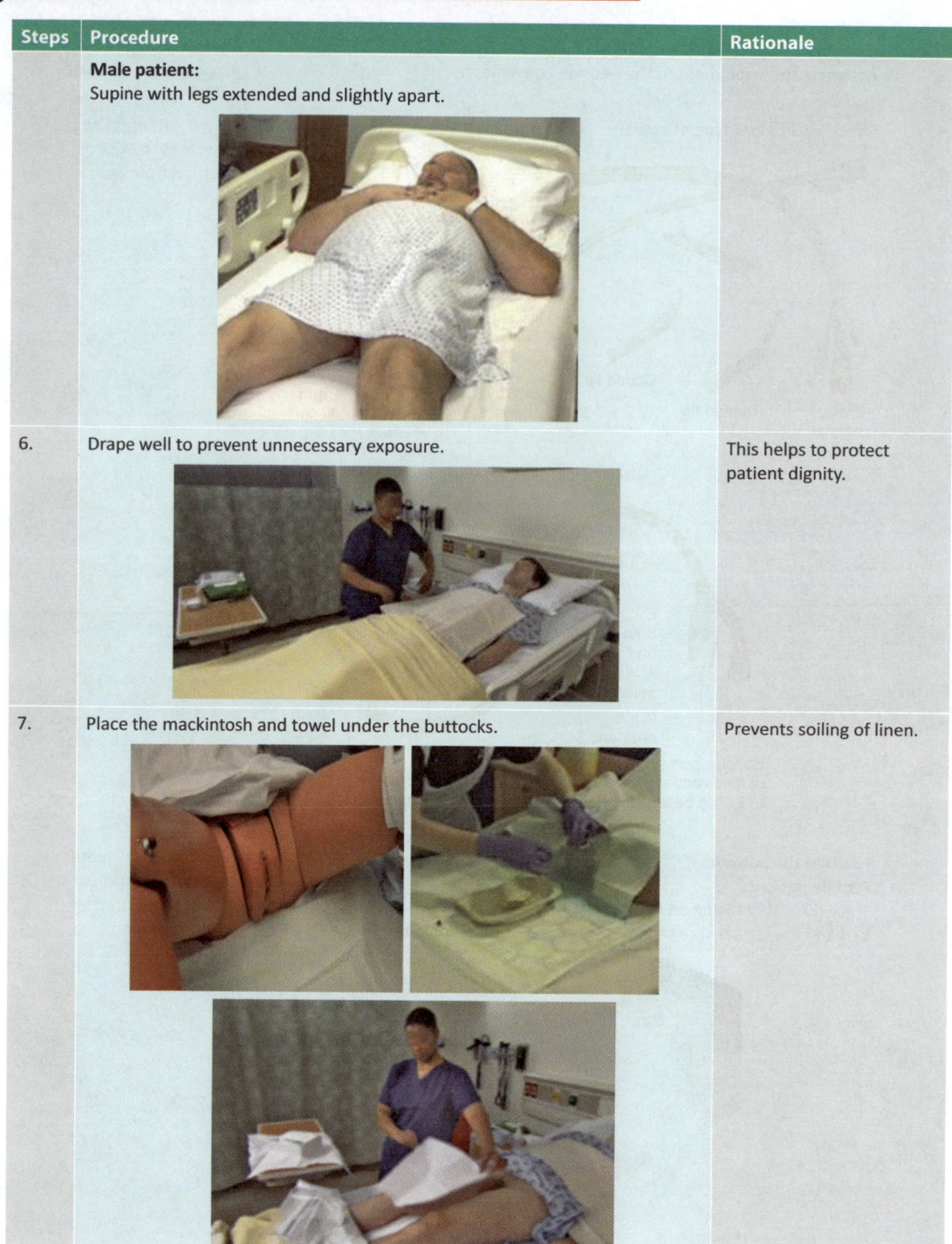	
6.	Drape well to prevent unnecessary exposure.	This helps to protect patient dignity.
7.	Place the mackintosh and towel under the buttocks.	Prevents soiling of linen.

Contd...

Steps	Procedure	Rationale
8.	Place the articles conveniently within reach of the nurse on a stool or table near the bed rather than on the bed itself. (If there is someone to assist the nurse, he/she can handle the unsterile articles) Add supplies and cleaning solution to catheterization kit, and according to agency policy.	This ensures preparation and organization for procedure.
9.	If using indwelling catheter and closed drainage system, attach urinary bag to the bed and ensure that the clamp is closed.	Urinary bag should be closed to prevent urine drainage leaving bag.
10.	Before leaving, explain to the patient the reason for leaving him/her after draping. Go and scrub hands as for a surgical procedure. After scrubbing, return to the bedside. Put on gloves.	Prevents transfer of micro-organisms
11.	Lift the draping sheet back with the elbow to expose the part. Place the sterile towel in position under the buttocks.	Patient should be comfortable, with perineum or penis exposed, for ease and safety in completing procedure.
12.	Using the artery forceps and swabs moistened in lotion, clean thoroughly the area (Labia majora and minora or the penis). Swabbing from above downwards using one swab only for one stroke and discarding the swab each time. (Throughout cleaning process use a gentle but firm downward motion)	Cleaning from more clean area to less clean area and this reduces the transmission of micro-organisms.

Contd...

Unit IV ❖ Basic Needs of the Patient

Steps	Procedure	Rationale

	• **In females:** Clean perineum from the mid-line outward in following order:
	  ▪ The vulva
	  ▪ The labia
	  ▪ Inside of labia on both sides
	  ▪ Outside of labia on both sides
	
	• **In males:** Using the forceps, clean the penis thoroughly with cotton moistened with antiseptic in a circular motion.	

13.	After cleaning, place the forceps in the unsterile kidney tray. 	The used forceps is considered unsterile and can be kept aside for cleaning.
14.	Place a swab lightly in the vaginal orifice. Place the sterile kidney tray in position on the sterile towel close to the vulva or penis. 	Helps prevent the spread of discharge upward and locates the urethra easily.

Contd...

Steps	Procedure	Rationale
15.	• Open the lubricant and eject the contents in the sterile bowl or tray. Add lubricant using sterile technique. 	Lubrication minimizes urethral trauma and discomfort during procedure.
	• Dip the tip of the catheter into the lubricant. Lubricate tip of catheter using sterile lubricant included in tray, or apply lubricant directly. 	This process helps visualize urethral meatus and relax external urinary sphincter.
16.	• **In females,** inspect the vestibule carefully for the urinary meatus by separating the labia minor with the thumb and forefinger of the non-dominant hand. With the non-dominant hand retract the foreskin in exposing the meatus in the centre of the glans. ▪ With the dominant hand, take the catheter from the tray, grasp it 7.5 cm away from the eye end. 	

Contd...

Steps	Procedure	Rationale
	• **In males,** lubricate the catheter. Insert it gently into the meatus, stretching the penis with the left hand lifting into an angle 90° in order to straighten the urethral canal as much as possible. (Insert the catheter about 20 cm or until urine begins to flow). 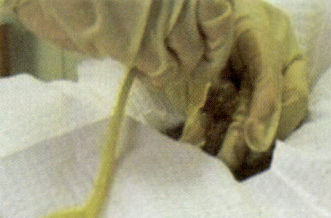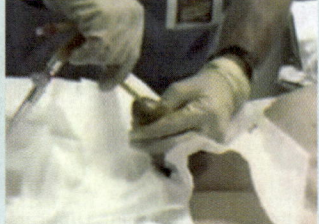 • **In female,** Insert gently and carefully about 5–7.5 cm into the meatus in an upward and backward direction (instruct the patient to breathe through the mouth). If any obstruction is felt, do not force the catheter; withdraw the catheter a little and again insert it slowly. If the catheter becomes unsterile before introducing, discard it and take the other sterile one. If gloves are not used, take the thumb forceps to pick up and insert the catheter. 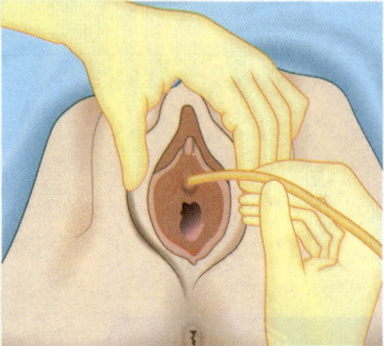	
17.	• The urine begins to flow freely into the sterile kidney tray. 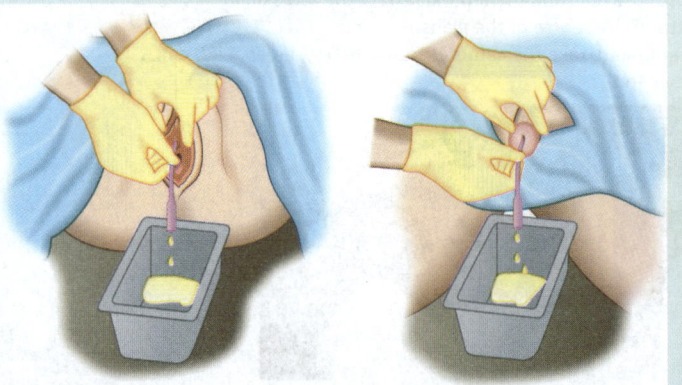	Urine specimen may be required for analysis.

Contd...

Steps	Procedure	Rationale
	• Collect the urine in the test tube or bottle by placing the end of the catheter directly into the bottle, if a sterile specimen is required. In case of culture, the last portion of urine must be collected as it is more likely to contain pus cells and microorganisms. 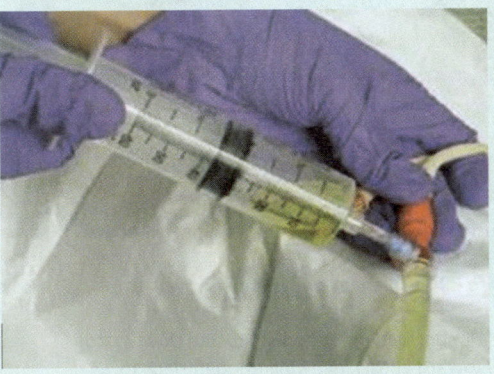	
18.	When the flow of urine stops, remove the catheter gently, after pinching, if it is a rubber one or after placing the finger over the tip of the catheter, if it is a metal one. Or slowly inflate balloon for **indwelling catheters** according to catheter size, using prefilled syringe. The size of balloon is marked on the catheter port. 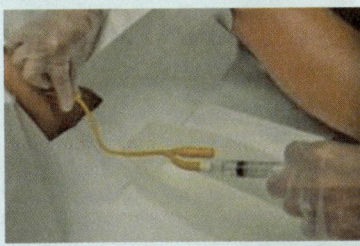 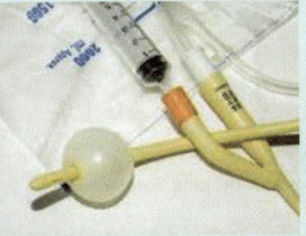	Catheter is removed in intermittent catheterization.
	After balloon is inflated, pull gently on catheter until resistance is felt and then advance the catheter again. 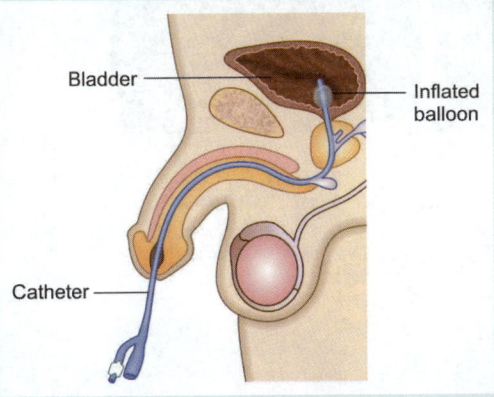	Moving catheter back into bladder will avoid placing pressure on bladder neck.

Contd...

Unit IV ❖ Basic Needs of the Patient

Steps	Procedure	Rationale
19.	Connect urinary bag to catheter using sterile technique. Keep urinary bag below level of patient's bladder. Do not lie on tubing Hang bag on frame of bed	This facilitates drainage of urine through gravity.
20.	Secure catheter to patient's leg using securement device at tubing just above catheter bifurcation. **Female patient:** Secure catheter to inner thigh, allowing enough slack to prevent tension. **Male patient:** Secure catheter to upper thigh (with penis directed downward) or abdomen (with penis directed toward chest), allowing enough slack to prevent tension. Ensure foreskin is not retracted.	Securing catheter reduces risk of CAUTI, urethral erosion, and accidental catheter removal.
21.	Swab the meatus with a moistened swab and dry the part. Wipe the external part with the towel used for draping. Replace the foreskin in a male patient at the end of the procedure.	For male patients, leaving the foreskin retracted can cause pain and edema.

Contd...

Steps	Procedure	Rationale
22.	Remove the mackintosh and other articles from the bed.	This reduces the transmission of micro-organisms.
23.	Adjust the bed clothes and leave the patient warm and comfortable. Evaluate catheter function.	Promotes comfort and well-being of patient.
24.	Take the articles to the utility room and measure the urine. Note the quantity and character of urine. See that the specimen is marked 'catheterized specimen' and send to the laboratory with requisition form if required so.	This reduces the transmission of microorganisms. Urine specimen may be required for analysis.

Contd...

Unit IV ❖ Basic Needs of the Patient

Steps	Procedure	Rationale
25.	Discard the urine and soiled swabs.	This reduces the transmission of microorganisms.
26.	Clean the used articles thoroughly. Set the tray and send it for sterilization. Keep the rest of the articles back in their proper places.	This reduces the transmission of microorganisms.
27.	Remove gloves and discard them. Perform hand hygiene.	Prevents cross-contamination.
28.	Document the procedure with date, time, size of catheter inserted, amount of water in balloon, patient's response to procedure, and assessment of urine	Documentation fosters quality care.

REMOVING AN INDWELLING CATHETER

Procedure

Steps	Procedure	Rationale
1.	Verify physician's order for catheter removal, perform hand hygiene, and gather supplies like a tray containing nonsterile gloves, sterile syringe, mackintosh and towel, garbage bag, and cleaning supplies for perineal care.	Organization of supplies ensures skilled procedure
2.	Explain procedure to the patient	Wins confidence and cooperation of patient
3.	Provide privacy	Prevents embarrassment
4.	Apply non-sterile gloves.	Reduces the transfer of microorganisms.
5.	Measure, empty and record contents of urinary drainage bag. Record drainage amount, color and consistency.	Timely and accurate documentation promotes patient safety.

Empty the drainage bag

Steps	Procedure	Rationale
6.	Remove gloves, perform hand hygiene, and apply new non-sterile gloves.	Always change gloves after handling a urinary catheter bag to prevent infection transmission.

Contd...

Steps	Procedure	Rationale
7.	Remove catheter securement/anchor device.	Facilitates easy removal of device.
8.	Insert syringe in balloon port and drain fluid from balloon. Verify balloon size on catheter to ensure all fluid is removed from balloon.	A partially deflated balloon will cause trauma to the urethra wall and pain.
9.	Pull catheter out slowly and smoothly. If resistance is felt, stop removal and reattempt to remove the fluid from the balloon. Attempt removal again.	This prevents mucosal trauma and promotes comfort to the patient.
10.	Wrap used catheter in waterproof packet. Unhook catheter tube from urinary bag. Discard equipment and supplies.	This prevents accidental spilling of urine from the catheter.

Contd...

Steps	Procedure	Rationale
11.	Provide comfortable position to the patient. Remove gloves, and perform hand hygiene.	Prevents transfer of microorganisms
12.	Document time of catheter removal, condition of urethra, and any teaching related to post-catheter care and fluid intake. Document time, amount, and characteristics of first void after catheter removal.	Documentation fosters quality care.

BLADDER IRRIGATION

It is the flushing or washing out the urinary bladder with a specified solution.

Purposes

- Helps to cleanse the bladder from decomposed urine, bacteria, excess of mucus, pus and blood clots.
- Helps in preventing urinary tract obstruction by flushing out small clots that form after the surgeries of prostrate or bladder
- Helps to relieve congestion and pain in case of inflammatory conditions by the application of heat.
- To promote healing.
- To maintain the patency of the urinary catheter.
- To arrest bleeding.
- To prevent and treat infections.
- To prevent the clot formation in case of bladder surgeries.
- Used to treat an irritated, inflamed, or infected bladder lining.

Solutions Used

- Sterile water
- Normal saline
- 5% dextrose solution
- Boric acid 2%
- Potassium permanganate 1:10,000
- Acriflavine 1:10,000
- Silver nitrate 1:5000
- Acetic acid 1:400 to treat pseudomonas infection.

Types of Irrigation

- Open irrigation
- Closed irrigation

Open Irrigation

In this the drainage must be opened to the environment to do the irrigation.

Closed Drainage

It is of two types:
1. Continuous
2. Intermittent

General Instructions

- Verify the order for irrigation method, type and amount of irrigant, as well as type of catheter in place.
- Palpate the bladder for distention and tenderness.
- Assess patient for abdominal pain or spasms, sensation of bladder fullness, or catheter bypassing.
- Observe urine for color, amount, clarity and presence of mucus, clots or sediment.
- Monitor intake and output.
- Assess patient's knowledge regarding purpose of performing a catheter irrigation.

Articles Required

A tray containing:

Articles	Purpose
Irrigating can with tubing and a clamp or sterile irrigation set with tray	For using as a reservoir for irrigation
Sterile Irrigating solution	For irrigating the bladder
Bulb syringe/60 mL piston type syringe	To instil solution into the bladder
Bath blanket	For providing privacy for the patient
Sterile collection basin	For receiving the return flow
IV pole	For adjusting the height of the irrigating can
A small bowl with antiseptic swab	To clean the lumen of the catheter
Mackintosh and towel	For protecting the bedding and the garments
Kidney tray and paper bag	For discarding the soiled wastes
Extra sheets and garments	For changing after the procedure
Screen	For providing privacy
Tape or elastic bandage	To rescue the catheter
Drainage tube clamping	To clamp the catheter

Procedure

Steps	Procedure	Rationale
1.	Explain the procedure to the patient	Allays anxiety and wins confidence and cooperation.
2.	Provide privacy with curtains. Close the doors and windows as needed.	Maintains clients self-esteem
3.	Wash hands. Wear appropriate PPE	Prevents transfer of micro-organisms.
4.	Determine the type of catheter in place.	Helps identify the type of irrigation to be performed.

Contd...

Steps	Procedure	Rationale
5.	Record the urinary output measurement and empty the drainage bag.	Allows more accurate measurement of urinary irrigation.
6.	Place the client in dorsal recumbent position and expose catheter junction.	Allows for proper performance of procedure.
7.	Place mackintosh and towel under the catheter	Protects from soiling of linen and clothes.
8.	Organize supplies according to type of irrigation prescribed.	Organization facilitates accurate skill performance.
9.	Wash hands. Wear appropriate PPE	Prevents transfer of micro-organisms.
	Closed irrigation system	
10.	Connect the irrigation tubing to the irrigating solution. Insert the tip of the irrigation tube into the irrigation bag using aseptic technique.	Flushing the tube removes air

Contd...

Steps	Procedure	Rationale
	• Fill drip chamber half full by squeezing chamber. Prime the tubing by flushing the tubing with solution without touching the tip of the tubing anywhere. • Once fluid has completely filled tubing, close clamp and recap end of tubing and hang on IV pole. 	
11.	Using circular motion, clean catheter port with antiseptic swabs. 	Prevents introduction of microorganisms into the tubings.

Contd...

Unit IV ❖ Basic Needs of the Patient

Steps	Procedure	Rationale
12.	Connect the irrigating tube into the catheter using aseptic technique. 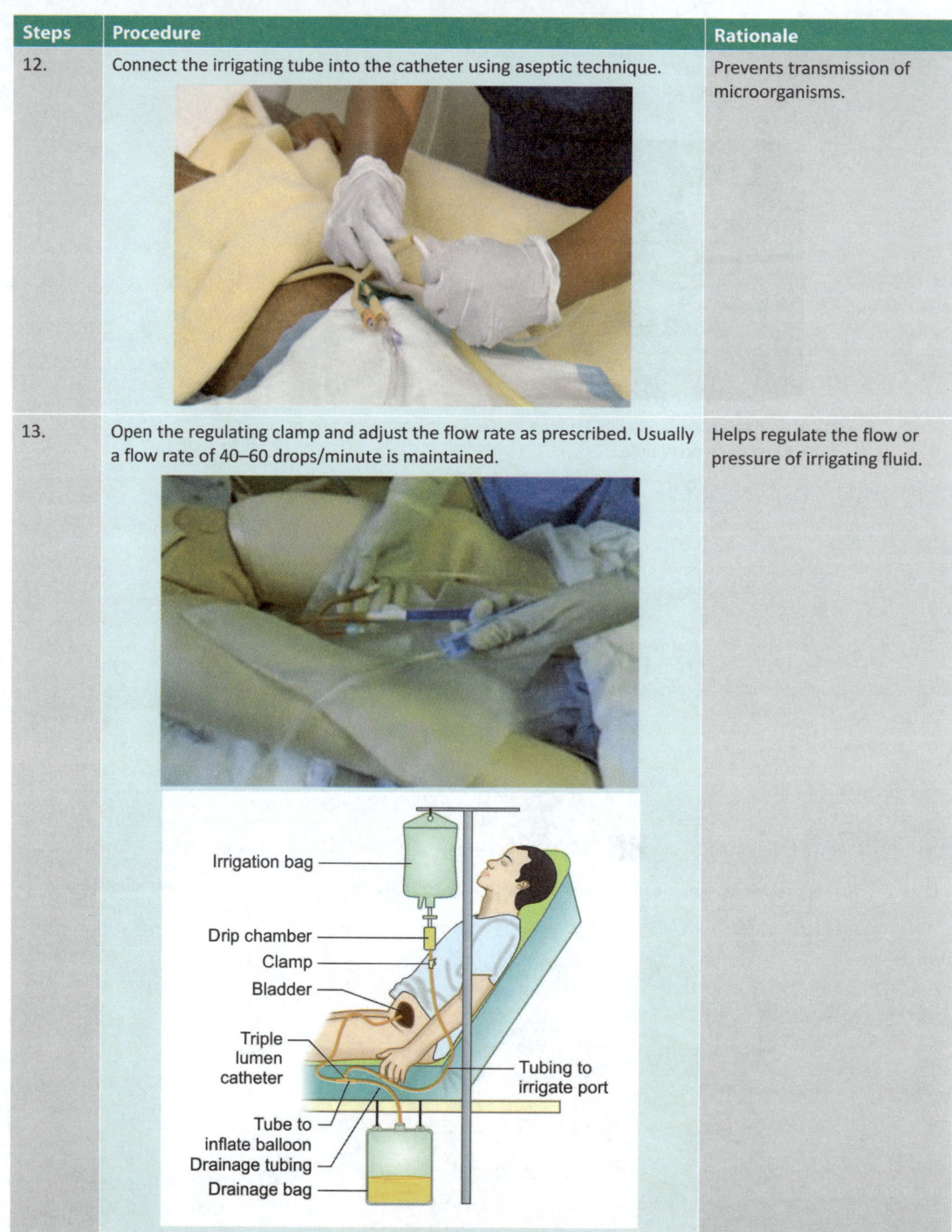	Prevents transmission of microorganisms.
13.	Open the regulating clamp and adjust the flow rate as prescribed. Usually a flow rate of 40–60 drops/minute is maintained.	Helps regulate the flow or pressure of irrigating fluid.

Irrigation bag

Drip chamber

Clamp

Bladder

Triple lumen catheter

Tubing to irrigate port

Tube to inflate balloon
Drainage tubing
Drainage bag

Contd...

Unit IV ❖ Basic Needs of the Patient

Steps	Procedure	Rationale
14.	Determine if the drainage is intermittent or continuous. • If it is continuous allow it to flow continuously and assess the drainage. • If it is intermittent, apply clamp for specified time and then release the clamp. 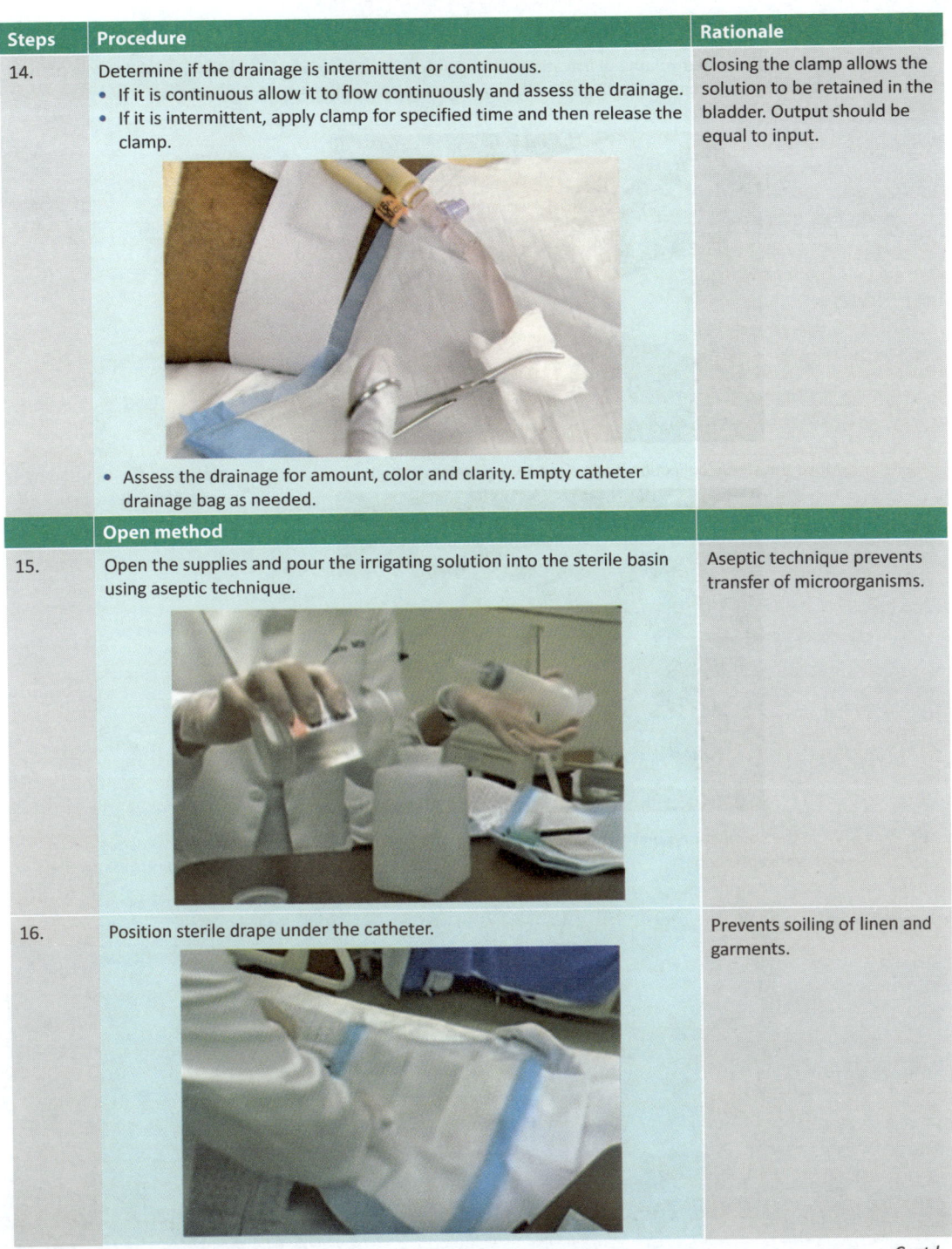 • Assess the drainage for amount, color and clarity. Empty catheter drainage bag as needed.	Closing the clamp allows the solution to be retained in the bladder. Output should be equal to input.
	Open method	
15.	Open the supplies and pour the irrigating solution into the sterile basin using aseptic technique.	Aseptic technique prevents transfer of microorganisms.
16.	Position sterile drape under the catheter.	Prevents soiling of linen and garments.

Contd...

Steps	Procedure	Rationale
17.	Aspirate prescribed volume of irrigation solution into irrigating syringe (usually 30 mL). Place the syringe into the sterile container until ready for.	Maintains the sterile nature of solution.
18.	Move the sterile collection basin close to the patient's thigh.	Helps drain the solution by gravity after cleansing.
19	Wipe the connection point between the catheter and drainage tubing with antiseptic wipes.	Prevents transmission of microorganisms into the bladder.

Contd...

Steps	Procedure	Rationale
20.	Disconnect catheter from drainage tubing allowing any urine to flow into sterile collection basin.	Maintaining sterility prevents introduction of micro-organism into the catheter.
	• Place the sterile cap at the end of the tubing and position tubing so it stays coiled on top of bed with end resting on sterile drape.	
21.	Insert tip of needleless syringe using twisting motion into port. Insert tip of syringe into lumen of catheter and gently push plunger to instil solution. Inject solution using slow, even pressure.	This minimizes the risk of trauma to the bladder.
22.	Remove syringe, lower catheter, and allow the solution to drain into a collection basin. The amount of drainage solution should be equal to or greater than the amount instilled. If ordered, repeat sequence of instilling solution and drainage until drainage is clear of clots and sediment.	Return solution drains by gravity.

Contd...

Unit IV ❖ Basic Needs of the Patient

Steps	Procedure	Rationale
23.	After irrigation is complete, remove protector cap from urinary drainage tubing end, clean end of tubing with antiseptic wipe and reinsert into lumen of catheter. Reconnect catheter to the drainage tube. Assess drainage for amount, color and clarity. 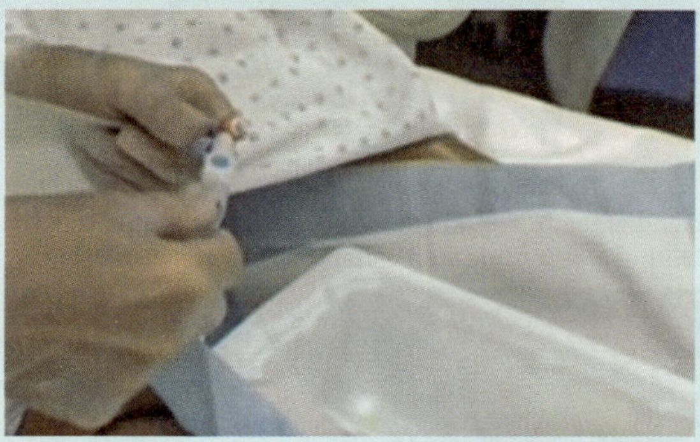	Amount of the drainage should be equal to the amount of entering the bladder.
24.	Anchor catheter with catheter securement device as shown in the figure below (female on left and male on right side). Help patient in staying at safe and comfortable position. Lower bed and place side rails accordingly. 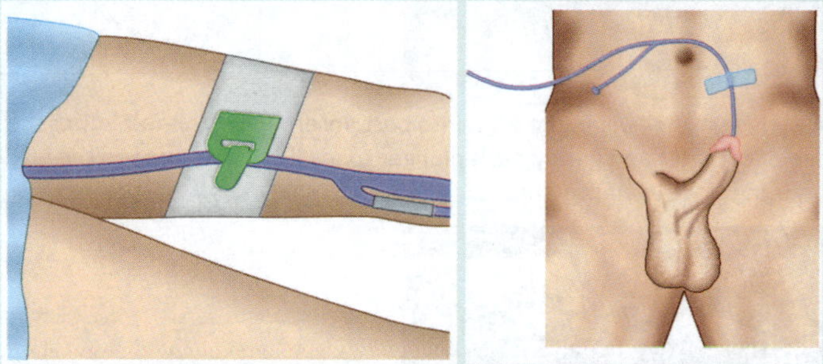	Prevents dislodgement or strain on the catheter.
25.	Measure actual urine output by subtracting total amount of irrigation fluid infused from total volume drained into basin. Inspect urine for blood clots and sediment and be sure that tubing is not kinked or occluded. 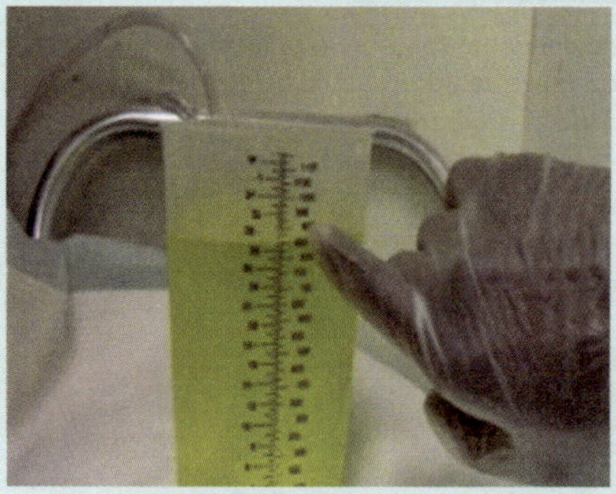	Helps to calculate fluid and electrolyte balance.

Contd...

Steps	Procedure	Rationale
26.	Dispose of all contaminated supplies in appropriate receptacle, remove gloves and perform hand hygiene	Prevents transmission of microorganisms
27.	Document the procedure and results, any abnormal constituents such as blood clots, pus or mucus shreds, amount of urine drained, type of irrigation done along with date, time and signature of the nurse.	Documentation fosters quality care.

CONDOM DRAINAGE

- Condom drainage is a method to collect and drain urine with the help of a catheter for men experiencing urinary incontinence.
- Condom catheters are external urinary catheters that are worn like a condom. A condom catheter is a urine storage device that can be used to treat short-term incontinence in men.

Purposes

- To provide urinary drainage when an indwelling catheter is not desired or needed
- Control incontinence in a male patient without the risk of urinary tract infection
- Greater comfort to the patient than an indwelling catheter

Preliminary Assessment

Measure the diameter of penis to determine the appropriate catheter size

Requisites

A condom drainage kit containing:

Articles	Purpose
Correct size of condom catheter (small, medium, large, extra-large) made of plastic or rubber.	For condom drainage application
Velcro, tape, or other kind of sheath holding material	To secure condom catheter
Urine bag with tube	For urinary drainage collection
Mackintosh/waterproof pad and bath towel	To protect the linen and clothes
Skin paste or tincture of benzoin or plasticized skin spray	For adhesive placement
A razor (if required)	To shave the pubic hair
Kidney tray	To discard soiled waste
Basin with warm water and soap	To clean the perineum

Contd...

Articles	Purpose
Disposable gloves	To protect from bodily secretions
Wash cloth/towel	To clean the perineum

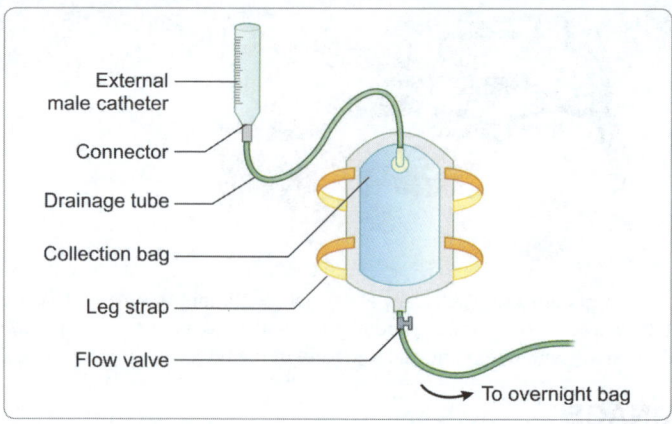

External male catheter

Connector

Drainage tube

Collection bag

Leg strap

Flow valve

To overnight bag

Figure 6: Condom catheter kit

Procedure

Steps	Procedure	Rationale
1.	Explain the procedure to the patient	Allays anxiety and wins cooperation of the patient.
2.	Place patient in either a supine or a bed sitting position with thighs slightly apart.	Positioning facilitates easy and comfortable application.
3.	Provide privacy, close door and drape the client's body with the bed clothes, with only penis exposed.	Provides privacy and reduces embarrassment.
4.	Place the mackintosh and towel under the perineal area.	Prevents soiling of linen and clothes.
5.	Wash hands and don gloves.	Prevents spread of microorganisms
6.	Take off old condom if the patient is already on condom drainage. Remove the tape, if it was applied and roll off the condom. Do not pull it off, as this could harm the skin. Inspect the penis for skin irritation excoriation, swelling or discoloration.	Careful handling prevents skin breakdown.

Contd...

Steps	Procedure	Rationale
7.	Shave or trim any hair on the base or the penis.	Presence of pubic hair may interfere while taping the adhesives.
8.	Clean the genital area by pulling the foreskin (if present) back and clean the head of the penis. **Two methods of washing:** 1. Wash directly with soap and water 2. Wash with the soapy wash cloth and rinse with the wet cloth. Roll the foreskin back down to cover the penis when done. Dry the area thoroughly.	Helps minimize skin irritation and excoriation after the condom is applied. Replacing foreskin prevents ischemia or necrosis to penis. Drying helps minimize skin irritation and excoriation
9.	Take condom out of package. Roll up the condom toward the funnel-shaped end. Place the funnel end of the condom over the head of the penis. Hold the penis at a 90° from the body in the nondominant hand. Gently roll the condom down over the head of the penis all the way to the base of the penis. Leave 1–2 inches leaving (2.5–5 cm) the condom catheter at the end of the penis. 	Proper placement of condom sheath facilitates urine drainage.

Contd...

Steps	Procedure	Rationale
10.	Securing the condom is done in any of the following methods: • In a self-adhesive type of condom, hold it in place after it is fully rolled down for 10 seconds. • If it is not a self-adhesive condom, secure the condom firmly but not too tightly to the penis by wrapping a strip of elastic tape spirally around the shaft of the penis (2/3rd the length of penis), making sure that the spirals do not overlap. • Get the condom holder out of the package. Wrap the condom holder about one inch above the base of the penis. Pull the strap over one finger to make sure the strap is not too tight. Fasten the condom holder and the elastic strap to the Velcro. 	Tape reinforcement prevents disconnection of tubing while the client moves.
11.	Attach the urinary drainage system securely to the condom. Make sure that the tip of the penis is not touching the condom and that condom is not twisted. 	Promotes comfort.

Contd...

Steps	Procedure	Rationale
12.	Attach the urinary drainage bag to the bed frame if the client is to remain in bed, or to the clients leg if he is ambulatory. Keep the drainage bag below the level of the condom and avoid loops or kinks in the tubing. 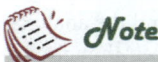 Condom catheter	Prevents disconnection of tubing while the client moves.
13.	Return bed to low position, cover the patient and make him comfortable. Confirm that the condom is secure and not leaking and observe the penis for swelling and discoloration after 30 minutes following application of condom.	Promotes comfort.
14.	Assess urine for color and characteristics. Wash and replace the articles.	Prepares for next use.
15.	Doff gloves and wash hands	Prevents spread of infection
16.	Document the procedure with date, time, response of patient, amount of urine collected, and characteristics of urine with signature.	Documentation fosters quality care.

Note

- Elastic tape is used to secure the catheter. Ordinary tape is contraindicated because it is not flexible and may stop blood flow.
- Change the condom daily, and assess the foreskin for signs of irritation, swelling and discoloration.

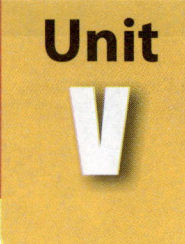

Unit V

Assessment of Patient

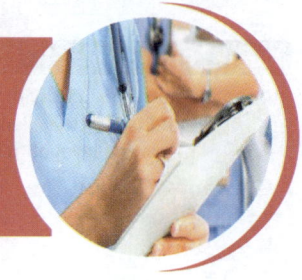

OBSERVATION NEEDS OF THE PATIENT

Definition

Observation: Observation is gathering data, recognizing and noting facts of occurrences. Observation refers to the gathering of information about the patient and the situation. It is the act of noticing something.

Importance of Observation

One of the vital factors in nursing care is intelligent observation of the patient. It is a chance to know the patient and to understand the condition of the physical, mental and spiritual being. Through observation, any change in condition improvement or regression may be detected. Specific information that will help in diagnosis may be obtained and results of treatment, medication and nursing care may be determined.

The art of nursing largely depends on the skill of observation. In the whole field of medical practice, there is nothing so difficult as diagnosis and nothing so essential to treatment. Observation and the analysis of observation is an essential factor in the diagnosis. Nothing can substitute observation. Even though the physician has many techniques in making accurate diagnosis, without an understanding of the symptoms, these techniques are futile. Physicians give great importance to what they can learn from the patients. Successful treatment depends on correct diagnosis and diagnosis depends to a great extent on the accurate observation of the patient and analysis of these observations. Doctor depends upon the nurse's alert and accurate observation in making the diagnosis and in prescribing treatment. The ability of the nurse in observation depends upon her knowledge, experience, interest and attention, and the development of skill in this method of gathering information.

Data obtained by observation might be the deciding factor between the life and death. Observation of patient is vitally important to the nursing care. It helps to plan his/her nursing care in a way which will bring the maximum benefit and comfort.

Physical Assessment

A thorough inspection or a detailed inspection of the entire body or some part of the body to determine the general physical condition or the conditions of some parts of the body or its function is called physical examination.

OBJECTIVES

- To detect disease at an early stage
- To determine causes and extent of disease
- For periodic check up
- To find out whether a person is physically fit

TYPES OF PHYSICAL EXAMINATION

- **Periodic health examination:** It is the kind of health examination which is done periodically at definite interval to see that the individual is keeping fit. It is the foundation stone of preventive medicine. The more complete the examination, the greater is its value as a preventive measure. It includes the inspection of the entire body. It is also done for patients as a follow up measure to watch the progress.
- **Physical examination for diagnostic purpose:** It is a medical examination done by the physician according to the patient's symptoms when illness occurs.

METHODS OF PHYSICAL EXAMINATION

- **Inspection:** It is the observation with naked eye, or observation of expression of patient to determine his general condition with naked eye, e.g., the presence of deformities or injuries, rashes or swelling.
- **Palpation** is feeling with the hands to note the size and position of the organs. The soft tissues are examined by palpation. The various organs of the abdomen and pelvis can be felt with the hands by applying pressure on the abdomen and pelvis.
- **Percussion:** Examination by tapping with the fingers on the body to determine the conditions of the internal parts by the sounds that are produced. It is done by placing a finger of the left hand firmly against the part to be examined as chest or abdomen and tapping with finger tips of the right hand over the finger kept on the part.
- **Auscultation:** It is listening to sounds within the body with the aid of a stethoscope or ear to patient's body. Stethoscope was discovered by an Englishman named Laennec in 1819. (Refer to Medical Encyclopaedia)
- **Manipulation:** Manipulation is examining a patient by moving certain parts of the body to note its flexibility or limitations in movement.
- **Testing of reflexes:** The response of the tissues to external stimuli is tested by means of the percussion hammer, a safety pin or hot and cold water.

ROLE OF THE NURSE IN THE PHYSICAL EXAMINATION

Preparation of the Environment and Equipment

- Maintain good ventilation and privacy
- Provide adequate light
- Arrange a separate examination room
- Provide a special examination table with mattress and pillow or an ordinary cot
- Articles should be arranged conveniently at the bedside

Unit V ❖ Assessment of Patient

Requisites for Examination

A tray consists of:

Sphygmomanometer	Specimen bottles
Stethoscope	Test tubes
Tongue depressor	Culture bottles and slides if needed
Flash light	Kidney tray
Tape measure and skin pencil	Ophthalmoscope for eye examination
Percussion hammer	Ear speculum
Safety pin	Cotton wool for ENT examination
Tuning Fork	Nasal speculum
Cotton applicators	Head mirror

(Screen for privacy if physical examination is done in the general ward)

Preparation of the Patient

Mental Preparation

The patient may be quite new to the hospital situation and he/she may be anxious and worried about his/her future life as well as his family. It is the duty of the nurse to allay his/her anxieties and fears by proper explanation of the advantages and purpose of the examination and treatment and try to win his/her confidence.

Physical Preparation

- Keep the patient clean.
- Help the patient to empty the bladder.
- Loosen the garments, expose only the needed areas and provide privacy.
- Keep the patient in a comfortable position and convenient to the doctor for examination.
- Avoid all unnecessary exposure.

Assistance for the Examination

- Never leave the patient alone during the physical examination, especially female
- Win the confidence and cooperation of the patient so that it will be easier for the doctor to do the examination
- Prepare the patient and get the equipment ready
- Secure privacy
- Keep the patient ready for examination
- Nurse should stand on the opposite side of the doctor to assist him. Adjust the position according to the need.
- Expose parts of the patient as needed for the examination
- Avoid unnecessary exposure
- Handle the equipment to the doctor as needed
- Turn the patient's head to the opposite side of the doctor especially during the chest examination.
- After finishing the examination, keep the patient in a comfortable position and replace the articles to the proper place after cleaning them.
- Send specimens to the laboratory immediately, if any taken.

Physiological Assessment—Vital Signs

Vital signs, or vitals are measurements of the inner workings of the human body. **Temperature, pulse, respiration** along with **blood pressure** reading are known as vital signs. Fifth vital sign is oxygen saturation.

One of the most common observations made by the nurse in relation to a patient's condition or progress is that of assessing his/her temperature, pulse and respiration. Because these findings are governed by the vital organs and often disclose even the slightest deviation from normal body functioning, assessment of vital signs is the most critical of observations regarding the condition of the patient. Significant variation in these findings may indicate problems relating to insufficient consumption or over consumption of oxygen, blood depletion, electrolyte imbalance, bacterial invasion or emotional distress.

A patient's vital signs are usually checked immediately on admission to a hospital or clinic and it is usually repeated at regular intervals during any acute stage and probably twice a day during his/her stay in the hospital.

BODY TEMPERATURE

Temperature is a measurement of heat expressed in degrees. Body temperature may be defined as the degree of heat maintained by the body. It is the balance between the heat produced and heat lost.

Temperature Range

Although the temperature varies from individual to individual, it can be classified as normal and abnormal.

Normal Temperature

- **Oral temperature:** 98.6°F (37°C). This may vary from 97° to 99°F (36°–37.2°C).
- **Rectal temperature:** 99.6°F (37.5°C).
- Axillary temperature: 97.6°F (36.4°C).

Abnormal Temperature

Subnormal: 97°F (95°–99°F) (36°–37.2°C)
- Hyperthermia is a temperature above 105°F (40.6°C).
- Hypothermia is a situation when the temperature falls below 95°F or 35°C
- Fever or pyrexia is a condition, in which the level of the body temperature rises uniformly above normal
- **Low pyrexia:** 99°–100°F (37.2°–37.8°C)
- **Moderate pyrexia:** 100°–103°F (37.8°–39.4°C)
- **High pyrexia:** 103°–105°F (39.4°–40.6°C)
- **Hyper pyrexia:** 105°F and over (40.6°C or over)

FEVER

Fever or pyrexia is a condition, in which the level of the body temperature rises uniformly above normal. Fever or pyrexia is defined as a rise in the body temperature above 99°F (37.2°C). The causes of fever are infections, diseases of the nervous system, certain malignant neoplasms, blood disease such as leukemia, embolism and thrombosis, heat stroke from exposure to hot environments, dehydration, surgical trauma and crushing injuries, skin abnormalities that interfere with heat loss, allergic reactions to foreign proteins and pyrogens, etc.

Unit V ❖ Assessment of Patient

Fever is not a disease but it is a sign. Fever is a protective function of the body, because the rise in temperature prevents the growth of organisms causing the disease. Fever if not too high, hastens the destruction of bacteria by increasing phagocytosis and by producing immune bodies. 34°–41°C (94°–105.8°F) is the normal range in the body temperature within which the cells can function efficiently. The central nervous system is extremely sensitive to the temperature variations. Irreversible changes may occur in the nervous system if the body temperature goes above 41°C (105.8°F) or below 34°C (93.2°F).

Types of Fever

- **Constant fever or continuous fever:** It is one in which the temperature remains constantly high throughout a period of days or weeks and there is only a variation of less than 2 degrees between morning and evening temperature and it does not reach normal till the course of disease is over, e.g., typhoid.
- **Remittent fever:** There is wide variation (more than 2 degrees) between morning and evening temperature but temperature does not reach normal, e.g., septicemia.
- **Intermittent fever or quotidian fever:** It is one in which the body temperature rises and returns to normal daily. There is a variation from normal or subnormal to high fever and back at regular intervals. When the difference between the high and low points is very high the fever is called hectic or septic or swinging fever.
- **Relapsing fever:** It is one in which there are brief febrile periods followed by one or more days of normal temperature. Usually fever tends to be higher in the evening, than in the morning. But sometimes fever is high in the morning and low in the evening. This is known as inverse type of fever. At other times fever is entirely irregular in its course, so that it cannot be classified under any special type of fever and is called irregular fever.

    The temperature of the body is a diagnostic aid. It is so important that with the pulse and respiration, it is termed as cardinal symptom. Many conditions are characterized by an elevation of body temperature and some by a fall.

Stages in the Course of Fever (Temperature Curve)

Fevers usually run a typical course, as a characteristic of a particular disease. In some diseases, the diagrammatic representation of the course of fever on the chart is so typical that the diagnosis is suggested at a glance.

- Onset or invasion of fever may be **sudden** as pneumonia or malaria or **gradual** as in typhoid.
- **Fastigium or stadium (height of fever or stage of advance):** The temperature rises and reaches its maximum. It remains fairly constant for a few days. This period of high fever is called fastigium or stadium.
- **Defervescence or decline** is the period of disappearance of fever. This may be gradual decline or decline by lysis.

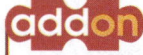

Lysis and Crisis are Situations

- **Lysis** is one in which the temperature falls step by step in a zigzag manner, little by little for 2 or 3 days or a week before reaching normal, during this time the other symptoms also gradually disappear, for example, typhoid. The fever may subside suddenly or by crisis.

    Crisis is one in which the temperature falls suddenly from high fever to normal or below normal within 24 hours as in pneumonia. This may be true crisis or false crisis.
    - **In true crisis** the temperature comes down and stays down and there is a general improvement in other symptoms and the patient's condition.
    - **In false crisis** the sudden fall in temperature is not accompanied by improvement in general condition. It may be a danger signal and not a sign of improvement.

Nursing Care of Patients with Fever

- **Regulation of the body temperature:** Care of the patients in fever focuses on reducing the elevated body temperature. Various methods of reducing the temperature may be started when a patient's temperature is moderately elevated.

  The various methods used for cooling the body are:
  - The room temperature should be maintained at a comfortable level. The room should be well ventilated.
  - The blankets and excess clothing should be removed but prevent the patient from getting draughts.
  - Exposure to cool air by an electric fan
  - Administration of cool drinks
  - Application of cold compress and ice bags
  - Cold sponging and cold packs
  - Cold bath
  - Ice cold lavages and enemas
  - Use of hypothermic blankets or mattresses

    When surface cooling is used, treatment is directed at not only cooling the body but also at preventing shivering. Prevent shivering as it increases metabolic activity, produces heat, increases the oxygen usage markedly, increases circulation, may cause hyperventilation and respiratory alkalosis. It takes longer time to reduce body temperature in a shivering patient.

- **Meeting the nutritional needs**
- **Providing rest and sleep**
- **Maintenance of personal hygiene**
- **Safety factors**
- **Observation needs of the patient**

THERMOMETER

The Clinical Thermometer

The clinical thermometer is a special instrument designed to measure the heat of the human body. It is made up of glass with a hollow tube in the center in front of which there is a scale in Fahrenheit or Centigrade degrees. It consists of an end bulb containing mercury and a stem. The heat of the body causes the mercury in the bulb to expand and rise through the fine column in the stem. The degree of temperature is indicated by the level of mercury. Just above the bulb there is a constriction which prevents the mercury from running back into the bulb after expansion unless it is shaken back.

Unit V ❖ Assessment of Patient

Parts of a Thermometer (Fig. 1)

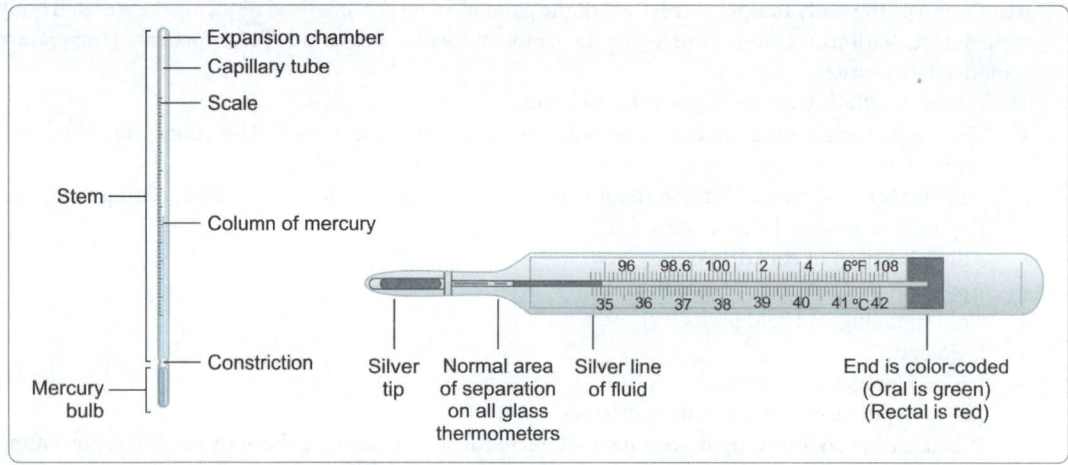

Expansion chamber
Capillary tube
Scale

Stem

Column of mercury

Constriction

Mercury bulb

Silver tip

Normal area of separation on all glass thermometers

Silver line of fluid

End is color-coded
(Oral is green)
(Rectal is red)

Figure 1: Different parts of a thermometer

The clinical thermometer is marked into degrees of Fahrenheit from 95° to 110° or 35° to 43.3°C. The long lines along the stem represent degrees and the short ones 2/10th of a degree (Fig. 1). An arrow marks the normal temperature 98.6°F or 37°C. The thermometer records temperature in 1–2 minutes depending on the make.

Thermometers are made with bulbs of different sizes and shapes. The long slender bulb is indicative of oral thermometer and those with short rounded or colored bulbs are used to take rectal temperature (Figs 2A to C).

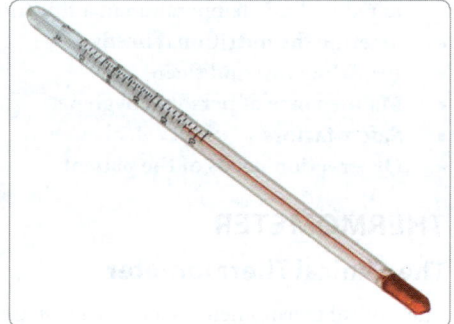

Figure 2A: Oral thermometer

Types of Thermometers

Oral Thermometer (Fig. 2A) and Rectal Thermometer (Fig. 2B)

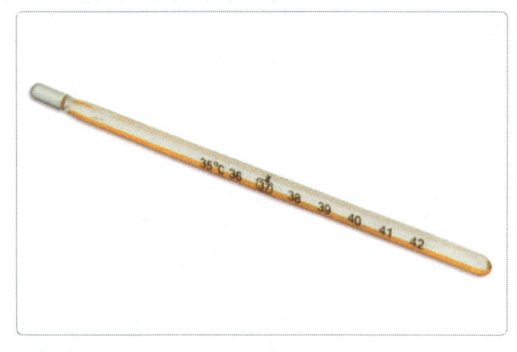

Figure 2B: Rectal thermometer

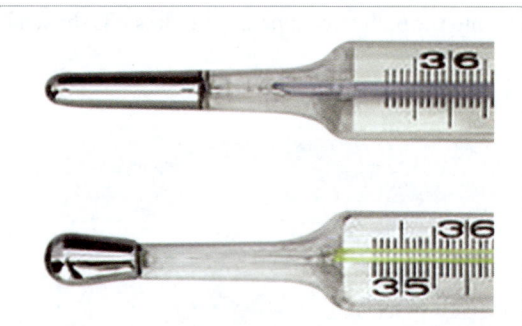

Figure 2C: Tip of thermometer oral (up) and rectal (down)

There are other types of thermometers available nowadays.

Digital Thermometer

It is a small hand-held device with a 'window' showing the temperature in numbers (Fig. 3).

Temporal Thermometer or Forehead Thermometer

It measures temperature of the skin surface over the temporal artery. These thermometers use an infrared scanner to measure the temperature of the temporal artery in the forehead (Fig. 4).

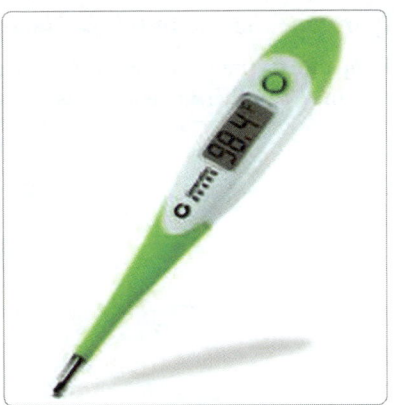

Figure 3: Digital thermometer

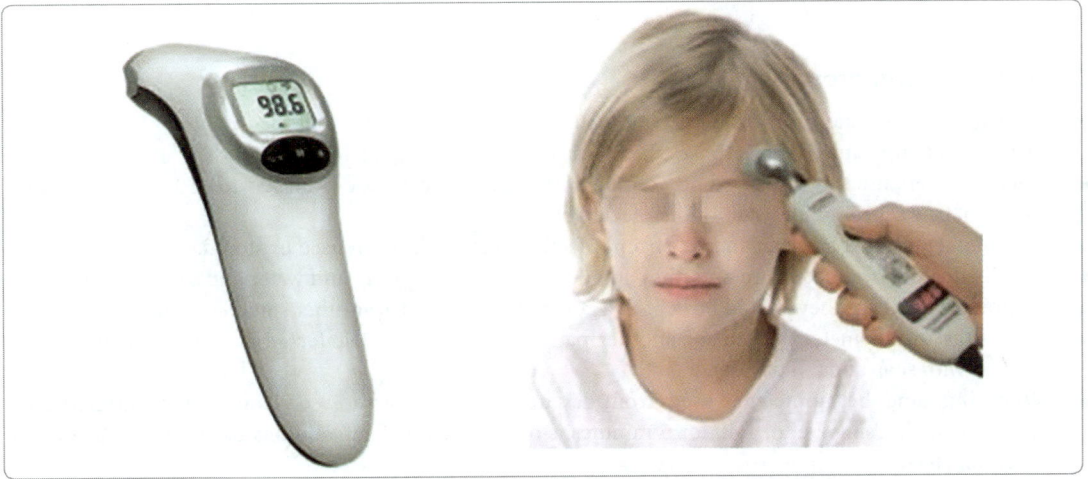

Figure 4: Temporal thermometer

Strip Thermometers

It contains heat-sensitive (thermochromic) liquid crystals in a plastic strip that change color to indicate different temperatures. Forehead Thermometer Strips are the fast, easy, and eco-friendly way to check for a fever or monitor temperatures for children (Fig. 5).

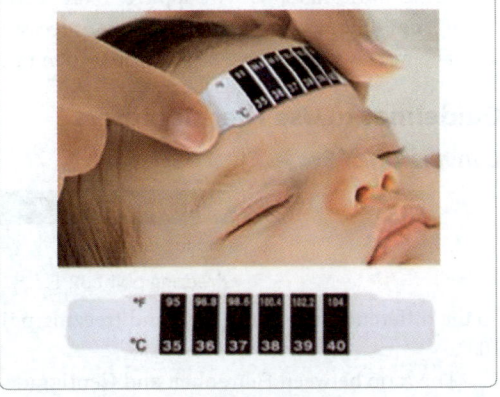

Figure 5: Strip thermometer

Unit V ❖ Assessment of Patient

Tympanic Thermometers or Electronic Ear Thermometer

Tympanic thermometers are usually small hand-held devices with a probe that is inserted into the patient's ear canal. This thermometer measures the temperature inside the ear by reading the infrared heat (Fig. 6).

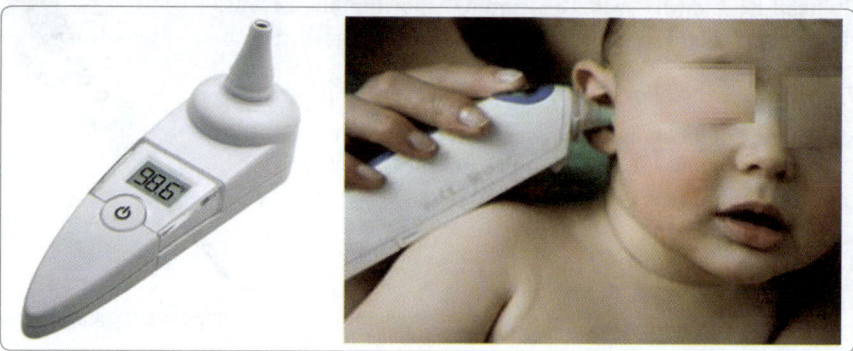

Figure 6: Tympanic thermometer

Care of Thermometers

- In using, cleaning and disinfecting thermometers, we must remember that the instrument, must not be exposed to temperatures above those which thermometer is designed to measure.
- Thermometers used to measure body temperature have a short scale from 95° to 110°F and therefore must not be washed in hot water or disinfected by heat.
- Thermometers must be clean and free from infectious materials when used or stored.
- If individual thermometers are used they should be washed with soap and water and dried after use.
- To prevent breakage they should be kept in a covered box, cylinder or other suitable containers.
- Before the thermometer is used for another patient, it should be disinfected chemically or in homes, washed with soap and tepid water.
- When the same thermometer is used, from day to day by two or more patients, it is disinfected each time it is used. Using Dettol 1:40 for 5 minutes is one of the efficient solutions used for disinfection of thermometers.
- The instrument should be thoroughly cleaned before disinfection.
- For esthetic reasons, rectal and mouth thermometers must never be kept in the same jar.
- Some lubricants should be applied to the rectal thermometers and should be wiped away after use to keep it from interfering with the cleaning process.
- The nurses should have clean hands when taking temperature.

Guidelines to Use Thermometers

Conversion of Scales

Fahrenheit	Centigrade (Celsius)
Boiling point 212°F	Boiling point 100°C
Freezing point 32°F	Freezing point 0°C

So the difference in boiling point and freezing point in Fahrenheit is 180°. Same difference in Centigrade is 100°.

The ratio between Fahrenheit and Centigrade is 180:100 = 9:5

The formula for converting Fahrenheit into Centigrade is:

$$C = (F - 32)\frac{5}{9} = (212 - 32) \times \frac{5}{9} \quad \text{That is } 180 \times \frac{5}{9} = 100°C$$

For converting Centigrade into Fahrenheit the formula is:

$$F = (C \times \frac{9}{5}) + 32 = (100 \times \frac{5}{9}) + 32 \quad \text{That is equal to } 212°F.$$

Celsius scale: A temperature scale on which the boiling point of water is 100° and the melting point of ice is 0°. This is the official scientific name of the temperature scale, which is also known as Centigrade. It was named after Anders Celsius, Swedish Astronomer (1701–1744).
(From Taber's Cyclopedic Medical Dictionary)

Sites and Time for Taking Temperature

Common sites: Mouth – 1–2 minutes
                 Axilla – 3–5 minutes
                 Rectum – 3–5 minutes
                 Groin – 3–5 minutes
                 Other thermometers—as per instructions in the manual
Common disinfectants used to disinfect thermometers after washing with soap and water.

Name of disinfectants	Strength	Time
Dettol	1:40	5 minutes
Savlon	1:20	do
Lysol	1:40	3 minutes
Carbolic	1:40	do

To get accurate measurement of the temperature of the interior of the body, the thermometer must be placed where it can be completely surrounded by body tissues and where there are large blood vessels near the surfaces. Temperature may vary if the bulb of the thermometer comes in contact with clothing, air or moisture.

Contraindications for Taking Temperature by Mouth

It is neither safe nor reliable to take temperature by mouth if patient is:
- Extremely nervous, delirious, unconscious, hysterical or mentally confused
- Mouth breather
- Patient having frequent convulsions
- Suffering from a parched, inflamed or injured mouth
- Suffering from extreme weakness and the thermometer may fall when the mouth is open while taking temperature
- Suffering from breathing difficulty and having frequent attacks of cough
- A child under 6 years of age or older unreasonable children
- Soon after drinks, smoking, bath, etc. temperature reading will not be correct. In all these conditions temperature should be taken by axilla or rectum

Frequency of Taking Temperature

Frequency of taking temperature is determined by the condition of the patient. It can be taken in the morning and evening for patients who are not seriously ill. For very ill patients, postoperative patients and patients who are running high temperature, the temperature needs to be taken every 4 hours or even half hourly according to the condition of the patient and the instruction of the doctor. If temperature is taken by axilla or rectum, it should be specified in the chart.

RIGOR

Rigor is an attack of intense shivering when the heat regulating center of the body is disturbed, usually seen in cases of certain acute infections or as the reaction of certain drugs, or during the administration of intravenous infusion of fluids or blood transfusion. The temperature rises rapidly following the chill and may stay either elevated or fall rapidly as profuse sweating occurs.

Stages of Rigor and Nursing Care

It has three stages:

Cold stage   –   First stage
Hot stage   –   Second stage
Perspiration stage –   Third stage

In the cold stage patient feels chill, extreme shivering and temperature rises in the hot stage, patient feels hot due to vasodilatation and feels thirsty. Patient perspires profusely and temperature falls down and patient again feels chill.

- **Cold stage or first stage:** There is uncontrollable shivering to the patient. Feeble and rapid pulse, skin becomes cold and face becomes pale. Rise in temperature occurs soon to 103°F (39.4°C) or even above.
  - **Nursing care:**
    - In this stage cover the patient with blankets
    - Apply hot water bags for additional warmth
    - Give warm drinks
    - Protect the patient from falling from the cot due to severe shivering

  This stage may last for a few minutes.
- **Hot stage or second stage:** The skin feels hot and dry and feels very thirsty. Shivering stops but the patient may be restless and anxious. Temperature may continue to rise.
  - **Nursing care:**
    - In this stage, remove the blankets and hot water bags.
    - Cover him/her with only a bed sheet.
    - Give him/her cold drinks.
    - Apply cold compresses to the forehead to relieve congestion and headache.
    - Monitor and record T.P.R. (temperature, pulse, respiration) every 15 minutes.
    - If the temperature goes high up to 105°F (40.5°C) cold sponging is given and watch for symptoms of perspiration.
- **Perspiration stage or third stage:** The patient sweats profusely. Temperature falls, pulse improves and acute discomforts are reduced. If patient is not cared properly, he/she may go to a stage of shock and collapse. His/her clothes may be wet due to profuse sweating or even due to cold application.
  - **Nursing care:**
    - During this stage, change his wet clothes without much disturbance to him/her. Give a sponge bath with wet towel and dry him/her soon. Do not expose the patient to draught. Put clean dry clothes and cover with a thin blanket or sheet.
    - Sweet drinks can be given to remove the fatigue. Make him comfortable and encourage him/her to sleep.
    - Watch him/her carefully and record TPR in every 15 minutes without disturbing him much.

- o Even though the temperature comes down, pulse will be rapid and feeble, which is to be considered as a false crisis. Patient should be watched carefully for any deterioration in the condition.
- o An occurrence of a rigor may cause great anxiety to the patient as well as the relatives. So the nurse should give psychological support as well as the physical care to the patient.
- o Do not leave the patient alone during the course of rigor. If it is due to reaction of some drugs, the doctor may order antidote for the same. If the rigor is during the administration of intravenous infusions of solution or blood transfusions, discontinue the procedure immediately, inform the doctor and do the care as mentioned above.

Charting a Rigor

Mark the maximum temperature on the graphic sheet by dots, connect it with the temperature taken at the regular time with the dotted line. Write specifically and neatly "Rigor at............." above the maximum temperature.

 Stimulant

> **Rigor mortis** is the name given to the stiffening of body occurring soon after death owing to coagulation of the muscle plasma, starts first in the muscles of the neck and jaw, then proceeds to those of the chest and upper extremities, finally reaching those of the lower limbs. The time of its appearance varies from 1 to 24 hours after death.

PULSE

Pulse is the alternate expansion (rise) and recoil (fall) of the arteries produced by the wave of blood forced into them as the heart's left ventricle contracts. As the blood is pumped out into the arteries, it causes the arteries to expand. The expansion goes on like waves throughout the arterial system, which can be felt by the fingers on a point where an artery crosses a bone, close to the surface of the skin. So pulse is the heartbeat conveniently felt at the arteries (Evelyn Pearce—A General Textbook of Nursing).

The pulse wave is felt during the contraction or systole of the heart and a recoil during the relaxation or the diastole of the heart. These two periods, constitute the 'pulse' and represent one heartbeat. In the average adult about 5 liters of blood is ejected from the left ventricle every minute, which is called the cardiac output. Cardiac output is the product of stroke volume and the heart rate, i.e., CO = SV × HR).

For example, in a healthy adult at rest, the stroke volume is about 70 mL and normal heart rate is about 70 per minute, consequently 4900 mL of blood is ejected every minute, which is little less than the volume of blood (5 L) in the circulatory system.

Normal Pulse Rate

Normal pulse rate for the healthy adult is 70–80 beats per minute. Pulse rate for an infant varies from 130 to 140 beats per minute. In old age, the normal pulse rate is decreased (60–70 per minute). The pulse rate for women is usually slightly more rapid than that of men.

Pulse deficit: The difference between apical and radial pulse is known as **pulse deficit and is tabulated as follows (Table 1).**

Unit V ❖ Assessment of Patient

Table 1: Pulse deficit

Pulse rate	Beats per minute
Before birth [fetal heart rate (FHR)]	140–150
At birth (newborn)	130–140
1st year	115–130
2nd year	100–115
3rd year	90–100
4–8 years	86–90
8–15 years	80–86
Adult	80–86
Old age	60–70

Characteristics of Normal Pulse

The study of the pulse is known as sphygmology.
- **Rate of pulse:** Rate is the number of pulse beats in a minute.
- **Rhythm or regularity:** Rhythm is the space or interval between two pulse beats.
  The pulse is usually regular in rhythm as heartbeats are heard at equal intervals and has uniform force.
- **Volume:** The volume or force is the strength of the beat. Normally the beats are equally strong as felt by the fingers at pressure points. If the volume of blood is normal, the pulse will be full or large. If the volume of blood is decreased as by hemorrhage, the pulse will be small, feeble, weak, thready or flickering. If the pulse is large or full and also rapid in rate, it may be described as bounding pulse.
- **Tension:** It indicates the amount of resistance the artery gives when the finger is pressing against it. The amount of tension present is due to the pressure of the blood in the arteries. Tension of pulse is usually expressed as high or low. A pulse of high tension is soft to touch and artery is difficult to compress. A pulse of low tension is soft to touch and artery is easily compressed where the walls of the arteries are relaxed.

Common Sites Where Pulse may be Felt: From Top to Bottom

- **Temporal artery:** At the temples (just above and to the outer side of the outer canthus of the eye)
- **Carotid artery:** On either side of the neck directly in front of the ear lobe
- **Brachial artery:** Above the elbow and in the antecubital fossa (anterior part of the elbow)
- **Radial artery:** At the thumb side of the wrist on the anterior surface of the forearm. This is the most common site
- **Femoral artery:** In the groin
- **Popliteal artery:** At the back of the knee
- **Posterior tibial:** Near the ankle joint
- **Dorsalis pedis artery:** Above the heels (Fig. 7).

Abnormal Pulse

- **Abnormal rate:**
  - **Tachycardia:** Rapid pulse—over 100 per minute may be caused by drugs such as stimulants or diseases like typhoid, heart disease, etc.

- • **Bradycardia:** Slow pulse—60 or less may be caused by drugs as sedatives or diseases like heart disease etc.
- ■ **Abnormal rhythm:** Irregularities in rhythm are called **arrhythmia**. The intervals between beats may be of different lengths or the beats may be of unequal force.

  Common irregularities in rate and rhythm include premature beats, pauses, tachycardia, bradycardia and chaotic pulse.

These conditions are seen in many apparently healthy persons and in some cases, the heart action is normal but in others this evidence indicates a serious arrhythmia. The nurse must report such changes in the rate and rhythm to the physician and at the same time include additional information gathered such as blood pressure, chest pain, dyspnea, apprehension and other changes in the patient's mental stage, change in color of the lips, nails and skin and headache. An electrocardiogram should be made to determine the origin of the irregularity.

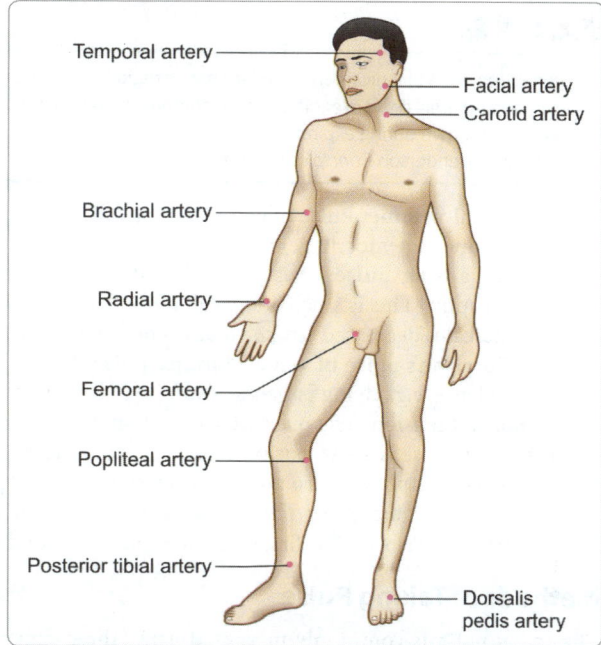

Figure 7: Common pulse points in human body

Chaotic pulse means an irregular pulse beats.

Other irregularities in rhythm and rate are:

- ■ **Intermittent pulse** is one in which pulse beats are missed at regular intervals.
- ■ **Tachycardia:** Rapid pulse is a fault in the rhythm causing change in the rate over 100 per minute.
- ■ **Bradycardia:** Slow pulse is a fault in the rhythm causing change in the rate 60 or less per minute.
- ■ **Extra systoles:** It is the premature contraction of the heart before the normal cardiac cycle, which is felt as the premature pulse.
- ■ **Atrial fibrillation:** It is the irregular contractions of the ventricles in rhythm and forces caused by the rapid contractions of the atrium.
- ■ **Ventricular fibrillation:** It is the term given to rapid chaotic electrical activity initiated by the ventricular ectopic. It is the rapid twitching of the ventricles. Dangerous arrhythmia may result from ischemia in the ventricles. It is fatal.
- ■ **Bigeminal pulse:** It is accompanied by an irregular rhythm in which every other beats come early. The second or premature beat feels weak. This is due to inadequate filling of the ventricles between the two beats. It may be so weak that it fails to produce a palpable pulse and it is called pulse deficit. It is seen in myocardial infarction and digitalis toxicity.
- ■ **Pulsus alternans:** The rhythm is regular but volume has an alternative strong and weak characters. This type of pulse is elicited in the left ventricular failure, heart block and digitalis toxicity.
- ■ **Bounding pulse:** Is an increased stroke volume usually seen in patients who perform exercises, who are anxious and in conditions such as anemia, hepatic failure, heart block and water hammer pulse.

Unit V ❖ Assessment of Patient

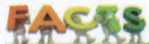

> • Arrhythmia is a technical term used for any variation from normal rhythm.
> • Sinus arrhythmia is the irregularity in the rhythm and rate of pulse in which the heart rate speeds up during inspiration and slows down during expiration. This is a beginning condition and does not require any treatment.
> (Ref: Virginia Henderson *Principles and Practice of Nursing* Chapter 6 and Shafer M. S. Nursing Chapter 21)

■ **Abnormal volume:** Pulse may be large or full volume, or may be of low or small volume (a fluttering pulse is due to hemorrhage)

　• **Collapsing pulse:** Weak/wiry/thready pulse—the one which is feeble to touch, then subsides abruptly. This is small and weak pulse that feels like a wire or thread while touching the arteries. It indicates decreased stroke volume and is seen in hemorrhage, shock or dehydration.

　• **Corrigan's pulse or water hammer pulse:** It is jerky pulse with full expansion followed by sudden collapse, e.g., dying patients. Running pulse is one with weak irregular beats.

■ **Abnormal tension:** The pulse may be of high tension (bounding) or of low tension.
A thready pulse is a low tension pulse, e.g., wiry pulse.

　• A dicrotic pulse is also due to low tension. Dicrotic pulse is one which has two marked expansions in one beat of the artery. The contraction is normal but in relaxation, a second sensation can be felt which resembles a beat. The first is stronger and the second sensation is weaker. For example, thyroid patients.

Methods of Taking Pulse

The radial pulse is commonly measured using three fingers. If the investigator uses his/her right hand to check the pulse while the patient is sitting in his right, then, the right index finger helps to fix the radial artery and also helps to assess the condition of the vessel wall, middle finger is used to feel the volume, rate and rhythm of the pulse, whereas the ring finger helps to diminish the impact of pulsations from nearby vessels (ring finger is used to nullify the effect of the ulnar pulse as the two arteries are connected via the palmar arches (superficial and deep)) and also judge the force of blood flow. It is used as:

■ Proximal finger to occlude and stabilize the artery.
■ Middle finger to check the parameters—rate, rhythm, volume, etc.
■ Distal finger to block retrograde pulsations from palmar arch.

Counting Apical Pulse

Place the stethoscope on chest under clothing. Auscultate the apex of the heart below left nipple. Move around a little at a time until the heartbeat is clearly heard. If there is difficulty in finding apical pulse, have patient lean forward while sitting, or turn to left side when lying down (Figs 8A to C).

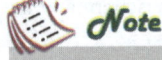

Lub-dub is one beat. Always count for one full minute.

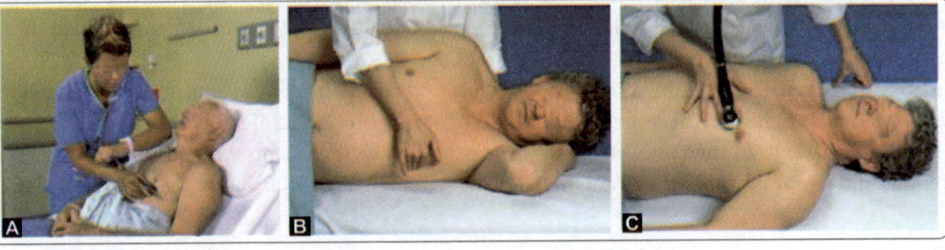

Figures 8A to C: Steps of taking apical pulse

Frequency in Taking Pulse

The pulse is taken usually along with temperature twice a day. It may be taken frequently in case of operations, heart diseases and seriously ill patients. Frequency depends upon the condition of the patient and also according to the doctor's orders. Change in pulse rate indicates the change in patient's condition.

RESPIRATION

Respiration is the act of breathing. It is the process of taking in oxygen and giving out carbon dioxide.

Respiration consists of an inspiration, expiration, and a pause. Respiration may be internal and external. The exchange of gases between the blood and the air in the lungs is called **external or pulmonary respiration.** The exchange of gas between the blood and the tissue cells is called **internal or tissue respiration.**

Regulation of Respiration

The respiratory center in the brain, the nerve fibers of the autonomic nervous system and the chemical composition of the blood are the factors that regulate respiration. The respiratory centre is situated in the medulla. To a limited extent respiration is under voluntary control.

Normal Respiration

It consists of a rhythmical rising and falling of the chest and abdominal walls occurring in a resting adult about 18 times in a minute. It is quiet and effortless. The usual ratio of respiration rate and pulse rate is approximately one to four (1:4).

Respiration rate: This is the number of full respirations in a minute. Average rate varies as follows:

Age	Respiratory rate in breaths per minute
At birth	30–40
1st year	26–30
2nd year	20–26
Adolescence	20
Adult	16–20
Middle age	14–18
Old age	10–24

Females tend to have a slightly rapid respiration than males.

What to Observe when Taking Respiration

- Rate
- Character of respiration, regularity and easiness
- Movements of the respiratory muscles, chest, nose, abdomen
- Color of the patient
- Position

Method of Counting Respiration

Count the number of respiratory cycles in 1 minute. One cycle is equal to the complete rise and fall of the patient's chest. Ensure that the patient is not aware about this as this may make him/her conscious of his/her breathing pattern and influence the accuracy of the rate. Place the hand on the patient's chest and count the number of respiratory cycles.

Unit V ❖ Assessment of Patient

Abnormalities in Respiration

- **Rate:** Fast respirations may be due to chest disease, fever, anemia, toxemia or drugs as atropine. Slow respirations may be due to coma (deep unconsciousness) or brain injuries.
  - Tachypnea (polypnea) means an increased respiratory rate over 24 breaths per minute.
  - Bradypnea means decreased respiratory rate to less than 10 breaths per minute.
- **Rhythm:** It is the regularity of respiration. In average condition rhythm is normal.

Stimulant

Cheyne-stokes respiration is a shallow respiration but it gradually get deeper and deeper, louder and louder and then, stops altogether for half to one minute. This is repeated. Critically ill patient may breathe in this manner when death is nearing. It is an irregular breathing.

- **Dyspnea means difficulty in breathing:** Labored respiration is the breathing in which the patient struggles for breath. This is caused by anything which slows down the amount of oxygen going to the lungs as in pneumonia and asthma. In this, the accessory muscles of respiration are used (sternocleidomastoid muscles). The breathing is quick, labored, noisy, the nostrils dilate, there is blueness of lips and finger tips as found in chest and heart diseases. Difficulty of breathing may be relieved to some extent by propping up the patients by means of back rest and pillows. Oxygen may have to be administered in certain conditions to relieve dyspnea.
  - **Orthopnea:** Difficult breathing in which patient can breathe only in an upright position and cannot get rest while lying down.
  - **Hyperpnea:** It is an increase in the depth of respiration.
  - **Anoxia (hypoxia):** It means lack of oxygen in the tissues.
  - **Anoxemia (hypoxemia):** It means lack of oxygen in the blood stream.
  - **Asphyxia:** It means a state of suffocation produced by prolonged interference with sufficient supply of oxygen.
  - **Cyanosis:** It is blueness of the skin and mucous membranes due to lack of oxygen in blood as in the cases of heart failure or in obstruction of the air passages. It is a serious sign and indicates the need for oxygen.
  - **Air hunger:** A characteristic symptom indicative of lack of sufficient oxygen for proper functioning of tissue cells. It is a form of dyspnea in which there are deep sighing respirations.
  - **Apnea:** Cessation of breathing for a short period. This may be periodic as seen in Cheyne-stokes respiration.
- **Noisy respirations:**
  - **Stertorous respiration:** It is a noisy breathing. These resemble snoring sounds due to air passing through secretions as in acute alcoholism or apoplexy or opium poisoning.
  - **Grunting:** The expiration is forced with a little grunt at the end of each breath.
  - **Stridor:** Inspiration is forced. There is frequently a whistling sound as in croup or diphtheria due to obstruction in the upper airway.
  - **Sighing and yawning:** The inspiration is forced as found in severe hemorrhage due to air hunger. Frequent sighs are signs of emotional tensions.
  - **Rales:** Bubbling noises caused by mucus in the air passages as in bronchitis.
  - **Wheezing respiration:** A type of whistling sound that occurs with the partial obstruction of the smaller bronchi and bronchioles in conditions like asthma or pulmonary emphysema.

- **Abnormal movements in respiration:**
  - **Shallow breathing:** Usually quick, may be due to painful breathing.
  - **Deep breathing:** It is usually slow.
  - **Restricted movement:** It is of either chest or abdomen, may be due to pain or paralysis of respiratory muscles.
  - **Hiccups** are due to spasm of the diaphragm and glottis and occasionally are found as postoperative complication.

BLOOD PRESSURE

The terms used here are:
- **Blood pressure (BP):** It is the force exerted by the blood against the walls of the blood vessels as it flows through them. Reading of BP is recorded as systolic and diastolic pressure.
- **Systolic pressure:** It is the highest degree of pressure exerted by the blood against the arterial walls as the left ventricle contracts and forces the blood from it into the aorta.
- **Diastolic pressure:** It is the lowest degree of pressure when the heart is in its resting period just before contraction of the left ventricle.
- **Pulse pressure:** It is the difference between systolic and diastolic pressure and represents volume output of the left ventricle. Pulse pressure is an indication of the tone of the arterial walls and is important in diagnosis and treatment.
- **Hypertension:** It is a condition of abnormally high blood pressure.
- **Hypotension:** It is a condition of abnormally low blood pressure.
  Heart action and blood pressure are not under man's control.

Normal Blood Pressure

The average blood pressure for the healthy adult is usually about 120/80 (systolic pressure 120 mm Hg and diastolic pressure 80 mm Hg with pulse pressure of 40 mm Hg). Normal venous pressure may range from 40 to 110 mm of water. BP is measured by an apparatus called sphygmomanometer or Erkameter (sphygmos = pulse) Mercury sphygmomanometer was developed by Riva-Rocci in 1896.

Factors Causing Variation in Blood Pressure

- **Age:** Blood pressure is much lower in children than in adults. The young adult will have a blood pressure of approximately 120/80 mm Hg and in older people, a blood pressure of 140/90 may be considered normal.
- **Sex:** The average blood pressure for men is slightly higher than that of women.
- **Posture:** BP is lower in lying position than in sitting position or standing. When the BP is decreased suddenly on standing posture, it is called orthostatic hypotension.
- **Time of the day:** BP is lowest in early morning to all people, it rises to a peak in the evening and it declines in the night during rest and sleep.
- **Body build:** The individual who tends to be obese will probably show higher than average blood pressure.
- **Exercise:** Muscular exertion will increase blood pressure.
- **Pain:** Severe pain may cause a temporary and marked increase in blood pressure.
- **Emotion:** Fear, worry, excitement and other emotions will cause blood pressure to rise sharply.
- **Disease:** Diseases affecting the circulatory system as arteriosclerosis and disease affecting the kidneys may increase blood pressure. Diseases that weaken the heart action may lower blood pressure.

Unit V ❖ Assessment of Patient

- **Hemorrhage:** Hemorrhage causes low blood pressure by decreasing the volume of blood in the vessels.
- **Intracranial pressure:** Pressure within the cranium will usually produce a rise in blood pressure.
- **Drugs:** Abnormal decreases are caused by drugs such as amyl nitrite and nitroglycerin and by lowered vitality of adrenal glands and certain drugs will increase blood pressure.
- **Race:** Certain races like Negroes will have high BP readings than other races.

Oxygen Saturation

Thomas Neff suggested inclusion of blood oxygen saturation as fifth vital sign. It is commonly referred to as 'SATS' and measures the percentage of hemoglobin binding sites in the blood stream occupied by oxygen.

When partial pressures of oxygen is low, most of the hemoglobin is deoxygenated.

Common causes of decreased oxygen saturation are:
- Heart ailments like heart defects
- Lung conditions such as asthma, emphysema and bronchitis
- High altitudes

- Normal level of oxygen is → 80–100
- Mild hypoxemia or mildly low blood oxygen is considered at → 60–80

PROCEDURES OF CHECKING TEMPERATURE, PULSE, RESPIRATION (TPR) AND BLOOD PRESSURE

General Instructions

- Privacy should be maintained. Use screen for privacy.
- Check patient's chart. Make sure that there is no order to take the patient's temperature using the rectal or axillary route.
- See that the rectum is empty before taking rectal temperature as the presence of faecal matter increases rectal temperature.
- Observe patient. Some information can be obtained by observing the patient as you approach him. For example, if you see that the patient is coughing constantly, you know that another method of obtaining the patient's temperature should be used.
- Enquire patient concerning contraindications. Ask the patient if he has smoked, eaten hot or cold foods, drank hot or cold fluid, or chewed gum within the last half-hour. If the patient has done any of these things within the last half-hour, then decide whether to wait and take his oral temperature later or take his temperature using a different site.
- Wait at least 20–30 minutes after the patient has eaten or had something to drink or smoked a cigarette
- Earwax, ear infections and ear tubes may interfere with getting correct readings.
- **Precautions to be observed while taking pulse**
  - See that the patient is at rest and usually kept in recumbent position.
  - Pulse should not be taken immediately after exercise, emotional stress or any painful treatment.
  - If patient is very nervous wait till he is calm and quiet. Place the tips of the first, second and third fingers on the artery for some time and when the patient is quiet, start counting the pulse.
  - Always concentrate when taking pulse.
  - Do not apply too much force or pressure but just enough to make the pulsation most distinct.

- Do not use the thumb to count the pulse as this may confuse our own pulse with that of the patient.
- Count the pulse for one full minute.
- It is wise to take pulse in both wrists of a new patient since in some conditions the pulse may be delayed on one side.

Articles Required

A tray consisting of:

Article	Purpose
Articles for hand washing	For reducing the number of micro organisms
Unsterile gloves (as per Institutions policy)	To prevent cross infection
Thermometers in a jar of Dettol 1:40 or Carbolic acid 1:40 with some cotton at the bottom of the jar/digital thermometer	For disinfecting the thermometers
Another jar containing Dettol or carbolic acid 1:40	If temperature is to be taken for several patients at a stretch
One jar with clean cold water	For dipping the thermometer that is removed from the disinfectant solution
Soap swabs in a container (Small pieces of cotton concentrated with soap solution)	For wiping the thermometer before and after checking temperature
Wet cotton swabs in a container	To remove the soap in the thermometer
Sphygmomanometer	For measuring blood pressure
Stethoscope	For measuring blood pressure
A bowl containing spirit swab	To wipe the bell and ear piece of the stethoscope
Vaseline in a container	For lubricating the rectal thermometer
Kidney tray or paper bag	For disposal of soiled swabs
Watch with second hand or Pulsometer	For checking pulse
Pen and temperature book or chart	For documentation

Other Preparations

Preparation of Patient

- Secure the cooperation of the patient by proper explanation
- Provide privacy
- Place the patient in a comfortable position
- Ensure that the patient has not taken anything orally for the past 30 minutes

Preparation of the Unit

- Ensure an area of good lighting
- Arrange all the necessary articles close to the bedside of the patient

Unit V ❖ Assessment of Patient

Procedure

Checking Temperature

Steps	Procedure	Rationale
1.	Perform hand wash	Prevents spread of microorganism.
2.	See that the patient is in a comfortable position. Explain the procedure to the patient and solicit his cooperation.	Encourages participation, allays anxiety and ensures accurate measurement
3.	Arrange the articles close to the bedside of the patient	Facilitates organized and skilled procedure
4.	Provide privacy	Decreases embarrassment
5.	Don gloves (as per Institution policy)	Reduces transmission of micro-organisms
6.	Take the thermometer from the jar touching the stem end of the thermometer and rinse it in cold water.	Cleansing removes disinfectant that can cause irritation to oral mucosa and prevents unpleasant taste of the disinfectant. Cool water prevents expansion of the mercury.
7.	Wipe the thermometer with the wet cotton swab from **bulb upward to the stem.** Avoid touching any part of the thermometer that goes into the patient's mouth.	Clean from the cleanest area to less clean area which prevents transfer of microorganisms.
8.	Hold the thermometer by the end opposite to the colored (red, blue, or silver) tip. Turn the thermometer in your hand until you see the red, blue, or silver line.	Turning the thermometer facilitates easy visualization of the mercury column.

98.6°

Oral glass thermometer

9.	Read the thermometer and shake the mercury column down to 95°F (35°C) or below, by grasping the thermometer between the thumb and first finger of the dominant hand. Shake the thermometer over a couch or bed by snapping the wrist in a downward motion.	Ensures accurate reading of the patient when the thermometer shows below normal temperature. This will keep it from breaking if it slips out of the hand.

Contd...

Steps	Procedure	Rationale
	Check the thermometer again to make sure it reads less than 96°F (35.6°C). 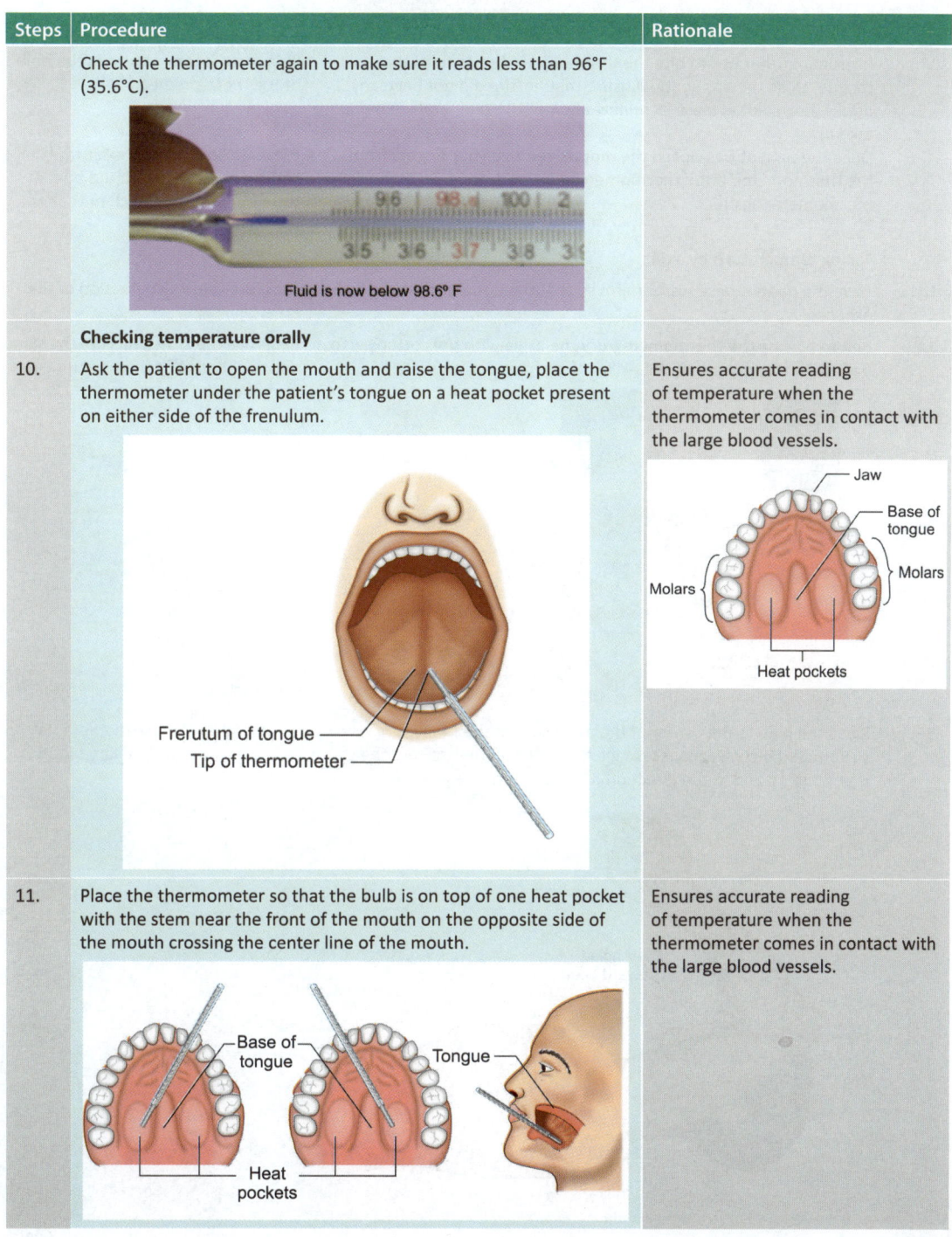 Fluid is now below 98.6° F	
	Checking temperature orally	
10.	Ask the patient to open the mouth and raise the tongue, place the thermometer under the patient's tongue on a heat pocket present on either side of the frenulum. Frerutum of tongue — Tip of thermometer — Jaw — Base of tongue — Molars — Molars — Heat pockets	Ensures accurate reading of temperature when the thermometer comes in contact with the large blood vessels.
11.	Place the thermometer so that the bulb is on top of one heat pocket with the stem near the front of the mouth on the opposite side of the mouth crossing the center line of the mouth. Base of tongue — Tongue — Heat pockets	Ensures accurate reading of temperature when the thermometer comes in contact with the large blood vessels.

Contd...

Unit V ❖ Assessment of Patient

Steps	Procedure	Rationale
12.	Instruct him/her not to bite the thermometer but to relax the tongue, close the lips gently (Ensure that he/she did not have any drinks (hot/cold) at least 15 minutes before the temperature being taken.) Once the patient has closed the mouth, remove your fingers from the thermometer. If the thermometer slips or droops, reposition the thermometer again.	Relaxing the tongue covers the bulb of the thermometer. Prevents environmental air from coming in contact with the bulb of the thermometer which may alter the reading.
	Taking temperature by axilla:	
13.	Have the patient raise his/her arm so that the underarm area is fully exposed.	Facilitates easy visualization of the area.
14.	Before placing the thermometer, dry the axilla with dry cotton swab or any cloth and see that the axilla is free from perspiration. 	Excessive moisture will cool the skin and could result in an inaccurate temperature reading.
15.	Place the bulb in the center of the axilla so that the bulb is surrounded by body tissues. Angle the thermometer so that the stem is pointed up and in the direction of the patient's head. Angled toward head	Ensures that the thermometer is in contact with the axillary blood supply.

Contd...

Unit V ❖ **Assessment of Patient**

Steps	Procedure	Rationale
16.	Keep it in position by placing the arm over the chest and the fingers on the opposite shoulder and leave it in position for 8–10 minutes. Do not allow the clothes to come in contact with the thermometer. 	Ensures proper positioning of thermometer in place which ensures accurate reading.
	Taking temperature by rectum:	
17.	Screen the patient and secure the co-operation of the patient if he is conscious.	Providing privacy avoids embarrassment
18.	Position the patient Infant Adult	Proper positioning facilitates easy visualization of anus.
19	Clean the part if indicated/soiled with tissue paper. 	Aids in visualization of anus.

Contd...

Steps	Procedure	Rationale
20.	Wipe the thermometer with the cotton swab and lubricate the bulb with Vaseline or any lubricant jelly. 2×2 Gauze — Lubricant jelly — Stubby tipped thermometer	Promotes ease of insertion into the rectum.
21.	With dominant hand grasp the thermometer and with the nondominant hand expose the anus by separating the buttocks.	Aids in visualization of anus.
22.	Ask the patient to take a deep breath and insert the thermometer about 0.5 to one inch into the rectum gently, by separating the buttocks by the thumb and forefinger of the left hand. Rectum	Deep breathing relaxes anal sphincter. Inserting the thermometer gently prevents discomfort to the patient and prevents mucosal damage.
23.	Hold it in position for 3–5 minutes. Slide gently into rectum without force, Hold in place Never leave the patient alone with the thermometer in the rectum.	Facilitates accurate reading The patient may move about and break the thermometer causing injury to the part.

Contd...

Steps	Procedure	Rationale
	Taking temperature by groin:	
24.	For infants the groin temperature is taken sometimes. For this: Dry the groin.	Excessive moisture will cool the skin and could result in an inaccurate temperature reading.
25.	The thigh must be well flexed over the abdomen. Place the thermometer between the two folds of the skin formed by the inner part of the thigh and lower abdomen.	Ensures that the thermometer is in contact with the blood supply in the groin.
	Taking tympanic temperature:	
26.	Place the patient in a comfortable position to expose the ear.	Promotes easy access to the ear
27.	Place a cover over the probe.	This protects the lens and prevents contamination of thermometer.
28.	Hold the thermometer in dominant hand. In the nondominant hand, slowly pull the upper part of the ear backwards and downwards in an infant and backwards and upwards in child over 1 year old and in adults	This straightens the ear canal and facilitates easy access of the thermometer probe
29.	Gently put the tip of the thermometer in the ear until it stops. The tip should point to the space between the eye and the ear on the other side of the head. Apply firm pressure into ear canal.	Gentle insertion prevents trauma to the external ear. Firm pressure ensures contact of the probe against the tympanic membrane

Ear drum

Contd...

Steps	Procedure	Rationale
30.	When you hear a beep in about 2 seconds, remove the thermometer and read the temperature. 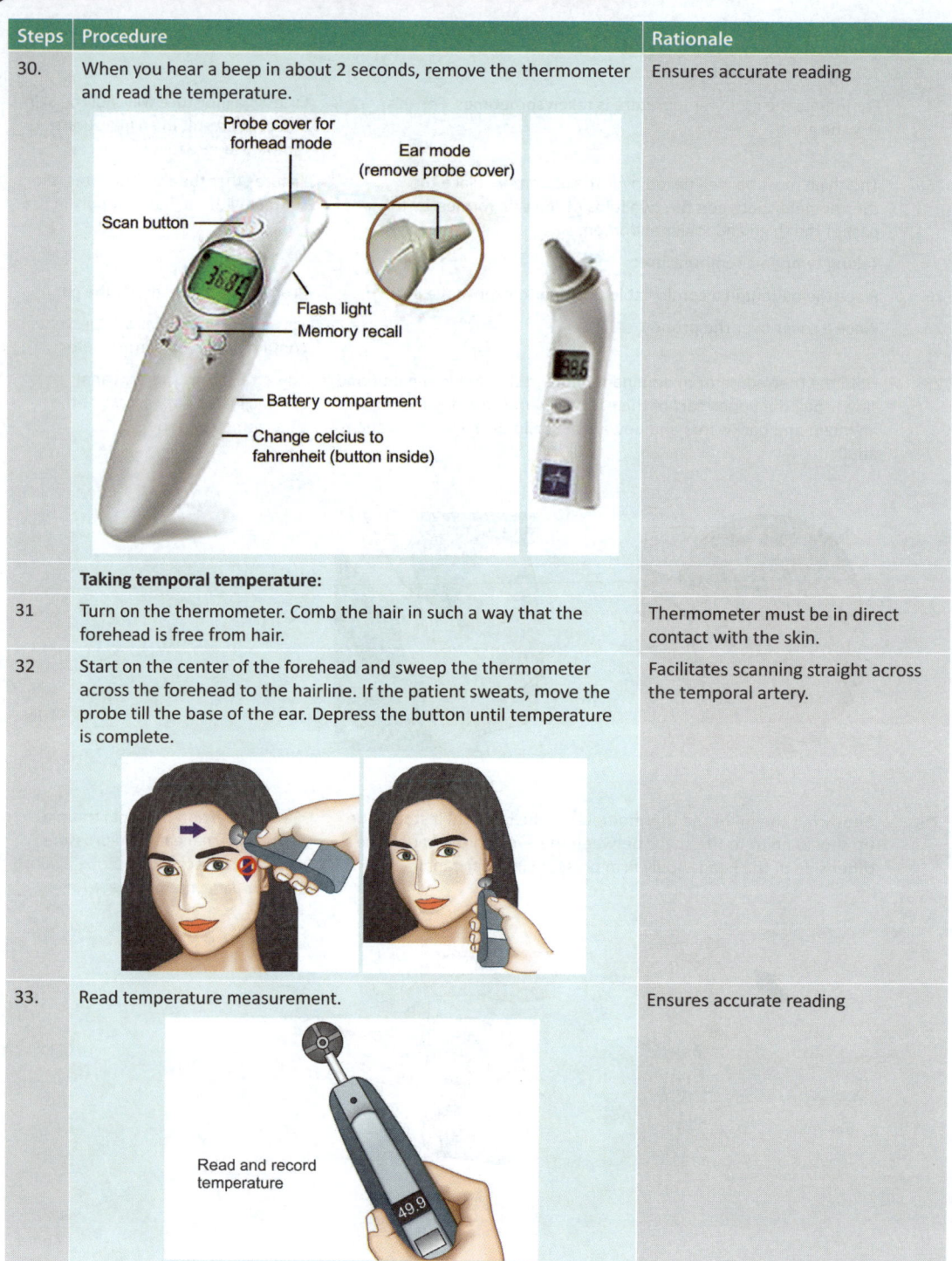	Ensures accurate reading
	Taking temporal temperature:	
31	Turn on the thermometer. Comb the hair in such a way that the forehead is free from hair.	Thermometer must be in direct contact with the skin.
32	Start on the center of the forehead and sweep the thermometer across the forehead to the hairline. If the patient sweats, move the probe till the base of the ear. Depress the button until temperature is complete.	Facilitates scanning straight across the temporal artery.
33.	Read temperature measurement.	Ensures accurate reading

Contd...

Steps	Procedure	Rationale
	Taking temperature by strip:	
34.	Ensure forehead is clean. Place temperature strips on the forehead. 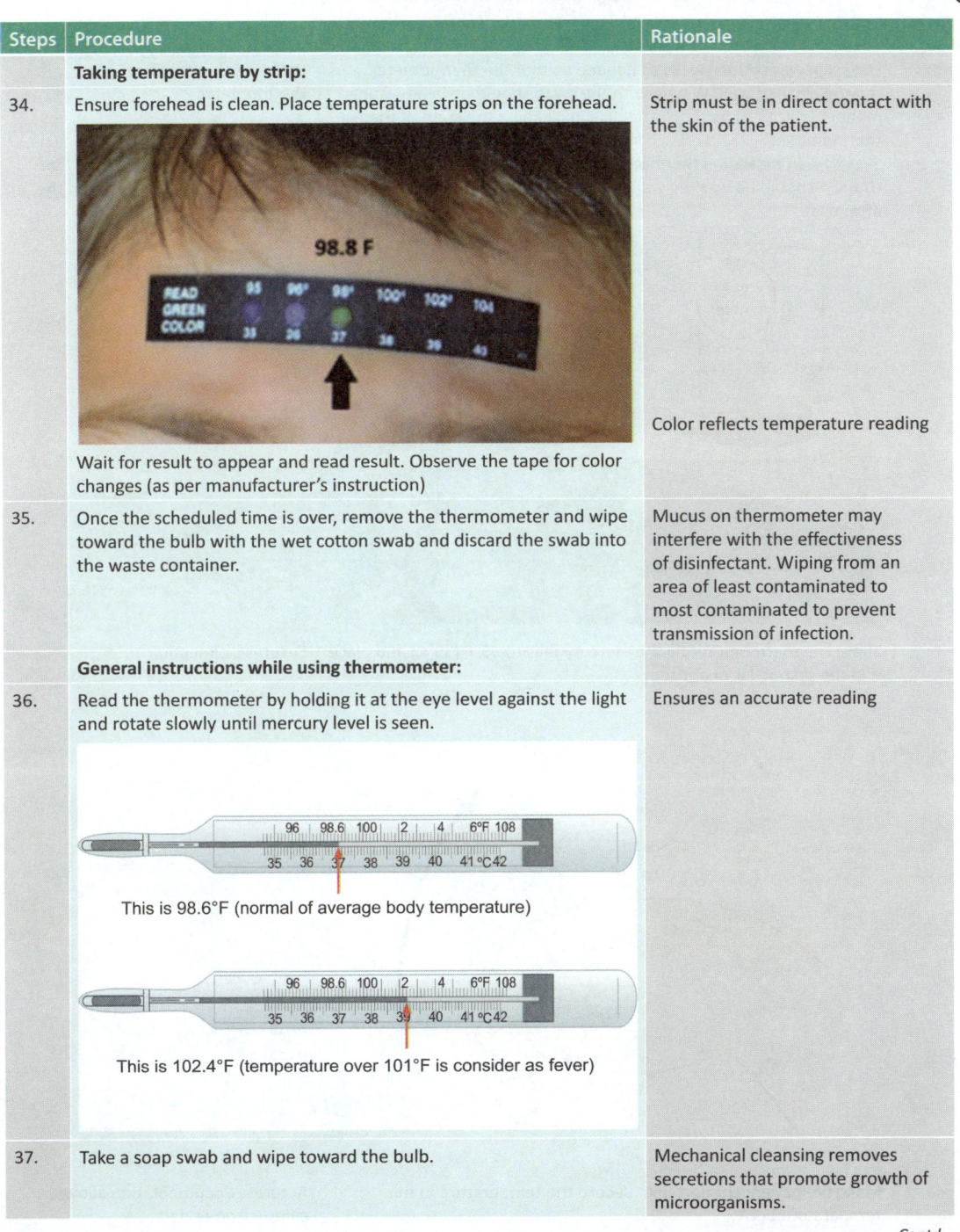 Wait for result to appear and read result. Observe the tape for color changes (as per manufacturer's instruction)	Strip must be in direct contact with the skin of the patient. Color reflects temperature reading
35.	Once the scheduled time is over, remove the thermometer and wipe toward the bulb with the wet cotton swab and discard the swab into the waste container.	Mucus on thermometer may interfere with the effectiveness of disinfectant. Wiping from an area of least contaminated to most contaminated to prevent transmission of infection.
	General instructions while using thermometer:	
36.	Read the thermometer by holding it at the eye level against the light and rotate slowly until mercury level is seen.	Ensures an accurate reading
37.	Take a soap swab and wipe toward the bulb.	Mechanical cleansing removes secretions that promote growth of microorganisms.

Contd...

Unit V ❖ Assessment of Patient

Steps	Procedure	Rationale
38.	Use plain wet cotton swabs as needed so that the thermometer may be cleaned well. Wiping with the swab should be in a twisting manner which will be more effective in cleaning the stem of the thermometer. (If individual thermometers are used as that of a private room, it should be washed well with soap and cold water and dried after use). 	Removes the soap from the thermometer. Hot water may cause coagulation of secretions and may expand the mercury.
39.	Shake the thermometer till the mercury falls to 95°F (35°C) and place it in the second jar of antiseptic. 	Ensures disinfection
40.	Make the patient comfortable. Record the temperature in the temperature book.	Accurate documentation allows comparison of data.

Contd...

Steps	Procedure	Rationale
41.	To take the temperature of a second patient, take the thermometer from the first jar, dip in clean water and continue the procedure as before, but before putting the used one. If there are more than one thermometer in the jar, remove the second thermometer from the first jar and put in the second jar, before putting the used one.	Prevents odd taste of the disinfectant
	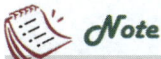	
	After care:	
42.	Wash and replace everything in proper place and discard the soiled swabs.	Facilitates preparation for next procedure
43.	Doff the gloves and wash the hands	Prevents transfer of microorganisms.
44.	Record the temperature in the chart in the appropriate column. Document temperature, including the date, time and method used as follows: 'O' for oral, 'R' for rectal, 'E' for ear, 'A' for axillary and so on.	Documentation fosters quality care

Taking and putting thermometers should be in rotation in the antiseptic lotion jars depending upon the number of patients. Tray setting for a single patient, only one jar with antiseptic lotion and one jar with clear water are required. For taking temperature of several patients there must be several thermometers, two lotion jars and one jar with clear water in the tray.

Note

- Keep the thermometer in the part for about specified period. Time of placing differs with different site and is based on the type of thermometer. (The time is adjusted, according to the instructions given with the thermometer).
- It ensures accurate measurement of temperature.

Unit V ❖ Assessment of Patient

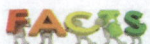

Various Sites for Taking Temperature

Site for taking temperature	Normal range °F/°C	Site for taking temperature	Normal range °F/°C
Oral	98.6°F/37.0°C	Axillary	97.6°F/36.6°C
Tympanic	99.6°F/37.6°C	Groin	97.6°F /36.6°C
Rectal	99.6°C/37.6°C	Temporal	99.6°F/37.6°C

Checking Pulse

- Place the wrist on the patient abdomen/chest until both the pulse and respiration are taken (if the patient is lying down).

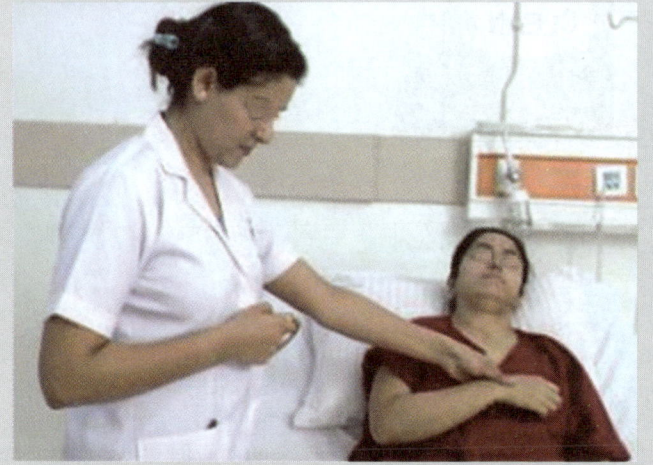

- If the radial artery is used, the arm must be well supported (the patient is in sitting position).

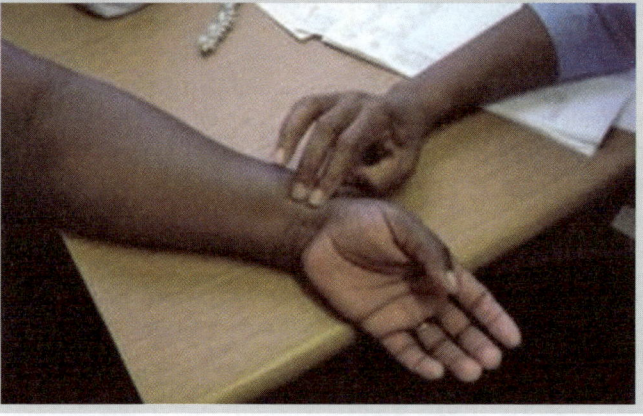

- Thumb is not used to take the pulse because the nurse might feel the pulsations of the radial artery of her own thumb.

Contd...

- Place the tips of the first three fingers over the radial artery on one hand at the anterior surface of the forearm just above the wrist and feel the pulsation.

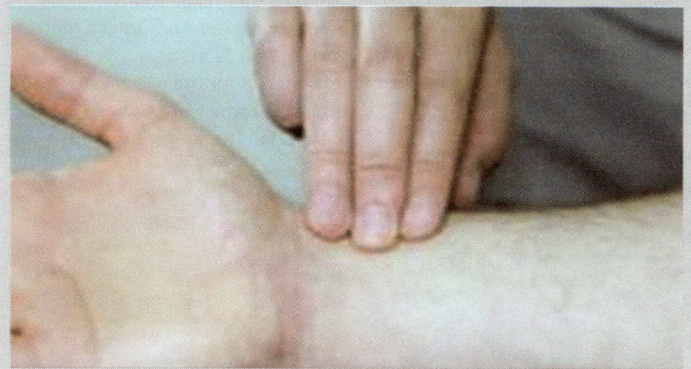

- To locate it place the fingers at the base of the thumb and slide down about 2 cm in the groove of the wrist pressing gently

Radial pulse is felt on the wrist, just below the thumb

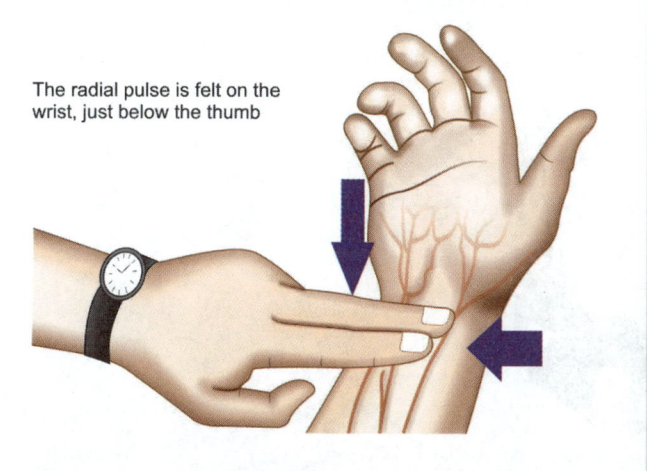

The radial pulse is felt on the wrist, just below the thumb

- Pressure should be exerted so that the wave may be felt, but care must be taken not to obliterate it.
- Note the rate, rhythm, volume and tension. Then count the number of beats for a full minute using a watch or pulsometer. If necessary, count longer, to be certain and accurate.

Checking Respiration

- Count respiration immediately after counting the pulse while fingers are still on the wrist.

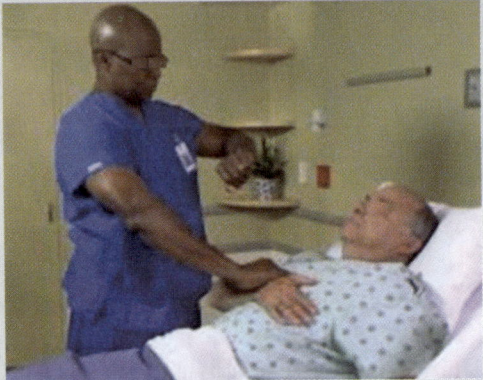

- This way the person does not know when his/her respirations are being measured—ensuring a more accurate measurement.
- It is difficult for the patient to breathe normally if he knows respirations are being counted.

- Do not relax fingers until finished.
- Watch the rise and fall of the chest as the patient breathes, without his/her knowledge.
- Count each inhalation and exhalation as one respiration and count for one minute.
- If patient's hand is resting on his/her chest, it is easy to count breaths when his/her chest rises and falls.

Checking Blood Pressure

Equipment for Taking Blood Pressure (Figs 9A and B)

- Sphygmomanometer

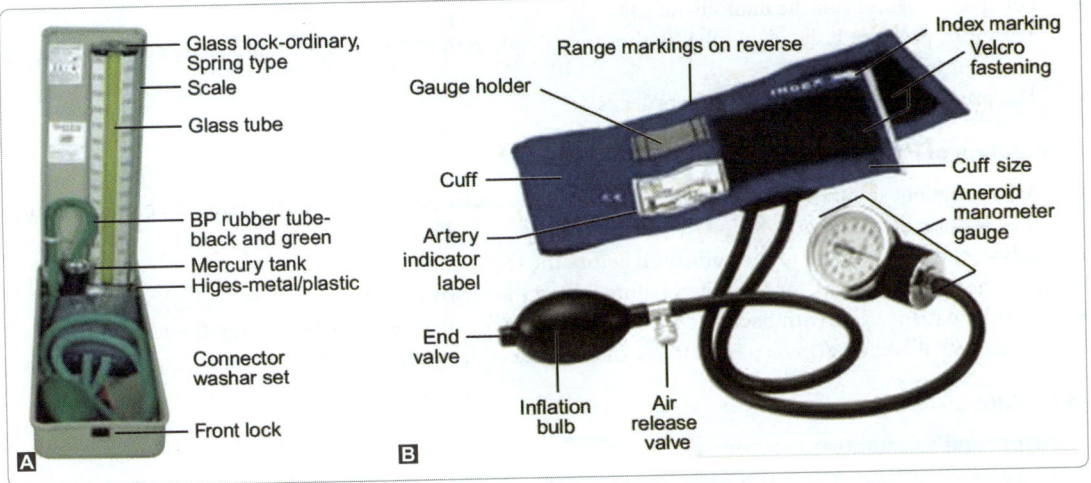

Figures 9A and B: (A) Net mercury sphygmomanometer; (B) Adult cotton Aneroid sphygmomanometer

- **Stethoscope (Fig. 10)**

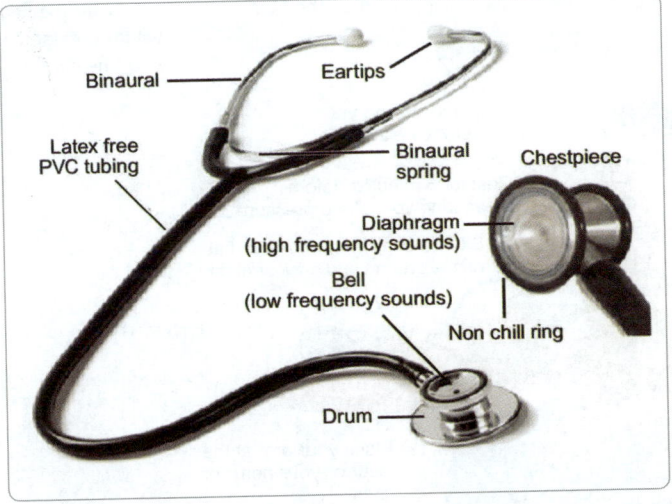

Figure 10: Labeled image of stethoscope

Guidelines for Checking Blood Pressure

Check apparatus:

- The level of mercury in glass tube should be zero.
- The meniscus should be a smooth, well-defined curve
- The mercury should rise easily in the tubing
- The mercury column does not bounce noticeably when the valve is closed
- The cap at the top of the calibrated glass tube to make sure it is securely in place

Unit V ❖ Assessment of Patient

- For spilled mercury in the manometer case
- The cuffs, pressure bulb, glass tube, stethoscope diaphragm and manometer and stethoscope tubing for cracks or tears
- The pressure control valve for sticks or leaks

Preparation of Patient

- Ask the patient about the history of smoking, drinking coffee 30 minutes before taking the blood pressure. If so wait for 30 minutes.
- Advice the patient to go to the bathroom before the test.
- Ask the patient to relax for 5 minutes before taking the measurement.
- Ask the patient to sit with back support (not to sit on a couch or soft chair). Keep the feet on the floor uncrossed. Place the arm on a solid flat surface (like a table) with the upper part of the arm at heart level.

Procedure

Palpatory and auscultatory method:

Steps	Procedure	Rationale
1.	Perform hand wash	Prevents spread of microorganism
2.	Instruct the patient to take a relaxed position either lying down with arm on bed or sitting with arm supported on the table at heart level to ensure accurate reading.	If the arm's position varies, or is not level with the heart, measurement values obtained will not be consistent with the patient's true blood pressure.

Position for taking your blood pressure at home

① Rest for 5 minutes before measuring your blood pressure

② Sit in a chair with both feet flat on the ground and back straight

③ Place your arm at the level of your heart or chest

④ Stay still and do not talk as your blood pressure machine apparatus

Contd...

Steps	Procedure	Rationale
3.	The apparatus is kept at the level of the heart of the patient in sitting or lying position. Measurement reading become lower — Correct measurement position — Measurement reading become higher — Incorrect — Correct	Positioning the apparatus facilitates to maintain the same hydrostatic component as that of the heart.
4.	Disinfect stethoscope earpieces and diaphragm using a spirit cotton swab.	Prevents transfer of microorganisms
5.	Roll sleeve above elbow about 5" [double prime] (12.5 cm), usually on left arm. Apply deflated cuff smoothly and evenly with rubber bladder over brachial artery (two tubes going toward palm of hand) lower edge about 2" (5 cm) above elbow and tuck loose end. 1/2" (1–2cm)	Clothing can impact a systolic blood pressure from 10 to 50 mmHg

Contd...

Steps	Procedure	Rationale
6.	• Fasten the cuff tightly and gently. Explain that the application of cuff may cause discomfort for a short time.	Ensures cooperation from the patient.
	• Tighten screw on rubber bulb of the apparatus. • Close the valve on the rubber bulb by turning the screw to the right. The screw will get shorter.	Prevents leakage of air
7.	Raise the mercury in the glass tube of the apparatus by pressing the bulb.	Bulb inflates the cuff for measuring the blood pressure

Contd...

Steps	Procedure	Rationale
8.	Palpate the radial artery and inflate the BP cuff by squeezing bulb until pulse disappears. 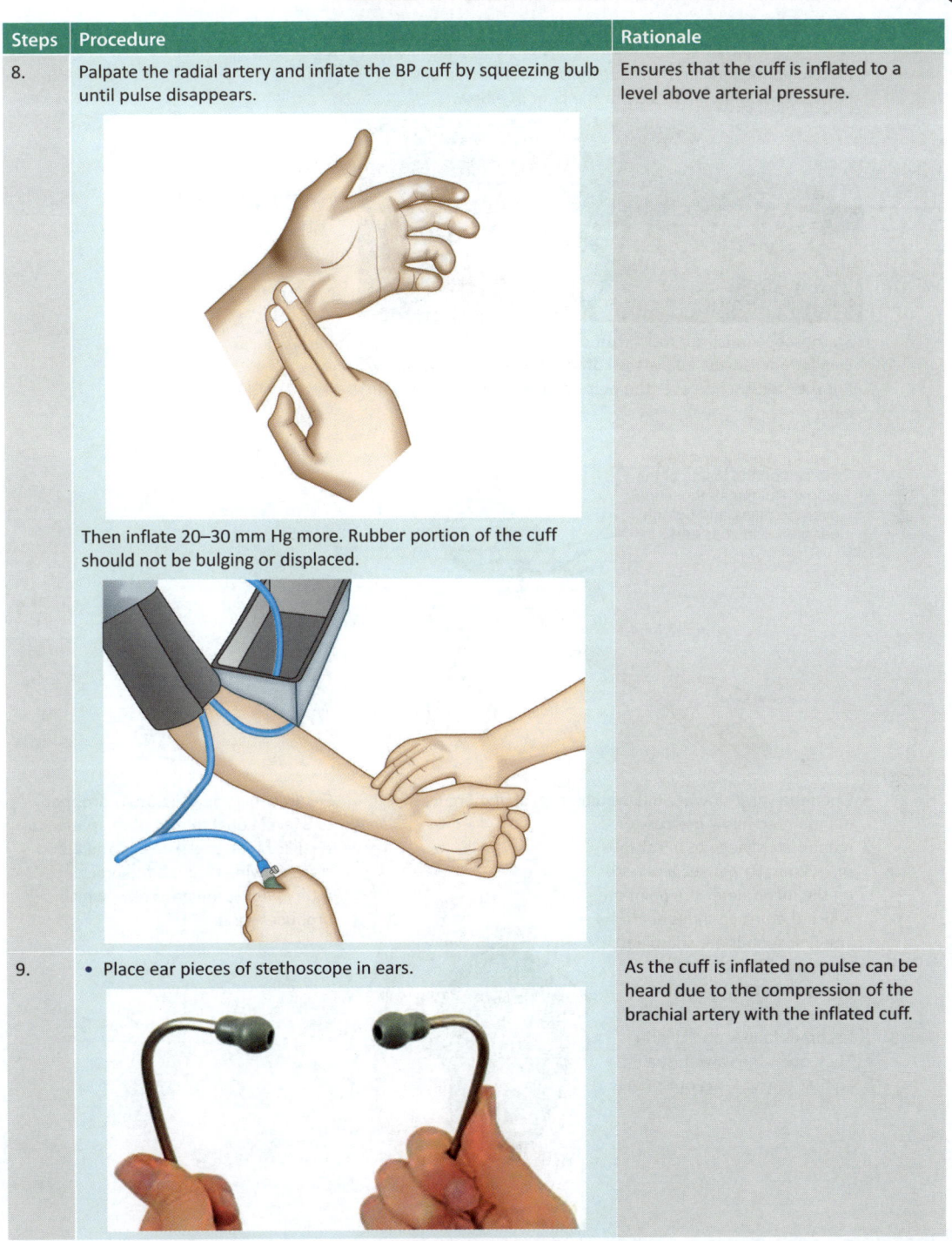 Then inflate 20–30 mm Hg more. Rubber portion of the cuff should not be bulging or displaced.	Ensures that the cuff is inflated to a level above arterial pressure.
9.	• Place ear pieces of stethoscope in ears.	As the cuff is inflated no pulse can be heard due to the compression of the brachial artery with the inflated cuff.

Contd...

Steps	Procedure	Rationale
	• Place diaphragm of stethoscope lightly but firmly in place. Pulse is felt on the inner side or the bent of elbow. 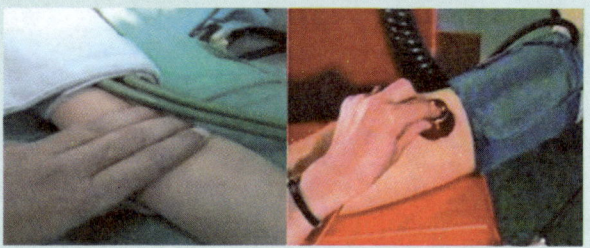 • Stethoscope must not touch cuff or tubes. • Feel for a pulse just below the cuff on the inside of the elbow. Put the stethoscope over the pulse and the ear pieces in your ears. Feel for a pulse just below the cuff on the inside of the elbow. Put the stethoscope over the pulse and put the ear pieces in your ears.	
10.	• Open the valve slowly while watching level of mercury in manometer. Allow mercury of manometer gauge to fall at rate of 2–3 mm Hg per sec and note on the manometer the point at which the first sound is heard. The first sounds are sharp and snapping. This is systolic pressure reading. As the air continues to escape, sound becomes louder and clearer. 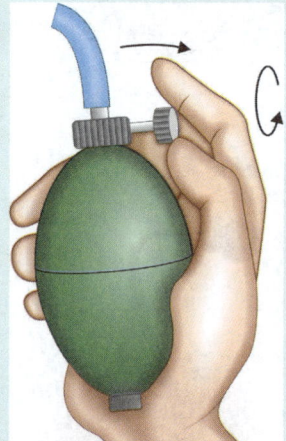 • Then open the valve just a little so that the air leaks out slowly.	Ensures that the pressure is dropped to a level equal to that of the patient's systolic blood pressure and the blood starts flowing through the brachial artery with turbulence flow, which produces thrill.

Contd...

Unit V ❖ Assessment of Patient

Steps	Procedure	Rationale
11.	Continue to release the air slowly. The sounds that heard louder and clearer becomes dull and disappears. Note the point of mercury column where the sound ceases. This is diastolic pressure reading. Allow all the air to escape and the mercury to fall to zero. 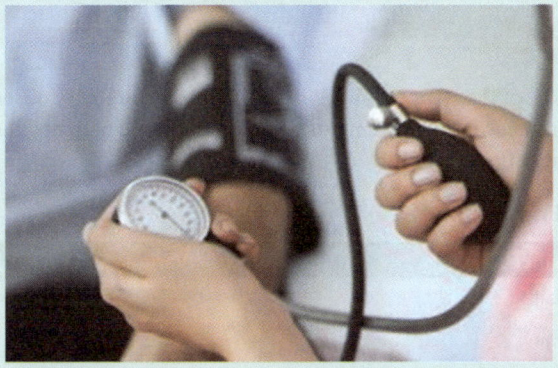	This ensures that the cuff pressure has dropped to a level of diastolic blood pressure and the flow becomes laminar flow and the thrill characteristic of pulse disappears or pulse becomes soft and then disappears very shortly. 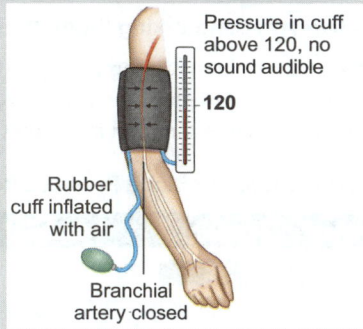 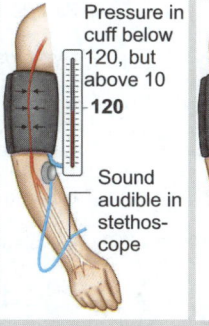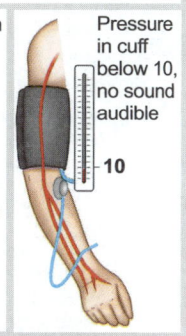
12.	Wait for one minute with the cuff deflated. Repeat the procedure if there is any doubt about the reading. Do not take blood pressure more than 3 times in succession on the same arm	Measuring more than 3 times may affect the venous flow of the forearm or it will falsely elevate the succeeding blood pressure reading.
13.	Remove cuff by rolling it off and replace it in box. Replace equipment. 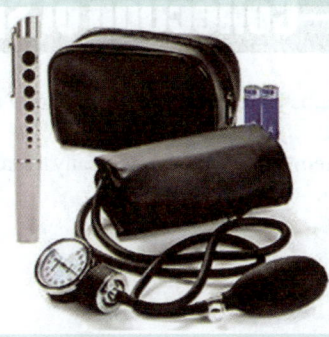	Facilitates subsequent measurement

Contd...

Unit V ❖ Assessment of Patient

Steps	Procedure	Rationale
14.	Leave the patient in a comfortable position.	Promotes comfort
15.	Wash hands	Prevents transfer of microorganisms
16.	Record reading immediately on paper or chart. Note any unusual observations.	Documentation fosters quality care

Factors Affecting Taking Blood Pressure

When taking blood pressure, it is vital that all of the steps involved in the process are properly observed. Small variations in technique can cause large variances in measurements, even on the same patient. The following chart shows some common issues that could affect readings:

Factors Affecting Blood Pressure Readings

Variance ↓ (mm Hg)	Cause of variance	Variance ↑ (mm Hg)
10–40	Cuff is too small	10–40
	Cuff over clothing	10–40
	Back/feet unsupported	5–15
	Legs crossed	5–8
	Not resting 3–5 minutes	
	Patient talking	10–15
	Labored breathing	5–8
	Full bladder	10–15
	Pain	10–30
	Arm below heart level	1.8/inch
1.8/inch	Arm above heart level	

Ref: https://www.adctoday.com

Laboratory Assessment—Collection of Specimens

A specimen may be defined as a small quantity of a substance or object which shows the kind and quality of the whole, e.g., blood or urine specimen.

Specimens sent to the laboratory are examined chemically or microscopically to aid in making a diagnosis or determining the line of treatment.

PURPOSES

- To make the diagnosis and prescribe the proper treatment
- To note the progress or recess of a disease
- To observe the effects of special treatments and drugs
- To ascertain the general health of the patient before surgery and anesthesia

KINDS OF SPECIMENS

- Urine
- Stool or feces
- Sputum
- Vomitus
- Vaginal secretions or tissue excretion
- Throat swab
- Eye secretions
- Wound discharges
- Blood
- Spinal fluid
- Fluids from body cavities

NURSE'S RESPONSIBILITIES

The collection of specimen is one of the important responsibilities of the nurses. The accuracy and reliability of findings depend on the correct method by which the specimens are collected and transported to the laboratory.

Inaccurate results may mislead the physician in making a correct diagnosis and giving prompt treatment. Hence, it is the responsibility of the nurse to see that specimens ordered are collected and sent in the appropriate manner. The responsibilities of the nurse may be divided under the following headings:

- **Preparation of the patient:** The nurse's responsibility varies according to the type of specimen to be collected. The patient should be prepared physically and mentally. Explain to the patient when to collect the specimen; what specimen is to be collected and how to collect and in what amount.

  Instruct the patient not to contaminate the outside of the bottle so that it may be safe for the workers to handle it.
- **Preparation of equipment to be used in collecting specimen:** A wide variety of containers are available for use in collecting specimens.

  The following containers are generally used:

Containers	Image
• **Glass bottle** or urine specimen container with wide mouth, for routine urine examination	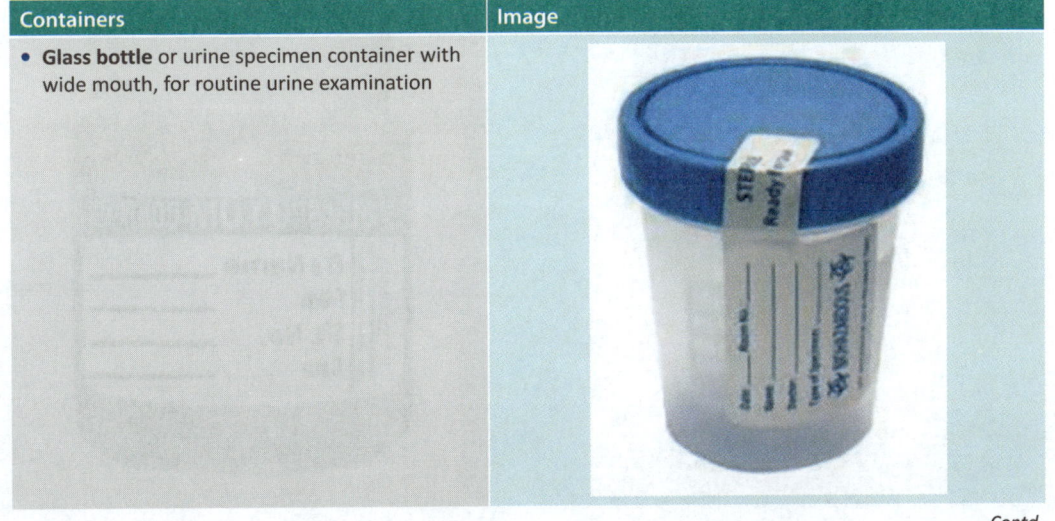

Contd...

Unit V ❖ Assessment of Patient

Containers	Image
• **Clean bottle** of small sizes for collecting stool specimen	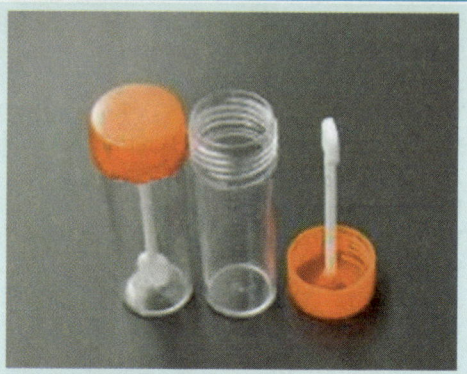
• **Large containers** (1 gallon) for 24 hours urine specimen	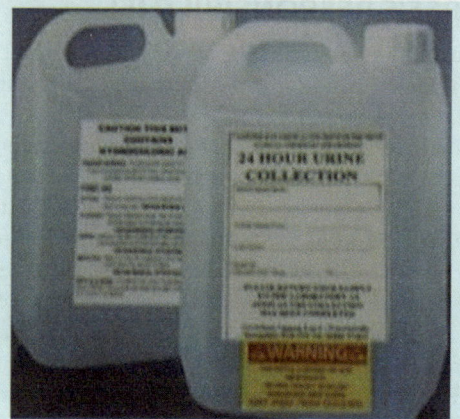
• **Glass jar** with cover or wax lined cardboard cup with cover for sputum or stool specimens	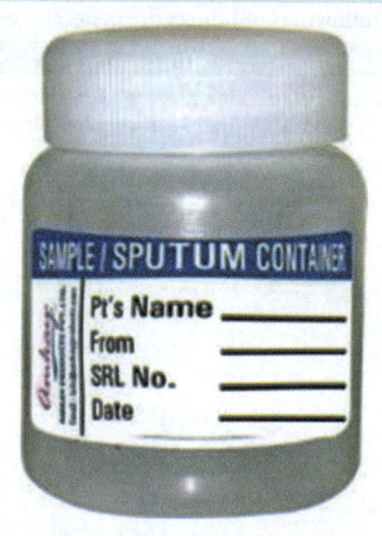

Contd...

Containers	Image
• **Sterile test tubes** (various sizes) for body fluids	
• **Sterile flask** with culture media for blood specimen when blood culture is to be done	
• **Clean slides** for smears.	
• **Vacutainers** for collecting blood sample	

The color guide for various blood sample collection in vacutainers is as follows:

Tube	Cap color	Additive	Determination
Sodium citrate	Light blue	Buffered sodium citrate 0.109 M (3.2%)	PT, APTT, D-dimer, lupus anticoagulant, anti-thrombin III, protein S and C, fibrinogen, factor assay, HLA B27
Red top pain	Red	Clot activator silicone coated	Cold agglutinins, abnormal blood group antibody screen, antibody identification and vitamin D2 and D3 (HPLC)
Plain	Gold	Colt activator and gel for serum separation	Biochemistry, virology, immunology, vitamin B12, folate, anticonvulsant drug monitoring, therapeutic drug monitoring (TDM) and other investigations that require serum (i.e., plain blood)
Royal blue plain	Royal blue (serum)	Trace element (with clot activator)	Zinc, copper, aluminum, selenium
Lithium heparin	Green	Lithium heparin	STAT biochemistry, plasma ammonia (in ice pack), CD34, blood alcohol, toxicological tests, chromosomes studies, electrolytes, renal function tests, TB spot
Lithium heparin	Light green	Lithium heparin and gel for plasma separation	STAT biochemistry, plasma ammonia (in ice pack), CD34, blood alcohol, toxicological tests, chromosomes studies, electrolytes, renal function tests
Royal blue EDTA	Royal blue (K_2 EDTA)	K_2 EDTA	Arsenic, cadmium, chromium, mercury, lead manganese
K_2 EDTA	Lavender	Spray-coated K_2 EDTA	FBC, PBF, MP, ESR, HBA1c, cyclosporine A, G6PD, RBC cholinesterase, ACTH, renin, HB electrophoresis, thalassemia screening, CD4/CD8, factor V Leiden
Sodium fluoride	Gray	Sodium fluoride	Glucose, lactic acid (in ice pack)

GENERAL INSTRUCTIONS

- Specimen containers should be clean. If the container is cracked, broken or damaged, it should not be used.
- All specimens for culture should be collected in sterile containers.
- There should not be any antiseptic present in any specimen bottle.
- The specimen should be sent to the laboratory while it is fresh with the requisition form properly filled in and signed (by the doctor).
- After the tests, reports are received from the laboratory and it is brought to the notice of the concerned doctor in time, for the proper diagnosis and treatment.

■ **Collection and transportation of specimen and receiving the reports:** Specimens are collected by nurses themselves or by doctors assisted by nurses or by the laboratory technicians. It is the responsibility of the nurses to see that the specified techniques are observed in collecting specimens. She/he also should see that the specimens are properly labelled with the following details:

Ward No:	Bed No:
Name and age of the patient:	IP.No...OP.No....
Address:	Name of specimen:
Nature of test to be done:	
Date and Time of collection:	
Date..........	Signature of the Doctor/Nurse/Technician

METHODS OF COLLECTING SPECIMENS

Blood Specimen Collection

Blood specimen collection is performed routinely to obtain blood for laboratory testing. Blood is most frequently obtained via a peripheral vein puncture (venipuncture).

Definition: Venipuncture involves puncturing a peripheral vein with a needle and collecting blood in a syringe or evacuated tube.

Purposes

Blood is usually drawn and collected in order to perform a variety of laboratory tests.
■ To help diagnose conditions such as electrolyte imbalances
■ To screen for risk factors like high cholesterol levels
■ To monitor the effects of treatments and medications.

Blood Collection Tubes

The following are the blood collection tubes that come with a variety of colored stopper caps and may contain additives.

Red Top (Fig. 11)

■ This tube contains no additives.
■ It is used for biochemistry tests requiring serum which might be adversely affected by the separator gel used in the yellow bottle.

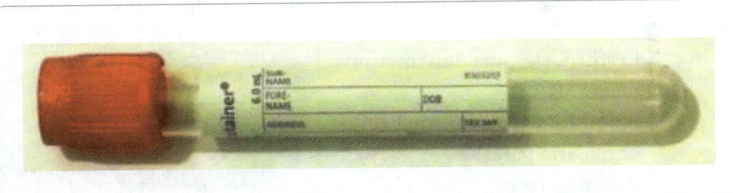

Figure 11: Blood collection tube with red top

■ This contains silica particle, which act as clot activators.
■ Commonly used for
The use of this bottle varies greatly as:
 • Some hospitals use it for many sensitive tests, including testing of hormones in toxicology, checking drug levels, bacterial and viral serology and antibodies, whereas others seem to only use it for a few very specific purposes and use the yellow bottle for most things.
 • Ionized calcium test.

Unit V ❖ Assessment of Patient

Dark Green Top (Fig. 12)

- This less commonly used bottle is for biochemistry tests, which requires heparinized plasma or whole blood for analysis.
- This contains sodium heparin, which acts as an anticoagulant.
- Commonly used for
  - Lithium and ammonia level
  - Insulin
  - Renin
  - Aldosterone

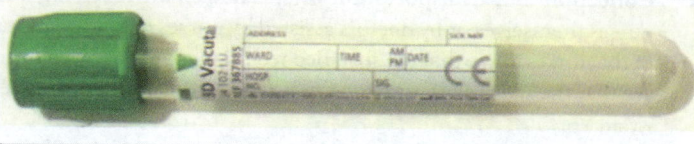

Figure 12: Blood collection tube with dark green top

Light Green Top (Fig. 13)

- This is used for biochemistry tests requiring separated heparinized plasma.
- It contains lithium heparin, which acts as an anticoagulant, and a plasma separator gel similar to that used in the yellow bottle, which acts to separate out the plasma layer.

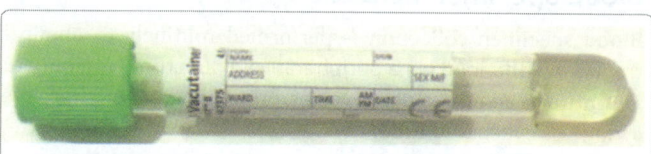

Figure 13: Blood collection bottle with light green top

- Commonly used for
  - It can be used for routine biochemistry, but most hospitals seem to use the yellow bottle for this purpose.
  - It can also be used for blood ethanol provided the sample is not for legal purposes.

Lavender or Purple Top (Fig. 14)

- They contain EDTA, an anticoagulant additive that chelates calcium (binds calcium in the blood).
- These tubes are used primarily for obtaining complete blood counts.
- Commonly used for
  - Erythrocyte sedimentation rate (ESR)
  - Blood film for abnormal cells or malaria parasites
  - Reticulocytes
  - Red cell folate
  - Monospot test for EBV
  - HbA1C for diabetic control
  - Parathyroid hormone (PTH)

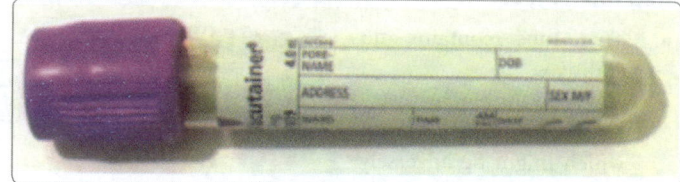

Figure 14: Blood collection bottle with purple top

Pink Top (Fig. 15)

- The pink bottles work in the same way as the purple ones, but are specifically used only for whole blood samples being sent to the

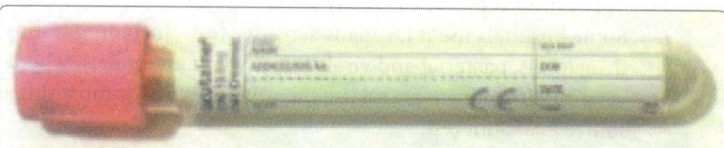

Figure 15: Blood collection bottle with pink top

transfusion lab.
- This tube also contains the anticoagulant EDTA.
- Commonly used for
  - Grouping
  - Crossmatching
  - Direct Coombs test (direct antiglobulin test) for autoimmune hemolytic anemia

Light Blue Top (Fig. 16)

- The light blue top tubes contain buffered sodium citrate, an agent that removes calcium.
- It acts as a reversible anticoagulant by binding to calcium ions in the blood and subsequently disrupting the clotting cascade.

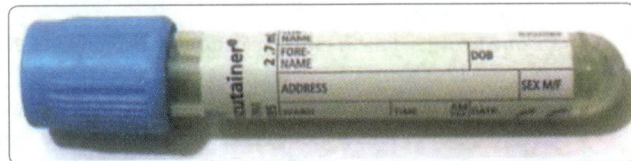

Figure 16: Blood collection bottle with light blue top

- Hence, it is used for hematology tests involving the clotting system, which require inactivated whole blood for analysis.
- Commonly used for
  - Coagulation screening including bleeding time for platelet function, prothrombin time (PT) for extrinsic pathway, activated partial thromboplastin time (APTT) for intrinsic pathway, and thrombin time (TT) or fibrinogen assay for the final common pathway
  - D-dimer for thrombosis, e.g., DVT or PE
  - INR for monitoring patients on warfarin
  - Activated partial thromboplastin ratio (APTR) for monitoring patients on IV heparin infusions
  - Anti-Xa assay for monitoring patients on high-dose low molecular weight heparins like tinzaparin

Light Gray Top (Fig. 17)

- This specimen tube contains sodium fluoride and potassium oxalate.
- Sodium fluoride acts as an antiglycolytic agent that preserves glucose for up to five days. It ensures that no further glucose breakdown occurs within the sample after it is taken.

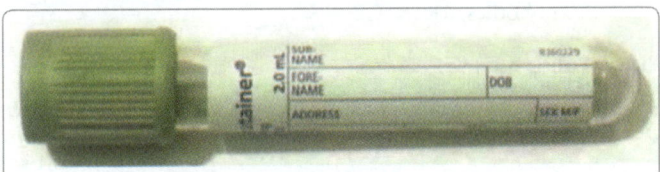

Figure 17: Specimen tube with light gray top

- Potassium oxalate acts as an anticoagulant.
- The tube is used primarily to obtain glucose levels.
- It is used for biochemistry tests requiring whole blood for analysis.
- Commonly used for
  - Glucose – this can be fasting or nonfasting, or part of a glucose tolerance test (GTT)
  - Lactate

Yellow Top (Fig. 18)

- These bottles are used for a huge variety of tests requiring separated serum for analysis, including biochemistry, endocrinology, oncology, toxicology, microbiology and immunology.

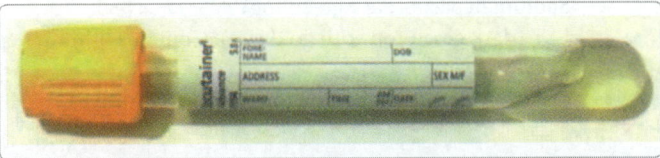

Figure 18: Specimen collection bottle with yellow top

Unit V ❖ Assessment of Patient

- This tube contains two agents; silica particles and a serum separating gel.
  - The silica particles work to activate clotting and cause the blood cells to clump together.
- Commonly used for Biochemistry tests like:
  - Urea, creatinine, sodium and potassium
  - C-reactive protein (CRP)
  - **Liver function tests (LFTs):** This includes bilirubin, ALP, AST/ALT, GGT, total protein and albumin
  - Amylase assay
  - **Bone profile:** This includes calcium, phosphate, ALP and albumin
  - Magnesium assay
  - **Iron studies:** These include serum iron, ferritin, transferrin saturation and total iron binding capacity
  - **Lipid profile:** This includes cholesterol, LDL, HDL and triglycerides
  - **Thyroid function tests (TFTs):** These tests include TSH, free T4 +/–free T3
  - Vitamins, e.g., vitamin B12
  - **Troponins:** This requires 2 samples to be taken at different times to assess the acute trend
  - Creatine Kinase (CK)
  - Urate
  - **Serum osmolality:** This requires a urine sample to be taken at the same time
  - **Endocrinology:** Beta-hCG, Calcitonin*, Cortisol, EPO, sex hormones, growth hormone, IGF-1
  - **Tumor markers:** PSA, CEA, CA-125, CA19-9, AFP, Lactate Dehydrogenase (LDH)
  - **Toxicology:** Ethanol, cannabis, opiates, benzodiazepines, other drugs, e.g., cocaine, amphetamines
  - **Drug levels:** Paracetamol, salicylates (aspirin), digoxin, lithium, gentamicin, carbamazepine
  - **Microbiology/virology:** Serology for a wide variety of bacterial, viral, fungal and parasitic infections including HIV and viral hepatitis
  - **Immunology:** Immunoglobulins, complement, autoantibody screen, rheumatoid factor, thyroid antibodies, α1at, ACE

Other Tubes having:

- **White:** Used for molecular diagnostics such as PCR and DNA amplification studies
- **Black:** For pediatric ESR

Order of Drawing Tubes for Blood Sample Collection

It is important that blood collection tubes be drawn in a certain order to avoid the cross-contamination of additives between tubes. It is recommended that tubes be drawn in the following order:

- **First:** Blood culture bottle or tube (yellow or yellow-black top)
- **Second:** Coagulation tube (light blue top).
- **Third:** Nonadditive tube (red top)
  - **Light-blue top:** This should not be the first tube drawn. If a coagulation assay is ordered alone, draw a nonadditive tube first (red or SST), then draw the light-blue top tube.
- **Last draw:** Additive tubes in the following order:
  - SST (red-gray or gold top). Contains a gel separator and clot activator.
  - Sodium heparin (dark green top)
  - PST (dark green top with gold rim). Contains lithium heparin anticoagulant and a gel separator.
  - EDTA (lavender top)
  - Oxalate/fluoride (light gray top) or other additives

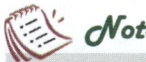

Note

- Tubes with additives must be thoroughly mixed. Clotting or erroneous test results may be obtained when the blood is not thoroughly mixed with the additive.

Sites of Venipuncture

- Veins in dorsal hands: The first choice for adult patients
- Median cubital vein.
- Cephalic vein.
- Basilic vein.
- Dorsal metacarpal veins.
- Veins in dorsal foot are commonly used for children but are avoided in adults because of the danger of thrombophlebitis.

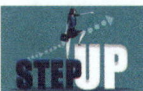

Four Patient's 'Rights'

There are four patient 'rights' the nurse should consider when collecting blood specimens. These rights are:

1. **Right specimen:** Make sure the specimen collected is the specimen ordered.
2. **Right time:** Certain blood tests must be obtained at specific times. For example, when drawing antibiotic levels, specimens should be obtained immediately prior to the next dose. The time to draw peak levels may be dependent upon whether the antibiotic is given intravenously, orally, or intramuscularly.
3. **Right patient:** Always verify the patient's identification before drawing a blood specimen. The person drawing the specimen should also label the container it is drawn into.
4. **Right method:** Always follow universal precautions when performing a venipuncture.

General Guidelines

- Avoid drawing blood from an arm affected by a stroke or neurological injury that has resulted in a loss of sensation. The patients may not be able to alert you if they experience pain or other problems.
- Avoid drawing blood from the arm on the affected side if a woman has had a mastectomy.
- Avoid areas with extensive scarring. Scar tissue is difficult to puncture.
- Attempt to collect the blood specimen from the opposite arm if a patient is receiving intravenous fluids, since fluid may dilute the blood sample.
- Do not use a site that is swollen, affected by certain skin conditions like eczema, or is infected.
- Use the right specimen tubes. Using the wrong tubes will cause the specimen to be rejected by the laboratory.
- Try using pediatric tubes when a patient has fragile veins that may not provide a large enough specimen. Though the smaller tubes store less blood, they will still give reliable results.
- Remove the tourniquet when the final tube of blood to be drawn is filling up.
- Send the specimen to the laboratory as soon as possible.

Unit V ❖ Assessment of Patient

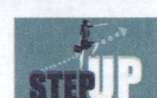

Vacutainer System in Venipuncture

- Venipuncture is usually done using a vacuum container (Vacutainer) system.
- This system consists of vacuumized specimen tubes, a needle and a plastic holder.

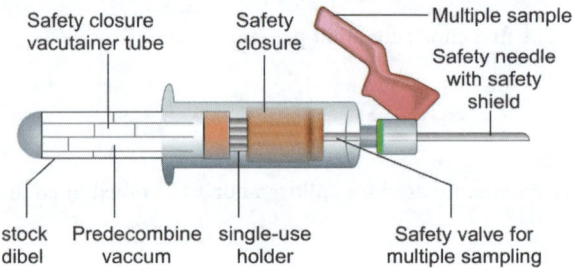

- When the tube is placed into the holder and pressed against the needle, negative pressure results, and blood is pulled into the tube.
- Normally, a 21-gauge needle is used to collect blood.

Articles Required

A clean tray containing:

Article	Purpose
Materials for hand wash	Aids in the removal of micro organisms
Sterile syringe and needle (needle 14–18 gauge) in a container or appropriate vacutainers	For proper collection of blood samples
A small bowl with cotton swabs or a pack of sterile swab.	To wipe the venipuncture site
70% alcohol (isopropyl alcohol or ethanol)	To wipe the venipuncture site
A small bowl containing dry gauze	To wipe the area after venipuncture and to secure the site from preventing bleeding
Tourniquet	Helps to make the vein swell
Mackintosh and towel	To protect linen from soiling
Non sterile gloves	To prevent cross infection
Kidney tray/paper bag	To dispose the soiled waste
Needle dispenser	To dispose the used syringes and needles
Adhesive tape	To secure the venipuncture site
Waste bin	To discard biomedical waste
Note pad and pen	To document the procedure
Laboratory forms and labeling	For proper documentation

Other Preparations

Preparation of Unit

- Ensure an area of good lighting
- Arrange all the necessary articles close to the bedside of the patient
- Provide privacy by closing the door, pulling the curtains and exposing only the site of venipuncture.

Preparation of Patient

- Explain the procedure and the reason for collecting the specimen and give the patient time to ask questions.
- Win the confidence and cooperation of the patient by giving proper explanation regarding the nature of the treatment.

Procedure

Steps	Procedure	Rationale
1.	Perform Hand wash and wear required PPE	Prevents spread of microorganism.
2.	Reassure the patient and explain the procedure. Place the patient in comfortable position.	Positioning mentally prepares the patient.
3.	Secure privacy by drawing curtains. Close windows and doors.	Prevents embarrassment.
4.	Before entering patient room, assemble all equipment. Label blood collection tubes with date of collection, patient name, and his/her identifier number. Fill out necessary laboratory form. Arrange the necessary articles near to the patient bedside along with the prepared medicine in a tray.	Facilitates skilful performance of the procedure.
5.	Wash hands. Wear required PPE.	Prevents spread of infection
6.	Select the site, preferably at the bend of the elbow. Uncover arm completely. Palpate the area; locate a vein of good size that is visible, straight and clear. The vein should be visible without applying a tourniquet.	Veins in the area of the arm are the safest for venipuncture and they are usually easier to find.

Contd...

Unit V ❖ Assessment of Patient

Steps	Procedure	Rationale
7.	Place a mackintosh under the extremity. Have the patient relax and support his arm below the vein to be used.	Protects the linen from soiling.
8.	Look for a suitable vein. Once finding a vein, place one finger over it. Use this finger to gently press up and down in a gentle bouncing motion for 20–30 seconds. 	This causes the vein to expand and become visible.
9.	Wrap an elastic tourniquet 2–4 in (5.1–10.2 cm) above the venipuncture site. Use a loose overhand knot or simply tuck the tourniquet ends into the band to secure it or apply the Velcro strap. 	This causes the vein to expand and become visible.
10.	Instruct the person to open and close his hands several times. Or the person can be asked to squeeze a stress ball and release it several times. Watch to see if the vein becomes more visible after about 30–60 seconds of this.	This causes the vein to expand and become visible.

Contd...

Steps	Procedure	Rationale
11.	Wait for the vein to swell. When using vacuum extraction system with holder, insert the blood collector tube into the holder.	Facilitates easy access
12.	Disinfect skin with an alcohol swab or gauze in a outward circular motion. Repeat 2–3 times. Do not touch the site once disinfected.	Prevents transfer of microorganisms

Steps	Procedure	Rationale
13.	Stabilize the vein by pulling the skin taut in the longitudinal direction of the vein. Use the nondominant hand to pull the skin taut against the vein, hold the needle with dominant hand.	Facilitates easy puncture into the vein.

Contd...

Steps	Procedure	Rationale
14.	Insert the needle at an angle of around 20–35 degrees with the bevel end up. Puncture the skin and move the needle slightly into the vein (3–5 mm). Hold the syringe and needle steady.	Facilitates puncture into the vein without piercing the vein.
15.	If blood appears hold the syringe steady, you are in the vein. If blood is not visible, try again.	Ensures that the needle is inside the vein. If the blood comes out with notable pressure and appears bright red and foamy, it affirms that the needle is inserted into an artery. Immediately pull the needle out and apply direct pressure to the site for at least 5 minutes to stop the bleeding.
16.	When blood starts to flow, ask patient to open his/her hand, aspirate, loosen tourniquet.	Facilitates free flow of blood and medicines that is injected.
17.	Once sufficient blood has been collected (minimum 5 mL), release the tourniquet before withdrawing the needle.	

Contd...

Steps	Procedure	Rationale
	If blood is required for multiple test replace appropriate vacutainer without removing the needle. 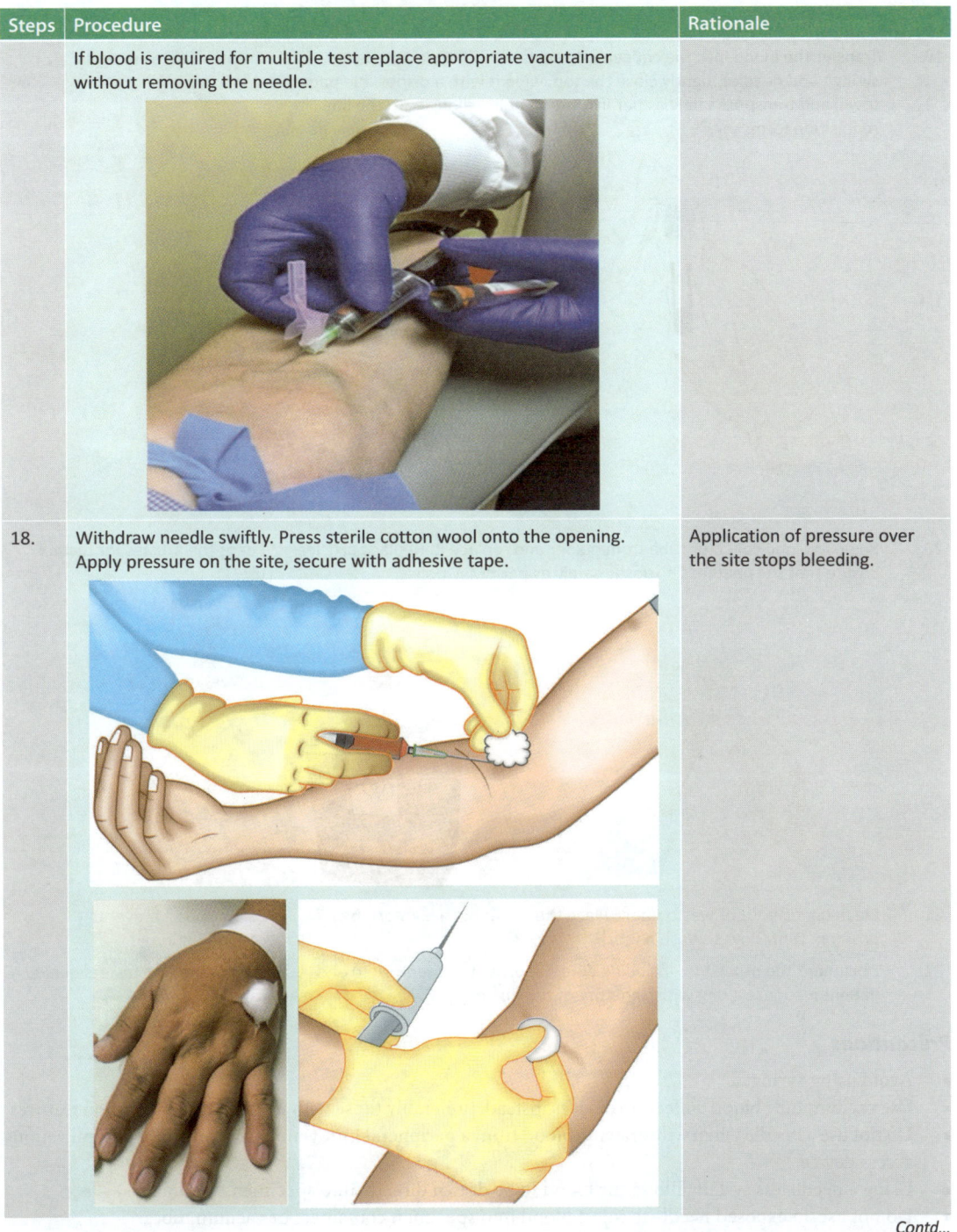	
18.	Withdraw needle swiftly. Press sterile cotton wool onto the opening. Apply pressure on the site, secure with adhesive tape.	Application of pressure over the site stops bleeding.

Contd...

Steps	Procedure	Rationale
19.	Transfer the blood into the concerned vacutainers (if collected using syringe and needle), tightly close the top, wipe it with a disposable paper towel and transport safely as per institution policy along with the lab requisition form. 	Ensures safe transport.
20.	Remove blood collector tube from holder and replace it. Replace articles. Ensure that the needle is disposed safely as per BMW policy. 	Keeps the articles for further use.
21.	Clean up; dispose of waste safely. Place the patient in a comfortable position. Doff Gloves. Wash hands.	Safe disposal prevents contamination.
22.	Document the procedure including date, time, lab tests requested and patient response along with signature of the nurse.	Documentation fosters quality care.

Assessment of Patient — Unit V ❖

Precautions

- Avoid using syringes.
- Use vacuum tube blood collection devices instead, preferably those with needle-stick prevention features.
- Do not use a needle when withdrawing blood from a peripheral intravenous line or from a central venous access device.
- Using a needleless system allows the blood to be drawn directly into specimen containers.
- Do not use an exposed needle to inject blood into specimen containers or vacuum tubes.

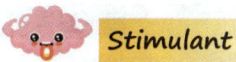

Stimulant

Techniques to Prevent Hemolysis in the Sample
- Mix all tubes with anticoagulant additives gently (vigorous shaking can cause hemolysis) 5–10 times.
- Avoid drawing blood from a hematoma; select another draw site.
- If using a needle and syringe, avoid drawing the plunger back too forcefully.
- Make sure the venipuncture site is dry before proceeding to withdraw.
- Avoid a probing, traumatic venipuncture.
- Avoid prolonged tourniquet application (no more than 2 minutes; less than 1 minute is optimal).
- Avoid massaging, squeezing, or probing a site.
- Avoid excessive fist clenching.
- If blood flow into tube slows, adjust needle position to remain in the center of the lumen.

Collection of Specimen of Feces

Stool is collected to determine the presence of blood, ova and parasites, bile, fat, pathogens, or substances such as ingested drugs. Additional studies include fecal urobilinogen, nitrogen, *Clostridium difficile*, fecal leukocytes, calculation of stool osmolar gap, food residues, and other substances requiring lab evaluation. Gross examination of stool characteristics, such as color, consistency and odor can reveal conditions such as gastrointestinal bleeding and steatorrhea (excess fat in feces).

Routine examination: Stool is collected in a clean bedpan and transferred to the specimen bottle by means of wooden spatula. Routine examination of stool consists of the examination for roundworm ova, hook worm ova and dysentery organism. In case of a dysentery stool examination, it should be sent to the laboratory in a covered container immediately after collection to investigate the living amoeba. Remember that stool being a contaminated material, other organism may grow soon in it.

Culture specimen of stool: Culture examination of stool is done usually to detect the presence of typhoid bacillus. The patient is instructed to pass stools in a clean bedpan. The specimen is taken from the center of the mass by means of a sterile cotton applicator. The sterile cotton applicator saturated with feces may be placed in sterile test tube, plugged with sterile cotton wool and may be sent to the laboratory with label accompanied by lab requisition.

If the examination is for tape worm or segments of tape worm, the entire stool should be sent to the laboratory in a wide-mouthed glass jar. Specimen from infants are collected and examined by sending the diaper containing the stool in a covered container. Stool specimens should not be mixed with urine, sometimes it is necessary to give a cleansing enema to collect the specimen. In such cases, saline or tap water is used for enema, as other solution may affect the characteristics of stool. Special note should be made for such fresh specimen.

Articles Required

A tray containing:

Articles	Purpose
Hand washing articles	For hand washing
Specimen container with lid	For collection of specimen
Identification label	For patient identity
Gloves	To prevent cross contamination

Contd...

Unit V ❖ Assessment of Patient

Articles	Purpose
Two tongue blades/wooden spatula	To collect the stool from bed pan or commode
Paper towel or paper bag	To spread in the bed pan or commode
Bedpan or portable commode	For fecal elimination
Dust bins according to BMW policy	For proper disposal of waste
Lab request form and lab biohazard transport bag.	For patient identity and safe transport

Procedure

To collect a random specimen:

Steps	Procedure	Rationale
1.	Arrange the articles. Label the specimen container after filling the identification details of the patient.	Facilitates a skilled procedure

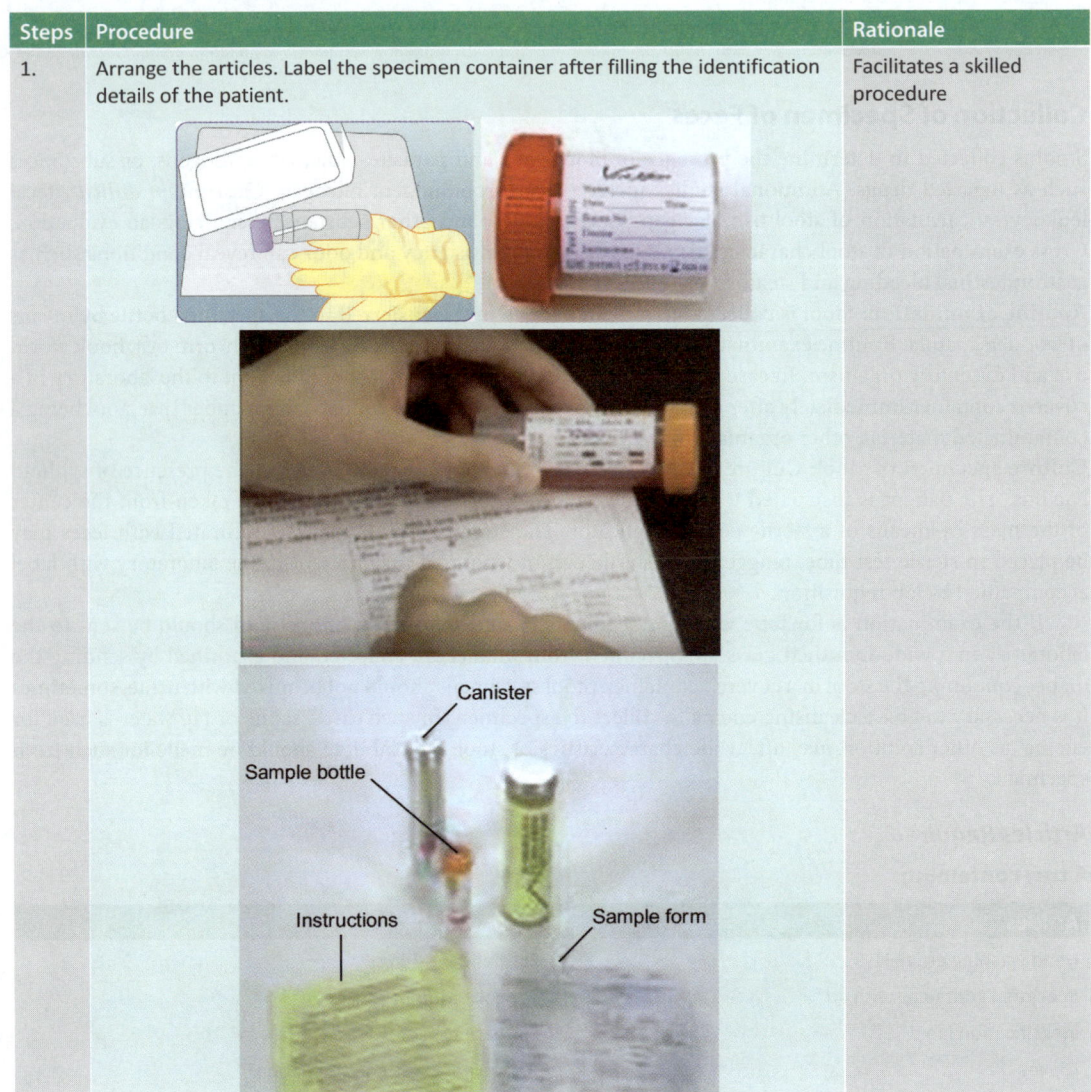

Canister

Sample bottle

Instructions

Sample form

Contd...

Steps	Procedure	Rationale
2.	Tell the patient to notify the urgency to defecate.	Helps to arrange equipment in advance
3.	Have him/her defecate into a clean, dry bedpan or commode. Instruct him/her not to contaminate the specimen with urine or toilet tissue. Spread a paper towel or paper bag over the commode. 	Facilitates easy collection of the specimen
4.	Wash hands	Helps to prevent cross infection
5.	Put on gloves.	Prevents cross - contamination
6.	Using a tongue blade/wooden spatula/spoon, transfer the most representative stool specimen from the bedpan to the container until the liquid reaches the fill line. If the patient passes blood, mucus, or pus with the stool, include this with the specimen. Spoon Fill line Liquid Stool Collect on plastic wrap and transfer to vial until liquid reaches fill line	

Contd...

Steps	Procedure	Rationale
7.	Remove the spoon or wooden spatula, Wrap the wooden spatula in a paper towel and discard it. Recap the container tightly. Shake the kit 2–3 times. Liquid to fill line Spoon Remove spoon from lid and discard Replace cap on vial tightly and shake for a minute. Place vial in refrigerator until ready to ship Garbage	Safe disposal prevents cross infection
8.	Transport the specimen in a safe biohazard sealed pack securely and at the earliest to the lab for further investigations.	Ensures safe transport of contents. Early transportation decreases multiplication of bacteria in the stool specimen container and may alter the test result.
9.	Remove and discard your gloves.	Prevents cross-contamination.
10.	Wash your hands thoroughly.	Prevents cross-contamination.
11.	Advice the patient to thoroughly clean his hands and perianal area. Make sure the patient is comfortable after the procedure.	Promotes comfort
12.	Document the date and time of the specimen collection in the patient's medical record along with instructions that the patient can resume his/her normal diet and medication regime unless otherwise specified	Documentation fosters quality care

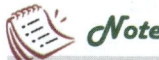 **Note**

- A single properly collected specimen is usually enough to identify the cause of acute bacterial diarrhea.
- To detect a carrier state, single specimens for three consecutive days are recommended.
- Only one specimen per patient per day will be accepted.
- All stool specimens for culture should be submitted in a transport media.
- Stool specimens should be collected in a clean, dry container.
- Stool specimens should not be contaminated with water, urine, barium, or mineral oil.
- Do not overfill the transport vial.
- Do not refrigerate.

Observations

Characteristics of Normal Feces

- **Color:** Normally the color of the feces is light to dark brown. This is due to the presence of bile pigments
- **Odor:** Normal stool has a pungent smell. This smell occurs because the stool is normally affected by the type of bacterial flora that is caused by the ingested food and medications.
- **Frequency:** One to two per day and it is painless.
- **Consistency and form:** In adult the stool is well formed and the consistency is semisolid.
- **Quantity:** Quantity depends upon the type and the amount of food taken. When the roughage in the diet is increased, the amount is also increased. Quantity varies from four to five ounces per day.
- **Composition:** The feces contains 30% water. The remaining portion consists of shed epithelium from the intestine, a considerable quantity of bacteria, a small quantity of nitrogenous matter mainly mucin, salts, calcium, phosphates, a little iron and cellulose, if present in the diet.

Characteristics of Abnormal Stool

- **Color:** Tarry black stools indicate bleeding in the upper gastrointestinal tract. The blood from the upper GIT gets altered by the intestinal juices. The occult blood test will be positive in such cases.
- When the stool appears black, it is termed as 'melena'. Black stools may also result from the administration of iron or charcoal.
- Clay colored stools indicate an obstruction to the flow of bile, because of the absence of bile pigment (stercobilin) that colors the stool.
- White stools may appear due to the presence of barium salts after barium tests.

Color of stool	Potential cause
Black	GI bleeding, iron, bismuth
Maroon	Gastrointestinal (GI) bleeding
Red - bright red blood	Hemorrhoids, anal fissure
Red - dark red/maroon, sometimes with clots or mucus	Inflammatory bowel disease (Crohn's disease, ulcerative colitis), infection, diverticular bleed, tumor, rapid upper GI bleed
Green	May be normal. A diet high in green vegetables is associated with diarrhea.
Brown	Normal color.
Yellow	Diseases of the pancreas, malabsorption, celiac disease, cystic fibrosis, Giardia infection
Clay, pale yellow, or white	Liver or biliary disease, lack of bile in the stool

Unit V ❖ Assessment of Patient

- **Odor:** In melena and dysentery, there will be foul smell. A strong smell results from diet containing plenty of meat.
- **Frequency:** It is increased in diarrhea and decreased in constipation or in patients who are on low residue diet.
- **Consistency and form:** In constipation, the stools are very hard.
  - Flattened and ribbon-like stools indicate some obstruction in the lumen of the bowel.
  - Watery stools are found in diarrhea, digestive upsets, due to bacterial invasions and after taking purgatives.
  - "Rice water stools" are typical of cholera.
  - "Pea soup stools" are typical of typhoid fever.
  - Pale, bulky, semisolid and frothy stools are characteristic of sprue.
- **Appearance:** Fresh blood in large amounts is suggestive of:
  - Bleeding piles
  - Stool with menstrual blood
  - Bleeding from the large colon
  - Malignant growths
  - Scurvy
  - Leukemia
  - Purpura.
- Other abnormal findings
  - The commonest cause of blood and mucus found in the stool is due to dysentery which may be amoebic or bacillary.
  - Stool may contain worms or segments of worms, e.g., round worm, thread worm, hook worm and tape worm.
    On microscopic examination, the stool is found to contain parasitic cysts, ova or larvae. The microorganisms commonly found are numerous such as amoebae, *E. coli, Vibrio cholera*, AFB, and salmonella group of organisms.

Collection of Sputum

Sputum is a material from the mucous lining of trachea and the bronchi. It is the recently discharged material from the bronchial tree, with minimal amounts of oral or nasal material.

- **Expectorated sputum:** Generated from a **deep** productive cough.
- **Induced sputum:** Produced with hypertonic saline if patient is unable to produce sputum on their own.

Indications for Sputum Collection

- To establish an initial diagnosis of TB
- To monitor the infectiousness of the patient
- To determine the effectiveness of treatment
  The consistency varies from a thin watery fluid to thick purulent material. An examination of sputum is made chiefly to know the presence of bacteria. Organisms commonly looked for, are tubercular bacilli, streptococci, pneumococci and diphtheria bacilli.

Collecting a Specimen from a Young Child

Specimens of sputum for examination are collected by having the patient cough up the material from the bronchi or lungs and expectorate into the container. The container most commonly used is the water proof waxed sputum cup because it can be destroyed easily after use. Specimens are usually collected in the

Unit V ❖ **Assessment of Patient**

morning before food is taken. The mouth should be rinsed with plain water before collecting the sputum. The patient should be given the container in the previous evening and instructed to raise material from the lungs by coughing and not simply expectorating saliva or discharges from the nose and throat. Antiseptics should not be poured into the container.

If a sterile specimen is required, the container used is a wide-mouthed glass bottle with a screw cap or a sterile petri dish. Sometimes the physician wishes to have the total sputum expectorated in 24 hours period. Then the size of the container depends upon the quantity of sputum.

A cotton applicator should be used to collect sputum from a very young child. The child may be made to cough by titillation of the back of the throat with a piece of gauze. If sputum is coughed up, the applicator can be used to mop up the amount needed for specimen. Take the applicator to which sputum has adhered and is dropped in a sterile test tube. The test tube should be closed with a sterile cotton plug.

Infants and children usually swallow the sputum when they have cough and expectoration. Therefore, physicians may sometimes order to collect, the specimen of sputum from the children or infants by aspirating the empty stomach early morning by a Ryle's tube.

Prerequisites

- Early morning sputum samples are preferable.
- For fungal culture—3 consecutively collected early morning specimens are recommended.
- For AFB—Collect 3 early morning specimens from a deep cough or 3 consecutively collected specimens, each collected in 8–24 hour intervals with at least one being an early morning specimen.

Preparation

Instruct patient to:

- Drink plenty of water the night before collection
- Remove dentures
- Not to eat, drink or smoke before coughing up sputum from the lungs.
- Go away from other people either outside or beside an open window before collecting the specimen. This helps protect other people from TB microorganisms when the patient coughs.
- Instruct the patient not to brush his/her teeth or use mouth wash.

Articles Required

A tray containing:

Articles	Purpose
Hand washing articles	For hand washing
Specimen container with lid	For collection of specimen
Identification label	For patient identity
Gloves, apron, facemask, eye protection (if required)	To prevent cross contamination
Nebulizer (if required)	To loosen the secretions
A glass with water	For rinsing the mouth
Kidney tray	For collecting the mouth rinsed water
Tissue paper	For wiping the mouth
Dust bins according to BMW policy	For proper disposal of waste
Lab request form and lab biohazard transport bag	For patient identity and safe transport

Contd...

Unit V ❖ Assessment of Patient

Procedure

Steps	Procedure	Rationale
1.	Arrange the articles. Label the specimen container after filling the identification details of the patient.	Facilitates a skilled procedure
2.	Explain the procedure to the patient and gain informed consent	Facilitates cooperation from patient
3.	Position the patient in an upright position in a chair, on the edge of the bed or well-supported by pillows in bed (high Fowler position)	Ensures maximum lung expansion
4.	Provide privacy to the patient	Prevents embarrassment
5.	Perform hand hygiene.	Prevents cross infection
6.	Have the patient rinse his mouth with water before the sample is collected. Provide kidney tray to spit the water if the patient is in bed. Place the tissues nearby.	Helps reduce the normal bacteria and cells that may interfere with the test results. Also it helps to avoid contaminating the sample with food residue and to remove dentures.
7.	Administer a prescribed sodium chloride 0.9% nebulizer (if required)	Helps to loosen secretions if they are thick and difficult to expectorate

Contd...

Steps	Procedure	Rationale
8.	Perform hand hygiene and put on an apron, non-sterile gloves and a facemask if you are likely to come into contact with bodily fluids. Wear eye protection if you have concerns about splash injury.	This reduces the risk of contamination of the specimen and the risk of cross infection.
9.	Ask the patient to take several deep breaths—breathing in through the nose and exhaling though the mouth	Helps to loosen secretions
10.	Ask the patient to force a deep cough	This ensures that the sample is obtained from the lower respiratory tract.
11.	Uncap the container but avoid touching the inside to ensure that it is sterile. Ask the patient to expectorate into the specimen collecting container carefully. Try not to touch the rim of the container. Repeat until there is 1–2 tablespoons of sputum in the tube.	Ensures adequate sample is obtained.

Steps	Procedure	Rationale
12.	Replace the cap tightly on the plastic tube. Secure the lid.	This prevents contamination
13.	Ensure the specimen is sputum rather than saliva, as samples may get contaminated with oropharyngeal secretions and saliva.	These are difficult to interpret and can be misleading.
14.	Replace the articles. Remove gloves, apron and facemask. Perform hand hygiene.	To reduce the risk of cross infection.

Contd...

Unit V ❖ Assessment of Patient

Steps	Procedure	Rationale
15.	Label the sample and complete microbiology forms. Place the specimen container in the clear plastic baggie that has the biohazard symbol imprint. Send the sample to the laboratory as soon as possible (within four hours).	Safe transportation on time facilitates accurate results
16.	Document the procedure in the patient's notes with date and time of collection along with the observations made including amount, consistency and color of the sputum collected.	Documentation fosters quality care.

Characteristic Points of Observation

What to Observe about Sputum?

- **Amount:** Normally no sputum is expectorated and in a disease in which sputum is produced, the amount may vary from a minute quantity to several hundred mL.
- **Color:** Varies considerably.
  - Bright red indicates presence of fresh blood.
  - Dark red shows that it was in the lungs for some time.
  - Rusty color is indication of pneumonia.
  - Greenish color is seen in bronchiectasis, lung abscess and carcinoma.
  - Brown is seen in gangrenous condition of the lungs.

- **Odor:** May have most unpleasant odor in lung abscess, gangrene, bronchiectasis and carcinoma of the lung.
- **Consistency:** Sputum varies from a thin-watery fluid to a thick purulent material (Figs 19A to D).

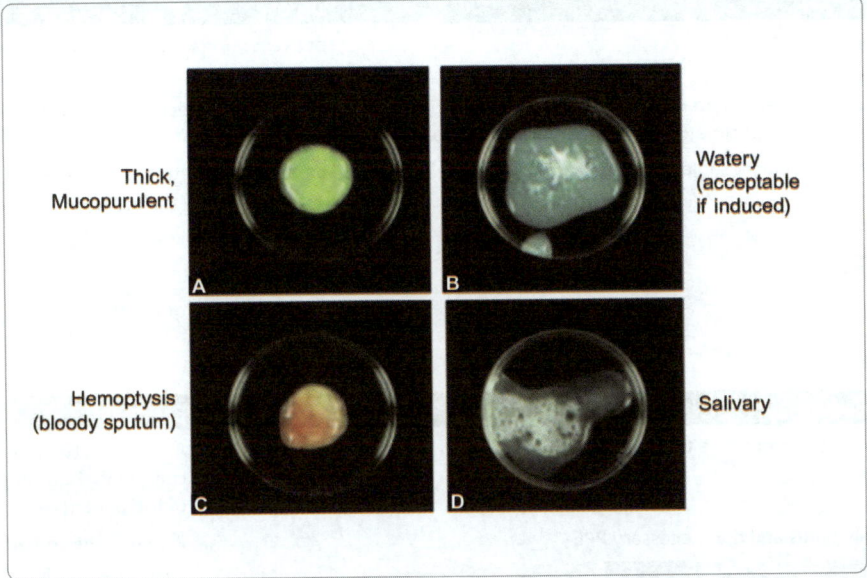

Figures 19A to D: Different characteristics of sputum

Throat Swab

A throat swab culture is a laboratory test that is done to identify microorganisms that may cause infection in the throat. It is most often used to diagnose streptococcal infection of throat.

A plain cotton wool swab should be used to collect as much exudates as possible from tonsils, posterior pharyngeal wall and other area that is inflamed or bears exudates.

Purposes

- To diagnose bacteria or fungal infection in throat
- Done to isolate and identify any pathogens
- To determine the effectiveness of drug against a particular organism

Preparation

Preparing the patient:
- Choose a well-lit room.
- Explain the procedure to the patient with its purposes.
- Stand directly in front of the patient.
- Place the patient in a comfortable sitting position facing a light source.
- Avoid touching the swab tip to any surface other than the tonsil area.

Unit V ❖ Assessment of Patient

Articles Required

A tray containing:

Articles	Purpose
Hand wash articles and PPE	For preventing transmission of micro-organisms.
Specimen bottle containing sterile throat swab or sterile cotton-tipped applicator in a specimen collection kit.	For collecting specimen from the throat
Tongue depressor or disposable wooden spatula	For easy visualization of throat by depressing the tongue
Kidney tray	For disposing soiled waste
Laboratory request form.	Legal document
Flashlight.	For visualization of the throat

Procedure

Steps	Procedure	Rationale
1.	Explain the procedure to the patient	Allays anxiety and wins confidence and cooperation of the patient.
2.	Wash hands and don necessary PPE	Prevents the spread of microorganisms.
3.	Remove the sterile swab from the protective packaging.	Organization promotes skilled performance. Helps to maintain the sterile nature of the content.

Contd...

Steps	Procedure	Rationale
	Hold the swab firmly by the handle. **Do not** place the swab on any surface once it is removed from the protective packaging.	
4.	Have the patient sit comfortably on a bed or chair and tilt her head back. Instruct patient to open mouth as wide as possible. Instruct patient to say 'ahh'. 	Proper positioning facilitates easy visualization and prevents discomfort.
5.	Use the flashlight to illuminate the back of the throat. Inspect the mouth and throat. The tonsil area may be reddened, swollen, or may have white patches. 	Ensures that the area to be swabbed is visible.

Contd...

Unit V ❖ Assessment of Patient

Steps	Procedure	Rationale
6.	Depress the tongue with a tongue blade or spoon or a wooden spatula so that the back of the throat can be seen.	Facilitates easy visualization of throat by depressing the tongue
7.	Touch the swab tip to the tonsil area. Rub the swab tip quickly and firmly with rotation on the back of the throat, over one tonsillar area of the soft palate and uvula, the other tonsillar area, finally the posterior pharynx and in any other area where there is redness, inflammation or pus and against any white patches. A gag reflex reaction is very common when a good sample is obtained.	Collecting swab in rotatory fashion facilitates easy coverage of specimen collection throughout the swab.

Contd...

Steps	Procedure	Rationale
8.	Remove swab from mouth (without touching any surface). Be careful not to touch the tongue, sides or top of the mouth with the swab. Do not lay the swab down. 	Touching other surfaces may contaminate the specimen.
9.	Replace the swab in the transport tube with care not to soil the rim. Seal tube tightly and label with patient name, date and initials of collector.	Ensures that the swab is not contaminated. Proper labelling acts as a legal document.
10.	Send the specimen to the laboratory with a completed on-line test order or with a test request form that indicates patient name, account number, medical record number, source, collection date and time, tests ordered, ordering physician's name, any antibiotics the patient is taking. If it cannot be transported immediately to laboratory it should be placed in a refrigerator at 4°C until delivery or preferably submitted in a tube of transport medium. The swab specimen should be processed as soon as possible after collection.	Safe transportation in an appropriate contains ensures accurate reading.
11.	Remove gloves and wash hands.	Prevents transfer of microorganisms.
12.	Document the procedure with date and time of collection, color and characteristics of specimen, patient response along with the signature of the nurse.	Documentation fosters quality care.

Note

If using the Virus/Chlamydia/ Mycoplasma Collection Kit swab, break off or bend swab shaft, leaving the tip in the tube.

Unit V ❖ Assessment of Patient

Disposable Nasopharyngeal Swabs

These are used for taking samples in COVID diagnosis too besides other respiratory infections. To take the nasopharyngeal swab, the patient must be seated comfortably with the back of his/her head against the headrest. The swab is inserted in the nose horizontally, along an imaginary line between the nostril and the ear (Fig. 20).

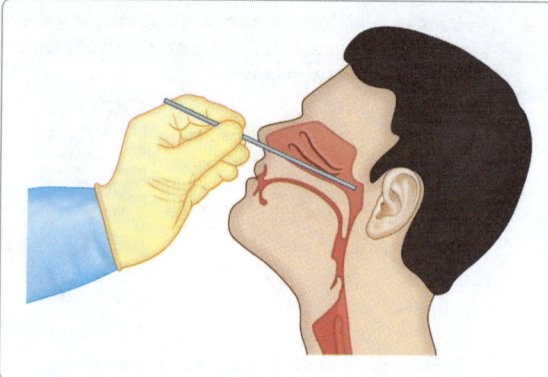

Figure 20: Taking nasopharyngeal specimen

Procedure

1. Tear open the sealed paper-plastic package and take out the swab.
2. Insert the swab into the nostril perpendicular to the nose and reach the nasopharynx so that the swab stays in the nasal cavity for 15-30 seconds. Gently rotate the swab in the nose for three times at the same time. Or extend the swab into the pharynx, wipe the swab on the bilateral pharynx tonsils and the posterior pharynx wall for 3–5 times
3. After the collection is completed, unscrew the whole collection cover and put the swab into the sample tube containing the preservation solution
4. Break off the redundant swab handle at the nozzle and leave the swab head in the sample tube.
5. Rotate the tube cover and label relevant sample information on the tube, and then take it back to the laboratory for testing.
6. Store specimens at 2-8°C for up to 72 hours after collection.

Collection of Vomitus

Vomiting is the forceful expulsion of contents of the stomach. If the person is vomiting at the time of the investigation, collect vomitus. Let the patient vomit directly into a specimen container. Take the specimen directly to the laboratory. If this is not possible refrigerate (do not freeze) the specimen (Figs 21A and B).

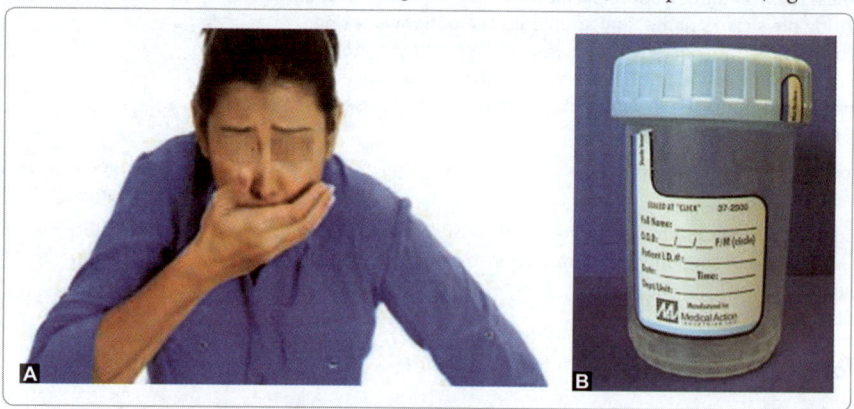

Figures 21A and B: Let patient vomit into specimen container

What to Observe

Color: Green, bright red, dark red, or brown.
Amount and consistency: Profuse, moderate, small, thin, watery, frothy, sour, clear, purulent, coffee colored or fecal.

Contents

- Presence of undigested food, mucus, blood and foreign body.
- Is the vomitus induced or brought out by the patient?
- Is the vomitus as a result of taste, smell or emotional upset?
- Vomitus is received in a bowl or kidney tray. It is covered and sent to the laboratory if needed to be examined.

BLOOD SMEAR

A blood smear is a blood test used to look for abnormalities in blood cells. A drop of blood is received on to a clean slide. This is smeared to render a thin film of blood by placing a second slide just beyond the drop of blood and slowly drawing it forward along the first. This is taken to:

- Determine the cell count.
- To find out the presence of certain parasites, e.g., malarial parasites, filaria parasites

Requisites

A tray containing:

Article	Purpose
Clean slides—2	For preparing the smear
Sterile needle in a container.	For capillary puncture
Cotton swabs in a bowl.	For application of disinfectant solution and to apply pressure after capillary puncture
Methylated spirit in a bottle.	For disinfecting the puncture site
Kidney tray or paper bag	For collecting the used swabs

Procedure

Steps	Procedure	Rationale
1.	Explain to the patient what is going to be done and its importance.	Proper explanation solicits cooperation and reduces anxiety.
2.	Make the patient seated or place him/her in a lying position.	Positioning promotes comfort of the patient

Contd...

Unit V ❖ Assessment of Patient

Steps	Procedure	Rationale
3.	Select two clean glass slides that are free of chipped edges and keep it ready along with the other articles in the bedside. Label the slide with the patient's name, date and identification number, following the protocol of the facility. 	Organization facilitates accurate skill performance.
4.	Wash hands and don gloves.	Prevents spread of microorganisms.
5.	Wipe one fingertip (Usually the third or fourth finger) of the patient with cotton swab dipped in methylated spirit. 	Prevents entry of pathogens.
6.	Press the fingertip with your fingers and give a gentle prick on the fingertip with a sterile needle, when the finger is dry from spirit. 	Squeezing the fingers causes pooling of blood at one site.

Contd...

Unit V ❖ Assessment of Patient

Steps	Procedure	Rationale
7.	Allow a drop of blood to fall on the slide and quickly make the smear evenly by the edge of the second slide. The drop should be in the center line approximately. 	A drop of blood that is too small may not be sufficient to prepare a proper smear. A drop of blood that is too large may cause the smear to be too thick.
8.	Apply a little bit of cotton on the finger tip of the patient and instruct him to give slight pressure over it for a short time with the thumb of the same hand.	Prevents further bleeding from the needle prick.
9.	Hold the slide with the drop of blood down with your non-dominant hand. Grasp the spreader slide with your dominant hand, letting the end of the slide rest at a 30° just in front of the drop of blood. 	The faster the spreader slide is moved, the longer and thinner the smear will be. The slower the spreader slide is moved, the shorter and thicker the smear will be. An angle greater than 30° makes the smear thicker. An angle less than 30° makes the smear thinner

Contd...

Steps	Procedure		Rationale
	Draw the spreader slide backward into the blood drop and allow the blood to spread from side to side, filling the space created by the 30°. Keeping the spreader slide at a 30°, push the spreader slide rapidly across the stationary slide in one, smooth even motion.	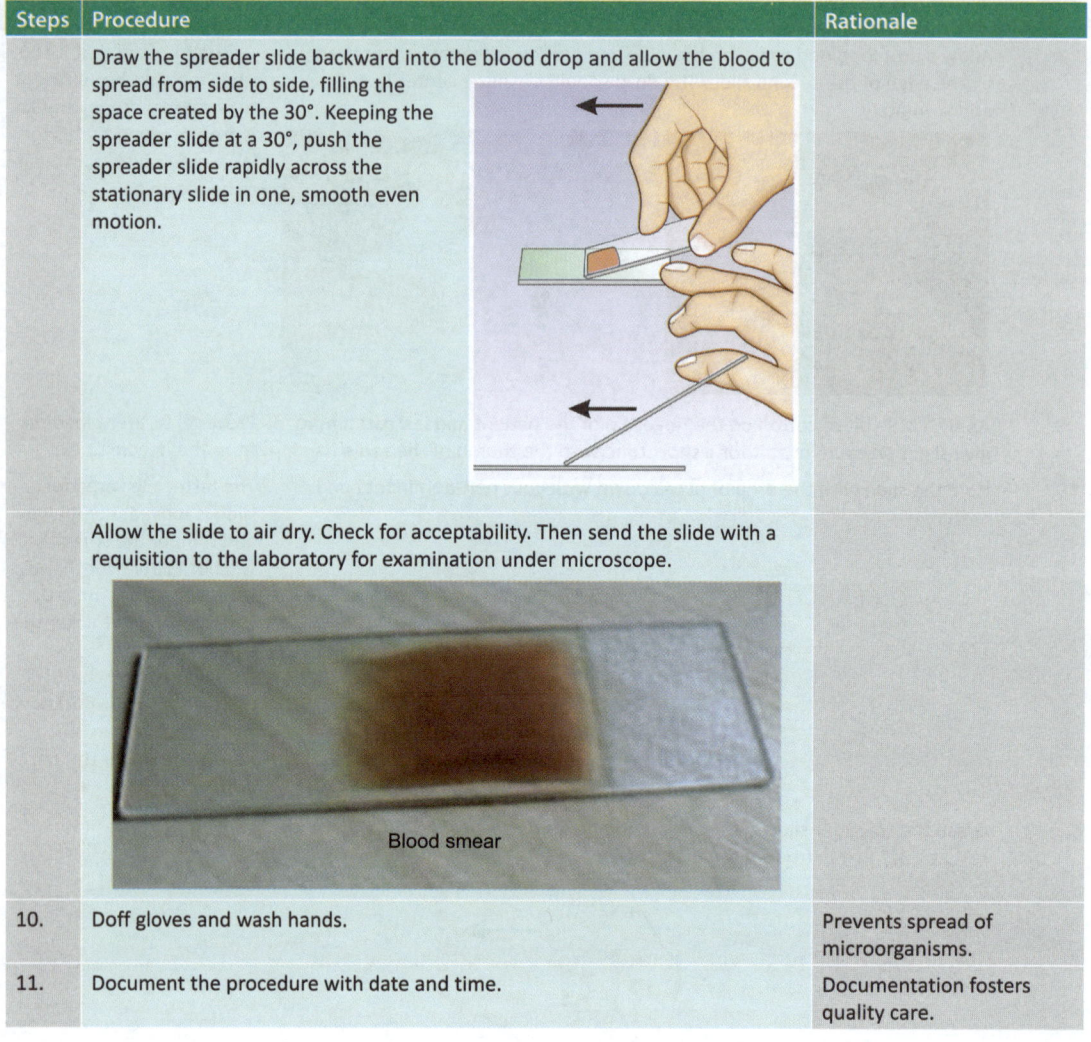	
	Allow the slide to air dry. Check for acceptability. Then send the slide with a requisition to the laboratory for examination under microscope.		
10.	Doff gloves and wash hands.		Prevents spread of microorganisms.
11.	Document the procedure with date and time.		Documentation fosters quality care.

Blood smear

Precautions

- Make the blood smear without delay. As soon as the drop of blood is placed on the glass slide, the smear should be made without delay. Delay in smearing the blood results in an abnormal distribution of the white blood cells, with many of the large white cells accumulating at the thin edge of the smear.
- Ensure that the spreader slide can only be used **once** to prevent carryover of patient's blood on to the next blood smear.
- Position your fingers on the spreader slide as down as possible and apply even, moderate pressure to the spreader slide. If the fingers are too high up on the spreader slide excess pressure will cause the slide to break, resulting in a cut.
- Any pressure exerted on the spreader slide should be directed across the slide in the direction that the film is made rather than down on the stationary slide.

URINE EXAMINATION

Article Required

A tray containing:

Articles	Purpose
Sterile cotton balls	For wiping
Antiseptic solution	For disinfecting
Sterile water or normal saline	For cleaning and as an diluent
Sterile specimen container, culture swab	To collect specimen
Clean gloves	To prevent self infection
Soap, water, wash cloth and towel	For cleaning

Procedure

Steps	Procedure	Rationale
	Collecting single urine specimen:	
1.	Prepare label for specimen with appropriate information and place it on specimen container, not the lid.	Label should be placed on the specimen container in the event the lid is misplaced or thrown away.
2.	Perform hand hygiene. Don gloves.	Protects from contamination by bodily fluids.
3.	Give the patient cleaning towel, wash cloth and soap. To collect a clean specimen of urine, the external genital area should be washed with soap and water and then rinsed with clean water.	For cleaning the perineum which prevents contamination of specimen.
4.	Open specimen container by maintaining the sterility of inside of specimen container. Place cap with sterile side inside up. Do not touch the inside of the container.	Prevents contamination of specimen container.

Contd...

Unit V ❖ Assessment of Patient

Steps	Procedure	Rationale
5.	**Male:** Hold penis with one hand using circular motion and antiseptic towel. Clean the meatus from center to outside 3 times. Or rinse the area with sterile water and dry with cotton balls or gauze pad. Ask the patient to pass the initial urine into the toilet and then pass the urine into the specimen container.	Initial urine flushes out the microorganisms that normally accumulates at urinary meatus and prevents transfer into the specimen.
	Female: Clean the urethral area using an antiseptic swab with dominant hand. Move from front (above urethral orifice) to back (towards anus). Clean 3 times using clean swab. Begin with the farthest end, then the closest and then down center or rinse the area with sterile water and dry with cotton balls or gauze pad. Ask the patient to pass the initial urine into the toilet and then pass the urine into the specimen container.	
6.	Cover the urine container with its lid. Do not touch the inside of the container. Wipe off the outside portion with a paper towel. Send the specimen container to the lab.	Prevents contamination of specimen.
7.	Doff gloves and wash hands.	Prevents spread of microorganisms.
8.	Document the procedure with date, time and signature.	Documentation fosters quality care.
9.	For collecting urine specimen for male baby	

For Collecting Urine Specimen from Male Babies

If a urine specimen is to be obtained from a male baby, attach a plastic bag with sticky edges to the penis and hold in position by strips of adhesive fastened over each buttock (Figs 22A and B).

Unit V ❖ Assessment of Patient

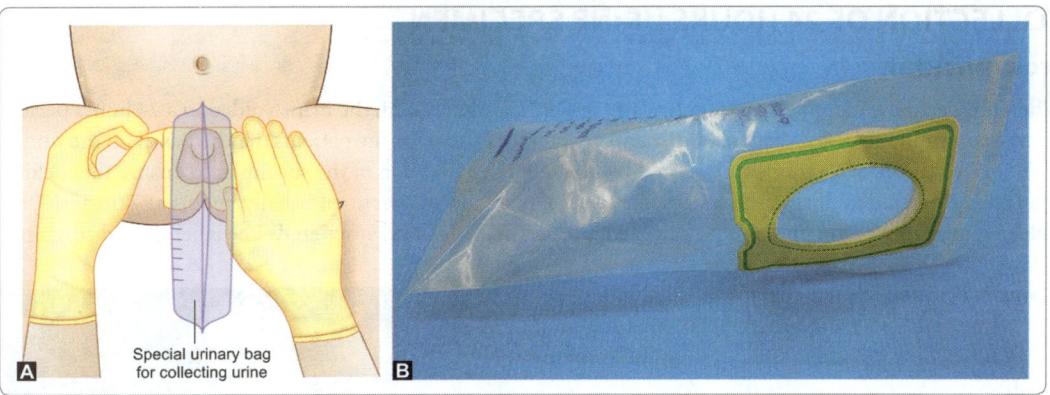

Figures 22A and B: Collecting urine sample in male baby

For Collecting Urine Specimen from Female Babies

Glass vessels that fit over the vulva can be held in place with a specially made T binder or sterile cotton wool and napkin and squeeze it to get urine or a simple way is to place a small tray or shallow pan under the buttocks, while the child is passing urine and collect it (Figs 23A and B).

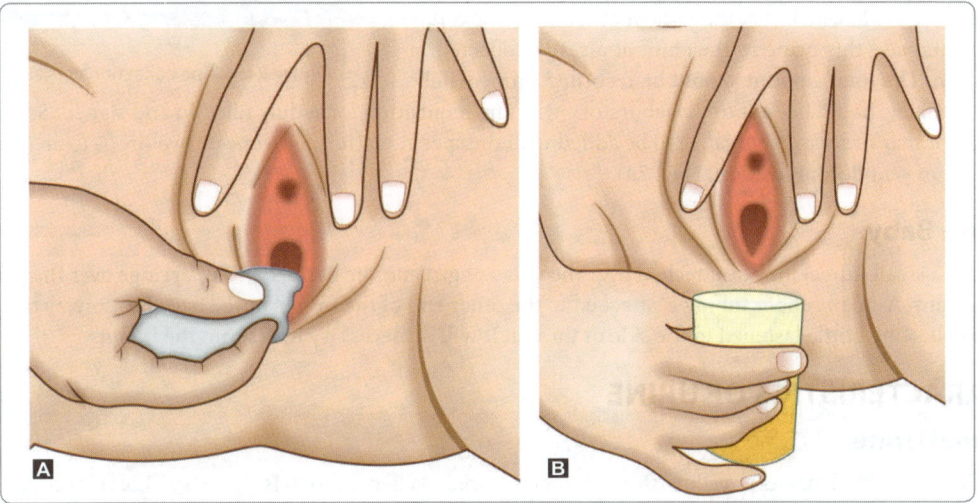

Figures 23A and B: Clean vulva and collect urine by fixing glass vessel over vulva

To collect a sterile specimen of urine: A sterile specimen of urine is obtained by catheterization and should be collected in a sterile specimen bottle or test tube. After introducing the sterile catheter into the bladder, allow 20–30 mL of urine to flow into the collecting basin, then the end of the catheter is held directly above the sterile specimen bottle till it is filled 3/4. Cover with sterile stopper. Label should contain in addition 'Catheterized Specimen'.

Unit V ❖ Assessment of Patient

COLLECTION OF 24 HOURS URINE SPECIMEN

From an Adult

When it is desirable to make a quantitative and qualitative analysis, all the urine voided in a 24 hours period is saved for examination. The diagnosis, diet and general treatment for the patients may be based on the findings of the examination. So extreme care should be taken in the collection of the specimen to ensure the inclusion of all the urine voided during the specified period. Collection of specimen usually begins at 7.00 am. This is collected in a large bottle preferably graduated, properly labelled and stoppered. The label should contain the following:

24 hours urine specimen chart:
1. Name and Age of the patient...
2. Address of the patient...
3. IP No.
4. Ward No...............Bed No...
5. Date and Time of Starting Collection..............................
6. Date and Time of Termination ....
7. Signature of the Doctor/Nurse ....
8. Date and Time ....

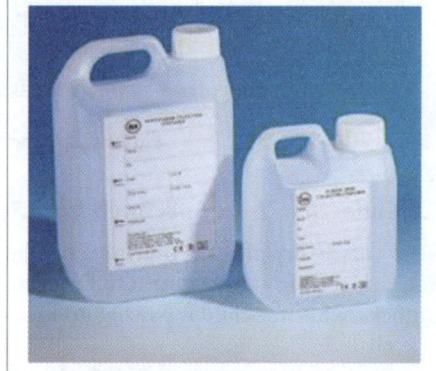

Figure 24: Urine collection container

Ask the patient to void at 7 am and discard the specimen. All the subsequent voiding should be measured and kept in the bottle, which is labelled. Ask the patient at 7 am the next day to void and add this urine to the amount already collected in the bottle. The total amount should be recorded immediately. The specimen should be sent to the laboratory with the requisition form duly filled in and signed. Sometime the doctor may order a preservative to be added with the specimen (formalin one or two drops to an ounce of urine to prevent decomposition) (Fig. 24).

From a Baby

For this, a small funnel may be attached over the vulva of girl and the barrel of a 5 cc syringe over the penis of a male baby. A small rubber tubing is attached to the other end of the funnel or the barrel to convey the urine to the collecting bottle fastened to the side of the cot. It will be necessary to restrain the infant.

CHARACTERISTICS OF URINE

Normal Urine

- **Color:** Normal urine is yellowish or amber colored. When output is increased color becomes pale yellowish. If decreased output color becomes deep yellow.
- **Volume:** Average urine excretion is 1000–2000 mL in 24 hours. Output depends on water intake. In hot weather it is decreased due to increased perspiration and in cold weather it is increased.
- **Appearance:** Normal urine is clear without any deposit.
- **Odor:** Normal urine has an aromatic odor. When kept for some time, strong aromatic smell comes due to the decomposition of urea in it.
- **Reaction:** Normally urine is slightly acidic (pH below 7)
- **Specific gravity:** It varies from 1.010 to 1.025 with normal fluid intake. But Sp: gravity varies due to the concentration of urine.

- **Constituents of urine:** Normal constituents of urine are:
  - Water 96%
  - Urea 2% (end product of protein metabolism)
  - The remaining 2% consists of uric acid, urate, creatinine, chlorides, phosphates, sulfates and oxalates.
    (Due to break down of tissues, uric acids and urates are formed; from the intake of sodium chloride in diet, chlorides are formed, other constituents like oxalates, phosphates and sulfates are derived from vegetable food)

Abnormal Urine

- **Volume:**
  - **Polyuria:** Abnormal increase in the volume of urine found in diabetes mellitus and diabetes insipidus
  - **Oliguria:** Decreased quantity of urine found in conditions like heart and kidney diseases and in shock
  - **Anuria:** Marked decrease in volume or even absence of urine
  - **Suppression:** Failure of the kidneys to secrete urine
- **Color:**
  Abnormal colors of urine can be seen due to the intake of certain medicines.
  - B complex capsules can cause yellow color in urine.
  - Green or brownish yellow color is due to bile salts and bile pigments.
  - Reddish brown is due to urobilinogen.
  - Bright red is due to large amount of fresh blood.
  - Pink color is due to small amount of fresh blood.
  - Smokey brown color is due to blood pigments.
  - Milky white color is due to chyluria which occurs because of filariasis.
  - Hematuria means presence of blood in urine.
- **Odor:**
  - In the presence of ketone bodies (Acetone and Diacetic acid) urine will have fruity or sweetish odor.
- **Appearance:**
  - In the presence of amorphous phosphates, urine may appear cloudy, which will disappear by adding few drops of acetic acid.
  - Presence of amorphous urates will cause cloudy appearance which will disappear on heating.
  - Presence of pus will cause turbid urine, which will be clear by filtering
- **Deposits:**
  - Deposits in urine is due to several substances

Mucus	–	Produce flocculent cloud
Pus	–	Produces heavy cloud and settles at the bottom
Stones	–	Seen as large sand particles of fine sand
Uric acid	–	Seen as grains of pepper
Blood clots	–	Seen as it is

- **Reaction:**
  - Urine may be alkaline in cystitis;
  - Stagnant urine will become alkaline due to formation of ammonia.

  So fresh urine should be tested for reaction.

Unit V ❖ Assessment of Patient

- **Specific gravity:**
  - Dilution or concentration of urine will change the specific gravity of urine, e.g., due to the presence of sugar in urine due to diabetes, specific gravity will be high.
  - Due to the inability of kidneys to concentrate urine by kidney diseases, the specific gravity will be low.
  - In diseased conditions specific gravity may range from 1.001 to 1.060 (1001–1060)
- **Abnormal constituents of urine:**
  - **Albuminuria:** Presence of albumin in urine due to kidney damage.
  - **Glucose:** Presence of sugar in urine due to diabetes. Any tumors in the pelvic cavity or even pregnancy which will cause pressure on ureters and the renal threshold is lowered, sugar is found in urine.
  - **Acetone** is seen in urine due to incomplete metabolism of fat usually seen in diabetic patients.
  - **Bile:** May be seen in urine of patients with jaundice or hemolytic diseases.

TYPES OF URINE EXAMINATION

- **Microscopic examination:** Such as deposits, pus cells, RBC, casts, epithelial cells, bacteria.
- **Physical examination:** As color, appearance, volume, reaction, specific gravity and odor.
- **Chemical examination:** Routine tests as tests for albumin and sugar; special tests as test for acetone bile pigments and bile salts.

Physical Examination

- **Color:** Collect urine in a clean glass jar and place it in a flat surface against light and note the color. Normally it is pale yellow or amber color.
- **Appearance:** Normal urine is clear. The whole urine collected in the glass jar is inspected for the presence of any sediments or turbidity.
- **Odor:** Normal urine has aromatic odor. Odor of the urine can be tested while collecting it for tests.
- **Volume:** It is measured by a pint measure by collecting the total urine for each voiding.
- **Specific gravity:** Normal specific gravity of urine is 1.010–1.030.

Microscopic Examination

Microscopic examination of urine is carried out for presence of pus cells.

Chemical Examination

Preparation of Articles for Chemical Tests

A tray containing:

Articles	Purpose
Several test tubes on a stand	To test urine for different tests
Test tube holder—1	For holding the test tubes
Spirit lamp—1	For heating the solutions wherever required
Matchbox—1 or a lighter	For igniting the spirit lamp
Kidney tray	To discard the waste
Duster or rag piece	To wipe outside of the test tube before heating
Acetic acid	To test albumin in urine

Contd...

Articles	Purpose
Nitric acid	To test albumin or bile in urine
Red and blue litmus paper	To test the urine for reaction
Urinometer	To test the specific gravity of urine
Benedict's solution or Fehling's solution I and II in separate bottles	To test the urine for sugar
Ammonium sulfate crystals, sodium nitroprusside crystals, liquor ammonia	To test the urine for acetone
White porcelain dish	To test bile pigments with nitric acid
Weak solution of tincture of iodine	To test bile pigments in urine
Sulfur powder	To test bile salt in urine
Glass jar	To rake urine to measure the specific gravity and to measure the amount of urine
Pippets—2 or dropper—2	To measure drops of urine and other reagents
Sulphuric acid	To clean the test tubes after testing urine for sugar in one test tube several times
A small bottle brush	To clean the test tubes

Test for Reaction

Reaction: Normal urine is usually acidic. When urine is exposed for some time it may become alkaline due to the production of ammonia. Certain type of bacteria (pathogenic) turn it into alkaline (Fig. 25).

Procedure:
1. Dip the end of blue litmus paper into the urine.
2. If the urine is acidic, blue litmus paper turns to red and remains the same.
3. If the urine is alkaline, the red litmus paper changes into blue.
4. No change in both litmus papers indicate neutral reaction.

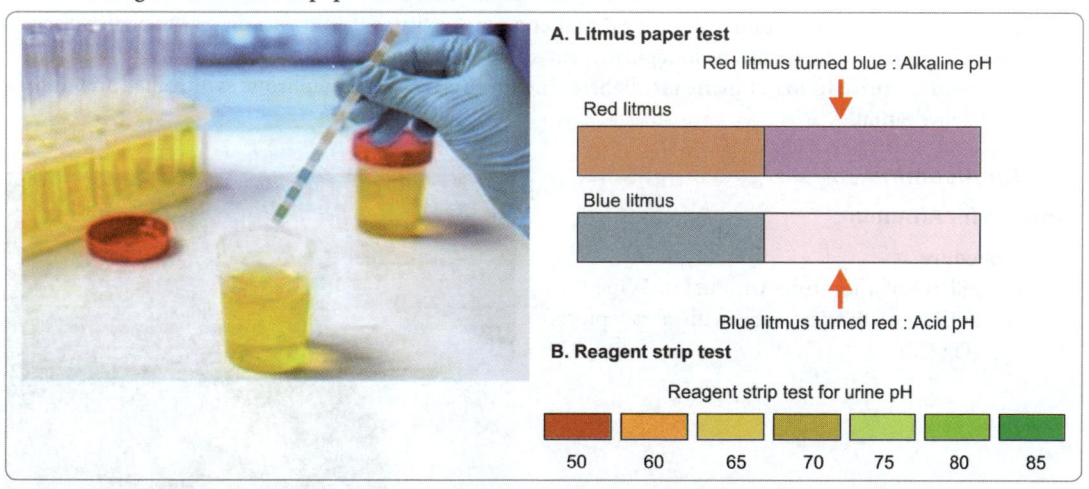

Figure 25: Litmus paper test

Unit V ❖ Assessment of Patient

Specific Gravity

- Specific gravity of urine is the relation of the weight of a known quantity of urine to the weight of an equal quantity of water.
- Specific gravity is measured by an apparatus called urinometer.
- Normal Specific gravity is 1.005–1.060 with normal intake of fluid. (This reading is from Taber's Cyclopedic Medical Dictionary). Slight difference in reading is seen in different books.

Procedure

1. Take sufficient amount of urine in a urine glass.
2. Lower urinometer gently into the urine and let it float freely.
3. Allow the urinometer to float in the urine taking care not to touch the sides.
4. Note the reading in the urinometer at the level of the urine by keeping the flask in a flat surface. Take the reading of SG on the scale (lowest point of meniscus) at the surface of the urine.
5. Specific gravity of urine varies with the substances dissolved in the urine. More concentrated urine have high specific gravity and vice versa (Figs 26A and B).

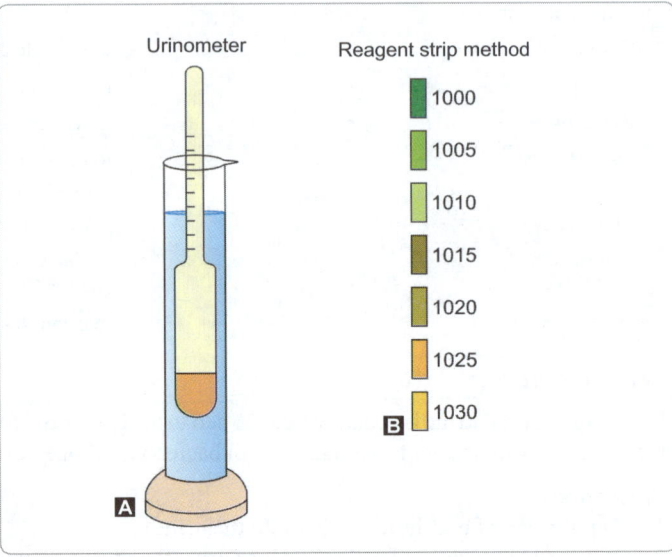

Figures 26A and B: Specific gravity test by urinometer and reagent strip

Low specific gravity (SG) (1.001–1.003) may indicate the presence of diabetes insipidus, chronic renal failure (low and fixed SG at 1.010 due to loss of concentrating ability of tubules) and compulsive water drinking. Low SG may also occur in patients with glomerulonephritis, pyelonephritis, and other renal abnormalities.

Causes of increase in SG of urine are diabetes mellitus (glycosuria), nephrotic syndrome (proteinuria), fever and dehydration.

Test for Albumin

Hot Test for Albumin

- **Procedure:**
    1. Fill 3/4 of a test tube with urine. Wipe the outside of the test tube with a rag piece (Fig. 27).

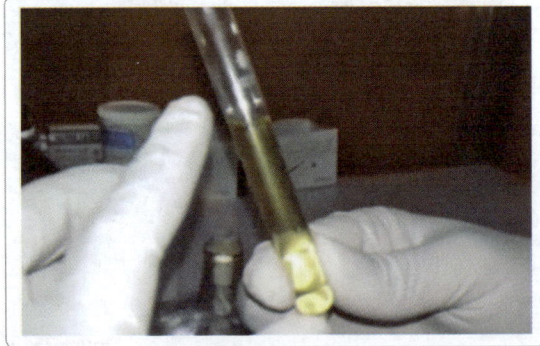

Figure 27: Fill 3/4 of test tube with sample and wipe outside

2. Heat the upper third of the urine and allow it to boil over the spirit lamp flame (Fig. 28).

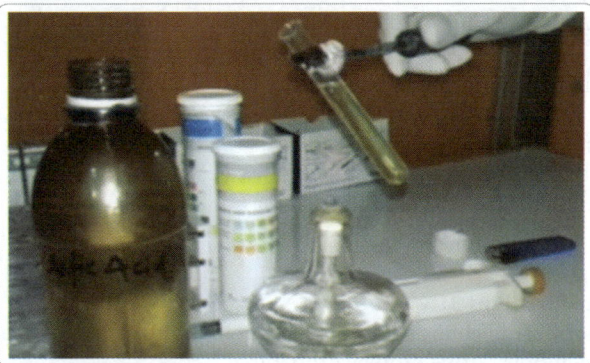

Figure 28: Heat upper portion to boil

3. A cloud may appear either due to phosphate or albumin (Fig. 29).

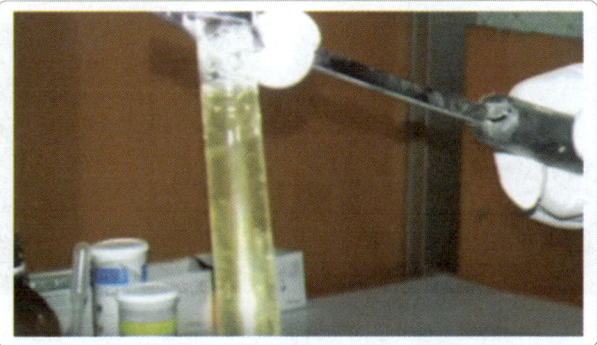

Figure 29: Cloud appears if test is positive

4. Add one or two drops of acetic acid into the test tube of urine. If the urine still remains cloudy it indicates presence of albumin and if it becomes clear it indicates that the cloudy appearance was due to phosphates. As the upper part only is boiled, the difference between the boiled urine and nonboiled urine is noted easily.
5. The thickness of cloud present indicates the quantity of albumin present in urine (Figs 30A and B).
6. Discard the urine and clean the test tube after use.

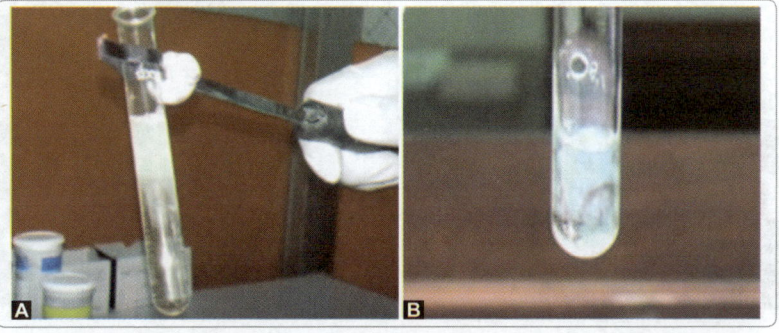

Figures 30A and B: Thickness of cloud indicates quantity of albumin

Unit V ❖ Assessment of Patient

Cold Test

Nitric acid test for albumin

- **Procedure:**
    1. Drop a small quantity of nitric acid into a clean test tube.
    2. Allow equal quantity of urine to trickle steadily down the side into the test tube.
    3. If albumin is present, a white precipitate will be seen where the two fluids meet.
    4. Precipitation of albumin using concentrated nitric acid.
    5. Discard the urine and clean the used articles.

Test for Sugar

- **Fehling's test: Procedure (Figs 31A and B):**
    - Take equal quantities of Fehling's solution I and II (3 mL) in a test tube and boil it.
    - Add an equal quantity of urine drop by drop into it.
    - Boil the mixture and allow it to cool.
    - If an orange red deposit appears, it proves the presence of sugar.
    - Discard the urine and clean the articles.

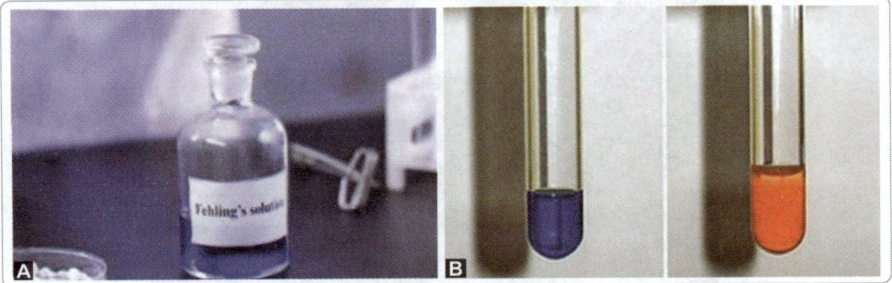

Figures 31A and B: Fehling test—red color proves presence of sugar in urine

- **Benedict's test: Procedure:**
    (Ref: Virginia Henderson Principles and Practice of Nursing Chapter 7).
    - Take 5 mL of Benedict's solution in a test tube (Figs 32A and B).
    - Add 8 drops of urine with pipette into the test tube and shake well.

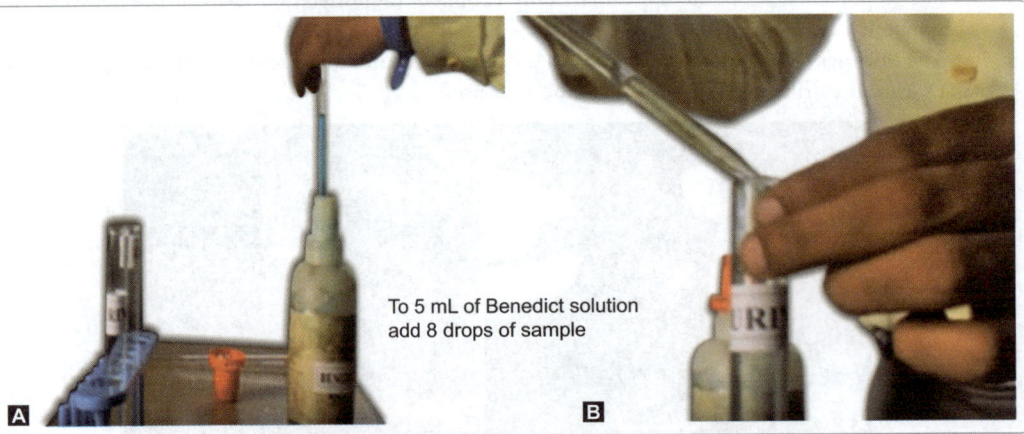

To 5 mL of Benedict solution add 8 drops of sample

Figures 32A and B: Benedict's test

- Check the color of the solution in the test tube (Figs 33A and B).
- Place the test tube over the spirit lamp flame for 2 minutes. Allow it to boil. Remove the test tube and allow it to cool (In certain books, it is written that solution alone should be boiled and observed, for any abnormalities, before pouring 8 drops of urine. It is a wise idea to get an accurate result.)

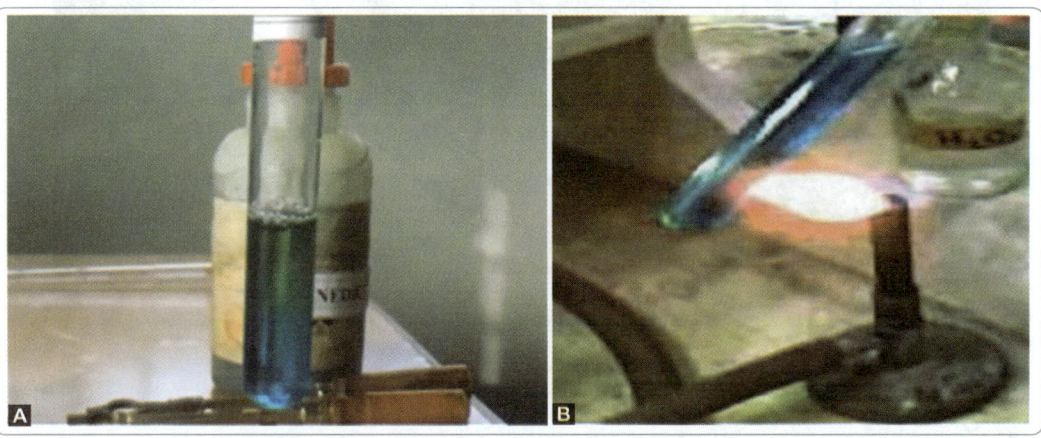

Figures 33A and B: Check the color and boil it

- **Result:** If there is no deposit, no sugar is present. The result may be recorded according to the color as blue, green, yellow, orange and brick red (Figs 34A and B).
  - Blue color indicates absence of sugar.
  - Green liquid without deposit denotes approximately 1% sugar.
  - Slight yellow deposit with greenish liquid indicates 2% sugar.
  - An orange deposit and liquid indicate 3% sugar.
  - Brick red color indicates approximately 5% sugar or above.

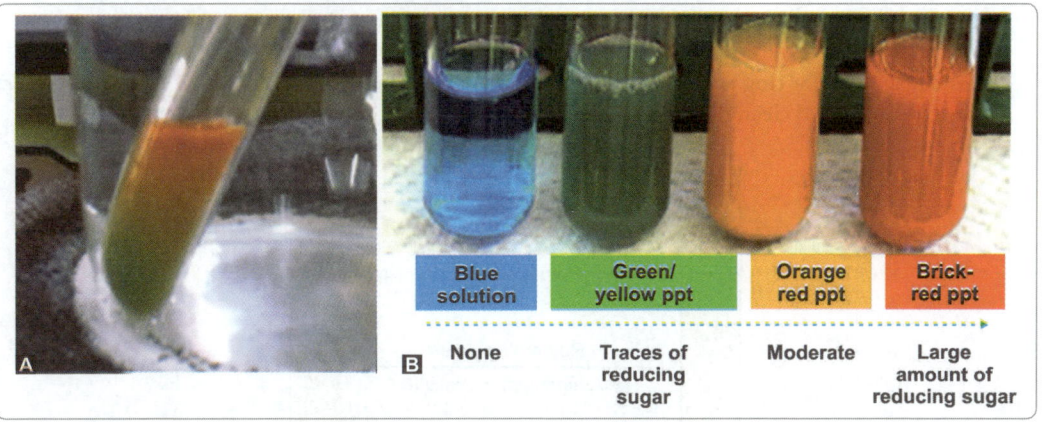

Figures 34A and B: Result of Benedict's test

- The amount of sugar present is determined by using a saccharometer or a reagent strip.
  - A color indicator can be used to estimate the amount of sugar in the liquid (Figs 35A and B).

Unit V ❖ Assessment of Patient

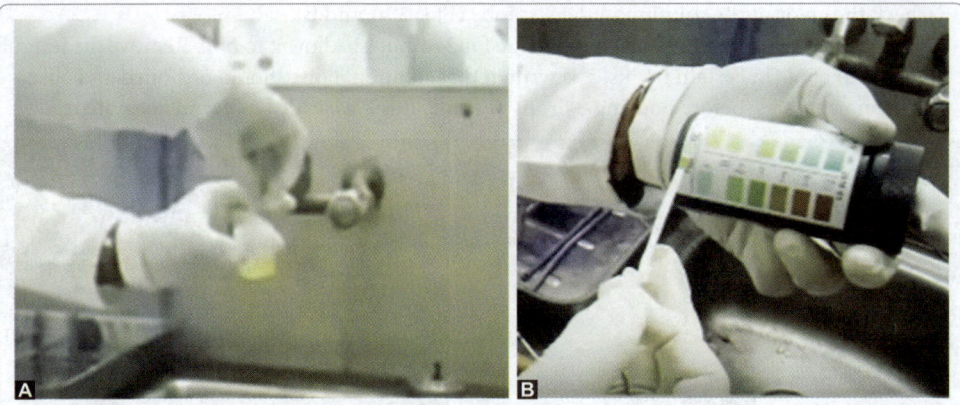

Figures 35A and B: Use of reagent strip to check sugar in urine

- Discard the urine and clean the used articles.

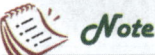 *Note*

One or two drops of sulfuric acid will make the test tube completely clean by dissolving the carbon in the tube when used several times to test the urine of a diabetic patient.

Test for Acetone (Rothera's Test)

Procedure:

1. Take about two inches of ammonium sulfate crystals in a test tube.
2. Add an equal volume of urine and one crystal of sodium nitroprusside.
3. Shake well till the crystals are dissolved in urine.
4. Add half inch of concentrated liquor ammonia into the test tube and allow to stand.
5. Read the result.
6. A permanganate color ring is formed at the junction of urine and liquor ammonia if acetone is present.
7. Discard the urine and clean the used articles (Fig. 36).

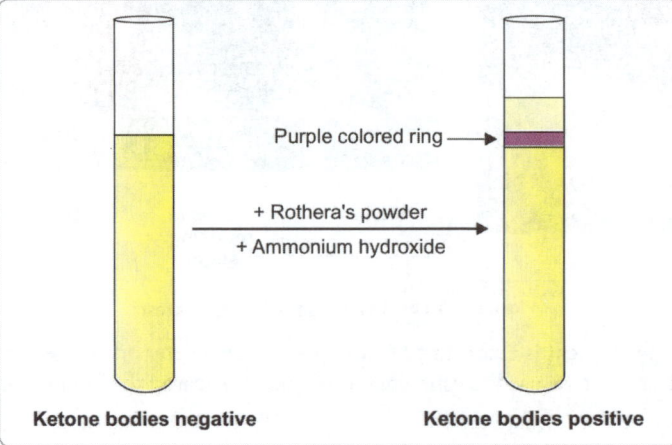

Figures 36: Rothera's test for acetone

Test for Bile

There are two types of test.

(i) Tincture Iodine Test (Smith's Test) (Figs 37A and B) to Test for Bile Pigment

- Fill 3/4 of a test tube with urine
- Add Tr. iodine, drop by drop to the urine along the side of the test tube so as to form a layer on the surface of the urine. (If the tincture iodine is concentrated, it will sink down in the urine so that no layer is seen on the surface).
- A green color at the junction of the two liquids indicates the presence of bile pigments.
- Discard urine and clean the used articles.

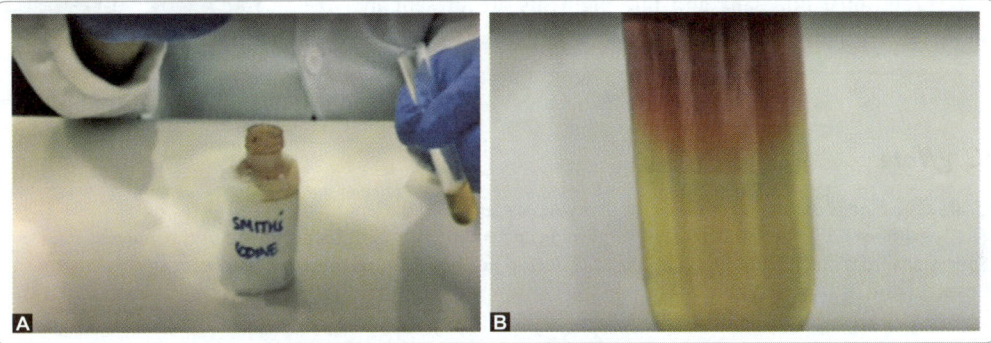

Figures 37A and B: Smith's test for bile pigment

(ii) Nitric Acid Test: (Gmelin's Test) (Fig. 38)

- Put a few drops of urine by means of a pipette in a white porcelain dish.
- Pour a few drops of nitric acid by the side of the container.
- When they meet there will be a play of colors of which, one will be green if bile is present.
- Discard the urine and clean the used articles.

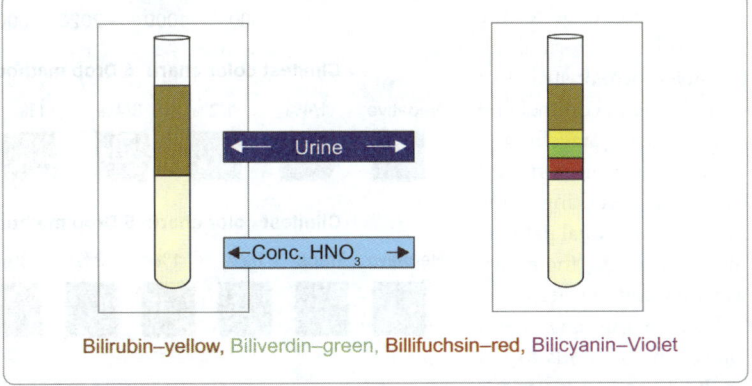

Bilirubin–yellow, Biliverdin–green, Billifuchsin–red, Bilicyanin–Violet

Figure 38: Gmelin's test for bile pigment

Unit V ❖ Assessment of Patient

Test for Bile Salts (Hay's Sulfur Test) (Figs 39A and B)

- Take a test tube half full of urine.
- Sprinkle sulfur powder on the surface of urine.
- If the powder sinks down in the test tube it indicates the presence of bile salts because bile salts reduce the surface tension of the urine and allows the sulfur powder to sink down.
- In the control, sulfur powder remains immiscible with the underlying liquid. In the positive test, the sulfur powder sinks to the bottom.
- After test, discard the urine and clean the test tube.
- **Interpretations:** Bile salts and bile pigments are present in urine in obstructive jaundice.

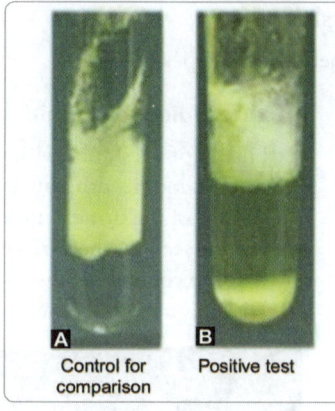

A　Control for comparison　　B　Positive test

Figures 39A and B: Test for bile salts

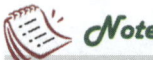 **Note**

- Urine specimen is obtained routinely for every newly admitted patient.
- The specimen should be fresh, always. A morning specimen is the best for complete urine analysis.
- Specimens from diabetic patients should be collected just before meal time to help doctor to regulate the insulin dose.

Few Modern Methods of Urine Tests

Although Benedict's test and Fehling's test are commonly done in the clinical laboratory to detect the presence of sugar in urine, several other tests are also conducted nowadays. The provision of exchange privileges of nurses and doctors in other countries have helped us to introduce some of the convenient and easiest method of testing urine for sugar and other abnormalities with reagents in the tablet form or stripes or as test-tape. They are simple to conduct and easy to carry with even during travelling, if available. Some of the very common tests are mentioned below. While working in the MC Hospitals we can see individual patients are using these methods to test their own urine when they are admitted in wards.

- **Clinitest method—using a reagent tablet:** It is one of the methods to test sugar in urine. It comes in a kit and is convenient to carry and store. A kit contains a test tube, a medicine dropper, caustic tablets, a small punch forceps and a color chart. When a tablet is put in the mixture of urine and water, it generates heat by itself and the color of the solution is graded against the color chart (Fig. 40).

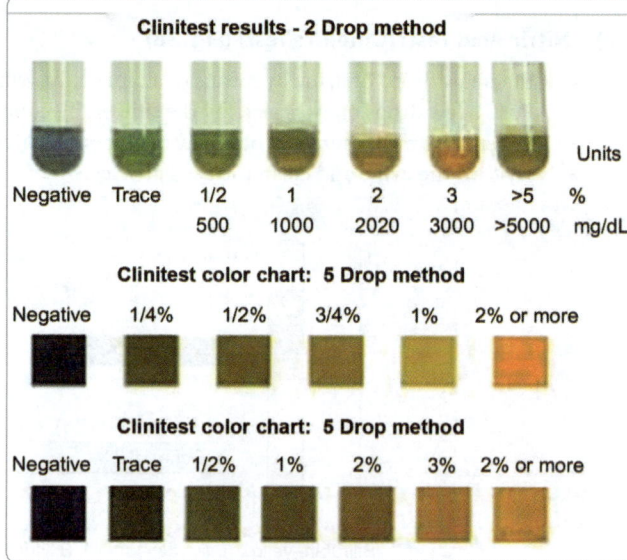

Figure 40: Clinitest

- **Two drops method: This method allows for an estimated concentration of sugar up to 5%.**
  This method allows for an estimated concentration of sugar up to 5%.
  - Hold dropper vertically and place 2 drops or 5 drops of urine in the test tube.
  - Rinse the dropper. Add 10 drops (0.5 mL) of water in the test tube.
  - Add one clinitest reagent tablet with the forceps. Do not shake test tube. It will produce heat and the mixture will boil.
  - Wait for 15 seconds after boiling stops (Heat produce by adding the tablet to urine water mixture to boil)
  - Compare color of urine with appropriate color chart.
  - Use only the 2 drop method color scale which has colors ranging in value from 0.5%. More details are obtained from.

  (*Ref: Medical Surgical, Nursing, Brunner and Suddarth, 3rd Edition; Med. Surg. Nursing Shafer's Seventh Edition*).

- **Dreypak:** It is another method used to detect sugar in the urine. A urine impregnated stripe of filter paper is dipped into boiling Benedict's Solution. Color changes are the same as for the Benedict's test (Fig. 41).

- **The Diastix and Testape:** There are reagent strip or tapes
  - The strip is merely moistened with urine and subsequently indicates the presence of glucose. The color on the reagent strip is compared to that of the color chart on the reagent strip container or separate chart.
  - Ketone bodies (acetone) are also tested for, by the use of reagent tablets (Acetest) or reagent stripes (Ketostix). There is also now available a combined ketone glucose reagent stripe (KetoDiastrix) (Figs 42A and B).

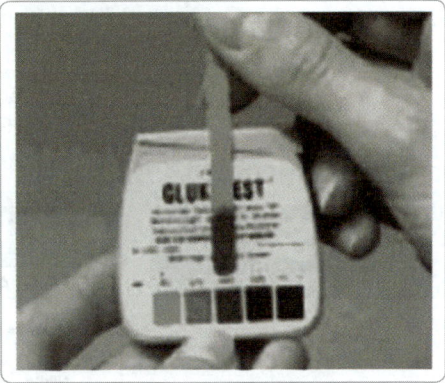

Figure 41: Dreypak method

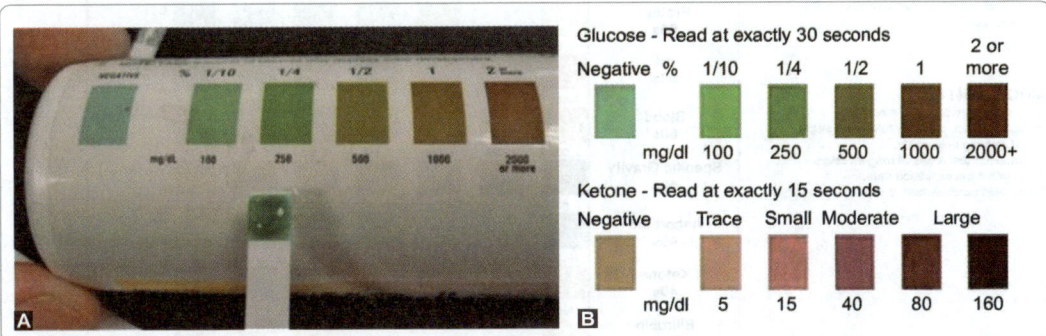

Figures 42A and B: Reagent strips with color codes for glucose and ketone

- **Combur test:** In this method 50 strips are packed in one container. The advantage of this method is that urine can be tested for bile, albumin and sugar with one stripe at a time. The strips are impregnated with reagent for testing these three abnormalities and color chart is marked on the outside of the container itself.

Unit V ❖ Assessment of Patient

Urine is taken in a small bottle and one strip is dipped into the urine for 30 seconds. After the prescribed time, the strip is taken out and matched with the color chart on the container. Color changes are noticed according to the presence of abnormalities. Instructions for the use of these strips are given on the Combur container itself along with the color chart (Fig. 43).

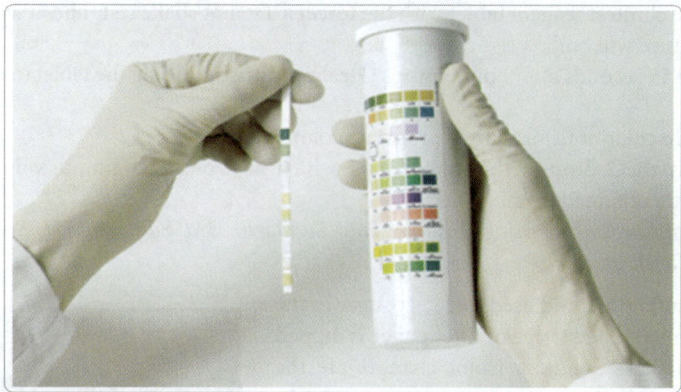

Figure 43: Combur test

- **Other similar reagent strips (Fig. 44):**

Courtesy: alibaba.com

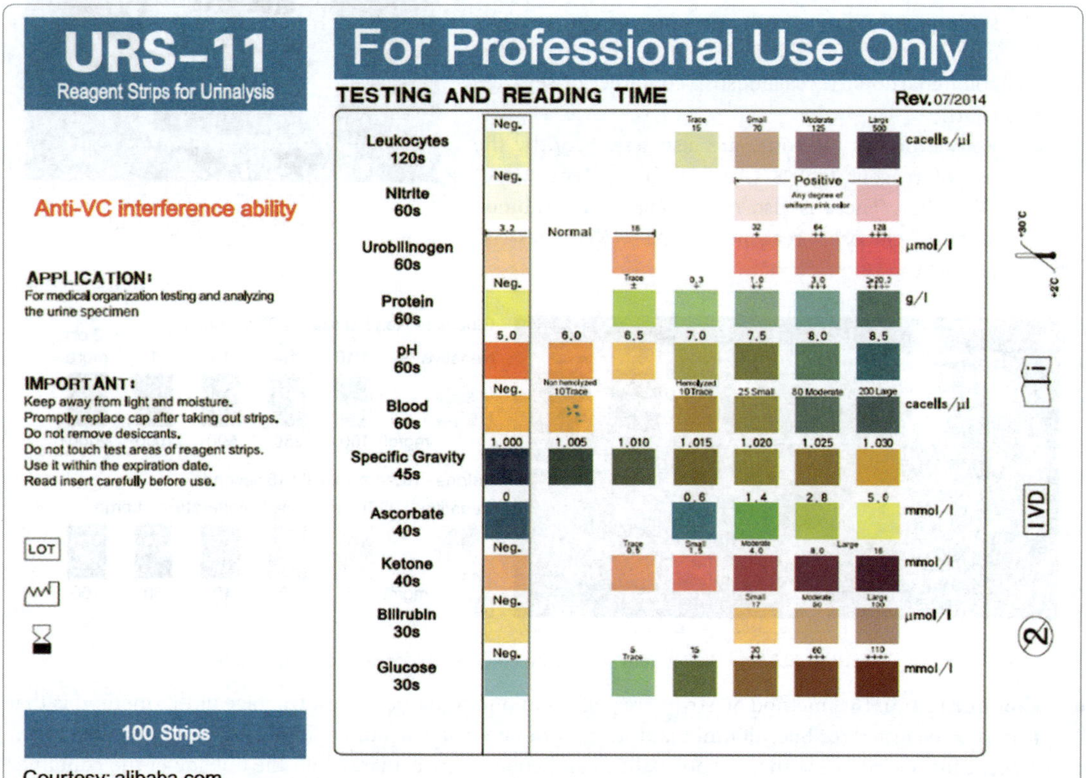

Figure 44: Other reagent strips

This cannot be denied that these kinds of advanced and costly reagents are not available in Indian general hospital practices especially in our Government. Hospitals. But people always search for convenience with minimum man power. We can observe that the individuals in our social circle like diabetic patients are using these types of advanced reagents to check sugar in urine. Moreover, the society expects professional nurses to remain updated of all new techniques. Therefore, it is a requirement for the future nurses to be informed of such advancements and to remain well-equipped with modern diagnostic knowledge.

PULSE OXIMETRY

Oxygen saturation sometimes referred to as 'the fifth vital sign,' is checked by pulse oximetry. Red blood cells contain hemoglobin. One molecule of hemoglobin can carry up to four molecules of oxygen after which it is described as "saturated" with oxygen. If all the binding sites on the hemoglobin molecule are carrying oxygen, the hemoglobin is said to have a saturation of 100%.

- Pulse oximetry is a painless, non-invasive method concerned with the monitoring of a patient's blood oxygen saturation level (SpO_2) intermittently and continuously.
- Pulse oximeter is a device that can detect a pulsatile signal in an extremity such as the finger or toe and can calculate the amount of oxygenated hemoglobin and the pulse rate producing a photoplethysmograph.
- Pulse oximeters often show the pulsatile change in absorbance in a graphical form. This is called the 'plethysmographic trace'.

Importance of Pulse Oximetry

Pulse oximetry helps us to ensure that the patient has an adequate supply of oxygen to the whole body. When patients do not have enough oxygen, 'hypoxia' can result.

Uses

Pulse Oximetry is used in a variety of situations:

- Throughout anesthesia during surgery
- During the recovery phase
- In intensive care during ventilation
- In wards and casualty departments
- When patients are sedated for procedures such as endoscopy
- In patients with long-standing respiratory disease

Principle

- The pulse oximeter consists of a probe attached to the patient's finger, toe, ear lobe, nose or forehead, which is linked to a computerized unit.
- Typically the probe has a pair of small light-emitting diodes (LEDs) that shines through a translucent part of the patient's body, usually a fingertip or an earlobe, onto a photodiode.
- One LED is red, with wavelength of 660 nm and the other is infrared, 905, 910, or 940 nm.
- These light wavelengths are absorbed differently by the oxygenated and the deoxygenated hemoglobin (HgB) molecules (Fig. 45).

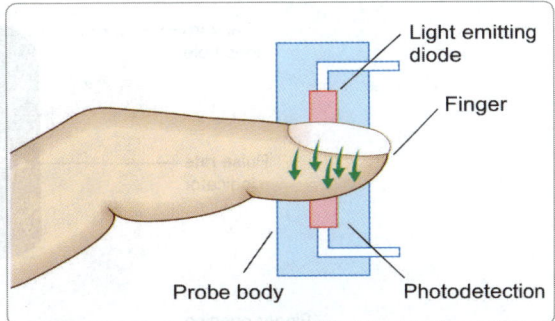

Figure 45: Principle of pulse oximetry

Unit V ❖ Assessment of Patient

- The receiving sensor measures the amount of light absorbed by the oxygenated and deoxygenated Hgb in the arterial (pulsatile) blood.
- Therefore, from the ratio of the absorption of the red and infrared light the oxy/deoxyhemoglobin ratio can be calculated, i.e. the blood oxygen saturation level (expressed as a %).
- The more HgB that is saturated with oxygen, the higher the SpO_2, which should normally measure above 95%.
- Pulse oximeters have an indicator of signal strength (such as a bar graph, audible tone, waveform, or flashing light) to show how strong the receiving signal is. Measurements should be considered inaccurate if the signal strength is poor (Fig. 45).
- Pulse oximeter will also indicate heart rate by counting the number of pulsatile signals (Fig. 46).

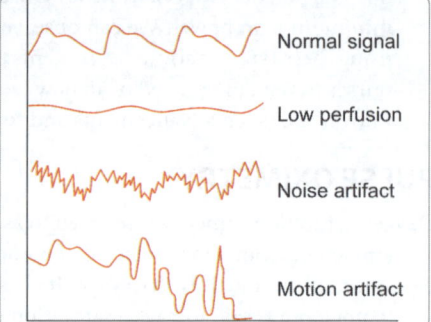

Figure 46: Pulse oximeter waveforms

Types of Pulse Oximeter (Figs 47A and B)

- Finger/mobile pulse oximeter
- Desktop pulse oximeter

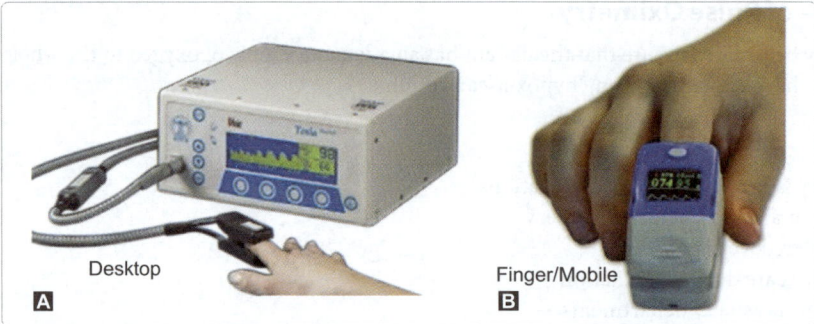

Figures 47A and B: Different types of pulse oximeters (A) Desktop; (B) Finger/Mobile

Parts of Pulse Oximeter (Fig. 48)

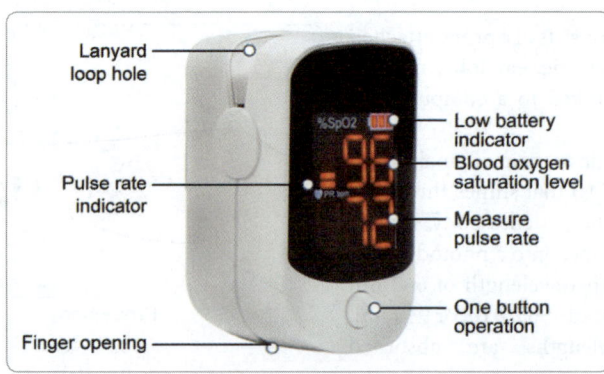

Figure 48: Parts of finger pulse oximeter

Limitations

- The most common cause of inaccuracy with pulse oximeter is motion artifact. Patient movement can cause pulsatile venous flow to be incorrectly measured as arterial pulsations, thus producing an inaccurate oximetry and pulse-rate reading.
- Another common cause of inaccuracy is poor peripheral perfusion. Poor peripheral perfusion can be caused by conditions such as hypothermia, peripheral vascular disease, vasoconstriction, hypotension, or peripheral edema. A forehead probe can be used for patients with decreased peripheral perfusion.
- Conditions such as jaundice, as well as intravascular dyes and carbon monoxide in the blood, can also influence oximetry readings.
- Anemic patients with low Hgb may have a normal SpO_2 reading, even though the available oxygen is not enough to meet the metabolic demands of the body.
- Patients with elevated bilirubin concentrations may also have falsely low SpO_2 readings.

Preliminary Assessment

- If measuring SpO_2 by attaching the probe to a finger or toe, check the radial or pedal pulse and capillary refill of the finger or toe you plan to use.
- If the patient's extremities are cold, try to warm his or her hands, or apply warm towels to improve perfusion.
- The patient's finger or toe should be clean and dry.
- Check that the patient does not have artificial nails or nail polish, as both will influence the light transmission and should, therefore, be removed before applying pulse oximetry.
- Check that the probe is positioned properly so that optical shunting (when light from the transmitter passes directly into the receiver without going through the finger) does not occur.
- Bright ambient light may also affect the accuracy of pulse oximetry readings.

Articles Required

A tray containing:

Articles	Purpose
Pulse oximeter	For measuring oxygen saturation
A bowl with alcohol swab	For cleaning the patient fingers and sensor
Kidney tray or paper bag	For discarding the soiled waste
Nail polish remover (If required)	For removing nail polish
Handrub	For hand washing
Required PPE	For preventing spread of microorganisms

Procedure

Steps	Procedure	Rationale
1.	Explain the procedure to the patient and the need for determining oxygen saturation. Explain that the values displayed may vary with patient movement, amount of environmental light, patient level of consciousness and the position of the sensor. Explain the need for an audible alarm system.	Enhances patient cooperation and decreases patient anxiety.

Contd...

Unit V ❖ **Assessment of Patient**

Steps	Procedure	Rationale
2.	Perform hand hygiene and wear required PPE.	Prevents the transmission of microorganisms.
3.	Choose pulse oximeter sensor and the type appropriate for the client's size and location to be used (finger, toe, ear) for the area with the best pulsatile vascular bed to be sampled.	Corrects sensor optimizes signal capture and minimizes difficulties. Inappropriate size or device may cause inaccurate results or pain.
4.	Select desired sensor site.	Adequate arterial pulse strength is necessary for obtaining accurate SpO$_2$ measurements.

If using the digits, assess for warmth and capillary refill.

Confirm the presence of an arterial blood flow to the area monitored.

Palpate the radial pulse (assess its course)

Avoid sites distal to indwelling arterial catheters, blood pressure cuffs, military antishock trousers (MAST) or venous engorgement like arteriovenous fistulas, blood transfusions.

Contd...

Steps	Procedure	Rationale
5.	Remove any finger nail polish or artificial nails on the fingers to be used if possible.	The sensor may be unable to provide an accurate reading through nail polish or acrylic nails.
6.	Before applying the sensor, use an alcohol wipe both on the site and the sensor should also be cleaned as per manufacturer's instruction. Allow alcohol to dry.	Using alcohol ensures that the site is clean and dry. Cleansing the device helps prevent the spread of infection
7.	Place the adhesive sensors and finger clip sensor for adults on the client's index, middle or ring finger. Adhesive wrap sensor Adhesive-free wrap sensor	Appropriate location ensures accurate reading.
	Adhesive sensor also can be placed on client's toe. A small earlobe clip is available for use on small adults, children's, and infants. If necessary, place newborn adhesive.	

Contd...

Unit V ❖ Assessment of Patient

Steps	Procedure	Rationale
8.	If any doubt arises about the chosen site, check the client proximal pulse and capillary refill.	Decreased circulation could skew oxygen saturation readings
9.	Check the sensor's markings to make sure that the light emitting diode and photo detector are correctly aligned. They should be opposite each other. Set appropriate alarm limits.	If sensors are not aligned, the sensor will give inaccurate reading.
10.	Attach the sensor to client cable and turn it on. The digital readout or light bar should show readings and alarm settings. The type will depend on the specific monitor being used	Readout or light bar indicates that the machine is working.
11.	Obtain a one time reading or keep the sensor in place and the monitor on continuous monitoring status.	Setting the alarm ensures notification to the nurse if the client values are out of the desired range, indicating the possible problem that requires intervention.

Contd...

Steps	Procedure	Rationale
	If continuous monitoring is ordered, make sure the alarm is on, before leaving the patient. The monitor has alarm limits that can be changed as per provider's order or Institution's policy. The continuous pulse oximeter gives audible and visual alarms and can be silenced for 60 seconds.	

Alarm indicator

Alarm silence

Steps	Procedure	Rationale
12.	Move an adhesive sensor every 4 hours and a clip type sensor at least every 2 hours. Watch for signs of tissue breakdown or irritation from adhesives or clips.	Moving the sensor helps to prevent tissue irritation and necrosis.
13.	Clean the sensor with alcohol wipes when it is removed. Evaluate sensor site every 4–8 hours.	Prevents cross transmission of micro organisms
14.	Remove PPE and perform hand hygiene.	This reduces the spread of microorganisms.
15.	Document the procedure including each oximeter reading and location of the sensor with the date, time along with the signature of the nurse. If the client is not on oxygen administration, the reading is documented as 'on room air' If the client receives supplemental oxygen document the quantity of oxygen administered (e.g. O_2 @ 3 LPM) Report any downward changes in oxygen saturation of 3%–5%.	Documentation fosters quality care.

Interpretation

The pulse oximeter gives a rapid estimation of the peripheral oxygen saturation. A normal healthy person should be able to achieve normal blood oxygen saturation levels (SpO_2) of 94%–99%. The readings of pulse oximeter are interpreted as:

What Does it Mean?	
SpO$_2$ reading (%)	Interpretation
95–100	Normal
91–94	Mild hypoxemia
86–90	Moderate hypoxemia
<85	Severe hypoxemia

Hazards of Pulse Oximetry

Pulse oximetry is generally considered to be a safe procedure. However, tissue injury may occur at the measuring site as a result of probe misuse. Pressure sores or burns are possible effects of prolonged application (>2 hours).

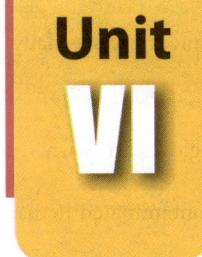

Unit VI Infection Control

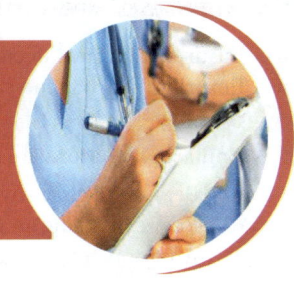

DEFINITIONS

- **Communicable disease** is a type of disease which may be transmitted directly or indirectly from one individual to another. It occurs due to an infectious agent or toxic products produced by it.
- **Infection control** is a process concerned with prevention of nosocomial or other health-threatening infections.

STANDARD PRECAUTIONS

Standard precautions are the measures taken to prevent the spread of infection among all patients whether they have a known infection or not. Standard precautions protect healthcare workers and patients from the spread of infection—secondary to contaminated blood and other bodily fluids.

The following are the types of precautions:
- Contact precautions
- Airborne precautions
- Droplet precautions
- Respiratory hygiene/cough etiquette
- Safe Injection practices

Precautions against Contact Infections

Contact precautions are defined as the measures taken to prevent the mode or means by which microorganisms move and get transmitted via direct or indirect contact with the infected person or an object that has been contaminated with the pathogen, respectively. It can be prevented by:
- Ensuring appropriate patient placement in a single patient space or room, if available.
- Using personal protective equipment (PPE) appropriately, including gloves and gown.
- Using gloves before providing care to patient.
- Using clean, nonsterile gloves for routine care of the patients.
- Changing gloves after contact with infective material.
- Removing gloves and washing hands after providing patient care.
- Following proper use of protective gown in case of direct contact with patient with potentially contaminated environmental surfaces and observe hand hygiene.
- Limiting the movement or transport of the patient from the room and also limiting the entry of visitors in the patient's room.
- Using disposable or dedicated patient-care equipment.
- Prioritizing cleaning and disinfection of the rooms of patients as per the policy of hospital.

- Ensuring that any infected or colonized areas are contained or covered.
- Ensuring that patient care items, bedsides equipment and frequently touched surfaces receive daily cleaning.

Contact precautions are essential, especially in situations like:

- Before and after any direct patient contact and between patients, whether or not gloves are worn.
- Before handling an invasive device.
- After touching blood, body fluids, secretions, excretions, nonintact skin, and contaminated items, even if gloves are worn.
- During patient care, when moving from a contaminated to a clean body site of the patient.
- After contact with inanimate objects coming to the immediate vicinity of the patient.

 Note

5 Moments of Hand Hygiene

The World Health Organization (WHO) recommends the '5 Moments of Hand Hygiene' to track hand hygiene performance of health care workers. Between the points of entering and exiting a patient's room, there are five critical moments when hand hygiene should be performed to ensure health and safety of patients and the staff members.

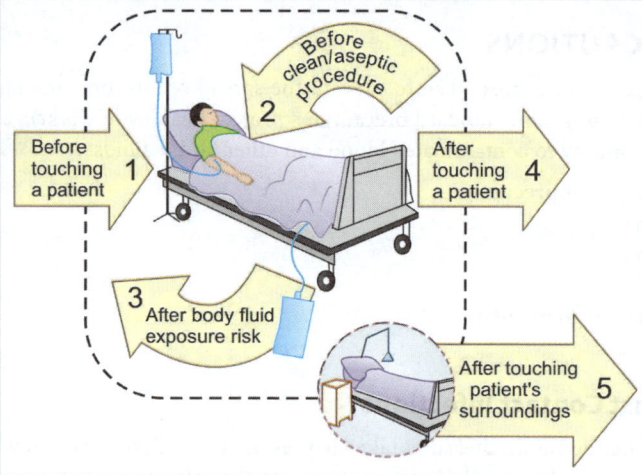

Precautions against Airborne Infection

Airborne precautions are indicated in the presence of a pathogen that is transmitted via the airborne mode of transmission:

- Used to prevent or reduce the transmission of microorganisms that are airborne in small droplet nuclei (5 μ or smaller in size) or dust particles containing the infectious agent.
- **Source control:** Ask the patient to put a mask.
- Ensure appropriate patient placement in an airborne infection isolation room (AIIR) constructed according to the guideline for isolation precautions.
- Restrict susceptible healthcare personnel from entering the room of patients known or suspected to have measles, chickenpox, disseminated zoster, or smallpox if other immune healthcare personnel are available.

- Use PPE appropriately, including an N95 mask or higher level respirator for health care personnel.
- Limit transport and movement of patients outside the room for medically-necessary purposes.
- Immunize susceptible persons as soon as possible following unprotected contact with vaccine-preventable infections (e.g., measles, varicella or smallpox).
- Place the patient in private room that has negative air pressure, with 6–12 air changes/per hour. If not available, cohort with patient with active infection with same microorganism.
- Use of respiratory protection.
- Keep the door of patient's room closed.

Precautions against Droplet Infection

- Used to reduce the risk of transmission of microorganisms transmitted by large particle droplets (larger than 5 µ in size).
- Ensure appropriate patient placement in a single room, if possible.
- Droplets usually travel 3 feet or less within the air and thus special air handling is not required, however newer recommendations suggest a distance of 6 feet be used for safety.
- PPE appropriately. Don mask upon entry into the patient room or patient space.
- Limit transport and movement of patients outside of the room to medically-necessary purposes. If transport or movement outside of the room is necessary, instruct patient to wear a mask and follow respiratory hygiene/cough etiquette.
- Room door may remain open.

Respiratory Hygiene and Cough Etiquette

- Education of health workers, patients and visitors regarding respiratory hygiene.
- Covering mouth and nose when coughing or sneezing.
- Hand hygiene after contact with respiratory secretions.
- Spatial separation of persons with acute febrile respiratory symptoms.
- Proper disposal of used materials, during coughing and sneezing.
- Use of surgical masks on coughing person when appropriate.
- Providing alcohol-based hand-rubbing dispensers and supplies for hand hygiene and educating patients and staff to use these.
- Encouraging hand hygiene after coughing or sneezing.
- Separating coughing persons at least 3 feet away from others in a waiting room or have separate seating arrangement.
- Instructing patients and providers not to touch eyes, nose, or mouth.

Safe Injection Practices

Safe injection practices include measures taken to perform injections in a manner that is safe for patients and providers.

- Use aseptic technique to avoid contamination of sterile injection equipment.
- Whenever possible, use of single-dose vials is preferred over multiple-dose vials, especially when medications will be administered to multiple patients.
- If multidose vials must be used, both the needle or cannula and syringe used to access the multidose vial must be sterile.
- Always use safety-engineered syringes.
- Correct disposal in appropriate container.

Unit VI ❖ Infection Control

- Do not recap needles. If recapping is necessary, use a one-handed technique.
- Discard packages if punctured, torn, or damaged by moisture.
- Use a sterile syringe and sterile needle for every injection.
- Avoid removing needle after injecting.
- Discard syringes as single unit.
- Avoid overfilling of discarded and unsterile sharps container.
- Never store cotton wet with disinfectant.
- Do not open glass ampoules with bare fingers.
- Do not store used sharps in an open container where they may be accidentally reused or cause needle-stick injuries when dumped.
- Seal boxes to prevent persons from removing needles to reuse them.
- Use puncture-proof containers to dispose of sharps and needles. Containers must be closed, puncture resistant, leak proof, color coded, and emptied routinely to prevent overfilling.
- Needle-sticks can occur if boxes are overfilled. Empty the boxes when it is ¾th filled.
- Provide postpuncture prophylaxis within two hours access to postexposure follow-up that confirms to CDC guidelines for testing and prophylaxis.
- Take utmost care when:
  - Handling needles, scalpels, and other sharp instruments or devices.
  - Cleaning used instruments.
  - Disposing of used needles and other sharp instruments.
- WHO recommends that health care providers should focus on the following 7 steps that make every injection safe.
  Step 1: Clean work space
  Step 2: Hand hygiene
  Step 3: Sterile and new syringe and needle, with reuse prevention and/or injury protection feature whenever possible
  Step 4: Sterile vial of medication and diluent
  Step 5: Skin disinfection
  Step 6: Appropriate collection of sharps
  Step 7: Appropriate waste management
- Employers need to maintain a **sharps injury log** for the recording of percutaneous injuries from contaminated sharps. The log must contain, at a minimum, the following information:
  - Date of the injury
  - Type and brand of the device involved
  - Department or work area where the incident occurred
  - Explanation of how the incident occurred

BARRIER NURSING

The nursing technique by which a patient with an infectious disease is prevented from infecting other people is called barrier nursing.

Barrier nursing was created as a means to maximize isolation care.

Types

- Simple barrier nursing consists of utilizing sterile gloves, masks, gowns, head-covers and eye protection.
- Strict barrier nursing, which is also known as 'rigid barrier nursing'.

Barrier Nursing Techniques in Infection Control

- Aseptic technique
- Isolation
- Safe handling of sharps
- Linen handling and disposal
- Waste disposal
- Handling biological spills
- Environmental cleaning
- Risk assessment
- Staff health

Aseptic Technique

Asepsis is the absence of disease causing organisms. The two types of asepsis are medical asepsis and surgical asepsis.

1. Medical Asepsis

Medical asepsis is defined as the absence of disease-causing microorganisms. Medical asepsis is often referred to as clean technique. It is based on principles of the infection control and practices that decrease the spread of infection. Medical asepsis reduces the number of pathogenic microorganisms and it also impairs the proliferation and growth of microorganisms, e.g., hand hygiene.

Special points in medical aseptic methods:
- Techniques for admitting patient, using gown, mask, gloves, glasses, using newspaper (or leaf mats), identification and use of clean surfaces, maintaining stock supplies, cupboards, etc. are dealt carefully and kept uncontaminated.
- Concurrent disinfection of articles used for more than one person.
- Cleaning and disinfecting everything when the patient leaves the room.
- Careful control of visiting hours and educating visitors and relatives.
- Educating the staff about health and hygiene.
- Vaccination, inoculation and use of medicines to prevent diseases and infection.
- Use of labor-saving devices and more efficient methods for careful aseptic practice.

Hand Hygiene
- Hand washing is the best and most effective way to prevent the spread of infection. Proper hand washing can be done with friction and regular soap and water or a special alcohol-based hand sanitizing antimicrobial solution.

Purposes
The purpose of medical hand washing is to:
- Reduce spread of disease from patient to patient
- Reduce spread of disease from patient to health care professional and vice versa
- Reduce spread of disease from health care professional to other health care professionals
- Reduce spread of disease to visitors in the health care facility

Principle: The basic principle of medical hand washing is to wash the hands thoroughly by holding the hands lower than the elbows—the clean area to a less clean area (the hands).

Prerequisites
- Ensure that watches are removed.
- Remove all jewelry (rings, bracelets).

Unit VI ❖ Infection Control

- Ensure that the nails are trimmed short.
- Remove artificial nails, if any.
- Remove nail polish, if any.
- Inspect the hands for any cuts, abrasions or open lesions.

Articles required

Article	Purpose
Antiseptic solution/Soap in soap dish	Aids in the removal of microorganisms
Running tap water with elbow or foot operated	For washing hands without contaminating the hands
Towels/Tissue paper	For wiping the hands after hand wash

Preparation of unit

- Ensure an area of good lighting.
- Arrange all the necessary articles close to the hand washing area.

Note

- Hand rubbing with alcohol-based hand rub is the preferred routine method of hand hygiene if hands are not visibly soiled.
- Hand washing with soap and water is essential when the hands are visibly dirty or visibly soiled (following visible exposure to body fluids)

Procedure

Steps	Procedure	Rationale
1.	• Turn on the water and wet hands and arms.	• Prevents wastage of water.
2.	• Once the hands are wet, apply enough soap or hand wash solution to cover all of the hands' surfaces and rub to produce lather.	• Soap facilitates removal of dust, microorganisms and aid protection.
3.	• Perform the steps of hand washing in the following manner for 40–60 seconds. ▪ Rub hands palm to palm.	• Ensures that all surfaces of hand are systematically washed to remove transient and resident microorganisms.

Contd...

Steps	Procedure	Rationale
	• Rub the back of both the hands with right palm over left dorsum with interlaced fingers and vice versa. 	
	• Interlace fingers with palm to palm and rub the hands together. • Interlock fingers and rub the backs of fingers to opposing palms. • Rub thumb in a rotating manner rubbing of left thumb clasped in right palm and vice versa followed by the area between the index and thumb finger. 	All surfaces of hand are systematically cleaned.

Contd...

Steps	Procedure	Rationale
	▪ Rotational rubbing, backward and forward with clasped fingers of right hand in left palm and vice versa, i.e., rub fingertips on palm.	• Cleans areas that are not easily reachable.
	▪ Rub both wrists in a rotating manner.	
4.	• Rinse hands thoroughly under running water, by **allowing the water to drain from the elbows to hands.**	• This allows water to drip from the elbows to hands, thus preventing the bacteria-laden soap and water from contamination.
5.	• Close the tap using the elbow or using paper towel.	• Prevents contamination of hands.
6.	• Dry the hands with the towels or tissue paper using a dabbing motion instead of a wiping motion from hands to arms.	• Drying helps to remove moisture, thus preventing growth of micro-organisms in a wet hand.

Duration

- **Hand washing with water and soap:** 40–60 seconds
- **Alcohol-based hand rubbing:** 20–30 seconds

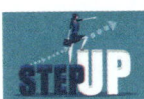

> Hand soap dispensers, hand sanitizer dispensers, hand dryers and paper towel dispensers placed at strategic points, throughout the medical facility, are invaluable in reducing cross infection.

2. Surgical Asepsis

Surgical asepsis is defined as the absence of all microorganisms. Surgical asepsis is often referred to as sterile technique. Surgical asepsis is used during all invasive procedures including surgical procedures and other invasive procedures such as endoscopy, for the administration of intravenous medications, for wound care and for the insertion of an indwelling urinary catheter as well as other internally placed tubes like central lines and peripheral intravenous lines.

Principles of Surgical Asepsis

Principles	Rationale
• Always face the sterile field. • Do not turn back or side on a sterile field. • **Never** lean over a sterile field.	• Sterile objects, out of vision are considered questionable and their sterility cannot be assured.
• Keep sterile equipment above waist level and table level.	• The margins of safety level are considered as the waist or above table level. This will promote maximum visibility of the sterile field.
• Do not speak, sneeze and cough over a sterile field.	• This helps to prevent droplet infection.
• Never reach across sterile field.	• When a nonsterile object is held above a sterile object. Gravity causes microorganisms to fall into the sterile field. So crossing across the sterile field questions sterility.
• Keep the unsterile objects away from the sterile field.	• Microorganisms may be transferred whenever a non-sterile object touches a sterile field.
• Keep the sterile field dry.	• Microorganisms do not pass easily through a dry surface. Microorganisms harbor easily on a wet surface.
• The edge of the sterile field is considered unsterile.	• Proximity to a contaminated area makes sterility questioned.
• Handle liquids cautiously near the sterile field or prevent drapes or wrappers from becoming wet.	• When liquid spills, it connects a nonsterile field with a sterile field.
• Sterile liquids must be poured carefully into sterile containers on the sterile field without the solution running over and obliterating the label on the bottle.	• When a liquid spills, it connects a nonsterile field with a sterile field.
• Each sterile supply should be clearly labeled about its contents, time and date of sterilization.	• Labeling helps to ensure sterility.
• Never assume that an object is sterile. Always check the expiry date of the sterile object.	• Sterility of an object wrapped in paper or cloth becomes doubtful after a month or as indicated.
• Avoid sweeping and dusting when the sterile objects are open.	• Microorganisms travel in the dust particles and thus the sterile object may become unsterile.

Unit VI ❖ Infection Control

Isolation

Isolation is defined as the separation of infected persons (persons suffering from infectious diseases) from noninfected persons for the period of communicability under conditions which will prevent the transmission of the infection to others.

Purpose of Isolation

Prevention of spread of infection to others.

Methods of Isolation

Isolation techniques are followed in the treatment and nursing care of patients suffering from communicable diseases, for preventing the spread of infection.

- A separate bed in a room protected from visitors (carriers). Exclusion of persons from the sick room and restricting those caring for the patient.
- Avoidance of contact with others by persons caring for the patient until every precaution has been taken to prevent the spread of infections.
- A washable outer garment should be worn by persons caring for the patient.
- Hands should be washed with soap and hot water after handling patient or contaminated objects in room.
- Outer garment to be removed on leaving the sick room and hung in the patient's room until disinfected.
- Disposal of paper bags, or soft tissue papers or clothes soiled with discharges from nose and mouth, with subsequent burning or disinfecting.
- Disinfection of objects contaminated by the patient prior to their removal from contaminated areas.
- Disposal of the patient's feces and urine containing the infectious agents according to appropriate instructions.
- Prophylactic immunization is done to contacts with appropriate vaccines.

Factors

Main factors about an isolated patients are:

- **Avoiding others coming in contact with patient**
  - The patient who is isolated will be kept in the isolated room or unit with separate articles for use.
  - The isolation room or unit should be provided with the minimum furniture and articles that are absolutely necessary only. All these things should be kept inside the room only.
  - Use old things as far as possible that can be destroyed after use, for example old linen, paper bag, etc.
  - No other things should be brought to the unit and nothing from the unit should be taken out until the terminal disinfection is done.
  - All those who attend the patient should protect themselves, by not coming in direct contact with the patient.
  - In order to achieve this, he/she can wear a gown, mask and cap to protect own clothes, etc. Important points to bear in mind in wearing the gown while attending a patient with infectious disease are:
  - The gown should be wide enough to cover the wearer's own clothing entirely
    - It should be wide enough to overlap in the back.
    - It should have either long or short sleeves, which can have fitting cuffs.
    - It should be made of strong and durable material (washable).
    - It should have belt at the waist.

- **Proper disposal of excreta of the patient**
  Aseptic disposal of discharges is necessary as discussed follows:
  - Disposal of untreated urine and feces by water carriage sewage is a safe practice.
  - Excreta must be disinfected before disposal. Lime water 1:8 or cresol 1:100 or carbolic 1:20 or Dettol 1:20 or Lysol 1:20 may be used in all cases.
  - The fecal matter should be broken up with a stick, which is kept in a disinfectant solution.
  - The disinfectant should be equal to the volume of excreta and the mixture should be left in a covered vessel for 2 hours at least.
  - The bedpan must be disinfected by chemicals or heat.

Forms of Isolation

- **Strict isolation:** Strict isolation is used in case of diseases that spread through the air and in some cases by contact. In this isolation technique, patients are kept in a special room equipped with a special lavatory and care giving equipment and a separate sink and waste bin.
- **Contact isolation:** Contact isolation is used in such cases to prevent the spread of diseases that can be spread through contact with open wounds.
- **Respiratory isolation:** Respiratory isolation is used for diseases that spread through particles that are exhaled. Those having contact with or exposure to such a patient are required to wear a mask.
- **Reverse isolation:** Reverse isolation often involves the use of laminar air flow and mechanical barriers. This helps to avoid physical contact with others and to isolate the patient from any harmful pathogens present in the external environment.
- **High isolation:** High isolation is used in patients in order to prevent the spread of unusually, highly contagious or with high mortality infectious diseases (e.g., smallpox, ebola virus and COVID 19). It stipulates mandatory use of:
  - Gloves (or double gloves if appropriate),
  - Protective eye wear (goggles or face shield)
  - A waterproof gown or PPE
  - A respirator
- **Source Isolation:** Airborne infection isolation room (AIIR) or negative pressure room.
- **Protective Isolation:** Positive pressure room with high-efficiency particulate air (HEPA) filter.
- **Isolation of patient in case of a particular diseases:**
  - **Respiratory diseases:** The most common respiratory diseases that occur in hospitals and for which isolation may be needed are:
    Influenza (sometimes isolated), diphtheria, whooping cough, pneumonia (sometimes isolated), meningitis, mumps, streptococcal sore throat, poliomyelitis, measles, tuberculosis and chicken pox.
    - **Purpose of disinfection:** To prevent the spread of infection through respiratory discharge and secretions.
    - **Procedure:** Gown technique, mask technique, disinfection of dishes, and linen and provide paper bag at the bedside. Dispose of nasal and throat discharges in the paper bag which should be burned.
  - **Intestinal diseases:** The most common ones that occur in hospitals are typhoid fever, dysentery (amoebic and bacillary) and cholera.
    - **Purpose of isolation:** To prevent the spread of disease by contact of contaminated excreta with other individuals.
    - **Procedure:** Gown technique, dishes disinfected, disinfection of excreta and disinfection of linen.

Unit VI ❖ Infection Control

- **Other diseases:** Most common ones are pediculosis, impetigo, scabies, erysipelas (Erysipelas is a skin infection caused by *Streptococcus haemolyticus* characterized by skin lesions, especially on face. These diseases commonly occur in persons of the age above 20 years and spread through direct contact), gonorrhea and syphilis.
  - **Purpose:** To prevent spread of disease by contact of skin, parasites and excretions with other individuals.
- **Puerperal sepsis:** (Sometimes) spread in maternity wards.
  - **Procedure:** Gown technique. Use precautions in disposing of soiled vaginal pads.
- **Purpose:** To prevent spread of tetanus, and gas gangrene caused by spore bearing organisms.
  - **Procedure:** Gown technique, protection of wounds, prophylactic inoculation in the proper time, disinfection of linen, precautions in changing dressings and disposing of soiled dressings.

Safe Handling of Sharps (As per WHO Guidelines 2014)

Safe placement of the sharps container is important in all health care settings.

- Choose containers that are designed to make one handed disposal possible and easy.
- Dispose of sharps immediately after use in a clearly labeled, sharps disposal container.
- Fill containers only to ¾ full, close the lid securely for disposal.
- Replace the used container with a new empty one.
- The container should have a tightly fitting lid that seals and prevents leakage.

Needles and Syringes

- Do not remove needles from syringes or other devices; always dispose of them as a single unit.
- Do not recap needles prior to disposal. Most needle stick injuries occur during recapping.
- Do not bend or break needles after use.
- Discard needles and syringes directly into a sharps container immediately after use.

- Do not leave a sharp protruding from the sharps container.
- Do not pour any disinfectants into the sharps container.
- Scalpels must be left intact and should be discarded directly into the sharps container.
- Discard disposable razors directly into sharps container.
- Pick up and discard broken contaminated glasses into the sharps container using forceps.

  Ref: https://www.who.int/water_sanitation_health/facilities/waste/module17.pdf?ua=1

Linen Handling and Disposal

- When removing linen from a bed or table, vigorous movements shall be avoided to prevent aerosols of microorganisms.
- All soiled linens should be bagged at the location where it was used, and the collection bag must be of sufficient quality to contain the wet/soiled linens and prevent leakage during handling and transportation.
- Linens must be placed and transported in labeled or color-coded bags or containers.
- Do not shake linen into the environment.
- Do not change linen during wound dressings in the same area.
- Use PPE when handling dirty linen.

Unit VI ❖ Infection Control

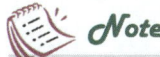 *Note*

- 6 Cs of handling soiled linen in a healthcare environment are shown in the following illustration:

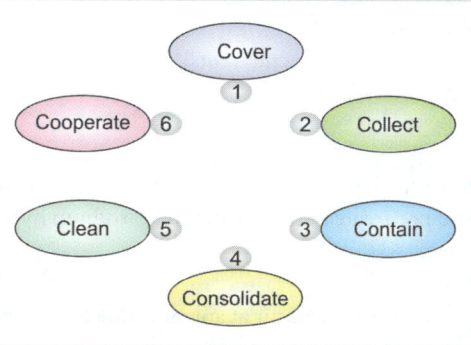

Waste Disposal

Waste management (or waste disposal) involves the activities and actions required to manage waste from its inception to final disposal.

Biomedical Waste Management (Amendment) Rules, 2018

Red bag

- Disposable contaminated waste, which can be recycled—will be disposed of by autoclaving treatment followed by shredding
- Tubing, bottles
- Intravenous tubes and sets, catheters, urine bags
- Syringes (without needles and fixed needle syringes)
- Vaccutainers with their needles cut and gloves.

Yellow bag

- Human anatomical wastes
- Body parts/tissues, etc.
- Cotton dressings, plaster casts, gauze pieces
- Antibiotics and other drugs
- Microbiology waste
- Culture devices, stocks or specimen of microorganisms
- Discarded linens, mattresses, dressings soiled with blood or body fluids, routine masks and gown.

Black bag

- General waste

Blue bag

- Puncture proof or leak proof containers
- Glassware—broken
- Contaminated glass
- Medicine vials, ampoules, etc.

Unit VI ❖ Infection Control

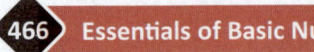

White puncture proof container

- White (L)—Waste sharps including metals—packed in puncture proof containers
- Needles, syringes with fixed needles
- Scalpels, blades, lancet
- Suture needle, aluminum foil
- Any contaminated sharp object causing puncture/cuts
- Handed over to waste agency when 2/3 full.

Chemical/Liquid Waste

- **Liquid waste:** To be treated with 1–2% Hypochlorite or to have an effluent treatment plant (ETP).
- Floor washing, etc. should be pre-treated onsite using 1–2% sodium hypochlorite or connected to ETP.

Handling Biological Spills

Spillage of blood, body fluids or chemicals can occur at any time due to broken or faulty equipment or human error. Hazmat is an abbreviation for 'hazardous materials'—substances in quantities or forms that may pose a reasonable risk to health, property, or the environment. Hazmats include substances such as toxic chemicals, fuels, nuclear waste products and biological, chemical, and radiological agents. Hazmats may be released as liquids, solids, gases, or a combination or form of all three, including dust, fumes, gas, vapor, mist and smoke.

Spill Management

- Put appropriate signage in the area.
- **Major spill:** Call the Hazmat (hazardous materials) activation team.
- Cover the area with gauze/pads soaked in 1% sodium hypochlorite. Keep it for 30 minutes.
- In case of minor spills, call unit housekeeping and clean the area using Hazmat kit.
- Hazmat Team shall clean the spill with appropriate PPE.
- Follow the hospital protocols.

Environment Cleaning

The role of environmental cleaning is to reduce the number of infectious agents that may be present on surfaces and minimize the risk of transfer of microorganisms from one person/object to another, thereby reducing the risk of cross-infection. There are three important factors that help to ensure the cleaning and disinfection practices. These include: chemicals, equipment and techniques.

Cleaning Chemicals

Appropriate care should be taken to ensure that the cleaning chemical is used appropriately and in accordance with the manufacturer's specifications.

- Ensure that the concentration of the cleaning solution is correct.
- Make sure that the cleaning solution was left with adequate contact time to ensure the effectiveness with maximal disinfection.
- Cleaning solutions should be regularly replaced in accordance with the manufacturer's specifications and more frequently. This includes in occasions such as when cleaning heavily contaminated areas, when solutions appear visibly dirty and immediately after cleaning blood and body fluid spills.

Cleaning Equipment

- All cleaning equipment used in healthcare facilities should be fit for use at any time, cleaned and stored dry between use, well-maintained and used appropriately.

- Equipment, which generates and disperses dust such as feather dusters and brooms should not be used within the healthcare facility as it may be a good source of transferring microorganisms.
- Vacuum cleaners, which are used to clean carpets close to clinical areas should be fitted with high-efficiency particulate air (HEPA) filters and undergo regular maintenance.
- Following a color-coding system for cleaning materials and equipment helps to ensure that materials and equipment used for cleaning purposes are not used in multiple different areas, therefore reducing the risk of cross-infection.

  For example:

  - **Red:** Bathrooms, washrooms, showers, toilets, basins and bathroom floors.
  - **Blue:** General areas including wards, departments, offices and basins in public areas.
  - **Green:** Catering departments, ward kitchen areas and patient food service at ward level.
  - **Yellow:** Isolation areas.

Cleaning of equipment (including buckets, mop heads, etc.) should be inspected regularly and changed when required.

The following basic principles should be followed:

- Equipment such as buckets and containers should be washed with detergent and disinfected after each use, stored upside down and allowed to dry in sunlight between uses.
- Buckets and containers should be inspected for cracks and replaced accordingly.
- Mop heads and cleaning clothes should be changed and laundered daily or after use (if used less frequently than daily) and changed when visibly soiled.
- Equipment such as clothes and mop heads, which are used to clean blood or body fluid spills or used in isolation rooms should either be disposable and discarded after use, or if re-usable, changed immediately after use and placed in a plastic bag for transport to the laundry.

Cleaning Techniques

The following points should form the basis of all standard operating procedures regarding cleaning in healthcare facilities:

- The flow of cleaning should be from areas which are considered relatively clean to dirty. This means that areas/elements, which are low touch or lightly soiled should be cleaned before areas which are considered high touch or heavily soiled. For example:
  - When cleaning a bathroom, the toilet should be cleaned last as it is likely to be the most contaminated element in that area.
  - In a patient room, items that are used commonly by the patient (high touch areas) include the patient bed, call-bell, locker, overway table, light switches, control knobs, hand basin, etc., while the low touch areas include the walls, windows and floors.
- The flow of cleaning should generally be from high to low reach surfaces. For example:
  - When dusting horizontal surfaces in a patient room, high areas such as those above shoulder height should be done first followed by all other elements.
- Dusting technique should not disperse the dust, (i.e., use damp cloths).
- When using clothes and bucket/solution system to clean:
  - Avoid 'double-dipping' used clothes into the bucket containing clean, unused clothes. This can contaminate the remaining clean clothes which are in the solution and result in spreading microorganisms to surfaces that are wiped thereafter.
  - To maximize the use of cleaning clothes, they should be folded and rotated in a manner so as all surface areas of the cloth, including the front and back, are used progressively as elements are cleaned
    - More clothes may be required to clean 'high-touch surfaces' compared to the same surface area of 'low-touch surfaces'.

Unit VI ❖ Infection Control

Concurrent Disinfection of Used Articles

- For nose and throat discharges; paper handkerchief may be used and must be disposed of waste receptacles, and burnt. Rag pieces may be used instead of paper handkerchief.
- Soiled dressings and similar refuses may be placed in waxed paper bags or wrapped in several layers of newspaper and burned.
- Liquid food waste should be disinfected with a chemical and solid can be burnt or buried.

Terminal Disinfection

- After a patient has recovered from a communicable disease, at the time of his discharge, the patient is given a good bath and shampoo and he is dressed in uncontaminated clothing and taken out of the isolated room or unit.
- In case of death, the body is prepared and carefully wrapped so that the outer surface is clean.
- The contaminated unit is then cleaned.
- The floor and furniture are washed well with soap and water by using a disinfectant.
- The walls are whitewashed if necessary.
- The mattress and pillows are brushed and aired in the sun for 6 hours or subjected to steam under pressure.
- All linen is disinfected and then laundered. Blankets are either washed or dry cleaned or sterilized in the autoclave.
- All enamel ware, glassware, instruments and rubber goods are boiled or treated with a disinfectant.

Risk Assessment

- No risk—routine care
- Low or moderate risk—wear gloves and plastic apron
- High risk (contact/splashing)—wear gloves, plastic apron, gown, eye/face protection, PPE.

Staff Health

- Immunization of whole staff
- Cover lesions with waterproof dressings
- Restrict nonimmune/pregnant staff
- Advice when suffering infection
- Report accidents/untoward incidents
- Follow hospital policy

PERSONAL PROTECTIVE EQUIPMENT

Personal protective equipment is specialized equipment and attire that is used by employees working in health care to protect themselves from against infections. Examples of personal protective equipment include gowns, gloves, masks, goggles and respirators.

Face Mask

Face masks are loose-fitting masks that cover the nose and mouth, and have ear loops or ties or bands at the back of the head.

Uses

- Face masks help limit the spread of germs.
- It prevents droplet infections when someone talks, coughs, or sneezes.
- It also protects the wearer's nose and mouth from splashes or sprays of body fluids.

Prerequisites

- Disposable face masks should be used once and then thrown in the trash.
- Make sure that the mask has no defects such as a tear, torn strap or ear loop, or contaminated.
- Don't wear if wet or soiled. Get a new mask.
- Don't criss cross ties.
- Don't leave a mask hanging of one ear or hanging around the neck.
- Don't reuse. Toss it after wearing once.
- Don't touch the front of the mask.

Types of Masks

There are many types of medical masks:

- **Ear loops:** Some masks have 2 ear loops that are normally made of an elastic material. This helps for easy stretching. To apply this, hold this type of mask by the loops, put 1 loop around one ear and then put the other loop around the other ear.
- **Ties or straps:** Some masks comes with pieces of fabric that are tied around the back of the head. Most masks with ties come with an upper and lower ties or straps. To apply this, hold the mask by the upper ties, place the ties around the back of the head and attach them together with a bow.
- **Bands:** Some masks come with 2 elastic bands that are placed over and around the back of the head (as opposed to around the ears). To apply these kind of masks, hold the mask in front of the face, pull the top band over the top of the head and place it around the crown of the head. Then pull the bottom band over the top of the head and place it at the base of the skull.

Articles Required

Article	Purpose
Hand washing solution or hand rub.	For hand washing.
Face mask.	For respiratory isolation.

Procedure of Wearing a Face Mask

Steps	Procedure	Rationale
1.	Clean the hands with soap and water or hand sanitizer before touching the mask.	Prevents transmission of microorganisms

Contd...

Steps	Procedure	Rationale
2.	Remove a mask from the box and make sure there are no obvious tears or holes in either side of the mask. 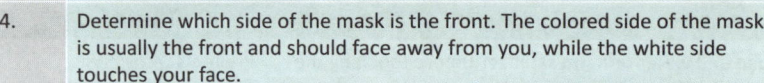	Proper assessment of mask beforehand eliminates the risk of infection transmission.
3.	Hold the side of the mask that has a stiff bendable edge as the top. Ensure this bendable side is facing upwards before applying the mask to face. 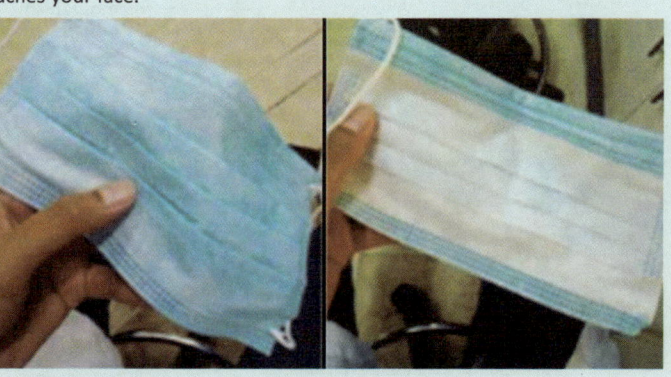	Stiff bendable edge helps to mold according to the shape of the nose.
4.	Determine which side of the mask is the front. The colored side of the mask is usually the front and should face away from you, while the white side touches your face.	Prevents cross infection.

Contd...

Steps	Procedure	Rationale
5.	Follow the instructions below for the type of mask you are using. **Face mask with ear loops** • Hold the mask by the ear loops. • Place a loop around each ear. • Put 1 loop around one ear and then put the other loop around other ear. **Face mask with ties** • Bring the mask to your nose level and place the ties over the crown of your head and secure with a bow. • Tie the upper strings at the top of the head with a butterfly knot. 	Facilitates proper fitting of the mask covering both mouth and nose and provides respiratory isolation.

Contd...

Unit VI ❖ Infection Control

Steps	Procedure	Rationale
	• Tie the lower strings at the back of the neck. 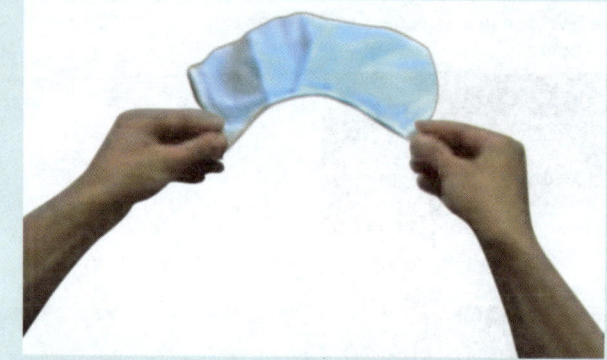***Face mask with bands*** • Hold the mask in your hand with the nosepiece or top of the mask at fingertips, allowing the headbands to hang freely below hands. 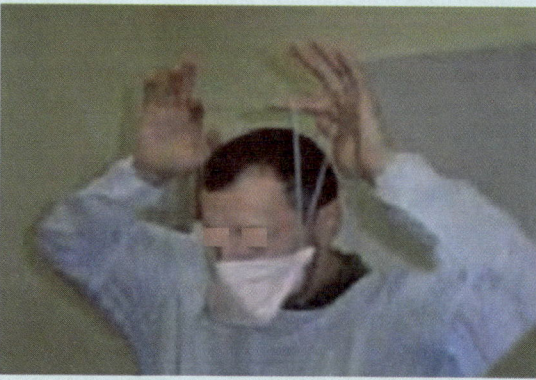• Cup the mask under the chin and pull the head bands up and over the head.	

Contd...

Steps	Procedure	Rationale
	• Bring the mask to your nose level and pull the top strap over your head so that it rests over the crown of your head. 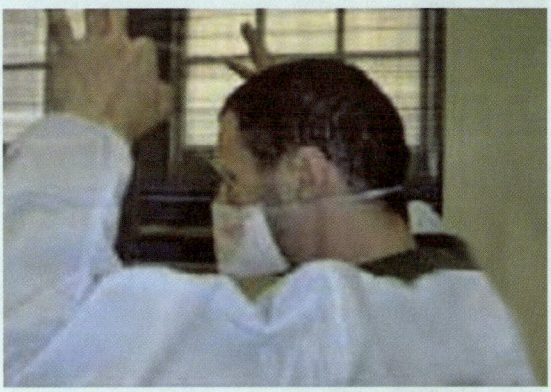	
	• Pull the bottom strap over your head so that it rests at the nape of your neck. 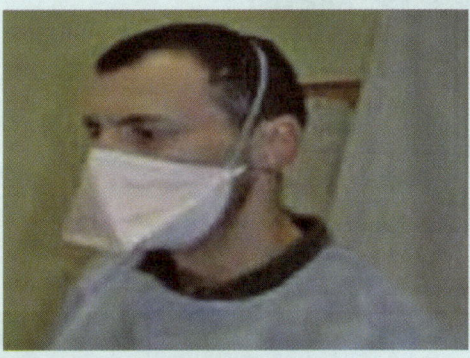	
6.	Mold or pinch the stiff edge to the shape of your nose. 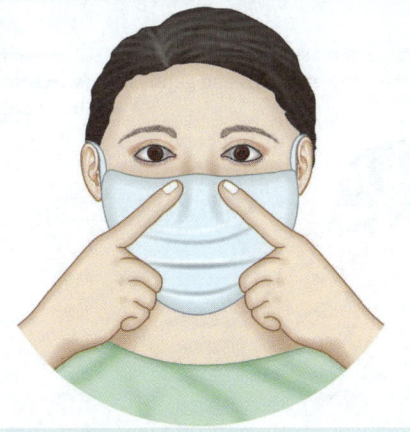	Prevents dislodging of the mask from its position.

Contd...

Steps	Procedure	Rationale
7.	Pull the bottom of the mask over your mouth and chin. 	Ensures that both the mouth and nose are covered securely.
8.	Ensure that the mask fully covers the nose, mouth and is stretched gently over the chin and fit snugly over the face. 	Ensures that proper respiratory isolations measures are taken.

Procedure for Removing a Face Mask

Steps	Procedure	Rationale
1.	Clean your hands with soap and water or hand sanitizer before touching the mask. Avoid touching the front of the mask. Only touch the ear loops/ties/band.	The front of the mask is considered the contaminated area.
2.	Follow the instructions below for the type of mask you are using. (i) *Face mask with ear loops:* Hold both of the ear loops and gently lift and remove the mask. 	Following the steps properly prevents transfer of microorganisms.

Contd...

Unit VI ❖ Infection Control

Steps	Procedure	Rationale
	(ii) *Face mask with ties:* Untie the bottom bow first then untie the top bow and pull the mask away from you as the ties are loosened. (iii) *Face mask with bands:* Lift the bottom strap over your head first then pull the top strap over your head.	
3.	Throw the mask in the trash as per Institution's policy.	Prevents cross infection.
4.	Clean your hands with soap and water or hand sanitizer.	Prevents transfer of microorganisms.

Gowning

Gowning and gloving will take place immediately after surgical hand antisepsis and the whole process is often referred to as scrubbing, gowning and gloving.

Gowning is the process of wearing special garments in order to control particulate contamination.

Purpose

To improve the perioperative outcome of interventions and procedures by enhancing and further promoting aseptic techniques.

Prerequisites

- This attire shall not be worn outside the change area
- **Gowns are considered sterile from waist level to chest level including sleeves to 2 inches above elbow.**
- Ensure that the gown is in a good state before wearing.
- Gown is worn after scrubbing the hands.

Procedure of Wearing Sterile Gown

Steps	Procedure	Rationale
1.	Perform surgical scrubbing and dry hands using a sterile towel and dispose it off.	Prevents transmission of microorganisms.

Contd...

Unit VI ❖ Infection Control

Steps	Procedure	Rationale
2.	Pick up gown which is folded with the inside uppermost by grasping at the neckline and lift it directly upward from the sterile package.	Inside portion of a gown comes directly in contact with your body.
3.	Step back from the table into an unobstructed area and gently shake it out, taking care not to let anything else touch it.	This ensures that the gown is not touching any other things in the surroundings.
4.	Let the gown unfold keeping the inside of the gown facing your body without touching the sterile exterior of the gown. If the gown does not unfold completely, the circulating nurse may assist by pulling down the unfolded bottom inside of the gown using a sterile forceps.	Exterior of the gown is considered sterile and ensures that it is not touching anywhere in the surroundings.

Contd...

Steps	Procedure	Rationale
5.	Carefully locate the neckband and hold the inside front of the gown just below the neckband with both hands. Open to locate sleeve or arm holes.	Holding over the neckband ensures that the sterile field is not disturbed.
6.	Hold the hands at shoulder level and slip both arms into the sleeves of the gown simultaneously until the hands reach the nearest edge of the cuff.	Maintains sterility of the gown.
7.	Keep your hands inside the sleeves.	This ensures that the hands are inside the sterile area.

Contd...

Steps	Procedure	Rationale
8.	Ask an assistant to help pull it up over your shoulders and fasten it up at the back by: • Reaching inside the gown. • Adjust the inside shoulder seam. • Bring the gown over the scrub person's shoulders. 	Proper securing prevents unnecessary disturbance during the sterile procedure.
	• Touch only the ties, snaps, or hook and loop fastener. • Secure the back of the gown at the neck and the waist. 	
	• Adjust the gown by grasping the bottom edge. • Pull it down to eliminate any blousing. 	

Contd...

Steps	Procedure	Rationale
9.	After donning the gloves, the unscrubbed person can assist with completing the gowning process by the following steps. Take the tab attached to the front tie that is presented by the scrubbed person. Hold it while the scrubbed person makes a three-quarter turn to wrap the back panel of the gown. 	Ensures that the scrubbed person is completely wrapped by the sterile gown.
10.	The scrubbed person then carefully retrieves the tie by pulling it out of the tab held by the unscrubbed person. Then the gown is secured by tying this tie to the short end of the waist tie. 	Ensures that the scrubbed person is completely wrapped by the sterile gown.

Removing Gown

At the end of the procedure, the gown is **always removed before the gloves** to prevent cross contamination of the wearer's scrub attire.

The circulating nurse assists by unfastening the neck and back closures of the gown.

The scrub person:

- Grasps the shoulders of the gown, pulls it downward from the shoulder and off the arms and turns the sleeves inside out;
- Folds the contaminates surface of the gown on the inside and rolls it away from the body; and
- Discards the rolled gown in the appropriate receptacle.

Unit VI ❖ Infection Control

Gloving

Sterile gloves are free from all microorganisms. Gloving is the procedure of donning sterile rubber gloves in such a way as to preserve asepsis before each surgical procedure.

Purposes

Gloves are worn for three important reasons in hospitals:

1. First, gloves are worn to provide a protective barrier and to prevent gross contamination of the hands when touching blood, body fluids, secretions, excretions, mucous membranes, and nonintact skin;
2. Wearing gloves reduces the likelihood of transmission of microorganisms present on the hands of personnel to patients during invasive or other patient-care procedures that involve touching a patient's mucous membranes and nonintact skin.
3. It also reduces the likelihood of transmission of microorganisms from a patient or a that harbors in the hands of personnel to another patient. In this situation, gloves must be changed between patient contacts and hands should be washed after gloves are removed.

Methods of Gloving

There are two methods of gloving, the closed-gloving technique and the open-gloving technique.

1. In the **closed-gloving technique**, the scrub person's hands remain inside the sleeves and should not touch the cuffs. The scrubbed person should use the closed gloving technique when initially donning a sterile gown and gloves.
2. In the **open-gloving technique**, the scrub person's hands slide all the way through the sleeves and out beyond the cuffs.

Prerequisites

- Choose the right size of gloves. Gloves come in multiple sizes. Make sure the gloves are tight enough so that objects are easy to pick-up.
- Sterile gloving does not replace hand washing because gloves may have small, apparent defects or may be torn during use, and hands can become contaminated during removal of gloves. Hands must be washed before and after any procedure.
- Failure to change gloves between patient contacts is an infection hazard.
- Remove jewellery, nail polish, artificial nails, extenders, or chipped nail polish.
- Ensure that the nails are short.
- Inspect hands for sores and abrasions. Cover or report to supervisor as required.
- Ensure sleeves are at least 2–3 inches above the elbows.
- Gather all supplies and prepare your patient for the procedure prior to applying gloves.
- Ensure the patient does not have a latex allergy prior to applying sterile gloves.

Procedure of Gloving

Steps	Procedure	Rationale
1.	Perform surgical or medical hand washing.	This decreases the bacterial count on hands and prevents contamination of sterile equipment.

Contd...

Steps	Procedure	Rationale
2.	Inspect package for sterility. Always examine sterile glove packaging for expiry date, intactness, and tears. The package should be dry. 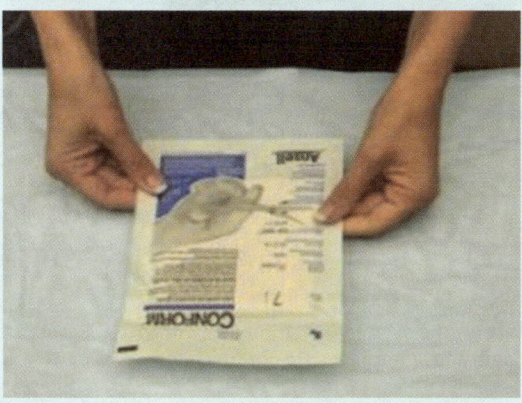	This ensures sterility prior to use.
3.	Open sterile packaging by peeling open the top seam and pulling down. Open sterile packaging without contaminating inner package. 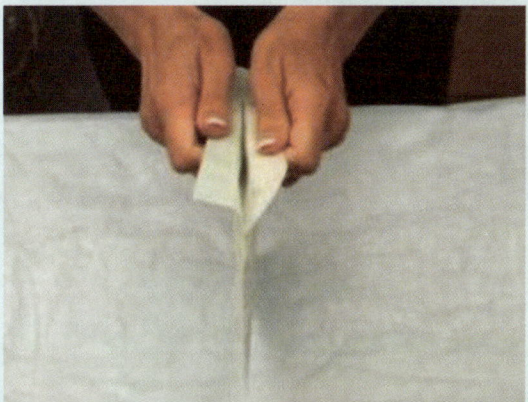	Prevents contamination of the inner package.
4.	Place inner package on working surface and open up to see right and left gloves. Start with dominant hand first. 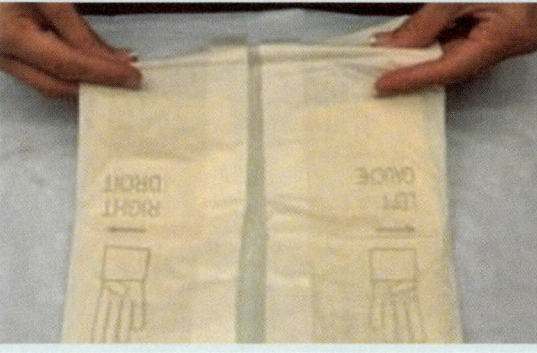	Facilitates easy donning of gloves.

Contd...

Steps	Procedure	Rationale
5.	Open packaging.	
6.	Pick up the left glove cuff, touching only the everted (i.e., turned down) edge of the cuff with his or her right thumb and index finger. Do not touch the outside of the glove.	Ensures that only the portion which comes in contact with the persons hand is touched.
7.	Insert hand into the opening and pull the glove onto the left hand up to the wrist.	Ensures that only the portion which comes in contact with the persons hand is touched.

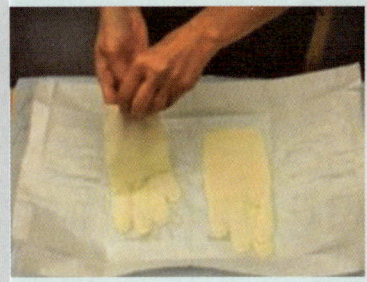
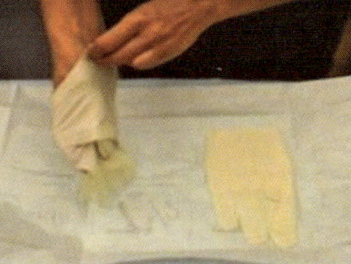

Contd...

Steps	Procedure	Rationale
8.	Pick up the right glove with the gloved left hand, keeping the gloved fingers under the everted cuff.	Ensures that the sterile portion of the gloved hand touches the sterile portion of the other glove.
9.	Slide fingers of the right hand inside the right glove cuff and pull the glove onto the right hand avoiding inward rolling of the cuff.	Ensures sterility.
10.	Pulls the right glove cuff by rotating the arm.	Ensures that the gloves fit perfectly.

Contd...

Steps	Procedure	Rationale
11.	Adjust gloves if necessary. Once gloves are on, interlock gloved hands and keep at least six inches away from clothing, keeping hands above waist level and below the shoulders. 	This prevents accidental touching of nonsterile objects or the front of the gown.

Procedure of Removing Gloves

Steps	Procedure	Rationale
1.	Grasp the outside of the cuff 1/2 inch below the cuff or palm of glove and gently pull the glove off. 	Prevents contamination of the hand.
2.	Turn the gloves inside out. 	Prevents contamination of the hand.

Contd...

Steps	Procedure	Rationale
3.	'Cup' it in your right hand	Prevents contamination of the hand.
4.	Take ungloved hand, place two fingers inside the other glove underneath the cuff.	Prevents the contamination of gloved hand touching ungloved hand.
5.	Pull glove off inside out.	Prevents the contamination of gloved hand touching ungloved hand.
6.	Throw your gloves away in a biohazard bag or bin.	Prevents transfer of microorganisms.

Contd...

Unit VI ❖ Infection Control

Steps	Procedure		Rationale
7.	Wash hands. 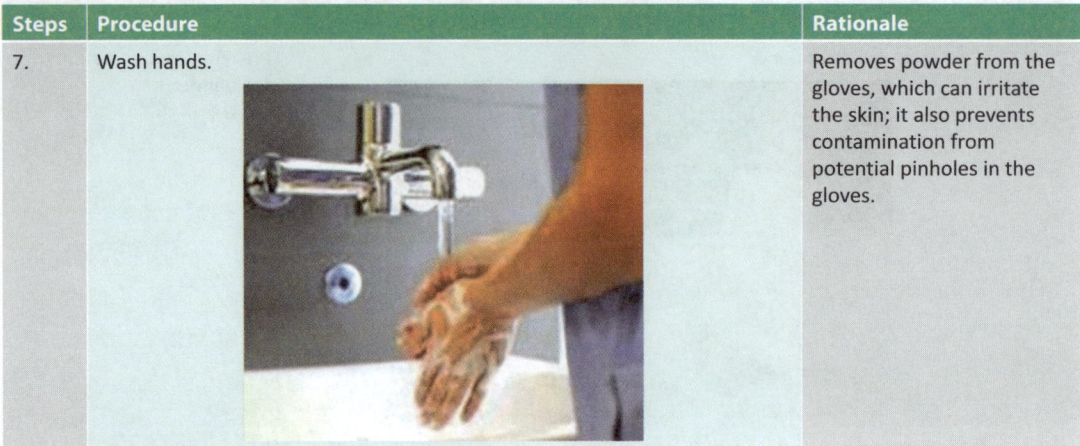		Removes powder from the gloves, which can irritate the skin; it also prevents contamination from potential pinholes in the gloves.

Surgical Caps

A surgical or scrub cap is a part of medical protective clothing and prevents germs from the hair or scalp of surgical personnel from contaminating the operating area. They are put on in the scrub room before entering the operating theatre and then later removed in the scrub room, as well.

Single-use surgical caps are most often made from a light, nonwoven fabric.

Purpose

The surgical cap minimizes the risk of hair falling and dandruff into the sterile area during surgery.

Procedure

- Perform hand hygiene.
- Pick up a cap and ensure that there are no defects found and the elasticity of the cap is persistent.
- Expand the cap in the area of elasticity and wide open it.
- Wear it on the head ensuring that all your hair is covered by the surgical cap before proceeding with scrubbing for surgery (Figs 1A and B).

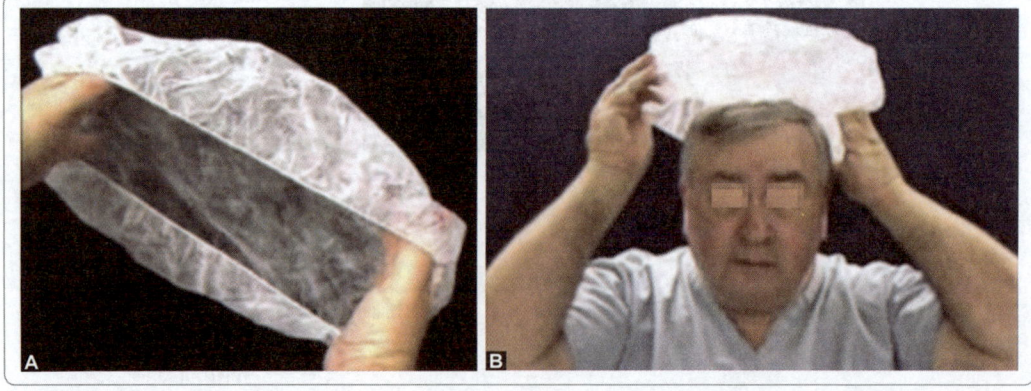

Figures 1A and B: (A) Check the cap for any damage; (B) Wear it by completely covering hair

Complete coverage of hair is necessary because uncovered hair acts as a filter and collects bacteria. These scrub caps are simply disposed of after use as per Institution's policy.

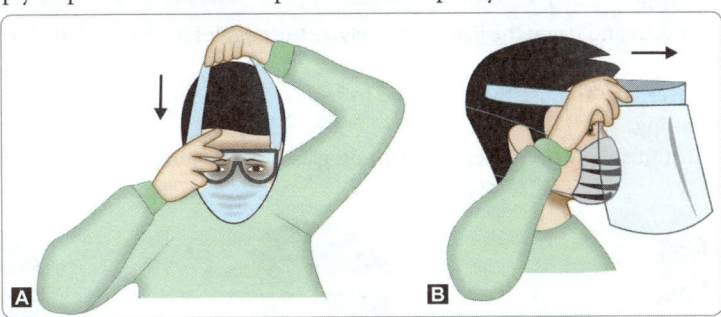

Figures 2A and B: (A) Goggles; (B) Face shield

Face Shields

Safety goggles do not provide protection against splashes and sprays to the whole face so they have limited application in irrigating wounds, suctioning secretions, and procedures where blood may spurt. Face shields are a preferred option. Outside of face shield and goggles are contaminated. They should be handled only by the headband or the sides.

After use, discard these into a lined waste bin or place into a receptacle for reprocessing or decontamination (Figs 2A and B).

Face shields are transparent sheets of plastic that extend from the eyebrows to below the chin and across the entire width of the persons head.

A face shield should wrap around the face till the ear protecting the face, nose, mouth, and eyes; should cover forehead, extend below chin and wrap around side of face which reduces the possibility of a splash reaching the eyes from the edges. It should also protect the crown and chin.

Purposes

- Face shields should be used during suctioning oral secretions, while responding to emergency where blood is spurting and when irrigating a wound.
- Face shields protect against nuisance dusts and potential splashes or sprays of hazardous liquids.
- It is always worn with the safety goggles.

Goggles

Goggles, or **safety glasses**, are forms of **protective** eyewear that usually enclose or protect the area surrounding the eye in order to prevent particulates, water or chemicals from striking the eyes.

These are tight-fitting eye protection that completely cover the eyes, eye sockets and the facial area immediately surrounding the eyes and provide protection from impact, dust and splashes.

Types of Goggles (Figs 3A to C)

- Indirectly-vented or **nonvented goggles prevent splashes,** sprays, and respiratory droplets.
- Anti-fog safety goggles offer the most practical and reliable use. It improves clarity PPE use in Healthcare Settings.
- Goggles with indirect airflow also reduces fogging.
- Some newer goggles also provide better peripheral vision.

Unit VI ❖ Infection Control

Procedure of Wearing Safety Goggles and Face Shield

- Perform hand hygiene.
- Place goggles over eyes and using the headband, secure the goggles to the head. It should fit snuggly over and around eyes.
- Place face shield over face and use the headband to secure it on the brow.
- Adjust for exact fitting.
- Safety goggles must fit snuggly even over prescription glasses with minimal gaps (Figs 3A to C).

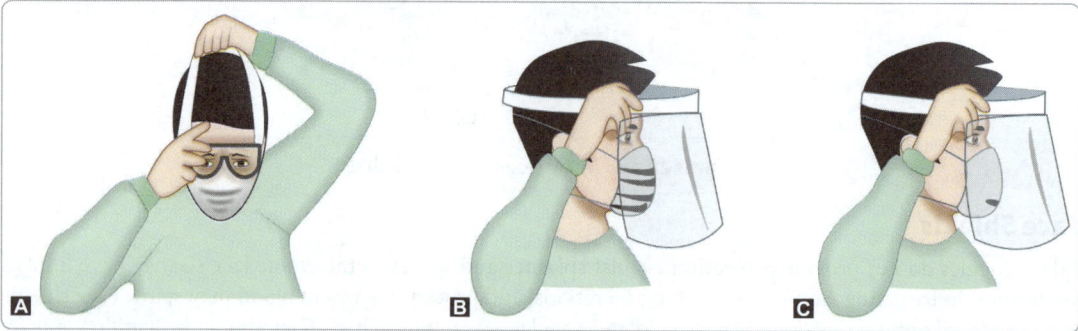

Figures 3A to C: Wearing goggles and face shield

Removing the Goggles and Face Shield

- Hold ear or head pieces with ungloved hands.
- Lift away from face.
- Dispose of the PPE in receptacles designated for that purpose.
- Wash hands or use an alcohol-based sanitizer after removing PPE, if your hands get contaminated during removal of PPE.

Shoe Covers

Shoe covers should be worn when exposure to blood or potentially infectious materials is anticipated.

Procedure

- Pick up a shoe cover (Figs 4A and B).
- Sit in a comfortable place which facilitates easy wear.

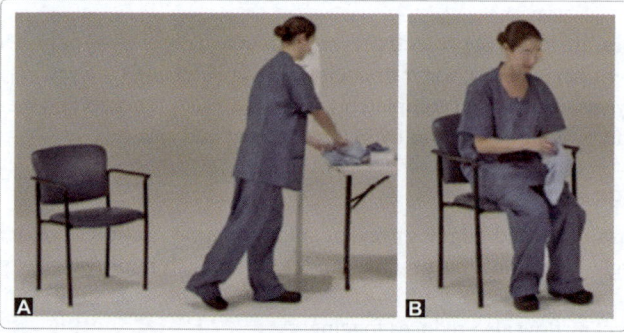

Figures 4A and B: Sit comfortably with a shoe cover

■ Wide open the shoe cover and put on your shoe covers. Make sure that all areas of the foot are covered and the boot or shoe covers are snug over your ankle and calf (Figs 5A and B).

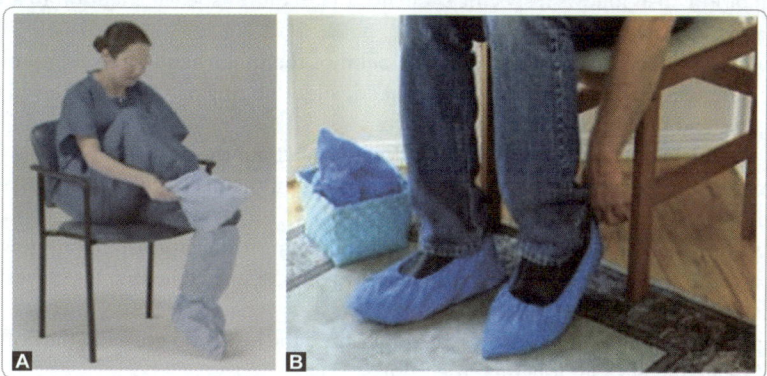

Figures 5A and B: Cover total area of the foot with shoe cover

■ If your shoes covers have a strap, wrap the strap around for a comfortable fit. Try not to touch the floor or other areas with your hands while putting the shoe covers on. If you do, disinfect your hands (Fig. 6).

Removal of Shoe Covers

■ Sit in the designated clean chair.
■ Once you sit down, be careful not to touch one leg with the other.
■ Then grasp the outside of the shoe cover and pull down toward your ankle with your gloved hand. Then, lift the

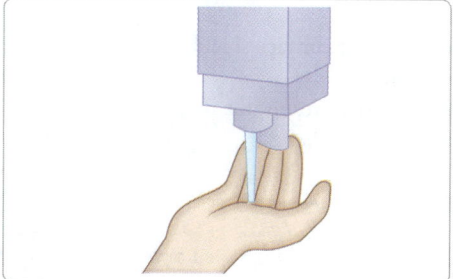

Figure 6: Disinfect hands

shoe cover over your heel, pull it off your foot and dispose of it correctly. The exact way to remove the shoe covers will vary based on the manufacturer's instructions (Figs 7A and B).

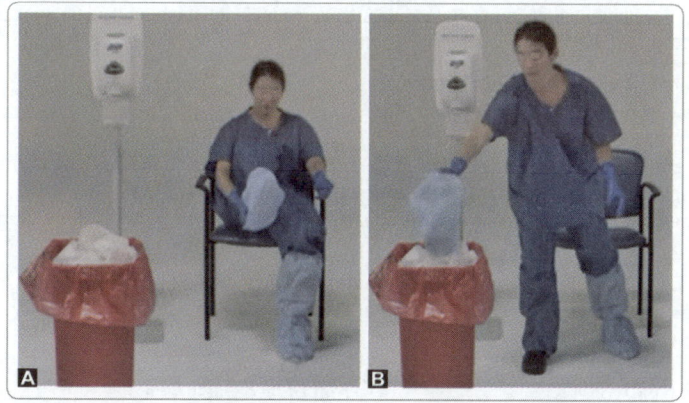

Figures 7A and B: Sit on clean chair and without touching one leg with other, remove and discard shoe covers in receptacle

■ Perform hand hygiene.

Unit VI ❖ **Infection Control**

General Instructions while Removing Personal Protective Equipment

The safe removal of PPE also follows a specific sequence that requires special attention to areas that are now considered contaminated:

- Gloves should be removed by first grasping the palm of the other hand and peeling off the first glove, keep hold of the removed glove in the gloved hand, slide the fingers of the ungloved hand under the remaining glove and peel it off over the first glove.
- Goggles or face shield should be removed by lifting from behind the head.
- Gowns should be untied and removed by pulling away from the neck and shoulders, turning the gown inside out and only touching the inside.
- Alternatively, the gloves and gown may be removed at the same time by grasping the gown from the front and pulling away from the body, rolling the gown into a bundle, and removing the gloves at the same time using the inside of the gown.
- Mask or respirator should be removed by reaching behind the head and grasping the bottom ties then the top ties, and removing without touching the front.

Order for Doffing (Removing) Personal Protective Equipment

- Gloves
- Goggles or face shield
- Gown
- Mask or respirator
- Perform hand hygiene

 **Note**

- If hands become soiled at any time while removing an article of PPE, stop and perform hand hygiene. Then, continue with PPE removal.
- Hand hygiene should be performed after removal of all PPE, and anytime during removal if they become contaminated.

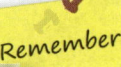 **Remember**

- Put on PPE before entering the patient's room.
- Keep hands away from face, and don't touch PPE.
- Avoid touching areas in the patient's room.
- Remove PPE at patient's doorway or outside of the room, and perform hand hygiene immediately.
- Remove the respirator outside of room after closing the patient's door.
- If hands become contaminated during PPE removal, stop and perform hand hygiene, and then proceed with PPE removal.

Clean Areas
- Inside of gloves
- Back of the gown
- Gown's ties
- Straps of face shield/goggles
- Straps of mask or respirator.

Contaminated Areas
- Outside of gloves
- Front of the gown
- Gown's sleeves
- Front of face shield/goggles
- Front of mask or respirator.

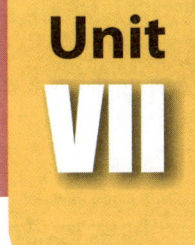

Unit VII

Therapeutic Nursing Measures

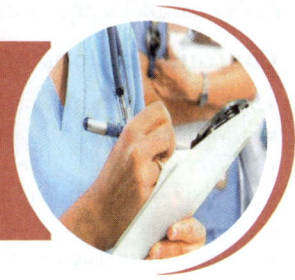

Hot Applications

Hot application means the application of an agent warmer than the skin.

THERAPEUTIC EFFECTS OF HEAT

The following are the therapeutic effects of heat:

Hemodynamic Effects

- Increases circulation twice than normal
- Increases inflammation, phagocytosis, wound healing
- Increases metabolism
- Decreases tissue stiffness (fluids less viscous and collagen releases)
- Decreases muscle spasm
- Decreases pain (analgesia); not as effective as cryotherapy for acute pain.

Neuromuscular Effects

- Inhibits muscle contraction
- Reduces muscle spasm
- Increases sensory nerve conduction.

THERAPEUTIC USES OF LOCAL HOT APPLICATIONS

- Provides warmth
- Stimulates peristalsis
- Softens the exudates
- Relieves deep congestion
- Promotes suppuration
- Promotes healing
- Decreases muscle tone
- Decreases pain.

Contraindications

- Impaired kidney, heart and lung functions.
- Malignancies
- Very old client and very young client
- Client with metabolic disorders.
- Headache
- Edema associated with venous or lymphatic diseases
- Open wounds
- Clients with paralysis
- Acutely inflamed areas
- Client with very high temperature.

Complications

- Hyperthermia
- Redness of the skin
- Burns
- Pain
- Pallor (secondary effect)
- Edema
- Maceration (with moist heat).

TYPES OF HOT APPLICATION

- **Local hot and dry:** Heat applied locally in the dry form, e.g., hot water bags, electric heating pads, electric cradles, heating lamps, diathermy.
- **Local hot and moist:** Heat applied locally in the moist form, e.g., fomentations, stupes, local baths, soaks, poultices, sitz baths.
- **General hot and dry:** Heat applied generally in the form of dry heat, e.g., hot dry packs, electric cradles to the whole body, blanket beds.
- **General hot and moist:** General application of heat in the moist form, e.g., hot wet packs, steam baths, hot baths.

Application of Local Dry Heat

Hot Water Bag

Application of hot water bag is a common method of applying local dry heat.

Purposes

- To relieve pain
- To reduce inflammation and congestion
- To supply warmth and comfort
- To aid in passing of urine, in case of retention of urine
- To stimulate circulation
- To relieve muscular spasm
- To promote healing
- To promote suppuration.

Requisites

A tray containing:

Articles	Purpose
• A jug or kettle with hot water at the right temperature.	• For pouring inside the hot water bag
• Bath thermometer, if available	• For checking the temperature of water
• Hot water bag and cover	• For hot application
• A duster	• For wiping the outside of the bag after pouring water
• A wash cloth or towel or a sheet	• To cover the bag before application
• Kidney tray	• For receiving waste

Procedure

Steps	Procedure	Rationale
1.	Explain the procedure to the patient.	Proper explanation allays anxiety and fosters cooperation.
2.	Prepare the equipment inspect the bag for any leakage and see that it has a good washer.	Organization facilitates accurate skill performance.
3.	Perform hand hygiene.	Prevents cross contamination.
4.	Test the temperature of the water by hand or using lotion thermometer. It should not exceed 149°F (65°C) for ordinary patient. For unconscious and paralyzed patients temperature should not exceed 120°–130°F (49°–55°C).	Hot water more than the prescribed temperature may cause burns.

Contd...

Unit VII ❖ Therapeutic Nursing Measures

Steps	Procedure	Rationale
5.	Fill 1/3 of the bottle or 1/2 with hot water. 1/3 or 1/2 depends upon the place where it is to be applied. 	Facilitates even heat transformation during application.
6.	Place the bag over a flat surface and expel air, cork it tightly. 	Air is a poor conductor of heat and cold. Corking tightly completely envelopes the water from the surrounding air.
7.	Test for any leakage by holding the bag upside down. 	Leakage in the hot water bag may burn the skin of the patient.
8.	Dry the outside with a duster.	Promotes comfort and protects clothing and linen.

Contd...

Steps	Procedure	Rationale
9.	Put on the cover (towel or pillow case) take it to the bedside. Never apply directly over the skin surface. 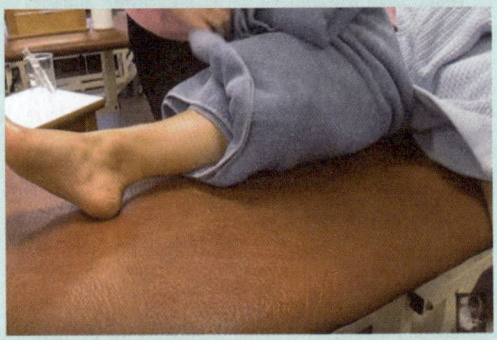	Ensures safety by protecting the skin from heat produced by hot rubber.
10.	Expose the needed part and apply it and cover with the sheet. If the application is to be continued it is refilled regularly and keep hot. In case of unconscious patient, patient in shock or an infant, the hot water bag should be placed outside the blanket covering the patient. 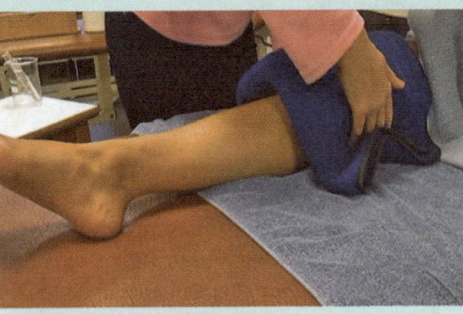	Ensures safety and prevents the risk of burns.
11.	Keep the bag in place for about 20–30 minutes, change the position in between as needed. Stand by the side of the patient and change the position of the bag often to avoid burning of the skin. Check the area for any redness, report it at once. Carelessness may lead to severe burns. Do not allow the client to lie on the hot water bag.	Promotes maximum therapeutic effect by convection to the surrounding space outside. Changing position prevents burns.

Contd...

Unit VII ❖ Therapeutic Nursing Measures

Steps	Procedure	Rationale
12.	Remove the cover, empty the bag, wash the outside with soap and water, dry it by hanging, fill it with air and keep in proper place. Wash the cover with soap and water, boil it and dry.	Prepares the equipment for next use.
13.	Perform hand hygiene.	Prevents spread of micro-organisms.
14.	Record whether it is applied for a therapy or comfort; also note the area to which it is applied, duration and the reaction of the patient with date, time and signature.	Documentation fosters quality care.

The temperature of the water depends upon the thickness of the cover used, the area to which the application is made and the condition of the patient and skin. Temperature may vary from 120°F to 149°F (49°C to 65°C).

Precautions

- Never apply the bag directly to the skin. There should be one or two layers of cloth between the patient and the bag.
- Note the temperature of the solution. Never give a hot water bag hotter than 149°F (65°C) to an ordinary patient and 120°F (49°C) to an unconscious patient. If it is for a baby, temperature should be 110°–115°F (40°–43°C)
- Test for leakage. The bag should have a proper cover.
- Change the position of the bag frequently when the patient is very serious or unconscious.
- When leaving a hot water bag to a very ill-patient report it to the ward sister while going off duty.
- Expel air when filling and avoid unnecessary weight.
- If the skin is reddened, report it at once and apply Vaseline or oil.
- The nurse who fills the bag is entirely responsible for refilling and keeping it at correct temperature.
- After application, record it in nurse's record.

Electric Cradle

- It is used to provide continuous dry heat from ordinary electric bulbs, especially for treatment of circulatory disturbances of lower extremities, to relieve tympanites, to dry plaster casts, etc.
- It is used when large body part is to be treated and covering of skin with gown or sheets is not possible.
- The cradle is equipped with several electric bulbs (25 Volts) which are enclosed in wire cages to prevent burns to the patient and accidental fire from contact with paper, linen or blanket.

Unit VII ❖ **Therapeutic Nursing Measures**

- A thermometer is hung inside the cradle to check the temperature.
- Sheet or blankets can be added over the cradle to maintain the heat at the desired levels.
- Duration of treatment is usually 20–30 minutes, after unit is warmed up, or can be used continuously to provide low temperature.

Hot Moist Local Applications

Hot moist applications are considered to be more penetrating than the dry applications.

Fomentations

Fomentations are moist applications of heat applied over an area by means of two thickness of flannel or other soft material wrung out from hot water or boiling water, protected by a water proof covering, wool and bandage. Fomentation can be prepared at the bedside or in the treatment room.

There are 3 types of fomentation:

1. Simple fomentation
2. Medicated fomentation
3. Surgical fomentation (when there is an open wound)

Simple Fomentation

Purposes

- To relieve pain and congestion by hastening the absorption of serous exudates
- To relieve inflammation by increasing hyperemia
- To relieve retention of urine
- To promote suppuration
- To stimulate the nerve endings and to increase peristalsis and relieve tympanites
- To relieve intestinal and renal colic
- To relieve muscular spasm
- To soften the crust and its easy removal
- To help in the absorption of exudates
- To relieve congestion in the internal organs.

Requisites: A tray containing:

Articles	Purpose
• A kettle of boiling water	• For moist heat application
• Fomentation pads or lint or flannel, large enough to cover the area, fomentation wringer and rods	• For application in the area
• Small mackintosh or jaconet larger than the fomentation pad. (Small mackintosh should be 1/2 inch (1.25 cm) larger than the fomentation pad all around and cotton pad should 1/2 inch (1.25 cm) larger than the Mackintosh all around)	• To prevent soiling of linen and clothes
• Cotton pad, binder, bandage and safety pins	• For securing the compress
• Two heated bowls	• One to keep the fomentation pad and wringer to prepare the heated pad and the other is to keep the prepared heated pad

Contd...

Unit VII ❖ Therapeutic Nursing Measures

Articles	Purpose
• Cotton balls and forceps	• To take the hot fomentation pad if required
• Hot water bag and cover	• To keep the fomentation hot
• Olive oil in a small dish	• For medicated fomentation
• Kidney tray or paper bag	• To dispose the soiled waste
• Bucket—1	• To discard the used water

Procedure

Steps	Procedure	Rationale
1.	Explain the procedure to the patient.	Allays anxiety and fosters cooperation.
2.	Screen the bed. Switch off the fan. Expose only the needed parts.	Provides privacy and prevents drought.
3.	Position the patient towards the edge of the bed. Place the mackintosh and towel under the body part.	Ensures proper body mechanics.
4.	Perform hand hygiene. Don gloves.	Prevents spread of microorganisms.
5.	Pour boiling water over the pad. Take the wringer and insert the rods. Place the fomentation pad in the wringer and keep it inside the bowl with free ends outside. Wring out the pad as dry as possible.	Wringers and the rods helps to remove excess hot water.

Contd...

Steps	Procedure	Rationale
6.	Keep the pad and wringer in the heated bowl and cover it with the other bowl after removing the rods. Take it to the patient. (To prepare the heated bowls, rotate the used boiled water in the same one and pour it to the other bowl and do the same rotation and discard the water to the bucket so that both the vessels become heated).	Prevents heat loss.
7.	Arrange the top bedding of the patient and expose the area to receive the fomentation.	Provides privacy and prevents chilling.
8.	Open the wringer, take out the pad with the forceps, and shake it well in order to allow some steam to escape. Test the temperature by applying it inside the wrist of your hand. Make sure that it should not burn the patient. Then apply it over the area.	Optimum temperature prevents burns.

Contd...

Steps	Procedure	Rationale
9.	Fomentation pad should be changed every 15 minutes. The procedure has been shown in figures. 	Prevents heat loss and maintains temperature constantly.
10.	Once the procedure is over, remove the fomentation. Dry the skin. Make the patient comfortable. Wash the pad and wringer, dry them well and keep them in proper place. 	Promotes comfort and prepares the articles for next procedure.

Contd...

Unit VII ❖ Therapeutic Nursing Measures

Steps	Procedure	Rationale
11.	After removal, the part should be dried gently and kept covered with that cotton pad for 10 minutes. Any reddening or blistering should be reported immediately. Olive oil may be smeared to protect the area from irritation.	Avoids chill.
12.	Doff gloves and wash hands.	Prevents spread of infection.
13.	Record date, time and duration and the effect of application along with the signature.	Documentation fosters quality care.

Medicated Fomentation

Turpentine stupes: It is a medicated local hot wet application.

Purposes

- To relieve tympanites by irritating the nerve endings of the intestinal wall.
- To increase peristalsis.
- To relax muscular spasm.
- To help the expulsion of gas from the intestines.

Requisites: A tray containing:

Articles	Purpose
• A kettle of boiling water	• For moist heat application
• Fomentation pad, fomentation wringer and rods	• For local application
• A small piece of water-proof sheeting or flannel 1" (2.5 cm) larger all sides than the fomentation pad.	• To prevent soiling of linen and clothes
• Cotton pad, binder or bandage (Cotton pad should be larger than water proof sheeting)	• For securing the compress
• Bowls—2	• Heated bowls to carry the foment to the patient as described in simple fomentation
• Cotton balls in a small bowl	• For application of medication
• Forceps—1	• For applying the warm cotton balls dipped in medication
• Kidney tray—1	• To receive the waste
• Hot water bag with cover	• To keep the fomentation hot
• A cup with turpentine and oil mixed in the correct proportion and kept in the bowl of warm water	• For medicated fomentation
• Bucket—1	• To receive the used water
• Articles needed to introduce the flatus tube in a separate tray. Flatus tube in a kidney tray with warm water	• For expulsion of gas from intestines
• Vaseline in a rag piece	• To apply over the skin
• Rag pieces in a bowl	• For application of Vaseline
• Mackintosh and draw sheet	• One each to put under the part
• Screen—1 (if the procedure is done in general ward)	• To provide privacy

Contd...

Procedure

Steps	Procedure	Rationale
Follow the steps of simple fomentation till step 1–6		
7.	Keep the pad and wringer in the heated bowl and cover it with the other bowl as described under simple fomentation. 	Prevents heat loss.
8.	Take the tray to the patient. Expose the needed part. Apply warm oil mixture over the part with cotton balls and forceps. 	Prevents unnecessary exposure.
9.	Open the wringer, take out the pad with the forceps, and shake it well in order to allow some steam to escape. Test it by applying it inside our wrist to make sure that it will not scald the patient. Then apply the foment over the area. 	Optimum temperature prevents burns.

Contd...

Steps	Procedure	Rationale
10.	Cover it with water-proof sheeting, if available, or flannel pad and apply cotton pads and secure it in position with binder.	Prevents heat loss.
11.	Place the hot water bag just above the binder to keep it warm otherwise the fomentation pad should be changed every 15 minutes; usually continued for 15–20 minutes. This may be ordered every 4 hours.	Prevents heat loss.
12.	Lubricate the flatus tube with Vaseline and insert it into the rectum. Keep the other end of the tube in a kidney tray containing water.	Ensures propulsion of gas.
13.	Keep the fomentation for 15–20 minutes and then remove it and allow the flatus tube to remain for another 10 minutes. Observe whether any flatus is coming out. After 10 minutes remove the flatus tube, rearrange the bed and make the patient comfortable. After removal of the pad, the part should be dried gently and kept covered with cotton wool for 10 minutes to avoid chill. Any reddening or blistering should be reported immediately.	Avoids chill.
14.	Wash the pad and wringer, dry well and keep them in the proper place. Remove the cover and empty the hot water bag, clean it and return it to the proper place. Wash the flatus tube, boil and dry it by hanging and then replace it in the proper place.	Prepares for next use.
15.	Doff gloves and wash hands.	Prevents spread of infection.
16.	Record the treatment, the time, date, effect of the application and signature of the nurse.	Documentation fosters quality care.

Precautions

- Great care should be taken to test the temperature of the pad to prevent scalding the skin. If the patient complains of any burning sensation before the prescribed period has expired, the treatment should be discontinued.
- Avoid chilling the part before, during or after the treatment.
- Oil the skin if very red.
- The ratio of turpentine to olive oil is 1:3 for adults and 1:6 for children. Ensure that they are well mixed before the application.

INHALATION

Inhalation is defined as the drawing of air or other vapors into the lungs through the mouth or nose. Drugs may be given by inhalation for either a systemic or a local effect. The systemic effect is produced immediately because of a large surface area of the lungs and the rich blood supply, e.g., inhalation of ammonia to overcome fainting, amyl nitrate to relieve pain in Angina pectoris.

Drugs used for local effect may be in the form of medicated steam or fumes, e.g., fumes from stramonium leaves to relieve spasm.

Types of Inhalation

- **Dry inhalation:** The inhalation of fumes from volatile drugs or burning drugs, e.g., anesthesia using chloroform, nitrous oxide, menthol, eucalyptus, and ammonia in spirit.
- **Moist inhalation:** The inhalation of plain steam or saturated with a drug. It is a hot wet application of heat. We will discuss it in detail.

Purposes of Moist Steam Inhalation

- To relieve inflammation and congestion of the mucous membrane in acute colds and sinusitis.
- To relieve inflammation, congestion and edema of the larynx.
- To soften thick, tenacious mucus and to relieve coughing.
- To warm and moisten the air following operations such as tracheotomy.
- To relieve irritation in bronchitis and whooping cough, by moistening the air.
- As a respiratory disinfectant.

Solutions used:

- Plain water
- Tincture Benzoin 4 mL (1 dr) to 500 mL of boiling water
- Menthol in alcohol few drops to 500 mL of boiling water
- Oil of eucalyptus 2 mL to 500 mL of boiling water
- A few camphor crystals to 500 mL of boiling water.

Methods

- Nelson's inhaler (Fig. 1)
- Jug method
- Continuous steam by a tent or canopy over the bed.

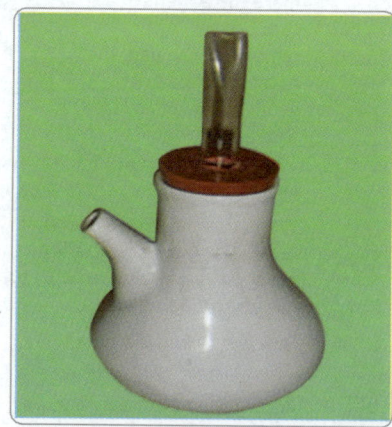

Figure 1: Nelson's inhaler

Medicated Inhalation by Using Nelson's Inhaler

Requisites: A tray containing:

Articles	Purpose
• Nelson's inhaler with glass mouth piece, passed through a cork which fits the neck of the inhaler. (Mouth piece should be boiled and cooled before use)	• To use as vaporizer
• A bowl with gauze pieces	• To wrap around the mouth piece
• A bowl with cotton balls	• To place at the steam exit or air inlet
• Tissue papers or face towel	• To wipe the secretion and to remove sweat from face during inhalation
• A deep basin	• To hold the inhaler
• A flannel or towel piece	• To cover the inhaler
• Inhalant in a bottle	• For inhalation
• Teaspoon or minim glass and pint measure	• For measuring the inhalant and water
• Boiling water in kettle. The temperature of water should remain between 120°F and 160°F or 54.5°–76.7°C	• To prepare the solution
• Sputum mug	• To cough and collect the sputum

Preparation of Patient and Environment

- Explain the procedure to the patient.
- Allow the patient to empty the bladder and bowel, if necessary give bed pan or urinal to bed-ridden patient.
- Provide Fowler's position with back rest, cardiac table and extra pillows.
- Observe the patient closely throughout the procedure for adverse effects.
- If volatile drugs are used (e.g., menthol), warn the patient to keep his/her eyes closed to prevent the drug irritating the conjunctiva.

Procedure

Steps	Procedure	Rationale
1.	Explain the procedure to the patient	Allays anxiety and wins confidence and cooperation of the patient
2.	Screen the patient. Close windows, door and put off the fans	Prevents draught
3.	Place the patient in semi Fowlers or sitting position if possible with a cardiac table in front is more convenient	Diaphragmatic excursion and lung compliance are more in this position and ensures deposition of aerosolized particles to basilar region of the lungs

Contd...

Unit VII ❖ Therapeutic Nursing Measures

Steps	Procedure	Rationale
4.	Wash hands	Prevents transmission of microorganisms
5.	Warm inhaler by pouring little hot water into the jug and emptying it	To maintain the temperature of the water constant for a longer period
6.	Pour the required amount of inhalant into the inhaler usually 4 mL to 1 pint. Fill 2/3 of the inhaler with boiling water or according to the instructions written on the inhaler	If the spout is filled with the water, it will not act as an air inlet, the patient will not get warmed air. It also prevents scalding of the patient
7.	Put the cork with the mouth piece and wrap the mouth piece with a gauze piece and cover the spout with thin layer of cotton. See that the mouth piece is in opposite direction to the spout	Prevents steam loss
8.	Cover the inhaler with a flannel or towel	Insulates the jug and prevents heat loss
9.	Place the inhaler in the basin and take it to the patient's bedside	Prevents burns
10.	Arrange the apparatus conveniently with the spout opposite to the patient. Remove cotton plug. Cover the head with blanket	Reduces the chance of burns. Removing cotton plug helps to keep up patency of spout for air entry

Contd...

Steps	Procedure	Rationale
11.	Instruct the patient to place his/her lips to the mouth piece and breathe in, to receive the steam and to breathe out through the nose removing his/her lips from the mouth piece. Place the sputum mug within the reach of the patient 	Relieves the congestion of mucous membrane
12.	Treatment is continued from 15 to 20 minutes. The patient should be instructed not to go out, but to remain in the same room for 15 minutes after inhalation. Wipe off the perspiration, make the patient comfortable	Prevents draught
13.	Clean and replace the articles. (Minim glass to be cleaned first with spirit swabs and then with soap and water). Empty the inhaler, clean its inside with spirit and finally with soap and water Mouth piece to be cleaned and boiled for next use after discarding the gauze piece	Prepares for next procedure
14.	Wash hands	Prevents transmission of microorganisms
15.	Document the procedure, inhalant used, reaction of the patient with date, time and signature	Documentation fosters quality care

Jug Method

An ordinary jug may be used if Nelson's inhaler is not available. But in this case, as there is no mouth piece; the patient may put a towel over his/her head in order to form a canopy under which to collect steam, or the mouth of the jug may be draped with a towel in a turban fashion to render the opening small enough for the patient to keep his/her nose and mouth to it or make a cone with a thick paper suitable to cover the mouth of the jug. Cover the jug with the base of the cone. Through a hole made on the top of the cone, the patient can breathe in the steam. In home situation, it is a good method (Figs 2A and B).

Unit VII ❖ Therapeutic Nursing Measures

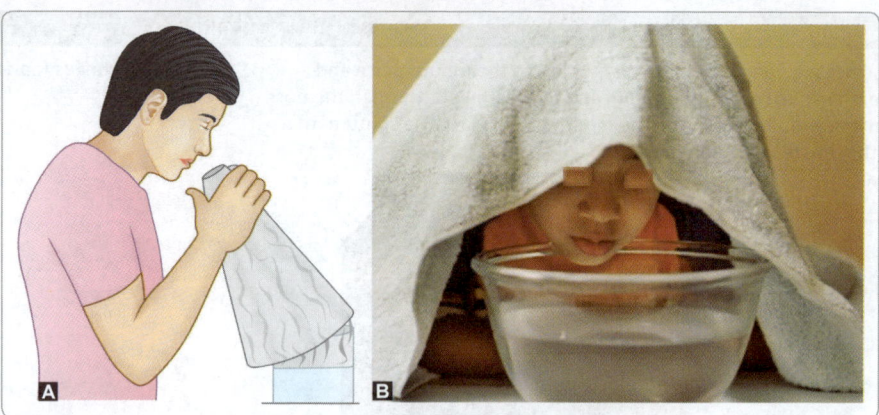

Figures 2A and B: Ask patient to inhale steam through cone or by making canopy

Steam Kettle

It is used to maintain a constantly moist warm atmosphere when required to supply steam for the treatment (Fig. 3).

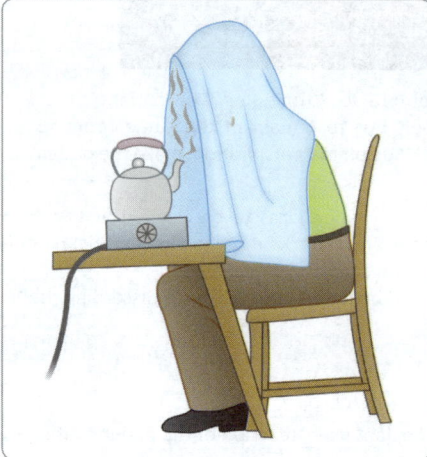

Figure 3: Steam kettle

Steam Tent

Aim is to keep the steam in a confined space so that the patient will get more of it for a continued period of time. When a high concentration of stream is required, a steam tent may be used. A canopy made from woolen blankets fastened with safety pins is arranged over the head of the bed over a special frame. The sides of the blankets are left hanging loose to aid in ventilation. Woolen blankets are preferred because they absorb much moisture and will not drip. The steam is directed away from the patient by inserting the spout of the kettle through an opening between the blankets at the side of the bed preferably from the back of the shoulders pointing upwards. Treatment should be continued for the length of time ordered. The steam may be given for 20–30 minutes at a time and it may be repeated every four hours (Figs 4A and B).

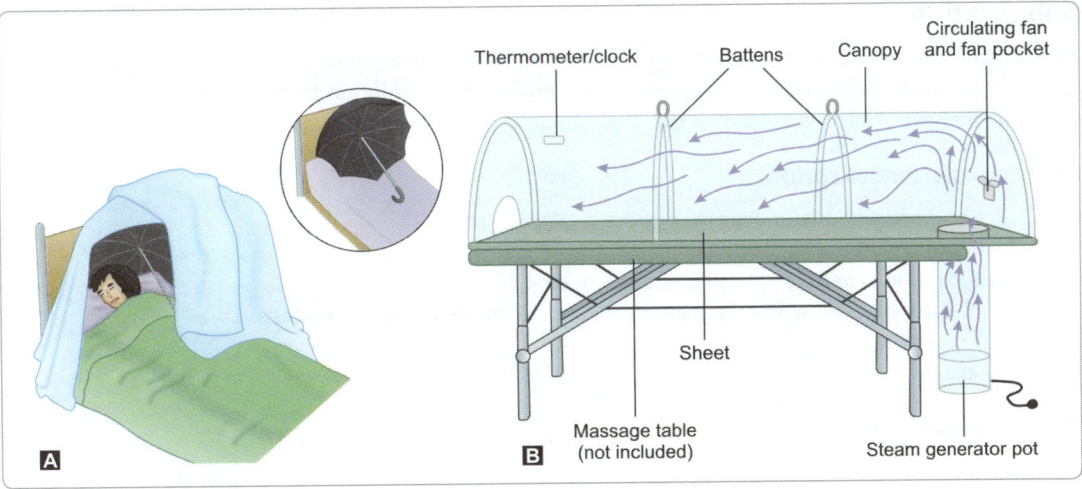

Figures 4A and B: Use umbrella or readymade steam tent

Electric Steam Inhaler

Small electric vaporizers can be used to give steam inhalation. It consists of a small jar with a heating element extending into the jar. The jar is filled with water. On the top of the jar is a removable perforated cup to which is attached a small metal spout (Fig. 5). Cotton saturated with medication is placed inside the cup and the metal spout is fitted over the cup. As the water boils, the medicated steam is directed through the spout which is inhaled by the patient.

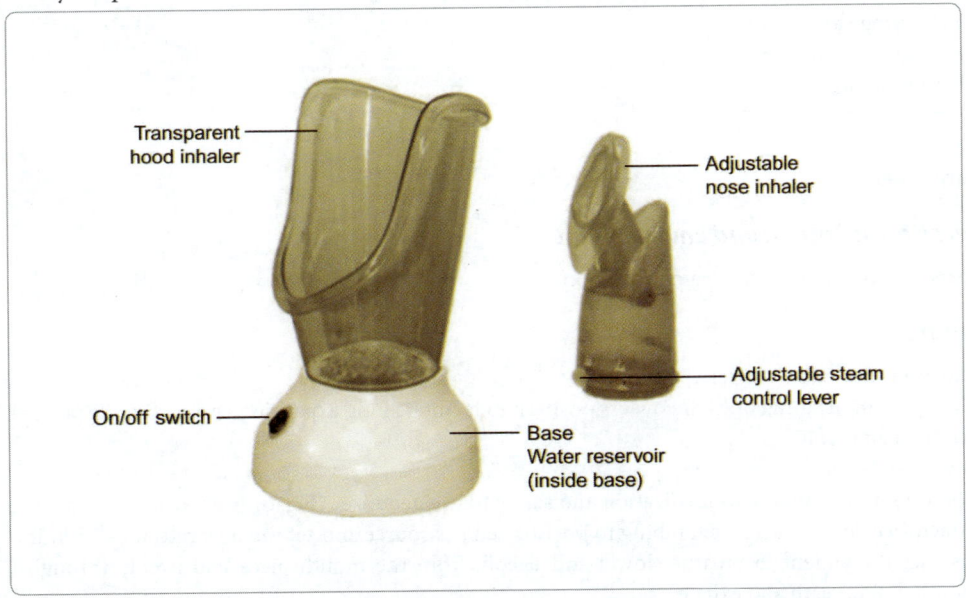

Figure 5: Electric steam inhaler

Nebulization

Nebulization means administering drugs by inhalation. A nebulizer is a small machine that turns liquid medicine into a mist. The equalizer present in this breaks up the solution to be inhaled into fine droplets which are then suspended in a steam of gas. The patient actively inhales this gas stream containing the drug.

Indications of Nebulization

- Delivery of bronchodilator drugs
- Infants and children with asthma
- Administration of antibiotics and antifungal agents.
- In some cases of resistant chest infections, e.g., cystic fibrosis or bronchiectasis
- To aid expectoration
- Local analgesia

Types of Nebulizers

- Jet nebulizers
- Ultrasonic nebulizers

Requisites

- Nebulizers
- Pressurized gas source
- Flow meter
- Oxygen tubing
- T-Piece mouthpiece or mask or other appropriate gas delivery devices
- Sterile normal saline solution or sterile distilled water
- 5 mL syringe and water
- Prescribed medication
- Flannel or a towel
- Sputum mug
- Kidney tray
- Face towel

Preparation of Patient and Environment

The steps are same as that for steam inhalation.

Procedure

- Explain procedure to patient.
- Place patient in sitting or high Fowlers position to facilitate lung expansion and aerosol dispersion to the basilar region of lungs.
- Wash hands before procedure.
- Add prescribed amount of medication and saline to the nebulizer (Fig. 6).
- Attach free end of the oxygen tubing to pressurized gas source and set the flow rate at 6–8 L/min.
- Instruct the patient to breathe slowly and deeply from the mouth piece and evenly through his/her mouth, hold breath and exhale.
- Remain with the patient during treatment (usually 15–20 minutes).
- Encourage the patient to cough out the sputum. Provide a sputum mug for spitting the expectoration.

- Make sure, the patient is comfortable.
- Document the time, date and duration of therapy, type, amount of medication added to nebulizer and the result of therapy such as loosened secretions, with signature.

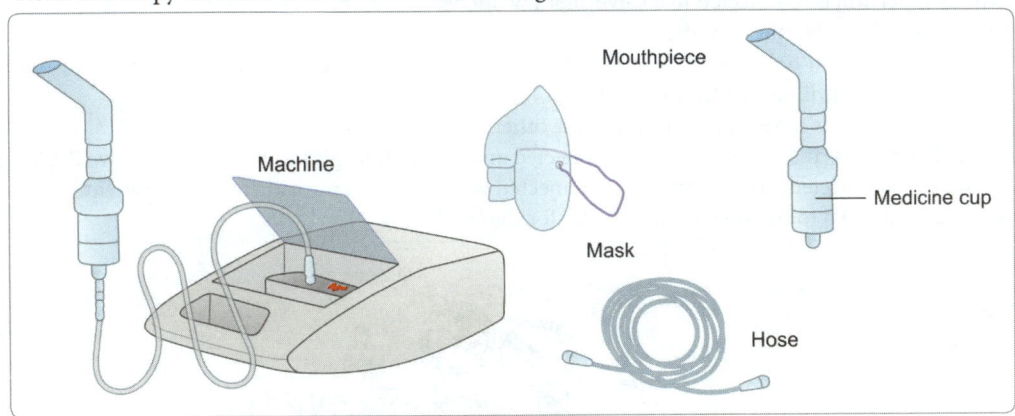

Figure 6: Nebulizer apparatus

Oxygen Inhalation

Oxygen is a colorless, odorless, tasteless gas heavier than air, a constituent of air and water, needed for all plant and animal life. It supports combustion, so it is kept away from inflammable material.

Oxygen is administered by inhalation to relieve anoxemia (deficiency of oxygen in the blood) and anoxia—a condition in which the body cells and tissues obtain insufficient oxygen to carry on the normal function.

Indications of Oxygen Therapy

- Any patient who is cyanosed or who has labored breathing.
- Shock and peripheral circulatory failure or patients under anesthesia.
- Poisoning with chemicals which alter the ability of the tissues to utilize oxygen in the body, e.g., cyanide poisoning.
- Hemorrhage and air hunger or psychologically induced dyspnea.
- Poisoning.
- In patients whose respiratory capacity is diminished by some disease as pneumonia or any operation on the lung or injury to the lung.
- To treat the diseases as congestive heart failure, coronary thrombosis, asthma and emphysema.
- Anemia and patients who are critically ill.
- An environment low in oxygen content like high altitudes.
- Asphyxia due to any reason like drowning, blockage of air passages by foreign bodies, electric shock, etc.

Methods of Administration

- Nasal or oral catheter
- Nasal or oral mask (Boothby, Lovelace and Bulbulian [BLB])
- Oxygen tent or chamber
- Nasal prongs or cannula
- Venturi mask

Unit VII ❖ Therapeutic Nursing Measures

Requisites

- Oxygen is supplied in cylinders of different capacity (or different sizes).
- This cylinder will be connected to a valve and flow meter.
- Key is needed to open the cylinder.
- A bottle with a two-holed cork through which 2 glass tubes are passed and with half full of water is connected to the cylinder with rubber tubings.
- Out of the two glass tubes, one is long and the other is short.
- To the longer glass tube, the cylinder is connected and to the short glass tube, which is above the level of the water is connected a rubber tubing is connected which leads to the catheter to the patient.
- A stand is attached to the side of the cylinder for the bottle (Fig. 7).

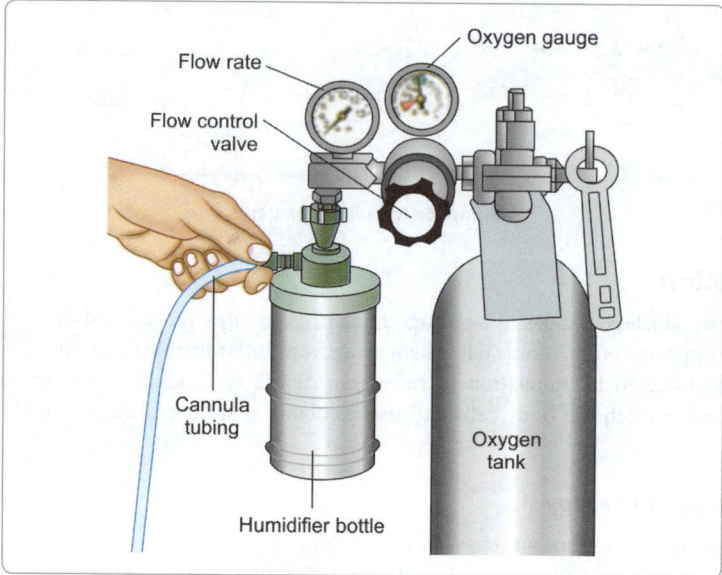

Figure 7: Equipment for oxygen therapy

 Stimulant

Important points to remember in handling the cylinder.
- Oxygen is irritating to the mucous membrane lining the nose and throat. Therefore, it is always passed through the water to humidify it. The bottle should be only half filled.
- It is never kept near an inflammable material.
- Never use oils or alcohol in the connections of the cylinder.
- Avoid electric pads. Turn off flow valve when cylinder valve is being opened and always check for leakage.
- 'NO SMOKING' board has to be displayed near the oxygen tent or chambers and smoking should be strictly prohibited.
- When cylinder is empty always, mark 'Empty'.
- The catheter should have three or four holes in the sides of the tip, to avoid the concentration of oxygen at one spot and also to prevent blocking by mucus from nose.

Preliminary Assessment of Patient and Situation

- Check the doctor's order and note the precautions in moving the patient, amount of oxygen to be given, etc.
- Get the instructions and help from the senior sister.
- Identify the patient and note the diagnosis, need for oxygen, amount of cyanosis, etc.
- Assess the response of patient to the therapy and breathing patterns.
- Check the vital signs and the type of pulmonary dysfunction.
- Assess the interior of the nose and surroundings.
- Check the patient's mood and ability to understand the instructions.
- Check the articles available in the unit.

Administration of Oxygen

Requisites

- Oxygen cylinder with all the accessories.
- A tray containing:

Articles	Purpose
• Nasal catheter/nasal prongs/oxygen mask in a cover	• To deliver oxygen
• Adhesive tapes and scissors	• To fix the catheter
• Bowl of water	• To check the flow of oxygen
• Flash light and tongue depressor	• To note the placement of catheter
• Cotton applicators and normal saline in a container	• To clean the nostrils
• Kidney tray and paper bag	• To receive the waste and tongue depressor after use
• Mackintosh and towel	• To protect the dress of the patient and bed
• Water soluble lubricating jelly	• For lubricating the nasal catheter
• Rag pieces or gauze pieces	• To wipe the secretions from nose and mouth during the procedure

Procedure

Steps	Procedure	Rationale
1.	Explain the procedure if the patient is conscious.	Allays anxiety and wins his cooperation.
2.	Check the doctor's order for flow rate and specific instructions.	Ensures safe administration.
3.	Perform hand hygiene and wear PPE.	Prevents spread of microorganisms.
4.	Assemble necessary articles near the bedside.	Organization facilitates skilful procedure.

Contd...

Unit VII ❖ Therapeutic Nursing Measures

Steps	Procedure	Rationale
5.	Prepare oxygen equipment by attaching the flow meter into the wall outlet or oxygen cylinder. 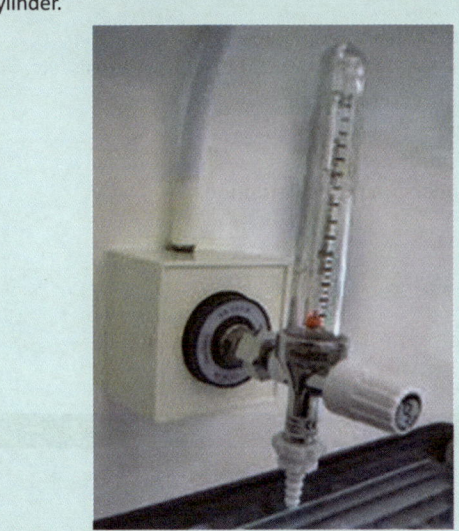	Humidification prevents drying of nasal mucosa Testing ensures appropriate flow of oxygen.
	Fill 1/3rd of the humidifier with sterile water. 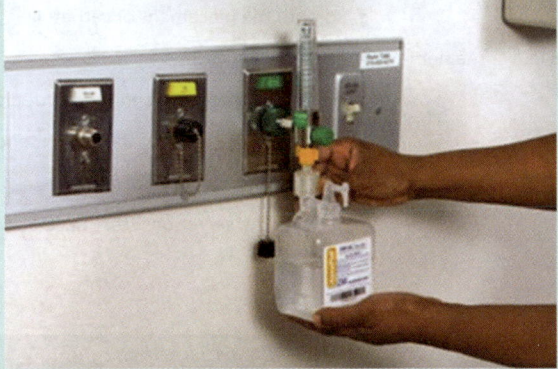	Proper tubing connection to facilitate correct flow of oxygen.
	Attaching the cannula/catheter/mask to the tubings. 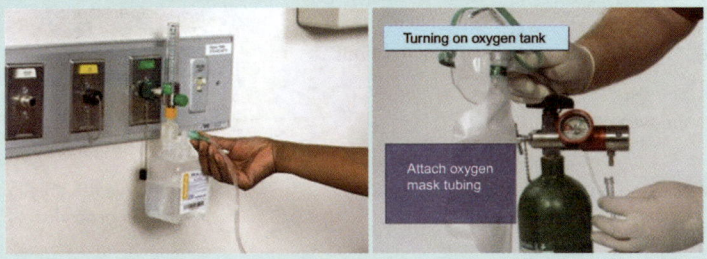 Turning on oxygen tank Attach oxygen mask tubing	
	Testing the flow of oxygen by opening the valve on your hand or by immersing the end of the catheter into a bowl of water.	

Contd...

Steps	Procedure	Rationale
6.	Open the cylinder before introducing the catheter into the nose. **Never open the cylinder after introducing the catheter in to the nose**. Adjust the flow rate and then introduce the catheter.	To avoid risk to patient.
7.	Now attach any one of the following to the patient for administering oxygen. **Oxygen administration through nasal catheter:** Lubricate the catheter before passing into the nose. Be careful that the tip of the catheter is not blocked by the lubricant. Hold the catheter, measure the distance between the nostrils and the lobe of the ear to make sure how much length is to be inserted into the nostril and mark it.	Lubricate catheter to avoid injury to mucus membrane.
	Gently introduce the catheter rotating as it is introduced up to the mark, slowly along the floor of the nasal cavity into the oropharynx. Observe the position of the catheter through the patient's mouth. Make sure that the catheter is in the position and not coiled up inside the mouth. This observation can be done only when the patient is conscious. Use flash light and tongue depressor to look in the mouth if needed. Fix the catheter in position to the cheek or to the fore head with adhesive tape. Uvula; Catheter tip placed behind uvula	To avoid any harm and to facilitate accuracy in procedure.

Contd...

Steps	Procedure	Rationale
	Administration of oxygen by using nasal catheter: • Oxygen flow can be regulated as desired according to the condition of the patient. • Oxygen may be given up to 4 L/min for adults or as prescribed by the physician. • Never leave an unconscious or struggling patient alone while administering oxygen. • Catheter should be changed every 12 hours if it is to be continued for a long time. • Always check the amount of oxygen in the cylinder at regular intervals throughout your duty time.	To facilitate accurate flow of oxygen.
	Oxygen administration through a nasal prongs/cannula:	
	Insert the nasal cannula into the client's nostrils and adjust the tubing behind the client's ears and slide the plastic adapter under the client's chin. Ensure if patient is comfortable.	Proper positioning allows unobstructed flow of oxygen.

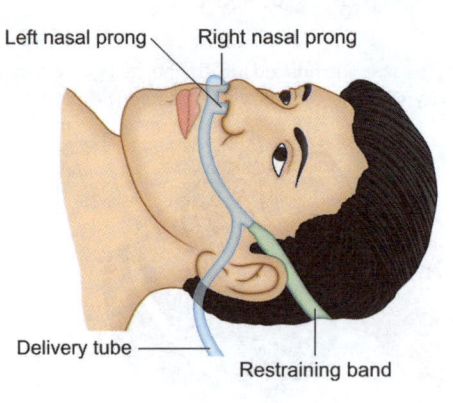

Left nasal prong

Right nasal prong

Delivery tube

Restraining band

Contd...

Steps	Procedure	Rationale
	Oxygen administration through a face mask:	
	Guide the elastic strap over the top of the client's head. Bring the strap down just below the client's ears. Gently and firmly, pull the strap extensions to center the mask on the client's face with a tight seal. 	For proper fitting.
8.	Encourage the client to breathe through the nose and expire from the mouth. 	Breathing through the nose inhales more oxygen into the respiratory system.
9.	Assess the patient's response to oxygen and the comfort of patient. Replace the articles	Anxiety stimulates the need for oxygen
10.	Doff gloves and perform hand washing	Prevents spread of infection
11.	Document the procedure with date, time, amount of oxygen administered, response of the patient, any adverse events and the signature	Documentation fosters quality care

Administration of Oxygen by Using BLB Mask

- This apparatus consists of a rubber mask joined by a metal-connecting device to a thin rubber bag similar to a football bladder.
- The usual type of mask is the oronasal one.
- The mask is fastened round the head by a rubber strap. Two tubes leading from the sides of the nose-piece pass around the sides of the mouth joining over the chin to form a single tube to which the metal tube connecting with breathing bag is attached.
- The connecting tube is fitted with an inlet tube for the oxygen.

Unit VII ❖ Therapeutic Nursing Measures

- With a flow of oxygen of 8–12 L/min an alveolar concentration of 25–60% oxygen can be attained.
- The rubber bag has capacity of 700 mL and should always be slightly distended while the apparatus is in use.
- When the patient breathes out, the expired air enters the bag and is mixed with the incoming oxygen.
- When the patient inspires the mixture of air and oxygen in the bag passes through the connecting tube into the mask.
- The bag should be tested to see for any hole.
- There should be no kinking in tubing.
- The size of mask should be suitable to the face.
- The nasal type of BLB mask allows the patient to eat and drink and to expectorate while wearing it.

Oxygen Tent

- It consists of a canopy which is made up of completely transparent material which covers the whole patient or part of the bed (Figs 8A and B).
- The canopy is attached to a frame and whole is mounted on wheels enabling the tent to be moved easily.
- The canopy has openings through which nurse's arms can be put to give attention to the patient.
- The aim of the tent is to have an oxygen content of 40–60% (average 50%) inside the tent.
- The excess carbon dioxide must be removed and air is prevented from becoming too hot and excessively humid.
- The cooling of the air inside the tent is effected by passing the air through an ice box or through a refrigeration unit and in some types of tents the carbon dioxide is removed by passing the air through a container of soda lime.
- A wall thermometer is hung inside the tent to check the temperature.
- It requires high volume of oxygen (10–12 liters) to use and hence it is not used ordinarily for adults.

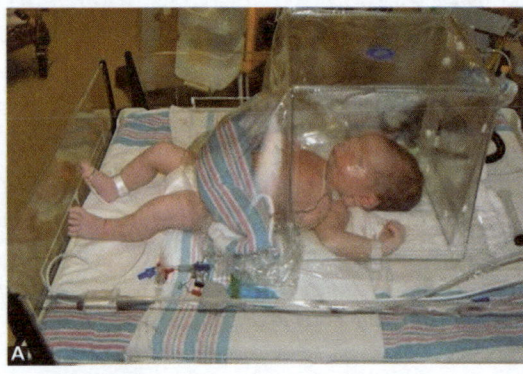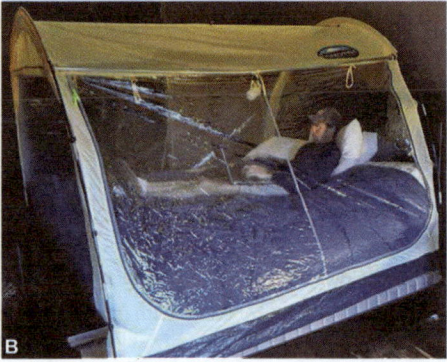

Figures 8A and B: Oxygen tent: (A) Partial type; (B) Whole type

Special Points

- The patient can be propped up in Fowler's position.
- The circulation of oxygen is maintained according to the doctor's orders. The concentration of oxygen in the tent should be checked at intervals.
- Nursing care should be planned so that the number of times the tent is opened should be minimum. Temperature in the tent should be maintained to 60°F.

- Care should be taken to prevent escape of oxygen by protecting the bed by rubber sheets.
- Since oxygen is a supporter of combustion 'No Smoking' label should be placed in the oxygen cylinder and no visitors should be allowed to smoke nearby.
- Any appliances or articles that sparkle should be kept away.
- Observe the general condition of the patient.
- The tent shall be inspected for any hole beforehand.
- After use the canopy should be washed well.
- Always follow the direction that is given on the tent for the use.

Cold Applications

Cold application is the application of dry or moist cold to a part of the body or to the total body surface

PURPOSES OF COLD APPLICATION

- To reduce fever
- To relieve pain and to prevent or reduce swelling
- To check hemorrhage
- To check inflammation and abscess formation.

EFFECTS OF COLD APPLICATION AND SCIENTIFIC PRINCIPLES

- **Vasoconstriction:** The constriction of blood vessels reduces circulation and thereby relieves pain caused by pressure. Tissue metabolism is decreased and also checks hemorrhage.
- **Numbness:** Intense cold is capable of affecting sensory nerves so that they are numbed and lose their ability to transmit sensations.
- **Check suppuration and inflammatory process:** Cold checks the activity of all living cells and checks the growth and activities of bacteria thereby the process of suppuration will be checked. As cold lessens the supply of blood in the part, the inflammatory process will also be checked.
- **Relief from pain:** Cold causes the involuntary muscles in the skin to contract and thus squeezes blood from capillaries of skin and thus relieves pain.
- **Sedative action:** Cold soothes nerve endings and gives a sedative action.
- **Vasoconstriction and vasodilatation:** Immediate effect of cold application is vasoconstriction but prolonged effect is vasodilatation.
- **Reduce body temperature and body resistance:** Prolonged application of cold reduces body temperature. So even death may result due to reduction of body temperature and lowered resistance.
- **Effect on internal organs:** Cold, when applied locally has action on the internal organs also. Due to reflex action, moist cold penetrates better than dry as water is a better conductor of cold than air.

    The effect of cold application depends upon the mode of application, the temperature, the duration, surface of the body where it is applied and the condition of the skin and patient.

CONTRAINDICATIONS OF COLD APPLICATION

- Do not apply cold pack if the patient shows symptoms of impaired circulation.
- When there is an infected wound where we want to drain off the pus, avoid cold application.

Unit VII ❖ Therapeutic Nursing Measures

- When we want to promote suppuration, cold application should be avoided.
- Cold application should be avoided on a part where there is poor nutrition.
- In anemic conditions and gastric disturbances, cold applications are contraindicated.

LOCAL DRY COLD APPLICATION

Ice Bag: Filling and Applying

Requisites

- A tray containing a bowl with ice pieces
- Hammer or something to break the ice
- Common salt in a cup and a spoon
- Ice bag with cover
- Small towel or duster
- Mackintosh and towel to protect the bed.

Action of Common Salt on Ice

While filling ice bag for local dry cold applications we add common salt in ice to make it a freezing mixture. A freezing mixture is formed by mixing a suitable soluble salt with ice. When common salt (NaCl) is added to ice, some ice melts in cooling the salt to 0°C and saturate solution of the salt at 0°C. But ice cannot remain in equilibrium with a saturated solution of the salt at 0°C, since the freezing point of a solution is always lower than the freezing point of the pure solvent. Hence, more ice melts taking the necessary latent heat from the solution, which in consequence gets further cooled. The cooling goes on until a temperature of –21°C is reached. Similarly, by mixing calcium chloride ($CaCl_2$) and ice, a temperature as low as –55°C can be produced.

Procedure

Steps	Procedure	Rationale
1.	Explain the procedure to the patient.	Allays anxiety and wins cooperation.
2.	Inspect the bag for holes and ascertain whether it is in good order. Assemble the equipment in the treatment room.	Organization facilitates skilled performance.

Contd...

Steps	Procedure	Rationale
3.	Perform hand hygiene. 	Prevents spread of microorganisms.
4.	• Break the ice into small pieces • Sprinkle with salt one teaspoon and put into the bag • Fill half of the bag with ice • Keep the bag on a flat surface and squeeze out the air • Screw the cap tightly • Test it for any leakage • Wipe the outside, put on the cover and place in the tray and take it to the bedside	Prevents melting of ice.
5.	Protect the bed with mackintosh and towel. Apply the bag to the part ordered. An ice bag should only rest lightly on the body. It should be suspended by a cradle or suspended on the head end of the bed so that no weight is on the part. When the ice has melted, remove it and refill if necessary and apply again. If there is an internal bleeding, the bag should be hung on a bed cradle touching slightly to the part. 	Prevents soiling of linen and clothes.

Contd...

Unit VII ❖ Therapeutic Nursing Measures

Steps	Procedure	Rationale
6.	After using the ice bag, empty it, wash it with soap and water. If it is greasy, wash with warm water and soap. After washing, dry it (inside and outside) powder it, blow in air and keep it in proper place. If it is to be disinfected, soak the bag in 1:80 Lysol or carbolic 1:20 for 1–2 hours. Then wash with soap and water and replace it as before.	Prepares for next procedure.
7.	Wash hands.	Prevents spread of infection.
8.	Record date, time of application and removal, place where applied and effect.	Documentation fosters quality care.

Precautions

- Protect the bed with mackintosh and towel
- Avoid weight of the ice bag on the part as far as possible by using cradles
- Empty all air from the bag before application
- Always use a cover for the bag.

Other Methods of Cold Application

- **Ice collar:** It is another method of applying dry cold locally. It is used to relieve pain following tonsillectomy and for other conditions affecting throat.
- **Leiter's coil:** It is made by coils of flexible materials such as plastic or rubber by means of which a continuous application of cold is made to a part ice water which constantly runs through.
- **Cold compress:** It is a local moist cold application made out of folded layers of gauze piece or lint or soft linen about half to 1 cm thick (1/6–1/3") wrung out of cold or ice water or some evaporating lotion and applied to the required area and left uncovered.
- **Ice poultice:** This is a form of cold application made to small area as in the case of an eye, instead of applying cold compress.

Purposes

- To relieve headache
- To reduce temperature
- Helps to prevent swelling around a sprained joint and relieves pain and congestion.

Requisites

A tray containing:
- A bowl with ice water, cold water or evaporating lotion (1 part of spirit to 3 parts of water)
- Piece of folded gauze, lint or folded soft old linen
- Rubber sheet and towel to protect the bed.

Procedure

- Explain the procedure to the patient.
- Protect the bed.
- Take the linen or gauze and immerse it in ice water, wring it and make sure that there is no dripping of water and apply it to the part.
- Change it as soon as it becomes warm.

- Time taken for procedure is 15–20 minutes.
- Do not cover the compress.
- If cold compresses are applied to a large area, hot water bottle is placed at the feet and all necessary steps to prevent sensation of chilling are taken. When the time is over, remove the compress, wipe the part and make the patient comfortable.

GENERAL COLD APPLICATIONS

Cold Pack

It is a general application of cold to the body by means of sheets or towels wrung out of cold water. It is used to reduce temperature and as a sedative to overcome insomnia.

Cold Sponging

Purposes

- To reduce temperature
- To relieve discomfort
- To soothe the nerves and promote sleep

    It is given only with the order of the physician and usually when the temperature of the patient is 103°F (39.5°C) or above.

Requisites

A tray containing:

Articles	Purpose
• A bed Mackintosh and sheet	• To protect the bed
• One top sheet	• To cover the patient
• Wash cloth or sponge cloths—8	• 2 to hold in the hands of the patient, 2 for the axilla, 2 for groin and 2 for alternate sponging
• One bath towel	• To put over the abdomen of the patient as cold compress
• Hot water bottle with cover	• To apply over the feet
• A large basin of water, temperature 60°–70°F (19.5°–21°C) and a Jug with cold water	• For cold sponging
• Bath thermometer	• To check the temperature of water
• Ice cap with cover	• For cold application
• Thermometer tray	• To monitor TPR
• A basin with ice	• To add to the basin if water temperature increases
• Two buckets	• One for dirty water and the other for the used linen
• A towel	• To dry the face and body
• Screen	• To provide privacy
• Feeding cup with water/any hot drinks	• For the patient to drink after the procedure

Procedure

Steps	Procedure	Rationale
1.	Explain the procedure to the patient.	Allays anxiety and wins cooperation.
2.	Screen the patient and offer bedpan if needed. Close the windows, doors and switch off the fans.	Provides privacy and prevents drought.
3.	Assemble all the equipment in a trolley.	Organization facilitates skilled performance.
4.	Fanfold the upper bed cloths, remove the gown and cover the patient with the sheet. Remove all extra pillows.	Facilitates easy access to all places and reduces temperature by exposing to air.
5.	Perform hand hygiene.	Prevents the spread of microorganisms.
6.	Protect the bed with mackintosh and sheet.	Prevents soiling of linen.
7.	Take TPR of the patient, continue to take it every 10 minutes.	Monitoring temperature helps to find the effectiveness in therapy.
8.	Mix the water with ice and note the temperature.	Reduces the temperature by conduction.
	Put the wash cloths in the water, squeeze gently and sponge the face first and dry it by the face towel. Apply cold compress to the forehead and hot water bottle to the feet. Place the wash cloths one on each axilla and give two wash cloths to the patient and ask him to hold them wet but water should not drip from it. It is better to keep two wet cloths in the groins also.	Promotes quick relief.

Contd...

Steps	Procedure	Rationale
9.	• Start with the face, back of the ears and then dry it. • Then sponge the arm, using alternate sponge, from the shoulder to the finger tips in long strokes. • Sponge the legs and back. Attend the back with spirit and powder Sponge the chest and dry properly. • Put the cold compress on the abdomen, sponge the general area also with cold water.	Reduces the temperature by conduction.
10.	During the procedure the temperature of the water should be maintained by adding chipped ice.	Maintains the temperature of water.
11.	• The treatment may last for 20 minutes. • When the treatment is completed, the cold compresses are removed. • Dry the patient's body thoroughly.	Prevents chilling.
12.	Remove the bed linen and mackintosh, hot water bottle and ice bag and remake the bed, make the patient comfortable.	Promotes comfort.
13.	If needed, give him/her hot drinks or stimulants after taking temperature.	Maintains temperature and prevents chilling.
14.	Wash and replace the articles. Wash hands.	Prevents spread of infection.
15.	Record the date, time and duration of treatment. TPR taken before, during and after sponging should be recorded. Any unusual symptoms should be recorded and reported.	Documentation fosters quality care.

Precautions

- Watch the condition of the patient. If the patient develops chill, stop the procedure. Cover him/her with a blanket. Give stimulants and inform the doctor.
- Apply cold compress to the forehead and hot water bottle near the feet.
- The environment should be warm.
- Do not rub the abdomen of a typhoid patient, as it may cause damage to the affected intestine.
- Temperature of the water should be 60°–70°F (19.5°–21°C).
- Give stimulant unless it is contraindicated.
- Protect the chest from getting chill.

Unit VII ❖ Therapeutic Nursing Measures

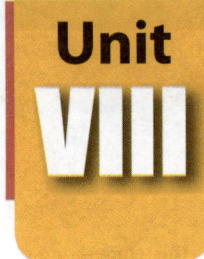
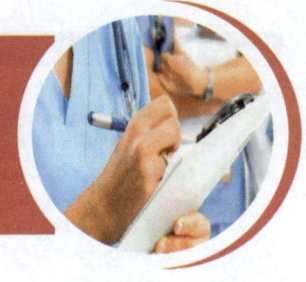

DEFINITIONS

- **Wound:** Disruption of the normal continuity of the body structure internally or externally is said to be a **wound**. It is a cut or break in the continuity of any tissue.
- **Injury:** It is the term usually applied to any damage affected to the body by an external force, e.g., mechanical injury, chemical injury, etc.

CLASSIFICATION OF WOUNDS

Wounds may be classified into three main groups according to the manner in which they are produced and according to their bacterial content.

According to Cause

- **Abraded wound or abrasion:** It is one produced by friction, which removes the superficial layers of the skin, e.g., falling in the sand or rough surface, etc.
- **Incised wound:** It is one made by a sharp cutting instrument which produces a clean and simple separation of tissues, e.g., operation wound.
- **Contused wound:** It is one made by blunt force which is characterized by considerable injury of the soft parts with hemorrhage and swelling, e.g., injury by a blow or falling weight on the body, etc.
- **Lacerated wound:** It is one in which the tissues are torn and the edges are irregular and jagged, e.g., injury by glass, metals, etc.
- **Penetrating wound:** It is one that has passed through deep lying tissues to enter in an important deep body cavity or organ, e.g., stab injury.
- **Punctured wound:** It is one made with a sharp pointed narrow instrument piercing beyond surface depth, but making only a small opening on the body surface, e.g., nail, bullet or glass pieces, etc. in leg.

According to Bacterial Contamination

Wounds are classified as:

- **Clean wound:** It is one in which no pathogenic organisms are present. When an incision is made under aseptic conditions, the wound remains clean. As the skin cannot be rendered sterile, it is impossible to produce a completely sterile wound. They are made harmless by the defensive mechanism of the body. Such wounds made in surgery usually heal without infection.
- **Contaminated wound:** It is one in which the number of organisms present in a wound is greater than clean wound. All wounds acquired by accident are contaminated since no preventive measures such as aseptic technique have been applied. Wound resulting from a hemorrhoidectomy is an example of such

type of wound. Although this type of wound is liable to infection, it may heal without manifestation of infection.

- **Septic wound:** It is one which is infected with pathogenic organisms. It contains a large number of pathogenic organisms which have caused the destruction of tissues in the affected area. A clean or contaminated wound may become infected very rapidly. In such situations, defensive reaction of the involved tissue becomes ineffective due to many reasons, like unsterile technique, poor resistance, etc. A wound made at the site where infection is already present makes the wound septic or infect it immediately, such as an incision made for drainage of an abscess.

According to the Extent of Tissue Injury

- **An open wound:** It is one in which there is cut or break in the continuity of skin or mucous membrane as caused by a sharp instrument or object and there is possibility for entry of organisms and foreign particles and loss of blood from the body.
- **A closed wound:** It is one in which there is cut or break in the continuity of skin and mucous membranes but accompanied by damage of tissues under the skin as caused by some blunt instruments or blow or by crushing. Blood vessels may be damaged or bleeding may take place under the skin.
- **Hematoma:** It is a significant localized bleeding under the skin.
- **Ecchymosis:** It is a discoloration due to extravasation of blood in the tissue.

WOUND CARE

Preparation of Sterile Handling Forceps

Take a wide-mouthed one pound size bottle (same size of steel jars also are available now) as shown in Figure 1. Clean the bottle or jar properly inside and outside. Boil it in the sterilizer for 20–30 minutes or autoclave it. If it is a bottle, cover the outside of the bottle with a rag piece while putting for boiling. Take a Cheatle forceps or long artery forceps and tie a long thread at its handle. Put it for boiling along with the bottle in such a way that the distal end of the thread should be hanging outside the sterilizer while closing it.

When the proper boiling time is over, allow it to cool. Open the sterilizer and take the forceps by handling on the thread with clean hands. Then hold on the handle of the forceps and with the forceps take the bottle or jar from the sterilizer. Remove the thread from the forceps. Prepare the lotion in the bottle or jar almost full, in the proper strength according to the type of chemical. Keep some sterile cotton at the bottom of the bottle to prevent the striking of the forceps while putting and taking. Keep the transfer forceps in it and place the bottle in the place where the sterile articles are to be handled.

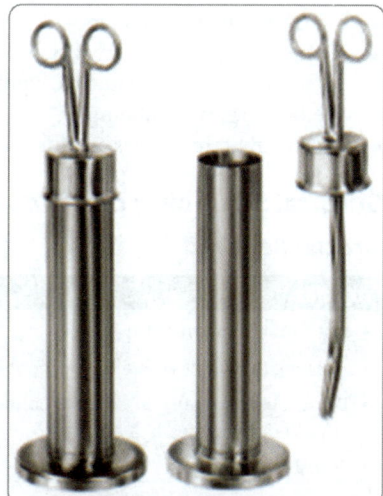

Figure 1: Sterile handling of forceps

Once the forceps is taken out for handling sterile articles, it should not be touched in any unsterile area. It should be placed carefully in the lotion without touching the outside of the bottle. The forceps should be handled only with clean hands. This kind of preparation of transfer of forceps in lotion in the ward should be repeated every morning and whenever we think the lotion, the forceps or the bottle is contaminated. Remember that there is no midway between sterile and unsterile.

Unit VIII ❖ Care of Wounds

SURGICAL SCRUBBING

Human hands are the most important tools for caring. However hands can also be a portal and transmitter of infection. 'Scrubbing in' dramatically reduces the risk of infection and significantly improves patient outcomes.

Purposes

The purpose of surgical hand scrub is to:
- Remove debris and transient microorganisms from the nails, hands and forearms.
- Reduce the resident microbial count to a minimum.
- Inhibit rapid rebound growth of microorganisms.
- Prevent the transfer or to reduce the amount of permanent flora of the hands, which would ultimately prevent surgical wound contamination from microorganisms found on the hands of the surgical team.

Principles

- The basic principle of the scrub is to wash the hands thoroughly and do it from a clean area (the hands) to a less clean area (the arm).
- A systematic approach to the scrub is an efficient way to ensure proper technique.

Prerequisites

- Remove all jewellery (rings, watches, bracelets)
- Ensure that the nails are cut short
- Remove artificial nails, if any
- Remove nail polish, if any
- Inspect the hands for any cuts, abrasions or open lesions
- Wear the personal protective equipment like cap, mask, etc. after performing medical hand washing and before surgical scrubbing
- Ensure that the sleeves are at least two to three inches above the elbows

Surgical Scrubbing of Hands with Brush: Needed in Maintaining Surgical Asepsis

Articles Required

Articles	Purpose
• Antiseptic solution/Scrub	• For reducing the number of microorganisms
• Running tap water with elbow or foot operated	• For washing hands without contaminating them
• Disposable nail brush in a sterile Container/brush sterilized and stored in a bin	• For thorough cleaning of the nails
• Transferring forceps	• For picking up nail brush from the sterile container or bin
• Sterile towels	• For wiping the hands after hand wash

Preparation of Unit

- Ensure an area of good lighting
- Arrange all the necessary articles near the hand washing area

Procedure

Steps	Procedure	Rationale
1.	Open out the sterile pack onto a clean table, only grabbing the outermost edges	This helps to maximize the sterile field and keep the required things after scrubbing ready such as sterile towel, gloves and gown.
2.	Open disposable brush impregnated with antimicrobial soap. If not available, use a transferring forceps to pick up the brush from the sterile bin	Helps to maintain sterile field.
3.	Turn on the water and adjust the flow. Wet hands and arms keeping the hands above elbows	Movement of water and dirt will flow from hands to less clean areas. This prevents contamination of the hands during scrub. (Refer to Principle)

Contd...

Steps	Procedure	Rationale
4.	Wet scrub brush and remove any gross debris from underneath fingernails using the nail cleaner	This removes debris hidden inside the nails and removes microorganisms with the help of friction.
5.	Apply the scrub solution as per the hospital policy and perform the steps of hand washing in the following manner. • Rub hands palm to palm • Rub the back of both the hands with right palm over left dorsum with interlaced fingers and vice versa	Ensures that all surfaces will be systematically scrubbed to remove transient and resident microorganisms.

Contd...

Steps	Procedure	Rationale
	• Interlace fingers with palm to palm and rub the hands together 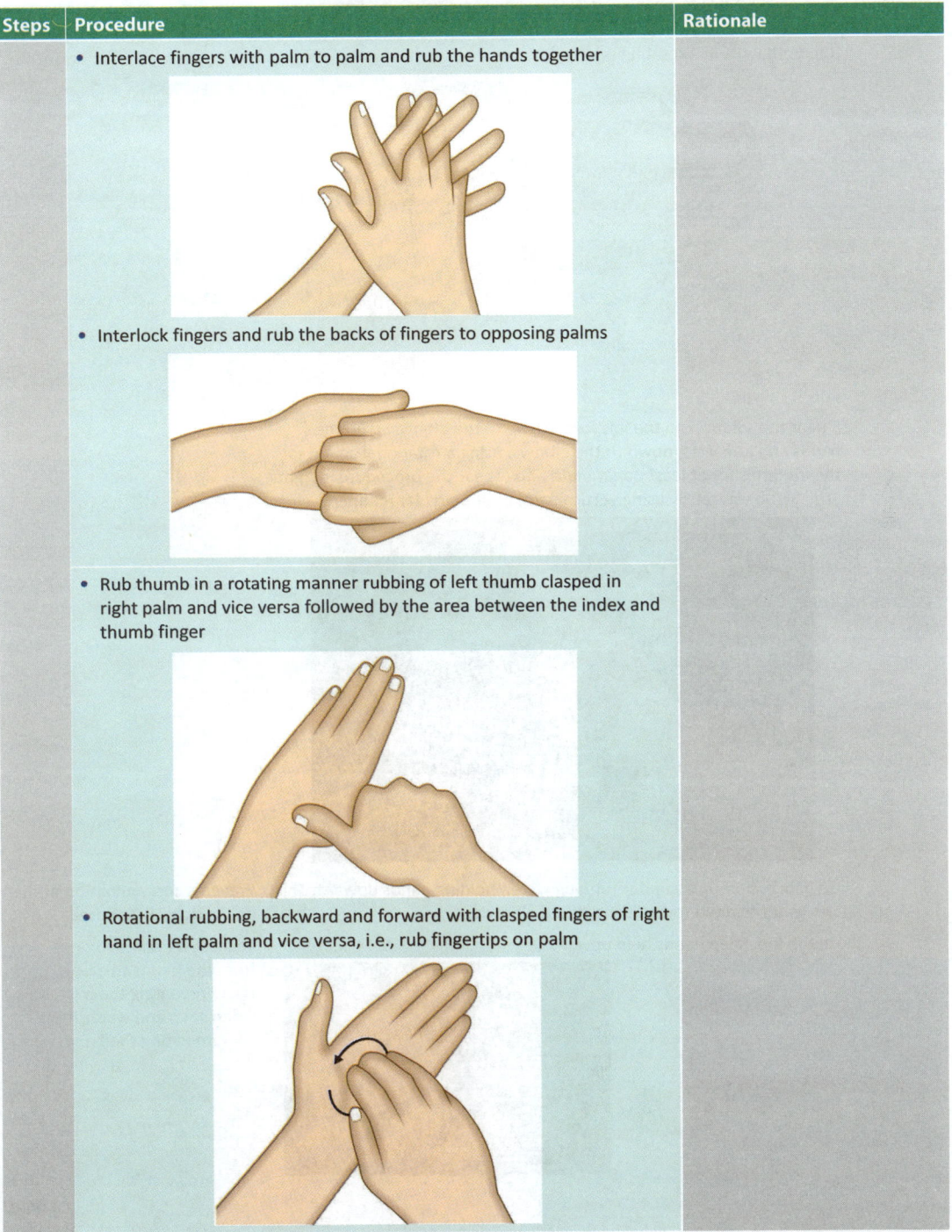 • Interlock fingers and rub the backs of fingers to opposing palms • Rub thumb in a rotating manner rubbing of left thumb clasped in right palm and vice versa followed by the area between the index and thumb finger • Rotational rubbing, backward and forward with clasped fingers of right hand in left palm and vice versa, i.e., rub fingertips on palm	

Contd...

Steps	Procedure	Rationale
	• Rub both wrist in a rotating manner • Smear the solution on the left forearm up to the elbow. Scrub the hands and forearms, down to the elbows, using a rotational action for the forearms for at least one minute and repeat the procedure in right arm. Scrub vigorously using vertical strokes in a circular manner	
6.	Rinse hands thoroughly under running water, holding hands upward. This allows water to drain towards the flexed elbows.	Prevents contamination of the hands from dirtier areas.
7.	Close the tap. Keep hands held upward	This allows water to drip from the hands to elbow, thus preventing the bacteria-laden soap and water from contaminating the hand.

Contd...

Steps	Procedure	Rationale
8.	Keeping the arms elevated, dry the hands and then the forearms with the sterile towels in the gowning pack, using a dabbing motion instead of a wiping motion. Use one side of the towel to dry one hand and reverse side for the other hand. If two towels are available, use separate towels for each hand. Discard towel without touching other objects in the surroundings	Prevents contamination. Touching non-sterile objects would mean the surgical scrub needs to be repeated again.
9.	Hold the hands and forearms away from the body and above waist and below neckline, until you put on a sterile gown and sterile gloves	Scrubbed hands and arms are considered contaminated once they fall below waist level.

 Stimulant

- Povidone iodine and chlorhexidine gluconate are the common solutions used in surgical hand washing.
- Recent experimental studies have demonstrated that the scrubbing technique frequently used in conventional surgical hand washing is not essential.
- Although the conventional brushing/scrubbing technique provides an effective antisepsis, it has been shown to increase complications such as cracks and scratches of the hand.

Unit VIII ❖ Care of Wounds

DISINFECTION AND STERILIZATION

The following are the means of reducing the number of destroying microorganisms. It is done either by physical or chemical means. All articles that can be sterilized by heat are treated by boiling, steam under pressure or dry heat.

- **Disinfectant:** For other things chemical disinfectants are used. If we use a disinfectant, it should satisfy the following:
  - It should be efficient.
  - It should be used in the correct strength.
  - It should be applied for a sufficient length of time.
  - It should not be injurious to the article.
  - The article should be fully immersed in it.
- **Sterilization:** It is the process of destruction of all microorganisms and their spores on a substance by exposure to physical or chemical agents.
- **Fumigation:** It is the term used when we use gas for disinfection. This method is largely used to disinfect books, rooms and flannels. The doors and windows including all devices are closed. The room and articles should be exposed to vapors for 12 hours. Formaldehyde is the agent most commonly used.
- **Disinfection:** It is the process of destroying all pathogenic organisms, except the spore bearing ones.
  - **Concurrent disinfection:** It is the immediate disinfection of all contaminated articles and body discharges during the course of disease of a patient.
  - **Terminal disinfection:** It is disinfection of patient's unit, that is, all articles including room, furniture and linen used by the patient on his/her discharge or release from isolation or death.
- **Isolation:** It is the separation of infected persons from non-infected persons for the period of communicability, under conditions which will prevent transmission of the infectious agent.
- **Barrier nursing:** It is a method of bed isolation, which enables a patient suffering from infectious disease to get nursed among those not so infected. In other words, it is the segregation of one infectious patient from the other type of patients in the general ward itself either in a corner bed with screens around or in a cubicle.

SURGICAL DRESSING

A surgical dressing is a protection with sterile covering of gauze or other materials applied over a wound after cleaning it with all aseptic precautions.

Types of Wound Dressing

Wound dressings are generally classified into three groups based on their functions.
1. Absorb exudates
2. Maintain moisture
3. Donate moisture

The choice of dressing will depend on the type, condition and location of the wound.

Advantages of Dressing

- Absorbs drainage.
- Prevents contamination from feces, urine, vomitus, etc.
- Splints or immobilizes the wound.
- Protects the wound from mechanical injuries.
- Promotes hemostasis as in a pressure dressing.
- Promotes mental and physical comfort of the patient.
- Provides protection for newly-formed tissue.

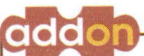

A New Trend in Dressing

In many hospitals we note that there is an increasing tendency to eliminate the dressings, shortly after operation or within immediate postoperative period, wherever it is possible. It is noted that in some other hospitals an initial dressing (applied in the operating room) is removed and usually it is not replaced. Some surgeons prefer to remove the initial dressings and it is replaced till the sutures are removed. It is believed that its purpose is more aesthetic than a necessary one. In the absence of dressing, a wound heals with fibrin.

The apparent advantages of no dressing are as follows. It:
- Eliminates the conditions for the growth of bacteria such as warmth, moisture and darkness.
- Allows better observation and early detection of abnormalities in the wound.
- Facilitates bathing of the patient.
- Tends to minimize the operation procedure.
- Avoids adhesive tape reaction.
- Appears to be more comfortable to the patient and facilitates his activity.
- It is more economical.

Disadvantages of no dressing method:
- Aesthetic view to the patient or relatives. The sight of a large wound and number of sutures may be fearful to the lay persons.
- The rate of contamination may be increased due to unhygienic environment and carelessness of the patient and relatives: such as dirty bed linen, scratching the incisional area itself.

Criteria of a Good Dressing

Certain criteria have to be applied to all kinds of dressings. These include:
- The assurance of positive sterilization of materials and the correct technique of their application.
- Economy in the use of materials and time.
- Durability of materials so that dressing will hold up even under the stress or motion including early ambulations.
- Simplicity in the mode of packing for the easy application without disturbing the principles of strict aseptic precautions.
- Physical and mental satisfaction of the patient with minimum pain and discomfort.
- Availability of materials in sufficient quantity in the wards at all times considering the fact that overstocking of sterile goods will increase the risk of loss of sterilization.
- Adequate means for the easy and safe disposal of used or contaminated dressings.
- Adequate facilities of proper hand washing for the protection of both the patient and the nurse.

General Instructions

- Strict aseptic technique is essential. Dressing should be done one hour after sweeping and dusting of the room. Close the doors if it is a room or screen the patient's bed before dressing, if it is an open ward.
- Clean wounds must always be dressed before those that are infected.
- External dressings are removed by grasping them so as not to remove the drains and packing if such are present.
- Dressings if contaminated with drainage are handled with forceps. Adhesive strips placed directly over the wound are not removed. But surgeon removes these.
- If possible, unpleasant dressings or painful dressing should not be done at the meal time.
- The patient should be instructed to keep away his eyes from the wound so that he does not get frightened.
- The person who does the dressing should be free from respiratory infection or should wear a mask.

Unit VIII ❖ Care of Wounds

Types of Dressing

Depending on the purpose, the dressings are of the following types:

- **Dry dressing:** Clean wounds are dressed by the application of 4 to 8 layers of gauze folded into suitable size and shape. The surroundings of the wound are cleansed by some antiseptic, dried and dry dressings are applied after the application of medicine to the wound.
- **Wet dressing:** It is used if wounds are infected and pus is in plenty to soften the discharge and to promote drainage. If wet compresses are hot, it stimulates the suppurative process. The dressings are made of many layers of gauze or cotton pad covered with gauze.
- **Pressure dressing:** This is done when there is bleeding or oozing from the wound. Have a thick pad of sterile gauze applied over the wound with a firm bandage or binder.

Preliminary Assessment of the Patient and Environment

- Check the doctor's order for specific instruction to note the types of dressings to be applied, about the type of lotions to be used, medicine to be applied, etc.
- Identify the patient, by name, bed no, etc.
- Check the nurse's record to note the condition of the wound in previous dressing.
- Check the diagnosis and general condition of the patient and the purpose of dressing.
- Ascertain whether there are any suturing or drainage tubes or what type of wound to be dressed and the type of dressing to be applied.
- Check the abilities of the patient for self-help, understanding and limitations.
- Get the instructions from the Senior Sister.
- Get the assistance, if required.
- Avoid the meal time of the patient and see that if the patient is tired of any other treatment or nursing procedure immediately before this.
- Find out the articles available in the ward.

Preparation of Unit

- Ensure an area of good lighting.
- Arrange all the necessary articles near to the bedside of the patient.
- Make sure the surrounding area is clean and tidy before you start.
- Dressings are not changed for at least 15 minutes after the room has been swept or cleaned. Sweeping and dusting of the room will raise the dust and the wound will be contaminated.
- See that the patient's room is in order with no unnecessary articles. Clear the bedside table or the overbed table, so that there is sufficient space to set up a sterile field and to arrange needed supplies and equipment.

Preparation of Patient

- Gain confidence of the patient by explaining the procedure to the patient
- Allow patients to ask questions and clarify their doubts.
- Provide privacy to the patient.
- Close the door and windows. Put on curtains to prevent drafts. Put off fan.
- Position the patient comfortably and adjust the height of the bed depending on the area to be dressed.
- Shave the area, if necessary to remove the hairs. Removal of the adhesive is more painful if the hair are present. So, the shaving should be done before the first dressing is applied.
- Give proper support to the body parts if the patient has to raise and hold it in position for a considerable time.
- Bring the patient to the edge of the bed.

Prerequisites

- Clean the trolley using soap and water, or disinfectant, and a cloth. Start at the top of the trolley and work down to the bottom legs of the trolley using single strokes with your damp cloth.
- Place the sterile dressing/procedure pack on the top of the trolley.
- Open the sterile dressing pack on top of the trolley. Open the sterile field using the corners of the paper.
- Open any other sterile items needed onto the sterile field without touching them.
- Call for assistance, if necessary, e.g., to do the unsterile procedure, to transfer sterile supplies, etc.

Requisites

Articles	Purpose
A sterile tray containing:	
• Sterile Dressing set	• For aseptic wound dressing
• Towel 1	• To spread around the wound
• Artery forceps 1	• To remove the soiled dressing
• Dissecting forceps or dressing forceps 2	• To clean the wound (if one is soiled the other one can be used)
• Scissors 1	• To cut the dead tissues if any and to cut the gauze, if needed
• Sinus forceps 1	• To open the sinus tract or to pack
• Probe 1	• To note the depth of the wound, if needed
• Small bowl 1	• To take the cleaning solution
• Safety pin 1	• To fix the short drain, if any
• Gown, Gloves, mask and other PPE 1	• To prevent cross infection
• Cotton swabs, gauze pieces and cotton pads	• As required for wound cleansing
An unsterile tray containing:	
• Transfer forceps kept in a sterile bottle with antiseptic lotion	• To handle the sterile articles
• Mackintosh and towel 1	• Protect the bed and to put under the wound
• Kidney tray and paper bag 1	• Collect the waste
• A large bowl with disinfectant	• To put the used instruments
• Swab stick in a sterile container	• To apply medication, if needed
• Bandages, binders, safety pins, adhesive plaster and scissors	• As required to fix the dressings
• Cleaning solutions in bottle	• As required for wound cleansing
• Ointments or powders or any other medicines	• As required to apply on the wound
• Ribbon gauze in sterile containers	• To pack a wound

Procedure

Steps	Procedure	Rationale
1.	Perform hand wash	Prevents spread of microorganisms
2.	Arrange the articles near the bed side	Facilitates performance of procedure in a systematic way
3.	Wear PPE	Prevents cross infection

Contd...

Steps	Procedure	Rationale
4.	Assist the client in comfortable position to have an easy access to the wound	Promotes comfort
5.	Place a Mackintosh and towel under the wound area	Prevents soiling of bed sheets
6.	Don non-sterile gloves	Protects from contamination
7.	Loosen tape of soiled dressing	Facilitates easy removal
8.	Remove soiled dressings carefully from clean to less clean area	Prevents transmission of infection
9.	Gently remove the dressing adherent to the wound using a sterile forceps without touching the wound	Lessens pain and prevents contamination of wound

Contd...

Steps	Procedure	Rationale
10.	If dressing is close to the skin, pour a small amount of normal saline solution onto it and then remove the dressing 	This moistens the dressing facilitating easy removal
11.	Assess wound. Note the type and the amount of drainage present 	Facilitates comparison of wound healing
12.	Discard the soiled dressing in waste bin as per BMW policy	Safe disposal prevents transmission of micro organisms
13.	Remove the soiled gloves and discard it in waste bin as per BMW policy	Safe disposal prevents transmission of micro-organisms
14.	Perform hand hygiene	Prevents transmission of microorganisms
15.	Place the sterile tray in the dressing trolley and other articles that are necessary for surgical dressing 	Arrangement of articles facilitates performance of skilled procedure

Contd...

Steps	Procedure	Rationale
16.	Open the sterile tray. Spread the sterile towel around the wound 	Creates a sterile field around the wound
17.	Prepare sterile field. Add necessary sterile supplies 	Ensures asepsis
18.	Perform surgical hand washing or scrubbing 	Prevents transfer of microorganisms
19.	Don sterile gown and gloves 	Ensures asepsis

Contd...

Steps	Procedure	Rationale
20.	Ask the assistant to pour small amount of cleansing solution into the bowl without touching the sterile area	Maintains asepsis
21.	• Clean the wound using one gauze per stroke from the centre to periphery, the incision then outer edges • From top to bottom • Discard the used swabs after each stroke in a kidney tray	Cleaning should be done from the cleanest area to the less clean area. Wound line is considered cleaner than the surrounding area even if the wound is infected
22.	Cleanse around drain (if present) using a circular stroke, starting with the area immediately next to the drain and continue this process to clean a little further out from the drain until the skin surrounding the drain is cleaned. Use one gauze per stroke	Cleaning should be done from the cleanest area to the less clean area

Contd...

Steps	Procedure	Rationale
23.	After thorough cleaning of the wound, dry the wound with dry swabs using the same technique. Discard the forceps in the bowl of lotion	Wet wound may act as a source of infection
24.	Apply medications if ordered. Apply a small portion on the dressing that goes directly over the wound	Applying the ointment directly to the wound may be difficult
25.	Apply the sterile dressings. Apply the gauze pieces first and then the cotton pads. Apply inner dressing to incision, then proceed to the drain site	Cotton placed directly onto the wound may stick on the wound, when the discharge dries
26.	Secure the dressing safely with placing cotton pads sufficiently. Apply outer dressing	This will prevent oozing of the drainage onto the bed of the patient

Contd...

Steps	Procedure	Rationale
27.	Cover the drain site and secure it	Prevents the spread of microorganisms
28.	Secure the dressings with bandage or adhesive tapes	Prevents dislodging of the dressing and secures the wound from contamination
	Aftercare of the patient and the articles:	
29.	Remove the mackintosh and towel	Safe removal protects the patients and the environment from infection
30.	• Help the patient to dress up and place the patient in a comfortable position in the bed • Change the garments, if soiled with drainage • Replace the bed linen	Promotes comfort of the patient

Contd...

Steps	Procedure	Rationale
31.	• Take all articles to the utility room • Discard the soiled dressings into a covered container and send for incineration • Remove the instruments and other articles from the disinfectant solution and clean them thoroughly. Dry them • Re-set the tray and send for autoclaving. • Replace all other articles to their proper places. • Send the soiled linen to the laundry bag for washing (remove the blood stains before sending them to washing)	Facilitates use for next patient
32.	Remove the gloves and discard into the BMW waste bin as per policy	Prevents transfer of microorganisms
33.	Wash hands	Prevents transfer of microorganisms
34.	Record the procedure on the nurse's record with date and time. Record the: • Condition of the wound • Size, type and amount of drainage, type of cleaning solution, and dressing applied • Condition of the sutures • Tolerance of the patient during the procedure • Any unusual findings or concerns • Report to the surgeon if abnormalities are found	Documentation fosters quality care
35.	Return to the bedside to assess the comfort of the patient. Special instruction regarding the wound care to be communicated to the patient	Promotes confidence of the patient
36.	Tidy up the bed and the unit of the patient	Promotes comfort

Special Points to be Considered during Wound Dressing

■ During the procedure the nurse has to make sure that he/she is not contaminating the articles and dressing materials.

■ If there are more than one wound on a patient, do the cleanest one first and follow the rest.

■ Usually two persons are needed to do a surgical dressing, one person to remove the outer dressing, and bandage and other one to hand over the sterile articles to the person who dresses the wound.

- During the period when the dressings are in progress, precaution should be taken to keep the number of bacteria in the air as low as possible. Domestic activities such as sweeping and bed making should be completed at least one hour before starting dressings.
- A treatment room large enough to accommodate a patient in bed and the necessary equipment will enable such procedures to be carried out with greater safety of the patient and less disturbance of the ward routine.
- Use mask during the procedure.
- Wards should be closed to all unnecessary traffic unless dressings are carried out in treatment room close to the ward.
- Hands whether wet or dry, scrubbed or unscrubbed are to be regarded as dirty and should not be allowed to come in contact with wounds or any material directly applied to wounds. If necessary, gloves should be worn, wash hands before and after each dressing.
- Wounds should be kept covered except during the actual dressing procedure. The skin around the wound should be treated with the same care as the wound itself. Create a sterile field around the wound by spreading sterile towels.
- Precautions should not be relaxed when dealing with wounds that are already infected.
- For cleaning, spirit should not be used directly over the wound or on granulation tissue but use only on the skin around.
- Avoid talking, coughing and sneezing when a wound is opened.

Recent Updates

Current Trends in Wound-Care Products

There are many wound-care products available including simple protective layers, hydrogels, metal ion-impregnated dressings and artificial skin substitutes, which facilitate surface closure like topical negative pressure and hyperbaric oxygen therapy, Alginates (if exudates present), Foams, Hydrocolloids, Hydrogels, Transparent films, Wound fillers, etc. Nurses need to have a sound knowledge on various types of dressing materials available and should be abreast of the recent developments.

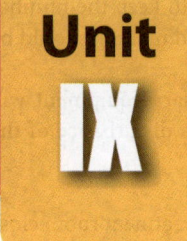
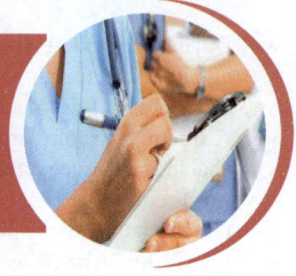

Medicine may be defined as a drug used to promote health, to prevent, diagnose, treat or cure a disease. Medicine is a term also used to designate the science of preventing or treating disease or injury.

ADMINISTRATION OF MEDICINE

Purposes of Medicine Administration

- To diagnose disease, e.g., barium which is used to visualize a part opaque to X-ray.
- To treat a disease. Various drugs are used in the treatment of diseases and they are classified according to their desired effects such as:
  - Drugs which are given for palliative effect or for temporary relief of distressing symptoms but such drugs neither remove the cause nor cure the condition. For example, injection Morphine in relieving pain in carcinoma.
  - Drugs for restoring normal function, e.g., administration of digitalis in heart disease.
  - Drugs used to supply a substance which is deficient in the body, e.g., insulin in diabetes mellitus.
  - Drugs used to cure disease. They are known as specific drugs, e.g., quinine for malaria.
  - To prevent a disease, e.g., vaccines and serum. For example, ATS in tetanus, smallpox vaccine, TAB vaccine, etc.

Factors Modifying the Dosage and Effect of Drugs

- **Age:** Infants, children and aged persons require small dosage of a drug than that of an average adult. Young's rule is usually used in calculating the dosage of medicine ordered for children up to 12 years.

  Formula: $\dfrac{\text{Age in years} \times \text{adult dose}}{\text{Age} + 12} = \text{Dose}$

  e.g, adult dose of castor oil is 1 oz (8 dr) or 30 mL.

  For a 4-year-old child, the dose to be administered $= \dfrac{4 \times 30}{4 + 12} = 7.5$ mL.

- **Weight:** A person who is overweight will require larger dose than the usual dosage. A person who is considerably underweight requires a smaller dose than the average dose.
- **Sex:** Males require larger dose than females.
- **Physical condition:** When pain is great, larger dose of morphine may be ordered. In shock and collapse the dose of stimulants ordered may be larger than usual. When drugs are given as antidotes for poisoning, larger doses are ordered.
- **Excretion of the drug and cumulative action:** The frequency of administration and the dose of certain drug depend upon the rate of excretion from the body. Drugs such as penicillin and sulfanilamide have to be administered every few hours because they are excreted rapidly from the body. Some drugs are

excreted at a slower rate, e.g., digitalis, sodium bromide, etc. Repeated dose may cause accumulation in the body and produce symptoms of toxicity. The nurse should recognize and report symptoms of toxic effect.

- **Tolerance:** Patients who possess a tolerance (i.e., capability of taking excessive doses of dangerous drug without producing toxic symptoms) for certain drugs will require larger doses to be effective.
- **Habituation:** Patients are said to be habituated to a drug when they have used it continuously for a longer period of time and it adds to the development of a tolerance. If the drug is withdrawn, they may develop a craving for the drug and show definite symptoms, e.g., persons who are in the habit of taking hypnotics (drugs which produce sleep) over a long period of time may be unable to sleep without them even though there may be no definite cause or reason for insomnia.
- **Addiction:** Prolonged use of alcohol and of narcotics may produce an extreme form of habituation and result in the condition termed addiction. In such patients if the drugs are withdrawn they may show psychic craving for them and show definite organic symptoms. For them, the dosage of drugs given to relieve pain may need to be increased because the drug must be effective enough to overcome tolerance, satisfy the psychic craving, supply the psychological need created by addiction and afford relief from pain.
- **Idiosyncrasy:** It is defined as a peculiar susceptibility of an individual to some drugs, protein and other substances. Such people react violently to certain drugs in some unusual way. The effect may be quite opposite to that ordinarily produced in other persons or an average dose may have a toxic effect, e.g., vomiting and ringing in the ears after taking soda salicylic; rashes, and abdominal pain after taking aspirin.
- **Effect desired:** The method by which a drug is administered will help to determine its effect. So the nurse should know whether the drug is being given for local effect or for a general systemic effect. A drug used for its local effect is applied directly to the site where its action is limited to the area to which it has been applied. A drug used for its general effect must be absorbed into the blood stream to produce the desired effect in various parts of the body, remote from the site of application. Drugs given orally for local effect should not be diluted and should be given after meals so that absorption is delayed and local effect is produced.

  Drugs given orally for general effect should be diluted and given at a time when the stomach is comparatively empty. Then drug is readily absorbed and general effect is produced.
- **Method of administration:** The effectiveness of drug sometimes depends on the method by which it is administered. Drugs given by rectum are absorbed slowly and only in part, therefore larger doses are required. Drugs given by intravenous route have a very quick and immediate action, therefore the dose given is slightly less than those of oral administration.

Routes of Administration

- Medicines may be given by various routes depending upon:
  - The effect desired (local or systemic effect)
  - The rapidity of the action needed
  - The nature and amount of drug to be given
  - The condition of the patient
- The speed of action of a drug depends on route of administration (from the most rapid to the least rapid):
  - **Injection:** The term "injection" is defined as the forcing of a fluid into a cavity, a blood vessel or to body tissues through a hollow tube or needle, e.g., intravenous, intraspinal or intrathecal, intramuscular, intraperitoneal, subcutaneous and intradermal.

Unit IX ❖ Medication Needs of the Patient—Pharmacology

- **Ingestion:** The word "ingestion" means the act of taking food, medicines etc. into the body by mouth. Medicine given by mouth may be swallowed or administered sublingually, e.g., mixtures, tablets, capsules, powders and syrups.
- **Inhalation:** It is defined as the drawing of air or vapors into the lungs by inhalation, e.g., ammonia and amyl nitrate.
- **Instillation:** It means the act of pouring a liquid medicine drop by drop into a cavity, e.g., eye drops, nasal drops and instillation of medicine into the urinary bladder.
- **Inunction:** It is defined as the process of applying an ointment or medicine to a part or area by rubbing it into the skin, e.g., ointments and liniments.
- **Insufflation:** It means administration of drugs in the form of powder, vapor, gas or air by blowing with an insufflators into a wound or a body cavity, e.g. Nebasulf powder into wounds, cranial insufflations, endotracheal insufflation, insufflation of the lungs, perirenal insufflation and tubal insufflation.
  - Forcing of air into the subdural space or cerebral ventricles is called the **cranial insufflations**.
  - Introduction of air into the trachea through a tube passed into the larynx, employed to avoid collapse of the lung in intrathoracic operations is called **endotracheal insufflation**.
  - The act of blowing air into the lungs for the purpose of artificial respiration is called the **insufflation of lungs**.
  - Injection of air around the kidneys for the purpose of X-ray examination is called **perirenal insufflation**.
  - Introduction of air into the fallopian tubes to test the patency in 'Rubin's test' is called the **tubal insufflation**.
- **Insertion:** It means inserting a medicine forcefully in to the body cavity.
  - **Rectal medication:** It means the administration of drugs through rectum, e.g., retention enema, suppository, proctoclysis.
    (Suppository means an easily fusible medicated mass to be introduced into an orifice of the body, e.g., glycerin suppository for rectal evacuation and slow injection of large quantities of liquid into the rectum is called proctoclysis.)
  - **Vaginal suppository:** Solid forms of drugs are introduced in vagina for local effects.
- **Implantation:** It means planting or putting of solid drugs into body tissues, e.g. Prosthesis to reshape the breast, plastic lens in eyes after lens extraction.
- **Forms of drugs used are:**
  - **Liquids:** Oils, mixtures, alcoholic solution as extracts and tinctures
  - **Solids:** Tablets, pills, capsules, powders
  - **Gases:** Oxygen, anesthetic gases, inhalations

Responsibilities of the Nurse in Administration of Medicine

Administration of the medicine is one of the greatest responsibilities of a nurse. He/she should see that all medicines are administered promptly and accurately in such a way as to obtain the best result. For this, he/she should know the following.
- **The nature of drug:**
  - Physical and chemical properties of the drugs
  - The expected effect–local and systemic actions and the best ways to attain them
  - Maximum and minimum dosage
  - The most effective means of administration
  - The signs and symptoms which would indicate an idiosyncrasy (susceptibility to some drugs).

- **Other factors:** He/she should know the various factors that modify the action of the drug.
  - He/she should be familiar with the habit forming drugs and the measures and means of restricting their use.
  - He/she should know the factors, which must be considered in determining the method and time of administration.
  - He/she should know the abbreviations and symbols used in writing orders for administering, e.g., TDS, BD, etc.
  - He/she should be familiar with the drugs, which are continually appearing in the market by reading the pamphlets, journals, etc.
  - **Dose:** A dose is the amount of drug administered at one time to produce an effect without harm to the patient.
    - Minimum dose is the smallest amount that will produce an effect in a body.
    - Maximum dose is the largest amount of drug that can be administered at one time without producing harm to the body.
    - Over dose is larger than the maximum dose and will have some poisonous effect.

Care of Medicine Cabinet and Drugs

The senior sister is entirely responsible for the cupboard. A register should be maintained to keep the account of all the drugs. To give proper care of drugs, each ward should be provided with a medicine cabinet.

- It should be large enough to accommodate all drugs to be stored there.
- As far as possible the medicine cabinet should be kept in a separate room near the nurse's room.
- A sink with running water should be provided in that room as a part of the unit.
- Adequate lighting should be provided within the cabinet to read the labels clearly.
- It should have separate compartments for mixtures, tablets, powders and ointments.
- Drugs for external use should be kept separate.
- Shelves of the cabinet should be narrow so that not more than two rows of bottles or other containers can be placed on them.
- Bottles should be arranged alphabetically so that it is easy to handle the drugs if the bottles are equal in size.
- Poisonous drugs should be kept in a separate cupboard which must have separate lock and key.
- Bottles, boxes and other containers should be kept closed. Liquid medicines such as alcoholic preparations may evaporate if bottles are kept open. Tablets and pills tend to disintegrate if exposed to air.
- Bottles should have proper labels (legible and neat).
- Drugs that are unusual in color, odor and consistency should be returned to the pharmacy to be discarded.
- Oils such as castor oil, serum, vaccines and antibiotics such as penicillin should be kept in refrigerators. Extreme cold prevents them from becoming rancid (decomposed due to liberation of fatty acids) and makes the oil preparations little more palatable.
- Emergency drugs such as stimulants should be kept in a box or tray where they are readily obtainable for emergency use.
- If medicines are sent home with patients, complete and definite instructions should be given about the use of the drugs.
- When indenting for drugs, indent only the required quantity.
- The medicine cabinet should always be kept neat and clean and all equipment after use should be thoroughly cleaned, returned to its proper place and kept ready for use again when needed.
- The medicine cabinet should be kept locked at all times and the keys should be kept where only doctors and nurses have access to them.

Unit IX ❖ Medication Needs of the Patient—Pharmacology

ORAL ADMINISTRATION OF MEDICINE

Oral administration of drugs is the most convenient and the most common method used. It is the most simple and economic method of administration of medicine. Drugs may be given by this method for:

- Local effect, e.g., cough syrup to relieve throat irritation.
- Systemic effect, e.g., digitalis to influence heart action.

  While administering oral medicine, it is important to know the following factors:
  - The effect desired and how to get it
  - Nature of the drug
  - How to protect the mouth and teeth from injurious action of the drug
  - How to make the drug acceptable to the patient

Rules for Oral Administration

Regarding Labels

- Give medications only from a clearly labelled container.
- Poisonous drugs should be labelled as "poisons" in red ink.
- Select the right drug from the cupboard. Read the label of the medicine container and the name of the medicine in the medicine card three times:
  - Before removing the bottle from the shelf
  - Before pouring the drug
  - Before replacing the bottle in the shelf
- Pour medicine from the bottle on the side opposite to the label.
- Never administer medicine from an unmarked bottle, or when in doubt about the nature of its contents.

Regarding Measuring Medicine

- Hold the medicine bottle in the right hand and open the cork or lid with left hand.
- Always use a calibrated measure in order to measure the accurate dose.
- Always give exactly what is ordered. Never give minims when drops are ordered and drops when minims are ordered.
- Avoid conversation or anything that prevents concentration on the task in hand.
- Make sure that medicine glasses are dry before pouring or measuring the medication.
- Shake the fluid medication before pouring it into the ounce glass.
- Hold the ounce glass at eye level and place thumb nail of the hand holding the glass at the height on the ounce glass to which medicine is to be poured.
- Wipe the mouth of the bottle and record it after use.

 Stimulant

Ten Rights of Medication Administration
Observe the ten rights in giving each medication.

1. Right Medication	6. Right Client Education
2. Right Dose	7. Right Documentation
3. Right Time or Frequency	8. Right to Refuse
4. Right Patient	9. Right Assessment
5. Right Route	10. Right Evaluation

Regarding Administration

■ Give medicine if there is a written and signed order only. If the order is not clear or not signed by the doctor, consult the head nurse.

■ Verbal orders should be accepted only in case emergencies.

■ When giving pills or tablets, place in proper container directly from bottle. Do not touch them with your hands. At least a piece of paper can be used.

■ Once the medication is poured out, it should not be returned to the bottle.

■ Do not use a drug that differs in color, odor or consistency.

■ Never give more than one drug at a time unless they are ordered.

■ Know minimum and maximum dose for the medication being given.

■ Give the medication at the time for which it is ordered.

■ Always identify the patient before giving medication by calling his/her name.

■ Always provide a drink or fresh water to the patient immediately after giving an oral medication, unless water is contraindicated.

■ Stay with patient until he/she has taken the medication but try to avoid the impression of compulsion and haste. The drug should not be left with the patient but a fresh dose is taken if the medication is to be given later.

■ An error in medication must be reported immediately to nurse in charge.

■ The nurse who prepares the medication should give and do the necessary recording.

■ Never give drugs in the dark or in the dim light.

■ Never allow one patient to carry medicine to another patient.

Regarding Recording the Drugs

■ Record each dose of medicine soon after it is administered.

■ Record if an ordered medication is refused or if it cannot be administered.

■ Use standard abbreviations in recording medications.

■ Record time, dose and kind of drug given.

■ Record only those medicines which "**You**" have administered.

■ Record effects especially any unusual effect of medication.

■ Never record a medication as "**Given**" before it has been administered.

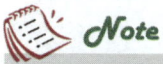 *Note*

Special Points to be Noted in Administering Oral Medicine

• Special drugs which should be given with plenty of water include diaphoretics, diuretics and narcotics.

Exceptions: Syrup, cough mixtures and sedative lozenges should be given without water and should not be followed by food or water.

• Tonics to stimulate appetite and secretion of gastric juice should be given before meals.

• Drugs administered to prevent deficiency of digestive fluids such as enzymes should be given with the meal or immediately after meal but diluted well with water before giving.

• Aperients are given at night if they are slow in taking effect, e.g. Liquid paraffin. Certain drugs are given early morning before food if rapid in action, e.g. Magnesium sulfate.

• Most drugs are given with cold water. Carminatives may better be given with warm water.

• Irritation of the mucous lining of the stomach by irritating drugs may be reduced by diluting with plenty of water or giving after food, such drugs include Iron, Arsenics, Salicylates, Aspirin, Iodides, Bromides, etc.

• Medicines which have a bad taste may be followed by bread or milk to remove the taste.

• Powders for children may be mixed with sugar or honey and given with a spoon.

• Tablets which cannot be swallowed may be crushed and powdered and dissolved in water.

Unit IX ❖ Medication Needs of the Patient—Pharmacology

Medication Calculation

$$D/H \times S = A$$

(**D** or desired dosage/**H** or Dose in hand × **S** or stock = **A** is amount prepared)

Prerequisites

Do not crush:

- Time release capsules as this may interfere with its absorption
- Enteric coated tablets as this may irritate the stomach's mucosal lining.

Assess the patient for:

- Impaired conscious state
- Swallowing ability
- Developmental disorders
- Psychiatric disorders
- Age of the patient—infants and children, old age
- Language barriers
- Cognitive impairments
- Sensory disorders

Requisite

A clean tray containing:

Article	Purpose
Materials for hand wash	Aids in the removal of microorganisms
Prescribed medications as per order	For curative, preventive, palliative or other purposes
Drinking water in a jug or permitted fluids	For swallowing tablets or capsules
Medication order	Prescription for verification of medicines
Pill crusher device/mortar and pestle	Aids in people with swallowing difficulties for crushing the medicines into powder form
Medicine cup	To keep the medicine ready for administering
A bowl of clean water	To wash the medicine glass
Ounce glass or measuring cup, minim glass, tea spoon, dropper, metal graduated oz measure, feeding cup	For measuring the amount of medications
Glass tubes or straw	For medications which stains the teeth
Mackintosh and towel	To prevent soiling of linen and patient's clothes
A towel or gauze	To wipe the mouth of the bottle and the medicine glass
Towel	To wipe the mouth of patient after taking medication
Kidney tray and paper bag	To dispose the waste
Non sterile gloves (as per Institutions policy)	To prevent cross infection
Waste bin	To dispose the waste

Preparation of Unit

- Ensure an area of good lighting
- Arrange all the necessary articles close to the bed side

Preparation of Patient

- Explain the procedure, the medication and its effects and give the patient time to ask questions.
- Position patient appropriately for medication administration.

Procedure

Steps	Procedure	Rationale
1.	Perform hand wash	Prevents spread of microorganism.
	Take the medicine card. If there is no card, make one after referring to the doctor's prescription on the patient's chart. Write patient's bed number name, age, drug, dose and frequency. For example: Bed No.6, Thankamma 24 years Mixt. Carminative 1 oz (30 mL) TDS. Tab: Vitamin C: 100 mg TDS	
2.	**DRUG CARD** _____ Patient's name Drug _____ _____ Generic Name Trade Name Classification _____ Action/Therapeutic Effect _____ _____ Therapeutic Drug Range _____ All Possible Routes _____ Side Effects _____ _____ Contraindications _____ _____ Nursing Implications _____ _____ _____ Source (including page number) _____ _____	Reduces the chance of medication errors
3.	After making the medicine card, proceed to the medicine cupboard with the card in a tray. Read the card. Locate the drug and read the label and see that it agrees with the medicine ordered 	Comparing the medication with the written orders helps to prevent medication errors.

Contd...

Steps	Procedure	Rationale

4.	Prepare medication in patient's bedside or in medication area as per the Institution's policy
	• Select proper medication from drawer or stock and compare with Kardex or order. Proceed from top to bottom of the Kardex.
	• Check expiration dates and perform calculations if necessary
	• Recheck each medication package or preparation with the order as it is taken
	
	• When all medications for one patient have been prepared, recheck once again with the medication order before taking them to patient
	• Place the prepared medications in the medication cup
	• Crush the medication using mortar and pestle if the client has swallowing difficulties. Grind tablets in a pill crusher until smooth
	
	• Ask patient's preference regarding medications
	  ▪ To be taken by hand or in cup
	  ▪ One at a time or all at once
	  ▪ With water or other permitted fluids
		This ensures that no medication order is missed
		
		Ensures that the correct dose of medicine is administered
		Reduces the chance of medication errors
		
		Crushed medicines helps easy swallowing by the patient

5.	Follow ten rights of medication administration at least three times before administration	Prevents medication errors

Contd...

Steps	Procedure	Rationale
6.	**Preparation of solution:** • Take the bottle in the right hand, shake it and read the label and medicine card a second time	Ensures proper mixture of the contents
Shake well	
	• Remove the cork, hold it between the 3rd and 4th finger of the left hand or take the cork using the small finger and the medial ulnar side of the inner palm of left hand. Screw cap can also be opened and kept upside down in the medication tray	Placing the cork in the medication tray prevent soiling of the cork as it is a multidose bottle
Onfi (clobazam) Oral Suspension	
	• Hold the medicine glass (with the left hand) so that the mark of the prescribed amount is on a level with eye, marking it with the thumb of the left hand	Ensures accurate measurement
	• Pour the exact amount of medicine from the bottle through the side opposite to the label. Place the ounce glass with the drug in the tray	Pouring away from the label keeps the label readable

Contd...

Steps	Procedure	Rationale
		Ensures safety of the medication during next use
	• Wipe the mouth of the bottle with the towel or a gauze, recork the bottle and place the bottle back in its place, after reading the label on the bottle and medicine card, a third time	
7.	Arrange the articles required at the bedside of the patient	Facilitates accurate skill performances
8.	Once again check the 10 rights of medication administration	Prevents medication errors
9.	Complete necessary assessments before giving medications	Ensures safety of the patient based on the medication action
10.	Assist patient to have an upright position	This makes swallowing easier and prevents aspiration
11.	Place the mackintosh and towel under the chin of the patient	Prevents soiling of linen and patient's clothes
12.	Don gloves as per the Institutions policy (if required)	Prevents cross infection
13.	Offer water or other permitted fluids	Facilitates easy swallowing of medication

Contd...

Steps	Procedure	Rationale
14	Place the prescribed medications in a: • **Medication cup:** Open the prepared medications and hand over it to the patients hand as per his or her preference either one by one or as a whole or • Use a spoon to hold the medicine after opening and give to the patient using the spoon • **Discard any medication that falls on the floor**	Facilitates easy administration of medicine as per patient preferences
15.	Remain with patient until each medication is swallowed	Ensures that the patient has taken the medicine
16.	Replace the tray to the utility room, wash, dry and replace all, in the cupboard	Prepares the articles for next use
17.	Perform hand hygiene	Prevents transfer of microorganisms
18.	Record each medication given on medication chart or record using required format along with: • Date and time of administration • Sign after administration of medicine • If drug was refused or omitted, record this in appropriate area on medication record 	Documentation ensures professional accountability
19.	Check patient within 30 minutes of drug administration to verify response to medication and for any adverse side effects	Helps to take further action

Unit IX ❖ Medication Needs of the Patient—Pharmacology

Advantages

- Oral medicines are more convenient to give
- More economic and time saving
- More safe if given with care

Disadvantages

- Drug cannot be given to patients with vomiting
- Patient may not like to take the drug with bad taste or irritating to the tongue
- Oral medicine takes time for action
- It cannot be given to unconscious or mental patients and patients who are not cooperative
- The actions of certain drugs are destroyed by digestive juices, e.g., Insulin

Contraindications for Oral Administration

- When there is nausea and vomiting
- When the patient is unconscious
- When urgency is required
- In case of oral surgery
- When the drugs are destroyed in the stomach and intestines by the action of the digestive juices, e.g., insulin and adrenalin

SUBLINGUAL ADMINISTRATION OF DRUG

In sublingual administration, the medicine in the tablet form is placed under the tongue and is allowed to dissolve in the mouth. Thus the medicine is absorbed through the mucous membrane under the tongue.

Advantages

- Absorption is uniform and fast
- The action of the drug is not destroyed in the stomach by the digestive enzymes. For example, Tab. Nitroglycerine in angina

Disadvantages

- Unpalatable and bitter drugs
- Few drugs are absorbed
- Large quantities not given
- Irritation of oral mucosa

Prerequisites

- Do not eat or drink when administering medication.
- Do not smoke for at least an hour before you take sublingual medication.
- Be aware of the possible risks like patients with open mouth sores may experience pain or irritation.

Procedure

Step	Procedure	Rationale
Follow the steps of oral medication administration procedure from step 1–12 as applicable.		
1.	Place the medication under the tongue on either side of the frenulum	Helps in quick absorption
2.	Tilt head forward to avoid swallowing medication.	Swallowing sublingual medication may cause erratic or incomplete absorption and could lead to improper dosing
3.	Wait for at least 5 minutes with the tablet under the tongue to allow the tablet to fully dissolve.	Helps in absorption of medicine

BUCCAL ROUTE OF ADMINISTRATION OF DRUG

Buccal administration is placement of medication between gums and inner lining of the cheek (buccal pouch) absorbed by buccal mucosa (Fig 1).

Advantages

- Avoids first pass effect
- Rapid absorption
- Drug stability

Disadvantages

- Inconvenience
- Advantages lost if swallowed
- Small dose limit

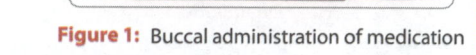

Figure 1: Buccal administration of medication

SPECIAL ACRONYMS

Latin Abbreviations Regarding the Time of Administration of Medicines

Abbreviation	Derivation	Meaning
TID	Three Times a day	9 am, 1 pm, 5 pm
QID	Four Times a day	9 am, 1 pm, 5 pm 9 pm

Contd...

Unit IX ❖ Medication Needs of the Patient—Pharmacology

Abbreviation	Derivation	Meaning
BID	Two Times a day	9 am, 5 pm, (BD)
OD	Once a day	8 am
HS		At bed time 9 pm
Q. 4 H	Once in four hours	8 am, 12 noon, 4 pm, 8 pm, 12 noon, 4 am
Q. 6 H	Once in 6 hours	10 am, 4 pm, 10 pm, 4 am
Q. 8 H	Once in 8 hours	6 am, 2 pm, 10 pm
Q. 12. H	Once in 12 hours	8 am, 8 pm

Medical Abbreviations Indicating the Time of Administration of Medicine

Abbreviation	Derivation	Meaning
AC	Ante cibum	Before meals
PC	Post cibum	After meals
am	Ante meridian	Morning
pm	Post meridian	Afternoon
Alt die	Alternis diebus	Alternate days
Alt noct	Alternis noctes	Alternate night
Alr hor	Alternis horis	Alternate hours
M et N	Maneet nocte	Morning and night
OM	Omni mane	Each morning
O D	Omni die	Daily
O N	Omni nocte	Each night
HS	Hora somni	At bed time
HN	Hac nocte	To night
CM	Cras name	Tomorrow morning
Hd	Hora decubitus	At bed time
H	Hora	Hour
PRN	Prorenate	When required
Qh	Quaque hora	Every hour
Rep	Repetatur	Repeat
BID (BD)	Bis in die	Twice a day
Q.	Quaque	Every
Q 2h, Q 3h, Q4h		Every two, three or four hours
QID or 4, d	Quarter in die	Four times a day
Stat	Statim	At once
SOS	Si opus sit	If necessary in emergency
TDS	Ter in die	Three times a day
TID	Ter in die	Three times daily

Abbreviation Regarding Types of Drugs

Abbreviation	Derivation	Meaning
aq	Aqua	Water
aq dest	Aqua destillatu	Distilled water
comp	Compositum	Compound
dil	Dilutis	Dilute
et	et	And
fl	Fluidum	Fluid
inf	Indusum	Infusion
Lin	Linementum	Liniment
empl	Emplastrum	Plaster
Liq	Liquor	Liquid
Lot.	Lotio	Lotion
mist	Mistura	Mixture
ol	Oleum	Oil
Pil	Pilula	Pill
pulv	Pulvia	Powder
sp	Spiritus	Spirit
Syr	Syrupus	Syrup
tinct of Tr.	Tincture	Tincture
ung	Unguentum	Ointment

Abbreviation Regarding the Amount or Dosage of Drugs

Abbreviation	Derivation	Meaning
aa	Ana	Of each
add	Adde	Add to
add part. dol	Adde partes dolents	To the painful part
ad lib	Ad Libitum	As much as desired
gal	Gallon	Gallon
C	Centigrade	Centigrade
C	Cum	With
c.c		Cubic centimeter
gm	Gram	Gram, grams
gr.	Granum, grana	Grain
gtt.	Gutta	A drop, drops
garg	Gargarisma	Gargle
kg.	Kilogram	One thousand grams
I. L.	Liter	One liter

Contd...

Abbreviation	Derivation	Meaning
Lb	Libra	Pound
m.	Minimus	Minim
mL	Milli liter	1 cc
no	Numero	Number
O	Octarius	A pint
part vic	Partitis vicibus	In divided doses
q.s.	Quantum sufficit	As much as is sufficient
Rx.	Recipe	Take thou
S	sine	Without
S.O.S	si opus sit	If necessary
SS	semis	On half
tsp	Tea spoon	Tea spoon full
tbsp.	Table spoon	Table spoon full
z	Drachma	Dram
oz	Uncial	Ounce

Miscellaneous Abbreviations and Measurements

Common Medical Abbreviation	
Hypo	=	Hypodermic
IM	=	Intra muscularly
Per	=	Through or by means of
PV	=	Per Vagina
SC	=	Subcutaneously
IV	=	Intravenously
PR	=	Per Rectum
i.e.	=	That is

Household Measures	
60 drops	=	Teaspoon
2 teaspoon	=	1 desert spoon
2 desert spoons	=	1 tablespoon
4 table spoons	=	1 wine glass
3 wine glasses	=	1 drinking glass

Sometimes it is necessary to change from one type of measure to another. Some of the approximate comparative measurements of the three systems are given below.

Household Measures

15 grains	=	1 gram
15 minims	=	1 cubic centimeter
1 dram	=	4 grams
1 dram	=	4 mL (cc) = 1 tea spoon
1 ounce	=	30 grams
1 ounce	=	30 cubic centimeters. It is seen as 25 mL (cc) in certain books.

Weights and Measures

There are several systems of measuring medicines: the apothecary, imperial, metric and household measures.

Combination of Apothecary and Imperial Systems

Table of weights	Table of measures
60 grains = 1 dram	60 minims = 1 dram
8 drams = 1 ounce	8 drams = 1 ounce
16 ounce = 1 pound	20 ounces = 1 pint
	2 pints = 1 quart
	4 quarts = 1 gallon

The Metric Systems

Table of weights	Table of measures
10 milligrams = 1 centigram 10 centigrams = 1 decigram 10 decigrams = 1 gram 10 grams = 1 dekagram 10 dekagrams = 1 hectogram 10 hectograms = 1 kilogram	10.cubic centimeters = 1 centiliter 10 centiliters = 1 deciliter 10 deciliters = 1 liter

Common abbreviations used in nursing	
WHO	World Health Organization
C	Centigrade (Celsius)
F	Fahrenheit
BCG	Bacille Calmette Guerin
CNS	Central Nervous System
CO_2	Carbon dioxide
O_2	Oxygen
Vol	Volume
U	Units
IU	International Unit
SC	Subcutaneous
IM	Intramuscular
IV	Intravenous
mm Hg	Millimeters of Mercury
MM	Millimeter
mL	Milliliter
Mg	Milligram
PR	Pulse Rate
PR	Per Rectum
PV	Per Vagina
BP	Blood Pressure
TC and DC	Total Count and Differential Count

Contd...

Unit IX ❖ Medication Needs of the Patient—Pharmacology

Common abbreviations used in nursing	
TPR	Temperature, Pulse and Respiration
LOC	Level of Consciousness
Sp Gr	Specific Gravity
Wt	Weight
Ht	Height
Hb	Hemoglobin
ESR	Erythrocyte sedimentation rate

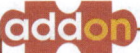

Classification of Drugs According to the Action

- Analgesics are drugs which relieve pain, e.g., aspirin.
- Anesthetics are drugs, which cause loss of sensation or insensibility to patients, e.g., ether, etomidate, ketamine and propofol.
- Antipyretics are drugs, which reduce fever, e.g., crocin, paracetamol, etc.
- Antihelminthics are drugs, which destroy and expel worms, e.g., quassia, mebex and albendazole.
- Antidotes are substances used to counteract the effects of poison, e.g., large quantity of dilute alkali for acid poisoning, e.g., activated charcoal for most poisons, e.g., activated charcoal for most poisons.
- Anticoagulant is substance that prevents or inhibits the coagulation of blood, e.g., heparin and warfarin.
- Antiemetic or antemetic is an agent used to prevent or relieve nausea or vomiting, e.g., dimenhydrinate.
- Antacid is a substance, which counteracts acidity or neutralizes acids, e.g., milk of magnesia.
- Antihistamine is a drug that counteracts the effects of histamine and has been used successfully in the treatment of certain allergic conditions, e.g., cetirizine.
- Anodyne is any drug used to relieve pain, e.g., opium, henbane, hemlock, tobacco, nightshade ("stramonium"), and chloroform.
- Blood coagulant is a substance used to hasten blood coagulation, e.g., desmopressin and vasopressin.
- Carminatives are drugs, which cause expulsion of gas from the stomach and intestine, e.g., ginger and mixture carminative.
- Cathartics are drugs, which cause intestinal evacuation. They are subdivided as follows:
- Laxatives or aperients have a mild action, e.g., liquid paraffin, magnesia.
- Purgatives are more powerful, e.g., magnesium sulfate and castor oil.
- Drastics have violent action, e.g., croton oil.
- Hydragogues produce loose watery stools, e.g., magnesium sulfate.
- Cholagogues are drugs, which are supposed to increase the amount of bile secretion, e.g., oxgall and ursodeoxycholic acid.
- Coagulant is an agent which acts to change a substance from a liquid state to a semi solid jelly - like form.
- Diaphoretics are drugs which increase perspiration, e.g., oxybutynin and aspirin.
- Diuretics are drugs which increase the flow of urine, e.g., lasix.
- Emetics are drugs which produce vomiting, e.g., ipecac and apomorphine.
- Ecbolics are drugs which stimulate uterine contraction, e.g., ergometrine, pitutrin.
- Expectorants are drugs which increase the bronchial secretion and help in expulsion of mucus, e.g., cough expectorants.
- Hypnotics are drugs which produce sleep, e.g., cough veronal, e.g., zopiclone.
- Histamine is a chemical factor which excites the flow of gastric juices and acts in addition to nerve stimulation of psychic factors involved and it is considered to be one of the causes of allergy.

Contd...

Unit IX ❖ Medication Needs of the Patient—Pharmacology

- Mydriatics are drugs which dilate pupils of the eye, e.g. drosyn, AK-Pentolate, altafrin, atropine ophthalmic.
- Miotics are drugs which contract the pupils, e.g. eserin, pilocarpine and carbachol.
- Narcotic is any drug which produces sleep or stupor and relieves pain, e.g. opium, heroin and codone.
- Sedatives are drugs which exerts a soothening or tranquilizing effect. They may be general, local, nervous or vascular opium and benzodiazepines.
- Specifics are drugs which have a special curative action in certain disease, e.g. quinine in malaria, streptomycin in tuberculosis.
- Stimulants are drugs which increase the functional activity of an organ, e.g. caffeine stimulates central nervous system.
- Stomachics or gastric tonics are drugs, which increase appetite, e.g. B complex.

PARENTERAL ADMINISTRATION OF MEDICINE

Parenteral administration of drugs is the term used for giving therapeutic agents including foods, besides the alimentary tract, e.g., injections, IV (intravenous) infusions, total parenteral nutrition (TPN).

Injections

The term "Injection" is defined as the forcing of fluid into a cavity, a blood vessel, or body tissue through a hollow tube or needle.

Purpose of injections

- To get rapid or a systemic effect of the drug, e.g., IV injections.
- To give a drug when other routes are undesirable, e.g. excessive vomiting or having gastric suction.
- To obtain local effect at the site of injection, e.g. local anesthetics such as novocaine infiltration, tuberculin test, etc.

Advantages of Injections

- It prevents the destruction of the effect of drugs in the alimentary canal.
- It is useful when the patient is unconscious.
- It is used in cases of vomiting and diarrhea.
- Drugs which are not absorbed in the small intestines can be given by injection.
- Drugs which are irritating to the stomach can be given by injection.

Disadvantages of Injections

- Infection due to careless handling and improper sterilization of syringes, needles and the fluids used for injection.
- Self-administration is difficult.
- More expensive.
- Pain on the site.
- Improper site of injection is dangerous.
- Keeping the correct time of injection is more important than oral administration.
- When a drug is taken by oral route, it can be removed to a certain extent, by stomach wash or bowel wash, if required. But when an injection is given in the tissues or blood vessels it cannot be removed from the body. And another injection of antidote has to be given to remove the effect of the drug.

Unit IX ❖ Medication Needs of the Patient—Pharmacology

Possible Complications of Injections

- Infection
- Allergy to drugs
- Injuries to the tissues
- Psychic trauma to the patient
- Pain
- Nerve injury and foot drop
- Overdose or under dose of medicines

  Stimulant

Common Solutions used for Injections
- Diagnostic drugs, e.g. dyes and histamines
- Preventive drugs, like toxoids, vaccines, etc.
- Curative drugs or remedial drugs, like antibiotics and other specific drugs
- Protein varieties, like minerals and vitamins

Solutions given in the Veins
- Saline solutions, like normal saline, glucose saline, etc.
- Glucose solutions of different strength
- Distilled water
- Blood and serum varieties
- Drugs for anesthesia, like pentothal

Types of Injections or Different Routes of Injections

- Intradermal injection drugs injected just under the skin or into the dermis
- Hypodermal or subcutaneous injection drugs injected in the subcutaneous tissue or areolar tissue (just below the skin)
- Intramuscular injection drugs injected into the muscles
- Intraosseous drugs injected in the bone marrow
- Intravenous injection drugs injected in the veins
- Intra-arterial injection drugs injected in the arteries
- Intraspinal or intrathecal injection drugs injected in the spinal cavity
- Intraperitoneal injection drugs injected in the peritoneal cavity

Medication Administration Safety

The nurse should ensure that safety measures are taken related to:
- Look-alike/sound-alike medications
- High-alert medications

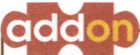

Syringes and Needles used for Injections

There are the following two types of syringes:
1. **Disposable syringe:** These can be used only once and should be discarded
2. **Reusable syringes:** These can be used again after proper sterilization.

Parts of Syringe and Needle

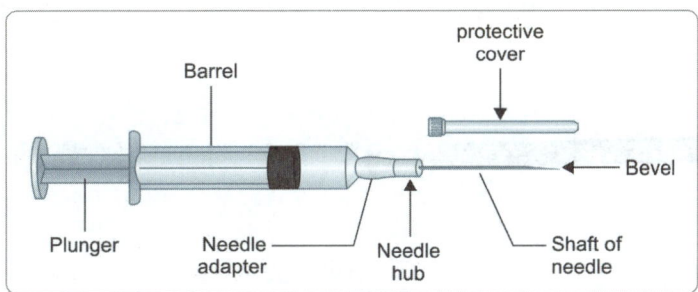

Figure 2: Disposable syringe and needle

- Syringes are made up of two parts. The outer part is called barrel and the inner part is called piston or plunges (Fig. 2)
- The measurements are recorded in c.c. or mL on the barrel of the syringe.
- The usual sizes of syringes are 2, 5, 10, 20, 30 and 50 mL.
- The insulin and tuberculin syringes are special syringes. The scale on the insulin syringe is marked in units according to the concentration of the insulin being used like U/40, U/80, etc. There will be 40 or 80 division in the barrel in 1 mL. It indicates that 1 mL contains 40 or 80 units of insulin.
- There is another type of small syringe used to give tuberculin, in which the scale on barrel shows 100 divisions. This can be used for giving insulin also. But proper calculation is required according to the unit of insulin in 1 mL. 1 mL is divided into 100 parts. 1 mL is marked as ten large divisions and each large division is again divided into ten small divisions. That means a small division is equal to 1/100 of 1 mL. It is used for measuring small amount of drugs such as tuberculin test and penicillin test dose, etc.

Various Types of Syringes

- Based on the size of syringes (Figs 3 and 4):
  - Smaller volumes mostly used for subcutaneous and intramuscular injections.
  - The larger the syringe size, the lower is the pressure flow.
  - 10–12 mL commonly used for central lines, catheters, medical tubing.
  - 20–70 mL commonly used for irrigation.

Unit IX ❖ Medication Needs of the Patient—Pharmacology

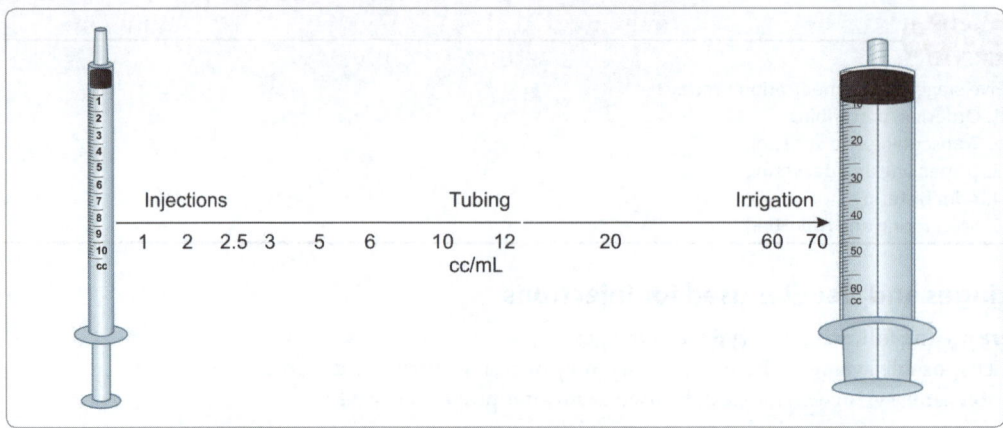

Figure 3: Syringe size continuum

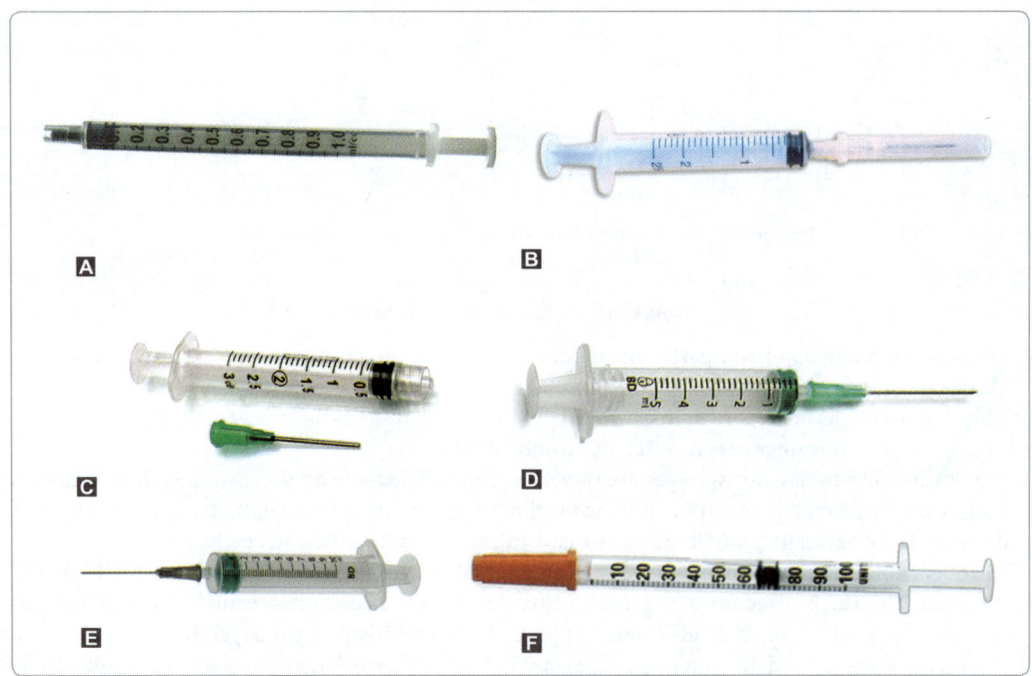

Figures 4A to F: Different types of syringes

These syringes can be used for giving insulin also if insulin syringe is not available. **But proper calculation is needed.** For example, if doctor instructs to give 20 units from a U/40 in 1 mL insulin. The nurse has to see that the syringe is marked 100 parts in 1 mL.

So find out that $\dfrac{20}{40} \times 100 = 50$ points in the syringe, should be given to the patient to get 20 units of U/40 insulin. If the syringe is real insulin syringe, there is no need of any calculation.

Unit IX ❖ Medication Needs of the Patient—Pharmacology

- **Based on the syringe tip (Fig. 5):**

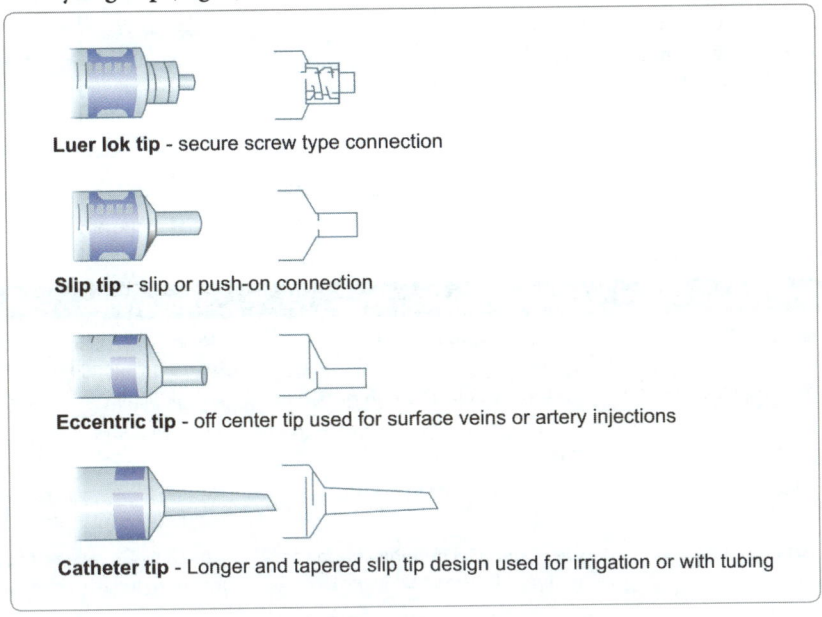

Luer lok tip - secure screw type connection

Slip tip - slip or push-on connection

Eccentric tip - off center tip used for surface veins or artery injections

Catheter tip - Longer and tapered slip tip design used for irrigation or with tubing

Figure 5: Types of syringe tips

- **Based on the type of plunger (Figs 6A and B)**

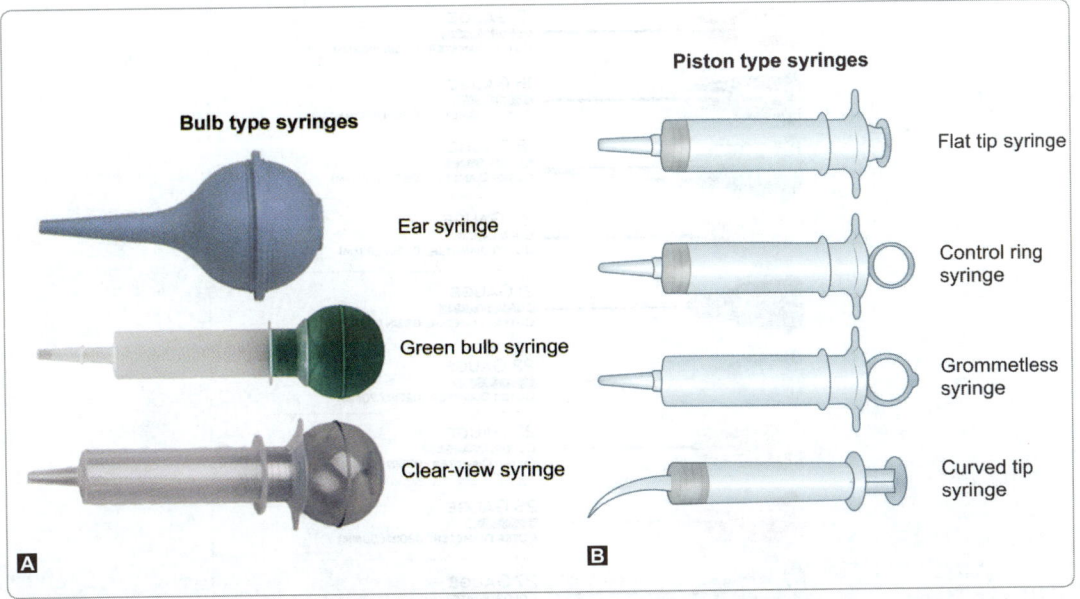

Bulb type syringes

Ear syringe

Green bulb syringe

Clear-view syringe

Piston type syringes

Flat tip syringe

Control ring syringe

Grommetless syringe

Curved tip syringe

A

B

Figures 6A and B: (A) Bulb type syringes; (B) Piston type syringes

Needles

Needles are made up of steel or any other metals. Like the syringes, needles may be disposable or reusable. Reusable needles and syringes are sterilized after use, for administering injection to another patient (Fig. 7). The various parts of the needle are:

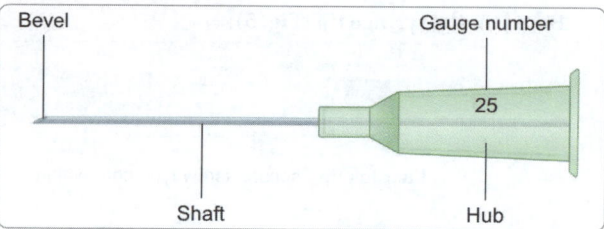

Figure 7: Parts of the needle

Table 1: Common syringes and needles

Routes of administration	Size of syringe	Size of needles
Intradermal injection	1 mL syringe marked 100 points	No. 26 or 27 gauge diameter and 3/8 to 5/8 inch length
Subcutaneous or hypodermal injection	1 mL marked in 40 or 80 Units (insulin syringe) or 2 or 3 mL syringes marked in 0.1. mL.	No. 25 gauge and ½ to 5/8 inch or same as above
Intramuscular injection	2 or 5 mL marked in 0.2 mL	No. 21, 22, 23, gauge needle 1 to 2 inches length
Intravenous injection of infusion	Size of needles depends upon the amount of fluid to be given	No. 18 to 21 gauge needle 1 to 2 inches in length

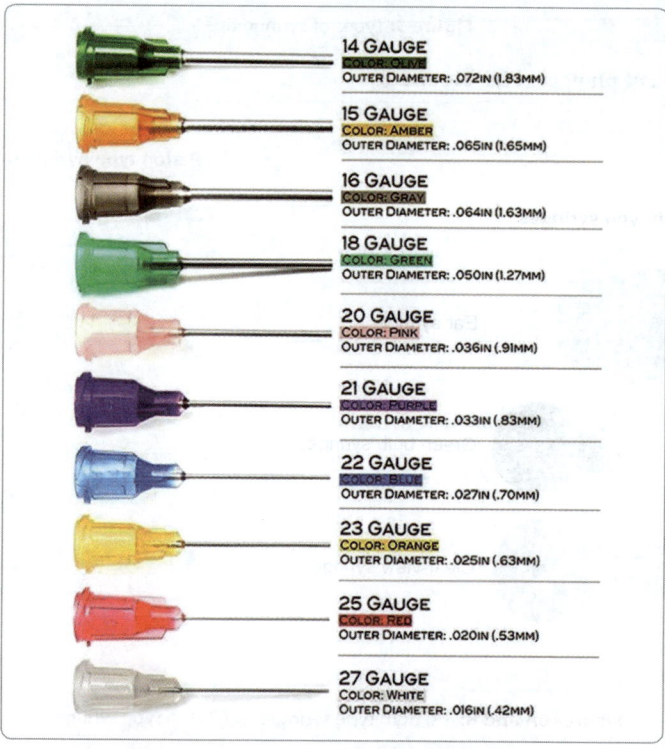

Figure 8: Size chart of needle Gauges for injections

METHODS OF WITHDRAWING MEDICATION

Medication preparation from a vial is the method of preparing a drug contained in a vial into a usable form.

Principles

- Be vigilant when preparing medications
- Avoid distractions
- Check for allergies
- Be diligent in all medication calculations
- Ensure medication has not expired
- Always clarify an order or procedure that is unclear
- Report all near misses, errors and adverse reactions
- Keep the injection preparation area free of clutter so all surfaces can be easily cleaned

Requisites

A clean tray containing:

Article	Purpose
Materials for hand wash or hand rub	Aids in the removal of microorganisms
Medication vial or ampule	To withdraw prescribed medicine
A small bowl with cotton swabs or a pack of sterile swab	To wipe the vial after opening its metal cap
70% alcohol (isopropyl alcohol or ethanol)	To wipe the vial after opening its metal cap
Ampule cutter or file (if required)	To open the ampule
Syringe with needle	For administration of injection
Sharps container	To dispose the ampule glass top
Waste bin	To discard biomedical waste

Withdrawing Medication from a Vial

Steps	Procedure	Rationale
1.	Wash your hands well and dry with a clean towel	Prevents spread of microorganism
2.	Confirm the 10 rights of medication administration	Prevents medication error
3.	Arrange the articles required	Helps to reduce anxiety and saves time and energy
4.	Inspect the medication for name, dose, expiry date, any particles in the solution	Prevents medication error
5.	Take the vial and keep in the tray. Flip the metal cap of the medication vial	Helps in easy access of the rubber stopping for medication withdrawal

Contd...

Unit IX ❖ Medication Needs of the Patient—Pharmacology

Steps	Procedure	Rationale
6.	Wipe the access diaphragm (septum) with 70% alcohol (isopropyl alcohol or ethanol) on a swab or cotton-wool ball using a circular motion for 15 seconds before piercing the vial and discard the swab in the paper bag. Allow to air dry before inserting the syringe into the bottle 	Prevents spread of microorganism
7.	Open the package in front of the patient. Remove the syringe and needle from the sterile pack and uncap the needle from its cover. Ensure that the tip of the needle doesn't touch anywhere as it is sterile. Take the needle, holding on the hub of it and fix it on the tip of the syringe. 	Ensures the patient that the syringe is not used for someone else. Ensures that the needle doesn't get dislodged.
8.	Pull back the plunger of the syringe and withdraw air into it. The amount of air should be equal to the amount of medication to be withdrawn from the vial. To prevent the syringe from slipping down, hold the first finger (thumb) on one side, next three fingers on the other side of the barrel and the small finger at the almost tip of the piston with a little force 	If very little air is introduced to the vial it interferes the flow of drug to the syringe and if too much air is introduced, the pressure in the vial increases and the piston is pushed down suddenly.

Contd...

Steps	Procedure	Rationale
9.	Take the vial with the left hand and check the name of the drug and other details again holding it in the eye level. Insert the needle into the center of the vial and gently pull back the plunger 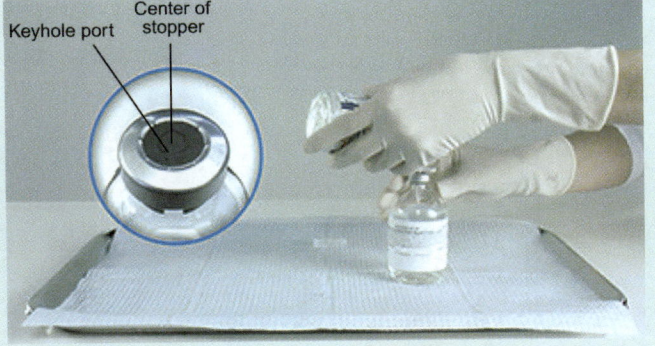 Push the air into the vial slowly 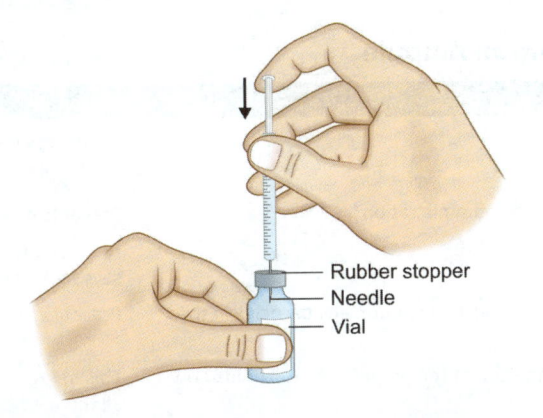	Aids in correct dispersion of medicine into the syringe
10.	Turn back the vial upside down and pull back the plunger. When the bottle is inverted, prevent it from falling down by holding near its neck between the index finger and middle finger of the left hand and holding on the barrel of the syringe with the ring finger and small finger in one side and first finger (thumb) on the other side of the left hand. Withdraw the required amount of medication as per the order 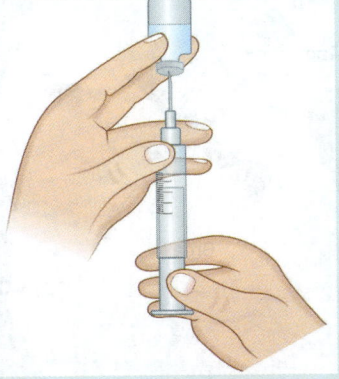	The air inside the syringe pushes the medicine inside the syringe which is supported by the action of the plunger

Contd...

Steps	Procedure	Rationale
11.	Remove the syringe from the vial and gently tap the syringe and push all the air from the syringe by pushing the plunger. Now the medication is ready for administration. Place the medicine in the tray (or as per hospital's policy)	Injecting the medicine with air bubbles may cause adverse effect on the patient.

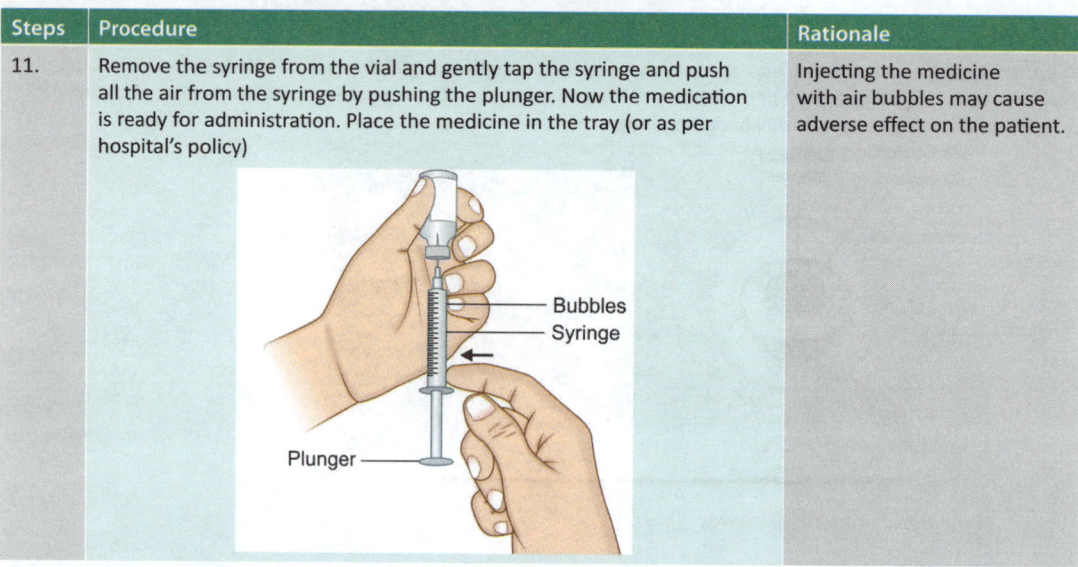

Withdrawing Medication from an Ampule

Steps	Procedure	Rationale
1.	Perform hand wash	Prevents spread of microorganism.
2.	Confirm the 10 rights of medication administration	Prevents medication error
3.	Arrange the articles required	Helps reduce anxiety and saves time and energy
4.	Inspect the medication for name, dose, expiry date, any particles in the solution	Prevents medication error
5.	Take an ampule and gently tap the top of the ampule until all fluids flow into the bottom chamber	This helps to make sure that all the medication is in the bottom part of the ampule.

Contd...

Steps	Procedure	Rationale
6.	Wrap an antiseptic wipe using the thumb and index finger around the neck of the ampule. If the drug is in a glass ampule, file is required to make a mark on the neck of the ampule where it is to be broken. The outside of the ampule and the file is cleaned with the swab moistened with alcohol	Prevents spillage of medication
7.	Using a file or an ampule cutter, firmly grasp the neck of the ampule at the area of demarcation to snap off the top by facing it away from you. Discard the top into the sharps, container	Directs shattered glass top of ampule away from the face.
8.	Open the package in front of the patient. Remove the syringe and needle from the sterile pack and uncap the needle from its cover. Ensure that the tip of the needle doesn't touch anywhere as it is sterile.	To reassure the patient that the syringe and needle have not been used previously.

Contd...

Unit IX ❖ Medication Needs of the Patient—Pharmacology

Steps	Procedure	Rationale
9.	Insert the needle into the opening of the ampule and draw the required amount of medication by pulling back the plunger. Withdraw by inverting the ampule slowly. Ensure that all the drug from the bottom of the ampule is withdrawn by tapping the tip until the liquid leaves it. **Never push in air into the ampule**	Ensures that no drug is wasted.
10.	Remove the syringe from the ampule. Discard the empty ampule into the sharp's container. Gently tap the syringe and push all the air from the syringe by pushing the plunger. Now the medication is ready for administration. Place the medicine in the tray (or as per hospital's policy).	Injecting the medicine with air bubbles may cause adverse effect to the patient.
11.	**Never** leave the medication unsupervised once prepared.	Medications left unattended may lead to medication errors.

ADMINISTRATION OF INJECTIONS

Intradermal Injection (ID)

Injection of a substance that is administered into the dermis layer of the skin, which is just between the epidermis and the hypodermis is called intradermal injection.

Purpose

- Diagnostic purpose, e.g., Schick test in diphtheria, tuberculin test.
- To note whether there is any allergic reaction, e.g., penicillin, AT serum, etc.
- Local treatment, e.g., local anesthetics before any invasive procedure, chaulmoogra oil in patients with leukoderma.

Sites of Injection (for Diagnostic and Allergic Reactions)

- Inner surface of the forearm midway between wrist and elbow as the skin is thin and free from hair.
- Directly to the patches in cases of leukoderma (Fig. 9).

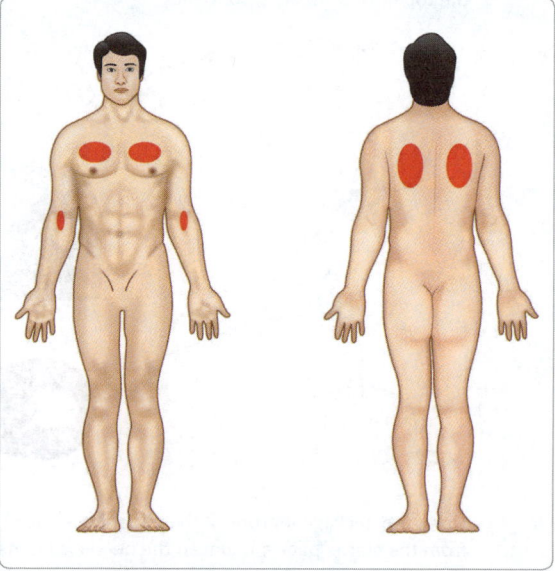

Figure 9: Sites for intradermal injection

Prerequisites

- Check the 10 rights of medication administration.
- Prepare the medication and keep it ready. The dosage of an intradermal injection is typically below 0.5 mL.

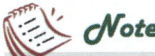 *Note*

- Do not pre-soak cotton wool in a container—these become highly contaminated with hand and environmental bacteria.
- Do not use alcohol skin disinfection for administration of vaccinations.

Articles Required

A clean tray containing:

Article	Purpose
Materials for hand wash	Aids in the removal of microorganisms
Sterile syringe and needle in a container. Special syringe and needles may be used (Needle 26 or 27 gauge, 1 cm long)	For easy administration of injection
Ampule or vial	To administer medication
A small bowl with cotton swabs or a pack of sterile swab	To wipe the injection site
70% alcohol (isopropyl alcohol or ethanol)	To wipe the injection site
A small bowl containing dry gauze	To wipe the area after administration of injection
Non-sterile gloves	To prevent cross infection
Kidney tray	To dispose the waste
Syringe dispenser	To dispose the used syringes and needles
Waste bin	To discard biomedical waste
Dot pen	To draw a circle around the site of ID injection
Note pad and pen	To document the procedure

Preparation

Preparation of Unit

- Ensure an area of good lighting.
- Arrange all the necessary articles close to the bedside of the patient.
- Provide privacy by closing the door, pulling the curtains and exposing only the site of injection.

Preparation of Patient

- Explain the procedure and the reason for administering the medication and give the patient time to ask questions.
- Win the confidence and cooperation of the patient by giving proper explanation regarding the nature of the treatment.

Unit IX ❖ Medication Needs of the Patient—Pharmacology

Procedure

Steps	Procedure	Rationale
1.	Prepare the injection from the vial or ampule as per the steps given earlier (Refer to method of withdrawing injection from vial or ampule)	Aids in easy administration of injection
2.	Perform hand hygiene	Prevents the transmission of microorganisms
3.	Place the patient in comfortable position	This prepares the patient for injection
4.	Don non-sterile gloves	Prevents cross infection
5.	• Locate correct site using landmarks. Choose an injection site that is free of hair, moles, rashes, scars, and other skin lesions • If patient's inner forearm is chosen, then position their arm with their palm facing up. The arm should be relaxed with elbow flexed • Apply a 60–70% alcohol-based solution (isopropyl alcohol or ethanol) on a single-use swab or cotton-wool ball • Wipe the area from the center of the injection site working outward using a circular motion, without going over the same area • Apply the solution for 30 seconds, then allow it to dry completely	Facilitates easy administration of injection Promotes comfort to the patient Prevents transfer of microorganisms Allowing the site to dry prevents stinging during injection and also prevent alcohol and other pathogens from entering the skin when the needle is inserted

Contd...

Steps	Procedure	Rationale
6.	Hold the syringe containing the medication in the dominant hand. With the non-dominant hand, grasp the client's dorsal forearm and gently pull the skin taut on ventral forearm	This prevents the movement of the skin while administration
7.	Insert the needle with bevel side up at 10–150 angle until resistance is felt. Move the needle approximately 3 mm below the skin surface. Ensure that the tip of the needle is visible under skin surface	Resistance indicates that the needle tip is in subcutaneous region
8.	Administer the medication slowly. Observe for a wheal	Ensures that the medication is injected intradermally
9.	Withdraw the needle at an angle that is the same as the insertion angle	This minimizes damage to the tissues at the injection site and discomfort to the patient

Contd...

Unit IX ❖ Medication Needs of the Patient—Pharmacology

Steps	Procedure	Rationale
10.	Cover injection site with sterile gauze. Do not massage the area	Massaging the area may cause the medication to spread to the underlying subcutaneous tissues
11.	Do not recap the needle and discard syringe and the needle as per the biomedical waste management (BWM) policy	Facilitates safe disposal of syringes thus preventing needle stick injuries
12.	Draw a circle around the wheal formed at the site. Re-adjust the patient's position, instruct the patient not to wipe or scratch the site	This helps to identify adverse reactions, if any
13.	Replace articles, discard supplies, remove gloves and perform hand hygiene	Prevents transfer of micro-organisms
14.	Document the procedure with date and time including the name of medication, time, route, site, date of administration, any adverse effects, unexpected outcomes and interventions applied, if any	Recording the procedure acts as a legal document.
15.	Assess patient's response to the medication after the appropriate time frame	Ensures that the patient does not have any adverse effects and if any appropriate actions can be taken immediately

Hypodermic or Subcutaneous Injection

It is the introduction of a small quantity of drug to the subcutaneous tissue.

Therapeutic uses or Purposes

- To give drug when other routes are undesirable.
- To prevent the drug from being destroyed or ineffective by the action of the digestive juice.
- To obtain the effect of the drug at the site of the injection.
- To obtain the prompt action. The drugs act more quickly or more effectively if absorbed through the subcutaneous tissue.

Selection of Site

Any of the less sensitive area of the body where no bones or large blood vessels on the surface are present, e.g., it could be outer surface of the arm 5 cm below the shoulder or the outer aspect of the thigh and around the umbilicus, muscular areas of the body, the outer aspect of the upper arm, the abdomen below the costal margins to the iliac crests, the anterior aspect of the thigh, the ventrodorsal gluteal area, or as an alternative, the scapular area (Fig. 10).

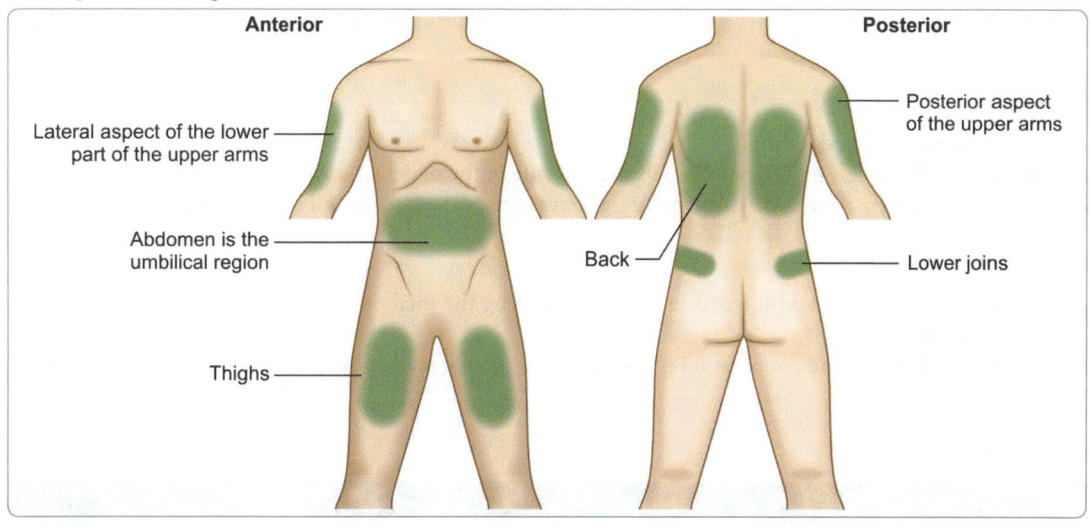

Figure 10: Sites to administer subcutaneous injection

Areas to give subcutaneous injections are, for example shoulders, around the umbilicus and outer aspects of the thighs.

Prerequisites

- Check the 10 rights of medication administration.
- When a patient is frequently given hypodermic injection, the sites of injection should be rotated, to avoid puncturing of the same spot too often.

Articles Required

A clean tray containing:

Article	Purpose
Materials for hand wash	Aids in the removal of microorganisms
Sterile syringe and needle in a container. Size of syringe 2 mL or 5 mL. Size of needle - No.25 and length 5/8 inch (1.83 cm)	For easy administration of injection
Ampule or vial	To administer medication
A small bowl with cotton swabs or a pack of sterile swab	To wipe the injection site
70% alcohol (isopropyl alcohol or ethanol)	To wipe the injection site
A small bowl containing dry gauze	To wipe the area after administration of injection

Contd...

Unit IX ❖ Medication Needs of the Patient—Pharmacology

Article	Purpose
Non-sterile gloves	To prevent cross infection
Kidney tray	To dispose the waste
Syringe dispenser	To dispose the used syringes and needles
Waste bin	To discard biomedical waste
Note pad and pen	To document the procedure

Preparation of Unit

- Ensure an area of good lighting
- Arrange all the necessary articles close to the bed side of the patient
- Provide privacy by closing the door, pulling the curtains and exposing only the site of injection.

Preparation of Patient

- Explain the procedure and the reason for administering the medication and give time to the patient to ask questions.
- Win the confidence and cooperation of the patient by giving proper explanation regarding the nature of the treatment.

Procedure

Steps	Procedure	Rationale
1.	Prepare the injection from the vial or ampule as per the steps given above (Refer to method of withdrawing injection from vial or ampule)	Aids in easy administration of injection
2.	Perform hand hygiene	Prevents the transmission of microorganisms
3.	Place the patient in comfortable position	This prepares the patient for injection
4.	Don non-sterile gloves	Prevents cross infection
5.	• Locate correct site using landmarks. Choose an injection site that is free of hair, moles, rashes, scars, and other skin lesions • Apply 60–70% alcohol-based solution (isopropyl alcohol or ethanol) on a single-use swab or cotton-wool ball • Wipe the area from the center of the injection site working outwards using a circular motion, without going over the same area • Apply the solution for 30 seconds, then allow it to dry completely	Facilitates easy administration of injection Prevents transfer of microorganisms Allows the site to dry, prevents stinging during injection and also prevents alcohol and other pathogens from entering the skin when the needle is inserted

Contd...

Steps	Procedure	Rationale
6.	Hold the syringe containing the medication like a pencil or a dart between the thumb and forefingers in the dominant hand. With the thumb and forefinger of the non-dominant hand, pinch the subcutaneous tissue.	This prevents the movement of the skin while administration.
7.	• Insert the needle quickly with bevel side up at 45° or 90° angle. Release the subcutaneous tissue and grasp the barrel of the syringe with non-dominant hand. • Using the dominant hand aspirate for blood by pulling back the plunger gently.	Inserting quickly causes less pain to the patient. Subcutaneous tissue is abundant in well-nourished, well-hydrated people and hence has to be inserted at 90°. In patients with little subcutaneous tissue, it is best to insert the needle at a 45° angle.
8.	If no blood appears, inject all of the solution gently and steadily by pushing down the plunger. Administer the medication slowly at a rate of 10 seconds per mL. Avoid moving the syringe.	Ensures that the medication is injected subcutaneously
9.	Cover injection site with sterile gauze, using gentle pressure. Gently massage the area. If an anticoagulant is administered, do not massage the area.	Promotes dispersal of the medication and facilitates absorption. Massaging after a heparin injection can contribute to the formation of a hematoma

Contd...

Unit IX ❖ Medication Needs of the Patient—Pharmacology

Steps	Procedure	Rationale
10.	Do not recap the needle and discard syringe and the needle as per the BMW (Biomedical Waste Management) policy.	Facilitates safe disposal of syringes thus preventing needle stick injuries.
11.	Replace articles, discard supplies, remove gloves and perform hand hygiene.	Prevents transfer of micro-organisms.
12.	Document the procedure with date and time including the name of medication, time, route, site, date of administration, any adverse effects, unexpected outcomes and interventions applied, if any.	Recording the procedure acts as a legal document.
13.	Assess patient's response to the medication after the appropriate time frame.	Ensures that the patient does not have any adverse effects and, if any appropriate actions can be taken immediately.

Intramuscular Injection (IM)

It is the introduction of a drug into the muscles with a syringe and needle. Quantity may range from 2 mL to 10 mL.

Purposes

- To give drugs which are not suitable for IV administration but from which quicker effect is desired than that is obtained by hypodermic or subcutaneous route.
- To give drugs, which are irritating to other tissues.
- To give drugs when the amount of solution is more, to be given subcutaneously.
- To give drugs, which are suspended in oil.

Complications

Intramuscular injections involve more risk than subcutaneous injection since there is a greater likelihood of striking nerves and large blood vessels.

- Complications that may occur include abscess, cyst, necrosis and sloughing of tissue, scar formation, pain, accidental intravascular injection and nerve injury.
- Injury of the sciatic nerve can occur after one injection in the buttock in any age group although the new-born infant, especially the premature infant is more likely to experience this complication.
- Foot drop and persistent paralysis in the lower leg and foot are signs of nerve injury, most often observed.

Site for an Intramuscular Injection

The selection of site for the injection is of utmost importance and requires an understanding of the anatomy of the area in which the injection is to be given. Sites for intramuscular injections include the dorsogluteal **ventrogluteal**, **vastus lateralis**, and the **deltoid site**.

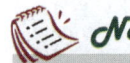 *Note*

Since the total gluteal region is small in the infant, the preferred site of injection is the mid-anterior aspect of the thigh with the quadriceps muscle as the recipient of the injected substance.

For adults, gluteal muscle of the buttock, deltoid muscle of the upper arm are considered safer.

Dorsogluteal

The dorsogluteal site is used most frequently for intramuscular injection in adults because the gluteus maximus, which is a big muscle is there, and it can absorb large quantities of solution, making irritating drugs less painful. Since there is danger of trauma to the sciatic nerve and the superior and inferior gluteal artery, it is necessary that the site should be located anatomically so that the needle is not be misplaced.

- The patient should be placed either in a prone position with the feet internally rotated and in plantar flexion, or sitting or lying down on his side with his buttock exposed. The position should be such as to relax the muscle of the area and to avoid tenseness of the body as a whole. These positions ensure the relaxation of the muscle as the injection is given.
- In standing or sitting position, the relaxation of the muscle is impossible and there is danger of a sudden jerking movement that may break the needle.
- Divide the buttock into four regions by imaginary lines:
  - **The upper and outer quadrant of the gluteal area is the recommended site and may be located by drawing line from the posterior superior iliac spine to the grater trochanter of the femur.**
  - Any injection given **lateral and superior to this line** will be at some distance from the sciatic nerve - Select the site at the upper and outer quadrant for the intramuscular injection (Figs 11A and B).

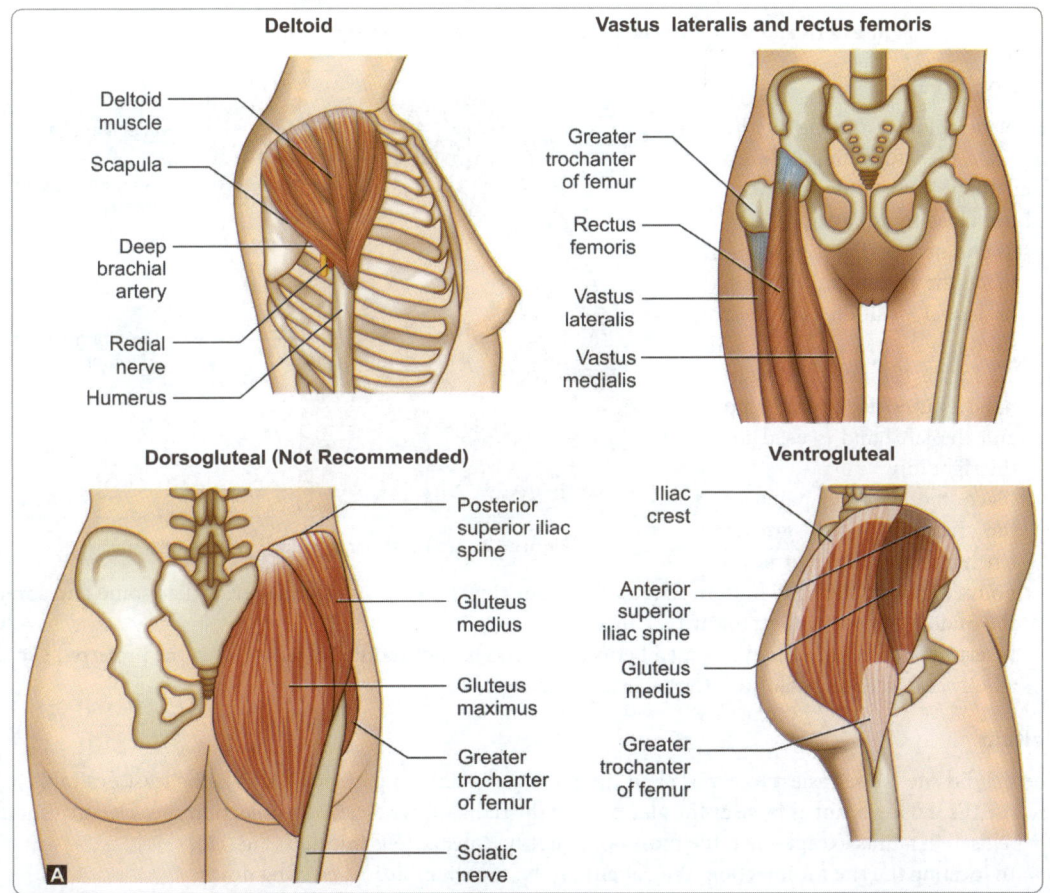

Figure 11A:

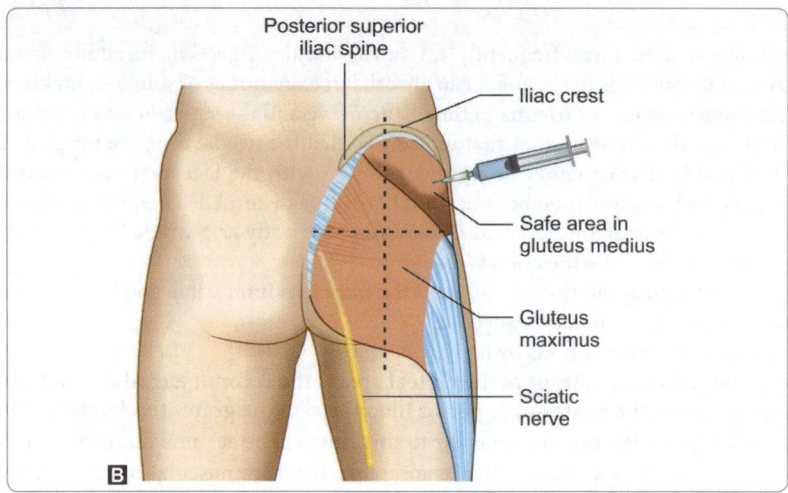

Figures 11A and B: (A) Selection of site for IM; (B) Method of administering IM injection

Ventrogluteal

The ventrogluteal muscle is the safest site for adults and children older than 7 months. It's deep and not close to any major blood vessels and nerves (Fig. 12).

- Place the patient in a supine or lateral position (on their side).
- To locate the site, the right hand is used for the left hip and the left hand is used for the right hip.
- Place the heel or palm of the hand on the greater trochanter, with the thumb

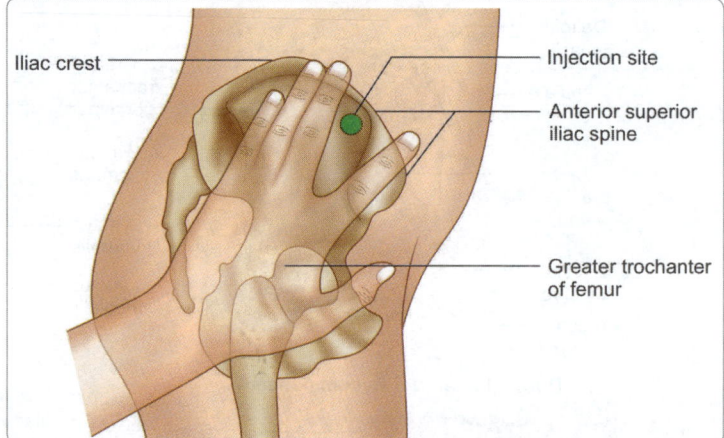

Figure 12: Intramuscular by using ventrogluteal site

pointed toward the belly button. Extend the index finger to the anterior superior iliac spine and spread the middle finger pointing toward the iliac crest.

- Insert the needle into the 'V' formed between the index and middle fingers. This is the preferred site for all oily and irritating solutions for patients of any age.

Deltoid

The deltoid site is the easiest to expose and the most acceptable to patients. But it is the least desirable area because the muscle is not as large as the gluteals and the radial nerve is near the injection site. The area should not be used in adults except when the most nonirritating substance is injected (Fig. 13).

- In locating the site for injection, the patient can be standing, sitting, or lying down.
- Expose the upper arm and find the acromion process by palpating the bony prominence.
- The site of injection is 2.5–5 cm (1–2 inches) below the acromion process.

- To locate this area, lay three fingers across the deltoid muscle and below the acromion process.
- A triangle is drawn on the lateral arm beginning with the lower edge of the acromion (Point where the scapula articulates with clavicle) on the top and ending at the point opposite to the axilla on the bottom. Inject into the middle of this triangle.

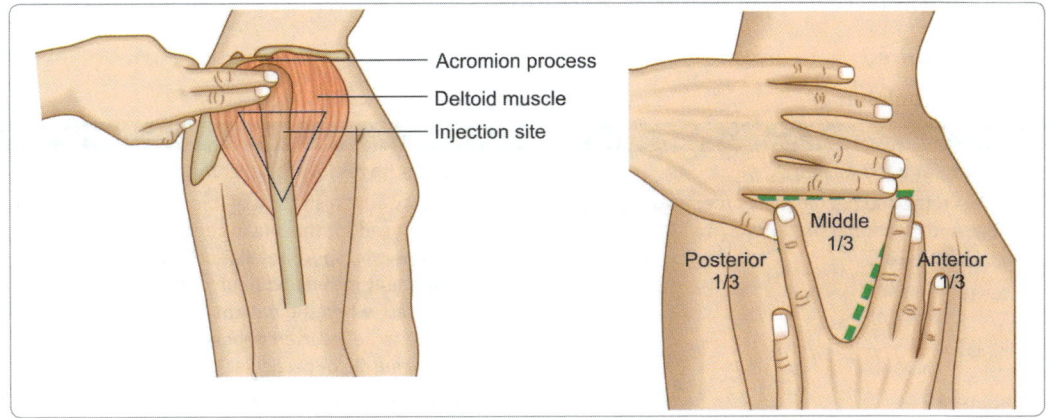

Figure 13: IM by using deltoid muscle site

This site may be used for small doses (not to exceed 1 mL) of nonirritating drugs when other sites are not available. Needle is inserted at 90° angle for intramuscular injection.

Vastus Lateralis

The vastus lateralis is commonly used for immunizations in children from infants and to toddlers. This muscle is located on the anterior lateral aspect of the thigh (Figs 14A and B).

- Ask the patient to lie flat with knees slightly bent, or have the patient in a sitting position.
- Divide the thigh into 3 equal parts.

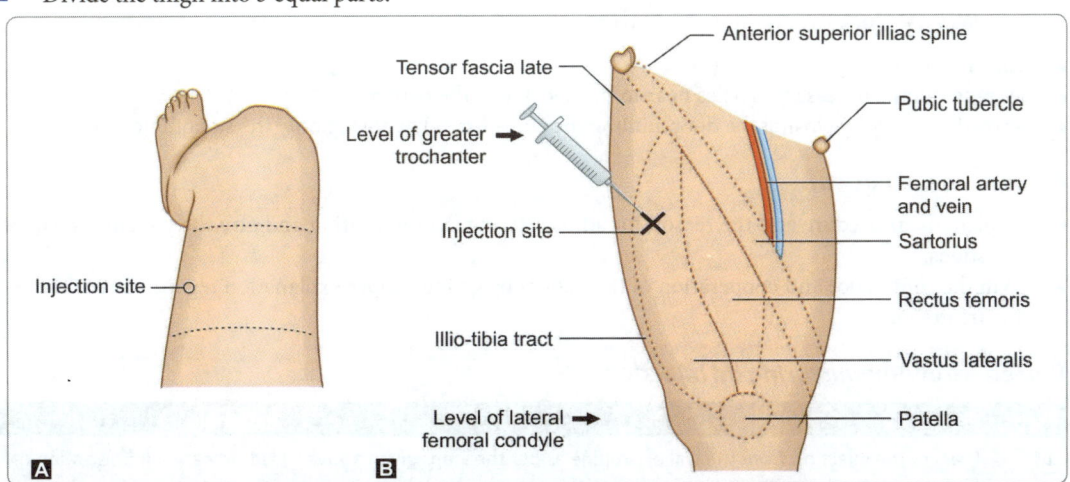

Figures 14A and B: (A) Locating site for injection; (B) Administering IM injection by using vastus lateralis muscle

- Locate one hand's breadth above the knee to one hand's breadth below the greater trochanter. The middle third is where the injection will be given.

Unit IX ❖ Medication Needs of the Patient—Pharmacology

Prerequisites

■ Check the 10 rights of medication administration.
■ When a patient is getting IM injection frequently, the sites of injection should be rotated, to avoid puncturing of the same spot very frequently.

Articles Required

A clean tray containing:

Article	Purpose
• Materials for hand wash	• Aids in the removal of microorganisms
• Sterile syringe and needle in a container. Larger syringe and longer needle 1–2 inches (2.5–5 cm) long. Size 21–23 G	• For easy administration of injection. Fine needles can be used for thin liquids and thicker ones for suspensions. Short needles are satisfactory when the patient is thin and flabby. Longer needles are necessary when the patient is obese. The length of needle to be inserted depends upon the thickness of the muscle of particular patient
• Ampule or vial	• To administer medication
• A small bowl with cotton swabs or a pack of sterile swab	• To wipe the injection site
• 70% alcohol (isopropyl alcohol or ethanol)	• To wipe the injection site
• A small bowl containing dry gauze	• To clean the area after administration of injection
• Non-sterile gloves	• To prevent cross infection
• Kidney tray	• To dispose the waste
• Syringe dispenser	• To dispose the used syringes and needles
• Waste bin	• To discard biomedical waste
• Note pad and pen	• To document the procedure

Preparation of Unit

■ Ensure an area of good lighting
■ Arrange all the necessary articles near to the bedside of the patient
■ Provide privacy by closing the door, pulling the curtains and exposing only the site of injection.

Preparation of Patient

■ Explain the procedure and the reason for administering the medication and give the patient time to ask questions.
■ Win the confidence and cooperation of the patient by giving proper explanation regarding the nature of the treatment.

Procedure of Administering IM Injection

Steps	Procedure	Rationale
1.	Prepare the injection from the vial or ampule as per the steps given above (Refer to method of withdrawing injection from vial or ampule)	Aids in easy administration of injection
2.	Perform hand hygiene	Prevents the transmission of microorganisms

Contd...

Unit IX ❖ Medication Needs of the Patient—Pharmacology

Steps	Procedure	Rationale
3.	Place the patient in comfortable position according to the site chosen.	This mentally prepares the patient for injection
4.	Don non-sterile gloves	Prevents cross infection
5.	• Locate correct site using landmarks. Choose an injection site that is free of hair, moles, rashes, scars, and other skin lesions • Apply a 60–70% alcohol-based solution (isopropyl alcohol or ethanol) on a single-use swab or cotton-wool ball • Wipe the area from the center of the injection site working outward using a circular motion, without going over the same area • Apply the solution for 30 seconds, then allow it to dry completely	Facilitates easy administration of injection Prevents transfer of microorganisms Allowing the site to dry prevents stinging during injection and also prevents alcohol and other pathogens from entering the skin when the needle is inserted
6.	Remove needle cap by pulling it straight off the needle 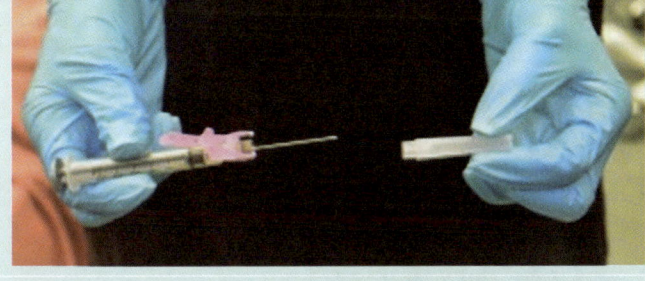	This prevents needle from touching side of the cap and prevents contamination
7.	Hold the syringe containing the medication like a pencil or a dart between the thumb and forefingers in the dominant hand. With the thumb and forefinger of the non-dominant hand, stretch the muscle tissue 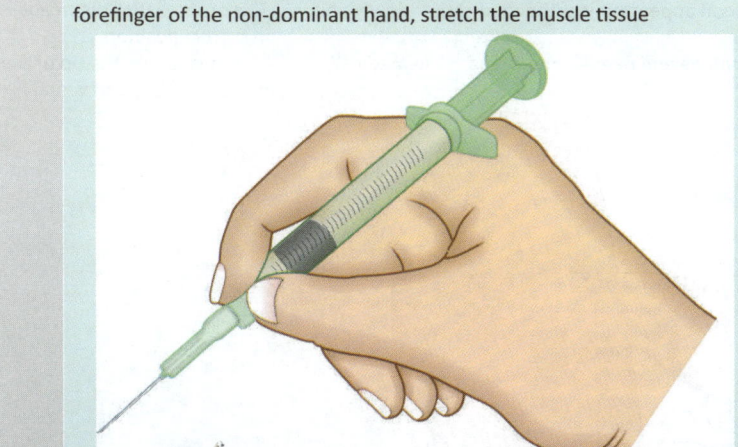	This prevents the movement of the site while administration

Contd...

Unit IX ❖ Medication Needs of the Patient—Pharmacology

Steps	Procedure	Rationale
8.	While communicating the patient, stretch the skin tight and then bunch up the muscle with the dominant hand, inject the needle quickly into the center of the muscle at 90° placing the bevel side up, using a steady and smooth motion	Inserting quickly causes less pain to the patient
9.	After the needle pierces the skin, use the thumb and forefinger of the non-dominant hand to hold the syringe	Movement of the needle can cause additional discomfort for the patient
10.	Aspirate for blood. If no blood appears, inject the medication slowly and steadily If blood appears, discard syringe and needle, and prepare the medication again Blood	This ensures that the needle is in correct position This means that the tip of the needle is in a blood vessel

Contd...

Steps	Procedure	Rationale
11.	Administer the medication slowly by pushing down on the plunger to inject the medicine. Do not force the medicine by pushing hard. Some medicines hurt. Avoid moving the syringe 	Ensures that the medication is injected
12.	Once medication is completely injected, remove the needle using a smooth, steady motion. Remove the needle at the same angle at which it was inserted 	Using a smooth motion prevents any unnecessary pain to the patient
13.	Cover injection site with sterile gauze, using gentle pressure. Gently massage the area	Promotes dispersal of the medication and facilitates absorption
14.	Do not recap the needle and discard syringe and the needle as per the biomedical waste management (BWM) policy	Facilitates safe disposal of syringes thus preventing needle stick injuries
15.	Replace articles, discard supplies, remove gloves and perform hand hygiene	Prevents transfer of micro-organisms
16.	Document the procedure with date and time including the name of medication, time, route, site, date of administration, any adverse effects, unexpected outcomes and interventions applied, if any	Recording the procedure acts as a legal document
17.	Assess patient's response to the medication after the appropriate time frame	Ensures that the patient does not have any adverse effects and, if any appropriate actions can be taken immediately

Unit IX ❖ **Medication Needs of the Patient—Pharmacology**

Stimulant

Z-Track Technique of Administering Intramuscular Injection

- Any intramuscular injection may be given.
- This method prevents seepage of the medication into the needle track.
- Reduces pain and discomfort.
- Advised for elderly patients who have decreased muscle mass.
- Some agents, such as iron, are best given via the Z-track method due to the associated irritation and discoloration.
- The skin is pulled down or to one side (about 2.5 cm) and held in this position with the left hand (for a right-handed person).
- The needle is inserted and the nurse aspirates carefully to detect the presence of blood.
- The medication is injected slowly, the needle is steadily withdrawn and the displaced tissue is released and allowed to return to its normal position.
- Apply gentle pressure with a dry sponge.

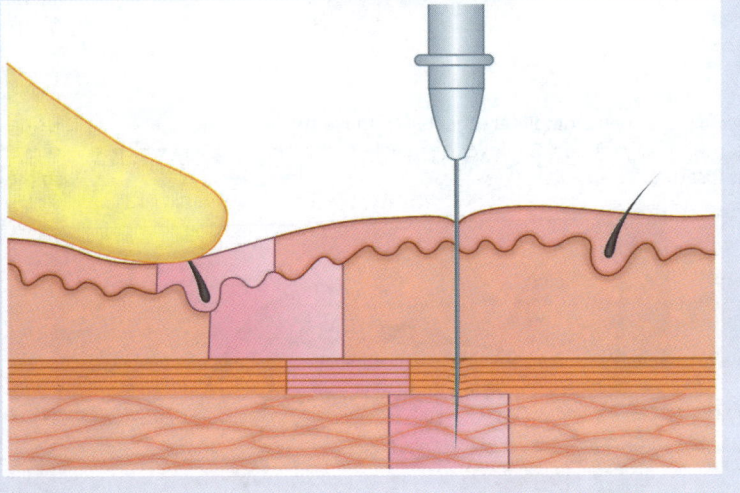

Intravenous Injection

Intravenous injection is given into a vein: Intravenous injections involves needle insertion directly into the vein and this way, the substance is directly delivered into the bloodstream.

Sites of Venipuncture

Veins in dorsal hands: The first choice for adult patients:

- Median cubital vein
- Cephalic vein
- Basilic vein
- Dorsal metacarpal veins

Veins in dorsal foot are commonly used for children but are avoided in adults because of the danger of thrombophlebitis.

Prerequisites

- Always label the IV syringe with the patients name, date, time, medication, concentration of the dose, dose, and your initials.
- Once the medication is prepared, never leave it unattended.
- **Never administer** an IV medication through an IV line that is infusing blood, blood products, heparin IV, insulin IV, cytotoxic medications, or parenteral nutrition solutions.

Articles Required

A clean tray containing:

Article	Purpose
• Materials for hand wash	• Aids in the removal of microorganisms
• Sterile syringe and needle in a container. (Special syringe and needles may be used) Needle is of 14–18 gauge	• For easy administration of injection
• Ampule or vial	• To administer medication
• A small bowl with cotton swabs or a pack of sterile swab	• To wipe the injection site
• 70% alcohol (isopropyl alcohol or ethanol)	• To wipe the injection site
• A small bowl containing dry gauze	• To wipe the area after administration of injection and to secure the site from preventing bleeding
• Tourniquet	• Helps to make the vein swell.
• Mackintosh and towel	• To protect linen from soiling
• Nonsterile gloves	• To prevent cross infection
• Kidney tray	• To dispose the waste
• Syringe dispenser	• To dispose the used syringes and needles
• Adhesive tape	• To secure the injection site
• Waste bin	• To discard biomedical waste
• Note pad and pen	• To document the procedure

Preparation of Unit

- Check the 10 rights of medication administration
- Ensure an area of good lighting
- Arrange all the necessary articles near to the bedside of the patient
- Provide privacy by closing the door, pulling the curtains and exposing only the site of injection.

Preparation of Patient

- Explain the procedure and the reason for administering the medication and give the patient time to ask questions.
- Win the confidence and cooperation of the patient by giving proper explanation regarding the nature of the treatment.

❖ **Medication Needs of the Patient—Pharmacology**

Unit IX

Procedure

Steps	Procedure	Rationale
1.	Perform hand wash	Prevents spread of microorganism
2.	Reassure the patient and explain the procedure. Place the patient in comfortable position	Positioning mentally prepares the patient
3.	Arrange the necessary articles near to the patient bedside along with the prepared medicine in a tray	Facilitates skillful performance of the procedure
4.	Uncover arm completely	Veins in the area of the arm are the safest to inject into and they are usually easier to find
5.	Place a mackintosh under the extremity. Have the patient relax and support his/her arm below the vein to be used	Protects the linen from soiling
6.	Look for a suitable vein. Once finding a vein, place one finger over it. Use this finger to gently press up and down in a gentle bouncing motion for 20–30 seconds	This causes the vein to expand and become visible

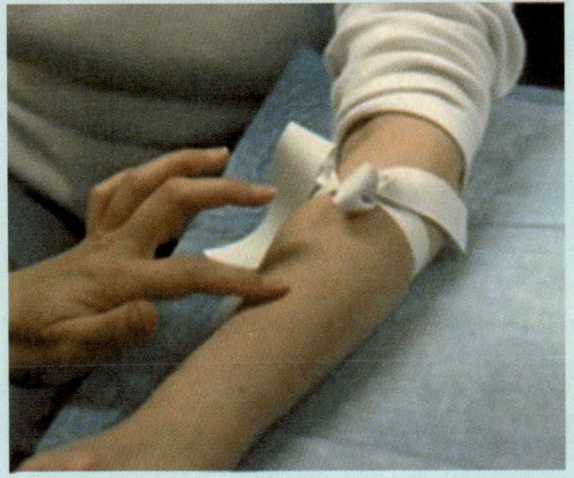

7.	Wrap an elastic tourniquet 2–4 in (5.1–10.2 cm) above the injection site. Use a loose overhand knot or simply tuck the tourniquet ends into the band to secure it or apply the Velcro strap	This causes the vein to expand and become visible

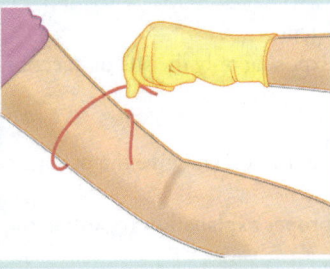 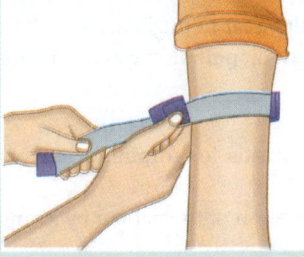

Contd...

Steps	Procedure	Rationale
8.	Instruct the person to open and close the same hand which has tourniquet in the arm hand several times • Or the person can be asked to squeeze a stress ball and release it several times • Watch to see if the vein becomes more visible after about 30–60 seconds of this	This causes the vein to expand and become visible
9.	Don gloves	Prevents cross infection
10.	Wait for the vein to swell	Facilitates easy access
11.	Disinfect skin with an alcohol swab or a gauze	Prevents transfer of microorganisms
12.	Stabilize the vein by pulling the skin taut in the longitudinal direction of the vein. Use the non-dominant hand to pull the skin taut against the vein, hold the needle with dominant hand	Facilitates easy puncture into the vein

Contd...

Unit IX ❖ Medication Needs of the Patient—Pharmacology

Steps	Procedure	Rationale
13.	Insert the needle at an angle of around 20–35 degrees with the bevel end up. Puncture the skin and move the needle slightly into the vein (3–5 mm). Hold the syringe and needle steady	Facilitates puncture into the vein without piercing the vein
14.	Aspirate. If blood appears, hold the syringe steady, you are in the vein. If it does not come, try again	Ensures that the needle is inside the vein. If the blood comes out with notable pressure and appears bright red and foamy, it affirms that the needle is inserted into an artery. Immediately pull the needle out and apply direct pressure to the site for at least 5 minutes to stop the bleeding
15.	Loosen tourniquet	Facilitates free flow of blood and medicines that is injected

Contd...

Steps	Procedure	Rationale
16.	Check for pain, swelling, hematoma; if in doubt, aspirate the vein again 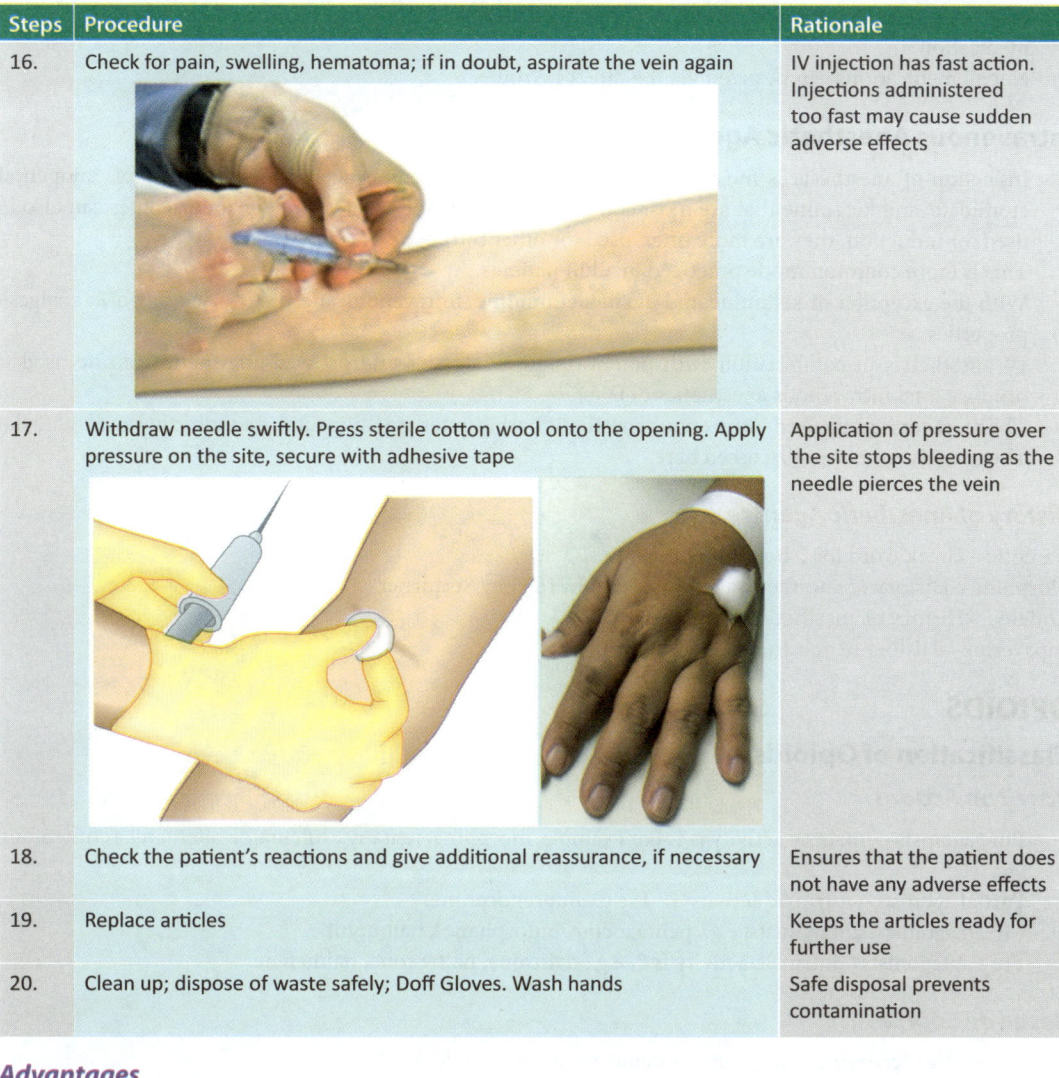	IV injection has fast action. Injections administered too fast may cause sudden adverse effects
17.	Withdraw needle swiftly. Press sterile cotton wool onto the opening. Apply pressure on the site, secure with adhesive tape	Application of pressure over the site stops bleeding as the needle pierces the vein
18.	Check the patient's reactions and give additional reassurance, if necessary	Ensures that the patient does not have any adverse effects
19.	Replace articles	Keeps the articles ready for further use
20.	Clean up; dispose of waste safely; Doff Gloves. Wash hands	Safe disposal prevents contamination

Advantages

- Intravenous medications can deliver an immediate, fast-acting therapeutic effect, which is important in emergent situations such as cardiac arrest or narcotic overdose.
- There is minimal or no discomfort for the patient in comparison to SC and IM injections.
- They provide an alternative to the oral route for drugs that may not be absorbed by the GI tract.
- IV direct route provides a more accurate dose of medication because none is left in the intravenous tubing.

Disadvantages

- Extravasation of certain medications into surrounding tissues can cause sloughing, nerve damage, and scarring.
- There is an increased risk of phlebitis with highly concentrated medication.

Unit IX ❖ Medication Needs of the Patient—Pharmacology

- Any toxic or adverse reaction will occur immediately and may be exacerbated by a rapidly injected medication.
- Not all medications can be given via the direct IV route.

Intravenous Anesthetic Agents

- Induction of anesthesia is most often achieved using intravenous agents such as propofol, thiopental, etomidate, and ketamine that are most commonly used. While opiates and benzodiazepines can also be used for induction, they are more often used for other purposes.
- This is more common mode practiced in adult patients.
- With the exception of ketamine and dexmedetomidine, intravenous anesthetics lack intrinsic analgesic properties.
- IV anesthetics in combination with potent opioid analgesics and/or local anesthetics can be used to produce total intravenous anesthetics (TIVA).
- The most commonly used intravenous anesthetic barbiturates are thiopental, methohexital and thiamylal. The opioids have been discussed here.

History of Anesthetic Agents

Narcotic—Greek word for "stupor"
Morphine—History of anesthetic agents isolated in 1803 by Serturner
Codeine—History of anesthetic agents – in 1832
Papaverine—History of anesthetic agents – in 1848

OPIOIDS

Classification of Opioids

Based on Actions

- Pure agonists—intrinsic activity is 1, For example, morphine, fentanyl, sufentanil, alfentanil, remifentanil, etc.
- Partial agonists—intrinsic activity 0–1, e.g., Buprenorphine.
- Mixed agonist—antagonists, e.g., pentazocine, butorphanol, nalbuphine.
- Pure antagonists—intrinsic activity is 0, e.g., naloxone, naltrexone, nalmefene.

Based on Source

- **Naturally Occurring:** Morphine, codeine, papaverine, thebaine.
- **Semisynthetic:** Heroin, dihydromorphone/morphionone, thebaine derivatives, e.g., etorphine, buprenorphine.
- **Synthetic:** Morphinan series, e.g., levorphanol, butorphanol; diphenylpropylamine series, e.g., levorphanol, butarphanol; benzomorphan series, e.g., pentazocine, phenylpiperidine series, e.g., meperidine, fentanyl, sufentanil, alfentanil, remifentanil.

Opioid Receptors

- G. protein coupled with seven membrane spanning regions
- Phosphorylation and glycosylation sites are responsible for effects
- Summary of some opioid receptors has been given in Table 2 as follows.

Table 2: Opioid receptors

	μ₁	μ₂	δ	κ
Actions	Analgesia (supraspinal, spinal) Euphoria Miosis Bradycardia Nausea and vomiting Hypothermia	Analgesia (spinal) Respiratory depression Constipation (marked) Physical dependence	Analgesia (supraspinal, spinal) Constipation (minimal) Urinary retention Physical dependence	Analgesia (spinal, supraspinal) Dysphoria Diuresis Miosis Sedation Low abuse potential
Endogenous ligands	Endorphins	Endorphins	Enkephalins	Dynorphin
Antagonists	Naloxone, nalmefene, naltreoxone			

Mechanism of intravenous analgesics has been depicted in Figure 15 as follows:

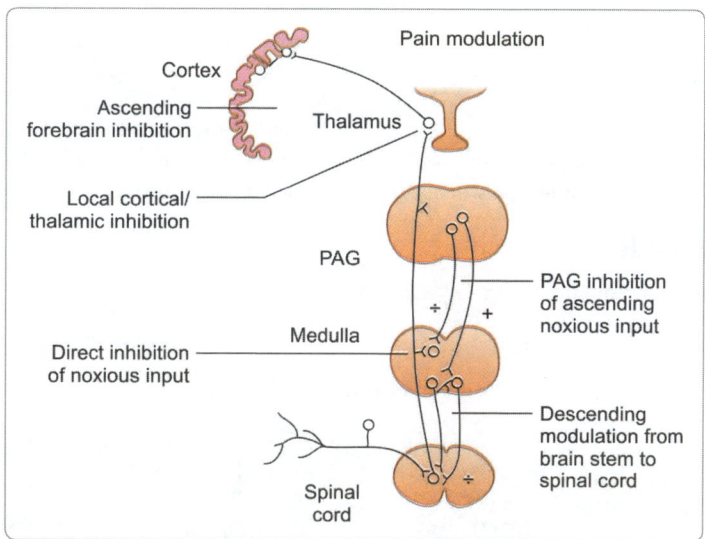

Figure 15: Mechanism of analgesics

Morphine

- Rigid pentacyclic T-shaped structure
- Tertiary +vely charged basic nitrogen
- Quaternary carbon
- Phenolic hydroxyl group or a ketone group

Anti-nociceptive Mechanism of Morphine in Central Nervous System

- Ascending forebrain inhibition
- Local cortical/thalamic inhibition
- Direct inhibition of noxious input

Unit IX ❖ Medication Needs of the Patient—Pharmacology

- PAG inhibition of ascending noxious input
- Descending modulation from brain stem to spinal cord (Fig. 16)

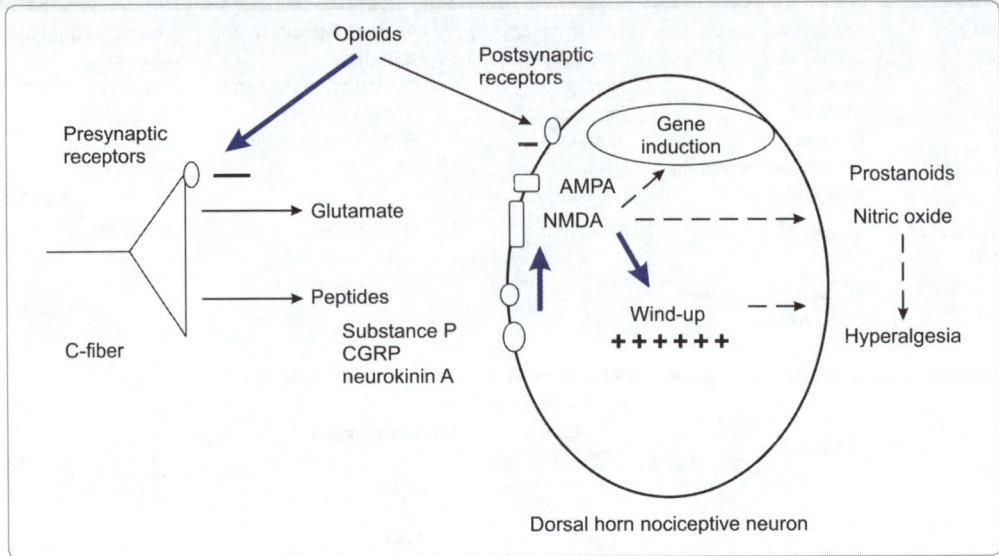

Figure 16: Antinociceptive mechanism of morphine

Endogenous Opioids

The common amino acid sequence is Tyr-Gly-Gly-Phe

Biosynthesis

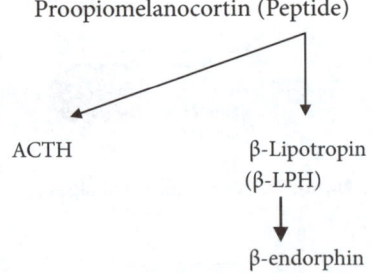

- *β-endorphin:* Present in anterior and intermediate lobes and hypothalamus
  - Outside CNS in small intestine, placenta, plasma
  - Modulates nociception during stress, midbrain periaqueductal gray stimulation and acupuncture
- *Enkephalins*

Proenkephalin (peptide)

↓

Met-enkephalin and other enkephalins

  - Widely found in CNS
  - Depress ventilation

- ***Dynorphins***

  Prodynorphin => Dynorphin
  - Found in hypothalamo-neurohypophysial axis and perioperative gray area, limbic system, thalamus, laminae I and V
  - Functions as neuromodulator in CNS by interacting with μ-δ- and κ⁻, receptors
  - Central control of cardiovascular system

Local Spinal Mechanisms

- Spinal cord presynaptic substance P inhibition by μ, κ, σ agonists
- Excitatory post-synaptic potential summation in dorsal horn is blocked by opioids => blocking development of dull persistent pain
- Local anesthetic-like effect on the surface of excitable cell membranes
- Inhibit early expression of DNA, integral to transforming cellular characteristics for development of chronic pain

Hormonal Mechanisms

- Morphine and meperidine cause histamine release and sympathoadrenal activation
- Effects—Dilatation of terminal arterioles
  - Direct positive cardiac chronotropic and inotropic
  - Increase cardiac index, decreases BP, decrease SVR
- Fentanyl, sufentanil, alfentanil and remifentanil do not produce increases in plasma histamine.

Pharmacodynamic Effects of Opioids

Neurophysiologic Actions

- Intravenous opioids produce dizziness, drowsiness, lethargy, apathy and sleep.
- Initially may stimulate coughing followed by cough depression.
- **Anesthetic action**
  - Consistent reduction in range of 60–70% in MAC of potent inhalational agents
  - Potency ratios for fentanyl/sufentanil/alfentanil/remifentanil based on MAC reduction 1: 12: 1/16: 1.2
  - Opioid anesthesia can be unpredictable and inconsistent
  - Intraoperative awareness may or may not be reported
  - Electroencephalogram (EEG) Opioids produce alpha ceiling effect when increased doses are given. No further change is observed in EEG once ceiling effect is reached.
- **Cerebral actions**
  - Modest decreases (10–25%) in cerebral metabolic rate and ICP
  - Mild to moderate decrease in cerebral metabolic rate
- **Advantages as neuroanesthetic**
  - Promotion of intraoperative systemic hemodynamic and cardiovascular stability
  - Rapid but smooth emergence
- **Neuroexcitatory phenomena**
  - Fentanyl and sufentanil can cause neuroexcitation
  - Delirium to grand mal seizures
  - Focal CNS excitation in subcortical and limbic system
  - Meperidine => normeperidine => CNS excitation and convulsions
- **Mechanism:** Alterations in central catecholamine concentration in dopaminergic pathways. Opioid induced increases in glutamate- activated secretes disinhibition of pyramidal cells of hippocampus.

Unit IX ❖ Medication Needs of the Patient—Pharmacology

Respiratory Actions

- **Therapeutic Effects**
  - Impair ventilation, decreased compliance but can improve synchronous breathing and decrease voluntary muscle tone

    ↓

    Improved dynamic total respiratory compliance in awake and mechanically ventilated patients in ICU
  - Antitussive action: Central action

    Fentanyl, sufentanil, alfentanil elicit brief cough when given IV

    ↓

    Pulmonary chemoreflex by J-receptor is responsible
  - Excellent agents for depressing upper airway, tracheal and lower respiratory tract reflexes
  - Blunt or eliminate somatic or autonomic responses to tracheal intubation – no coughing/ bucking
  - Decrease bronchomotor tone
    - ○ Fentanyl—Antimuscarinic, antihistaminergic, antiserotonergic actions

- **Nontherapeutic Effects**
  - Ventilatory depression through direct action on brain stem respiratory center
  - Decrease stimulatory effects of CO_2 on ventilation
  - Decrease hypoxic ventilatory drive
  - Eliminate spontaneous respiration without producing unconsciousness
  - Respond to verbal commands and breathe when directed to do so
  - Opioids effects on respiratory pattern:
    - ○ Increased respiratory pauses
    - ○ Delays in expiration
    - ○ Irregular/periodic breathing

Factors Affecting Opioid—Induced Respiratory Depression

- Increased dose
- Increased intermittent bolus
- Increased brain penetration/drug delivery
- Decreased reuptake from the brain
- Decreased clearance
- Secondary peaks in plasma opioid levels
- Sleep
- Increased age
- Metabolic alkalosis and respiratory alkalosis

Cardiovascular Actions

Large doses of opioids administered as sole or primary anesthetic result in hemodynamic stability throughout operative period.

- Nucleus solitarius (NS) is the primary central synapse for baroreceptor mediated reflexes
- Nucleus solitarius and parabrachial nucleus—Hemodynamic control of vasopressin secretion
- Ventrolateral periaqueductal gray region—Hemodynamic control
- Most opioids reduce sympathetic nervous system and enhance vagal and parasympathetic tone—Hypotension may result in volume depletion or individuals on high sympathetic tone.
- **Bradycardia:** Stimulation of central vagal nucleus—morphine directly affects SA and AV node.

- **Contractility:** May increase or decrease depending on pre-existing myocardial function.
- Cardiac conduction is decreased – Slow AV conduction
  – Can prolong QT interval
- Baroreceptor reflexes are minimally affected.

Renal Effects

- μ-*receptor activation—Antidiuresis and decrease electrolyte secretion*
- κ-*receptor activation—Diuresis and better change in electrolyte secretion*
- Inhibition/alteration of ADH secretion
- Disturbances in micturition characterized by urinary retention

Gastrointestinal Effects

- Opioids decrease GI motility => Antidiarrheal agents
- Gastric emptying delayed => Delayed passage of intestinal contents through colon => Increased H_2O absorption => Constipation
- Opioids increase tone and decrease propulsive activity in most of intestine

Biliary Tree Effects

- Increase biliary duct pressure and sphincter of Oddi tone
- Can be reversed by naloxone, glucagon, glyceryl trinitrate

Intestinal Circulation

- Fentanyl increases intestinal blood flow in dose-dependent manner
- Dose-related decrease in intestinal O_2 uptake and increased intestinal blood flow--->luxury perfusion

Nausea and Vomiting

- Opioids increase incidence of nausea and vomiting
- Stimulate *CTZ* in area postrema of medulla through δ receptors
- Factors increasing incidence of nausea and vomiting:
  - Age (inc in pediatric)
  - Females
  - Obesity
  - History of motion sickness
  - Duration of surgery and ambulation
  - Laparoscopic surgery
  - Gastroparesis
- Antiemetic prophylaxis should be considered before opioid anesthesia
  - Scopolamine IV/IM/ Transdermal patch
  - Droperidol 0.005–0.07 mg/kg IV
  - Metoclopramide 0.1–0.3 mg/kg
  - Ondansetron
  - Acupressure (P-6)

Muscle Rigidity

- Increase muscle tone and may cause muscle rigidity.
- Fentanyl 0.6–0.8 mg IV causes chest wall rigidity within 60–90 sec.

- Clinically - Wrist flexion
  - Hoarseness
- **Wooden chest syndrome**
  - Rigidity of abdominal or thoracic muscles and difficulty to ventilate.
  - Vocal cord closure is responsible for difficult ventilation.
- **Mechanism of muscle rigidity**
  - Catatonic state produced by altering dopamine concentrations and stimulation of GABAergic interneurons.
  - Nucleus pontis raphae is the center.
- Problems associated with opioid-induced muscle rigidity.
  - Hemodynamic – $\uparrow CVP$, $\uparrow PAP$, $\uparrow PVR$.
  - Pulmonary – $\downarrow$ compliance, $\downarrow FRC$, $\downarrow$ ventilation, hypercarbia, hypoxia.
  - Miscellaneous – $\uparrow O_2$ consumption, $\uparrow ICT$, dislodged IV lines.
- **Prevention and treatment**
  - Pretreatment/concomitant use of non-depolarizing muscle relaxants.
  - Succinylcholine.
  - Avoiding rapid administration of a large dose of opioid.

Pruritis

- Most common side effect of opioids.
- Localized to face, neck or upper thorax.
- **Mechanism**
  - Cephalad migration of opioid in CSF and subsequent interaction with opioid receptors in trigeminal nucleus.
  - Histamine release is **NOT** causative.

Thermoregulation and Shivering

- Opioid anesthesia reduces thermoregulatory thresholds to similar degree as by inhaled anesthetics.
- Antishivering effects are countered by reduction in shivering threshold by meperidine.

Obstetrics

- Fentanyl clinically useful during harvesting human ova for subsequent in vitro fertilization
- Alfentanil has been recommended as useful in providing analgesia for oocyte retrieval
- Labor analgesia – Opioids with or without local anesthetics can be used for painless labor.

Ocular Effects

- Fentanyl, sulfentanil and alfentanil during induction of anesthesia can help to prevent increases in intraocular pressure

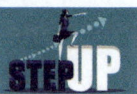

Viral Reactivation
- Reactivation of herpes simplex labialis virus in obstetric patients with use of epidural morphine.
  - Occurs in 2–5 days of opioid administration.
  - Mechanism involves cephalad migration of opioid in CSF and subsequent interaction with the trigeminal nucleus.

INDIVIDUAL OPIOID AGONISTS

Meperidine (Pethidine)

- Synthetic opioid agonist at μ and κ opioid receptors (Fig. 17)
- Structurally similar to atropine
- Analogues of meperidine—fentanyl, sufentanil, alfentanil, remifentanil

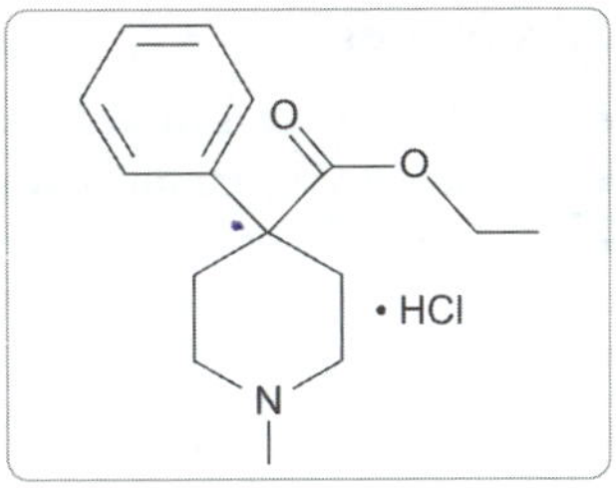

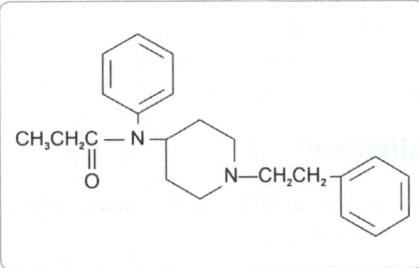

Figure 17: Meperidine

Pharmacokinetics

- 1/10th as potent as morphine
- Duration of action—2–4 hours
- Hepatic metabolism—90% drug metabolized to normeperidine
- Normeperidine produces CNS stimulation, meperidine-induced delirium
- Elimination half-life—3–5 hours

Clinical Uses

- Analgesia during labor and delivery
- **Postoperative analgesia:** Dose 1.0–2.0 mg/kg
- Postoperative shivering (κ-effect)

Adverse Effects

- Orthostatic hypotension in therapeutic doses

Fentanyl

- Phenylpiperidine-derivative synthetic opioid agonist (Fig. 18)
- 75–125 times more potent than morphine

Pharmacokinetics

- Greater potency and rapid onset of action due to increased lipid solubility
- Lungs exert a significant first pass effect and transiently take up 75% of IV dose of fentanyl
- Metabolized in liver by N-demethylation to norfentanyl
- Relatively long acting due to widespread distribution in body tissues
- **Effect:** Site equilibration time 6–8 minutes

Figure 18: Fentanyl

Clinical Uses

- Analgesia—1–2 μg/kg IV
- Anesthetic induction with sedative-hypnotic 2–6 μg/kg (loading dose)
- Maintenance of anesthesia with 60–70% N_2O with low inhaled anesthetics 25–50 μg every 15–30 minutes or a constant infusion of 0.5–5.0 μg/kg/hr
- As a sole anesthetic—50–150 μg/kg IV
- *Oral transmucosal fentanyl citrate (OTFC)*—Decrease anxiety in children used preoperatively
- Transdermal Fentanyl preparations—75–100 μg/hr

Advantages

- Lack of direct myocardial depressant effects
- Absence of histamine release
- Suppression of the stress responses to surgery

Disadvantages

- Patient awareness
- Postoperative ventilatory depression

Sufentanil

- Thienyl analogue of fentanyl (Fig. 19)
- Analgesic potency is five to ten times that of fentanyl

Pharmacokinetics

- Twice as lipid soluble as fentanyl and highly bound (93%) to alpha$_1$-acid glycoprotein
- First-pass pulmonary extraction, retention, release similar to fentanyl
- High hepatic extraction ratio – 0.8
- Metabolized by N-dealkylation and O-demethylation
- Effect-site equilibration time 6.2 minutes

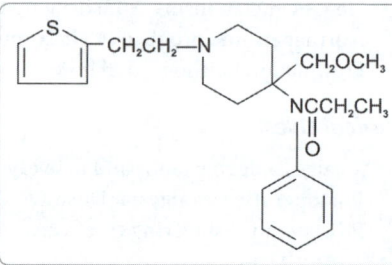

Figure 19: Sufentanil

Clinical Uses

- To blunt pressor response 0.25–1.0 µg/kg minutes prior to induction
- Anesthetic induction with sedative hypnotic
- Maintenance of anesthesia with N_2O (60–70%) 0.10–0.25 µg/kg intermittent bolus
- Constant infusion 0.5–1.5 µg/kg/hr

Alfentanil

- Analogue of fentanyl (1/5th to 1/10th) as potent as fentanyl (Fig. 20)
- Duration of action 1/3rd that of fentanyl

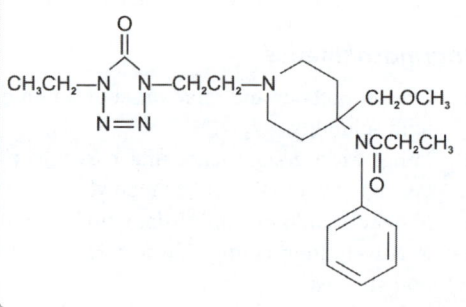

Figure 20: Alfentanil

Pharmacokinetics

- Shorter elimination half-life compared with fentanyl and sufentanil
- Rapid onset of action/or/rapid effect site equilibration time of 1.4 minutes after IV administration (Reason: low pKa, mostly unionized so widely diffusible/crosses BBB)
- **Metabolism:** N-dealkylation and O-demethylation

Clinical Uses

- To supplement a sedative-hypnotic induction—5.0–50 µg/kg
- Maintenance of anesthesia—0.5–2 µg/kg/min or intermittent boluses 5–10 µg/kg

Remifentanil

- Selective µ opioid agonist with an analgesic potency similar to fentanyl (Fig. 21)
- 15–20 times as potent as sufentanil
- Structurally unique because of its ester linkage

Pharmacokinetics

- Small volume of distribution, rapid clearance, low variability
- Extraordinary clearance—3 L/min
- Context-sensitive half time is nearly independent of infusion duration in 4 minutes
- Highly lipid soluble; highly bound to alpha$_1$ acid glycoprotein

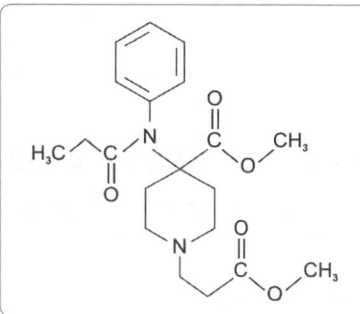

Figure 21: Remifentanil

Clinical Uses

- Profound analgesic effect is desired transiently, e.g., performance of retrobulbar block
- Suppression of pressor response to laryngoscopy and intubation
- Longer operations when a quick recovery is required
- Analgesic component of GA—0.05–2.00 µg/kg/min IV
- Anesthetic induction—1 µg/kg IV over 60–90 sec or Infusion 0.5–1.0 ug/kg for 10 minutes

Advantages

- Brevity of action
- Precise and rapidly titrable effect due to its rapid onset and offset
- Noncumulative effects
- Rapid recovery after discontinuation of its administration

Metabolism

- Unique metabolism by nonspecific plasma and tissue esterases
- Not influenced by renal or hepatic failure

OTHER OPIOID AGONISTS

Tramadol

- Synthetic 4-phenyl-piperidine analogue
- Racemic mixture of two enantiomers
    - Inhibition of NE uptake
    - Inhibition of 5HT uptake and facilitation of its release
- One fifth to 1/0th as potent as morphine

Unit IX ❖ Medication Needs of the Patient—Pharmacology

Mechanism of Action

- μ-agonist and lesser extent δ-& κ-receptors
- Activates spinal inhibition of pain by ↓ NE & 5HT uptake

Dosage: 50–100 mg every 4–6 hours with a maximum daily dose of 400 mg in a 24-hr period

Side Effects

- If used intraoperatively causes intraoperative awareness
- High incidence of nausea and vomiting
- Seizures are associated with tramadol administration when combined with drugs lowering seizure threshold

OPIOID AGONIST—ANTAGONISTS

- Binds to μ-receptors and produce limited responses or no effect
- Partial agonists at κ & δ receptors

Pentazocine

- Benzomorphan derivative
- Opioid agonist with weak antagonist actions
- Agonist at κ & δ receptors

Pharmacokinetics

- Extensive first pass metabolism
- Elimination half-life is 2–3 hours

Clinical Uses

- 10–30 mg IV or 50 mg orally for relief of moderate pain
- Sequential analgesic anesthesia. Fentanyl 10–15 mg/kg followed by pentazocine 1 mg/kg

Side Effects

- Sedation is most common side-effect and limited analgesia
- Diaphoresis, dizziness, nausea and vomiting
- Dysphoria and fear of death
- High risk of physical dependence
- Depresses myocardial contractility, ↑BP, ↑HR, ↑SVR, ↑Pulmonary artery pressure, ↑LV work index

Nalbuphine

- Agonist—antagonist opioid
- Binds to μ-receptors as well as κ-and δ-receptors
- Antagonist at μ-receptor and agonist at κ-receptors
- Provides good analgesia for mild to moderate but not severe postoperative pain

Pharmacokinetics

- Onset of effect is rapid (5–10 minutes)
- Duration is long—3–6 hours

- Long plasma elimination life 5 hours
- Hepatic metabolism

Clinical Uses

- Premedication—0.1 mg/kg
- Analgesic supplement for conscious sedation or balanced anesthesia (0.3–0.5 mg/kg)
- Analgesic for postoperative and chronic pain syndromes

Butorphanol

- Agonist at κ-receptors and antagonist or partial agonist at μ-receptors
- 5–8 times potent than morphine, used only parenteral

Pharmacokinetics

- Onset rapid after IM injection, peak analgesia in 1 hour
- Plasma $t_{1/2}$ is 2–3 hours

Clinical Uses

- For analgesia when used as supplement in N_2O-opioid-O_2 anesthesia
- Relief of acute rather than chronic pain
- Epidural analgesia 1–2 mg

Side Effects

- Drowsiness, sweating, nausea and CNS stimulation
- ↑BP, ↑PAP, ↑Cardiac output—Risky in patients with cardiac disease

Buprenorphine

- Thebaine derivative
- μ-receptor partial agonist; 33 times more potent than morphine
- Insignificant activity at κ-receptors

Pharmacokinetics

- Highly lipophilic but opiate receptor association and dissociation are slow
- Slow onset of action
- Peak effect at 3 hours
- Duration of effect <10 hours
- Hepatic metabolism

Clinical Uses

- Premedication 0.3 mg IM
- Analgesic component in balanced anesthesia 4.5–12 µg/kg
- Postoperative pain control 0.3 mg IM

OPIOID ANTAGONISTS

- Substitution of an alkyl group for a methyl group on an opioid
- Pure μ opioid receptor antagonists with no agonist actions—naloxone, naltrexone

- **Clinical Uses**
  - Treat opioid-induced depression of ventilation, e.g., postoperatively. Dose: 1–4 µg/kg/hr
  - Treat opioid-induced depression of ventilation in neonate due to maternal administration of opioid
  - Facilitate treatment of deliberate opioid overdose
  - To detect suspected physical dependence
- **Pharmacokinetics**
  - Short duration of action—30–45 minutes; onset is rapid 1–2 minutes
  - Requires continuous infusion of naloxone 5 µg/kg/hr
  - Elimination half-life—60–90 minutes
- **Side Effects**
  - Nausea, vomiting, pruritis
  - ↑BP, & ↑HR after naloxone reversal of opioids
- **Contraindications**
  - Whenever ↑ in BP and HR are detrimental, e.g., coronary artery disease.
  - Pheochromocytoma/chromaffin tissue tumors
- **Other Applications**
  - For alcoholism
  - Septic and hemorrhagic shock
  - Post anesthetic apnea in infants
  - Primary apnea and periodic breathing associated with hypoxia
  - BZD, Barbiturate and alcohol reversal
  - Role in heat stroke, Alzheimer's, schizophrenia, thalamic pain syndrome, intractable pruritis

Naltrexone

- µ,δ, and κ-opioid receptor antagonist
- Longer $t_{1/2}$ 8–12 hours
- Decreased first-pass metabolism
- Stimulates cardiovascular system
- Frequency and severity of relapses in alcoholics are decreased

Nalmefene

- Pure opioid antagonist similar to naloxone and naltrexone
- Greater preference for µ than δ or κ receptors
- Long acting but equipotent to naloxone
- Dose: Oral 0.5–3.0 mg/kg
- Parenteral 0.2–2.0 mg/kg
- Hepatic metabolism

TOTAL INTRAVENOUS ANESTHESIA (TIVA)

- The availability of drugs with short blood–brain equilibration times enables the clinician to use intravenous anesthetics and analgesics where controllability is easy and recovery rapid.
- Total intravenous anesthesia offers some important advantages over inhalation anesthetics, including rapid recovery with minimal hangover and a low incidence of nausea and vomiting. TIVA may be the technique of choice for some operations.
- The most common combination used for TIVA is propofol and remifentanil.

- It has added advantage in neurosurgery of decreasing **Intracranial** pressure.
- It has added advantage in thoracic surgery of having drugs which maintain pulmonary vasoconstriction reflex.
- It is safely used in patients with **Malignant Hyperthermia** gene.
- It decreases the risk of environmental pollution.

SPECIAL POINTS TO BE NOTED DURING ANY INJECTION

- Administer injections only with doctor's orders.
- Strict aseptic precautions are to be taken when giving injection.
- The syringe, needle and drug used should be sterile, and not contaminated.
- Nurse should wash hands thoroughly and dry it.
- Area is cleaned before injection.
- Remember to dip the forceps in the jar of sterile water after removing it from the lotion, to wash out the particles of chemical from the forceps before it is used for taking the needles and syringe.
- Once the forceps, is taken and dipped in water it should be placed in the lotion jar, only after its use for the procedure. Never talk, cough or sneeze over sterile syringe and needle or the drug.
- Syringe and needle for injection of drugs should be kept separate. Never use them for aspiration or an aspiration syringe and needle for injection of drugs.
- Always use sharp straight needle.
- Always make sure that syringe is air tight and check the needles for any blockage and leakage.
- Check the drug and dosage with the patient's name in the order sheet three times.
- Check the label on the bottle of the drug for the strength of drug and its date of expiry.
- Be careful to take the correct drug, the correct dose and correct patient.
- Never use a drug that is out of date.
- Always check the drug and the dose with the Senior Sister in the ward.
- Never allow the patient to walk soon after an injection and he/she should be watched for any reaction.
- Never give an injection to the patient while standing but give only when patient is sitting or lying in a comfortable position.
- Never inject air.
- Always expel air before injecting the drug.
- When injection is given, inject at the correct site.
- Needle is inserted gently and quickly and the drug is injected slowly. The needle is withdrawn gently and quickly.
- After inserting the needle in intramuscular injection, always withdraw the piston to see whether it is in the proper position and not in blood vessel.
- If there is any trace of blood inside the barrel, always withdraw the needle and insert it in another area, with another needle.
- Massage the area at the site of injection to aid the absorption of drug, but not in intradermal injection.
- Massaging is prevented when thick solutions are injected, e.g., interferon, uniferon PAM, etc.
- Injection should be charted immediately after giving and should be signed.
- After injection, replace the articles.

Unit IX ❖ Medication Needs of the Patient—Pharmacology

Stimulant

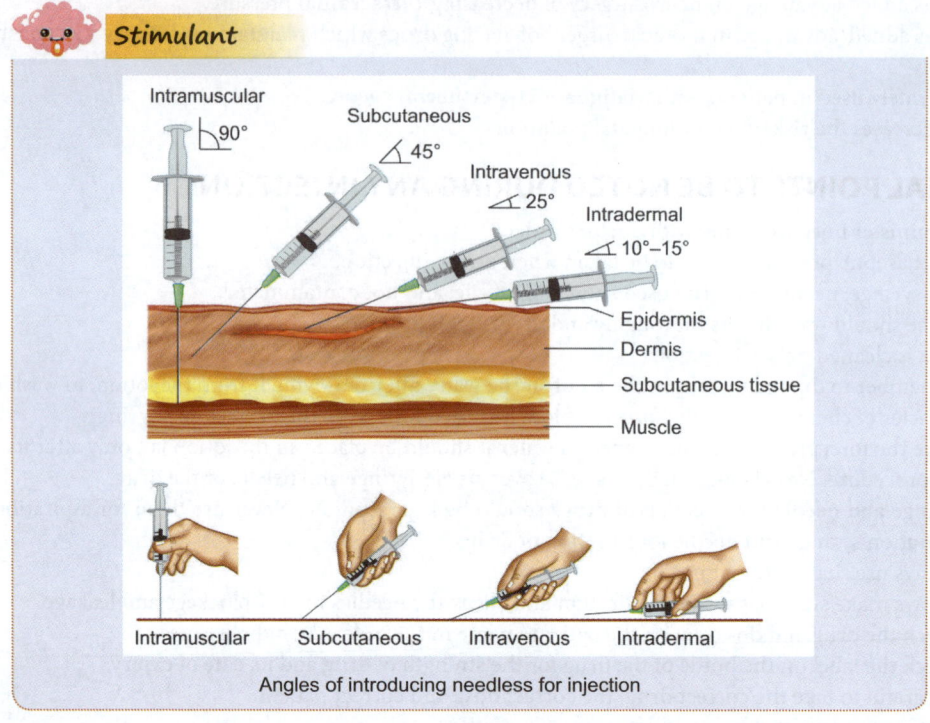

Angles of introducing needless for injection

DIABETES MELLITUS—SPECIAL CONSIDERATION

Diabetes is a very common disease for which nurses are to give care in hospitals as well as in homes. So knowledge about this disease and administration of insulin is a must for every nurse. In view of this idea, it is detailed below.

Diabetic mellitus is a metabolic disorder of the body, characterized by an increased amount of glucose in the blood and excretion of this glucose in the urine. The basic defect is the disturbance in the production, action or the rate of use of insulin, which is a hormone secreted by the Islets of Langerhans in the pancreas. The insufficiency of insulin may be due to failure in its production, blockage of its use or its destruction by the body, so that carbohydrate metabolism is disturbed.

Signs and Symptoms of Diabetes Mellitus

- Polyphagia (increased appetite)
- Polydipsia (increased thirst)
- Polyuria (increased urination)
- Glycosuria (presence of sugar in urine)

When the amount of sugar is increased more than normal it is called **hyperglycemia** and when it is less than normal it is called **hypoglycemia**. Diabetes is a hereditary disease. When it is diagnosed early it can be controlled by regulating the food. When the condition is advanced and not controlled by food, treatment is started with tablets along with regulation of carbohydrate food. Further, nowadays diabetes and insulin therapy are very common and insulin reaction and diabetic ketoacidosis are medical emergencies. Information about these aspects is most useful for any health team member. Therefore, these topics are put in a nutshell, as follows.

Blood Glucose Monitoring

People with diabetes require regular monitoring of their blood glucose to help them achieve close to normal blood glucose levels.

A glucometer is a medical device for determining the approximate concentration of glucose in the blood.

Prerequisites

- Review the patient's medical history for the type of diabetes, medications and/or anticoagulant therapy.
- Determine if the test requires special timing; for example, before or after meals.
- Blood glucose monitoring is usually done prior to meals and the administration of antidiabetic medications.
- Determine, if blood glucometer needs to be calibrated.
- Assess patient's sites for skin puncture.
- Avoid having the patient stand during the procedure to reduce the risk of fainting.
- Do not milk or massage finger site. Milking or massaging the finger may introduce excess tissue fluid and hemolyze the specimen.

Articles Required

A clean tray containing:

Article	Purpose
Glucometer	To determine the concentration of glucose in the blood
Lancing device	Contains a release button and holds lancet/needle for pricking
Glucostrip container	To store the biosensors strips
Reagent strips	For checking glucose
Lancet	Needle used to prick
Carry pouch	To keep all contents
Nonsterile gloves	To prevent cross infection
A small bowl with cotton swabs or a pack of sterile swab	To wipe the site
70% alcohol (isopropyl alcohol or ethanol)	To dip the swab for wiping the site
A small bowl containing dry gauze	To wipe the area after pricking
Kidney tray	To dispose the waste
Waste bin (as per BMW)	To dispose the waste

Preparation of Unit

- Ensure an area of good lighting
- Arrange all the necessary articles near to the bedside of the patient

Preparation of Patient

- Explain the procedure and the reason for performing the test and give the patient time to ask questions.
- Win the confidence and cooperation of the patient by giving proper explanation regarding the test.
- Place the patient in comfortable position.

Unit IX ❖ Medication Needs of the Patient—Pharmacology

Procedure

Steps	Procedure	Rationale
1.	Perform hand hygiene	Prevents the transmission of microorganisms
2.	Place the area to be punctured in a dependent position. Do not milk or massage finger site	Dependent position will increase blood flow to the area
3.	Select appropriate puncture site. Clean the site with the alcohol cotton swab in a circular motion and allow it to completely dry prior to skin puncture	Prevents entry of microorganisms
4.	Remove a reagent strip from the container and reseal the container cap. Do not touch the test pad portion of the reagent strip	Closing the container tightly keeps strips safe from any environmental factors
5.	Switch on the glucometer and place the test strip into the slot to turn on the meter	This prepares meter for accurate readings

Contd...

Steps	Procedure	Rationale
6.	Apply nonsterile gloves	Prevents cross infection
7.	Fit the lancet in the lancing device and calibrate the points for piercing	Calibration helps to adjust the depth of skin penetration for various skin thicknesses
8.	Perform skin puncture using the lancet and gently squeeze the finger above the site of puncture to produce a large droplet of blood	A large droplet of blood covers the test pad on the reagent strip
9.	Apply the drop of blood in the test chamber of the reagent strip ensuring that it is filled with blood completely. The meter gives a beep to indicate that the test is starting. Read the results on the display	Smearing the blood will alter results

Contd...

Steps	Procedure	Rationale
10.	Apply pressure, or ask patient to apply pressure, to the puncture site using a gauze pad	This will stop the bleeding at the site
11.	Turn off the glucometer and dispose the test strip, gauze and lancet according to hospital policy. Replace the articles	This reduces contamination by blood to other individuals
12.	Remove the gloves, dispose them in the appropriate waste bin	Reduces transmission of microorganisms
13.	Perform hand hygiene	Prevents cross infection
14.	Document the test results with date and time of procedure	Recording the procedure acts as a legal document

Insulin

Insulin is a specific drug given as injection to diabetic patients subcutaneously in the areolar tissues. It cannot be given orally as the effect of the drug will be destroyed by the digestive enzymes.

Advancement of the condition of the diabetes needs insulin therapy.

Types of Insulin

There are different types of insulin:

- **Rapid-acting:** These include Apidra, Humalog, and Novolog. They have an onset in less than 15 minutes, peak in 30–90 minutes and duration of 3–5 hours.
- **Regular (short-acting):** These include Humulin R and Novolin R. They have an onset of a half an hour to one hour, a peak of 2–4 hours and duration of 3–5 hours.
- **Intermediate-acting:** These include Humulin N and Novolin N. They have an onset of one to three hours, a peak of eight hours and duration of 12–16 hours.
- **Long-acting:** These include Levemir and Lantus. They have an onset of one hour, minimal or no peak, and duration of 20–26 hours.
- **Combinations/pre-mixed:** These combine intermediate-acting insulins with regular insulin and are convenient for people who need to use both. These include mixtures of Humulin or Novoline, Novolog Mix, and Humalog Mix.
- **Inhaled insulin:** Afrezza has an onset of 12–15 minutes, a peak of 30 minutes, and duration of 180 minutes.

Depending upon the duration and intensity of the disease and the amount of sugar present in the blood, Doctor prescribes the type of insulin. This injection can be administered by the nurses who have learned the basic nursing procedures. Some patients themselves take this injection under the supervision of technically qualified persons or doctors.

Different types of insulin are available and prescribed by doctors. It should be given in the correct time and the correct dose. Periodical examination of sugar in the urine and blood should be conducted and reported to the doctor to make the required changes in the dose of insulin. Depending upon the type and strength of insulin, it is marked on the vial as 20, 40 and 80. That means 20 units of insulin in 1 mL, 40 units in 1 mL, and 80 units in 1 mL. (20-U/mL, 40-U/mL, 80-U/ 1 mL). *When the vial is taken for injection, the name of the drug, date of manufacture, strength of insulin in 1 mL and the date of expiry should be checked.* The name and age of patient and the prescribed dose should be verified. All 10 rights of medication administration should be observed.

Precautions to be Observed while Administering Insulin

- Insulin should be administered only according to the prescription of a doctor. For regular insulin patients urine should be received. Periodical examination of blood is conducted.
- Insulin is administered half an hour before or after taking food. Depending upon the action time of insulin, adjustments are made and patient is observed.
- The nurse who administers the insulin should be aware of the type of insulin, time of starting and terminating its action.
- Be punctual about the time and dose of insulin.
- Clean the hands of the nurse properly and use only sterile articles.
- Better to use insulin syringe or make sure about the amount taken in the syringe and the needle suitable for subcutaneous injection.
- For those who take insulin regularly, rotate the points of inserting the needles to prevent the hypertrophy of tissues and malabsorption of drug.
- Advise the patient to carry some sweets while travelling after injection, to use in case of hypoglycemia.
- Site of insulin injection should not be massaged after injection as it will hasten the absorption.

All patients who get insulin or hypoglycemic drug should be taught about personal hygiene, foot care and especially the importance of diet in controlling diabetes. Too much insulin for the available glucose in the blood will cause a condition called **insulin reaction or hypoglycemic reaction** or even known as insulin coma. One cup of sweet drink in the concentrated form may usually relieve the condition.

Hypoglycemic Reaction or Insulin Reaction

All patients with diabetes and their immediate relatives should be informed about the signs and symptom and treatment of hypoglycemia. Even if patients follow their usual schedule of medication for diabetes and the prescribed diet, they may have slight reaction at times. Severe reactions are usually caused by too large dose of insulin or oral antidiabetic drug or too little food. Reactions may occur in between meal and bed time supplements of food that have been prescribed but have been omitted. Vomiting, diarrhea, added exercise or added emotional stress may also cause insulin reaction. Persons who have diabetes should carry a card having their name and address of physician, the fact that they have diabetes and the daily insulin or oral hypoglycemic drug dosage or wear Medic Alert bracelets or necklace.

Unit IX ❖ Medication Needs of the Patient—Pharmacology

Signs, Symptoms and Management

- If a person feels weak, slightly nervous, perspires, irritable or feels dizzy after taking insulin, additional food should be given. These are the initial signs of too much insulin. Weakness, hunger, headache, palpitation, tremor, blurring of vision, or numbness of lips or tongue may occur.
- Persons taking insulin should carry concentrated sugar forms to be eaten in such emergencies.
- If it happens at home, patient should drink a glass of orange juice, other fruit juices or any other readily available sources of glucose.
- Giving concentrated form of glucose by mouth will prompt the patient to take the sweet drinks as the mucous membrane of the mouth will easily absorb the given sweets.
- If impending hypoglycemia is not treated immediately the patient becomes stuporus and unconscious because hypoglycemia interferes with the oxygen consumption of nervous tissues, there can be irreparable brain damage, if sugar is not administered promptly.
- The insulin reaction varies with the type of insulin taken and with the individual patient.
- Usually, the patient can recognize that they are becoming hypoglycemic. Immediately blood is tested for blood sugar, if possible and sugar is given in any form. In home, do not wait to test the blood but sugar is given orally in concentrated form.

Diabetic Ketoacidosis and Diabetic Coma (DKA)

Diabetic ketoacidosis occurs when there is no sufficient insulin available in the body to metabolize glucose, which if allowed to continue, results in diabetic coma and death. In untreated patients of diabetes the carbohydrate metabolism of the body is disturbed and body is unable to use carbohydrate satisfactorily, so that the body attempts to compensate by an increased appetite. Due to the inability of the body to metabolize carbohydrate, a large amount of body fat is oxidized for the energy, leading to weight loss. Fats on oxidation, large amount of fatty acids (ketone bodies) are released, which in normal amount gets neutralized with the base like tricarbonate in the blood to maintain the normal acid base balance of the body. When excessive amount of fat burns, the bases in the blood plasma may be exhausted and a condition called acidosis (ketosis) develops, consequently acetone bodies are excreted in the urine. Weakness and fatigue are common because of the difficulties in meeting the energy requirement. Onset in children is rapid and in older obese patients, it is usually gradual. Sugar in the urine will be very high and fasting blood sugar will also be very high. Normal blood sugar range is 80–120 mg/100 mL of blood.

Signs and Symptoms

- The signs and symptoms of diabetic ketoacidosis is linked to severe dehydration, loss of essential electrolytes and acidosis. If untreated, it will lead to diabetic coma and death due to insufficient insulin to metabolize glucose. All the glucose is excreted through urine and fat is burnt for energy and ketosis results.
- The signs and symptoms include weakness, dull headache, fatigue, general malaise, severe thirst, epigastric aching pain, nausea and vomiting.
- Accompanying physical findings are severe dehydration and acidosis; mucous membranes are dehydrated, there is loss of skin turgor, eye balls will be soft or sunken, lips and tongue are red and patched, face is usually flushed and hyperpnea (Kussmaul's breathing) is present.
- The temperature is elevated at first and then may go down with resultant hypovolemia. Hypovolemic shock is common and systolic blood pressure may be as low as 60–70 mm Hg. Sometimes the patient becomes anuric; acetone may be present in urine and circulatory collapse may occur. In elderly patients, myocardial infarction may occur as coronary circulation is interfered.

Management

- Diabetic ketoacidosis is a medical emergency, which needs intensive treatment and care. Therapy is directed toward correcting acidosis, dehydration, electrolyte disturbances, and other factors such as infection.
- Blood is tested and insulin is ordered by physician intravenously, or subcutaneously according to the amount of ketone bodies present in the blood.
- Dehydration is treated with a large amount of normal saline or SC Usually 4 liters or more may be needed in the first 24 hours. Depending on the severity of ketosis, treatments are carried out and nursing interventions are planned.
- Vital signs are monitored and level of consciousness is assessed frequently. Blood and urine tests are carried out, results are reported to the doctor and necessary alterations are made accordingly.
- Blood is drawn frequently to test for ketones, sugar and electrolyte levels.
- If patient is unconscious, an indwelling catheter is put. **Fluid intake and output chart is maintained.**
- When the patient's condition improves, ketone level of the blood drops and blood sugar returns back to normal. It is the time when the patient is carefully watched to prevent insulin reaction. It should be remembered that ketone and sugar return to normal level before the urinary level. When the patient is able to take fluid by mouth, fruit juices, broth, cooked cereals and milk are given. Solid foods are given as soon as possible to improve gastric tone. As patient recovers, the cause of acidosis is reviewed so that he/she understands how to avoid a recurrence.

  Ref: Shafer's Med Surg Nursing Seventh Edition.

Table 3: Differences between hypoglycemia and hyperglycemia

	Hypoglycemia	Hyperglycemia
Onset History	Onset rapid Taken insulin ½–4 hours previously, but has not eaten/has eaten but had unusual burst of energy	Slow (2–3 days) Has not taken insulin/acute infection
Patient's reactions	Irrational, bad tempered, disoriented (may be mistaken for drunk)	Thirst, nausea, abdominal pain, constipation, vomiting.
	Respirations normal, no drowsiness, BP normal, pulse normal, skin moist, tongue moist	Ketoacidosis, drowsiness, BP low, pulse weak and rapid, skin dry, tongue dry
Leads to	Coma	Coma
Needs	Glucose	Insulin and Restoration of fluid balance

These conditions are avoided by recognizing the early symptoms and taking appropriate action.

Unit IX ❖ Medication Needs of the Patient—Pharmacology

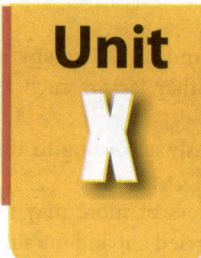

Unit X

Care of Dying Patient and Care of the Body after Death

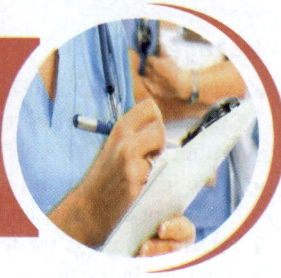

SIGNS AND SYMPTOMS OF APPROACHING DEATH

Sometimes death may come suddenly. A few moments earlier, the individual may seem to be in good health and in a fraction of a second the person may die. In other cases, the person may be on the border line between life and death for hours, days or even weeks or more.

In sudden death, the symptoms are few as compared to the death that occurs at the end of a specific illness.

There are two phases, which arise prior to the actual time of death: The "preactive phase of dying", and the "active phase of dying". On an average, the proactive phase of dying may last approximately for two weeks, while on average, the active phase of dying lasts about three days. The general signs are:

- First, there is general slowing of circulation. The feet first, later the hands, ears and nose are cold to touch.
- There will be excessive sweating.
- Skin gets pale and mottled due to congestion of blood in the vein.
- There is loss of one of muscles, the jaw sags while the dying man breathes through the mouth with the lips and cheeks sucked in and blown outward in each respiration.
- The reflexes gradually disappear.
- The pupils fail to react to light.
- The ability to swallow is lost.
- The respiration may be rapid and shallow or abnormally slow.
- Breathing may be noisy due to the presence of mucus in the throat and drying of the upper part of the respiratory tract due to open mouth.
- Eyes get sunken and half closed and sometimes a film is seen over the eyes.
- Speech becomes difficult and hearing is thought to be dulled in most cases.
- There may be restlessness, tossing movements and pulling of the bed clothes, crying, moaning and talking incoherently.
- Usually, there is an expression of anxiety and fear.

Some of these signs of death are distressing and indicate to either mental or physical suffering and this can be relieved to a certain extent by proper care.

Always remember that your loved one can often hear you even until the very end, even though he or she cannot respond by speaking. Your loving presence at the bedside can be a great expression of your love for your dying relative and can help him/her to feel calmer and more at peace, at the time of death.

THE STAGES OF DYING

Dr Elizabeth Kubler suggests that there are five stages most people go through when they understand that they are going to die. These are:

1. **Stage of denial:** It is the first stage of death that is the nonacceptance of the situation. Person thinks that this is not going to happen with him/her surely and there must be some sorts of miscalculations in the opinion of the doctor. So the patient seeks reassurance from the nurse and questions him/her regarding it, like "What the doctor has said". In this matter, the nurse can seek guidance from the doctor in order to know what the patient and family members have been told by the doctor so that he/she can provide support to them, accordingly.

2. **The stage of anger and hostility:** After the period of denial, the patient goes through an understandable period of anger and hostility. He/she will think why should this happen to him/her and what should he/she do to avoid this punishment. At this stage, the patient starts neglecting the people who come close to him, like physician, nurse, hospital and his family. He/she is angry to even God. The nurse should have patience and tolerance to the patient. Even the relatives may go through anger and hostility and blame the staff. The nurse should realize that these are all normal reactions. Practice tolerance in such situations.

3. **The stage of bargaining:** It is the third stage. From early childhood, one is taught that good behavior is rewarded and bad actions are punished. He/she may promise to self that he/she would be very good, repent for his/her sins and make up the errors if he/she can just live a little longer or have a day free of pain. It is just like a student who promises that he/she would study every night faithfully in future if he/she could just pass the examination. In this stage, the nurse cannot change the patient's prognosis, but can do something for the relief of pain and keep the patient as comfortable as possible.

4. **The stage of depression:** When the patient realizes that his/her bargaining is of no use, usually the person enters into a stage of depression. It is only a normal reaction that he/she contemplates that he has to take care of kith and kin in his life and moans its loss. At this stage, patient is concerned about family that how they are going to manage when he/she is gone and he/she may be anxious "to put all affairs in order". Sometimes, it may be difficult for him/her to discuss these matters with his/her family members who may react very emotionally to any talk of death. Also at this stage, the patient may not want to talk a great deal. He/she may wish only to see the nearest and dearest. In this case, a third person such as the chaplain, social worker or a close friend may be the best person to deal with the practical concerns of the family. The presence of someone who sympathetically cares for him/her is reassuring. Some hospitals allow important members of the family to stay with the seriously ill patient or the family members to visit the patient as often as they wish. A terminally ill patient is placed in a single room so that the patient and family may have privacy. Perhaps this contributes to the patient's sense of isolation. The presence of the nurse can overcome the patient's feelings of isolation.

5. **The stage of acceptance:** The final stage of the dying process comes when the patient accepts that he/she will die soon and is prepared for it. By this time, the patient is tired and at peace. At this stage, the family requires the most support. The family members react to death and dying in a variety of ways. They too go to the same stage as the patient does but not always in the same time. Relatives are often at a loss as what to say and how to react. An imminent death even may be denied by the family. The nurse can help the family by such actions as ensuring them privacy, permitting them access to patient and showing them some kindness for their comfort as well as to the patient's comfort. Make the relatives feel that the patient is getting the best possible care. Helping the patient to die in a dignified and peaceful manner is perhaps one of the most valuable contributions the nurse can make for the comfort of the patient and relatives.

Unit X ❖ Care of Dying Patient and Care of the Body after Death

NEEDS OF THE DYING PATIENT AND HIS/HER RELATIVES

It is the responsibility of the nurse to relieve the physical distress and to report any changes, which indicate that death is near.

- Privacy should be provided for the patient by keeping him/her in private room. When private rooms are not available, screens should be arranged around the bed because the sight and sounds of death affect the other patients.
- The nurse must be very sympathetic and kind toward the patient and his/her relatives.
- In some cases, the dying patient may ask the nurse questions about his/her condition. The nurse should always be truthful, she should satisfy the patient by her wise answers.
- Never whisper anything about the dying patient in front of him/her.
- Make the patient understand that you are always there for any help at any time.
- Put the patient in a comfortable position with the head turned to one side and protect the bed with mackintosh and draw sheet.
- Head may be elevated on pillows if there is dyspnea as it may relieve breathing difficulties.
- As the patient gets weaker, the amount of fluid given should be reduced and mouth and lips are moistened by giving sips of water at frequent intervals.
- The mouth needs careful attention.
- If there is any discharge in the eyes, it should be cleaned.
- Bedpan and urinal should be put in position periodically.
- If there is distension of the bladder, catheterization should be done.
- If there is any dentures, that should be removed and kept safely.
- Prevent disagreeable odors in the room by keeping the environment clean.
- The room must be well-ventilated and provided with good light.
- The position of the lower extremities should be changed frequently. The pillow under the knee should be removed, fluffed and replaced.
- Never leave the patient in wet clothes and never leave him/her alone.

IMMEDIATE SIGNS OF DEATH

- Cessation of heart's action and of respiration.
- Opaqueness of cornea.
- Absence of reflexes.
- Manifestation of rigor mortis.
- Discoloration of the body is the important immediate sign of death. These signs lead to complete stopping of breathing.

When the patient's breathing ceases, it should be reported to the physician immediately so that the death can be certified by him/her.

After death being certified and the proper care is given, the body is allowed to be removed from the ward through the back door.

PHYSIOLOGICAL CHANGES AFTER DEATH

- **Rigor mortis:** Otherwise called **postmortem rigidity** is the stiffening of the body that occurs about 2–4 hours after death. This is often referred to as the third stage of death and results from lack of Adenosine triphosphate (ATP), which causes the muscles to contract, and in turn immobilizes the joints. It starts in the involuntary muscles (heart, bladder) then progresses to head, neck, trunk and extremities.
- **Algor mortis:** Algor means—coldness. It is gradual decrease of the body temperature after death when the individuals no longer produce body heat. When blood circulation terminates and hypothalamus ceases to function, body temperature falls down.

- **Livor mortis:** It is the bluish–purple discoloration of body after death, which occurs due to the gravitation of blood after death. After blood circulation has ceased, the RBCs are broken down leading to discoloration of surrounding tissues.
- **Decomposition:** Tissues after death become soft and eventually liquefied by bacterial fermentation. The hotter the temperature, the more rapid the change. So bodies are stored in cool places or embalming is performed.

CARE OF THE BODY AFTER DEATH

Purposes

- To prepare the body for the morgue
- To prevent discoloration or deformity of the body
- To protect the body from postmortem discharge

Procedure

1. Check orders for any specimens.
2. Ask for special requests from family (e.g., shaving, a special outfit a religious book in hand).
3. Wash hands and put on the required PPE.
4. As soon as the patient has breathed his/her last, nurse should gently close his/her eyes and mouth if they are not already closed.
5. Replace dentures.
6. Lead the relatives from the room.
7. If possible, get the help of another nurse so that the body can be handled more easily and more reverently.
8. The body is placed flat on the bed with legs quite straight and arms laid at the sides.
9. All pillows, bolsters and air rings are removed except one pillow under the head.
10. A folded towel is used to prop up the chin in position for a short time or bandage can be used to hold the jaw firm.
11. Ankles are securely fastened together with a bandage to prevent it falling apart or kept on position by means of sand bags.
12. Then ask the relatives to remove all the jewelries (except wedding ring, if the relatives are particular), then list them, keep in separate package and pack along with other valuables.
13. Soiled dressing should be replaced and adhesive marks to be removed.
14. Drainage tubes if any, should be removed.
15. Then the patient's body should be given a complete bath and hair combed and dressed.
16. The rectum and vagina are packed to prevent the escape of urine and feces from the relaxed meatus and anus.
17. Body is covered with a sheet.
18. An identification tag containing the patient's name, age, address, ward no., bed number and date and time of death is attached to one wrist.
19. The body is moved to the mortuary in a stretcher after half an hour, if the relatives are not present.
20. If present, the body is handed over to them with the permission of the doctor.
21. The body should be removed through the back door.
22. If autopsy is to be done, permission should be obtained from the relatives.
23. All clothing and other personal belongings of patient should be listed and wrapped neatly in a bundle, properly tagged and taken to the office or given to the family according to the regulations of the institution.
24. The room should be cleaned as early as possible. The physician fills the death certificate before the body is taken home and the certificate is sent to the office.

Unit X ❖ Care of Dying Patient and Care of the Body after Death

25. The nurse should fill in the nurse's record with all details of death. He/she should see that the records are complete and sent to the office or record section for filing.
26. If the death is caused by incidences, like accident, suicide, homicide, murdering or poisoning, the body should not be handed over to the relatives but is moved to the mortuary for autopsy.
27. When death occurs following certain communicable diseases as smallpox, plague, etc. and the body requires special handling, then nurse should help in preventing the spread of the disease.

PLACING AND RELEASING BODY FROM MORTUARY

Mortuary is an important and integral part of every hospital as it deals with the preservation of the dead body.

Definitions

- A mortuary is the place used for the storage of human corpses awaiting identification or removal for autopsy or respectful burial, cremation or other method.
- Morgue is a place where dead bodies are kept in the refrigerated body store and examined in the post-mortem room.

Purposes

- To keep the dead body till the relatives claim and take over the body for disposal.
- To keep unclaimed bodies until disposal (burial or cremation) is arranged by the hospital authorities.
- To allow viewing and identification by relatives, police and other people.
- To receive dead bodies requiring pathological postmortems pending final disposal.
- To receive dead bodies brought to the hospital for medicolegal postmortem work and store in the mortuary pending further disposal.
- To impart teaching programs for undergraduates as well as postgraduates.

Types of Dead Bodies Preserved In Mortuary

The types of dead body preserved in the mortuary can be classified as:
- **Nonmedicolegal**
  - Identified
  - Unknown
- **Medicolegal cases (MLC)**
  - Identified
  - Unknown

Disposal of Dead Body

Death Occurring in the Hospital

- Once death occurs in hospital ward or casualty, the doctor (Registered Medical Practitioner) who has attended the deceased in his/her last offices should issue the death certificate in a prescribed format issued by the government.
- In an MLC, death occurring in any of the clinical areas viz. inpatient wards/ICU/Emergency, the dead body will be mandatorily sent to the mortuary.
- In case of the death of a non-MLC patient, if the relatives of the patient want to receive the dead body without delay, then the sister I/C senior most sister on duty will hand over the body to the relatives (against receipt in the death register) along with the dead body receipt slip of the patient, against clearance received from the admission office (after clearing bills, etc.) from where he/she will get a dead body receipt slip with stamp "Body may be handed over".

- However, in all such cases, the relatives have to be gently advised to complete the formalities and remove the patient's body within one hour of the declaration of the death; otherwise the body may be sent to the mortuary.
- The ward sister will keep one copy of dead body receipt slip and one of the death report forms in his/her records.
- Ideally, there should be 4–5 copies of death certificate for non-medicolegal case and medicolegal case respectively (a) for relative, (b) for medical record, (c) for municipal board for issue of formal death certificate, (d) for autopsy request, if required, (e) for police, if MLC
    - In AIIMS, the death certificates are made in two copies for non-MLC and in three copies for MLC. One copy is given to the relatives and one is retained by the hospital, which is forwarded to municipal body. The third copy for MLC is given to police.
- The doctor is legally bound to report all the medicolegal deaths to the nearest magistrate or police officer in the jurisdiction.
- All bodies (MLC and non-MLC) are kept in the mortuary cold storage till it is handed over to the relatives or the police.
- The doctor on duty or nurse on the behalf of the doctor should intimate the mortuary technician and send the body to mortuary along with a copy of death certificate.
- The body should be transported by stretcher.
- It should be covered by a shroud and then wrapped in a sheet.
- A standard label must be fixed to the winding cloth over the upper part of the body, so that when it is taken out of the mortuary cold storage room, head first identification is easy.
- The death certificate and the label should be marked "MLC" in bold letters for medicolegal cases.
- The label should have the following information on it:
    - Patient's name
    - Father's name
    - Age and sex
    - Hospital registration number
    - Ward
    - Date and time of death
    - Date and time of placement of body in the mortuary cold storage.
- The body should also have identity wrist bands, which serves as a ready means of identification. The best label in a plastic waterproof covering is clipped on the patient's wrist.
- In case of MLC bodies, two police officers who have seen the dead body in position in which it was found and are competent to detect any attempt at substitution or tampering with the body or its coverings, shall accompany the body to the mortuary and remain in charge of it until examination is complete.
- The officer who has accompanied the body from the spot shall hand it over personally to the medical officer conducting the postmortem examination together with all reports and articles sent by the investigating officer to assist the examination and shall receive and convey to the investigating officer the postmortem report.
- As soon as the civil surgeon intimates that his/her examination is complete, the police shall, unless they have received order from a competent authority to the contrary, hand over the body to the deceased's relatives or friends. If there are no relatives or friends, or they decline to receive it, the police shall decide whether the body to be buried or burnt according to the rules framed in this behalf by the district magistrate.

Unit X ❖ Care of Dying Patient and Care of the Body after Death

Death Occurring Outside Hospital

- The non-MLC bodies from outside maybe permitted to be kept in the mortuary for storage on the request of the relatives on the following conditions:
  - Cold storage room must be in working condition.
  - Space must be available for the body.
  - Proper application along with a copy of death certificate, embalming certificate, if embalmed and no objection certificate from police.
- The body shall be kept at the risk of the concerned relatives.
- In case of the MLC the investigating officer should come with an application along with a copy of death certificate.
- The body should be handed over to the police or relatives after proper identification.

Unclaimed Body

- If a body is unidentified, the officer making the investigation shall record a careful description of it, giving all marks, peculiarities, deformities, other distinctive features and shall take the finger impressions.
  - In addition to taking all other reasonable steps to secure identification he shall, if possible, have it photographed.
  - Unidentified body should be handed over to any charitable society, who is willing to accept it and if no such society comes forward, it should then be buried or burnt.
- The police sends telegram message called 'Hue and Cry Notice' to various police headquarters of the country. The 'Hue and cry notice' contains brief description of the identification features of the deceased.
- The body is preserved in the mortuary for 72 hours, from the time telegram message is sent.
- If there is no one to claim the body after 72 hours, the police is legally authorized to dispose of the body.
  - But if the police think that the body maybe identified by the relatives, it should be preserved for longer time till relatives come and claim the body.
- The expenditures on the disposal of body in unidentified case are borne by the police department. This is applicable in medicolegal cases expired outside hospital or inside the hospital.
- In case of unclaimed bodies in hospital, and if such kinds of deaths have occurred due to the natural cause, the hospital authority is lawfully in charge of such bodies.
- Police should send telegram messages to whatever address of the deceased is available.
- If the body is unclaimed even after 72 hours, police are legally authorized to dispose of the body bearing this expenditure.
- As per Human Transplant Act 1994, the hospital authority is authorized to give permission for removal of any human organ from the unclaimed body after 48 hours.

add·on

The primary legislation related to organ donation and transplantation in India, Transplantation of Human Organs Act, was passed in 1994 and was aimed at regulation of removal, storage, and transplantation of human organs for therapeutic purposes and for prevention of commercial dealings in human organs. In India, matters related to health are governed by each state. The Act was initiated at the request of Maharashtra, Himachal Pradesh, and Goa (who therefore adopted it by default) and was subsequently adopted by all states except Andhra Pradesh and Jammu and Kashmir. Despite a regulatory framework, cases of commercial dealings in human organs were reported in the media. An amendment to the Act was proposed by the states of Goa, Himachal Pradesh, and West Bengal in 2009 to address inadequacies in the efficacy, relevance, and impact of the Act. The amendment to the Act was passed by the Parliament in 2011, and the rules were notified in 2014. The same is adopted by the proposing states and union territories by default and may be adopted by other states by passing a resolution.

- The unclaimed MLC bodies in hospital should be handed over to the police who shall dispose of the body after postmortem.

Embalmed Body

- The body taken for embalming should be identified properly beyond doubt and proper consent from a near relative or from the person in lawful possession of the dead body is necessary.
- It would also be accompanied by death certificate, postmortem certificate, if postmortem was done and no objection certificate from police.
- In the case of foreign nationals, clearance from respective embassy is necessary.
- Embalming should not be done before autopsy (where autopsy is necessary) as it destroys the medicolegal evidence, especially in poisoning death, by hindering its detections in viscera.
- On completion of embalming, a certificate is issued by a competent authority (embalmer). This certificate is prerequisite for transportation of the body.
- Embalming is necessary to prevent putrefaction in case the relative wants to keep the body for longer time.

Cadavers for Anatomical Dissection

The Anatomy Act, 1959 provides for the collection of an unclaimed dead body for teaching purpose, only if death occurs in a state hospital or in a public place within the prescribed zone of medical institution, provided the police has declared a lapse of 48 hours that there are no claimants for the body and it could be used for medical purpose [anatomical examination, dissection and removal of healthy organs from the deceased for transplantation in living persons].

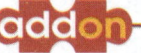

Mass Disaster Plan to Take Care of Dead Bodies
- The mass disaster plan must have a proper guideline for proper identification, preservation and disposal of the dead body taking into consideration all medicolegal formalities.
- To take care of the dead bodies, the disaster plan must include setting up of temporary emergency mortuaries like air conditioned tents
- The medical person has an important role such as:
  - Proper scientific numbering and tagging of the dead bodies for future identification purpose by the relatives
  - Identification of body as far as possible by noting down the identification features
  - Issuing of death certificates
  - Conduction of medicolegal autopsy

Transport of Dead Body from Hospital

- After death, the body should be properly labeled mentioning the name, father's name, admission number, ward, date and time of death, etc. by nursing staff on duty.
- In addition, in medicolegal cases the letters 'MLC' should be put on the label prominently.
- Nursing staff on duty in the ward should ensure that the body is wrapped in leak-proof sheets/plastic bag and handed over to next of kin or mortuary attendant.
- The mortuary attendant on duty is informed that a pick up or removal is necessary from the wards.
- The hearse van service is provided free of cost for transportation of the body from the hospital to the Mortuary.
- The morgue attendant will receive the duly wrapped and labeled bodies in a courteous, sensitive and professional manner, along with the relevant records including death slip.

Unit X ❖ Care of Dying Patient and Care of the Body after Death

INTAKE PROCEDURE AND MAINTENANCE OF MORTUARY REGISTER

- The morgue attendants will receive the 'Death Slip' from the hospital along with the dead body.
- Identity of the body should be confirmed by matching the label on body by the death slip particulars and should be matched with ID band.
- The morgue attendant will note the complete details of the death slip in the register and ensure that the details in the dead body tag are matched with the death slip.
- Custody of MLC bodies: It is the responsibility of the police personnel for taking 24 hours care of all such dead bodies of MLCs and maintaining safe legal custody of the MLC corpse.

Procedure

Steps	General procedure	Rationale
1.	Once death is confirmed by the physician, the nursing staff completes all the required formalities including Last offices Documentation with due signatures	Ensures dignity and respect. Documentation ensures accountability
2.	Complete mortuary cards (A sample card is given below)	Ensures correct and easy identification of the body in the mortuary

Ward & Site		Fiscal Case	Yes/No/Unknown
Name		Infective	Yes/Unknown
CHI Number		Religion	
Address		Jewellery/ items on body	Yes/No If Yes, list below: ....
Sex	M/F	Height & Weight	If known H.............. W..............
Date of Birth	.../.../...		
Date of Admission	.../.../...	Patient's named Consultant	
Date of Death	.../.../...		
Time of Death	...... hours	Time collected	...... hours
Names of persons removing body			
Any other comments:			

Steps	General procedure	Rationale
3.	Contact portering staff to arrange removal of the body from the ward and transfer to mortuary. Provide the portering staff with information on the patient's weight and size when requesting transfer to mortuary	Enables staff to make informed choices regarding equipment required and staff available to assist
4.	Handover the mortuary request form to the mortuary in charge or the concerned, as per the Institution's protocol	Ensures readiness for safe and discrete transfer of the deceased

Contd...

Steps	General procedure	Rationale
5.	On arrival, porters should pick up the necessary documents from the staff and ensure that ID band is in place	Ensures that all necessary documentation has been completed before transferring the deceased to the mortuary
6.	Raise sides of the trolley and place cover over the deceased and moves to the mortuary	Ensures safe and discrete transfer of the deceased
7.	On arrival at mortuary, porters will transfer the deceased into an appropriate location or fridge compartment. All necessary transfers in the mortuary should be carried out with a sufficient number of handlers, using appropriate handling equipment	Facilitates a safe system of work for handling the deceased within the mortuary
	Mortuary staff—Procedures for receiving, storing and releasing bodies	
8.	Mortuary staff must check that fully completed ID bands are attached to wrist and ankle. If ID bands are missing or incomplete, a member of ward staff must be summoned to identify the deceased and complete/attach the ID bands. In MLC cases, the police officer logging the body into the mortuary should ensure that it is labelled correctly	Ensures correct and easy identification of the body
9.	Details of deceased's name and fridge number are recorded on the mortuary notice board and on the register located in the body storage area	Ensures correct and easy location of the body
10.	Bodies will only be released to appropriate persons as directed by the family. All necessary paperwork must be completed and should be in the possession of the mortuary staff before the body can be released	Ensures that the body is released to bonafide persons
11.	Mortuary staff and concerned family members (any other as per Institutional policy) **Must Double Check and Confirm** the deceased's identity on wristband	Ensures that correct body is handed over
12.	Mortuary staff should handover the relevant paperwork to the family member and both should sign the mortuary register and only then will the body be released	Ensures accountability and traceability of staff involved in every transaction
13.	On some occasions the family may request, for religious, or other reasons that the body be removed directly from the ward. The ward staff must ensure that all necessary paperwork has been completed before they release the body from the ward with due entry in mortuary register	Allows the relevant details to be entered into the mortuary register
	Procedure for unclaimed bodies	
14.	If a body is lying in the mortuary and even after 5 days no contact has been made by anyone about disposal/removal, the following procedure should be carried out and the attached form is to be completed in all cases. Ensure that there were no relatives for the deceased from the ward staff. Then they raise the claim form for unclaimed bodies and necessary action will be taken as specified above	Ensures that appropriate action is taken when bodies are not claimed by family or when there are no known relatives

Contd...

Unit X ❖ Care of Dying Patient and Care of the Body after Death

Steps	General procedure	Rationale
15.	**Documentation in mortuary:** The maintenance of a full and accurate record of the body brought to the mortuary and its effect is one of the most important tasks of the mortuary technician. All morticians should keep a mortuary register. It is preferred to have a large heavy book that cannot be easily lost or removed. The following details of everybody brought into the mortuary should be recorded in this book. • Give a number to each body. These numbers run consecutively from January 1 to 31 December in each year • Name, sex, age of the deceased person • Date and time of death • Identification marks of the deceased and finger impressions may also be noted • Details of close relatives, e.g., name, relationship, address and phone number should be noted • Whether or not an autopsy was carried out • If autopsy done, then date and time of autopsy and name of the autopsy surgeon • Date and time when the body is placed in the cold storage • Length of the body and breadth across the shoulder (helps in making coffin of correct size) • A list of valuables, which have not been removed from the body such as rings, bangles and others • Signature of the mortuary technician who allows body to be taken away • Date and time when the body is removed • Documentation if feasible should be computerized • Name of the relatives or police personnel collecting the body	Documentation fosters quality care.

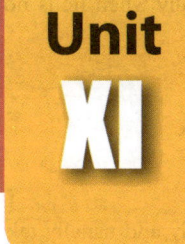

Geriatric Nursing

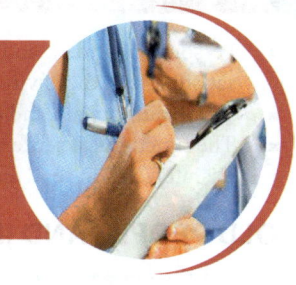

GERIATRICS

Geriatrics is a branch of medicine covering all aspects of old age and the disorders arising from it. Geriatric nursing is the nursing care given to the aged people.

OLD AGE

Usually the period of retirement is considered to be the starting of old age. But tremendous variations exist in this concept. Chronological age is related to old age but not identical with the term 'aging' because individual and personal variables are seen in people. The US department of health education and welfare has defined aging in terms of three classes.

1. **Biological aging:** It means aging occurs when body gradually accumulates damage of various cells and tissues.
2. **Psychological aging:** It occurs, when a person's capacity for adapting to his/her environment is reduced.
3. **Social aging:** That is, when a person's role in the family and community is lowered, his interests and activities become down and he reaches aging.

   Because of any of these reasons, some people may be old at 45 years of age whereas others are not old even at 80.

   Some gerontological experts define three groupings within the age group 65 years to 100+ years:
   - Young old, aged 65 years to 75 years
   - Old, aged 75 years to 85 years
   - Oldest old aged 85 years and older

   The problems and needs of these groups may be different. The 'old old' group has more physical changes, typical of aging and more social problems such as loss of friends and loss of independence than the young old.

CHARACTERISTICS OF AGING

Aging is a normal process in which certain anatomic and physiologic changes take place. These changes are associated with a decline in the effectiveness and functioning of the body.

- Heart rate may be reduced but blood pressure may be increased
- Body temperature and pulse rate may be slightly reduced and respiration rate also may be reduced
- Due to the weakness of the brain, the power of memory may be declined
- The power of muscles will be reduced and muscles start looking flabby
- The smoothness of the skin is lost and it looks rough
- Sexual interest diminishes

- Person looks weak and disinterested in everything, but irritated and angry, especially when he is not satisfied with the environment and experiences from others
- Complains of pain and discomfort in the body
- The functions of sense organs, especially eyes and ears get reduced
- Disinterested in food and may have constipation or diarrhea, dyspepsia and flatulence

OLD PEOPLE AND ILLNESSES

Most of the old people suffer from chronic illness. These illnesses have developed slowly and usually take time to alleviate. Heart disease, cancer, renal disease, vascular disease such as cerebrovascular accidents, chronic pulmonary diseases, asthma, arthritis, and skin disorders are some of the common conditions seen in old age. When elderly persons become ill, they may be particularly apprehensive and worried because their security is affected by illness as compared to younger persons. They prefer hospitalization because of real fear. Many of the illnesses of old age may be real physical disabilities and some of the illness may be reflections of psychological problems. Whatever is the cause these are all problems to the person.

PROBLEMS, NEEDS AND CARE OF OLD AGE

- **Hygienic needs**
  - Oral hygiene
  - Care of nails and hair
  - Prevention of bed sore
  - Exercise, rest and sleep
  - Elimination
    The needs and care required for the old age patients are more or less same as mentioned here:
    - There should be a safe and convenient room to give treatment and nursing care to any patient.
    - The room for keeping an aged patient should be very convenient for walking without any obstructions on the floor, easy to go to the toilets and the bed should be comfortable and safe.
    - If the house is a two-storied building, the aged persons should be accommodated on the ground floor with bath and toilet facilities as it may cause hazards to the aged.
    - Toilet articles such as bedpan, urinal, sputum cups, etc. should be placed within the reach of the aged persons.
    - If there is any chance of spoiling the mattress or pillows by any discharges from the body, it should be protected with rubber or plastic sheets and covered with bed sheets.
    - If there are any electric fittings in the room, it should be protected safely against electric shock.
- **Nutritional needs of the aged:** Food is one of the important factors of health. One cannot live without food for long period. Most of the aged people suffer from the diseases due to lack of proper food. So the nurse, giving care to the aged should take special attention in the feeding of the particular client.
  - Nurse should understand the food habits of the patient.
  - As the activities of the body being reduced in the old age, the calorie requirements also may be lessened. But the supplements like, proteins, vitamins and minerals should be supplied in plenty.
  - Due to the limitations of the taste buds in the old age, the taste of foods may be reduced and dyspepsia will be common and it may affect the digestion also.
  - The digestive enzymes will not be working properly, which may be one of the causes for loss of appetite.
  - Whatever is the cause for loss of appetite, it is not desirable to make a sudden change in the routine of food habits.

- The nurse should tactfully understand the knowledge of the patient and relatives about the balanced diet. She and help them to realize the needs of required food factors and try to remove their knowledge deficits.
- Small meals of simply prepared, easy to chew and digestible foods should be given several times in a day.
- As mentioned above, most of the old people may be suffering from chronic digestive troubles which need a great deal of food control. For such people certain food factors may be restricted.
- Apart from that, financial deficiency, mental depression, lack of loving relatives for encouragement, knowledge deficiency of required food, inability of preparing food, individual bias about certain foods, misconception of limiting food in the old age, loneliness in life, etc. are some of the causes for rejecting or reducing food in the old age. We can see many old people who are taking only one cup of tea with few pieces of bread per day. The reason may be any one or many of the causes mentioned above.
- The nurse who looks after the aged people should observe and consider their individual likes and dislikes and their health status should be ascertained and diet is adjusted accordingly.

■ **Emotional needs:** The important emotional needs of his/her old people are acceptance and communication with others. The nurse should recognize the emotional needs of his/her patients. Most of the time, old people are left alone. So they suffer from the trauma of loneliness. A nurse should pay special attention to exclude these conditions. Old people are much interested in talking than listening, especially about their past experiences. The nurse should find out some time, to listen to their talk. They will appreciate discussing religious and social leaders. Even though they like to talk about the good memories and experiences of their past life, they will be interested in listening to the current trend of the society and the performances of the youngsters. Even if there are limitations in the eye sight and hearing, they will expect and like to know the current news from newspapers or periodicals. Old men like the good listeners than the best speakers.

Very old patients like to see and talk with their grandchildren. If they are not in a position to go and meet the grandchildren, they will appreciate talking to young ones through telephone or if possible face to face. Occasional visits of dearest and nearest ones will be a happy time for them and gives mental satisfaction. In sickness or weakness, old people should be hospitalized, if required. It not only helps to relieve the sickness but also it will be an opportunity to meet, talk and exchange the ideas and experiences with the friends and relatives. Old patients who have fulfilled all their responsibilities in the life by bringing up and educating the children and resolved all the responsibilities of a family in an appropriate manner are to be really respected. So the elders who have spent their strength, side-lining their own enjoyment and working for the betterment of their children and family, really deserve tender care in their vulnerable old age. The present youngsters are enjoying the essence of the effort, blood and sweat of their old parents. They are repaying the old parents with negligence instead of acceptance and rejections instead of respect. The type of experiences they are getting from the youngsters are clearly reflected and understood by their talk, expressions, reactions and behaviors to others. An intelligent nurse should recognize, and realize these reactions while living in the company of the old parents and represent himself/herself as a loving kin in the place of those thankless youngsters and try to satisfy them in the last part of their life.

This is not the complete picture of our society. There is other side of the coin as well. In spite of such genuine, trenchant and pathetic instances, few aged lucky old people are enjoying life with their children and grandchildren. They consider that old parents are a blessing, they are loved, respected and accepted; their needs and likes are recognized and even anticipated and fulfilled; they live and mingle with them. Those youngsters believe that old parents are the glitter of the house and such a family with peace, prosperity and providence is a heaven in the world. During day time, when the young parents go for their work and grandchildren go to school, home nurses are posted as the only help and support to the old patients. Such helpers should be capable of anticipating and recognizing the priorities of the old parents just like their loving children.

- **Diversional therapy:** Those aged people, who are capable of reading, watching television or listening to radio should be provided with such conveniences and reading materials like newspapers, periodicals or books, which they like as religious books. If small letters are difficult for them to read, sufficient big letters should be provided. For those who are blind, but interested in surroundings, the nurse should read the matters loud enough for the patient to hear. Spend some time to listen to the aged carefully instead of speaking to them so that they may have the sincere feelings to the nurse. Those who are able to see and hear, may be provided with television or radio which may be a diversional therapy and relieve some of their mental tension.

  Aged people always like to do some useful small work at home as a diversion. There are many simple works at home suitable to the aged if their illness is not serious. Aged ladies always like simple works like stitching, knitting, preparing vegetables, drying dinner plates and so on.

  Aged male may like to spend time at home if they are able, by making or repairing toys for their grandchildren or repairing small home appliances. Drawing and painting are easy and interesting hobby to all aged people. They may be very slow and take much time to do all such works. When they perform their routines or works very slowly, we should not make them hurry up or should not show any impatience towards the work. If one is impatient or impertinent towards the 'aged', they will lose their interest and alertness and refuse to do such diversional works.

- **Spiritual needs:** Most of the aged people are always conscious about their death. Especially those who are rejected, dejected, deluded, derelicted and despised by others and desperate by the experiences in the last part of their life, expect and welcome the death eagerly. The nurse should not neglect this matter and not only that, he/she should be provided with opportunities to express his/her opinion and belief about death. An old aged patient may desire to meet and discuss with their religious advisers, spiritual experts, legal advisers, responsible relatives or any of his/her capable and good friends to get the spiritual advice or to talk about some important matters, which are not fulfilled according to his/her own satisfaction. More than that of treatment and nursing care, nurse is the person who stays with the patient most of the time for comfort and dealings, this is the reason that he/she may find nurse as a suitable and sincere person for fulfilling his/her needs. Nurse should tactfully understand the reaction of the family and his/her relatives, about his/her demise. It is one of the important duties of the nurse to give comfort and console the patient and relatives in such critical situations.

  For a person, who is living in a comfortable environment, old age is really a best period of life for him because it is an opportunity for him/her to think and to be happy about the good experiences and success of the past life or repent about the disasters happened. In this phase of life the elderly has enough time to correct them in the best possible way, reconsider any particular performances, pray and meditate till the last breath in which all the worldly ties are cut off. There are some old people who spent their youthful life without minding anyone or anything and they were concerned only with their own affairs in their own way, without bending the head before any one self-contained and imposing his/her might and power upon others. But all the splendid victory will be declined in the old age and naturally people will turn to the spiritual side of life depending on the 'Almighty' as any Science cannot prevent one's death. When one is nearing to his/her last days, his/her spiritual needs become more intense and prominent. Whatever is the caste and religion of the individual, it is the fundamental right of every critical patient aged or not, to consult their religious advisers and get their advices and help for one's own satisfaction and peaceful death. The nurse should recognize and understand the need of the patient in time and provide opportunities for the same.

- **Social needs:** The old people must be allowed to live in their own homes, and in their familiar neighborhood. But institutionalization is a risk the elderly face. Studies specify that elderly people who live in old age homes often experience morbidity and mortality in excess when compared with elderly living in their own homes. This is because of the lack of adequate contact with family and friends and the tendency for excessive custodial attention. This can result in depression and withdrawn feeling.

    Respect for the elderly is not only the responsibility of individual families. It is also a society's function to promote such respect. Care of the elderly by the family is generally in line with society's norms and sanctions. Nurses should understand that in the care of the elderly, maintaining quality of life and optimum health status are important. Living in the community and receiving community-based long-term care are advantageous to the elderly. Hence, it is also important to train community members including family members, neighbors and friends to take care of their elderly at home.

    Although gerontological nurses work in a variety of settings, including acute care hospitals, rehabilitation, nursing homes (also known as long-term care homes and skilled nursing facilities), assisted living facilities, retirement homes, community health agencies, and the patient's home, their main responsibility is as a caregiver.

NURSING ASSESSMENT OF ELDERLY PATIENTS

Health assessment of elderly is similar to that of any adult health assessment. However, special considerations and some essential skills are required when assessing geriatric patients in any clinical setting.

Obtaining the Health History

Before the physical assessment begins, collect the health history by interviewing the patient (and family members, if needed). Speak louder if required. Elderly people may have sensory deficits, which may hinder them in giving appropriate and necessary information.

Physical Examination of Elderly: Special Considerations

- Skin wrinkling is a common skin condition of the elderly which results from loss of elasticity and turgor. With age, the skin gradually thins and loses density. This makes the skin more susceptible to bruising and tears. Observe for any skin tear and bruising.
- Also observe the skin for lesions and moles. When examining moles, look for irregular shapes; ask the patient if any moles have gotten bigger or any change in color.
- Excessive sun exposure exacerbates age-related changes. This may predispose to skin cancers such as melanoma.
- Observe for pressure ulcers. Pressure ulcers are most common on the sacrum, heels, and trochanters. These pressure ulcers are preventable and occur primarily from decreased mobility and activity, insufficient caloric intake and incontinence.
- Observe the hair color. Decline in melanin production makes the hair less vibrant in color, leading to graying. Also, the hair thins; many older adults lose their hair altogether and become bald.
- Some men are genetically predisposed to baldness and may experience hair loss at younger ages. This is due to the diminished dermal vascular beds with age, altering hair distribution patterns.
- Note the color, length and cleanliness of nails. Check for abnormalities of nails. For instance,
    - Clubbing may indicate a cardiac or pulmonary disorder.
    - Pitting in the nails and transverse groves may be present in peripheral vascular disease, arterial insufficiency, or diabetes.
    - Brittleness may stem from decreased vascular supply.
    - Yellow or brown nails may signal a fungal infection.

Unit XI ❖ Geriatric Nursing

- Limited range of motion (ROM) commonly occurs from arthritis or muscle weakness, and can cause pain and discomfort in older adults.
- When assessing the ROM of neck, the person may have complaints of pain or dizziness or jerky and abnormal movements; these may indicate health problems such as fractured vertebrae, Parkinson's disease, a transient ischemic attack, or stroke.
- Note whether the patient's eyes, eyebrows, nose, and mouth are centered and symmetrical. Asymmetrical features suggest a stroke.
- Look for appropriateness of affect and behavior.
- Check facial skin for dryness, sagging, looseness, and wrinkling, which occur due to the changes related to aging like decrease in skin elasticity, subcutaneous fat and moisture.
- Vision can deteriorate with age. Older adults should have 20/40 vision or better. Conditions such as changing eye shape (presbyopia), cataracts and glaucoma typically worsen with age. Older adults may be more sensitive to glare because of structural changes in the eye. This may result in increased risk of falls and result in injury. Encourage them to get annual eye examination.
- Hearing loss is common in older adults and usually affects both ears. In general, older adults find more trouble in hearing high-frequency sounds, such as consonants (especially p, s, and t) than low-frequency sounds, such as vowels. Advise these patients with hearing difficulty to consult an audiologist.
- Investigate for abnormalities such as loss of balance, gait disorders, postural abnormalities, or inability to transfer from a chair to a standing position.
- Evaluate muscle groups for atrophy, tremors, and involuntary movements.
- If the patient is weak, with poor coordination, perform functional examination, in depth.
- Assess the patient's ability to perform activities of daily living (ADLs), including self-care activities like bathing, dressing, toileting, continence and feeding.
- Evaluate the patient's fall risk.
- Other systems assessment should be carried out as routine.

Nursing Procedures Related to Geriatrics

Routine nursing care procedures create risks for elderly patients to a greater extent because of the physiological changes. For example:

- Starting an IV line and blood sample collection are often difficult due to small and fragile veins.
- Intravenous fluid administration poses the risk of fluid overload. Fluid balance is more delicate with elderly persons. The elderly are particularly vulnerable to dehydration which may be manifested as confusion.
- Fragile skin is easily torn during removal of plasters.
- Moving in bed can injure fragile skin causing increased risk of pressure ulcer.
- Fractures may result from very minor trauma due to osteoporosis.
- Medications may cause special risks because of slowed metabolism, relatively more body fat, compromised renal function and alterations produced by disease conditions. Older adults are highly sensitive to the effects of drugs. A narrow margin of safety—between minimal effective dose and toxic dose—is often a factor.

Ref: Safers Med Surg Nursing Seventh Edition.

Maternal and Newborn Care

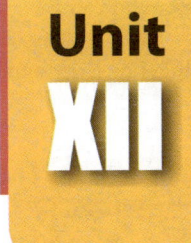

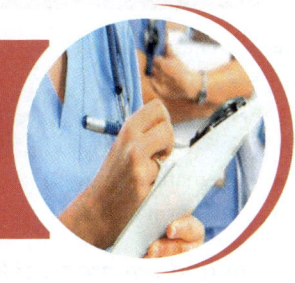

Maternal Care

INTRODUCTION

In every country mothers and children constitute a priority group. In India 65% percent of the total population are mothers and children. They are not only the larger group, but mothers and children are vulnerable or special risk groups. Risk for the women is concerned with child bearing and in case of infants and children, growth and development are risk factors. Most of the risk factors are preventable by proper treatment and care. By improving the health of mothers and children, we contribute to the health of the total population. Because of this consideration, provisions of special health care to the mothers and children are developed all over the world. Recently, maternal and child care are being integrated with family welfare services in most of the countries.

MATERNITY CYCLE

The stages of maternity cycle are:

- Fertilization
- Antenatal care
- Intranatal care
- Postnatal care

Health supervision and care is required in all these stages. The main objective of maternity care is the delivery of a healthy child without any injury to the mother.

Fertilization

The ovum is released from the ovary about the 14th day of the menstrual cycle and it is caught up by the fimbriated end of the fallopian tube. The spermatozoa reaches the uterine cavity and travels to the fallopian tube and fuses with the ovum. The union of a sperm with a mature ovum in the fallopian tube is called *fertilization*.

Once the fertilization has taken place, the ovum becomes impenetrable to any other sperm. Segmentation of the fertilized ovum begins at once at a rapid rate.

Growth of embryo and fetus: The fertilized ovum reaches uterus by 8–10 days and burrows in the uterine endometrium. Cell division proceeds rapidly and differentiation of all organs and tissues of the body are formed. The periods of growth have been divided as follows:

- Prenatal period
  - Ovum   0–14 days
  - Embryo   14 days to 9 weeks
  - Fetus   9th week to birth
- Premature infant   27th to 37th week
- Full term birth   280 days (average)

Signs and Symptoms of Pregnancy

The main signs and symptoms of pregnancy are divided into three main groups:
1. Presumptive signs
2. Probable signs
3. Positive signs

1. Presumptive Signs

- Amenorrhea
- Morning sickness
- Breast changes
- Bladder irritation
- Quickening

2. Probable Signs

- Pelvic signs: Goodell's sign, Hegar's sign, Chadwick's sign
- Abdominal enlargement

3. Positive Signs

- Fetal heart sounds
- Fetal movements
- Fetal parts
- X-ray or scanning evidences

Antenatal Care or Prenatal Care

It is the care given to the women during pregnancy, which normally starts from the time of conception and continues throughout pregnancy.

Objectives

- To promote and maintain the health of the mother during pregnancy
- To detect the high risk factors and give special attention
- To assure the mother to receive the best care during pregnancy
- To prepare the mother physically, mentally and materially for delivery
- To reduce maternal and infant morbidity and mortality
- To have a healthy baby born
- To teach the mother to look after the newborn and infant during the first month of life.

The objectives of promotion and maintenance of health during pregnancy is achieved by:

- **Routine antenatal examination:** The expectant mother should attend the clinic once a month during the first 7 months, twice a month during the next two months and thereafter once in a week if everything is normal.
- **Prenatal advice**
  - **Diet:** In India, prevalence of malnutrition is seen among pregnant ladies, especially of poor classes. So advices regarding diet are important. Diet should be adequate and balanced. It should provide:

Calories	3,300 kcal
Protein	55 grams
Iron	40 mg
Calcium	1 gram

    Besides vitamins, daily intake of green leafy vegetables, fruits, milk, eggs and meat should be encouraged to meet the dietary needs.
  - Care of nipples
  - Personal hygiene such as personal cleanliness, rest and sleep, bowels, exercise, dental care and restriction of sexual intercourse.
- **Specific health protection:**
  - Correction of anemia
  - Prevention of nutritional deficiencies
  - Protection against tetanus
  - Protection from toxemia of pregnancy
  - Protection from syphilis
- Mental preparation
- Mother craft
- Family Planning

Routine Antenatal Examination

- **Clinical examination:** It includes:
  - Medical history
  - Recording blood pressure
  - Recording weight
  - Physical examination of heart, lungs and other systems
  - Obstetrical examinations - Such as abdominal examination for height of the uterus, fetal movements, etc.
- **Laboratory examinations such as:**
  - Urine
  - Stools
  - Blood examination
  - Blood grouping
  - Test for syphilis (VDRL test) and HIV
- **Maintenance of records:** The antenatal card is prepared during the first examination, which contains Registration number, identifying data, previous history and main health events. This card is kept in the mother and child health care (MCH) center. The antenatal patients should be given full information about the *warning signs of toxemia* of pregnancies, and instructions are given to report any such signals, immediately to the doctor.

Unit XII ❖ Maternal and Newborn Care

Warning signs:
- Swelling on feet
- Fits
- Headache
- Blurring of vision
- Bleeding or discharge per vagina
- Any other unusual symptoms

- **Antepartum hemorrhage:** Bleeding after 28th week of pregnancy or during first or second stages of labor is called antepartum hemorrhage. Main causes are placenta previa and accidental hemorrhages.
  Effects in baby: Intrauterine asphyxia evidenced by fetal distress, malformations of the baby and premature birth.

- **Detection of pelvic deformities:** This may create difficulty to the fetus if not detected early and treated properly.
  Effects in baby are excessive moulding of fetal head during labor, fracture of the fetal skull, hemorrhage and fetal asphyxia.

- Exposure to the radiation is dangerous to the fetus during early pregnancy and during the first four months, X-rays should be avoided as far as possible. Nowadays scanning is preferred in pregnancy.

- **Use of drugs:** The use of certain drugs such as hypnotics may cause malformations to babies. Therefore in the early period of pregnancy, drugs should be minimized and in unavoidable conditions, medical advices should be obtained.

Intranatal Care

Intranatal care is the care given to the mother at the time of delivery. The objective of intranatal care is to ensure that the mother receives the best available care during labor to prevent maternal and child mortality and morbidity.

The principles of good intranatal care are:
- Thorough asepsis
- Safe delivery with minimum injury to the infant and mother
- Readiness to deal with complications such as antepartum and postpartum hemorrhage and asphyxia of the newborn.

Normal Labor

About 95% of the labor cases are normal. On admission to the labor room, the nurse should receive the patient pleasantly with a smiling face, which gives an emotional support to the woman during labor and help to relieve much of her tension and anxiety. After taking her obstetrical history, an abdominal examination is done.

- If the patient is in labor, the preliminary preparation is shaving the vulva followed by a warm enema.
- A warm soap and water enema not only evacuates the bowel, but also stimulates the labor pain.
- After the enema has worked well, the patient is examined in the labor room for the progress of labor pain.
- Vital signs are checked and recorded. Fetal heart sound is counted and recorded. If it is more than 160/minute or less than 100/minute, the matter is brought to the notice of the doctor.
- A sample of urine is tested for albumin and sugar, heart, lungs and other system are examined by the doctor followed by an abdominal palpation to note the presentation, position, lie and attitude of the fetus. If needed, a vaginal examination is performed with strict aseptic precautions.

Stages of Normal Labor

Normal labor is divided into three stages (Fig. 1 and Table 1).

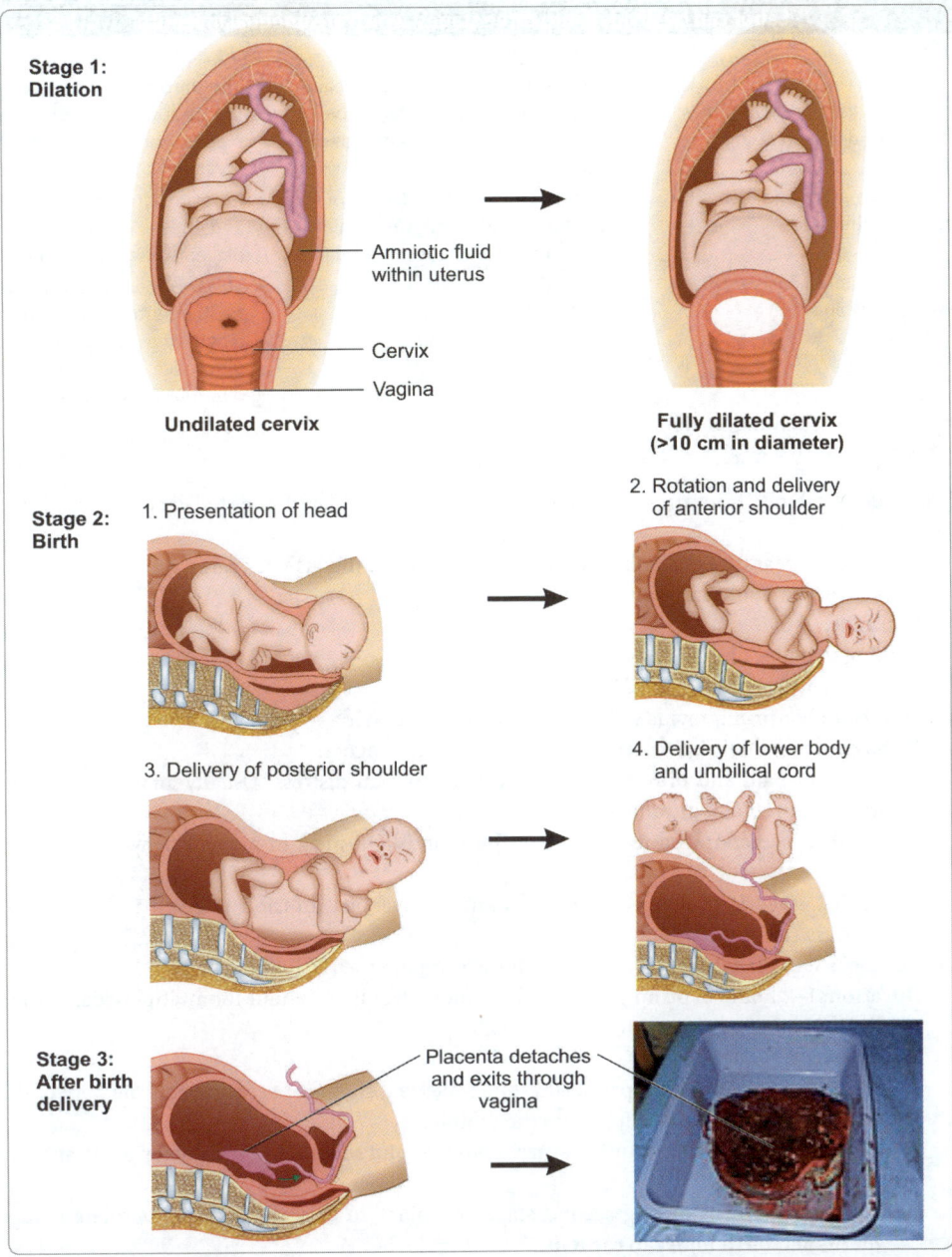

Figure 1: Stages of normal labor

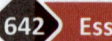

Table 1: **Normal labor and delivery**

Stages of Normal Labor		
Labor can be divided into three stages, which are unequal in length		
First stage	**Second stage**	**Third stage**
• It begins with the onset of true labor contractions and ends when the cervix is fully dilated (10 cm)	• The second stage of labour begins with complete dilatation of the cervix and ends with the birth of the baby	• The third stage is that of separation and expulsion of placenta and membranes and also involves the control of bleeding
• Cervical effacement and dilatation occur in the first stage	• The duration is about 1–1½ hours in primipara and about 30–45 minutes in multiparous women	• It begins after the birth of the baby and ends with the expulsion of the placenta and membrane
• First stage of labor consists of two phases: Latent and active		• This the shortest stage, lasting up to 30 minutes, with an average length of 5–10 minutes. There is no difference in duration for primi and multiparous women
The first stage of labour is the longest for both nulliparous and parous women		

■ **First stage:** It extends from the onset of true labor to the full dilatation of the cervix. Onset is indicated by:

- Show, i.e., appearance of small quantity of blood stained mucus per vagina
- Painful rhythmic uterine contractions
- Backache
- Leaking of liquor amnii
- Dilatation of the cervix
- **Duration:** For primigravida—12–16 hours for multigravida—6–8 hours
- **Management:** Chief aims of management in the first stage is:
  - Relief of pain and prevention of maternal and fetal distress. Usually analgesics like injection pethidine100 mg. intramuscular is ordered.
  - Mother is encouraged to take sweet fluids and light meal to prevent dehydration in the later stages.
  - If first stage is prolonged, glucose saline intravenous infusion is given to prevent maternal distress.

■ **Second stage:** Starts from the full dilatation of the cervix to the birth of the baby.

- **Duration:** 1–2 hours in primi patient and not more than half an hour for multigravida. In the second stage pain is more intense with short intervals.
- **Management:**
  - Mother is more anxious, panic and sometimes cry, shouts or screams. It is the duty of the nurse to give good emotional support to the mother.
  - Fetal heart sounds are counted every 5 minutes and reported to the doctor if any abnormalities are noted.
  - Common hazards during second stage are injury to cervix, vagina or perineum, rupture of uterus and birth injury to the fetus.
  - An episiotomy is performed in primigravida if required, when the head reaches the perineum. When the head is seen at the vulva, i.e. 'crowned', flexion is maintained during each contraction to allow the smallest diameter while the head is extended.

   o If the umbilical cord is encircling the neck, it should be slipped over the head or over the shoulders. If it is too tight, it should be clamped and cut. When the head comes out, nostrils are cleared of mucus and eyes are swabbed and cleaned before opening.

- **Third stage:** Begins with the birth of the baby and ends with expulsion of placenta. Usually half an hour is allowed. Immediately after the birth of the baby 0.25 mg of ergometrine is given intramuscularly and placenta is separated and expelled within few minutes with strong contractions. Symptoms of separation are strong uterine contractions, lengthening of the cord, gushing of fresh blood and the uterus becomes hard and round.
  - **Management:**
    - o Uterus is massaged and pressed downwards and backwards to expel the placenta.
    - o When expelled, membranes are examined to ascertain if expulsion is complete.
    - o Pillow is removed under the head of the patient.
    - o Vulva is washed and swabbed.
    - o Episiotomy incision is sutured, if any, dressing and pad are applied. Patient is dressed and kept comfortable, warm sweet drinks are given.
    - o BP and pulse recorded half hourly for the rest two hours.
  - **Complications in the third stage are:**
    - o Postpartum hemorrhage, shock, retained placenta and asphyxia neonatorum.
    - o The nurse should observe for any unusual symptoms and report immediately to the doctor and should be ready to deal with any of these complications.

Domiciliary Care

Mothers with normal obstetric histories can have their confinement in their own homes under the supervision of a junior public health (JPH) nurse. A single JPH can manage a population of 2500 or 100 deliveries in a year.

Institutional Care or Hospital Delivery

The confinement of the following women should be conducted in hospitals:

- Primi paras or grand multi paras
- Difficult labor cases
- Mothers with history of complications
- Where conditions at home are not suitable for delivery

Postnatal Care (Puerperium)

Puerperium commences after the delivery of the placenta and membranes and lasts up to 6 weeks. It is the post partum period in which the uterus and other generative organs return to normal. The important change is 'involution' of the uterus. Uterus weighs about 1000 grams at the end of labor which reduces in size till it is reached about 2 ounces at the end of the puerperium. The maximum involution occurs during the first week and is completed by the end of 6 weeks. Cervix regains its form by the end of 2 weeks.

Management of Puerperium

The management of puerperium is shortly described here:

- **Daily observations** of the following matters should be done on postpartum patient.
- **Observation of vital signs:** Temperature, pulse and respiration (TPR) and blood pressure (BP) are checked and recorded ½ an hour basis during the first 2 hours and after that twice daily.
- **Fundal height:** The uterus is palpated for assessing the height of fundus. This is measured above the symphysis pubis everyday at a fixed time daily. Ensure that the bladder and bowel are empty while measuring. Clinically, the fundus lies about 5 inches (12.5 cm) above the symphysis pubis after delivery.

Unit XII ❖ Maternal and Newborn Care

During the first 24 hours, there is no descent of the fundus. From the second day onwards up to 11days, the fundus descends by about 1–1.25 cm per 24 hours on an average. If there is no descent of fundus, it should be reported to the medical officer.

- **Lochia:** Lochia is the vaginal discharge that occurs after child birth. It contains blood, mucus, and uterine tissue.

  Lochia progresses through three stages:
  1. **Lochia rubra** (or **cruenta**): This is the first discharge and is red in color because of the large amount of blood. It is composed of blood, shreds of fetal membranes, decidua, vernix caseosa, lanugo and membranes. It typically lasts for 3–5 days after birth.
  2. **Lochia serosa:** In this, the lochia has thinned and turned brownish or pink in color. This is due to the presence of serous exudate, erythrocytes, leukocytes, cervical mucus and microorganisms. This stage continues until around the tenth day after delivery.
  3. **Lochia alba** (or **purulenta**): It is the lochia, which is whitish or yellowish-white. It typically lasts from the second through the third to sixth week after delivery. It is white in color because it contains fewer red blood cells and is mainly made up of leukocytes, epithelial cells, cholesterol, fat, mucus and microorganisms.

- **Perineal care:** Perineum should be washed with warm Dettol lotion after each urination and defecation.
- **Breasts:** Nipples should be cleansed with sterile swab before and after each breastfeeding. Cracked nipples should be observed and treatment given.
- **Bladder:** For the first few days it will be difficult for the mother to pass urine. She should be encouraged to pass urine in every 7–8 hours. In extreme difficulties catheterization is done with the permission of the doctor, under strict aseptic measures. Regular emptying of the bladder will encourage the involution of uterus and full bladder will interfere with the involution.
- **Constipation:** Postnatal mother may suffer from constipation for the first few days due to lax in abdominal muscles. In many hospitals it is a routine care to give an ounce of milk of magnesia on the second night followed by a simple enema on the following morning. It is better to give one ounce of milk of magnesia every night for a few days to ensure daily bowel action.
- **Ambulation:** Ambulation should be initiated as early as possible. In many hospitals, the mother is allowed to take rest on the first day of delivery and from the next day, she is ambulated. Usual practice is to discharge the mother and baby after delivery within 2–3 days if everything goes normal.
- **Blood examination:** If the mother is anemic after delivery, her blood is tested for hemoglobin and treatment is given according to the result.
- **Advice to mother:**
  - **Diet:** Mother should have liberal intake of milk and fluids during the first 24 hours with light meal during meal time. She can eat her normal diet as soon as possible.
  - **Exercise:** Mother should be told about the importance of exercise to tone up the abdominal and pelvic muscles. For mothers who are working, gradual household duties is good enough. For others, exercises involving deep breathing, contracting and relaxing of abdominal and pelvic muscles should be taught.

Family Planning

Advise the mother about family planning. Permanent family planning methods are advised to those who are already having 2 or 3 living children. Tubectomy or intrauterine devices (IUD) should be advised. Tubectomy operation is best done on 4–7 days after delivery.

Postnatal Visits

Mothers are advised to have a follow up visit in the clinic after the first 2 weeks and a final visit at the end of 6 weeks to ensure the involution of uterus is complete. For home delivery, the JPHN should give the nursing care and advices for the first 10 days, which is a time span of secondary infection. Health worker or JPHN should visit the mother and baby twice a day for the first 3 days and once a day till the umbilical cord drops off. At any cost, JPHN or health visitor should be responsible for the mother and baby during first 10 days.

Care of Newborn

RESUSCITATION

The prime importance of respiration is a clear airway to the baby. As soon as head is born, liquor and vaginal materials are wiped off from the mouth and nose of the baby. Soon after birth, the baby must breathe and cry well. In a normal new born, the baby may be held upside down by his/her feet to allow the swallowed secretions to flow out and to clear the airway. Then the mouth and nose are wiped with a piece of sterile gauze wrapped around the little finger of the nurse or doctor. Resuscitation is required, if natural breathing fails to be established.

The steps in resuscitation techniques are:

All labor rooms should be equipped with resuscitation equipment, which consists of a mucus extractor, suction apparatus, a plastic esophageal airway, an infant laryngoscope, an endotracheal tube and oxygen. An infant mask should also be provided:

- Clear the airway with mucus extractor (Figs 2A and B).

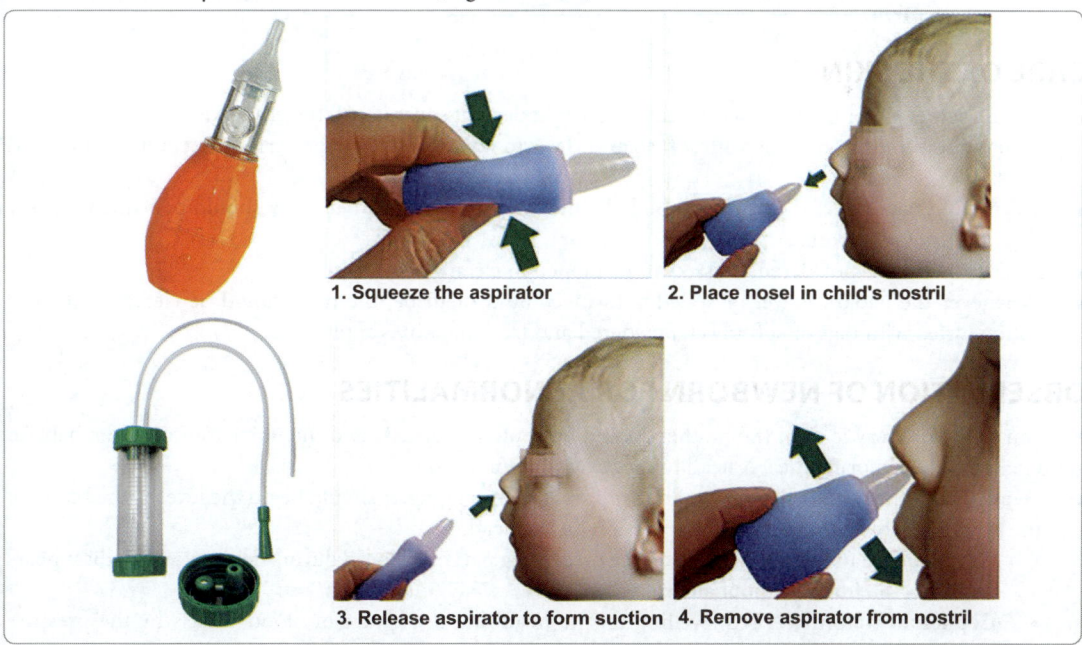

1. Squeeze the aspirator
2. Place nosel in child's nostril
3. Release aspirator to form suction
4. Remove aspirator from nostril

Figures 2A and B: Mucus extractor for newborn babies

- If respiration is not established within 1–1½ minutes, Oxygen is administered by oropharyngeal airway.
- If respiration is not established within 4 minutes, pass an endotracheal tube via a laryngoscope and suck the mucus from the air passages and give intermittent positive pressure ventilations (IPPV) at the rate of about 40 per minute.
- In rural areas, a simple procedure is used as resuscitation. That is, the infant is kept on a cot and the head is kept low by keeping him/her on a pillow. Then blow into the mouth of the baby slowly and gently once in 2–3 seconds. This procedure is followed for 10 minutes or until the baby breathes himself/herself. If spontaneous breathing is delayed, the ideal is to administer oxygen by a competent person.

CARE OF UMBILICAL CORD

- In normal infant, the umbilical cord should be tied and cut when the pulsation on the cord is stopped.
- After the pulsation is stopped, one clamp is applied about 4 inches away from the umbilicus and the second clamp is applied 2 inches away from the first one.
- Then the cord is cut in the middle of the two clamps and separated. Cord ties and instruments should be sterilized properly to prevent tetanus and other infections to the infant.
- The cut end of the cord is tied once again with a sterile tape or thread and treated with Tiruture iodine and wrapped in sterile gauze.
- The cord should be cleaned daily with rectified spirit and dressing is applied till it drops within one week.
- The cord drops off spontaneously within one week leaving a small clean ulcer, which disappears soon.

CARE OF THE EYES

- At birth, the eyes are cleaned with sterile cotton swabs before they are opened.
- Some doctors prefer to drop freshly prepared silver nitrate 1% solution in the eyes to prevent the infection.
- Any unusual discharge from the eyes of an infant in the first few days is pathological and needs immediate medical attention.

CARE OF THE SKIN

- Some doctors prefer not to bath the baby on the first day but cover in soft towel and keep near the mother. Others allow to bath the baby with soft soap and warm water to remove the vernix, meconium and blood clots.
- Warm oil is applied on the head and body before bath. In cold weather, baby should be bathed quickly and not exposed to chill.
- After bath, baby is powdered, dressed and wrapped in clean warm towel.
- Whenever the napkin is wet or soiled with meconium or urine, the part should be cleaned with wet cotton, dried with rags or soft towel, powdered and fresh napkin is applied.

OBSERVATION OF NEWBORN FOR ABNORMALITIES

As soon as the delivery is over, the mother should be kept comfortable and the nurse examines the baby in good light for any abnormalities. A head to foot examination is done.

- **Head:** Check the head, whether fontanels are sunken or bulging. It should be on the level as the bones of the head. Look for any swelling or depression on the head.
  - **Caput succedaneum:** A swelling on the presenting part of the head during delivery, which disappears within 24–48 hours without any treatment.
  - **Cephalohematoma:** A red swelling on the head due to rupture of blood vessels by the pressure during delivery, which gradually disappears within a few weeks or months.

- **Eyes**: Any discharge from the eyes shall be pathological, which needs treatment. Any red spot on the white of the eyes shall be ignored as it will gradually disappear.
- **Mouth**: Examine for hare lip or cleft palate. If any of these is present, feeding should be adjusted. It shall be corrected at about the age of 2 years to the baby.
- **Esophagus** is checked for esophageal atresia. A few drops of sterile water is given to check the swallowing reflex before the baby is put to breast, in suspicious case.
- **Chest:** Heart is examined by the pediatrician for any murmurs.
- **Respiration:** Note the normal breathing rate immediately after birth, which is 40/minute.
- **Spine:** Examine the spine with a finger to exclude spina bifida.
- **Arms and legs:** Baby should be able to move his/her arms and legs. Failure to do this indicates paralysis or dislocation. Look the feet for any talipes.
- **Anus:** If the baby has not passed any meconium already, try to pass a rectal thermometer into the anus to find out any imperforated anus.
- **Penis:** Check the penis when the baby passes urine. Any ballooning of the prepuce is a medical indication.
- **Skin:** Examine the skin for any discoloration like jaundice and for any growths or any abnormalities.
- **Reflexes:** The central nervous system of the infant can be examined by eliciting the following reflexes.
    - **Startle reflex:** When a loud voice is made at the side of the bed or even placing a cold hand on the baby, it responds by suddenly throwing out its arms and then immediately withdrawing. Absence of this reflex shows cerebral damage or depression.
    - **Sucking reflex:** It is checked by placing a teat or mother's nipple by touching at the corner of the baby's mouth when the baby will search for it with its lips.
    - **Grasp reflex:** When the nurse attempts to touch inside the palm of the child, the baby extends his fingers and closes them over the examiner's fingers.

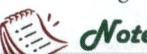 *Note*

Emergencies if Found on Examination

The following abnormalities if found on examination should immediately be reported to the doctor.
- Cyanosis of the skin and lips
- Any difficulty in breathing
- Persistent vomiting
- Imperforated anus
- Signs of cerebral irritation such as twitching, convulsions, rolling of eyes, neck rigidity, bulging of anterior fontanel, instability in temperature, pulse or respiration.

- Details of weight of the baby
    - The birth weight of the baby is noted and recorded immediately after birth.
    - The normal birth weight of an Indian baby is 2.8 kg. (6.16 lbs).
    - Weight less than 2.5 kg is said to be premature baby or 'low birth weight baby'.
    - During first 4–5 days most babies loses weight by about 10%.
    - From 10th day onwards they gain weight at the rate of ½ kg per month in the first 3 months and thereafter 1/ 4 kg per month.
    - At the end of 5 months, the baby doubles its birth weight and at the end of one year baby gains three times of the birth weight.
    - Weight is an index of the growth and development of the baby.
    - After the initial improvement in weight during the first few months, some decline may be seen in the weight chart of some babies due to malnutrition resulting from inadequacy of mother's breast milk or infant feeding. Therefore, weighing the baby at regular intervals and recording on the weight chart is an important health measure to the babies for early detection and prevention of growth failure like kwashiorkor and marasmus.

Unit XII ❖ Maternal and Newborn Care

BABY BATH

Objectives

- To keep the baby's skin clean
- To refresh the baby
- To stimulate circulation
- To prevent any skin infection

Types of Bath

- **Lap bath:** Bathing the baby by keeping him/her on the lap. Here, the mother sits on a stool. She can sponge and change his/her dress on her lap itself. So, therefore, there is no need of having additional table.
- **Sponge bath:** Bathing the child in bed
- **Oil bath:** Oil is applied all over the baby's body. After finishing, wipe off any oil that remains, with fresh pieces of rags or cotton and dress the baby.
- **Tub bath:** This is the common method of giving bath to a baby. Here, we use small tub or basin.

Routine Time for Bath

Ideal time for bathing baby is before the second feeding but make sure that the baby is not tired or hungry.

- Baby should not be bathed within an hour after he/she is fed because moving may cause him/her vomit and also soon after feeding most of the babies may go to sleep.
- There should be a fixed time for the bath, which will help the baby to form a habit on an orderly schedule.

Preliminary Assessment of the Child and Situation

- Identify the child and check the Doctor's order for any specific instructions about bathing the baby.
- Get further instructions from the ward sister.
- Assess the general condition of the baby and his need for bathing.
- Find out from the mother whether the child had his feeding within the previous one hour.
- Decide the type of bath to be given and find out the proper place for the same.
- Check the articles available in the unit.
- Collect the individual soap powder and dress, etc. from the mother itself if possible.

Requisites

A tray containing:

Articles	Purpose
• Screen—1	• To provide privacy and to prevent drought
• Buckets—2	• One to collect dirty water and the other for disposing soiled linen
• Jugs—2	• One for cold water and the other for hot water
• Basin—1	• To bath the baby
• Big towel—1	• To wrap the baby
• Soap in a soap dish	• To clean the baby
• Kidney tray or paper bag—1	• To receive the waste
• Bath blanket—1	• To keep the baby warm
• Small towel—1	• To keep the baby

Contd...

Articles	Purpose
• Oil in a bottle	• To apply on the body
• Small pieces of rag in a container	• To clean the baby
• Cotton balls in a container	• To wipe the cord stump, if any
• Spirit and cord powder	• To dress the cord stump, if any
• Swab sticks or cotton cones in a container	• To clean the nose and ears
• Mackintosh	• To prevent soiling of linen and clothes
• Cotton apron for the nurse	• To protect the dress of the nurse
• **Dress for baby:** Baby frock and napkin	• To dress the baby

Procedure

Steps	Procedure	Rationale
1.	Explain the procedure to the mother	Reduces anxiety of the mother and wins her co-operation
2.	Close doors and windows. The room should be warm	Keeps off draught and provides privacy
3.	Collect all the articles in readiness before beginning the procedure **Arrangement of equipment on the table:**	Organizations facilitates skill performance
4.	Keep the table against the wall, place the tub or basin on one end of the table and the toilet tray and clothing on other end conveniently so that the baby will be protected on 3 sides and there is less chance for the baby rolling off the table. If it is in a corner of the room two sides of the table are protected with walls. Place the mackintosh and towel over the table	Protects the baby from falling
5.	Wash hands and wear gloves and apron	Prevents transfer of microorganisms
6.	See whether the baby is wet with urine or motion, If so, clean the part	Prevents contamination

Contd...

Unit XII ❖ Maternal and Newborn Care

Steps	Procedure	Rationale
7.	Undress the baby and smear oil on the head and body as required 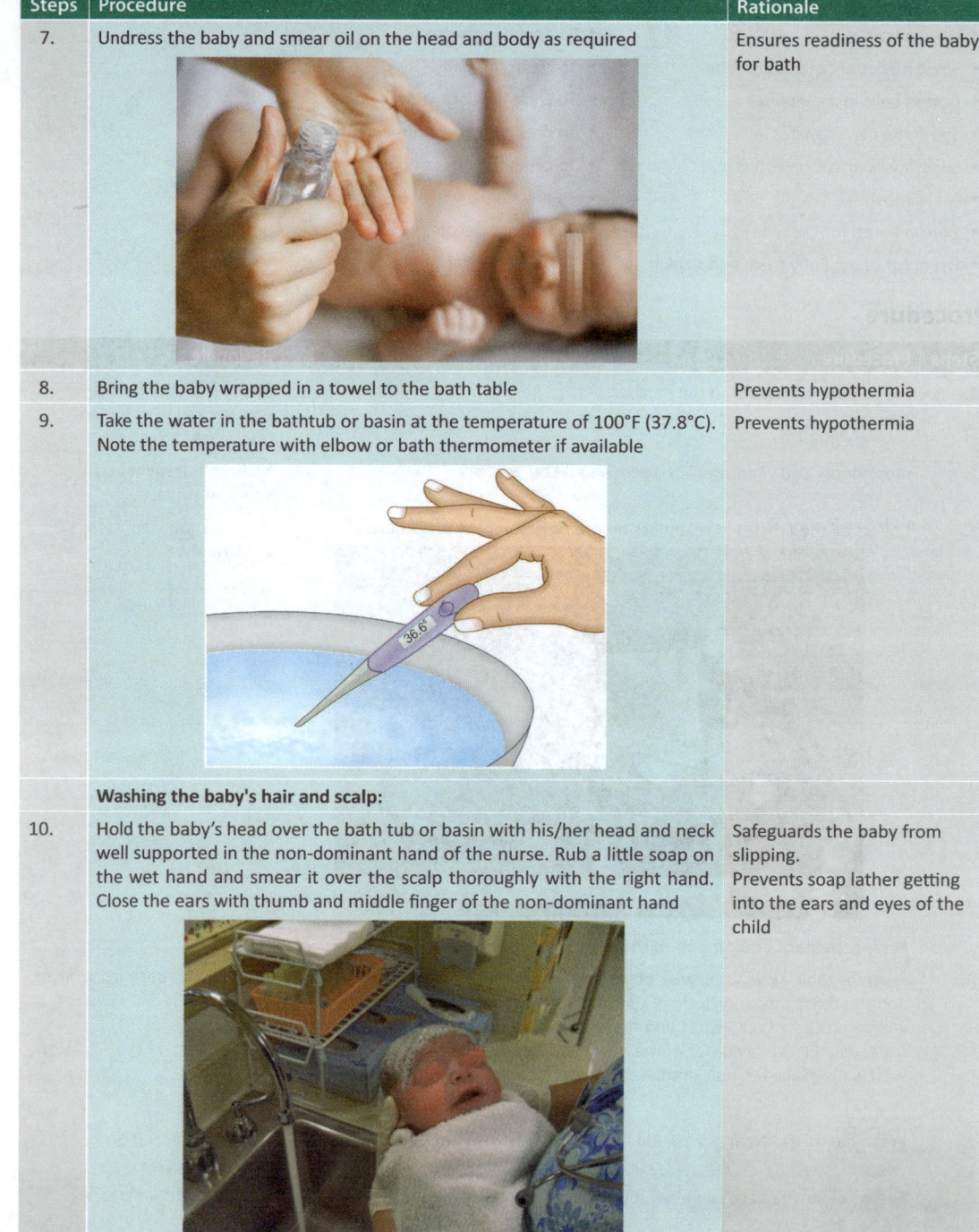	Ensures readiness of the baby for bath
8.	Bring the baby wrapped in a towel to the bath table	Prevents hypothermia
9.	Take the water in the bathtub or basin at the temperature of 100°F (37.8°C). Note the temperature with elbow or bath thermometer if available	Prevents hypothermia
	Washing the baby's hair and scalp:	
10.	Hold the baby's head over the bath tub or basin with his/her head and neck well supported in the non-dominant hand of the nurse. Rub a little soap on the wet hand and smear it over the scalp thoroughly with the right hand. Close the ears with thumb and middle finger of the non-dominant hand	Safeguards the baby from slipping. Prevents soap lather getting into the ears and eyes of the child

Contd...

Steps	Procedure	Rationale
11.	Rinse the head with water. Dry his/her head gently with a soft towel	Prevents hypothermia
12.	Discard the water in the bucket or in the wash basin. Exchange the warm water	Replacing dirty water protects the baby from dirt and infection
	Cleaning the face:	
13.	See that the eyes, nostrils, ears and mouth are clean. Wipe the eyes from inner canthus to outer canthus using a cotton swab. Wipe the face, dry gently. Do not use soap on the face. Attend the parts if necessitated	Cleans from less contaminated to more contaminated area

Contd...

Steps	Procedure	Rationale
	Cleaning the body	
14.	Unwrap the body. Hold the baby so that his head is supported on the wrist and fingers of the hand and hold him securely in armpit. Dip the body in water in the basin. Be careful that the head of the baby in the hands of the nurse is above the water. Soap the body. Special attention is to be given to the creases in his/her neck, arms and axilla	Prevents slipping of the baby
15.	Rinse the baby carefully. Fresh water should be used for this. Be careful not to leave any soap anywhere on the skin, especially in the creases and folds. If the baby is a girl, separate the labia and clean. When the bath is finished take him from basin and keep on the bath towel spread on the table. Dry the baby thoroughly by patting and not rubbing	Soap left behind might cause irritation to the baby's skin
	Cleaning the baby's nose:	
16.	Arrange the soft face towel under the baby's chin. Steady the baby's head with the left hand to prevent moving about. Take a cotton cone and then introduce just inside the nostril and turn it gently. If mucus has collected, the baby may sneeze. Then remove the mucus with a clean swab stick. Do not use same swab stick for both nostrils. Discard the soiled swab each time to prevent infection from one to the other	Sneezing brings out the mucus and any dry particles outside

Contd...

Steps	Procedure	Rationale
	Cleaning the baby's ears:	
17.	Steady the baby's head in the same manner as when nose is cleaned. Take the swab stick, clean the creases of the outer ear and behind the ear where the skin surfaces are tough. A clean swab is used for each ear	Prevents the possibility of water entry during washing into the baby's ears
	Care of the umbilical cord:	
18.	Clean the cord stump, if any, using cotton balls	Prevents umbilical cord infection
19.	Dress him/her (first napkin and then dress). Better to use loose back open frock. Feeding is given after bath. Then take the baby to the cradle and leave him comfortable	Promotes comfort
20.	Wash and replace the articles in the proper place. Remove PPE and wash hands	Prevents transfer of microorganisms
21.	Record the procedure in the nurse's record with date, time and signature of the nurse	Documentation fosters quality care

Contd...

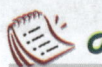

Note

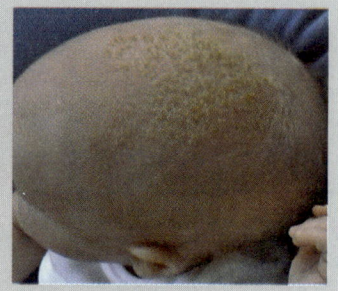

- Careful soaping and rinsing of the scalp is necessary to prevent a condition called 'cripcap' or cradle cap'. (It is a greasy looking crust which sometimes appears on the baby's head. If it is present, rub with oil each night to remove the crust and wash his head thoroughly in the morning.)
- A baby's mouth need not be cleaned. The saliva always being produced in the mouth keeps it clean. If there is mucus, clean it with a fine rag piece moistened with water. At times during the bath, the baby usually cries. This is an opportunity to observe the condition of the mouth. If any white spots or red areas are noticed on the lips, gums, edges of the tongue or inside the cheeks, the condition may be called thrush and should be reported at once to the sister in charge of the ward.

BREASTFEEDING

Breast milk is the best food for the baby. It not only gives nourishment but also satisfies the baby's emotional needs. The newborn baby should be put to breast as soon as the mother is fit to receive him/her, usually 6–8 hours after birth or even before this time. The present trend is to start the breast feed to the baby as early as possible after birth.

Advantages of Breastfeeding

- Breastfeeding develops bonding and makes the mother feel close to the baby (sense of satisfaction)
- Gives the baby a sense of security or feeling of oneness with the mother.
- Saves the mother's time in preparing a formula
- It is economic.
- Protects the child from communicable diseases because the breast milk is sterile and it contains protective antibodies.
- The mother's nipples satisfy the sucking reflex more adequately than the artificial nipple and the infant is less likely to be a thumb sucker
- Breastfeeding aids involution of uterus
- Breast milk is of correct temperature suitable for the baby.
- Breast fed baby is said to have better tissue and bone development and resistances to infection.

Points to Remember in Breastfeeding

Mother should take bath daily and wear clean clothes.

- Cleaning of breast should be done before and after feeding (clean the breast from the nipple towards the periphery). Hands of the mother should be washed before each feed and nails must be cut short.
- The mother and baby should be in a comfortable position, mother sitting and leaning slightly forward. Support the breast in the palm of the hands, allowing the nipples into the baby's mouth and she must keep the breast away from the baby's nose.
- Maximum time for feeding the baby is 20 minutes. Both breasts must be given for each feed (10 minutes on each breast)
- Air is swallowed while sucking. To release the air from the stomach, the child is put over the mother's shoulders and gently patted over the back, which helps to produce eructation—that is burping.
- Baby should be dressed in clean clothes before feeding.

Contraindications to Breastfeeding

Conditions Relating to the Mother

- Diseases of the breast, e.g., breast abscess, mastitis, cracked nipples.
- Active tuberculosis, cancer, cardiac diseases, advanced nephritis, acute contagious diseases.
- When the mother is unconscious and suffering from mental diseases.
- When another pregnancy ensues.

Conditions Relating to the Baby

- If the baby is premature, removal from the warm crib or incubator may chill the baby and he will be more exposed to infection.
- Babies with harelip and cleft palate.

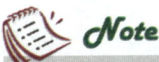 **Note**

How to find out the Quantity of Breast Milk Taken by a Baby
Weigh the baby before and after breast feeding. The difference in weight gives the amount of milk taken. This is called test feed.

WEANING

Switching an infant from breastfeeding to normal feeding is called weaning. When baby is 5–6 months old, the mother tries to stop breastfeeding by introducing other foods. Breast feeds should not be stopped all sudden. Weaning can start from the age of 5th or 6th months. The process should be gradual. Child can be completely weaned by the end of 9th or 10th month. The feed can be replaced by cow's milk and some solid foods.

Artificial Feeding of Infants

It is the feeding of an infant with other foods in the absence of breast milk. The milk of each species seems especially adopted by nature to the needs of the young ones of the same species. Since it is not always possible to provide human milk for the human infant, milk of another species of animal may be used. Earlier cow's milk was considered as best substitute for human breast milk. But there are observations that as cow's milk contains high concentration of proteins and minerals, it can harm baby's kidneys. Moreover, cow's milk does not have right amount of iron, vitamin C and other nutrients for infants (Table 2).

Table 2: Difference between human milk and cow's milk

	Carbohydrate	Fat	Protein
Human milk	7%	3.5%	1.5%
Cow's milk	4%	4%	4%

Cow's milk can be humanized by diluting, boiling, and adding sugar, e.g., for a feeding of 150 mL: take 105 mL of milk, add 45 mL of water and 4 grams (one teaspoon) of sugar. As the infant grows, the strength of the mixture should be increased. By 6–8 month, he may have undiluted milk. Cow's milk may be diluted according to the age and weight of the baby.

Cow's milk can be substituted by evaporated milk, dried milk or other milk formula.

Unit XII ❖ Maternal and Newborn Care

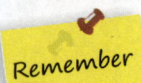

Important points to remember when artificial feeds are given to babies:
- Calculate the formula according to the nutritional needs of the baby as per the age and weight.
- All the articles needed for the actual feeding should be sterilized properly.
- Milk to be given should be warm. Temperature is tested by dropping a little milk on the inner aspect of the arm of the nurse.
- Mother and baby should be seated comfortably and the teat is always filled with milk by keeping the bottle at 45° slanting position when it is in the mouth of the baby to prevent the entrance of air in the mouth.
- The hole on the teat should be of a moderate size prepared with red hot needle so that a slow and steady flow of milk is ensured to the mouth of the baby.
- 'Break the wind' (burp) from the stomach of the baby in between feeds and at the end of feeds.
- Mother should not show any tension or hurry to feed.
- Feed should be given at regular intervals.
- Change the napkin if soiled, before feed and dress the baby with fresh dresses.
- The mother should wash her hands well before preparing the feed and before feeding the baby.
- Give a small quantity of sterile water at the end of each feeding.
- Never press the nose of the baby to make him/her to open the mouth but press on his cheeks, in case it is needed.

Different Ways of Feeding Infants

- By feeding bottle and teat
- By dropper
- By using a spoon
- By using a tube (nasal feed)
- By Belcroy feeder

Feeding the Baby with a Feeding Bottle

Preliminary Assessment of the Baby and Environment

- Check the doctor's order for the specification of feed and type of feeding.
- Note the weight and general condition of the baby and prepare the formula.
- Find out the nutritional need of the baby and the time of last feeding.
- Note the digestibility of the baby by noting the amount and times of passing urine and meconium, the size of abdomen and the ability of sucking.
- Get the instructions from the ward sister about feeding as well as the preparation of formula.
- Find out the articles available in the ward.

Requisites

A tray containing:
- Feeding bottle and teat in a sterile container
- Required amount of feed in a mug kept in bowl of warm water
- A bottle with sterile water
- A piece of flannel to cover the feeding bottle
- A towel
- Another tray containing baby's frock, baby sheet, napkin and bib, mackintosh and towel, gown and mask

Procedure

1. Assemble the equipment at the bedside.
2. Wash the hands and use gown and mask if available (if the baby is premature)

3. Then pour milk into the bottle. Fix the nipple carefully so that it will not get contaminated. Wipe the outside and cover it with a flannel or lint or old clean cloth. Temperature of the feed should be 100°F.
4. Change the frock and napkin if wet and wash the hands.
5. Protect the lap with mackintosh and towel and protect the neck of the baby with bib.
6. Test the temperature once again by pouring a few drops over the wrist of the nurse.
7. Hold the baby in a position similar to that of breast feeding. Hold the bottle in an angle of 45° and bring the nipple to the lips and then to the mouth of the baby. When holding the bottle, it should be tilted so that the milk is against the neck of the bottle during the feeding time. Otherwise baby may suck in air.
8. Feed should last for 10–20 minutes and see that the bottle is not empty. Break the wind in between the feed.
9. When finished, give little sterile water to clean the mouth of the baby. Keep the baby on mother's shoulder and pat over the back, to expel the air from the stomach which is called burping.
10. Remove the mackintosh and towel. Lay the baby in the cradle on the right side, after removing the bib.
11. Wash the bottle and nipple with cold running water. Then wash with hot soap solution and boil it. While boiling, add some salt which will give a smooth surface to the nipple.
12. Record the details of feeding in the nurse's record with signature.

Precautions

- Absolute cleanliness should be observed in preparing the feed and feeding the baby.
- The feed should be at correct temperature.
- If the child is sleeping wait till he/she wakes up.
- Hold the bottle while feeding, in such a way that the nipple gets filled with milk.
- Never introduce an empty nipple into the mouth of the baby.
- After feeding the baby, expel air by patting the baby over the back.
- Never hold baby's nose to make him/her open the mouth, but press on his/her cheeks to open the mouth.

If we prepare the feed for a single baby, it is better to prepare the milk formula for the whole day and keep it in separate bottles in refrigerator. If it is not possible, keep some milk and then the required amount of boiled water. Add sugar and warm the mixture again according to the need.

After Care of Infant and Articles used for Feeding

- Keep the baby to the shoulder of the mother and pat over his back for burping.
- After the air has been expelled through the mouth, take him to the lap of the mother, wipe his face, remove the bib, put his dresses properly, cover him with a towel as if the mother holding him in her hands near to her chest and keep him in the cradle moving as little as possible, because vigorous movements may cause vomiting.
- Record the feeding with time, date and amount given.
- Take the articles to the utility room. Empty the feeding bottle, wash it with cold water and then with warm soap water using soft brush.
  - Clean the bottle and teat thoroughly under running water.
  - Place the bottle in cold water and heat it to the boiling point. Better to wrap the bottle in a small towel before putting for boiling.
  - Put the teat in the boiling water for few minutes.
  - After boiling, take it out, allow it to dry and keep in the proper container, ready for the next use
  - Clean all the other used articles and replace them in the proper places.
- Wash the hands.
- Observe the baby whether he/she is comfortably lying, sleeping or had any nausea or vomiting and care him/her accordingly.

Unit XII ❖ Maternal and Newborn Care

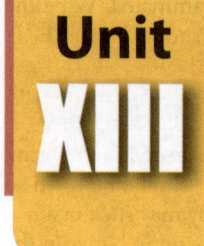
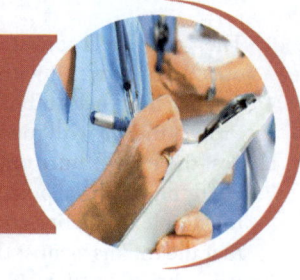
LET'S DISCUSS SOME COMMONLY USED OPERATION THEATER INSTRUMENTS

Cheatle Forceps or Handling Forceps or Transfer Forceps or Crocodile Forceps

Specifications

- It is a large heavy metal forceps with remarkably curved blades (Fig. 1).
- Inside the blades there are large serrations which help to get firm grip while taking instruments, vessels or linen.
- There is no lock.

Uses

- It can be used to select and pick up sterilized articles, like drapes, instruments and vessels or even bottles from sterilized drums or autoclave.
- As it is heavy, long and well serrated, sterile articles can be safely transferred from one tray to another.
- Usually it is dipped in an antiseptic solution like Dettol lotion or carbolic lotion for ready use. It is also called transfer forceps.

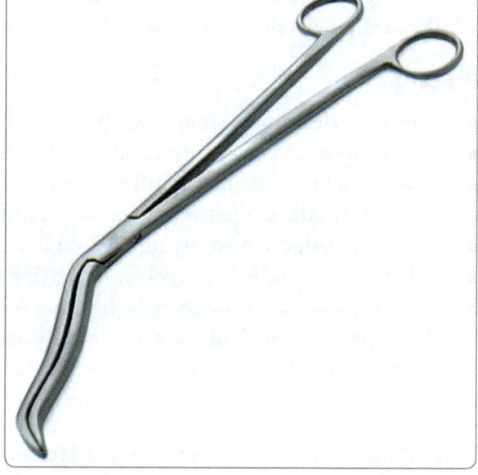

Figure 1: Cheatle's forceps

Rampley Sponge Holding Forceps (Fig. 2)

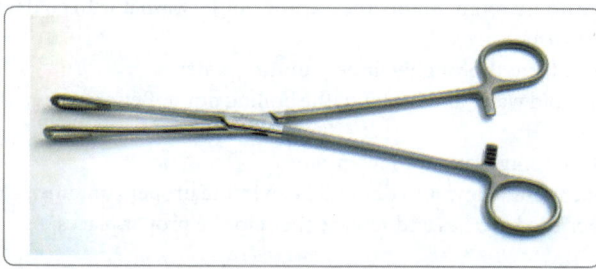

Figure 2: Rampley sponge holding forceps

Specifications

- It is a heavy metal instrument 23–75 cm in length.
- Shafts are thin, blades are fenestrated at its distal end.
- The inner aspects of the blades are serrated.
- It has a catch lock which gives firmness while holding anything.

Uses

- Very common use is for cleaning the operative field.
- For swabbing or packing body cavities, like vagina.
- It can be used to catch soft organs of the body, like ovary, soft cervix in pregnancy, etc.
- Used for blunt dissection in deeper area.
- Substituted in the place of ovum forceps.
- Used for deep mopping to clear the area during manipulating works on organs.

Towel Clips

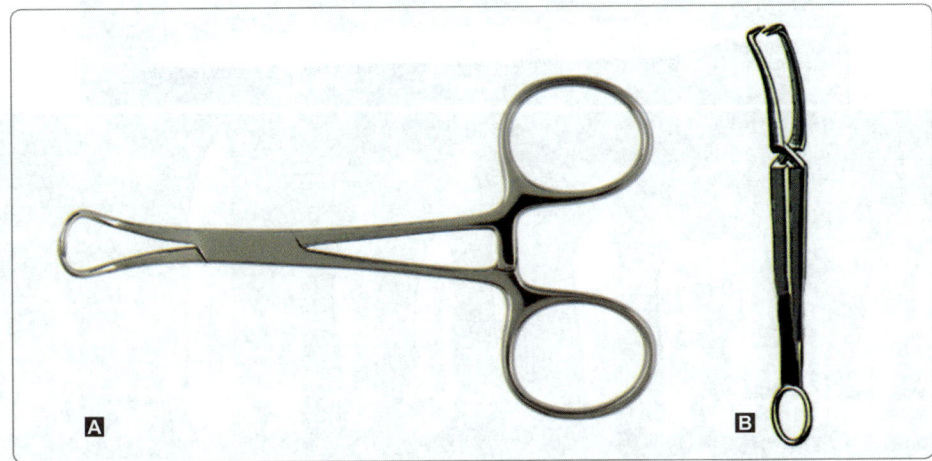

Figures 3A and B: (A) Mayo's towel clip; (B) Doyen's towel clip

The common types are:
- Mayo's towel clip (Fig. 3A).
- Doyen's towel clip (Fig. 3B).

Specifications

- It is a metal instrument, light but strong, in different length.
- It has a catch lock nearby the proximal end to fix the grip of drapes.
- The distal ends are curved to two sharp points as teeth, to catch the drapes firmly with the pointed tips.
- Shafts are short and its handles are curved.

Uses

- To fix the drapes in any manner to expose only the required area.
- To fix the tubings (like suction tubes) to the drapes preventing displacement.

Unit XIII ❖ Common Operation Theater Instruments

- To hold or elevate the ribs in chest injuries.
- Can be used as tongue holding forceps, but the disadvantage is that it perforates the tongue.
- It may be used to hold and retract the cord during hernia repairing operation.
  (There are other types of towel clips also in use).

Bard Parker Knife Handle and Blades (BP Handle) (Figs 4A to C)

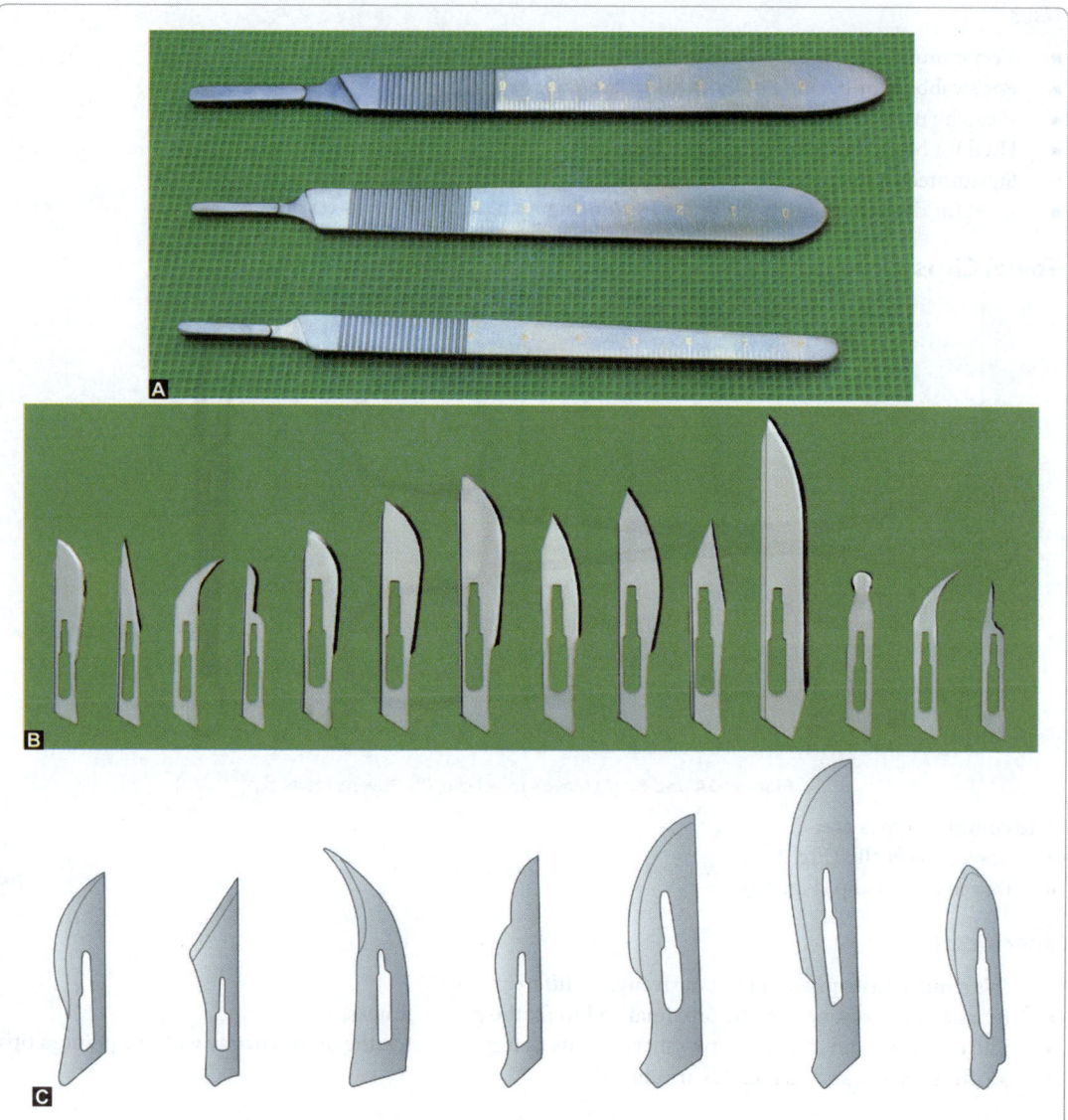

Figures 4A to C: (A and B) Bard Parker knife handles; (C) Blades of the different types of the BP handles

Specification

- It is a metal instrument used to attach different types of blades at the distal end.
- Handles are of different sizes. Blades can be attached according to the size of the handles. Blades are selected according to the use.
- Shaft is flat with 1 cm breadth at the middle.
- The distal end is narrow enough to fix the blades with an adjustment to fit on the handle.
- The proximal flat end is round.
- Different sizes of handles are required to fix different sizes of blades according to their uses.
  There are scalpel handle combined with blades and scalpel handle with detachable blades.

Uses

- Scalpel BP handle with blades are the most important instrument in surgery.
- Some BP handle can be used for opening the skin and to cut the fascia or to open the peritoneum by changing the blades then and there.
- The round proximal end of the BP handle may be used to dissect the muscles on the abdomen after cutting the fascia over it.
- Handling the BP handle and blades may be in the 'dinner knife' position, 'writing position' or in 'Fiddle bow position' while putting the incision.

Scissors

Scissors are of different sizes and designs for the particular uses (Figs 5A to E).
A. Straight scissors (Mayo's) may be blunt or sharp
B. Curved on angle (episiotomy scissors)
C. Curved on flat scissors (Mayo's)
D. Suture cutting scissors—may be curved or angled or straight fine pointed tips
E. Bandage scissors, dressing tissue forceps and curved mayo scissors

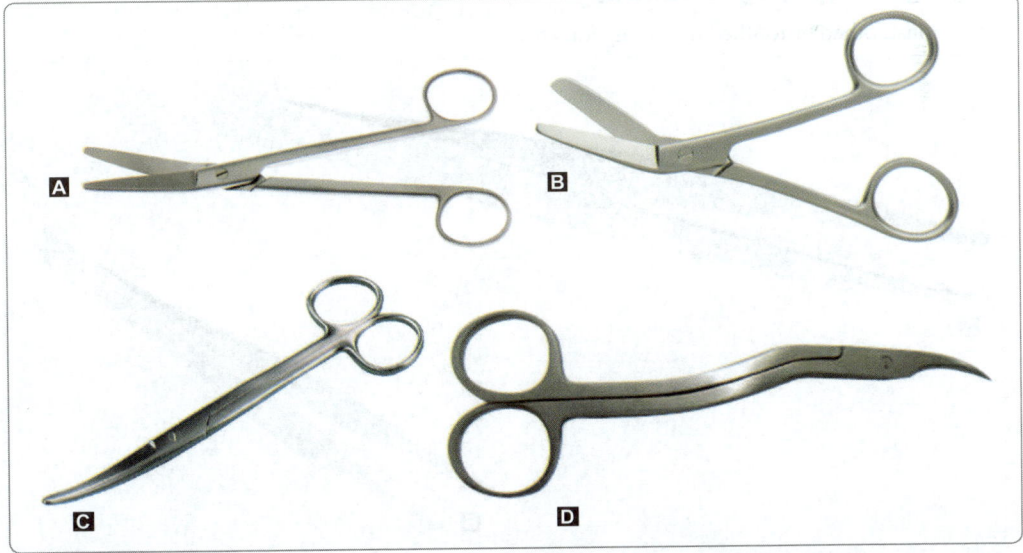

Figures 5A to D:

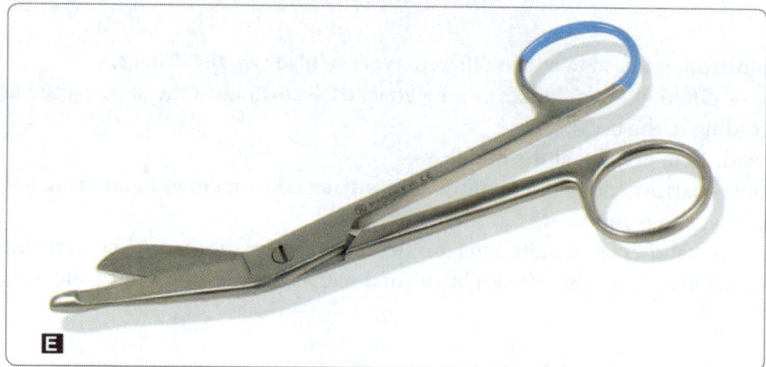

Figures 5A to E: (A) Straight Mayo scissors; (B) Curved Mayo scissors;
(C) Episiotomy scissors; (D) Suture cutting scissors; (E) Bandage cutting scissors

Uses

- Scissors can be used for blunt or sharp dissection.
- It is used for cutting the tissues in various structures.
- Helps in cutting the ligatures and sutures.
- Gauze or bandage scissors are used only for cutting the gauze or bandages in required size and length.
- Straight or pointed curved scissors are used for removing the sutures of the incisions.
- Curved on flat scissors are used to cut the ligatures or other suture material during operation by the assistant surgeon or scrubbed nurse.
- Straight or curved Mayo scissors which are very smooth at the ends are used to cut the tissues and internal organs so that adjacent tissues are protected while using.

Dissecting Forceps (Figs 6A and B)

It may be non-toothed or toothed dissecting forceps.

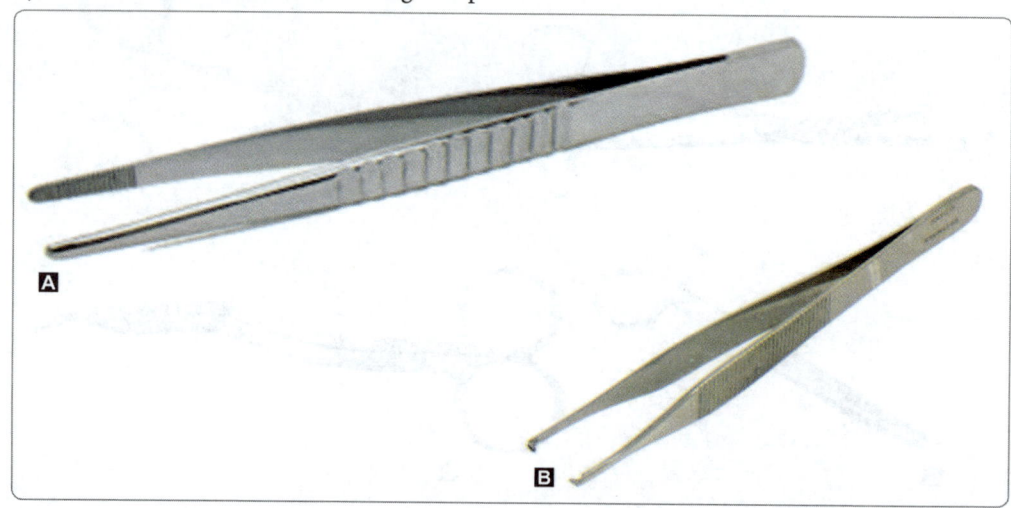

Figures 6A and B: Dissecting forceps: (A) Non-toothed; (B) Toothed

Specifications

■ Dissecting forceps has two equal flat wings joining by a sharp curve at the middle which is the proximal end.
■ On pressing their shafts or limbs the pointed tips are well opposed so that they do not slip against each other.
■ The outer surfaces of the shaft are made rough and irregular to get the firm grip while holding in hands.
■ Toothed dissecting forceps has tooth in the inner surface of the distal end.
■ There is a special type of Russian forceps; fenestrated clubbed tip with a serrated inner surface to have firm hold over the soft tissues preventing damage.

Uses

■ Plain dissecting forceps is used to hold the delicate structure, like intestine, skin over the face and cartilages for stitching purposes.
■ It is used in dissecting soft friable structures
■ Toothed dissecting forceps is used to hold the tough structures, like skin, fascia, rectal sheath, etc. while suturing.
■ To lift the knots of sutures put on the incision while removing the same after wound healing.
■ Russian forceps is used to hold the skin for suturing or to hold the soft tissues preventing the damage to the organs.

Hemostats (Artery Forceps) (Figs 7A to C)

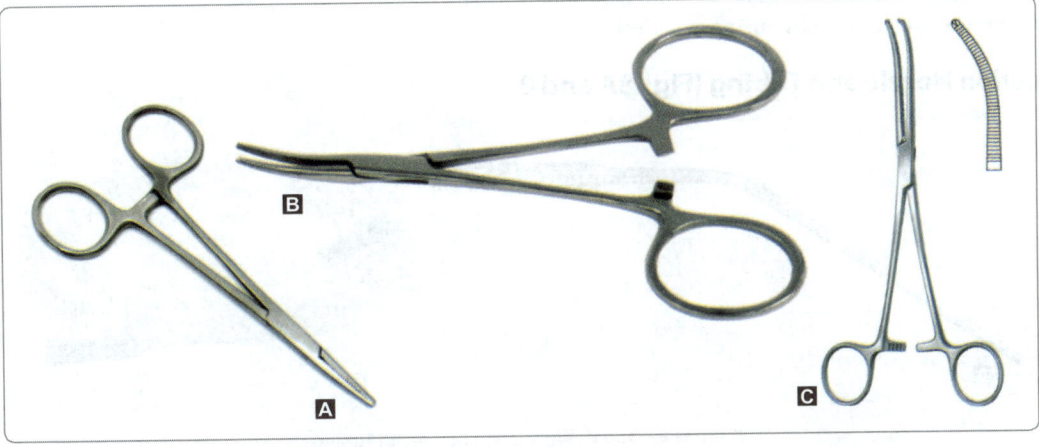

Figures 7A to C: Hemostat: (A) Straight artery forceps; (B) Curved artery forceps; (C) Kocher's forceps

Artery Forceps

■ Small often called mosquito forceps (straight or curved)
■ Medium
■ Large or pedicular
■ When it is single toothed at distal end it is called Kocher's artery forceps or lane's artery forceps
■ Non-toothed type may be Spencer Well's or Halstead's artery forceps

Unit XIII ❖ Common Operation Theater Instruments

Specifications

- It is a straight or curved strong metal instrument.
- Blades are tapering to the distal end but blunt.
- It has a catch lock to bring the blades together and lock it.
- The inner surface of the blades are serrated.
- Locking the blades are well in a position.

Uses

- It stops the bleeding by holding the vessel.
- It is used as a clamp for the pedicles of internal organs, like kidney, spleen, ligaments of uterus, etc.
- It is used to hold the appendix and crush the base of the appendix.
- It is used as a substitute in the absence of sinus forceps to enlarge the opening of an abscess.
- It is used to introduce small plug or drain in a small cavity.
- It is used as a substitute in the place of a needle holder.
- It is used to hold the incised edges of skin, fascia, etc. but rarely used due to crushing of tissues.
- It is used to hold the free end of sutures at the beginning of sutures and hold the cut ends of tension sutures before tying.
- It is used to hold the tape in the abdominal pads or sponges during operations to prevent missing it in the cavity.
- It is used to hold the free end of thread or catgut during anastomosis of intestines.
- Mosquito forceps are used to hold the small bleeding points
- It is used for blunt dissection by holding peanut or swabs.
- It is used to hold swabs during mouth cleaning.

Suction Nozzle and Tubing (Figs 8A and B)

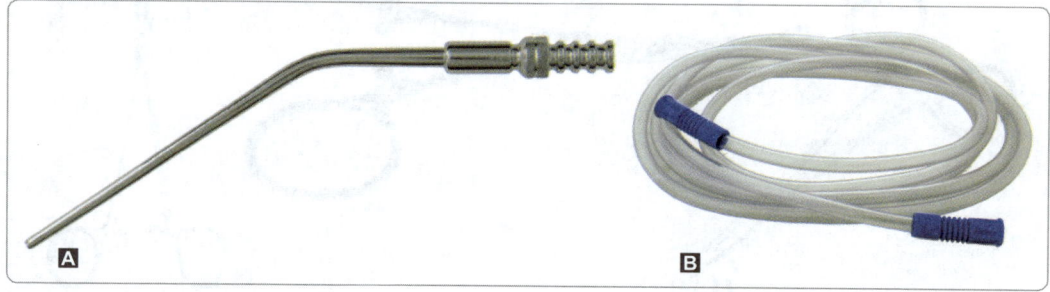

Figures 8A and B: (A) Suction nozzle; (B) Tubings

Specifications

- Suction nozzle is a metal instrument attached to the distal end of the rubber tubing.
- The proximal end of the rubber tubing is attached to the suction bottle or the reservoir. Usually the suction apparatus is foot operated.
- The distal end of the suction nozzle is protected with perforated tips to prevent the sucking of tissues during functioning or at least a small rubber tube is fitted at the tip.

Uses

- It is used to suck off the blood or fluids from the cavities, like mouth, abdomen or fluids from a large ovarian cyst, etc. during operations so that the field of operation is cleared.
- Being made up of metal and rubber, it can be sterilized along with other instruments to be reused in the sterile field. While a vacuum is produced in the suction bottle, the fluid or blood is sucked through the nozzle to the rubber tube and collected in the bottle.

Lister's Sinus Forceps (Fig. 9)

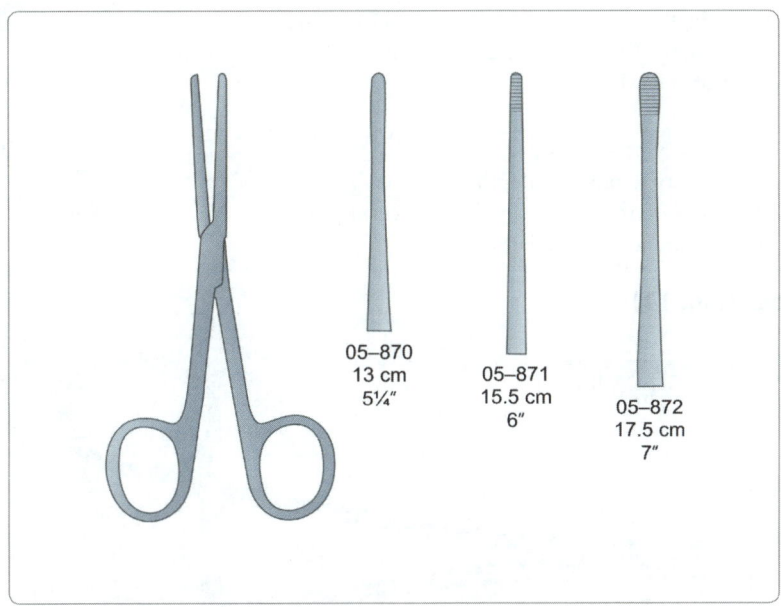

05–870
13 cm
5¼"

05–871
15.5 cm
6"

05–872
17.5 cm
7"

Figure 9: Lister's sinus forceps

Specifications

- It is a metal instrument with about 24 cm long.
- It has two blades, shaft and handles.
- The distal tip is round, blunt and smooth with serrations inside the tip. There is no lock for the grip.

Uses

- Used to enlarge the opening in incising an abscess.
- To introduce rubber drainages or gauze plugs freely in any cavity, like ears, nose and cavity of abscess. As there is no lock, the material can be introduced in the cavity without strain and pain to the patient.

Unit XIII ❖ Common Operation Theater Instruments

Probe

Specifications

- It is a very thin and long metal instrument about 4 cm or more in length (Fig. 10).
- The distal end is round and smooth to introduce in any cavity smoothly. Usually there is an eye in the proximal end through which a long thread can be introduced, which helps to find out the probe when put in deep cavity. If the probe is fully immersed to the depth of a cavity there is chance for missing it inside. In that case the thread will be seen outside so that the metal probe is located easily.

Uses

- To introduce in a cavity to note the depth
- To identify the hole of the cervix in pinhole cervix before introducing the uterine sound or dilator.

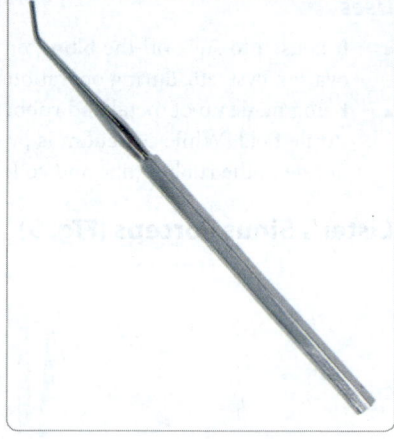

Figure 10: Probe

Needle Holder (Fig. 11)

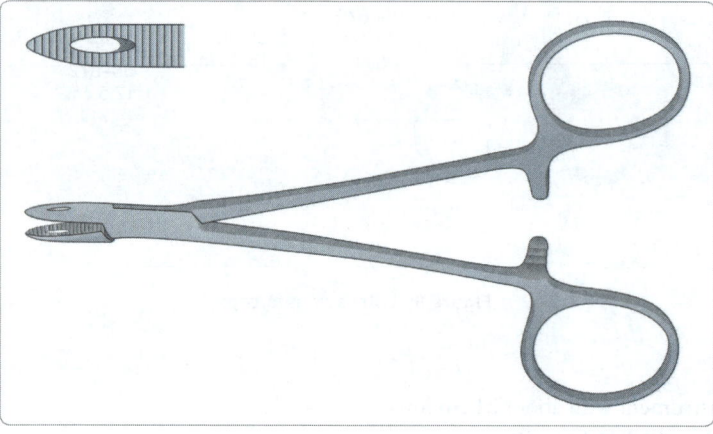

Figure 11: Needle holder

Specifications

- It has got long handles and small blades that resemble artery forceps.
- The blades have very good cross serrations.
- It has a groove for catching the needle on its inner surface.
- It may be straight or curved.

Uses

- To hold the needle for suturing.
- Straight type is used for holding needles while suturing flat surface; curved type is used to work at depth or inside the cavity.

Suture Needles (Figs 12A to D)

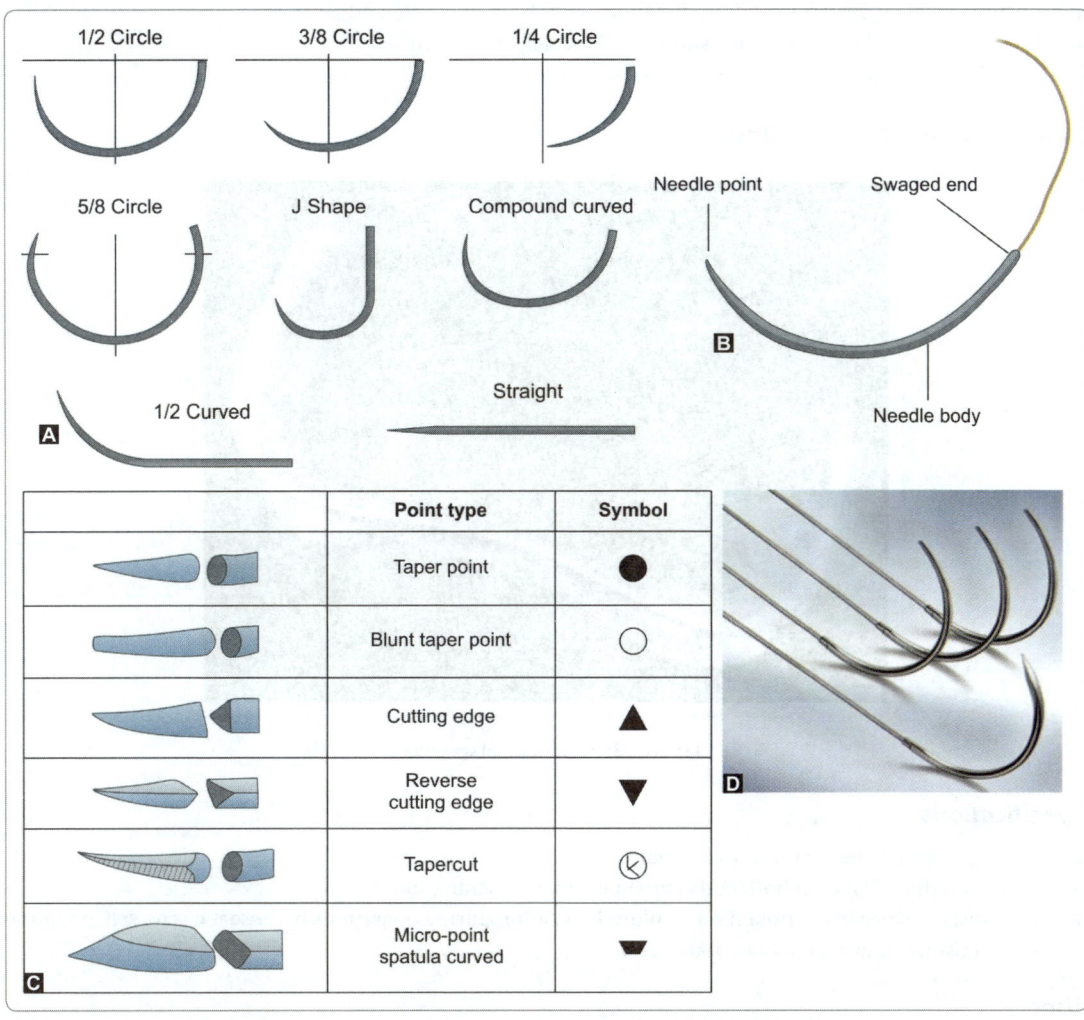

Figures 12A to D: Needles: (A) Curved round bodied; (B) Curved cutting; (C) Straight cutting needle; (D) Atraumatic needle

Specifications

- Suture needles may be specified
  - On the basis of its edge
  - On the basis of its curvature
  - On the basis of its eye
  - Atraumatic eyeless needle is that the suture material is swaged into the blunt end of the needle so that no injury to the tissue occurs due to the doubling of the suture material at the eye end. It can be used only once

Unit XIII ❖ Common Operation Theater Instruments

Uses

■ Cutting needle is used for stitching the tough structures, like skin and fascia.
■ Round body needles are used for suturing of the delicate structures.
■ Straight needles are used for giving mattress sutures in the skin.

Sims' Vaginal Speculum (Fig. 13)

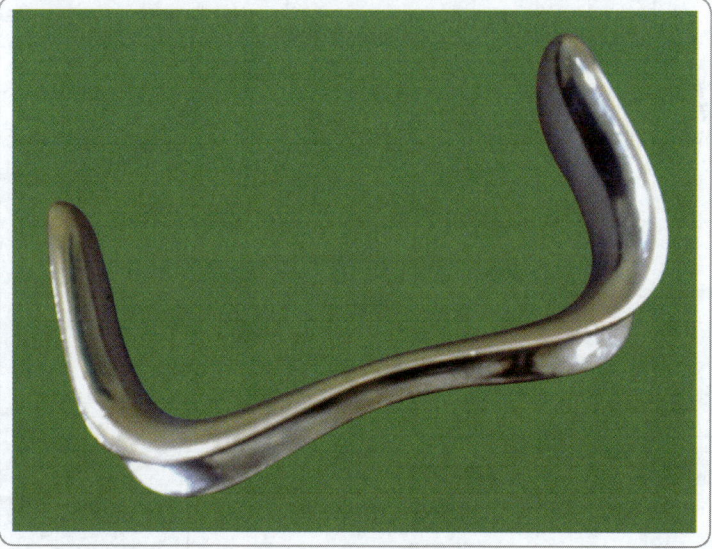

Figure 13: Sims' vaginal speculum

Specifications

■ It is a moderately heavy metal instrument.
■ It has two thick blades at both ends curved laterally to same side.
■ An assistant is needed to hold the speculum in position during operations because it has no self-retaining mechanism. It is available in various sizes.

Uses

■ It is used in vaginal examinations and operations of the cervix and vagina in lithotomy position.

After placing the patient in lithotomy position with the buttocks at the edge of the bed, one blade of the speculum is introduced along its edge with the blade lying vertically in anteroposterior diameter of the vagina and then rotated to adjust the blade in the vagina. Then the assistant holds at the lower blade and gives enough traction downwards according to the required space to be retracted.

Guedel's Oropharyngeal Airway (Fig. 14)

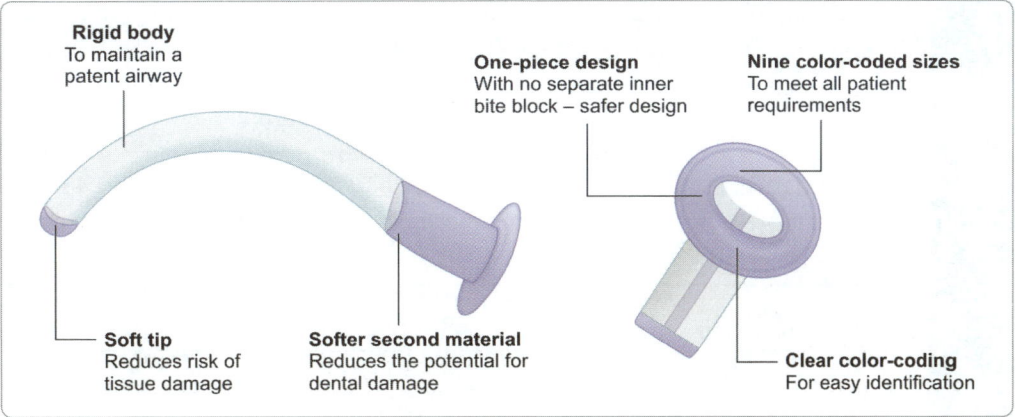

Rigid body
To maintain a patent airway

One-piece design
With no separate inner bite block – safer design

Nine color-coded sizes
To meet all patient requirements

Soft tip
Reduces risk of tissue damage

Softer second material
Reduces the potential for dental damage

Clear color-coding
For easy identification

Figure 14: Guedel's oropharyngeal airway

Specifications

- Oropharyngeal airway is made up of hard rubber or plastic which is the widely used airway nowadays (Fig. 14).
- It is a hollow plastic or rubber tube, bend at the shaft according to the curve of the oropharynx with full opening of the tube at the tip.
- At the proximal end there is a round metal connection joining the plastic tube to provide easy handling during introduction and prevent collapse of the tube between the teeth.

Uses

- Used to prevent biting and obstruction of endotracheal tube.
- To prevent obstruction of natural air passage by relaxed tongue and soft pharyngeal tissue during induction and recovery from anesthesia.
- It also facilitates suctioning of pharyngeal secretions through the hole of the airway.

Unit XIII ❖ Common Operation Theater Instruments

NOTES

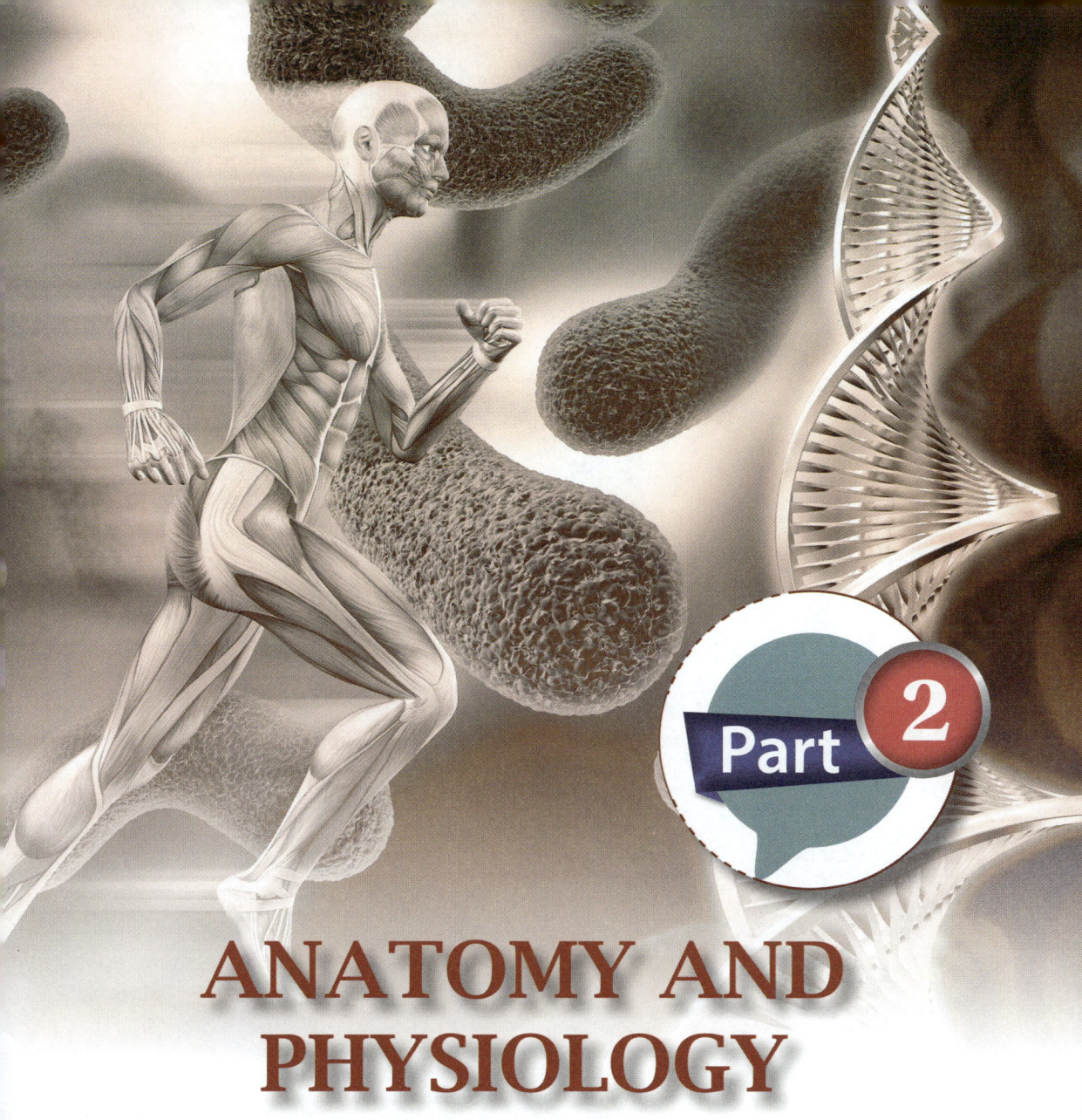

ANATOMY AND PHYSIOLOGY

ANATOMY AND PHYSIOLOGY

Unit 1

Introduction

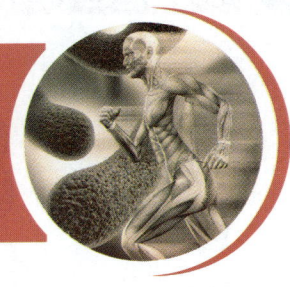

DEFINITIONS

- **Anatomy:** It is the science, which deals with the structure of the human body and the relationship of its constituent parts to each other.
- **Physiology:** It is the study of the functions and mechanisms which work in the normal human body.

HUMAN BODY

The human body is made up of many tissues and organs. Each organ has its own particular function to perform. One organ cannot perform the function of other organ but their functions are related to each other. The cell is the *unit* or the smallest element of the body by which all parts are made up of. The cells of an organ are adapted to perform the special functions of that particular organ. So *cell* is the basic structural unit of living organisms. Organic tissues are made up of numerous cells. Group or layer of similarly arranged cells together forms a tissue to perform certain special functions. An organ consists of numerous tissues for the special functions of that organ. A system consists of many organs to perform its particular function. Thus a human body consists of different systems. Each system situated in different parts of the body is related to each other and functions effectively and regularly in a living individual. The functions of each organ and system continue simultaneously and independently like a machine without interfering with each other. Therefore, we can say that human body is a wonderful and highly sophisticated machine.

Levels of Constitution

Different levels of constitution (Fig. 1) of a human body are as follows:

- Cellular level
- Tissue level
- Organs level
- Systems level
- Organism level (individual)

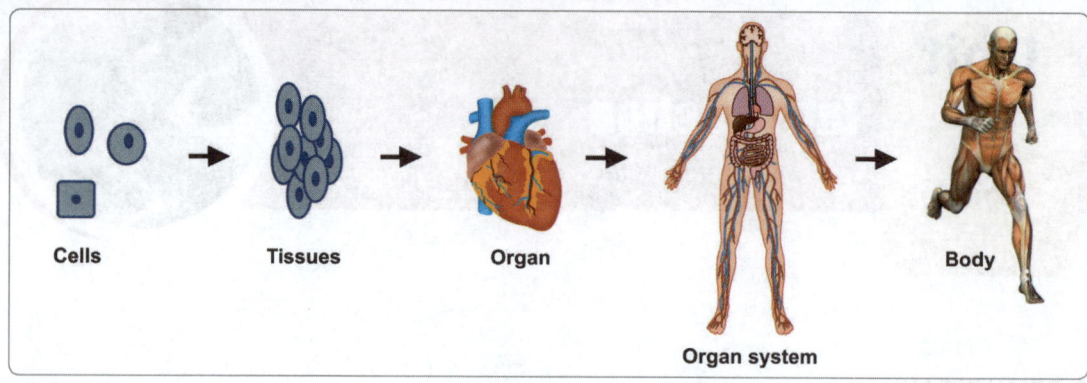

Figure 1: Levels of constitution of a human body

We can observe the structure of a human body and explain the functions carried out by them by studying from the basic unit level to the complete organism level.

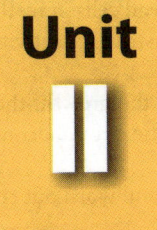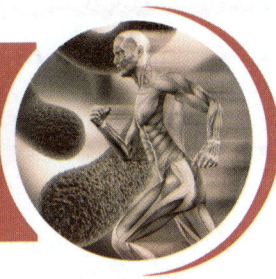
THE CELL

The components of cells have been shown in Figure 1.

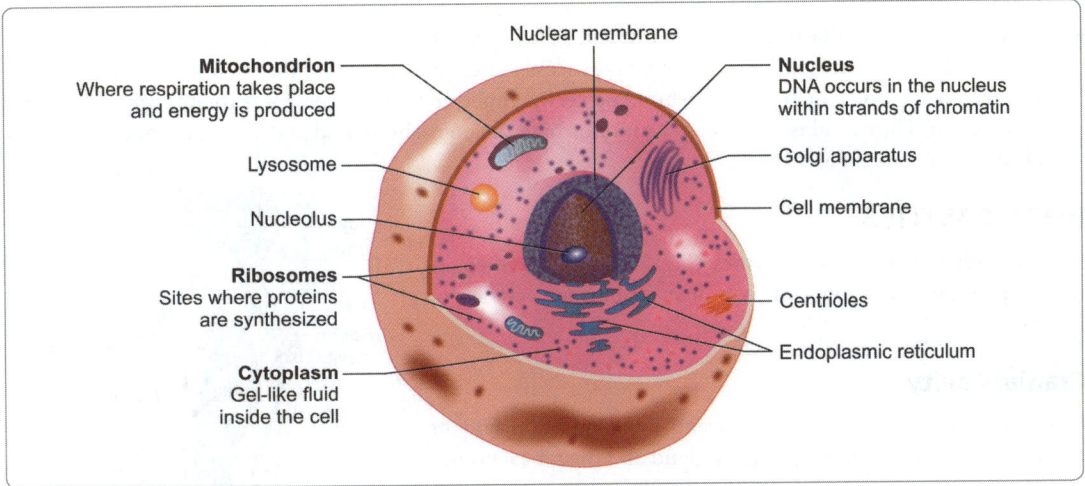

Figure 1: Internal structure of cell

A cell is a minute (jelly-like) mass of protoplasm containing a nucleus and is bounded together by a cell membrane. Its component include a plasma membrane, cytoplasm, ribosomes, and deoxyribonucleic acid (DNA). These carry out its function.

Characteristics of Cell

Cells possess the qualities of all living matters, including self-preservation and reproduction. The qualities of cells are as follows:

- **Metabolism:** Metabolism includes catabolism and anabolism. Cell needs energy for its activities. For this, food is broken down (catabolism) and energy is stored in the form of adenosine triphosphate (ATP) to provide heat and make up or build up the complex molecules in cell (anabolism). Therefore, metabolism is the chemical changes that take place in the body, necessary for the fulfillment of its vital function.
- **Responsiveness (irritability and conductivity):** Cells respond to the internal and external environments with the help of receptors located in the cell surface.
- **Movement:** Cells possess the quality of movement at cellular, tissue level, organs and systems level to a specified limit. The energy obtained from food is used for movement of body as whole.

- **Growth and repair:** Cells multiply and grow in all systems and replace the worn out dead cells. It further helps in body's physiological function. Cells increase in size that is, it *grows*. These constructive activities of growth and repair are the anabolic functions of the cell or anabolism.

- **Differentiation:** Developed cells are different from growing cells. Depending upon the growth, there is difference in the structure and functions of cells. For example, after fertilization, the ovum becomes zygote, embryo, fetus, baby and as an individual.

- **Reproduction:** Cells multiply by mitosis and meiosis. New cells are formed, develop and worn out cells are replaced and this way human life continues.

- **Respiration:** Respiration takes place when oxygen is circulated to the cells and tissues from the lungs through hemoglobin in blood and the gaseous waste product called carbon dioxide is removed. This process is essential for the functioning and survival of the cell.

- **Excretion:** The waste materials of catabolism are eliminated from the cell into the interstitial fluid and then carried away by the blood. The blood transports the carbonic acid waste to the lungs where it is removed from the body as carbon dioxide. Other waste substances are eliminated by the kidneys in the form of urine.

- **Ingestion and assimilation:** Ingestion is intake of food and assimilation is the process by which nutrients are absorbed in the form of energy. For this process to happen, cells select the chemical substances such as amino acids which help the cell to build up very complicated substances, e.g., proteins, which make up protoplasm. Thus a cell is a very active unit in which the nourishing food materials consumed by man is absorbed and assimilated.

BODY CAVITIES

Human body has four main cavities (Fig. 2). These cavities are made up of bones or muscles to protect important systems or organs.

Cranial Cavity

It is mainly formed by skull bones and contains brain and its covering. It also contains the pituitary gland and the pineal body.

Thoracic Cavity

It is situated at the upper part of the trunk and made up of bones, ribs and intercostal muscles, sternum in front, vertebral column in backside, 12 pairs of ribs and 11 pairs of intercostal muscles. The thoracic cavity contains the lungs and the heart, which is located in the mediastinum.

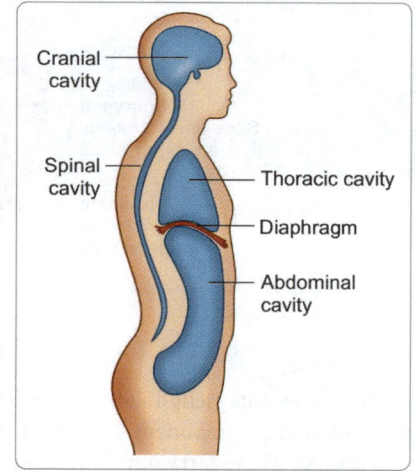

Figure 2: Body cavities of human body

Thoracic cavity contains vital organs such as lungs, heart and its blood vessels—thoracic aorta, inferior vena cava, esophagus and vagus nerve that passes through it.

Relations of boundaries of thoracic cavity are as follows:

Superior	-	The structures forming the neck
Inferior	-	The diaphragm
Anterior	-	The sternum, front portion of ribs with intercostal muscles
Posterior	-	The thoracic vertebrae with their intervertebral discs, back portion of the ribs with their intercostal muscles
Sides	-	Sides of the ribs with their intercostal muscles.

Abdominal Cavity

This is the largest cavity in the body. It encloses most of the digestive organs and kidneys.

Relations

Superiorly—the diaphragm separates it from thoracic cavity.

Inferiorly—the pelvic cavity is continuous with abdominal cavity.

Anteriorly—the flat muscles of anterior abdominal wall.

Posteriorly—the vertebral column and the muscles forming the posterior abdominal wall.

Organs enclosed in the abdominal cavity are as follows:

The greater part of the alimentary canal, i.e., the stomach, small and large intestines, liver, gallbladder, pancreas, spleen, kidneys and adrenal glands, ureters, abdominal aorta, inferior vena cava, receptaculum chyli, part of thoracic duct, lymphatic vessels, glands, nerves, peritoneum and fat.

Pelvic Cavity

It is roughly funnel-shaped, situated in the lower part of the abdominal cavity, mainly formed by the bony structure with hip bones, sacrum, coccyx and the muscles of the pelvic floor. The pelvic cavity encloses the bladder and reproductive organs.

Organs enclosed in pelvic cavity are as follows:

- **In females:** The urinary bladder and the ureters, pelvic colon and rectum, uterus and ligaments, fallopian tubes and ovaries.
- **In males:** Urinary bladder and ureters, pelvic colon and rectum, the prostate glands, seminal vesicles, vas deferens and ejaculatory ducts.

Pelvic blood vessels, lymphatic vessels, glands and nerves are present in the pelvic cavity.

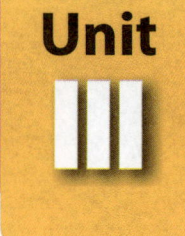

Unit III

Major Systems of the Human Body

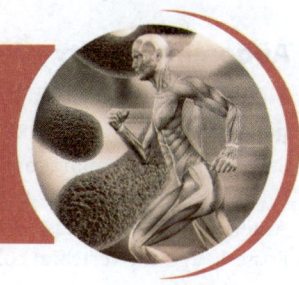

INTRODUCTION

The major systems in the human body are as follows:

- Integumentary system (skin)
- Skeletal system
- Muscular system
- Endocrine system
- Cardiovascular system (heart, blood vessels and blood)
- Lymphatic system
- Respiratory system
- Digestive system
- Urinary system
- Reproductive system
- Nervous system (brain and nerves)
- Special sense organs

Let's discuss these in detail.

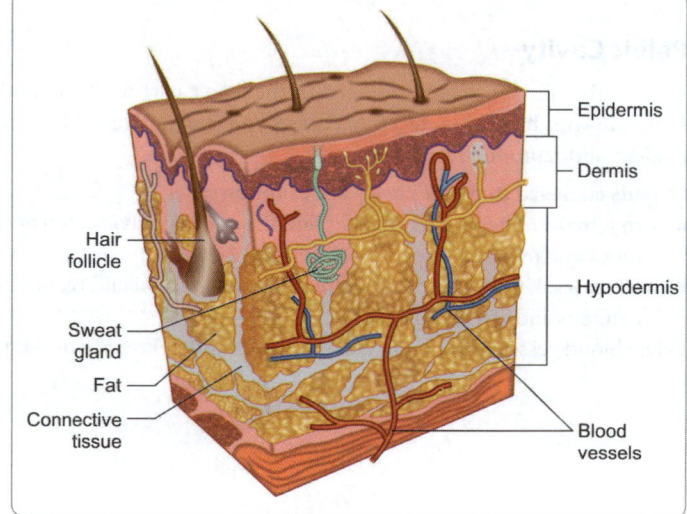

Figure 1: Internal structure of skin

INTEGUMENTARY SYSTEM (SKIN)

The skin is the largest organ of our body. It covers the entire body. The skin is made up of three layers. Each layer has certain functions:

1. **Epidermis:** It is the thin outer layer of the skin. It consists of three types of cells:
   i. **Squamous cells:** The outermost layer of the skin, consisting of keratinized cells is called the stratum corneum.
   ii. **Basal cells:** Basal cells are found just under the squamous cells, at the base of the epidermis.
   iii. **Melanocytes:** Melanocytes are also found at the base of the epidermis and make melanin. This gives the skin its color.
2. **Dermis:** It is the middle layer of the skin. The dermis contains blood vessels, lymph vessels, hair follicles, sweat glands, collagen bundles, fibroblasts, nerves and sebaceous glands
3. **Subcutaneous fat layer (hypodermis):** The subcutaneous fat layer is the deepest layer of skin. It consists of a network of collagen and fat cells. It helps conserve the body's heat and protects the body from injury by acting as a shock absorber (Fig. 1).
   - Appendages of the skin are: Nails, hair, sweat glands and sebaceous glands.

Functions of Skin

- **Regulation of body temperature:** The body temperature is constant at about 36.9°C or 98.4°F.
- **Protection:** Skin protects the deeper structures against the invasion of microbes and other harmful agents. Skin is the covering of the body.
- **Skin has excretory, secretary and absorptive:** By perspiration waste materials are excreted. Sebaceous glands secrete a fatty substance called sebum which keeps the skin soft and smooth and the hair glossy. Medicines or oily substances are absorbed by the skin when applied externally.
- **Formation of vitamin D:** The ultraviolet rays from sun convert the fatty substance of the skin into vitamin D.
- **Sensory organ:** Skin carries sensory impulse of pain, temperature and touch to the brain.
- **Storage:** Skin acts as storage of water and the adipose tissue beneath the epidermis. It is one of the fat depots of the body.
- **Immunity function:** Certain epidermal cells protect the body against foreign invaders thus act as a part of immune system.
- **Reservoir of blood:** The dermis carries 8–10% of the total blood flow in a resting adult. Blood flow to the skin increases in moderate exercise. The blood vessels in the skin constrict during strenuous exercise and thus allow more blood to circulate through contraction of muscles.

SKELETAL SYSTEM (FIG. 2)

The study of bones is called osteology. There are movable and immovable bones in the human body. The knowledge about the movements of the bones, types and other details of bones is necessary for a nurse to give proper care to the patients.

Functions of Bones

- Provide support and protection for some of the soft organs, particularly skull and pelvis
- Acting as levers in movements of the body
- Producing blood cells
- Storing the minerals
- Providing attachment to the skeletal muscles

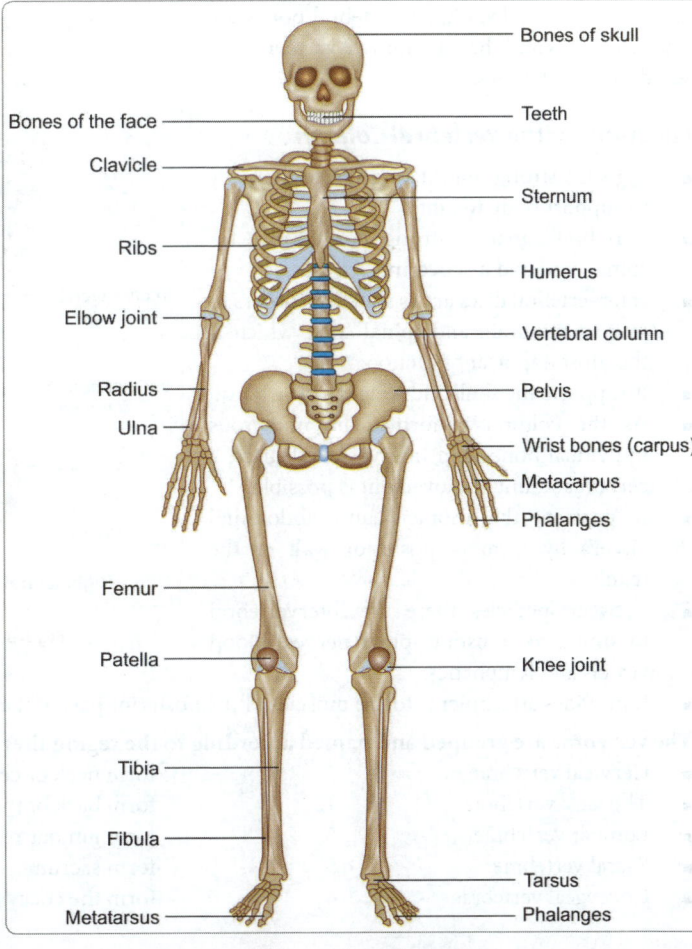

Figure 2: Skeletal system

Classification of Bones

There are 206 bones in a human body in total.

Classification of bones according to their shape:

- Long bones   e.g.   bones of the limb like femur, humerus
- Short bones   e.g.   bones of wrist—carpus—tarsus
- Flat bones   e.g.   posterior part of the shoulder girdle, namely scapula
- Irregular bones   e.g.   bones of the hip joints – hip bones
- Sesamoid bones: They are developed in the tendons of muscles and are found in the vicinity of a joint, e.g., **Patella is the largest sesamoid bones** in the body.

Vertebral Column (Fig. 3)

Bones of the Vertebral Column

There are 33 vertebrae in the body. The adult vertebral column measures about 60–70 cm (24–28 inches) in length, 24 vertebral bones are separate bones and the remaining 9 vertebrae are fused to form 2 bones.

Functions of the Vertebral Column

- It gives a strong central long axis to the body to support body weight.
- Vertebral canal is strong bony canal for spinal cord and its covering.
- Intervertebral discs act as shock absorbers to protect the brain and spinal cord, which is the most important function.
- It supports the skull and weight of the body.
- As the column is formed by numerous individual bones and intervertebral discs, a certain amount of movement is possible.
- It protects the thoracic and abdominal viscera by forming posterior wall of the trunk.
- Between pedicles there are intervertebral foramina to transmit spinal nerves, blood vessels and lymphatics.
- It provides attachments to the muscles of the posterior part of the body.

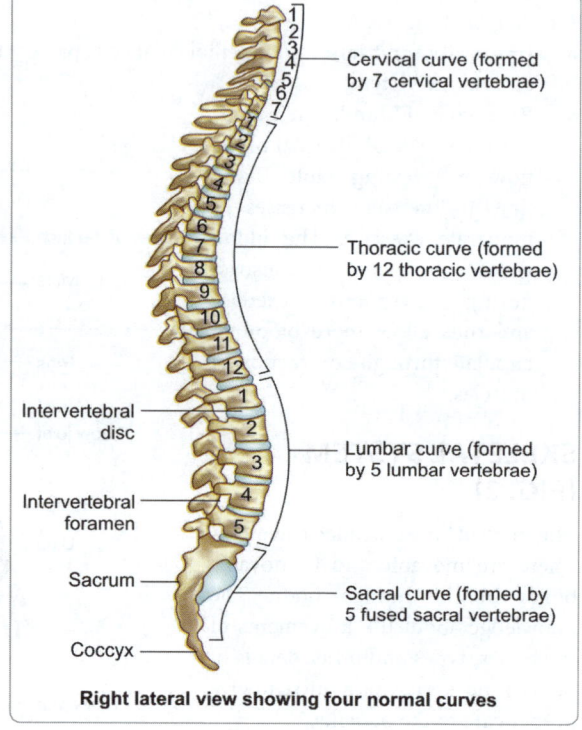

Right lateral view showing four normal curves

Figure 3: Curves of vertebral column

The vertebrae are grouped and named according to the region they occupy:

- Cervical vertebrae   -   7   -   form neck or cervical region
- Thoracic vertebrae   -   12   -   form back of the thorax or chest
- Lumbar vertebrae   -   5   -   form lumbar region or loin
- Sacral vertebrae   -   5   -   form sacrum
- Coccygeal vertebrae   -   4   -   form the coccyx or tail

Curves of the Vertebral Column

When one looks from the side, the vertebral column presents four anteroposterior curves (Fig. 3).

- The cervical curve in the neck, which is convex forwards
- The thoracic curve or dorsal curve – convex backwards
- The lumbar curve - convex forwards
- The pelvic curve - convex backwards

Skull

The skull is a bony framework of the head, arranged in two parts: the cranium also called calvaria consists of eight bones and facial skeleton of fourteen bones (8 + 14 = 22). Total bones in skull are 22 (Fig. 4).

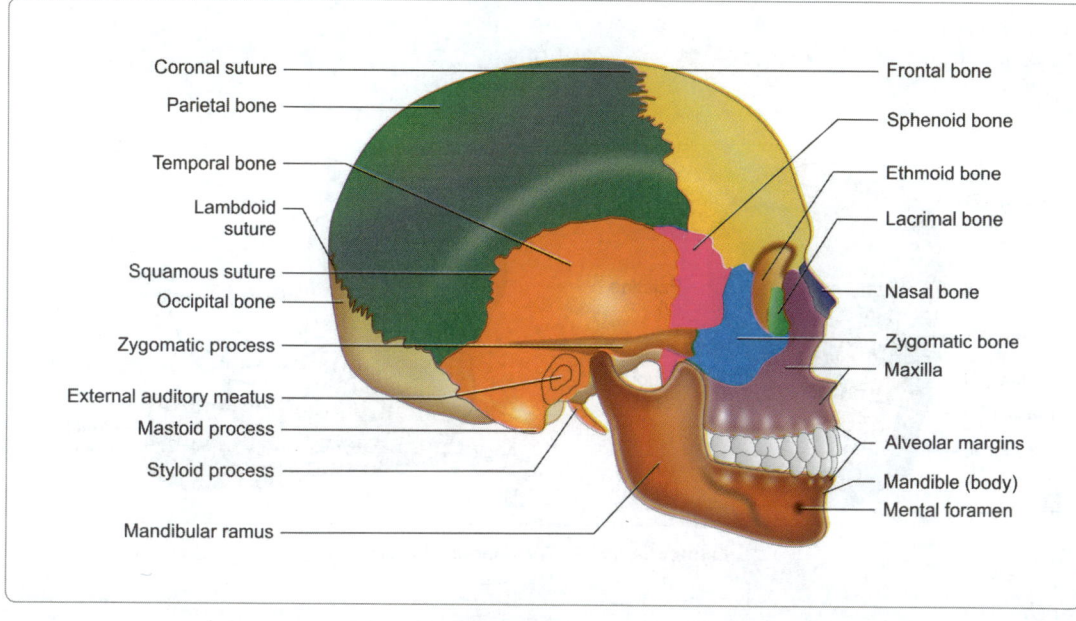

Figure 4: The skull

Bones of Cranium

Cranial bones	
Occipital bone	1
Parietal bones	2
Frontal bone	1
Temporal bones	2
Sphenoid bone	1
Ethmoid bone	1
Total	**8**

❖ Major Systems of the Human Body

Unit III

Bones of the Face

There are 14 facial bones. All are united by sutures and they are immovable except mandible bone (Figs 5A and B).

Facial bone	
Nasal bones	2
Lacrimal bones	2
Zygomatic bones (cheek bones)	2
Maxilla	2
Vomer	1
Palatine bones	2
Inferior Conchae	2
Mandible bone	1
Total	**14**

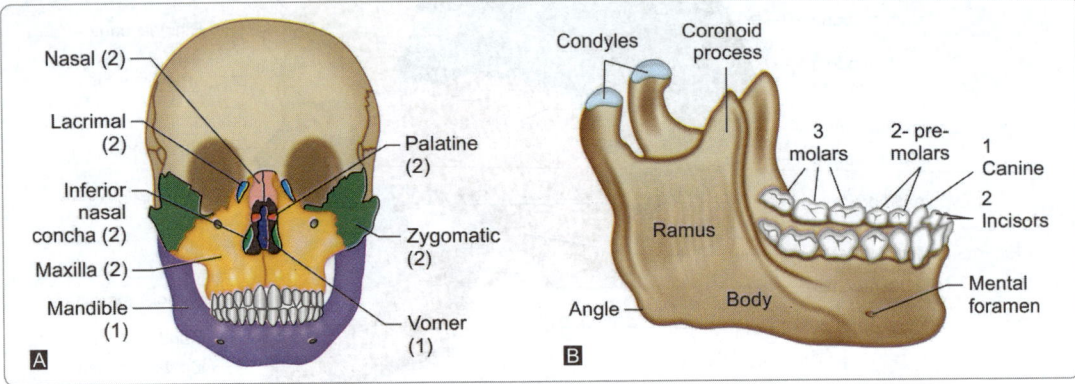

Figures 5A and B: The bones of the face

Teeth

There are 32 teeth in the mouth of an adult. Teeth come in two sets–the temporary set and the permanent set. **Temporary sets or milk teeth** are 10 in each jaw named from the middle line on each side.

Incisors - 2   5 in right side
                and
Canine - 1   5 in left side
Premolars - 2

The permanent teeth are 32 in number. Sixteen in each jaw. They are named from the center as shown in Figure 6.

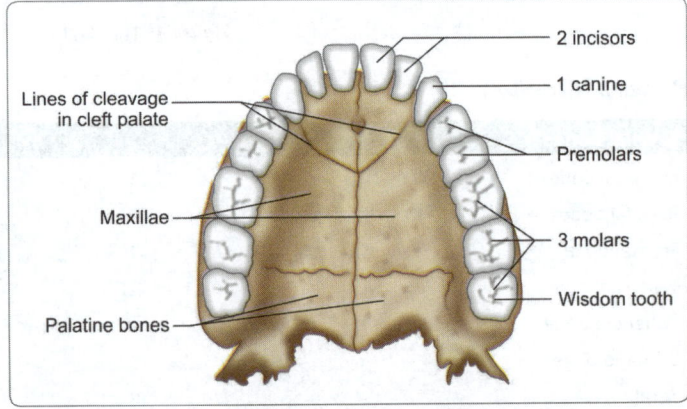

Figure 6: The upper teeth and bony palate

Incisors   - 2
Canine   - 1
Premolars - 2
Molars   - 3 (the last molar is the wisdom tooth)

The permanent teeth begin to replace the temporary ones at about the age of six years (Fig. 6).

Skeleton of the Upper Limb

The skeleton of the upper limb is attached to the skeleton of the trunk by means of the shoulder girdle which consists of the clavicle and scapula.

Below this are, the following bones that form the skeleton of the arm, forearm and hand, making a total of 30 bones.

Humerus	1
Radius	1
Ulna	1
Carpal bones	8
Metacarpals	5
Phalanges	14
Total	**30**

Bones of Shoulder

- **Clavicle or collar bone**: It forms the anterior part of the shoulder girdle.
- **Scapula**: It forms the posterior part of the shoulder girdle–lies at the back of the thorax–triangular and flat with two surfaces and three angles and three borders (upper, lateral and medial).
- **Humerus**: It is a long bone–longest of upper limb and bone of the upper arm above the elbow joint.
- **Radius**: It is a long bone–lateral bone of the forearm shorter than ulna.
- **Ulna**: It is a long bone–medial bone of the forearm longer than radius.
- **Wrists or carpal bones**: Short bones form wrists–total 8 bones.
- **Metacarpals**: Small long bones form the skeleton of the palm, 5 in number.
- **Phalanges**: Phalanges or bones of fingers or small long bones—14 in number—3 in each finger and 2 in the thumb (Fig. 7).

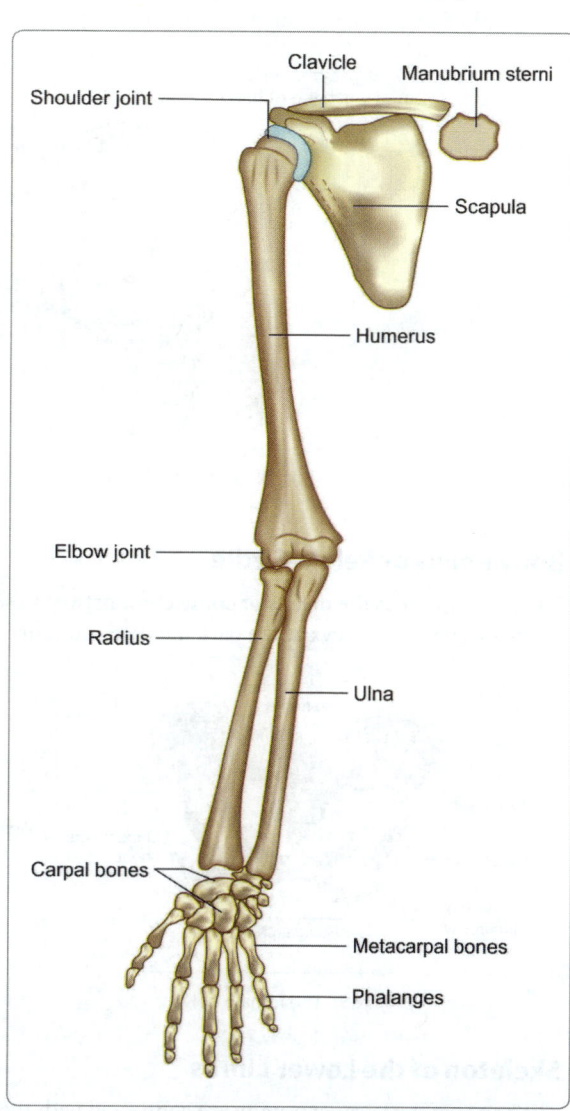

Figure 7: The joints and bones of the right upper limb

Unit III ❖ Major Systems of the Human Body

Bones of the Thoracic Cage

The bones of the thoracic cage is made up of bones and cartilages. It is formed by the thoracic vertebrae (12 in number) at the back–the sternum in front and 12 pairs of ribs at the sides.

- **Sternum:** Sternum or the breast bone is a flat bone which lies in the anterior part of the chest.
- **Ribs:** There are 12 pairs of ribs which are attached to the thoracic vertebra at the back. Interiorly the first seven pairs of ribs are attached directly to the sternum with the help of inter costal cartilages. The first one is the shortest rib. From the last lower five pairs, three pairs are attached indirectly to the sternum by means of attachment of their costal cartilages to the cartilage of the rib above. The last two pairs are not attached and they are called floating ribs (Fig. 8).

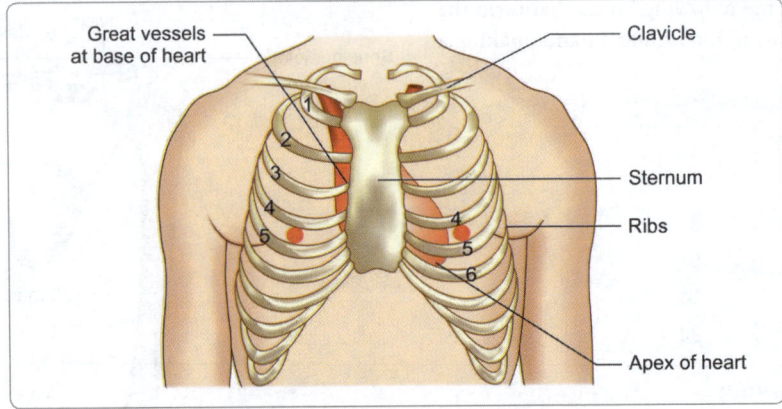

Figure 8: Sternum, ribs, intercostal cartilage and position of the heart

Bony Pelvis or Pelvic Girdle

The pelvic girdle is the means of connection between the trunk and lower extremities. This girdle is formed by the sacrum and coccyx at the back and two innominate bones at the sides (Figs 9 and 10).

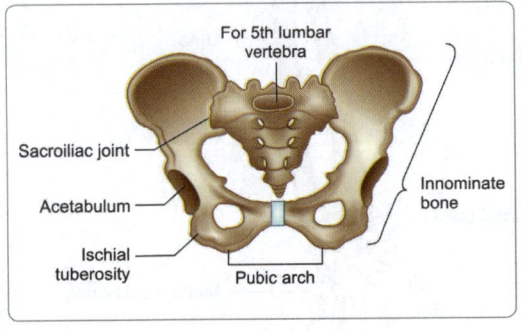

Figure 9: The female pelvis

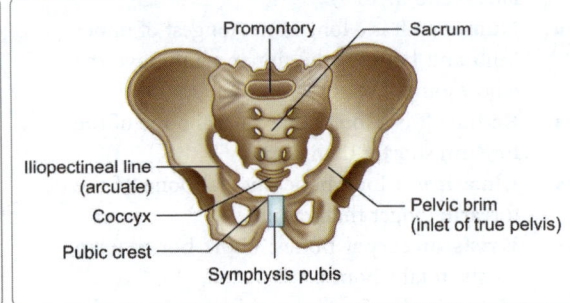

Figure 10: The male pelvis

Skeleton of the Lower Limbs

The bones of the lower extremity are connected with the trunk by means of the pelvic girdle. The lower extremity consists of 31 bones.

Unit III ❖ Major Systems of the Human Body

Innominate bone	1
Femur	1
Tibia	1
Fibula	1
Patella	1
Tarsal bones	7
Metatarsal bones	5
Phalanges	14
Total	**31**

- **Innominate bone:** The innominate bone is an irregular flat bone formed by the union of three bones that help to form the pelvic girdle. The names of the three bones are: the upper most one is ilium, the front one is pubis and the most posterior one is ischium (Fig. 11).

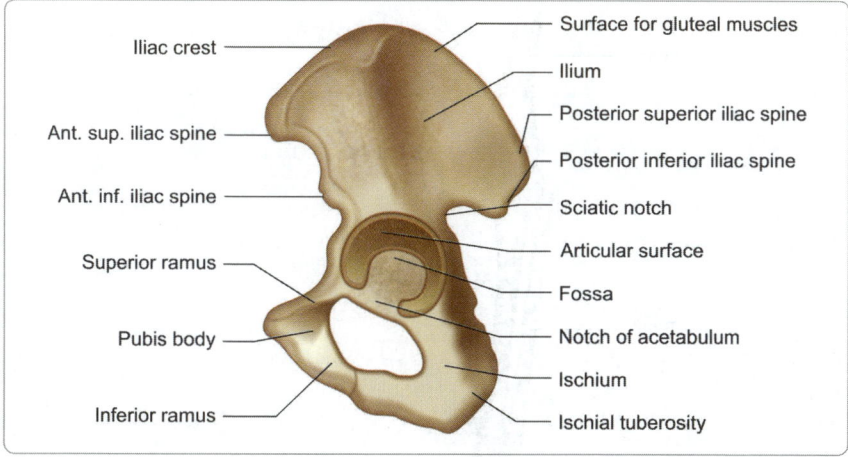

Figure 11: The external surface of the left innominate bone

- **Femur: The longest bone of the body**–articulates above with the pelvic girdle and below with knee joint of the leg.
- **Patella:** It is a sesamoid bone which lies in front of the knee joint of the leg – almost triangular in shape.
- **Tibia:** It is a long bone – forms the main skeleton of the leg and lies medial to the fibula.
- **Fibula:** It is a long bone – lateral bone of the leg – deeply embedded in the muscles of the leg.
- **Tarsal bones:** They are short bones – 7 in number form the ankle joint of the foot.
- **Metatarsal bones:** They are long bones – 5 in number – articulates above with tarsal bones arid below with phalanges of foot.
- **Phalanges of the toes:** They are long bones but shorter than phalanges of the fingers. Similar to those of the fingers; 14 in number (Fig. 12).

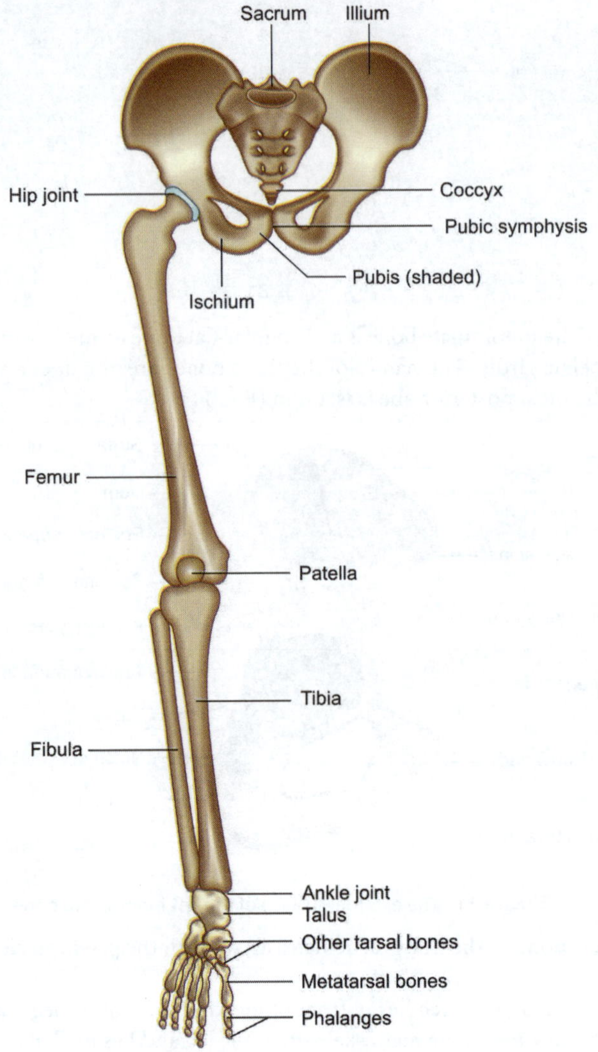

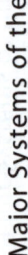

Figure 12: The lower limb with joints

MUSCULAR SYSTEM

Muscles are formed by a large number of strong tissues (Figs 13 to 16).

Types of Muscles

- Voluntary muscles, e.g., skeletal muscles.
- Involuntary muscles, e.g., cardiac muscles and smooth muscles.
  - Skeletal muscles are under voluntary control, e.g., limbs.
  - Cardiac muscles form the muscular layer of the heart called myocardium.

- Smooth muscles line the respiratory, alimentary and urinary system and found in blood vessels, eyes and other such viscera.

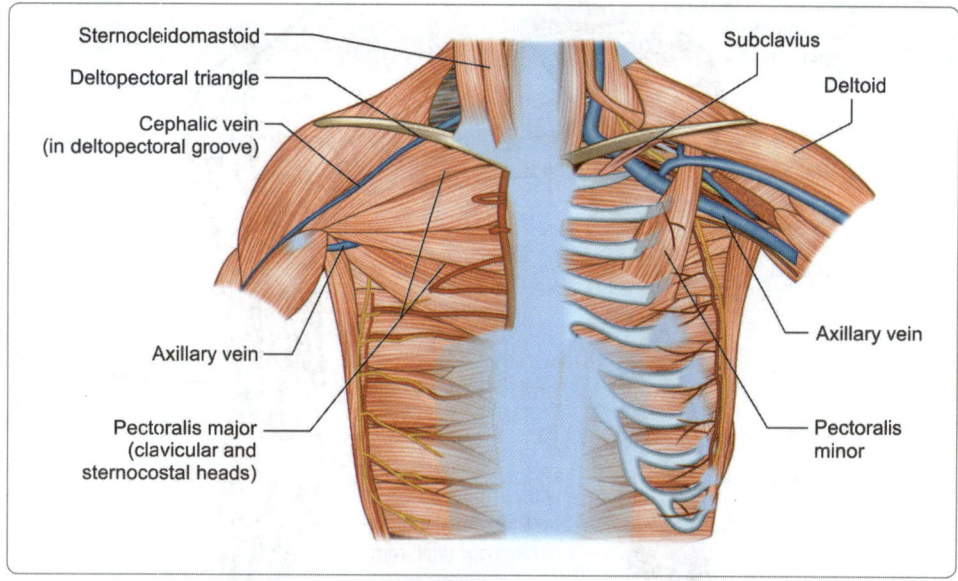

Figure 13: Muscles of the anterior aspect of the shoulder and chest wall

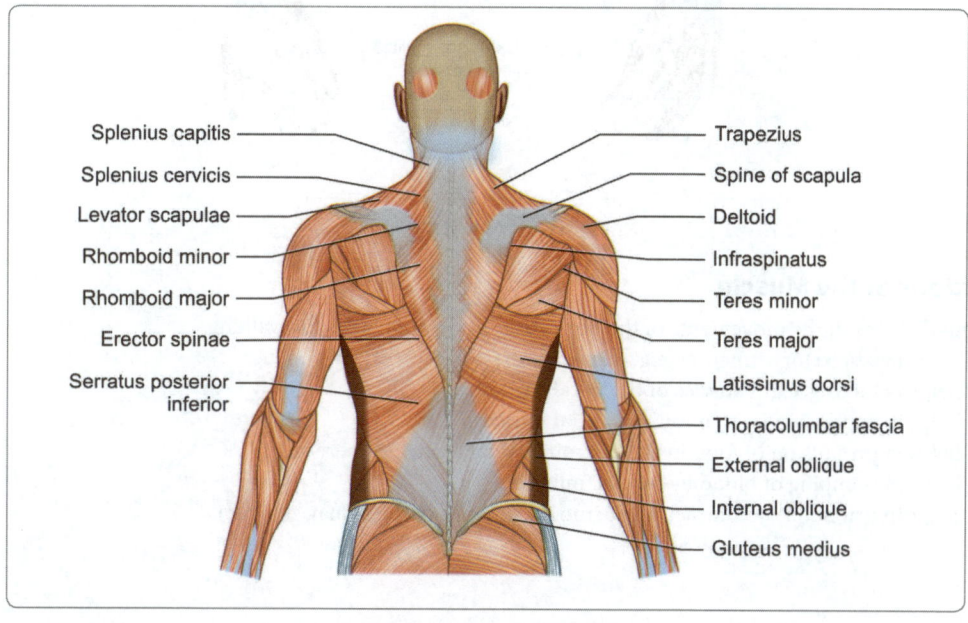

Figure 14: Muscles of back

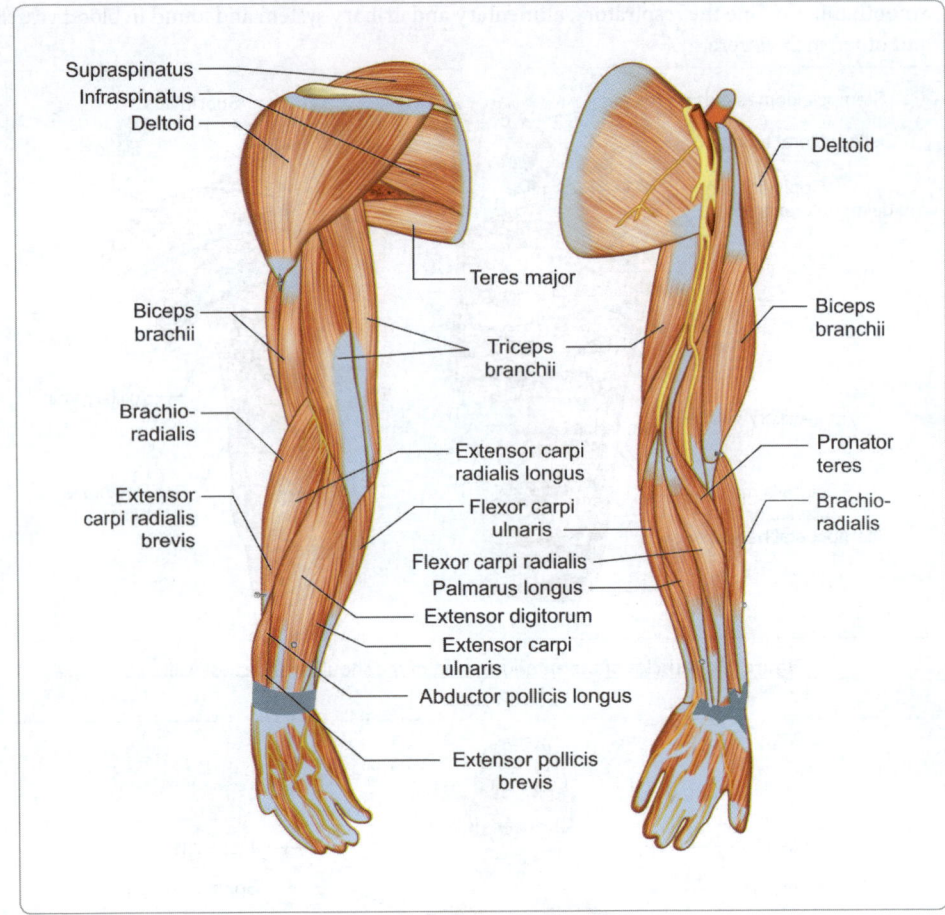

Figure 15: Muscles of arm

Functions of the Muscle

- Muscle helps in the movements of the bones, e.g., skeletal muscles for walking.
- It helps in respiratory function, e.g. diaphragm.
- It helps in talking, e.g., muscles of the vocal cord.
- It helps in expression of emotion, e.g. facial muscles.
- It helps in propulsion of food in the gastrointestinal tract, e.g., peristalsis.
- It helps in pumping of blood by cardiac muscles.
- It helps in urination by contraction of smooth muscles of the urinary bladder.

ENDOCRINE SYSTEM

The endocrine organs or ductless glands are grouped together under this name because the secretions called hormones are passed directly into the blood by circulating substance of the gland and not through the ducts and hence they are called ductless glands. The word endocrine means 'internal secretion' and these are the hormones. Some endocrine glands produce a single hormone and others produce more. For example, pituitary gland produces a number of hormones, which control the activity of many other endocrine organs and because of this reason the *pituitary gland* has been described as the *master gland of the body* (Fig. 17).

The endocrine organs are:

Pituitary gland	1
Thyroid gland	1
Parathyroid gland	4
Thymus gland	1
Adrenal glands (Suprarenal glands)	2
Pineal body or gland	1
Pancreas	1
Ovaries in the female	2
Testes in the male	2

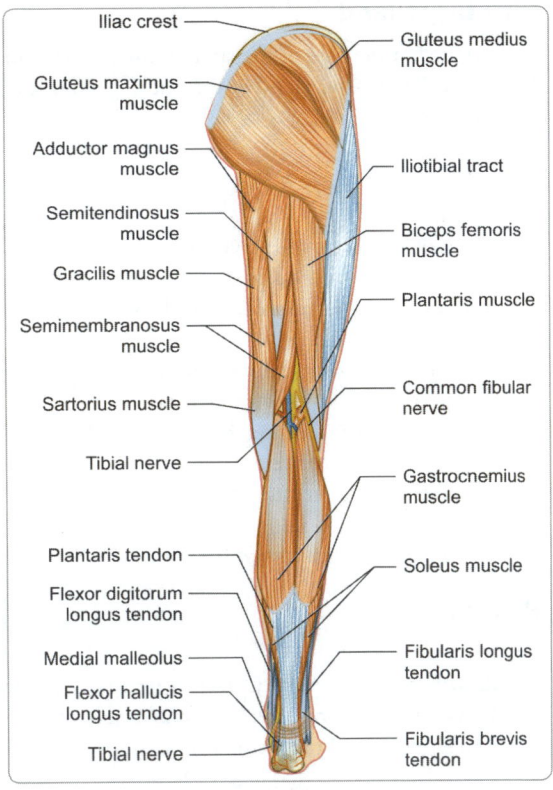

Figure 16: The muscles of thigh

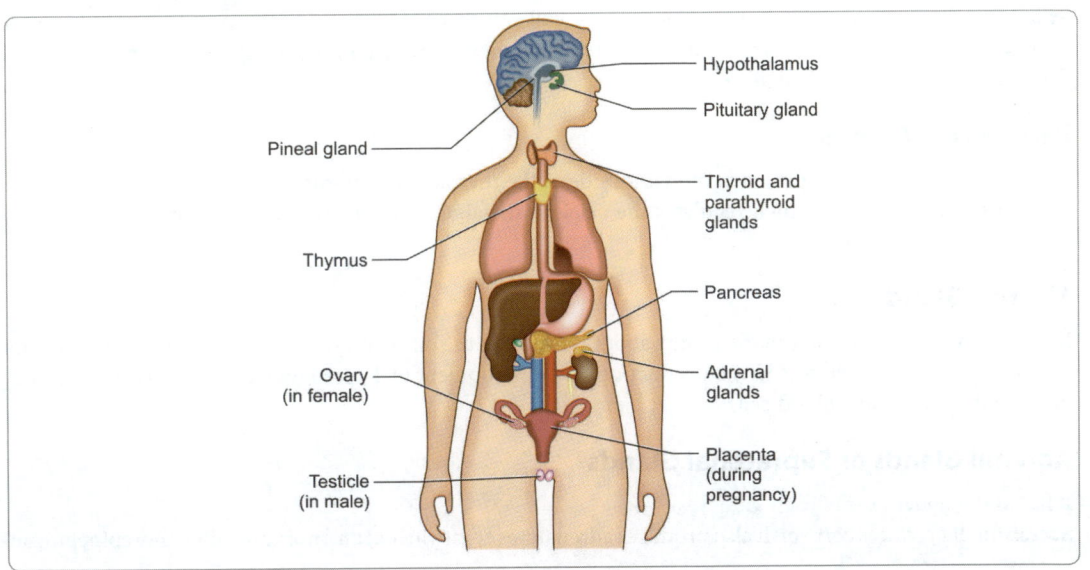

Figure 17: Endocrine glands in the body

Unit III ❖ Major Systems of the Human Body

Pituitary Gland

It is situated in the base of the skull in the pituitary fossa of the sphenoid. It has anterior and posterior lobes. It is also called master gland of the body. The hormones of the pituitary gland help regulate the functions of other endocrine glands.

Anterior Lobe

Anterior lobe secretes:

- **Growth hormone (GH):** GH is essential in early years for maintaining a healthy body composition and for growth in children. In adults, it aids healthy bone and muscle mass and affects fat distribution.
- **Thyrotrophic hormone (thyroid stimulating hormone) (TSH):** Stimulates the thyroid gland to produce hormones.
- **Adrenocorticotropic hormone (ACTH):** Stimulates the adrenal glands to produce hormones.
- Gonadotrophic hormones such as:
  - **Follicle stimulating hormone (FSH):** Works with luteinizing hormone (LH) to ensure normal functioning of the ovaries and testes.
  - **Luteinizing hormone (LH) (interstitial cell stimulating hormone):** LH works with FSH to ensure normal functioning of the ovaries and testes.
  - **Prolactin (luteotrophin)** stimulates breast milk production.

Posterior Lobe

Posterior lobe secrets:

- **Antidiuretic hormone (ADH):** Prompts the kidneys to increase water absorption in the blood.
- **Oxytocic hormone:** Involved in a variety of processes, such as contracting the uterus during childbirth and stimulating breast milk production.

Thyroid Gland

It consists of two lobes placed on each sides of the trachea in the neck.
Secretion: The thyroid secretes several hormones, collectively called thyroid hormones. The main hormone is thyroxine, also called T4. Thyroid hormones act throughout the body, influencing metabolism, growth and development and body temperature.

Parathyroid Glands

They are four small glands placed two on each side of the thyroid gland in the neck.
Secretion: Parathormone which regulates the calcium metabolism of the body and controls the amount of calcium in blood and bone.

Thymus Gland

It consists of two lobes. It lies in the thorax about the level of the bifurcation of the trachea in the neck region. The thymus serves a vital role in the production and development of T-lymphocytes or T cells, an extremely important type of white blood cell.

Adrenal Glands or Suprarenal Glands

It lies in the upper pole of each kidney.
Secretion: It produces cortisol. It also produces adrenaline (epinephrine) and noradrenaline (norepinephrine).

Pineal Body or Gland

It is situated near the corpus callosum in the brain. Researchers do know that it produces and regulates some hormones, including melatonin, which is known for the role it plays in regulating sleep patterns.

Pancreas

It lies behind the stomach and in front of the first lumbar vertebra. The pancreas has two main functions: an exocrine function that helps in digestion and an endocrine function that regulates blood sugar. The main secretion is insulin- an antidiabetic hormone.

Ovaries

Ovaries are placed one on each side of the uterus below the uterine tubes (fallopian tubes). The ovary is attached to the back of the broad ligament of the uterus.

Functions

Ovary has four functions:
1. To produce ova
2. To transport and sustain these cells.
3. To nurture the developing fetus.
4. To produce hormones - estrogen and progesterone, which control menstruation

Testes

Testis lies on both sides of the scrotum. Testes are the male organs of generation where spermatozoa are formed.
Function: In addition to their role in the male reproductive system, the testes also have the distinction of being an endocrine gland because they secrete testosterone—a hormone that is vital to the normal development of male physical characteristics.

CARDIOVASCULAR SYSTEM (HEART, BLOOD VESSELS AND BLOOD)

- The circulatory system consists of the heart, blood vessels, blood, and lymphatics.
- The heart is the great pumping organ that maintains the circulation throughout the body.
- The arteries carry blood from the heart.
- The veins carry blood to the heart.
- The capillaries uniting the arteries and veins form the 'capillary lake'. It carries nourishment to the tissues, takes off waste matter and interchange of gases.
- Lymphatics collect, filter and pass back the lymph through the minute capillary walls to bathe the tissues.

Heart

The heart is a cone-shaped muscular organ. The base of the heart is situated above and the apex below, which is inclined towards left side. The heart weighs about 300 g in adults.

Position of the Heart

Heart is situated in the thoracic cavity, between the lungs and behind the sternum and directed more toward the left than the right side. The apex of the heart is a point on the left side between the fifth and sixth left ribs or in the fifth left intercostal space 9 cm (3½ inch) from the midline (a little below the left nipple) is

Unit III ❖ Major Systems of the Human Body

the position of the pointed extremity of the ventricles. There will be slight variations in the measurements according to the body structure.

Structure of the Heart

The heart is about the size of a closed fist. The adult heart weighs about 220–260 g (8–9 oz). It is divided into two sides, right and left. Normally, there is no communication between these two sides after birth. Each side of the heart is further divided into the two chambers, an upper chamber called atrium and a lower chamber called ventricle. There are two atria, right and left and two ventricles, right and left. The atria and ventricles of each side communicate with each other by means of atrioventricular opening which are guarded by valves: on the right side by tricuspid valve and left side by or bicuspid valve (Fig 18). (The terms atrium and auricle are synonymous).

The atrioventricular valve permits the passage of blood in one direction only, i.e. from atrium to ventricle and they prevent the blood

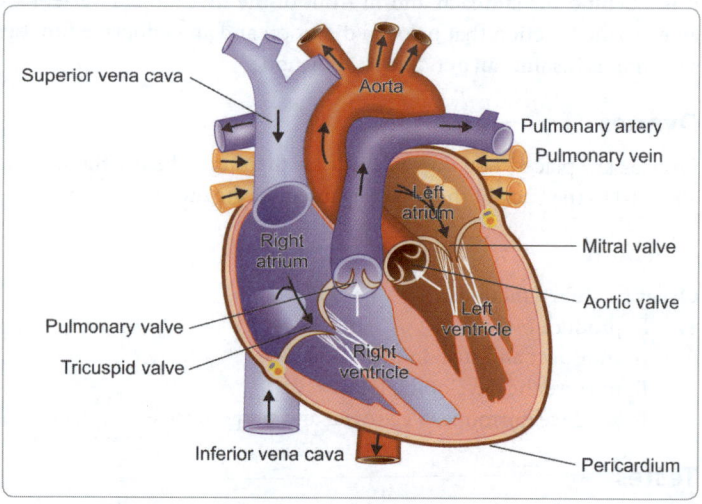

Figure 18: Anatomy of heart

flowing backwards from ventricle to atrium. The tricuspid valve has three flaps or cusps and the mitral valve has two flaps. The mitral valve has some resemblance to a Bishop's mitre and hence the name.

Layers of Heart

The heart is composed of the following three layers (Fig. 18).
1. **The pericardium** is outer covering with two layers. Inner layer is Parietal Pericardium and outer layer is Visceral Pericardium and in between these, there is thin layer of pericardial fluid.
2. **The myocardium** is a middle muscular thick layer
3. **The endocardium** is the inner thin layer

The muscular walls of the heart vary in thickness, the ventricles have the thickest walls, the walls of the left are thicker than right ventricle because the force of contraction of the left ventricle is much greater. The walls of atria are composed of thinner walls.

The circulation of blood in the body is carried out by heart, blood vessels and blood. Heart consists of four chambers, namely right and left auricles and ventricles composed of specialized muscle fibers capable of self-activity and thus it is a great pumping station of circulation. Blood flows through arteries and veins.

The pure blood (oxygenated blood) flows from the heart through all the arteries except pulmonary arteries and is supplied to all parts of the body. Pulmonary arteries carry the impure blood to the lungs for purification. The blood supplied by the arteries to all parts of the body is carried to the heart through veins except pulmonary veins. The pulmonary veins carry the pure or oxygenated blood from the lungs to the left atrium.

Blood Vessels Attached to the Heart and Circulation

The superior vena cava and inferior vena cava empty their blood into the right atrium and it reaches the right ventricle through the opening between them, guarded by semilunar valves of the heart. The pulmonary arteries take the impure blood from the right ventricle to the lungs for oxygenation. From the lungs the two pairs of pulmonary veins bring the oxygenated blood to the left atrium and from there to the left ventricle and then through the aorta—the biggest artery of the body—blood is pumped to all parts of the body. Heart valves permit the flow of blood in one direction only.

Blood Vessels Supplying Blood to the Heart

The right and left coronary arteries are the first vessels leaving the aorta. These then divide into small arteries which encircle the heart and supply blood to all parts of the organ. The returned blood from the heart is collected mainly by the coronary sinus and returned directly into the right atrium.

Nerve Supply to the Heart

Sympathetic nerves and vagus nerves modify the action of the heart. The sympathetic nerves accelerate the rate of heart but the vagus nerves which is a part of parasympathetic or autonomic system causes the action of the heart to be slowed or inhibited. Normally the heart rate is controlled by vagus nerves. But when the vagal tone or 'brake' is removed to meet the needs of the body during exercise or emotional excitement, the heart rate is increased and during physical rest and sleep, it is decreased.

Cardiac Cycle

The heart is a pump and the events occur in the heart during the circulation of blood are said to be the cardiac cycle (Fig. 19).

Atrial Events vs Ventricular Events

- Out of 0.7 seconds of atrial diastole, first 0.3 seconds (0.27 seconds accurately) coincides with ventricular systole.
- Then, ventricular diastole and it lasts for about 0.5 seconds (0.53 seconds accurately).
- Later part of atrial diastole coincides with ventricular diastole for about 0.4 seconds. So, the heart relaxes as a whole for 0.4 seconds.

This action has two parts:

i. Contraction of the heart is systole
ii. Relaxation of the heart is diastole

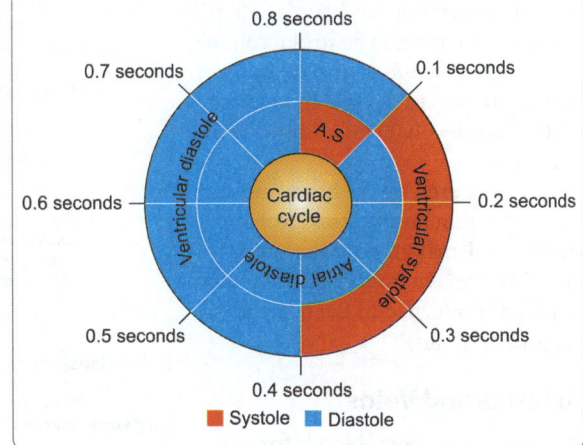

Figure 19: Cardiac cycle

The heart beats continuously, day and night, throughout life and the only rest the cardiac muscle gets is during ventricular diastole or relaxation. The systole and diastole occur at regular interval. The contraction and relaxation of atrium is called atrial systole and atrial diastole respectively. Similarly the contraction and relaxation of ventricle is said to be ventricular systole and ventricular diastole respectively. The ventricular contraction is short (0.3 seconds) and ventricular relaxation phase is long (0.5 seconds).

Unit III ❖ Major Systems of the Human Body

The contraction of the atria is shorter than contraction of the ventricles, which are strong, forcible and longer and that of left ventricle is most forcible than any other chambers as it has to force the blood through the aorta to all parts of the body. The right ventricle pumps exactly the same volume of blood. It sends blood to the lungs, where the pressure is much less. This action of the heart experienced in the arteries is the pulse. If the pulse rate is 70 per minute, it means the cardiac cycle occurs 70 times in a minute. This rhythmic action of the heart is involuntary and it is the special quality of the heart muscle.

The pumping rate of the heart varies in health under conditions of living, working, food intake, age and emotion. The pulse rate corresponds with cardiac cycle. If the pulse rate is 70, the cardiac cycle will occur 70 times in a minute (Table 1).

Table 1: **Pulse rate corresponding to age groups**

Age group	Normal pulse rate range
In the newborn	140 beats/min
During first year	120 beats/min
During second year	110 beats/min
At the age of 5 years	96–100 beats/min
At the age of 10 years	80–90 beats/min
In the adult	60–80 beats/min

Cardiac Output

In a resting person the heart beats 70 times per minute and pumps 70 mL of blood each time. (The stroke volume is 70 mL). Therefore, the amount of blood pumped each time in a minute is 70 × 70 mL = 4900 mL. A little below five liters.

During exercise the heart rate may be 150 per minute and stroke volume is over 150 mL making a cardiac output of 20–25 L/min. An exactly equal volume of blood is returned to the heart in the veins each minute.

Arteries and Veins

Arteries carry pure blood from the heart and supply to the different parts of the body. The biggest artery in the body is aorta. Veins carry impure blood from the different parts of the body to heart.

The arteries and veins are named according to their positions and routes or pathways, e.g. iliac artery, iliac vein (Figs 20 to 22). The blood supply to upper and lower limbs has been shown in Figures 23 and 24.

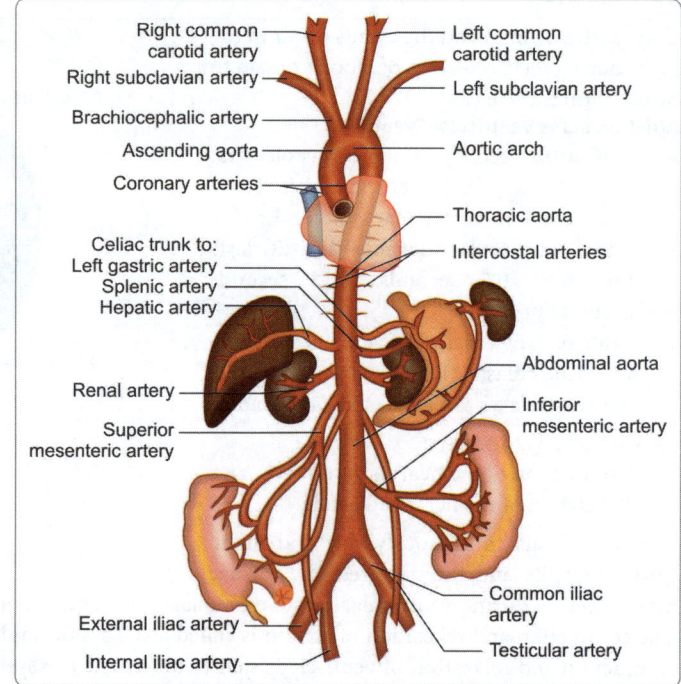

Figure 20: The aorta and its main branches

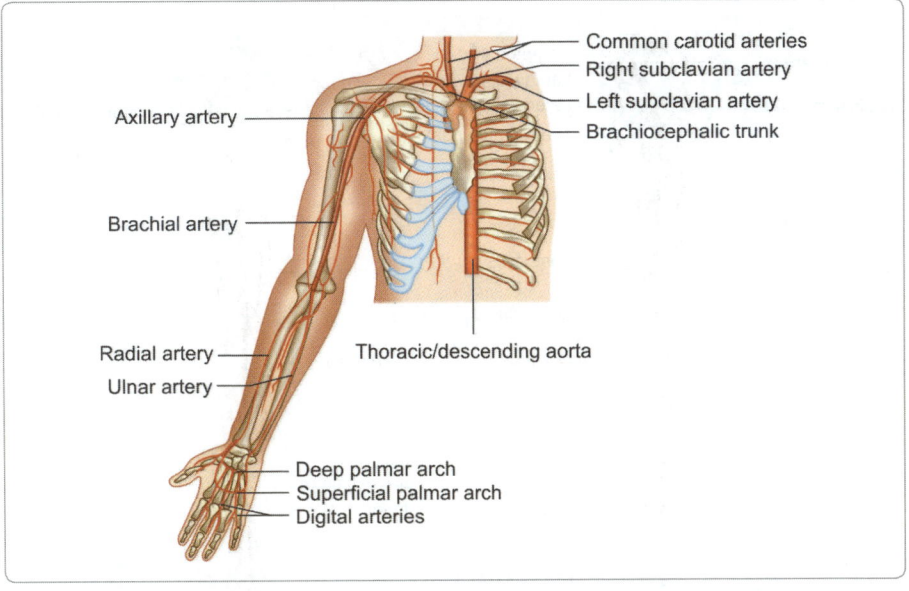

Figure 21: Main arteries of the upper limb

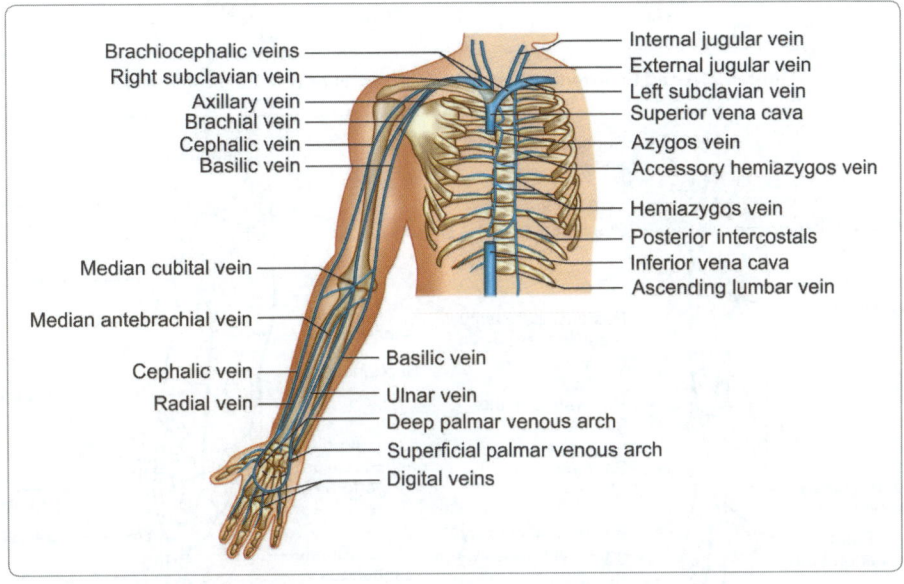

Figure 22: Superficial veins of the right upper limb

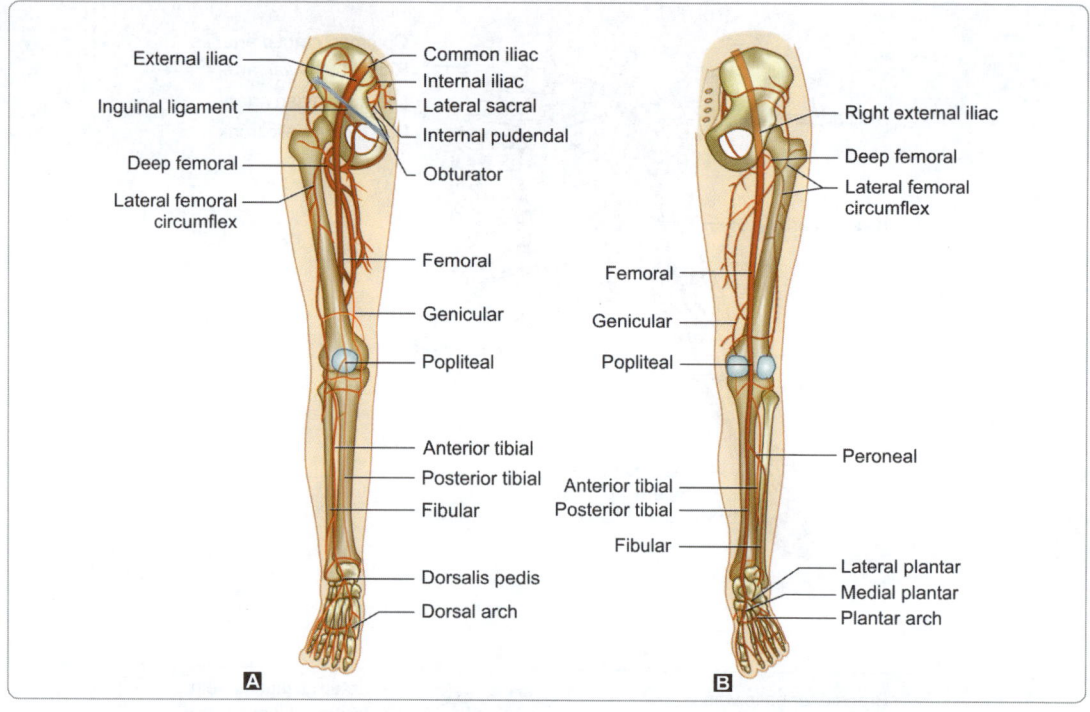

Figures 23A and B: Arteries of lower limb: (A) Anterior view; (B) Posterior view

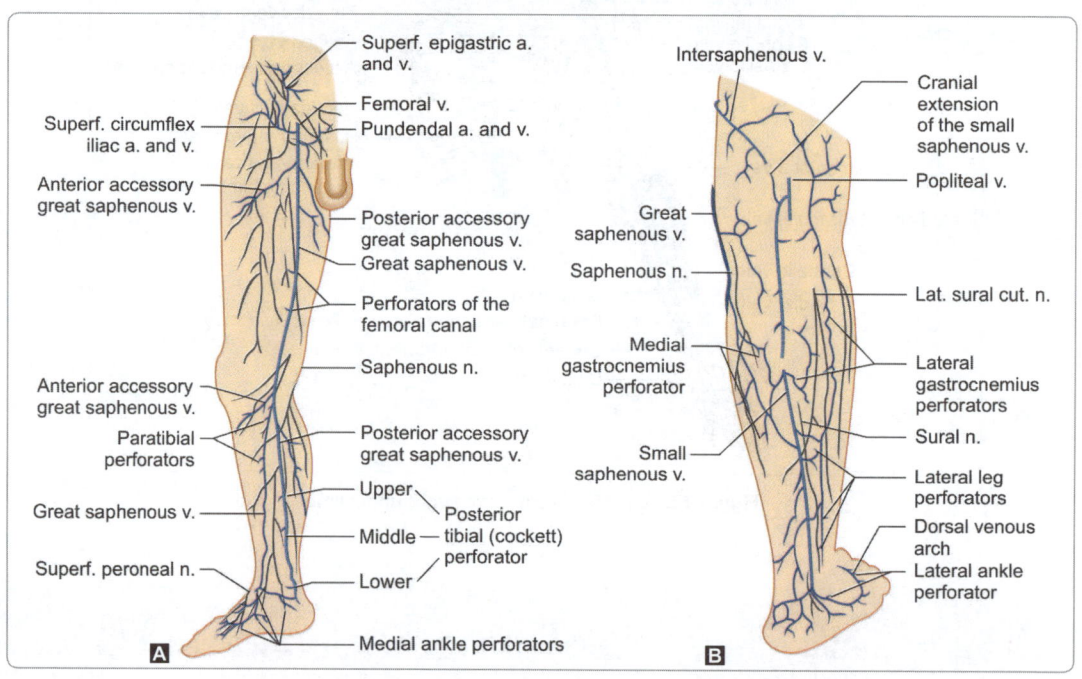

Figures 24A and B: Veins of lower limb: (A) Anterior view; (B) Posterior view

BLOOD

Blood is a fluid tissue composed of two parts. The fluid that occupies the intercellular substance is called plasma, in which the float formed elements are the blood cells or corpuscles. The total volume of blood forms about one-twelfth of the weight of the body or about five liters. About 55% is fluid and the remaining 45% is made up of blood cells. This figure is described as the hematocrit or packed cell volume, ranging from 40% to 47%.

Composition of Blood

Blood is a specialized body fluid. It has four main components as shown here in Figure 25.

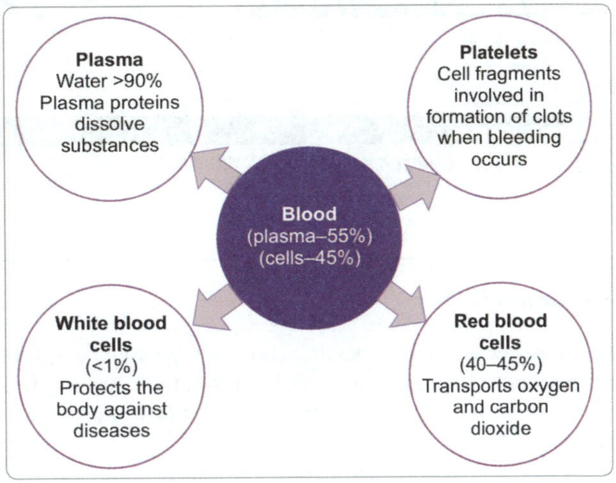

Plasma

Blood serum or plasma is made up of:

- Water 91%
- Protein 8% (albumin, globulin, prothrombin and fibrinogen)
- Salts 0.9% (sodium chloride, sodium bicarbonate, salts of calcium, phosphorus, magnesium and iron, etc.)
- Balance is made up of traces of a number of organic materials: glucose, fats, urea, uric acid, creatinine, cholesterol and amino acids.

Plasma also carries:

- Gases—Oxygen and carbon dioxide
- Internal secretions
- Enzymes and antigens

Figure 25: Components of blood

Blood Cells (Fig. 26)

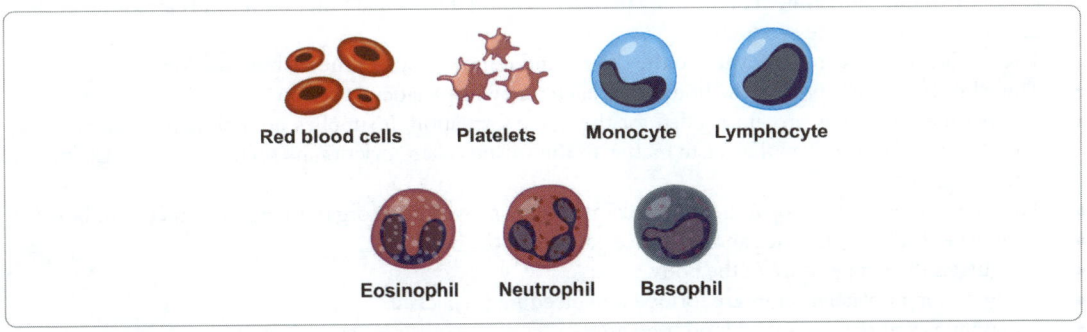

Figure 26: Different types of blood cells

Blood cells are of three types:

1. Erythrocytes or red cells
2. Leucocytes or white cells
3. Thrombocytes or platelets

Unit III ❖ Major Systems of the Human Body

FACTS

Summary of the number of blood cells in each cubic millimeter of blood:	
The normal blood count or the number of cells per cubic millimeter of blood is approximately:	
Red cells	4,500,000 to 5,500,000 (average 5,000,000)
White cells	6,000 to 10,000 (average 8,000)
Thrombocytes or platelets	250,000 to 500,000 (average 350,000)

White Blood cells include (differential count):

Granulocytes	Percent	Average percent
Neutrophil cells	60–70	65
Eosinophil cells	1–4	3
Basophil cells	½–2	1
Agranulocytes		
Lymphocytes (large and small)	20–30	25
Monocytes	4–8	5
Total		**100**

Functions of WBCs

As the result of the phagocytic action of the white cells, inflammation may be entirely arrested. When the activity does not proceed to complete resolution, pus may be formed.

(The numbers of the differential count of white cell may be seen with very little difference in different books.)

The nurse should have a good knowledge about the average blood count of a normal person in normal condition. It may be different in diseased conditions. Testing the blood for total and differential count is one of the first and important measures of diagnosing the disease. Changes in the numbers and types of count are considered as one of the best indicators of diagnosis and prognosis.

Functions of Blood

- It acts as the transport system of the body, conveying all chemical substances, oxygen and nutrients required for the nourishment of the body in order to fulfill the normal functioning and carry away carbon dioxide and other waste products.
- The red blood cells convey oxygen to the tissues and remove some of the carbon dioxide.
- The white blood cells protect the body from bacteria by its phagocytic action.
- The plasma distributes protein needed for the tissue formation. It supplies nourishment to all cells and acts as a vehicle to convey the waste matter to the various excretory organs such as skin, lungs, kidney, etc. for elimination.
- The internal secretions, hormones and enzymes are conveyed from organ to organ by means of blood.
- It regulates the water balance and acid base balance of the body.
- It regulates the temperature of the body.
- By the action of platelets clots are formed and bleeding is checked.
- It maintains and regulates the blood pressure.

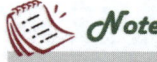 **Note**

Hemoglobin is a complex protein, rich in iron which gives the red color to the blood. It has an affinity for oxygen and combines with it forming oxyhemoglobin in red cells. By this function oxygen is carried to the tissues from the lungs.

Unit III ❖ Major Systems of the Human Body

Pregnant ladies and children need more hemoglobin in blood. In many forms of anemia, the amount of hemoglobin is diminished in blood. Anemia is of different types according to the deficiency of hemoglobin.

Blood Groups (Table 2)

Table 2: **Blood groups**

	Group A	Group B	Group AB	Group O
Red blood cell type	A	B	AB	O
Antibodies in plasma	Anti-B	Anti-A	None	Anti-A and Anti-B
Antigens in red blood cell	A Antigens	B Antigens	A and B Antigens	None

- The four main groups of blood are: AB, A, B and O. In considering the donors of blood, group 'O' can give blood to all people having other blood groups. So group 'O' is 'universal donor' for all groups'.
- As recipient, group 'AB' can receive blood from all other group. So group 'AB' is a universal recipient'.
- Usually, the blood of the same group is given to the patient and only in emergency the blood of a universal donor is given. It is important that before taking and administering blood to the patients, proper grouping and matching should be performed to prevent the complications.

LYMPHATIC SYSTEM

The lymphatic system is closely related to circulatory system. The blood leaves the heart by arteries and returned to heart by veins. Other fluids from capillaries are removed by the lymphatics by permeating the tissue space (Figs 27 to 29).

The parts of lymphatic system are:

- Lymphatic glands or nodes
- Lymphatic vessels
- Lymphatic ducts
- Lymphatic tissues and
- Lymphocytes (numerous white blood cells)

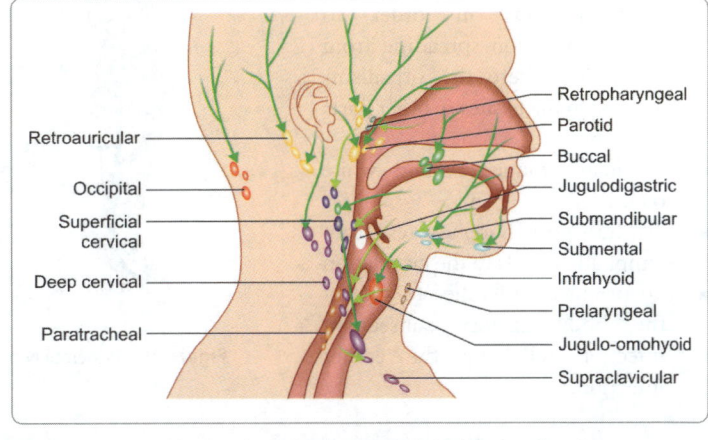

Figure 27: Lymphatic glands of the head and neck

Retroauricular

Occipital

Superficial cervical

Deep cervical

Paratracheal

Retropharyngeal

Parotid

Buccal

Jugulodigastric

Submandibular

Submental

Infrahyoid

Prelaryngeal

Jugulo-omohyoid

Supraclavicular

Unit III ❖ Major Systems of the Human Body

Organs of lymphatic system:

- **Spleen:** The major organ containing lymphoid tissue is spleen lying on the left side of the abdomen beneath the ninth, tenth and eleventh ribs, against the fundus of the stomach and its outer surface is in contact with the diaphragm.

  Other organs containing a large amount of lymphoid tissue are:

- **Tonsils** are situated one on each side of the pharynx in the neck.
- Villi of intestines in the abdomen.
- Payer's patches of the pancreas as solitary glands.

  Pancreas is 23 cm (7 inches) long situated in the abdomen extending from the duodenum to the spleen.

- Serous membranes like peritoneum which cover the abdomen contains numerous lymphatic nodes.

Function of lymphatics are:

- To return fluid and protein from the tissues to the circulation
- To carry emulsified fat from the intestines to the circulation
- To filter out and destroy microorganisms in order to prevent infection spreading from the point where the organisms entered in the tissues to other parts of the body
- To help produce certain white blood cells
- To transport lymphocytes from lymphatic glands to the circulation
- To produce antibodies to protect the body against subsequent infection following the earlier infection.

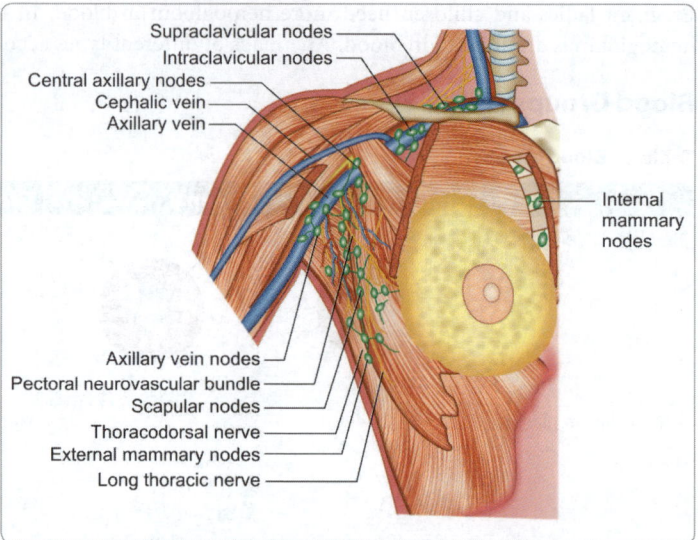

Figure 28: The Lymphatic drainage of right arm and breast

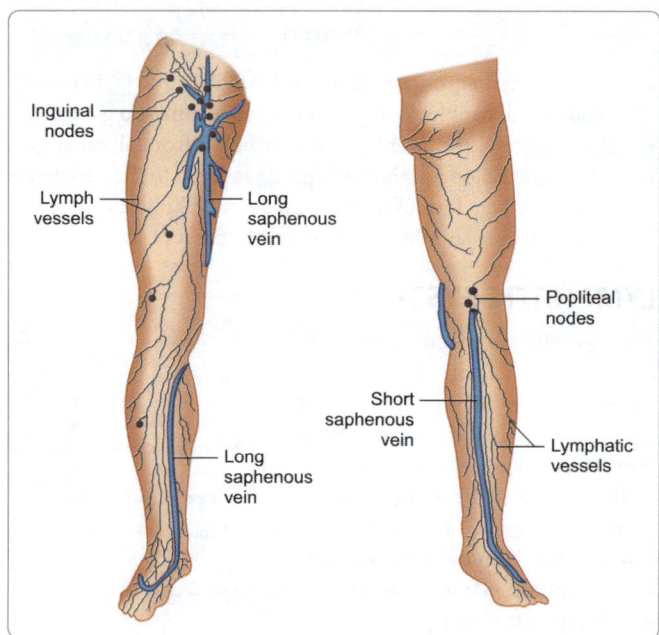

Figure 29: Principal lymphatic glands of the right lower limb

RESPIRATORY SYSTEM

Organs of respiratory system (Fig. 30) are:

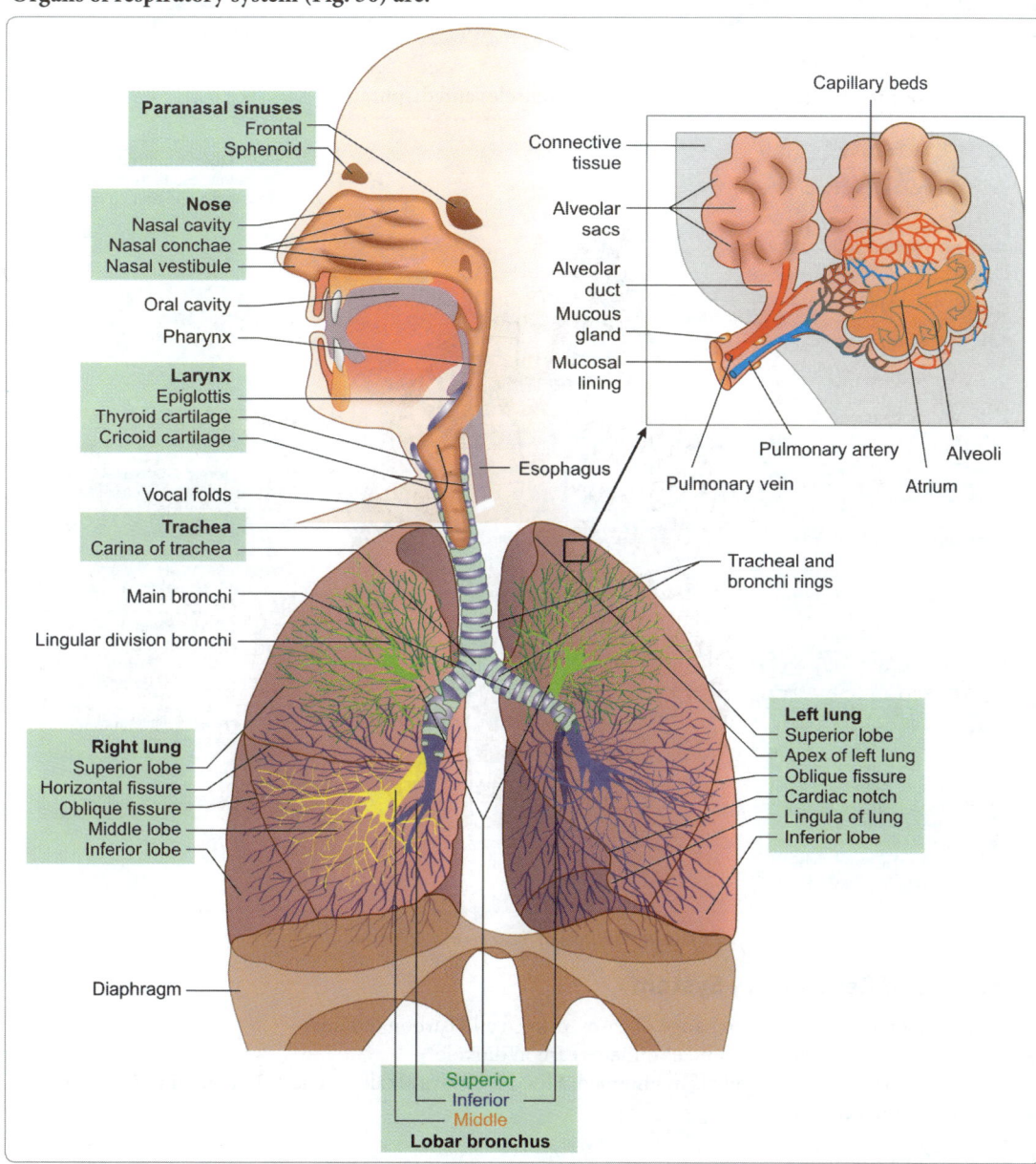

Figure 30: Organs of the respiratory system

Upper respiratory system:

- Nose and nasal cavities
- Pharynx

Lower respiratory system:

- Larynx
- Trachea
- Two bronchi
- Two lungs and their coverings—Pleura

Muscles of Respiration (Fig. 31)—The intercostal muscles and diaphragm

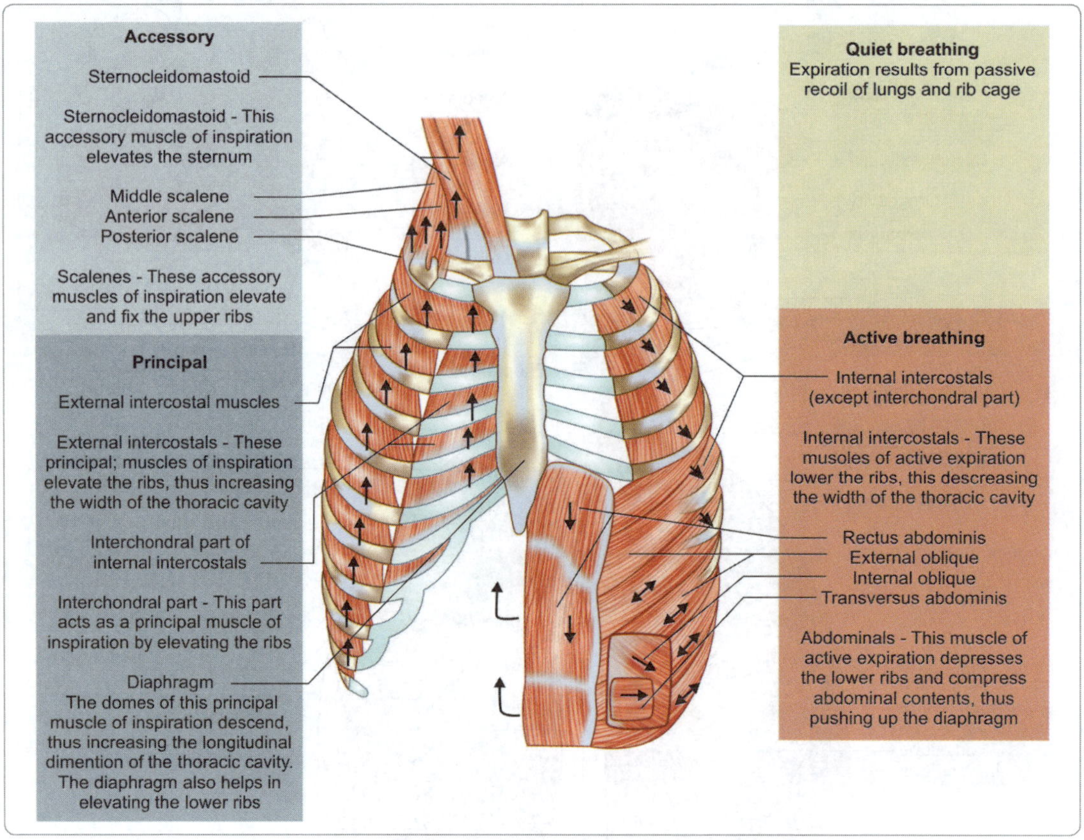

Accessory

Sternocleidomastoid

Sternocleidomastoid - This accessory muscle of inspiration elevates the sternum

Middle scalene
Anterior scalene
Posterior scalene

Scalenes - These accessory muscles of inspiration elevate and fix the upper ribs

Principal

External intercostal muscles

External intercostals - These principal; muscles of inspiration elevate the ribs, thus increasing the width of the thoracic cavity

Interchondral part of internal intercostals

Interchondral part - This part acts as a principal muscle of inspiration by elevating the ribs

Diaphragm
The domes of this principal muscle of inspiration descend, thus increasing the longitudinal dimention of the thoracic cavity. The diaphragm also helps in elevating the lower ribs

Quiet breathing
Expiration results from passive recoil of lungs and rib cage

Active breathing

Internal intercostals (except interchondral part)

Internal intercostals - These musoles of active expiration lower the ribs, this descreasing the width of the thoracic cavity

Rectus abdominis
External oblique
Internal oblique
Transversus abdominis

Abdominals - This muscle of active expiration depresses the lower ribs and compress abdominal contents, thus pushing up the diaphragm

Figure 31: Role of muscles in respiration

Functions of Respiratory System

The function of lungs is the interchange of gases, oxygen and carbon dioxide.

- Supplies oxygen to the body and eliminates carbon dioxide.
- Acid base balance of the body is maintained. Blood is always alkaline. The pH of blood is 7.35–7.45.
- Larynx produces voice.

 *Note*

The degree of alkalinity depends on the hydrogen-ion concentrations and this is expressed as PH of blood.
- The pH of 7 represents a neutral solution
- The pH from 1 to 7 is an acid solution
- The pH from 7 to 14 is an alkaline solution
Any change in the pH value of blood leads to certain diseases like acidosis and alkalosis.

The functions of respiratory system have been tabulated as follows:

Structure	Function
Nostril	It traps dust particles contained in the inhaled air from the atmosphere with the aid of the hairs in the nostril.
Nasal cavity	It is responsible for detecting smell. It also warms inhaled air and traps any microbes present in air with the help of its mucus living
Pharynx	It is lined with mucus and hairs which help to filter inhaled air
Trachea	It acts as a passage through which inhaled air gets to the lungs and exhaled air gets to the atmosphere lined with cilia and contains mucus secreting cells to filter air passing through it so as to protect the lungs. It is also called wind pipe
Lungs	They are the main organs for gaseous exchange which takes place in the alveoli
Larynx	Contains vocal cords, which vibrate to produce sound when one is speaking. It also lined with ciliated epithelium and mucus secreting cells which help to trap dust particles and microbes in the air.
Diaphragm	Relaxes and contracts to aid gas exchange during breathing.
Intercostal muscle	Regulates the variation of the movement of ribs to aid external respiration
Ribs	Protects the lungs and also aids in breathing
Bronchi	Strengthen by incomplete rings of cartilage to keep it open for passage of air in the alveoli

- Capacity of the lungs
  - The total capacity of the lungs is from 4500 mL to 5500 mL or 4%–5% liters of air.
  - **Vital capacity:**
    - The volume of air that can be respired by the lungs through the most forcible inspiration and expiration is termed as the vital capacity of the lungs.
    - It is measured by means of **spirometer.**
    - In normal man, it is 4–5 liters and in normal woman it is 3–4 liters.
    - The vital capacity is reduced in diseases of the lungs, heart and by weakness of the muscles of respiration.

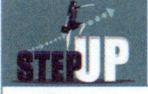

A normal adult has a vital capacity between 3 and 5 liters. The vital capacity depends on age, sex, height, mass, and may be on ethnicity.

The vital capacity represents the change in volume from completely emptied lungs to completely filled lungs. In human medicine, vital capacity is an important measure of a person's respiratory health.

DIGESTIVE SYSTEM

Parts of Digestive System (Fig. 32) are:
- Mouth including teeth, tongue and salivary glands
- Pharynx
- Esophagus—23–25 cm (9–10 inches) long
- Stomach
- Small intestine is about 2–4 m (8 feet) long in living condition. The usual figure of 6 meters (20 feet) is a postmortem finding when the muscle tone is lost. It has been divided into three parts—duodenum, jejunum and ileum.

- The large intestine or colon comes after small intestine about 1.5 m (5 feet) long and it starts from the place where the small intestine ends. It is divided into cecum, ascending colon, transverse colon, descending colon and sigmoid colon.
- Rectum is last part of large intestines. It is 13 cm (5 inches) long.
- The lowest part is anus, which is about 4 cm (1 inch) long.

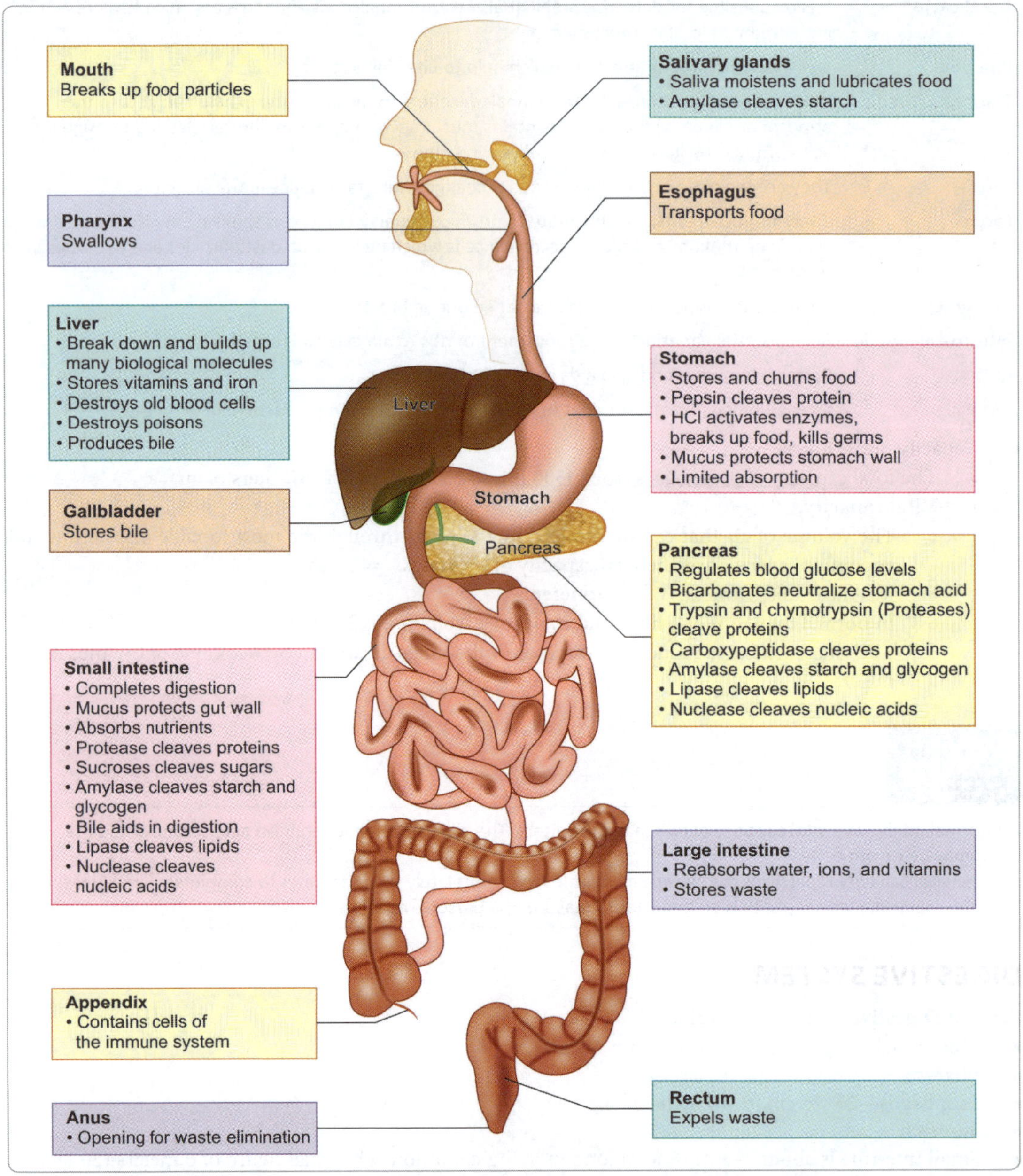

Mouth
Breaks up food particles

Salivary glands
• Saliva moistens and lubricates food
• Amylase cleaves starch

Esophagus
Transports food

Pharynx
Swallows

Liver
• Break down and builds up many biological molecules
• Stores vitamins and iron
• Destroys old blood cells
• Destroys poisons
• Produces bile

Stomach
• Stores and churns food
• Pepsin cleaves protein
• HCl activates enzymes, breaks up food, kills germs
• Mucus protects stomach wall
• Limited absorption

Gallbladder
Stores bile

Pancreas
• Regulates blood glucose levels
• Bicarbonates neutralize stomach acid
• Trypsin and chymotrypsin (Proteases) cleave proteins
• Carboxypeptidase cleaves proteins
• Amylase cleaves starch and glycogen
• Lipase cleaves lipids
• Nuclease cleaves nucleic acids

Small intestine
• Completes digestion
• Mucus protects gut wall
• Absorbs nutrients
• Protease cleaves proteins
• Sucroses cleaves sugars
• Amylase cleaves starch and glycogen
• Bile aids in digestion
• Lipase cleaves lipids
• Nuclease cleaves nucleic acids

Large intestine
• Reabsorbs water, ions, and vitamins
• Stores waste

Appendix
• Contains cells of the immune system

Anus
• Opening for waste elimination

Rectum
Expels waste

Liver   Stomach   Pancreas

Figure 32: Digestive tract

Unit III ❖ Major Systems of the Human Body

The accessary organs of digestion are:

- Salivary glands
- Liver
- Gallbladder
- Pancreas

Functions of Digestive System are:

- Digestion
- Absorption (assimilation)
- Elimination

Digestive system deals with the reception of food and with the preparation of it for assimilation by the body and elimination of waste products of digestion.

URINARY SYSTEM

Organs of urinary system (Fig. 33) are:

- **Kidneys 2,** which secrete urine
- **Ureters 2,** which convey urine from kidneys to bladder
- **Urinary bladder 1,** which acts as a reservoir
- **Urethra 1,** for discharges of urine from bladder

Functions of Urinary System

- Regulation of water balance in the body
- Regulation of concentration of salts in the blood
- Regulation of the reaction (acid base balance) of the blood
- Excretion of waste products and any excess of salt from the body

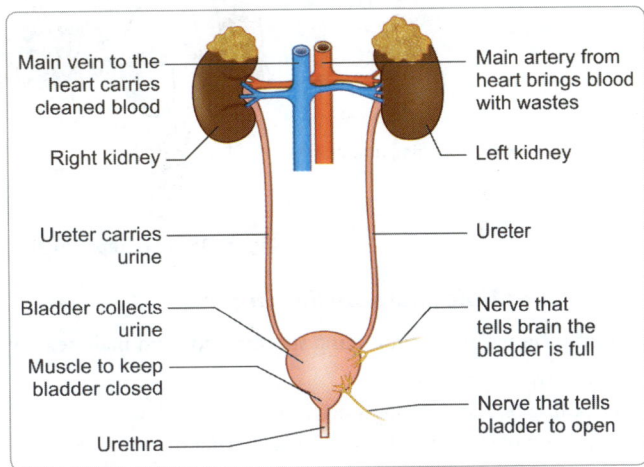

Figure 33: Parts and functions of urinary system

The functions of the kidneys are simple infiltration, selective reabsorption and secretion of urine.

REPRODUCTIVE SYSTEM

Male Reproductive System

Parts of Male Reproductive System

Organs of reproduction in males (Fig. 34) are:

- **Testes:** These are a pair of sperm-producing organs that maintain the health of the male reproductive system. The testes are known as gonads. It is the male organ, where spermatozoa and male sex hormone testosterone are produced. Testis lies in the scrotum.
- **Epididymis:** It is a small organ lying behind testis and attached to it.
- **Vas deferens:** It is a duct passing from the lower aspect of the epididymis.
- **Prostate glands:** It lies below the bladder, surrounding the urethra and is composed of glands, ducts and involuntary muscles.
- **Scrotum:** It is a pouch-like structure composed of skin devoid of subcutaneous fat; it contains a little muscular tissue. Testis lies in the scrotum.

- **Penis:** It is composed of spongy tissue and is expanded to form the glans penis at the part where the urethra opens. The male urethra is 17–23 cm (7–9 inches) long.

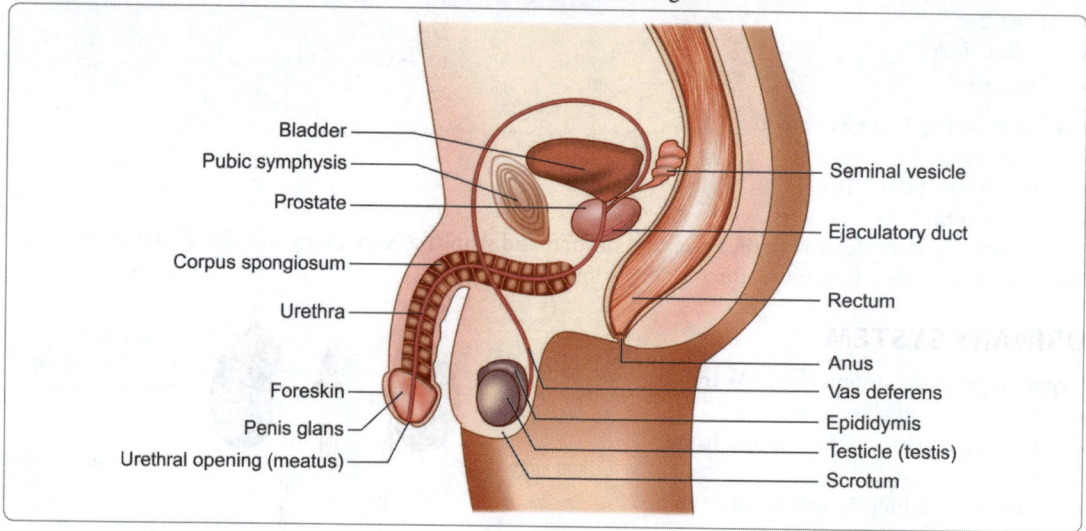

Figure 34: Male reproductive organs

Functions of Male Reproductive Organ

Reproduction: Organs producing spermatozoa and male sex hormone that is testosterone.

Penis has two functions:
1. Voiding of urine through urethra.
2. Ejection of semen which contains spermatozoa.

Female Reproductive System

Parts of Female Reproductive System

Organs of reproduction in females (Fig. 35) are:
The organs of generation in females may be divided into external organs and internal organs.

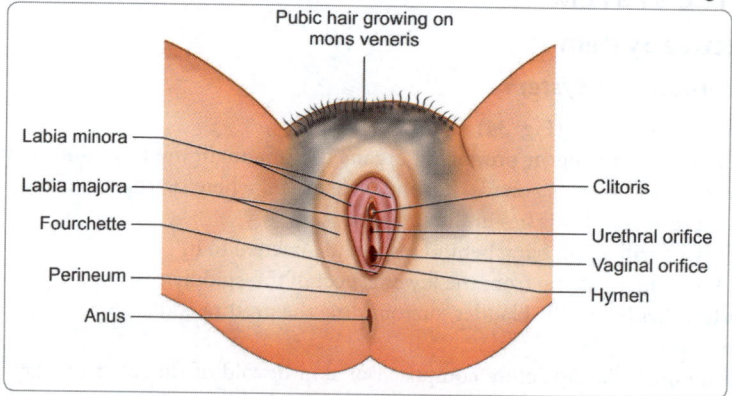

Figure 35: A diagram showing female external genitalia

External Organs

The external organs are collectively known as vulva and are comprised of the following parts:

- **The mons veneris:** It is a pad of fat lying in front of the symphysis pubis, it gets covered with hair at puberty.
- **The labia majora:** These two thick folds form the sides of the vulva. The length of labia majora is about 7.5 cm (3 inches).
- **The nymphae or labia minora:** These are two small folds of skin situated between the upper parts of labia majora.
- **The clitoris:** It is a small erectile body which corresponds with the penis in male.
- **The vestibule:** It is limited on either sides by the labial folds and leads to vagina. The urethra also opens into the vestibule in front of the vagina just behind the clitoris.
- **The hymen:** It is a thin membranous diaphragm which is perforated centrally to allow the menstrual discharge to drain away. It is situated at the orifice of the vagina thus separating the external and internal genitals.
- **The vagina:** It is a muscular tube, lined with membrane composed of special type of stratified epithelium rich in blood vessels and nerves. The vagina is in relation with the base of the bladder and urethra anteriorly and with rectum posteriorly.

Internal Organ

The internal generative organs of reproduction are situated in the pelvis namely the uterus, ovaries and uterine (fallopian) tubes.

- **The uterus:** It is a thick muscular pear-shaped organ in the pelvis. Uterus is 5–8 cm (2–3 inches) long and weighs 30–60 g (1–2 oz). It is situated between the rectum posteriorly and the bladder anteriorly.
- **The ovaries:** They are two almond-shaped glands placed one in each side of the uterus, just below the fallopian tubes (uterine tubes).
- **The uterine tubes (fallopian tubes):** They pass one on each side from the upper angles of the uterus outwards, below the uterine tubes, attached to the back of the broad ligament, toward the sides of the pelvis. They are about 3 cm long 2 cm wide and 1 cm thick and their uterine ends are narrow. The other end is bend downwards to form a fimbriated margin (Fig. 36).

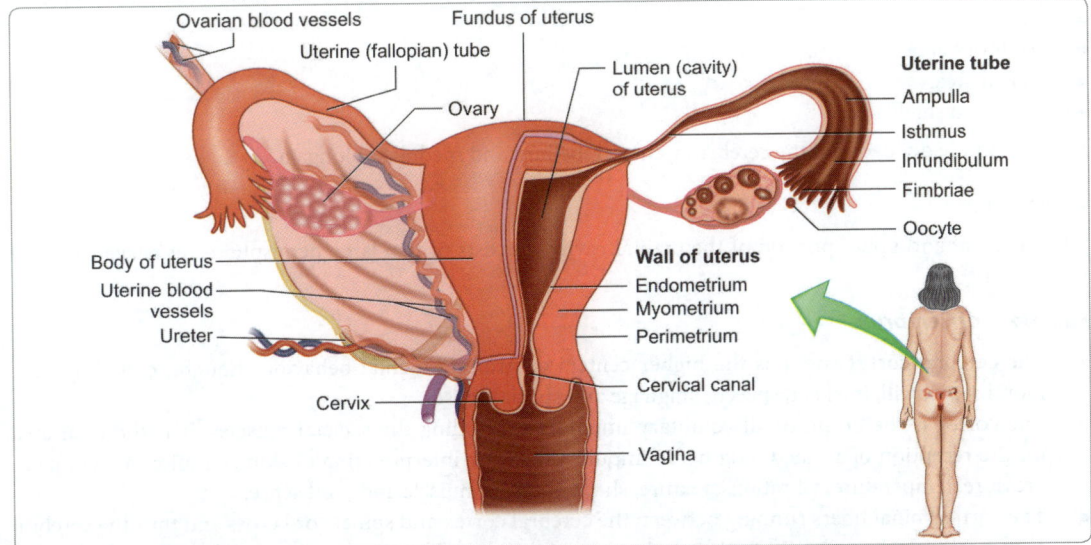

Figure 36: Female reproductive system showing escape of an ovum from the ovary

Unit III ❖ Major Systems of the Human Body

Function

Reproducing and sustaining human species.

The Mammary Glands (Breasts)

- The mammary glands or breasts are accessory female reproductive organs. They secrete milk.
- Lactation or the secretion of milk and its discharge from the breast during suckling is the function of breast.

NERVOUS SYSTEM

Nervous system includes central or cerebrospinal nervous system and autonomic nervous system (sympathetic and parasympathetic nerves).

- **Central nervous system** includes brain, spinal cord and the nerves given off from these – the peripheral nerves. This group is also called cerebrospinal nervous system.
- **Autonomic nervous system** consists of sympathetic and parasympathetic nerves.

    To study the functions of nervous system in detail, one has to learn about the nerves in its entirety. Some valuable information is given about the nervous system in the following section.

Central Nervous System

Brain

The brain lies within the cranial cavity of the skull. It develops from a single tube which initially shows three enlargements, the fore-runners of the brain, forebrain, mid-brain and hindbrain. Brain is divided into: cerebrum, the brain stem, and the cerebellum

- Forebrain is called cerebrum and thalamus.
- Midbrain is also called mesencephalon
- Hindbrain is called pons, medulla oblongata (brain stem) and cerebellum.

There are different areas in the brain to control the functions of different organs in the body. For example:

- Sensory area
- Auditory area
- Visual area
- Taste and smell area

Brain is mainly divided into the cerebrum, the cerebellum and medulla oblongata.

Cerebrum

Fills the front and upper portion of the cranial cavity, consists of two large hemispheres of nerve cells and nerve fibers.

Functions of Cerebrum

- The cerebral cortex contains the higher centers controlling mental behavior, thought, consciousness, moral sense, will, intellect, speech, language and special senses.
- The cortex is the origin of all voluntary impulses controlling the skeletal muscles. It is the final area for the reception of all incoming nerve impulses for their interpretation of skin sensation, touch, pain, pressure, temperature, vibrations, texture, shape and size, muscle and joint sense.
- The corticospinal fibers running between the cerebral cortex and spinal cord cross and thus the cerebral cortex controls the movements of opposite sides of the body. The sensory cortex of the right side controls the movements of left side and the sensory cortex of the left side controls the movement of the right side.

Cerebellum

Is the largest portion of the hind-brain, occupies the posterior cranial fossa.

Functions of Cerebellum

- Regulates posture and postural activities, muscular coordination and maintenance of balance.

Medulla Oblongata

Forms the lower portion of the brain stem linking the pons and joins the spinal cord (Fig. 37).

Functions of the Medulla Oblongata

- It contains certain vital centers which control respiration and cardiovascular system. Injury to this part of the brain stem is liable to have serious consequences.

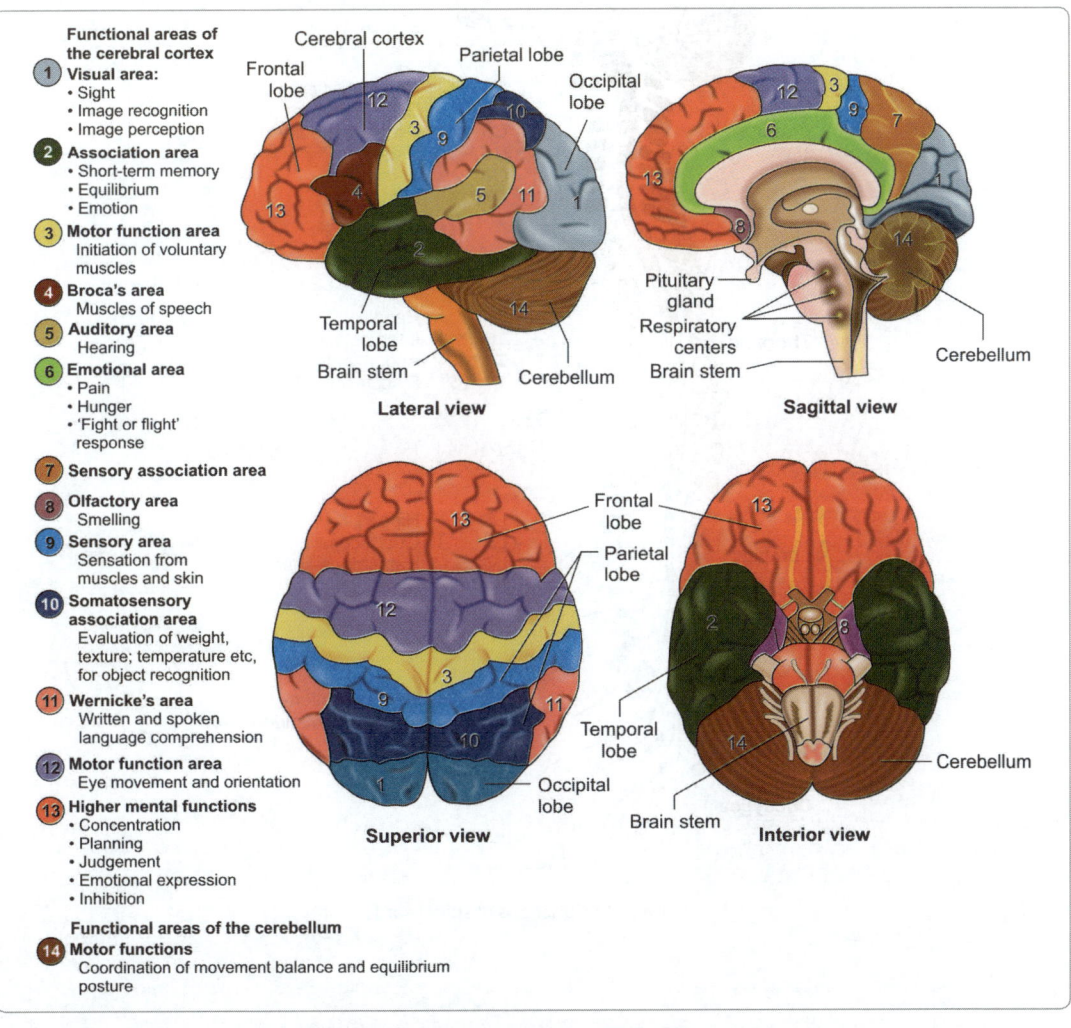

Figure 37: Anatomy and functional areas of brain

Spinal Cord

Begins at medulla oblongata and ends between the first and second lumbar vertebrae.

Functions of spinal cord are (Fig. 38):

- Communication between brain and all parts of the body
- Reflex action stimulation by external environment and responding.

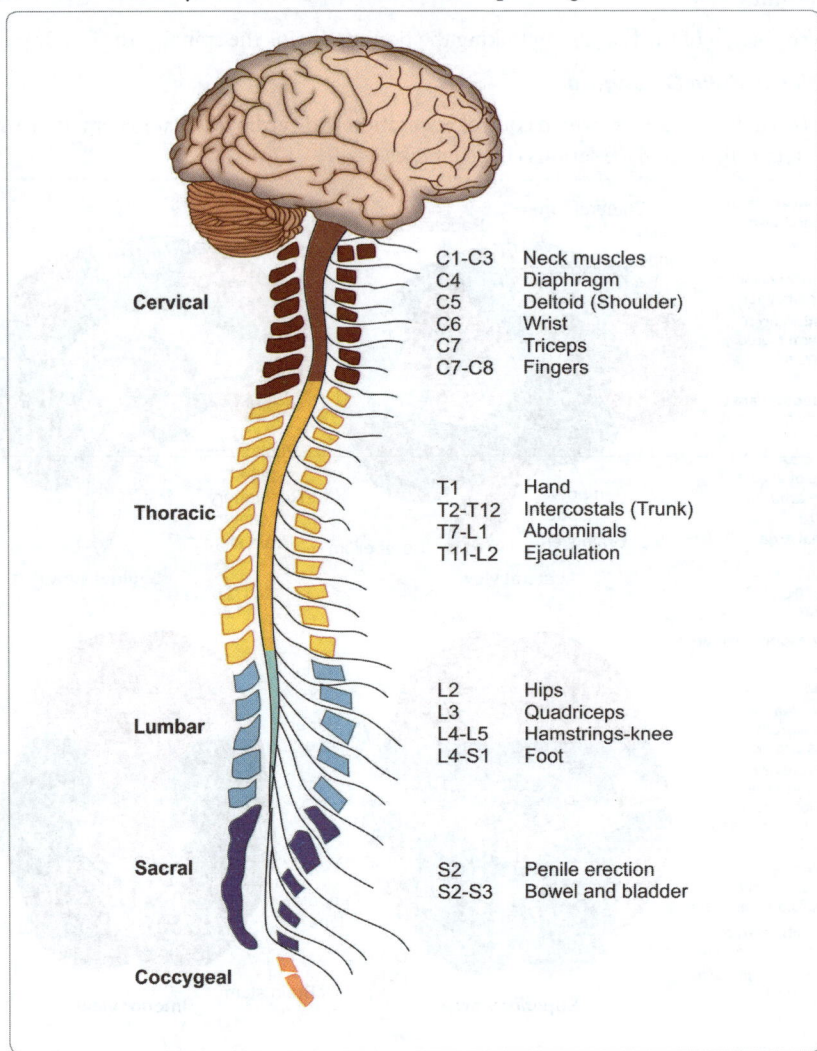

Figure 38: Functions of spinal cord

Nerves

The nerve trunk is formed by many nerve fibers. These nerve fibers are capable of recognizing, receiving and responding the physical, chemical, mechanical and electrical stimulations of inside and outside of the body. This quality is called the conductivity and excitability of the nerves.

There are separate nerves for functioning of the organs in the body. In total, 12 pairs of cranial nerves are present in the body.

Functions of Nerves

- The functions of the body are controlled by nerves. The functions carried by nerves have been listed in the table as follows:

	Name	Nerve type	Function
I	Olfactory	Sensory	Smell
II	Optic	Sensory	Vision
III	Oculomotor	Motor	Most eye movement
IV	Trochlear	Motor	Moves eye
V	Trigeminal	Both	Face sensation, mastication
VI	Abducens	Motor	Abducts the eye
VII	Facial	Both	Facial expression, taste
VIII	Vestibulocochlear	Sensory	Hearing, balance
IX	Glossopharyngeal	Both	Taste, gag reflex
X	Vagus	Both	Gag reflex, parasympathetic innervation
XI	Accessory	Motor	Shoulder shrug
XII	Hypoglossal	Motor	Swallowing, speech

- The nerve fibers possess the power of conductivity and excitability. It is capable of receiving and responding to stimuli from some outside agent. For example, the stimulus may be mechanical, electrical, chemical or physical. This gives rise to an impulse which is conducted along the nerve fibers.

SPECIAL SENSE ORGANS

The main sense organs are:
- Tongue
- Nose
- Eyes
- Ears
- Skin (it is another sense organ which is already explained as the integumentary system). Others are sense organs for the reception of certain kinds of stimuli.

Unit III ❖ Major Systems of the Human Body

Tongue

It is placed in the mouth. It has many taste buds so that we can recognize the taste of items which we put in the mouth. It also recognizes the heat and cold on touch. There are four true sensations of tastes: sweet, bitter, sour and salty. Tongue is capable of larger movements such as forming an important part of mastication and swallowing. It is needed for speaking as well (Fig. 39).

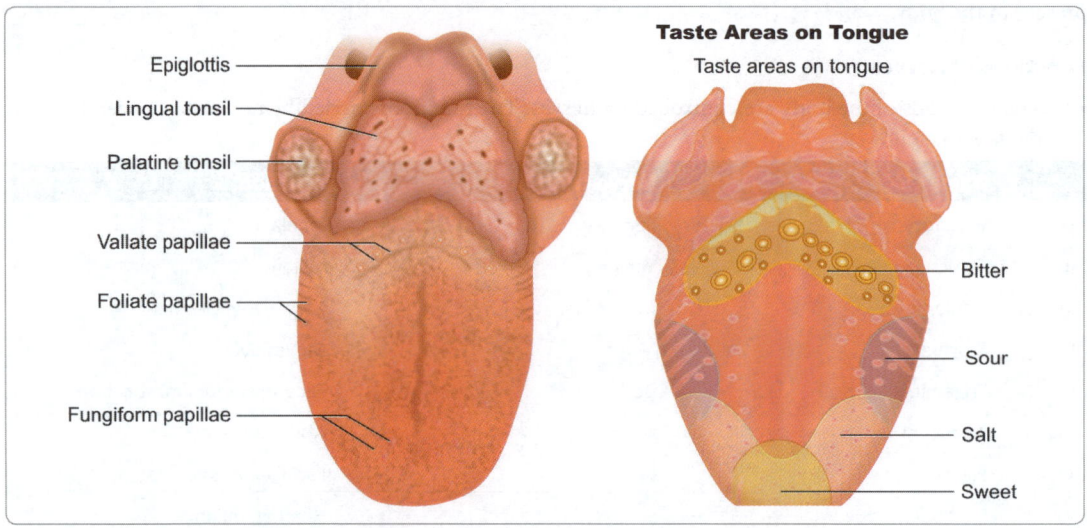

Figure 39: Tongue

Nose

It is placed in the middle of the face. It has two nasal cavities. Nose is required for breathing and to recognize the smell by the action of olfactory nerves. The sense of smell is stimulated by gases inhaled or by small particles of anything. Nose is a part of respiratory organ (Fig. 40).

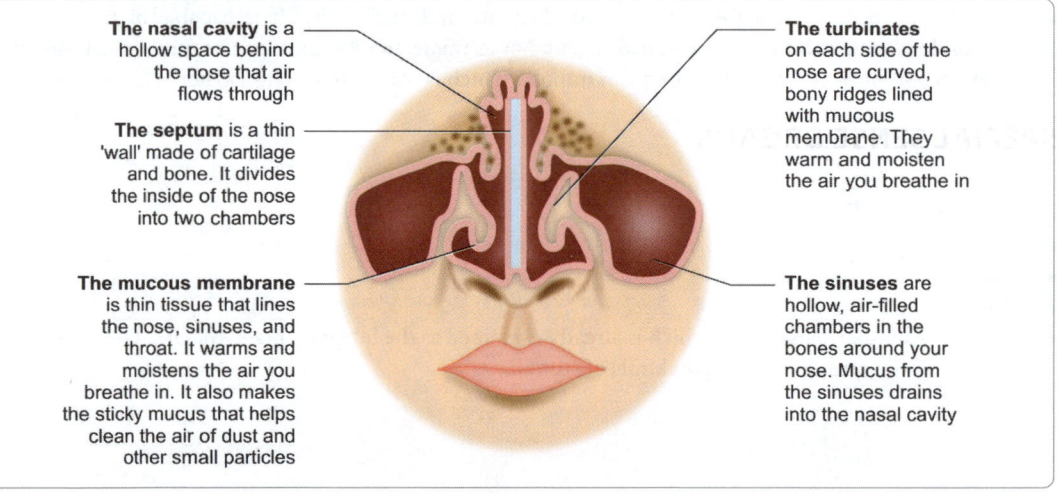

Figure 40: Anatomy and functions of nose

Eyes

- It is situated in the upper part of the face on both sides, in the orbital cavity. It is the organ of sight. It is described as a globe or sphere, but it is oval and not circular, about an inch in diameter, transparent in front.
- These are the special organs of sight (Fig. 41).

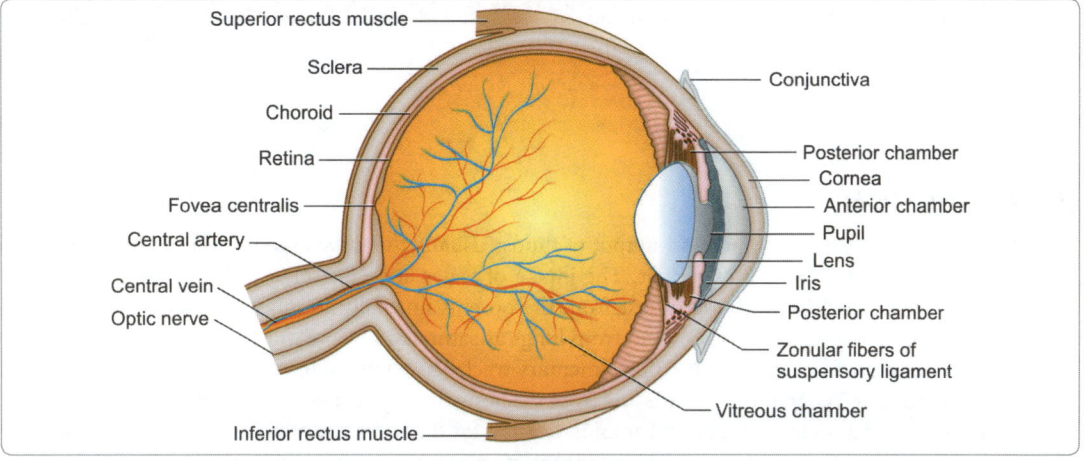

Figure 41: Anatomy of eye

Ears

These are the special sense organs of hearing placed in either sides of the skull, behind and near the face. It serves as the organ of hearing. It is the important organ for maintaining the equilibrium of the body (Fig. 42).

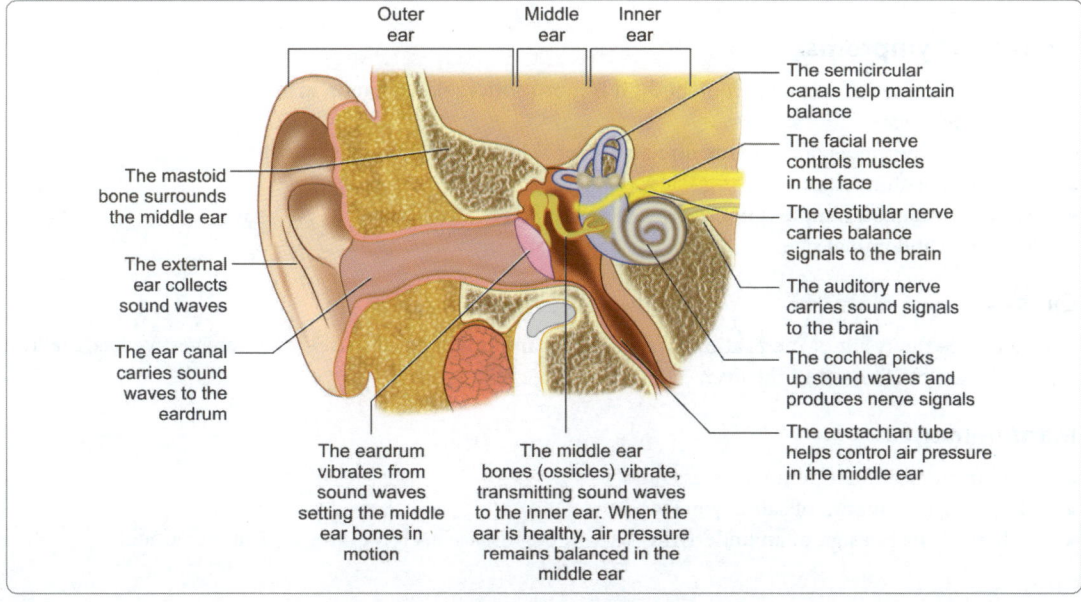

Figure 42: Anatomy and functions of ear

Unit III ❖ Major Systems of the Human Body

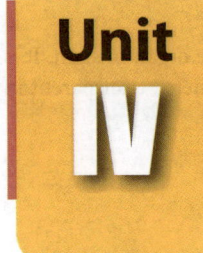

Fluid and Electrolyte Balance

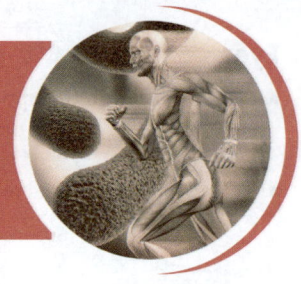

INTRODUCTION

Fluid balance is the balance of input and output of fluids. Usually the same amount of fluid taken as input, into the body is excreted from it as output. The intake of water and electrolytes in the body is usually as water, as other fluids and in food. Water lost from the body is normally from kidneys as urine, from skin as sweat, from alimentary canal as stools and from lungs as saturated air (breathed out). Electrolytes are lost from the body in urine, from the skin and the alimentary tract. The ability of the body to maintain electrolytic balance is only natural. When more water is lost from the body through urine, sweat, vomitus or diarrhea, the body needs increased amount of water and as an indication for the need, the patient feels more thirsty.

Managing patient's fluid and electrolyte balance is of great importance as either excess fluid (edema) or depletion (dehydration) can have serious consequences.

EDEMA

Edema is retention of fluid and salt in the tissues which may also is an abnormal condition which needs immediate medical attention.

Signs and Symptoms

Although edema can affect any part of body, it is more noticeable on hands, arms, feet, ankles and legs.
Signs are as follows:

- Swelling or puffiness of the tissue directly under skin, especially in legs or arms
- Stretched or shiny skin
- Skin that retains a dimple (pits), when pressed for a few seconds
- Increased abdominal size

Causes

Edema can be the result of medication, pregnancy or an underlying disease—often congestive heart failure, kidney disease or cirrhosis of the liver.

Management

- Taking medication to remove excess fluid
- Reducing the amount of salt in your food
- When edema is a sign of an underlying disease, the disease itself requires separate treatment.

DEHYDRATION

This condition can occur in the following two ways:

1. It may be due to too much loss of water by vomiting, diarrhea, bleeding, excess sweating, etc.
2. It may also occur in infants, helpless people, particularly the elderly and in unconscious patient who are not given enough water.

Signs and Symptoms

- Shrinking of the skin and tissues
- Faintness
- Loss of blood pressure
- Muscular weakness
- Sometime the patient may not feel thirsty, but tongue and lips become dry and coated.
- Patient may be emaciated and restless.

Management

- Inform the doctor immediately.
- Administer fluids by mouth if not contraindicated.
- If oral administration of fluid is possible, give oral rehydration salt, fluids which contain enough electrolytes and it is a readymade preparation in powder form with instructions on the packet to prepare. After consulting the doctor, instructions are carried out promptly. If immediate steps are not taken in dehydration, the patient may reach a condition called **shock**.

Shock

Shock is a disproportion of blood in the cardiovascular system and peripheral circulation. It is a condition which may lead to the slowing of the function of the heart, if not treated as an emergency. The causes of shock may be many such as dehydration, electric shock, damage to the brain, severe bleeding, salt depletion, strong emotions like fear, sudden injury or witnessing an injury or accident, etc. Whatever is the cause, shock is a medical emergency.

Signs and Symptoms

Rapid and weak pulse, skin clammy, the volume of circulating blood is decreased and blood pressure becomes low, fainting, weakness, restlessness lead to unconsciousness. The most common causes are severe bleeding and salt depletion.

Management

- Lay the person down, if possible
- Begin cardiopulmonary resuscitation (CPR), if necessary
- Treat obvious injuries
- Keep person warm and comfortable

ORAL REHYDRATION SOLUTION

A packet of powder prepared with special ingredients to use in emergency to save the life is called oral rehydration solution (ORS) packet. Infants or children suffering from moderate fever, vomiting or diarrhea

Unit IV ❖ Fluid and Electrolyte Balance

may be getting better only with the administration of ORS without much treatment. If we think that medical treatment is necessary even after the administration of ORS, medical advice should be resorted to.

Contents

Oral rehydration solution helps to prevent the further damages and save the patient. ORS contains:

Sodium chloride	3.5 g
Sodium bicarbonate	2.5 g
Potassium chloride	1.5 g
Glucose/dextrose	20 g
Boiled and cooled water	1 L

Oral rehydration mixture is readily and freely available in health centers. In case of difficulties, homemade oral fluids can be prepared by adding fistful of sugar and a teaspoonful of salt to one liter of boiled and cooled water.

In severe cases, when the patient goes into coma or shock, intravenous rehydration is administered till the patient is able to take oral rehydration fluid.

Stimulant

Oral rehydration therapy (ORT) does not stop diarrhea, but it replaces the lost fluids and essential salts thereby preventing or treating dehydration and reducing the danger. The glucose contained in ORS solution enables the intestine to absorb the fluid and the salts more efficiently.

Guidelines for Oral Rehydration

Degree of dehydration	Volume of fluid to be given per kg of body weight	Time of administration
Mild dehydration Patient: Thirsty Pulse: Normal Tongue: Moist	50 mL/kg of body weight	Within 4 hours
Moderate dehydration Patient: Thirsty Pulse: Rapid and weak Eyes: Sunken Tongue: Dry	100 mL/kg of body weight	Within 4 hours

Preparation of Solution from ORS Packet

Packets are available in different measurements. Certain packets should be mixed completely in measured amount of clean or sterile water. In some other packets there will be measuring spoons to take the powder for the mentioned amount of water. In preparing the mixture, the instructions given on the packet should be followed.

The instructions given on the cover of the packet should be considered.

- Take 5 glasses (1 L) of sterile water (water boiled and cooled) in a clean big vessel.
- Put the whole powder of one packet.
- Mix it with a spoon till it is dissolved in the water.

- Give to the patient one cup at a time to drink. For children, amount should be reduced each time. Depending upon the thirst and need, the amount can be increased gradually.
- Balance of solution should be kept covered in the same vessel for the day. Balance should not be used on the next day. If it has to be given on the next day new solution should be prepared.

Home Made ORS Preparation

Another type of solution, which can be prepared in home situation when ORS packet is not easily available: A nurse can try to save the life of a patient in home situation, to a certain extent, when ORS packet is not easily available.

- Take drinking water in a glass (200 mL)
- Put a pinch of common salt (sodium chloride) with the thumb and index finger in the water and stir it slowly till it is dissolved (powder the salt if it is big crystals)
- Taste the solution. It should be less salty in taste than our tears. If we feel it is more than that, leave it and prepare another glass of it.
- Put one teaspoon full of sugar in it and dissolve. If sugar is not available jaggery can be used.
- If teaspoon is not available the sugar can be measured with the four fingers of the hand holding together to put in the prepared salt solution in the glass.
- Stir it till the sugar is completely dissolved.
- Give the solution to the patient to drink depending upon the thirst and need. For children, the amount given should be small and increased gradually. For moderate vomiting or diarrhea, this solution can be given in between.

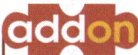

Our body fluids contain minerals like sodium chloride and potassium, etc. So when the fluids and electrolytes are lost by vomiting or diarrhea, such solutions are very useful to replace the lost fluids and salts. Such fluids may not cure the disease but it will help to replace the lost materials in the body. The replacement of the lost fluids and salt in children will help to prevent the weakness. If the child requests for more water to drink, it indicates that more water is needed in the body. So to prevent the loss of fluids and salts in the body, such solutions are helpful. For further treatment medical advice should be resorted to.

NOTES

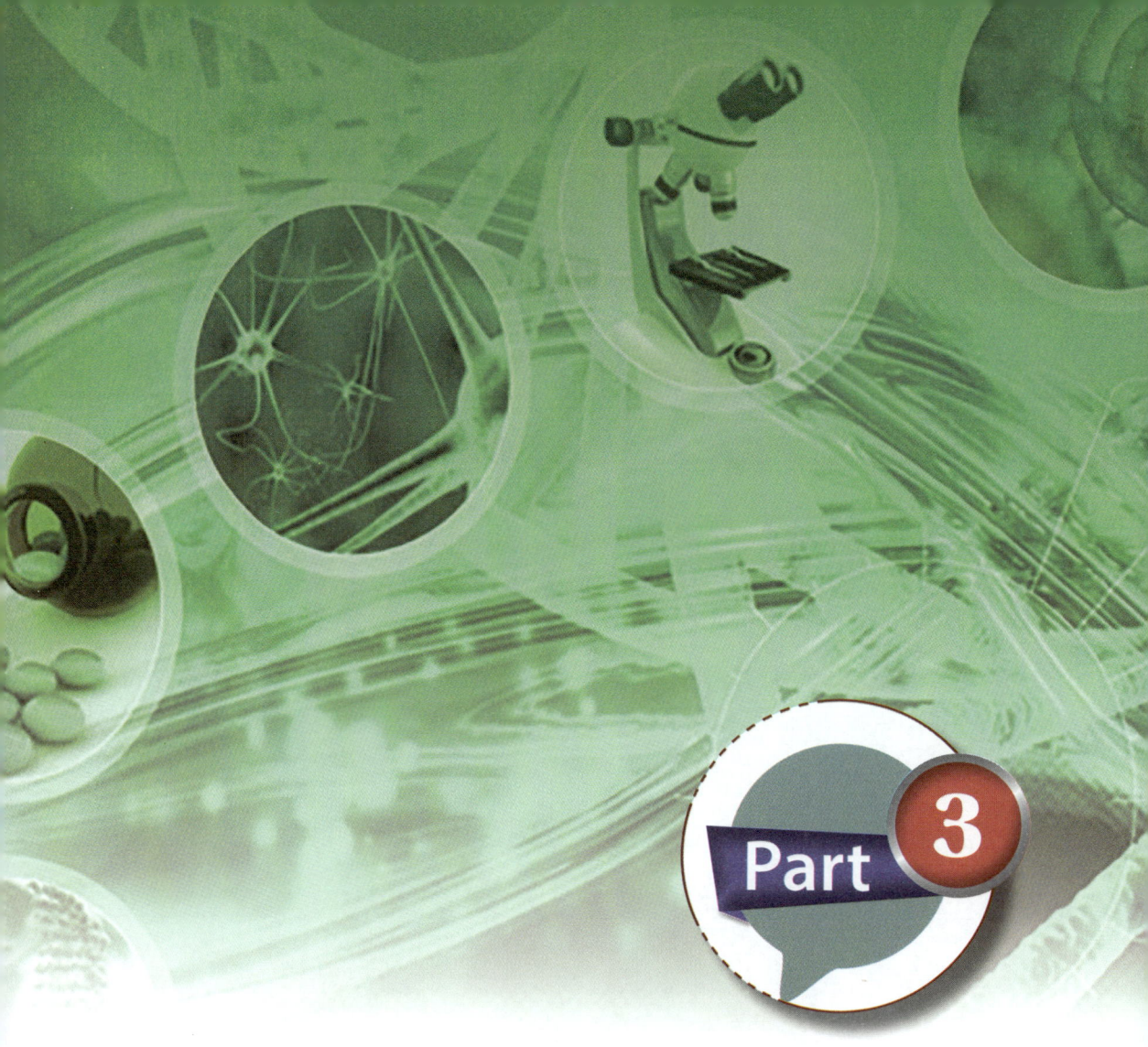

Part 3

Microbiology

Part Outline

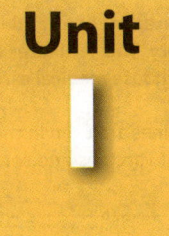

Unit
I
Introduction

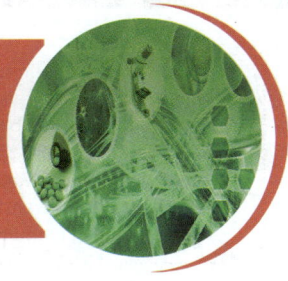

DEFINITION

Microbiology has been defined as the study of living organisms which are so minute that they can be seen only with the aid of a microscope. The basic principles of several nursing procedures are drawn from the science of microbiology. The knowledge of microbiology is of great value to every person because of the simple fact that even ordinary rules of cleanliness and hygiene are based on it. Microorganisms are of many diseases in human body. To prevent the spread of infection from the patient to the nurse and vice versa, all preventive measures are to be practiced by the nurse.

APPLICATION OF MICROBIOLOGY IN NURSING

In order to see how microbiology affects the practice of nursing and to get an insight into the study of the subject, few nursing situations are presented below. Each situation involves one or more basic principles of microbiology.

- The nurse washes her hands before and after doing any nursing procedures and before attending another patient.
- A clinical thermometer used for one patient should be disinfected before being used for a second patient or to the same patient again.
- Instruments and dressings required for surgical procedures are sterilized and kept sterile in suitable containers.
- Patients with communicable disease are isolated and precautions are taken to prevent the spread of infection to the nurse herself and others.
- Drinking water should be boiled and cooled before use whenever it is possible.

 Stimulant

The knowledge of microbiology helps the nurse in different ways to do her work properly. These are mentioned as follows:
- She learns how pathogenic organisms enter the body and how they are discharged from the body and how they spread from person to person. This knowledge further helps in controlling the spread of infection in surroundings.
- She understands the principles of using disinfectants and the action of certain drugs on microorganisms. This helps in applying aseptic rules in surgery and patient care.

Contd...

- She recognizes the importance of the proper collection of specimens for bacteriological examinations and is able to understand the deviations from normal, in the reports received from the laboratory. This facilitates a nurse to manage the biomedical waste in effective way. The reports enable a physician to choose medical care for patient.
- The knowledge of microbiology is necessary for the nurse to understand how sera and vaccines are used in the treatment and prevention of diseases and their effects on human body. The knowledge of vaccines and sera helps a nurse in immunization.

DISCOVERIES AND INVENTIONS

The scientists recognized that the communicable diseases are spread through microorganisms and hence they isolated the patients who are suffering from such diseases, like leprosy, plague and syphilis.

- In 1683 *Antonie van Leeuwenhoek* discovered microscope and described various types of bacteria.
- **Louis Pasteur** in 1857 introduced the theory of sterilization and developed a vaccine against rabies (hydrophobia) and because of his contributions, he is considered as the **father of bacteriology**.
- *Joseph Lister* introduced antiseptics in 1867 and he is known as the father of antiseptic techniques in surgery.
- *Robert Koch* (1843–1910) discovered the bacillus, causing anthrax, tuberculosis and vibrio cholera and he is known as the father of bacteriological techniques of culturing and staining for the study of bacteria. He gave postulates which are base for establishing a causative organism as a cause of disease (Fig. 1).

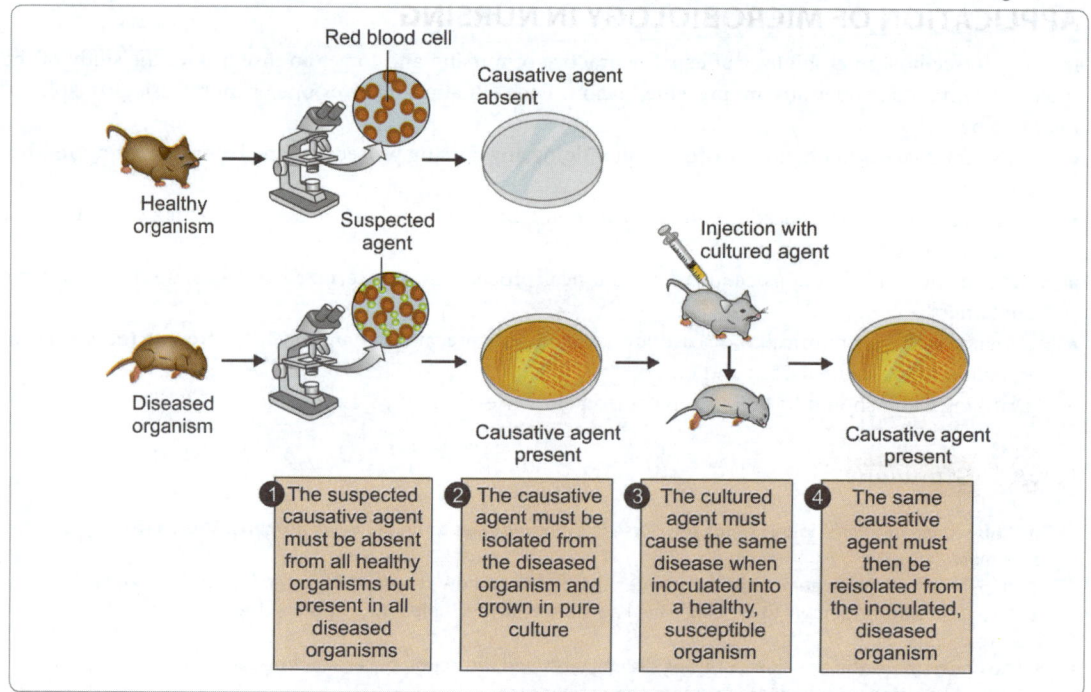

Figure 1: Robert Koch postulates

- *Edward Jenner* in England introduced vaccination against small pox using cow pox material in 1796.
- *Hans Christian Gram*, a Danish bacteriologist invented Gram staining (a method of staining bacteria that played a major role in classifying bacteria).
- *Dmitri Iosifovich Ivanovsky* Russian botanist discovered viruses, the tobacco mosaic virus in 1892.
- *Paul Ehrlich*, German hematologist, immunologist, and chemotherapist, was a Nobel prize-winning. He worked in the fields of hematology, immunology, and antimicrobial chemotherapy. He is credited with finding a cure for syphilis in 1909.
- *Walter Reed*, US Army physician discovered in 1900 that the yellow fever is transmitted by a particular mosquito species, rather than by direct contact.
- *Robert Hooke*, using an early microscope, discovered cells in living plant tissue.
- Thus, since centuries back, scientists discovered and differentiated microorganisms and their fact of contact in human beings. Infectious diseases spread from person to person through direct contacts with infected persons or through indirect contact of contaminated articles like cloths, vessels, remnants of foods, other materials, discharges from patients and also through air. It is proved that patients in labor room and operating room and wards are getting secondary infection due to the dirty hands and careless dealings of doctors and nurses working in those areas. Proper hand washing and disinfecting with antiseptics and practicing strict sterile techniques for doing the procedures will prevent or reduce the spread of infection. Once a person is infected and cured after smallpox or chicken pox is not usually reinfected by the same diseases, and based on this principle, small pox vaccination is given to people as a preventive measure.

Unit I ❖ Introduction

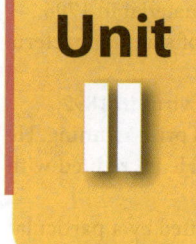

Microorganisms

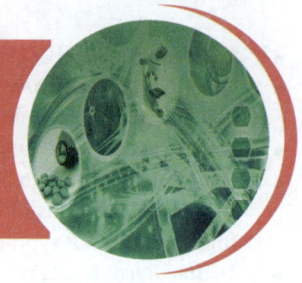

DISTRIBUTION OF MICROORGANISMS

Microorganisms are widely distributed in nature. They are found on the skin, in water, food we ingest and in the air we breathe. They are in plenty on the upper layer of the soil. Persons like nurses and doctors who are involved in the care of sick are supposed to think about microorganisms only in relation to their harmful effects to human body. They should be very conscious about the pathogenic organisms. Although enumerable species of microorganisms are there on earth, but only a small number of these organisms produce diseases in human which are said to be the pathogenic organisms.

According to a new estimate, there are about one trillion species of microbes on Earth, and 99.999% of them have yet to be discovered.

Finding the number of species has broader implications:
- How many species could have actually evolved in four billion years?
- What are the upper constraints of evolution on earth?
- How many species have evolved?
- How many species could have evolved?

Majority of microorganisms are helpful to mankind. The organisms in the soil carry on useful activities such as decomposition of dead animals and vegetable matters. The organisms live on decaying or dead organic matter causing putrefaction are called saprophytes. Some organisms ferment food stuffs and are used in industries to manufacture alcohol, lactic acid, butter, cheese and other substances.

CLASSIFICATION OF MICROORGANISMS

According to the mode of living and their study, microorganisms are classified as follows:
- Protozoa   -   It's study is called Protozoology
- Algae   -   It's study is called Phycology
- Fungi   -   It's study is called Mycology
- Bacteria   -   It's study is called Bacteriology
- Viruses   -   It's study is called Virology
- Archaea   -   This constitutes a domain of single-celled organisms. These microorganisms lack cell nuclei and are therefore prokaryotes.

Protozoa

These are the smallest-celled animals, much larger than bacteria. Most protozoa are saprophytes, living on dead organic matters while few cause diseases in animals and plants.

Some protozoa-caused human diseases include:

- *Plasmodium* causes malaria
- *Giardia* causes giardiasis
- *Leishmania* donovani causes kala-azar
- *Trichomonas* causes urogenital tract infection
- *Entamoeba histolytica* causes dysentery
- *Criptosporidia* causes diarrheal diseases.

Algae

These are simple forms of plant life. These form a slimy form of film on sand filter beds and aid purification of water.

Fungi

Fungi are microscopic saprophytic organisms without coloring matter and they reproduce sexually or by spore formation. Some fungi (molds) induce or cause disease in man and animals when the food items containing fungi are consumed. The toxic compounds produced by fungal contamination of food are termed *mycotoxins* and the resulting diseases are called *mycotoxicosis*. Fungal diseases may be superficial on the skin only or deep-seated (systemic). Deep-seated are usually pathogenic only as 'opportunists' taking advantage on patients with lowered resistance.

Bacteria

These are minute organisms, different from plants as they do not contain chlorophyll and some are actively motile. Nearly two billion average sized bacteria can be present in a single drop of water. Of the various groups of organisms, bacteria are the easiest to study and learn the principles of science.

Factors Affecting the Growth of Bacteria

- **Moisture:** Like all living things, bacteria are sensitive to living environment. Water is necessary for the growth of bacteria because they cannot absorb food materials unless it is in solution, e.g., preservation of food by drying such as fish, meat, fruits.
- **Food and metabolism:** Bacteria obtain their nourishment from organic and inorganic matter for growth and multiplication. The minimum nutritional requirements are a source of water, carbon, nitrogen and some inorganic salts. Some bacteria need vitamins to grow.
- **Optimum temperature:** Each species of bacteria requires a certain temperature range for its growth which is called optimum temperature. For most bacteria optimum temperature is 37°C and most of them are killed in 30 minutes at 56°C. Bacteria usually attack human body because body temperature suits them and provide them best habitat. Low temperatures inhibit the growth of most bacteria and high temperature destroys them. Refrigeration for preservation of foods and sterilization by heat are based on these principles.
- **Acidity and alkalinity:** (Hydrogen ion concentration) Most bacteria grow best in neutral or slightly alkaline medium (pH 7.2–7.6). An acid medium prevents the growth of bacteria. The preservation of fish, meat and vegetables by pickling in vinegar is based on the sensitivity of bacteria to the extreme acidity of the vinegar.
- **Oxygen:** Organisms that grow in the presence of free oxygen are called aerobes. Those cannot grow in the presence of free oxygen but obtain their oxygen from oxygen-containing compounds are known as anaerobes. A few pathogenic organisms such as those of tetanus and gas gangrene are anaerobic.

Unit II ❖ Microorganisms

- **Osmotic pressure:** Many bacteria are sensitive to a concentrated solution of salt or sugar because of their high osmotic pressure. Preservation of food in concentrated salt solution or thick sugar syrup is based on this principle.
- **Light and radiation:** Most bacteria grow well in darkness. Direct sunlight destroys many bacteria within few minutes or hours. It is therefore possible to disinfect articles by exposing them to sunlight. Mattresses, pillows and blankets used in hospitals are disinfected by sunlight. Ultraviolet rays and radiation also destroy bacteria. Special lamps which produce ultraviolet rays destroy bacteria. Such lamps are sometimes used in the treatment of skin infection.

Viruses

These are the smallest living units, filter passing and ultramicroscopic, and can be seen only through electron microscope. Virus cannot grow on lifeless media such as agar, but only within susceptible cells as egg yolk. Virus has no independent metabolic activity. Three methods are employed for cultivation of viruses:

i. Inoculation into animals
ii. Embryonated eggs
iii. Tissue cultures

Viruses are inactivated by sunlight, ultraviolet rays, radiations and chlorination, but are more resistant than bacteria to chemical disinfection. They are readily inactivated by heat. Antibiotics which are active against bacteria are completely ineffective against virus.

Viral diseases range from minor ailments such as common cold to highly fatal diseases like rabies, yellow fever, hepatitis B and Acquired Immunodeficiency Syndrome (AIDS). They may be sporadic such as mumps, endemic like rabies, epidemic such as measles or pandemic namely influenza.

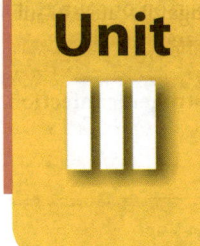

Unit III

Infection Process

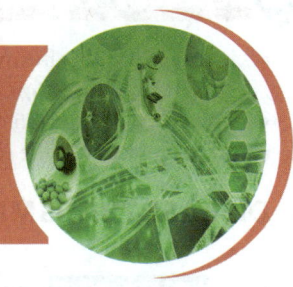

DEFINITION

When the pathogenic organisms enter and multiply in the tissues of a host (human or animal) it is known as infection. Although every instance of infection may not result in an infectious disease.

TYPES OF INFECTION (FIG. 1)

Infection may be of various types:

- The first infection by a parasite in a host is known as **primary infection**.
- If the same parasite infects the same person again it is called **reinfection**.

Concise picture of types of infections and their characteristics have been shown here in Figure 1.

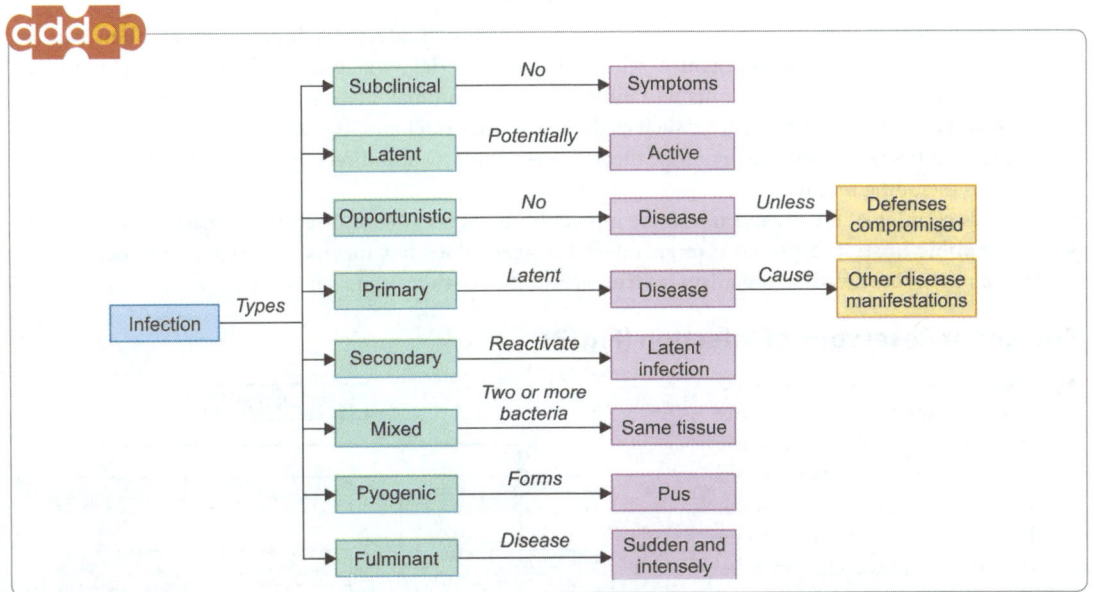

Figure 1: Types of infection

- When a person already suffering from one disease caused by a parasite is infected with a new parasite is said to have **secondary infection**.
- When the infection causes disease in a particular organ or site, it is termed as **focal infection**, e.g., appendicitis.

- When a patient already suffering from a disease gets a new infection from another person or source, it is called **cross infection**. Cross infection usually occurs in hospitals, boarding schools and hostels.
- When cross infection occurs in hospitals it is called **nosocomial infection**.
- If the infection is the result of treatment or investigative procedures it is known as **iatrogenic infection**.

DISEASE TRANSMISSION

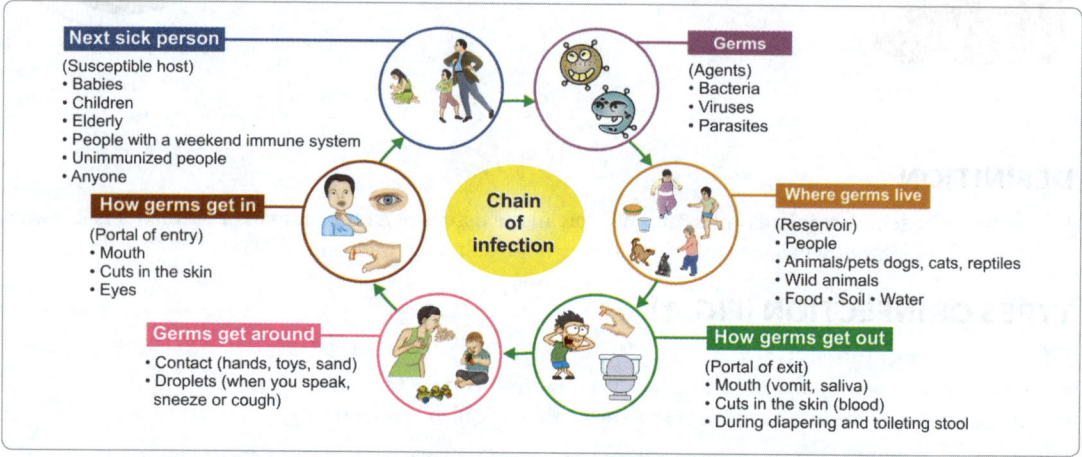

Figure 2: Chain of infection

A chain of events and factors are necessary for the transmission of infectious disease (Fig. 2). They are:

- **Causative agent** or invading organism which may be bacterial, viral, protozoal, fungal or helminthic.
- **Reservoir** is a place for the organism to multiply, human, animal, insects, soil, water or food.
- **A portal of exit** from the reservoir such as the respiratory tract and digestive tract.
- A **mode of transmission** which may be direct (direct contact) or indirect through animate and inanimate vectors including fomites.
- **Portals of entry** of the organism into the human body such as the respiratory and gastrointestinal tract.
- **Susceptible host:** The presence of an infectious agent does not inevitably produce disease. Infection results when the invading organism is virulent and the host's resistance is weak.

Sources or Reservoirs of Infection (Fig. 3)

- **Human beings:** A person who is a reservoir of such organisms may be a patient or carrier. A carrier is a person who harbors the pathogenic organisms in the body and shows no symptoms or signs of illness. They may be a convalescent carrier, chronic carrier, unhealthy or contact carrier.
- **Animals:** Many pathogenic organisms infect humans and animals. In some instances, the

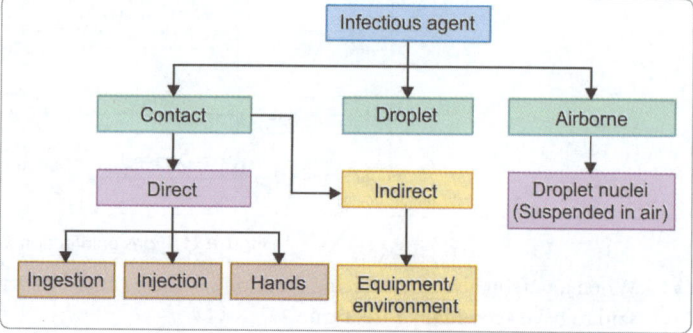

Figure 3: Sources of infection

infection in animals may not cause any disease but act as reservoir hosts. Diseases transmitted from animals to human are called zoonotic diseases. These diseases may be bacterial, like leptospirosis and plague from rats, viral such as rabies from dogs and protozoal, like leishmaniasis from dogs.

- **Insects:** Insects such as mosquitoes, ticks, mites, flies and lice that transmit disease are called vectors.
- **Soil and water:** The spores of some pathogenic organisms survive in soil for very long period, e.g., bacilli causing anthrax, tetanus and worm infestations, like hookworm, round worm, etc. Water is contaminated by pathogenic organisms such as *Vibrio cholerae* and Hepatitis A virus serves as source of infection.
- **Food:** Infected or contaminated food serves as a source of infection, e.g., infected meat and fish.

PORTALS OF ENTRY OF ORGANISMS

There are certain gates or pathways by which microorganisms enter the body (Fig. 4). They are known as portals of entry. Most of the organisms can cause disease only if they enter through their particular portal. For example, if dysentery bacilli are rubbed into a wound on the skin, it may not cause any trouble, but if the same organisms are swallowed, it is almost certain to cause dysentery.

- **Skin and mucous membranes:** A large number of organisms are present on the skin but most of them do not penetrate the unbroken skin. However, organisms, like staphylococci and some fungi are able to penetrate the skin under certain conditions and cause disease in deeper tissues. Insects and animal bites, injection with contaminated products, trauma, sexual contact with infected persons are other ways in which microorganisms enter the body through the skin, e.g., rabies, malaria, hook worm, etc.
- **Respiratory tract:** Air around us contains microorganisms which can spread widely while coughing, sneezing or talking and these may enter into the respiratory tract with air inhaled, e.g., organisms causing common cold, influenza, pneumonia and pulmonary tuberculosis.

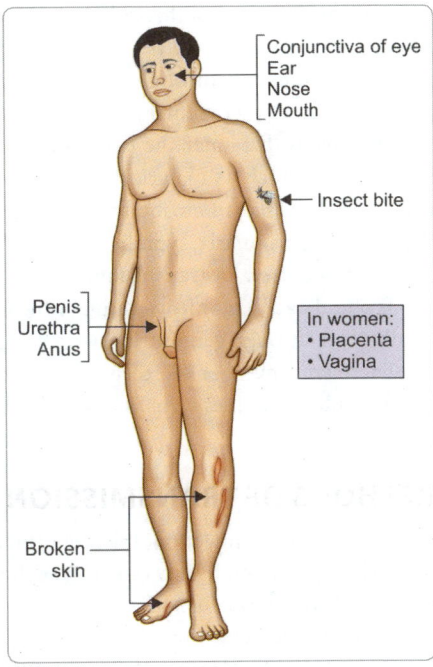

Figure 4: Portals of entry for organisms in the human body

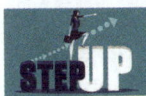

Update of March 17, 2020: An outbreak of respiratory disease caused by a novel coronavirus that was first detected in China and has now been spread in more than 100 countries worldwide, including the United States. The virus has been named "SARS-CoV-2" and the disease has been named "**coronavirus disease 2019**" (COVID-19). The disease has been declared as pandemic and spreads very fast through droplet infection. Till date 7175 mortalities have occurred worldwide. The casualty is higher in old people and very young people.

On January 30, 2020, the International Health Regulations Emergency Committee of the World Health Organization (WHO) declared the outbreak as pandemic.

- **Digestive tract:** Microorganisms enter the body along with food and water. The organisms causing typhoid, dysentery, cholera and hepatitis enter the body in this way.
- **Genitourinary tract:** Generally, urinary tract infection (UTI) is caused by bacteria from urethra, perineum, etc. going upwards (ascending infection) and sometimes introduced by catheterization.

Unit III ❖ Infection Process

UTI can also take place through the blood. Venereal diseases such as gonorrhea and syphilis are acquired through sexual contact and transmission.

- **Infection through inoculation:** Infection through inoculation may occur by the use of unsterile syringes, injuries allowing tetanus spores, blood transfusion and inoculation of infected blood by insects as in malaria.

PORTALS OF EXIT

Very often organisms leave the body through the same path they entered in. Organisms causing respiratory diseases usually come out through the nasal discharges and sputum. Pulmonary tuberculosis, pneumonia and diphtheria are examples of respiratory infections. Organisms which enter digestive system through mouth, usually leave the body through feces and rectum. Examples of microorganisms infecting digestive system are typhoid, cholera and dysentery.

Organisms that enter the body through skin often produce pus and leave the skin in through the pus. Some diseases such as malaria and yellow fever occur because the organisms enter through the skin into blood due to the bite of mosquito. These organisms leave the same way when a mosquito sucks blood from a diseased person. Malaria, syphilis, hepatitis B and acquired immunodeficiency disease can also leave the body through blood used for transfusion.

Typhoid bacilli may leave through the urinary tract. Organisms responsible for syphilis and gonorrhoea usually leave through genitourinary tract.

There are a number of exceptions where microorganism leaves the body by a route different to the one which it entered. Rabies virus is a good example which enters through the skin but leaves the body through the saliva.

METHODS OF TRANSMISSION OF MICROORGANISMS

In order to produce infection, the organism has to be transferred from one infected host to a new host. This may be brought about by any one of the following methods:

- **Direct infection:** Infection may be transmitted directly from person to person either by direct contact with infected person or by contact with the secretions and excretions of infected persons, e.g., organisms causing diphtheria, common cold and tonsillitis may be transferred by kissing. Sexually transmitted diseases including hepatitis B and AIDS are usually transmitted by direct sexual contact with the infected persons. A nurse may contact typhoid fever or dysentery by soiling her hands with feces of a patient and not taking care to wash her hands before eating food. A special type of direct infection is called **droplet infection**. Microorganisms are thrown out into the air from the mouth and throat while coughing or sneezing, along with fine droplets of saliva and mucus. They may be thrown as far as 3½ feet while talking and up to 10 feet while sneezing. Droplet nuclei and dust containing a variety of organisms may be carried by the air. This is a major way by which the organisms—causing cold, influenza, pneumonia, diphtheria and tuberculosis spread.
- **Indirect infection:** Infection may be acquired indirectly by articles which have been recently contaminated. These articles which are likely to carry the pathogenic organisms are called **fomites** which include bed linen, handkerchiefs, drinking cups and eating vessels. Organisms causing gastrointestinal and respiratory infections may be transferred through fomites, contamination of water by sewage and

contamination of milk by the milk handlers are other examples for indirect infection. Very often indirect infections are occurred through **food, feces, fingers, flies and other fomites (5F).**

- **Infection by inoculation:** This may occur by the use of unsterile syringe and needles, tetanus spores entering the body through injuries, blood transfusion and inoculation of infected blood by insects as in malaria.

COMMON TYPES OF HOSPITAL INFECTION (NOSOCOMIAL INFECTION)

Nosocomial infections are developed during hospitalization which is not present at the time of admission of the patient to the hospital. Hospital environment is heavy with pathogenic organisms, and not only that, the patients may come with lowered vitality and resistance power. Transmission of infection usually occurs through the hands of hospital personnel, respiratory droplets, food, drinking water, contaminated surfaces, catheters and equipment used in procedures and diagnostic measures. Infection can be transmitted from patients to nurses and from nurses to patients while doing procedures, if precaution is not taken.

Common types of hospital infections are:

- **Urinary tract infection:** *Escherichia coli* and other organisms from colon are the causative organisms. Infection usually results from catheterization and indwelling catheters. Strict aseptic technique minimizes the transfer of infection.
- **Respiratory infection:** Aspiration in unconscious patients and pulmonary ventilation or instrumentation may lead to nosocomial pneumonia. Antibiotic treatment is useful in prevention and management of such cases.
- **Wound infection:** Surgical wound infections are mostly due to organisms introduced during operative procedures, wound dressing, and labor rooms by using unsterile techniques and materials and careless handling of sterile materials.
- **Bacteremia and septicemia:** This may occur at any site of the body but are commonly caused by the infected intravenous cannula left in place for several days. Strict aseptic technique and minimized use of intravenous therapy will reduce the infection.
- **Hepatitis B and AIDS:** These serious conditions occur to the patients who are receiving blood transfusions or undergoing renal dialysis. It is one of the major risks to hospital personnel too. Proper grouping, matching and testing of blood before transfusion and strict preventive measures are the methods of reducing risks.
- **Food poisoning:** Acute gastroenteritis from food poisoning, contaminated cooked food and outbreak of diarrhea are the examples of acute gastroenteritis. Scrupulous cleaning of kitchen, dining hall and vessels, fresh items of food, proper supervision of preparation and serving and in-service education of workers, health talk to patients and relatives will help to prevent such complications in hospital.

Diagnosis and Control of Hospital Infection

Diagnosis of hospital infection is made by routine bacteriological methods of smear, culture, identification and sensitivity testing. Sterilization techniques have to be tested. There should be an infection control team in every hospital and every outbreak of infection should be investigated and isolation techniques should be practiced strictly. Education of the patients, relatives and menial staff regarding the control of infection is conducted frequently. Infection control should not be based on the antiseptics. According to Sir William Osler, soap, water and common sense are the best disinfectants to prevent infection.

Unit III ❖ Infection Process

The nurse can play a vital role in control of hospital infection (Fig. 5), this is summarized as follows:

Note

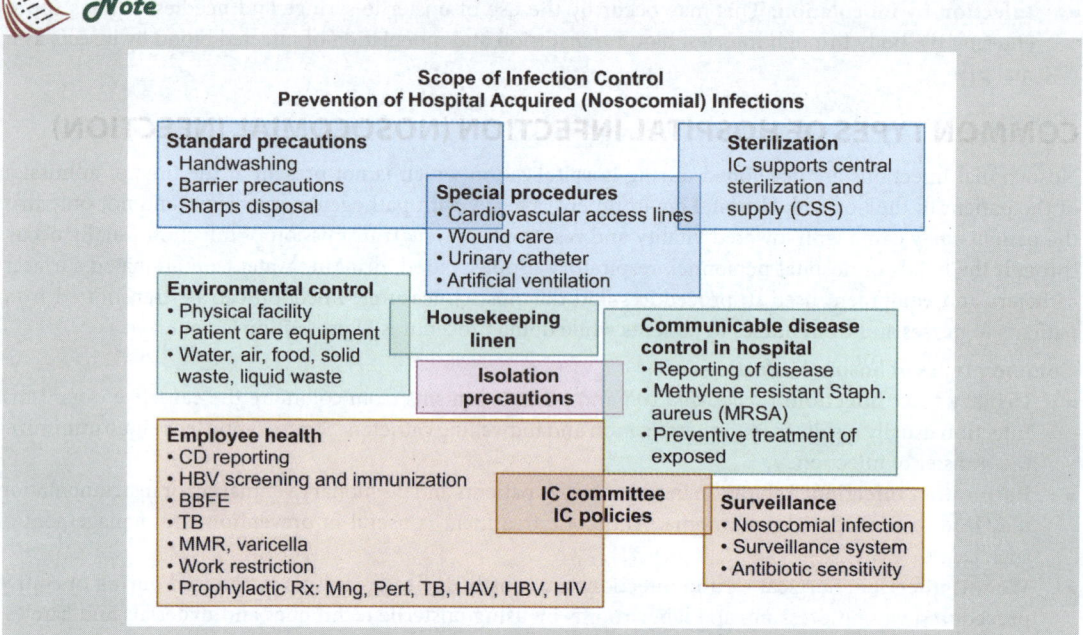

Figure 5: Control of hospital infection

Abbreviations: *IC, internal committee; HBV, hepatitis B virus; BBFE, blood body fluid exposure; TB, tuberculosis; MMR, vaccine against measles, mumps, and rubella; HIV, human immunodeficiency virus; HAV, hepatitis A virus*

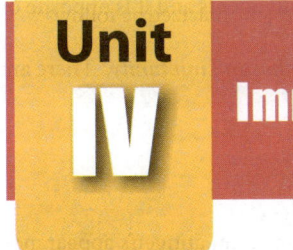

Unit IV — Immunity

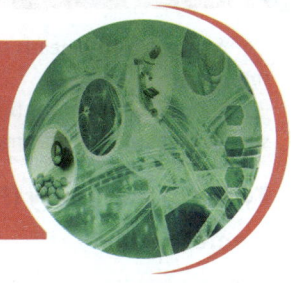

INFECTION AND RESISTANCE

Infection results from the successful entrance of microorganisms in the body; and their growth and multiplication in the body. The entrance of microorganisms in the body itself does not mean that infection will result. Infection occurs depending upon the following factors:

- The portal of entry
- The virulence or ability of the organisms to produce disease
- The number of organisms entered in the body
- The defensive power of the body

Microorganisms produce disease in the body by the following two ways:

1. Disease is produced by its mechanical effects such as filling up of tissue spaces and capillaries by the multiplying bacterial cells. This process of multiplication of microorganisms and spread in tissue is called invasion.
2. Infection due to the poisons known as toxins that are produced by the bacteria:
   - Endotoxins, which are present in the bacteria until the organism dies and breaks up as found in gonococci and typhoid bacilli.
   - Exotoxins, which diffuses out through cell membrane into the surrounding tissues as in diphtheria and tetanus bacilli.

Resistance is the opposing force or power of the body against infection. This kind of protection against bacteria can be *general defences,* like mechanical, physiological and chemical method of protecting itself against organisms. For example, skin is a very important protection.

Specific defence mechanism comes into play once microorganisms gain entrance into the body, breaking the general defense barriers by producing specific antibodies.

IMMUNITY

Immunity is the safety or security against diseases (Fig. 1). Immunity refers to the ability of an organism to recognize and defend itself against infectious diseases. Immunity gives the power to resist and overcome infections caused by particular organisms.

Susceptibility means the vulnerability of the man to get harmed by infectious agents and it is opposite of immunity.

There is some immunity in every individual at birth. This is called innate *or natural immunity*. There are several ways in which immunity develops in the body after birth.

Types of Immunity (Fig. 1)

Innate immunity

It refers to nonspecific defense mechanisms that act immediately or within hours of an antigen's appearance in the body. These mechanisms include physical barriers such as skin, protective agents in the blood, and cells of immune system that attack foreign cells in the body. The innate immunity is of two types: nonspecific and specific.

- It can be nonspecific or specific.
  - **Species immunity:** For example, many diseases of human species do not affect animal species.
  - **Racial immunity:** Certain groups of people are naturally resistant to some disease, e.g., Hebrews are more resistant to tuberculosis. It is a type of individual immunity.
  - **Herd immunity:** Which is developed in a community or in a group of people, e.g., filariasis is rare in people residing in hilly areas. Herd immunity helps to limit the epidemics.
  - **Individual immunity:** It is believed that some people have a strong natural resistance or immunity to certain diseases, e.g. certain people are not affected by common cold even in adverse climate.

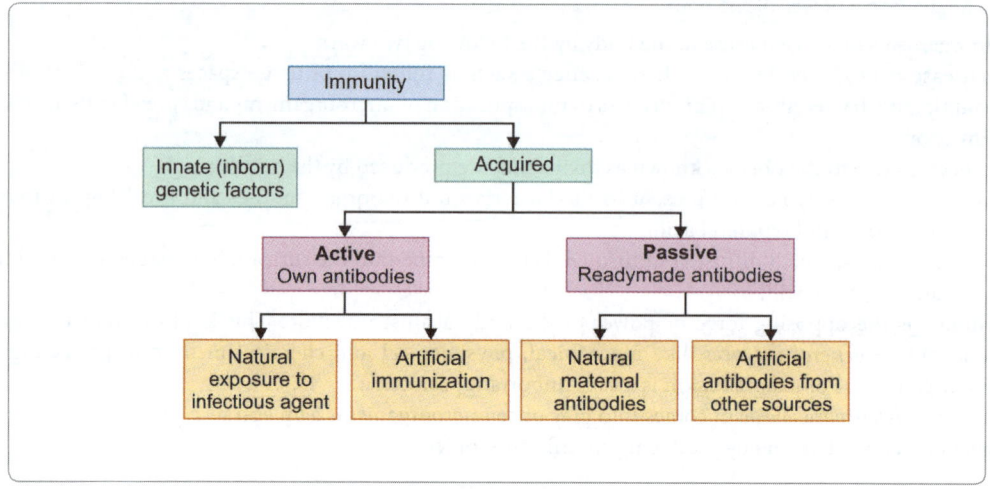

Figure 1: Types of immunity

Acquired Immunity

It is the specific immune system, of the overall immune system and is composed of highly specialized, systemic cells and processes that eliminate pathogens or prevent their growth. It is of two types:
1. Active immunity
2. Passive immunity

Active Immunity

It is the resistance developed by an individual as a result of an antigenic stimulus due to the active functioning of the person's immune system. For example, a person who had an attack of chicken pox, rubella or measles is not usually affected by the same disease again.

Passive Immunity

Immunity that develops after a person receives immune system components, most commonly antibodies, from another person. That is, antibodies produced in the body (human or animal) are transferred to another to induce protection against disease. Passive immunity is induced by administration of vaccines, immunoglobulin (antibodies) or antisera (antitoxins)

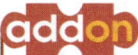

Expanded Program of Immunization (EPI)

- The expanded program on immunization (EPI) was initiated in India in 1978 with the objective to reduce morbidity and mortality due to diphtheria, pertussis, tetanus, poliomyelitis and childhood tuberculosis by providing immunization services to all eligible children and pregnant women by 1990.
- Expanded program on immunization (EPI) is a World Health Organization (WHO) Program with the goal to make vaccines available to all children.

The Ministry of Health of the Government of India has established the EPI program of WHO in 1974 as a national effort to immunize the children against 6 target diseases, namely tuberculosis, diphtheria, pertussis (whooping cough), tetanus, poliomyelitis and measles. The vaccines are centrally procured and supplied to the state-level EPI manager for implementation. Following the eradication of small pox globally, WHO started a program for eradication of poliomyelitis by the year 2000. Immunization against hepatitis B, rubella, MMR and rotavirus is also available now. The recently proceeding schedule is given as follows:

Unit IV ❖ Immunity

Immunization Schedule
Vaccination Chart (https://www.vaccinebox.com/types-of-vaccines/immunization-chart/)

Vaccine	Birth	6 wks	10 wks	14 wks	6 m	7 m	9 m	10-12 m	12 mnts	15 m	16-18 m	18 m	2 yrs	4-6 yrs	10-12 years
*BCG vaccine	Dose 1														
*Hepatitis B vaccine	Dose 1	Dose 2			Dose 3										
*OPV	Dose 0				Dose 1		Dose 2							Dose 3	
*IPV		Dose 1	Dose 2	Dose 3							Dose 4				
*DTP (DTwP/ DTaP) Vaccine		Dose 1	Dose 2	Dose 3							Dose 4			Dose 5	
*Hib vaccine		Dose 1	Dose 2	Dose 3							Dose 4				
Pneumococcal vaccine		Dose 1	Dose 2	Dose 3						Dose 4					
*Rotavirus vaccine		Dose 1	Dose 2	Dose 3											
Influenza Virus vaccine					Dose 1	Dose 2									
*MMR vaccine							Dose 1			Dose 2				Dose 3	
Typhoid conjugate vaccine								Dose 1					Dose 2		
Hepatitis A vaccine									Dose 1			Dose 2			
Chickenpox (Varicella) vaccine										Dose 1				Dose 2	
*Tdap vaccine															Dose 1
HPV vaccine															Dose 1 Dose 2
Legend	Routine oral drops	N	Routine injectable dose						N	Booster Injectable Dose					

Contd...

Recommended vaccination schedule, as per current Universal Immunization Program (UIP) by Government of India and Indian Academy of Paediatrics revised schedule 2019 (IAP), on the guidelines of WHO.

Vaccine	Routine dose (Should be given as per schedule)	Catch-up dose (Can be given if the doses as per schedule are missed)
BCG*	At birth or at 6 weeks of age	Up to 5 years
Hepatitis B*	• 1st dose of monovalent hepatitis B at Birth, followed by 2nd dose at 6 weeks and 3rd dose at 6 months of age (2nd and 3rd dose can be monovalent/pentavalent) • According to latest 2019 IAP update, it is mandatory to give Hep B dose within 24 hours of age of the baby • Alternatively, 3 primary doses of pentavalent vaccine, including Hep B at 6, 10 and 14 weeks after birth dose	• If a birth dose is missed, monovalent Hep B before 4 weeks of age • Next dose after 1 month, followed by a third dose after 6 months of first dose (0, 1, 6 months schedule)
OPV*	• Birth dose of OPV is a must • Complete replacement of OPV by IPV can be done for primary schedule • bOPV can be given for all the primary doses at 6, 10 and 14 weeks of age only if IPV is not available or feasible • No child should leave the health facility without polio immunization (IPV or OPV), if indicated by the schedule	• Additional doses of OPV on all pulse polio days for children till 5 years of age
IPV*	• Complete replacement of OPV by IPV can be done • 3 primary doses at 6, 10 and 14 weeks of age is recommended • If IPV is not possible for all the primary doses. Then 2 doses of intramuscular IPV instead of three, should be given starting at 8 weeks, with an interval of 8 weeks between the 2 doses at a government facility • If IPV is not available or feasible, the child should be given two fractional doses of IPV via intradermal route at 6 and 14 weeks or at least one full dose of IPV via intramuscular route, either standalone or as a combination vaccine at 14 weeks of age. • Booster dose of IPV at 12–18 months of age if primary doses of IPV are given	• Doses at 2 months gap followed by a booster dose at 6 months gap after the previous dose
DTP (DTwP or DTaP)*	• 3 primary doses (DTwP/DTaP) at 6 weeks, 10 weeks and 14 weeks of age • First booster at 16–24 months of age, followed by a second booster at 4–6 years of age	• Missed primary doses can be completed till 1 year of age • The 1st booster dose can be given up to 4 years • 2nd booster dose can be given before 7 years of age
Hib*	• 3 doses of Hib or Hib conjugate vaccine at 6 weeks, 10 weeks and 14 weeks of age • Booster dose at age 12–18 months	• For age <12 months; 2 doses at 4 weeks interval, with a booster at age 12–18 months • For child 12–15 months; 1 dose only followed by a booster dose after at least 4 weeks • Above 15 months; single dose • No catch up above 5 years of age

Contd...

Unit IV ❖ Immunity

Vaccine	Routine dose (Should be given as per schedule)	Catch-up dose (Can be given if the doses as per schedule are missed)
Pneumococcal Conjugate (PCV)	• 3 primary doses at 6 weeks, 10 weeks and 14 weeks of age • Booster dose at 15 months of age	• For infants of age 6–12 months, 2 doses can be given at 4 weeks gap followed by 1 booster dose. • For children of age 12–23 months, 2 doses can be given at 8 week gap. • For children of age 2–5 years, single dose can be given
Rotavirus*	• 3 primary doses at 6 weeks, 10 weeks and 14 weeks of age • The first dose of monovalent Rotavirus vaccine (RV1) can be given at 6 weeks and the second at 10 weeks of age in a two-dose schedule. Any of the available Rotavirus vaccine may be administered	• Missed doses can be given before 8 months of age at a minimum gap of 4 weeks • No catch-up after 8 months
Influenza	• 2 doses starting at 6 months of age at 4 weeks gap for the first time vaccination • Single dose every year for age group 1–9 years • Influenza vaccine should be given annually on the routine basis to the high-risk group of children below age of 5 years	• 2 doses can be given at 4 week gap at any time for children less than 1 year
MMR*	• 1 dose of MMR vaccine at a minimum age of 9 months (270 completed days) through 12 months of age • The 2nd dose at 15 months through 18 months of age or at any time 4–8 weeks after the 1st dose • 3rd dose should be given at 4–6 years of age • (According to IAP revised Schedule 2016–17) • Additional dose of MR vaccine should be given during MR campaign for healthy children of age 9 months to 15 years. This should be irrespective of previous vaccination status to support national programs	• All school children and adolescents who did not have natural infection or received the vaccine earlier should be immunized with 2 doses of MMR at minimum 4 weeks interval • Monovalent measles/measles containing vaccine can be administered to infants aged 6 through 8 months during measles outbreaks. However, this dose should not be counted.
Typhoid Vi PS Conjugate	• Primary dose at 9–12 months (an interval of minimum 4 weeks should be maintained with the MMR1 dose while following the schedule) • Booster dose at 2 years of age with either typhoid conjugate (Typbar-TCV®) or Typhoid polysaccharide • Booster doses every 3 years if Typhoid polysaccharide vaccine is used • No further boosters are required if Typhoid Vi PS Conjugate is used	• Doses can be given till 18 years of age

Contd...

Vaccine	Routine dose (Should be given as per schedule)	Catch-up dose (Can be given if the doses as per schedule are missed)
Hepatitis A	• Only one dose of hepatitis A live attenuated vaccine staring at 12 months through 23 months of age • First dose of Hepatitis A killed vaccine starting at 12 months through 23 months of age • 2nd dose of Hepatitis A killed vaccines at 18 months of age or at minimum interval of 6 months from 1st dose. Gap is flexible anytime between 6 and 18 months	• 2 doses for killed vaccine can be administered at minimum 6 months gap to unvaccinated persons • Only single dose of live attenuated H_2-strain need to be given to unvaccinated persons • Hepatitis A vaccine can be given till 18 years of age
Chicken pox	• First dose at 12–15 months • Second dose at 4–6 years	• For children aged 7–12 years, 2 doses can be given at a minimum gap of 3 months • For persons aged 13 years and older, 2 doses can be given at a minimum gap of 4 weeks
Tdap*	• 1 single dose at age of 11–12 years	• Can be given up to 18 years • Tdap can be given to 7–10 years old kids who are not fully immunized against pertussis
HPV	• Only 2 doses of either of the two HPV vaccines (HPV2/HPV4) for girls aged 9–14 years. The minimum interval between the two doses should be at least 6 months • 3 doses are recommended for girls aged 15 years and older. 2nd dose is given 1–2 months after the 1st dose and the 3rd dose 6 months after the 1st dose (at least 24 weeks after the first dose). Either HPV4 (0, 2, 6 months) or HPV2 (0, 1, 6 months) is recommended in 3-dose schedule	• Vaccination can be done till 26 years of age, maintaining the minimum intervals between the doses

*Mandatory vaccines: Vaccines to be administered compulsorily to each child in the country.

 Stimulant

- The human papilloma virus (HPV) vaccine helps to protect against certain types of HPV that can lead to cancer or genital warts. Also known by the brand name Gardasil 9, the HPV vaccine protects against: HPV types 16 and 18—the 2 types that cause 80% of cervical cancer cases. HPV types 6 and 11, which cause 90% of genital warts cases.
- The HPV vaccine is FDA-approved and is recommended for females of the age 19–26. The reason for not giving the vaccine to older persons is that by this time women (and men) have had enough sex and they will probably have already exposed to the virus and there will be no benefit.
- **Important:** HPV also prevent throat cancer often caused by oral sex.

Unit IV ❖ Immunity

Immunization of antenatal mothers with two doses of tetanus toxoid at one month's interval has become part of antenatal care now.

Vaccine	When to give	Dose	Route	Site
For pregnant women				
TT-1	Early in pregnancy	0.5 mL	Intramuscular	Upper arm
TT-2	4 weeks after TT-1	0.5 mL	Intramuscular	Upper arm
TT booster	If pregnancy occurs within three years of last tetanus shot	0.5 mL	Intramuscular	Upper arm

The above schedule should be used as a guideline only. Modifications may be made according to local conditions as per the state health department rules. BCG may be given at birth or at any age thereafter. If there is a break in the schedule due to any reason, there is no need to restart from the first dose. The break is to be ignored and immunization continued as if there is no break.

Every health team member is responsible to make the people, especially parents, understand the need and importance of immunizing the children to control the preventable diseases and complications, and to assure a better healthy future of next generation.

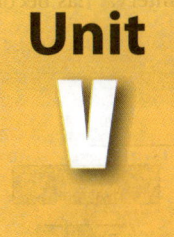

Unit V

Control of Bacteria (Methods of Disinfection and Sterilization)

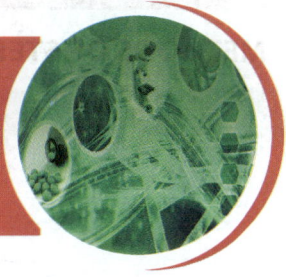

CONTROL OF BACTERIA

Although most organisms in the nature are harmless, it is necessary to realize that some pathogenic species are often mixed with non-pathogenic ones and special precautions have to be taken to destroy them in order to prevent the spread of infections. It is essential for the nurse to understand the fundamental principles of removal of microorganisms and to possess a good working knowledge of this procedure. It is already mentioned that bacteria are sensitive to drying, sunlight, high temperature and other physical and chemical conditions. This knowledge will be useful to destroy and remove bacteria. Before discussing the details of various methods of destroying microorganisms, it will be helpful to define some of the terms used for the removal of bacteria which are as follows:

TERMINOLOGIES

- **Antisepsis:** The prevention of infection usually by inhibiting the growth of bacteria is antisepsis.
- **Antiseptic:** The agent capable of producing antisepsis is antiseptic.
- **Asepsis:** It means the absence of infection or pathogenic organisms.
- **Bacteriocidal agents:** The substances which are able to kill bacteria are bacteriocidal agents.
- **Bacteriostatic agents:** These substances prevent the multiplication of bacteria and they may remain alive. These substances may check the growth and development of bacteria but do not necessarily kill them. A chemical substance which has bacteriocidial action at a specific concentration will be only bacteriostatic action at a lower concentration, that is why it is diluted further.
- **Cleaning:** Means removal of contamination such as dirt and dust.
- **Disinfection:** The destruction of all pathogenic organisms except spore-bearing organisms is disinfection.
- **Disinfectant:** The substance which kills pathogenic organisms is called disinfectant.
- **Sepsis or infection:** It means presence of pathogenic organisms.
- **Sterilization:** It is the process of making something free from bacteria, their spores or other living microorganisms.

METHODS OF STERILIZATION AND DISINFECTION

Disinfection and sterilization may be accomplished by the following methods (Fig. 1):

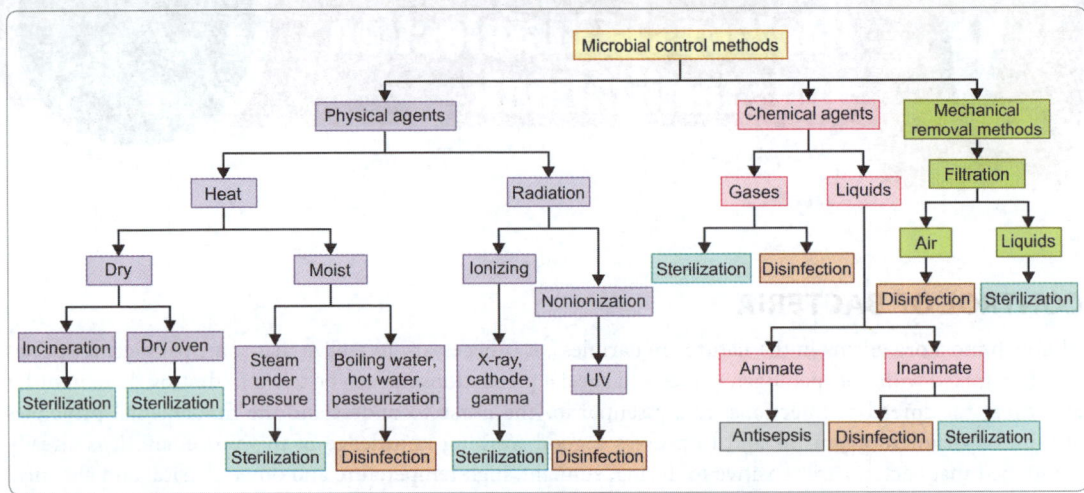

Figure 1: Controlling microorganisms

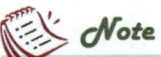 *Note*

The differences between disinfection and sterilization are given as follows:

Disinfection	Sterilization
This technique minimize the number of microorganisms but does not eliminate them completely	This technique is the elimination of all the microorganisms
This method does not eliminate bacterial spores	This method kills bacteria as well as vegetative spores
It is not an absolute condition	It is an absolute condition
Various types include chlorination, coagulation, and treatment with ozone, chlorine dioxide, ultra violet light, flocculation, sedimentation and filtration	Various methods include steam, heating dry heat, moist heat, chemical sterilization, ethylene oxide gas radiation sterilization, sterile filtration
Disinfection method is used for decontamination of surfaces and air	Sterilization process is used for decontamination of food, surgical equipment and instruments and several medicines
Disinfectants are commonly used in daily life	Sterilization used in surgical operations and various labs where sterile conditions are a prerequisite
Disinfection processes do not require a strict guideline to be followed	The sterilization processes are well laid down and follow a strict protocol to completely kill the pathogens
Disinfected objects has lesser number of the microorganisms	No viable organisms are present on sterilized items
Requires 10 minutes contact time	Requires 1 minute contact time

Mechanical Methods of Controlling Bacteria

- **Scrubbing** is usually done with soap and water. Washing is done either with hands alone or using brushes.
- **Filtration** is the process of passing a liquid through a material filter, in which the pores are so small that the bacteria cannot pass through cotton, gauze or other filters can be used.
- **Sedimentation** is the process by which the suspended particles in a liquid settle to the bottom of the liquid carrying with them bacteria which stick on to them. For example, purification of water in this method may be done along with other methods of chlorination.

Physical Methods of Controlling Bacteria

Moist Heat

- **Boiling:** Most of the organisms are killed within 3–5 minutes by boiling.
  - Boiling is a common method of sterilization. It is very easy, cheap and feasible method at anytime and anywhere for sterilization, provided the material is not damaged by boiling. But if boiling is to be effective, certain principles should be observed. The article should be scrupulously cleaned before putting for boiling. Bacteria will be killed by 5 minutes boiling except spores.
  - **Principles of boiling:**
    - The water should be boiled for full five minutes. The addition of cold metal instruments during boiling the water, will reduce the boiling point. The water must be boiled again for five minutes to get the effect if cold metal is added during the process.
    - All instruments or materials should be completely under water while boiling.
    - Used articles and instruments should be cleaned and boiled for five minutes and carefully dried before storing back.
    - Articles should be kept in dust proof cup board when not in use.
    - Material to be sterilized by boiling must be a good conductor of heat such as metal or so constructed that the boiling water can reach easily in all surfaces. Materials such as thread wound on reels require longer period of boiling because heat does not penetrate easily to the inner layers of such materials.
    - In case of suspected contamination with spore-bearing organisms such as anthrax or tetanus, all instruments and articles which have been used should be either autoclaved or subjected to prolonged and repeated boiling. The articles are boiled for one hour and equipment a cooling a period is allowed. The boiling is repeated for a further period of one hour. Any spores which have escaped destruction will revert to the vegetative form during the interval and are killed during the second boiling. This method is called *intermittent sterilization*.

- **Steam under pressure:** Sterilization in autoclave.
  - The structure and working of a simple autoclave is shown as follows (Fig. 2):

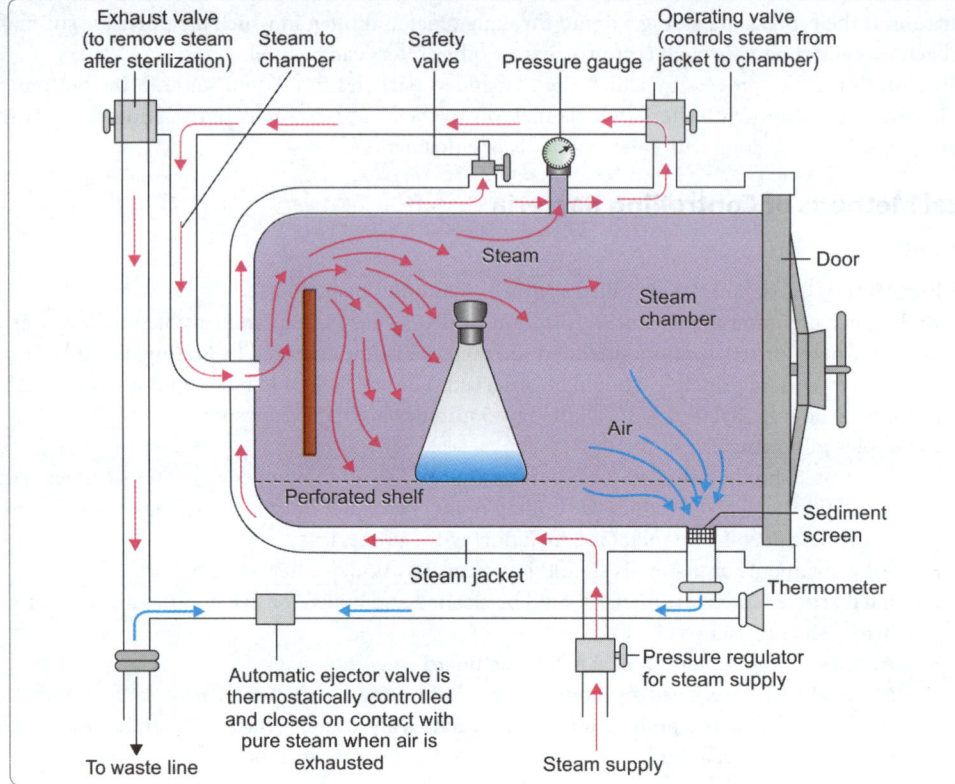

Figure 2: Autoclave

- **Uses of autoclave:** Autoclaves are used in hospitals by surgeons to sterilize surgical tools. They are also used in medical facilities and dentists' offices in order to sterilize instruments such as speculums, scopes, and scrapers.

 Stimulant

New Trends in Sterilization of Patient Equipment
Sterilization and Disinfection in Healthcare Settings
(CDC recommended guidelines)
The medical and surgical devices in healthcare settings are classified as critical, semicritical and noncritical.
- **Critical:** Medical/surgical devices which enter normally sterile tissue or the vascular system or through which blood flows should be sterile.
  All surgical instruments come under this category.
  Sterilization is the method adopted for making these items microorganisms free.
  - Steam sterilization
  - Hydrogen peroxide gas plasma ethylene oxide

Contd...

- Ozone and hydrogen peroxide
- Vaporized hydrogen peroxide

- **Semicritical:** Medical devices that touch mucous membranes or skin (that is not intact) require a disinfection process (high-level disinfection [HLD]) that kills all microorganisms and high numbers of bacterial spores like, Endoscopes, ENT scopes, endocavitary probes, laryngoscopes, cystoscopes. High quality disinfection is the control measure.
- **Noncritical:** Medical devices that touch only intact skin require low-level disinfection.
  Blood pressure cuffs, stethoscopes, wound vacuum like instruments come under this category.

New trends in sterilization of patient equipment
- Alternatives to ETO-CFC
  ETO-CO_2, ETO-HCFC, 100% ETO
  - New low temperature sterilization technology
  - Hydrogen peroxide gas plasma
  - Ozone and hydrogen peroxide
  - Vaporized hydrogen peroxide

Cleaning enhances effect of sterilization by:
- Cleaning removes salts and proteins and must precede sterilization
- Failure to clean or ensure exposure of microorganisms to sterilant (e.g., connectors) could affect effectiveness of sterilization process

- **Pasteurization**: It is a process of making milk or other foods safe by destroying all harmful organisms. It is a method of disinfection and not sterilization.

Dry Heat

- **Hot air oven:** A special oven which is similar to home-baking oven may be used for this method of sterilization.
- **Incineration:** Very badly contaminated materials such as sputum cups, infected dressings and garbage may be burnt in a furnace or in incinerator which is called incineration.
- **Flaming:** This is another form of burning by which an article is passed through an open flame.

Sunlight

A large number of organisms are killed in a few hours by exposure to bright sunlight owing to its ultraviolet rays. Blankets, mattresses and pillows are disinfected by this method.

Drying

Moisture is needed for the growth of bacteria. Drying has harmful effect in bacteria. Spores are not destroyed by drying. This method is unreliable for disinfection and sterilization.

Radiation

Special types of radiations are used for sterilization purposes. Infrared and gamma radiation and high energy electrons are useful for effective mass sterilization and therefore are used commercially.

Chemical Methods of Controlling Bacteria

There are many chemical compounds used as disinfectants or for antiseptic action.

A chemical disinfectant acts by coagulating the bacterial protein or by changing the composition of protein so that it no longer exists in the same form.

Unit V ❖ Control of Bacteria (Methods of Disinfection and Sterilization)

Common Chemical Compounds that are often used in Hospital Practice

Common chemical compounds that are often used in hospital practice are Phenol, Lysol, Hibitane, Cetrimide, Savlon, Dettol, chlorine, chloride of lime (bleaching powder), tincture of iodine, hydrogen peroxide, potassium permanganate, bichloride of mercury, metaphen, mercurochrome, gentian violet, acriflavine, formaldehyde (formalin is 37% solution of formaldehyde in water), alcohol, boric acid, hexachlorophene.

There are many other chemical compounds also used as disinfectant and antiseptics. The strength of solution depends upon the type of chemical, purpose of use and the type of material to be treated.

Dettol is nonpoisonous and nonirritating to the skin not so costly, therefore it is widely used in hospitals and homes as disinfectant and antiseptics.

Qualities of a Good Disinfectant

- It should destroy bacteria.
- It should not harm human tissues and the articles to be disinfected.
- It should act quickly and penetrate the material to be disinfected.
- It should get dissolved easily and quickly.
- It should be easily available and low in cost.
- It should not have any unpleasant odor.
- It should be easily removable on washing.

 Stimulant

The differences between disinfectant, sterilant, sanitizer, cleaner and virucidal agent have been given as follows:

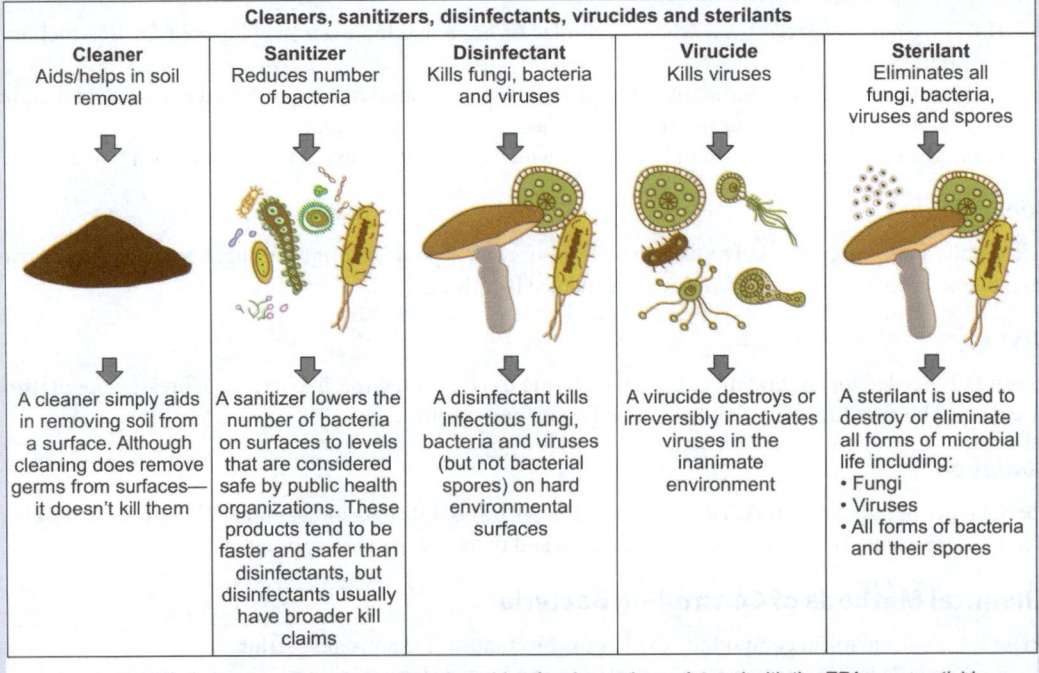

Cleaners, sanitizers, disinfectants, virucides and sterilants

Cleaner	Sanitizer	Disinfectant	Virucide	Sterilant
Aids/helps in soil removal	Reduces number of bacteria	Kills fungi, bacteria and viruses	Kills viruses	Eliminates all fungi, bacteria, viruses and spores
A cleaner simply aids in removing soil from a surface. Although cleaning does remove germs from surfaces—it doesn't kill them	A sanitizer lowers the number of bacteria on surfaces to levels that are considered safe by public health organizations. These products tend to be faster and safer than disinfectants, but disinfectants usually have broader kill claims	A disinfectant kills infectious fungi, bacteria and viruses (but not bacterial spores) on hard environmental surfaces	A virucide destroys or irreversibly inactivates viruses in the inanimate environment	A sterilant is used to destroy or eliminate all forms of microbial life including: • Fungi • Viruses • All forms of bacteria and their spores

Any product that claims to kill bacteria, viruses, mold or fungi must be registered with the EPA as a pesticide.

Factors Influencing the Action of a Disinfectant

- Concentration of the solution required
- Time required for the action of the solution
- Type and nature of material to be disinfected
- Kind of infecting organisms
- Temperature of the solution: The higher the temperature of the solution, the more active the disinfectant is likely to be effective (Fig. 3)

The main points have been presented in the figure as follows:

Important Points to Remember While using a Disinfectant

- The article to be disinfected should be completely immersed in the solution.
- Strong solutions act faster than the weak ones, but if time is available, a weak solution will be better as it is less expensive.

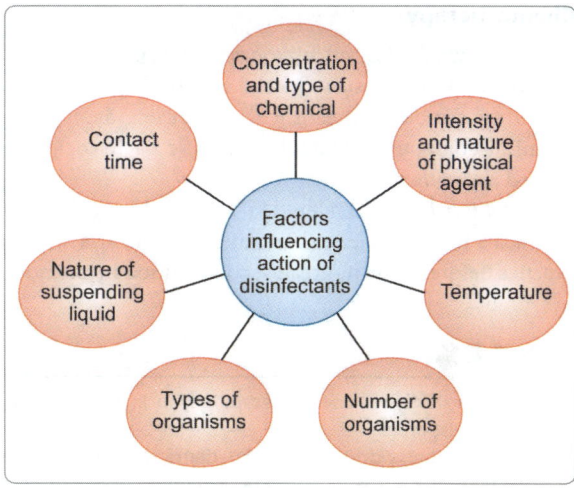

Figure 3: Factors influencing action of disinfectant

- A chemical which may be disinfectant in certain strength may act only as an antiseptic in a weaker solution and in a very weak solution it may even stimulate the growth of the organisms.
- It is better to prepare the disinfectant whenever it is required to be used rather than preparing large amount and keeping for longer period as certain type of chemical may change its color or quality if it is preserved for longer periods.

  But solutions for medical effect on human tissues, which are used only very little like, acriflavin, mercurochrome, Tr: iodine, etc. shall be prepared with proper strength and amount in airtight bottles, and be kept safely in cupboard and taken into small bottles for at hand use only. Such mild chemicals prepared in sterile water as weak solutions are used for irrigating body cavities like urinary bladder, or wound sinuses or as medicines in wounds with or without dressings.

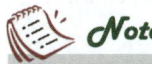 *Note*

- Hypochlorites are most recommended for decontamination of hepatitis and AIDS viruses. Organic material such as feces or blood inactivate chlorine based disinfectants, therefore, surfaces must be clean before their use.

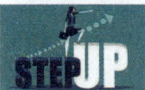

Gas plasma
- Plasma is a fourth state of matter which is distinguishable from liquid, solid or gas. In nature, plasma is widespread in outer space
- Gas plasma is generated in an enclosed chamber under deep vacuum using Radio frequency or Microwave emery to excite gas molecules are produced charged particles
- It can be used for hand sterilization

Gas plasma is safe as it helps in achieving sterilization at relatively low temperatures (≤50°C), preserving the integrity of polymer-based instruments, which cannot be subjected to autoclaves and ovens. Moreover, plasma sterilization is safe, both for the operator and the patient.

Unit V ❖ Control of Bacteria (Methods of Disinfection and Sterilization)

CONTROL OF MICROORGANISMS IN THE HUMAN BODY

Chemotherapy

Chemicals which destroy microorganisms on the skin are not satisfactory for destroying them in the internal organs and deeper tissues. Special chemical compounds are required, which can be taken into the body and carried by the blood stream without causing damage to any part of the body. The treatment of disease by chemical compound, which has specific bacteriocidal or bacteriostatic actions against microorganisms is termed *chemotherapy*.

Paul Ehrlich is considered to be the **father of chemotherapy** who is the first person to put effort in finding chemicals to treat diseases. Treatment of Malaria with quinine and amebic dysentery with emetine was in practice before. Ehrlich's greatest contribution in chemotherapy is the discovery of Salvarsan for the treatment of syphilis.

FACTS

- The era of cancer chemotherapy began in the 1940s with the first use of nitrogen mustards and folic acid antagonist drugs.
- Sidney Farber, world-renowned pediatric pathologist, made major contributions to his field but is acknowledged as the father of the modern era of chemotherapy. He recognized that folic acid stimulated leukemic cell growth and enhanced disease progression.
- Dr Suresh Advani is known to be the first oncologist in India to have successfully done a bone-marrow transplant. He used chemotherapy in a 9-year-old girl down with myeloid leukemia. He was also a part of clinical trials to help children with lymphoblastic leukemia.

Antibiotics

Antibacterial substances produced by living cells are known as antibiotics. This term is used for synthetically-produced agents also. First antibiotic discovered by Alexander Fleming in 1928 was penicillin produced by a mold *Penicillium notatum*. Penicillin was in use from 1940. By the end of World War II, penicillin was in wide use. Streptomycin is specifically effective against tuberculosis and chloramphenicol against typhoid. Further developments are erythromycin, gentamicin, terramycin and others.

Some antibiotics act effectively on different organisms at a time and these are called *broad spectrum antibiotics*. They are therefore useful in the treatment of a number of diseases. Chloramphenicol, erythromycin, etc. are examples for broad spectrum antibiotics.

Untoward Effects of Antibiotics and Chemotherapy

Even though the antibiotics and chemotherapy have created great are the hopes in treating diseases, they have two untoward effects, which are as follows:

- **Resistance of microorganisms to the drug and allergic reactions in some people:** Resistance to drug is developed due to inadequate dosage or failure of maintenance of adequate concentration of drugs in tissues. To prevent the allergic reaction, the antibiotic sensitivity should be tested in patient before administering any one of them.
- **Super infections:** It is important to remember that antibiotics are given for long time to a patient, it will kill or remove the normal organisms in the body and other organisms grow and multiply producing other infections to him. This is known as *super infection*.

PRECAUTIONS TO BE OBSERVED WHILE ADMINISTERING ANTIMICROBIAL AGENTS

Because the antimicrobial agents produce adverse reaction in people, we should always try to get a history of previous sensitivity to the drug. It is most important in the case of penicillin. On no account should penicillin be given to a patient without testing his sensitivity or to a patient with history of sensitivity. It may result in death. Sensitivity test should be done with a very small dose of penicillin. Adrenalin should be ready at hand to administer immediately even during performing the sensitivity test. The adverse reaction may be of varying severity, like anaphylaxis, serum sickness or contact dermatitis. Nurses are prone to develop contact dermatitis because of the constant contact with such drugs. Antibiotics should not be administered without specific instruction from a physician and the instructions should be strictly followed.

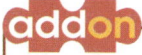

Penicillin sensitivity has been summarized as follows:

Penicillin allergy

- In severe penicillin allergy (e.g., anaphylaxis, bronchospasm, urticaria, angioedema), avoid all penicillins, cephalosporins and other beta-lactam antibiotics
- In non-severe penicillin allergy (e.g., mild rash) use cephalosporins and carbapenems with caution
- Some reactions (e.g., nausea) are not considered allergies and do not warrant prohibiting penicillin use

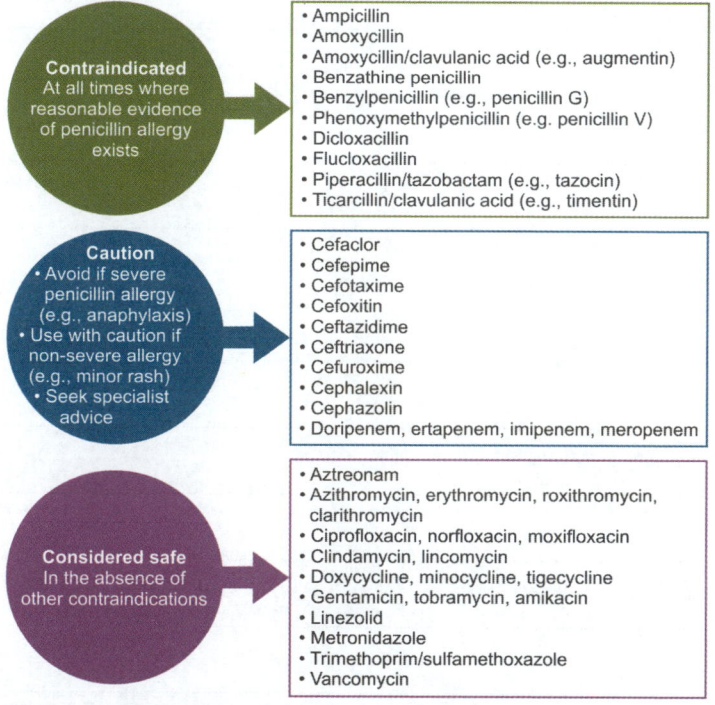

- Record allergy alert in the patient health record allergy section
- Record details of allergy incident including drug name, description of reaction, severity date, and name of the person making the report
- In hospitals, contact ward pharmacist, infectious diseases or immunology consultant for any concerns/queries
- Immunology consultation for formal testing and/or desensitization may be indicated

Unit V ❖ Control of Bacteria (Methods of Disinfection and Sterilization)

NOTES

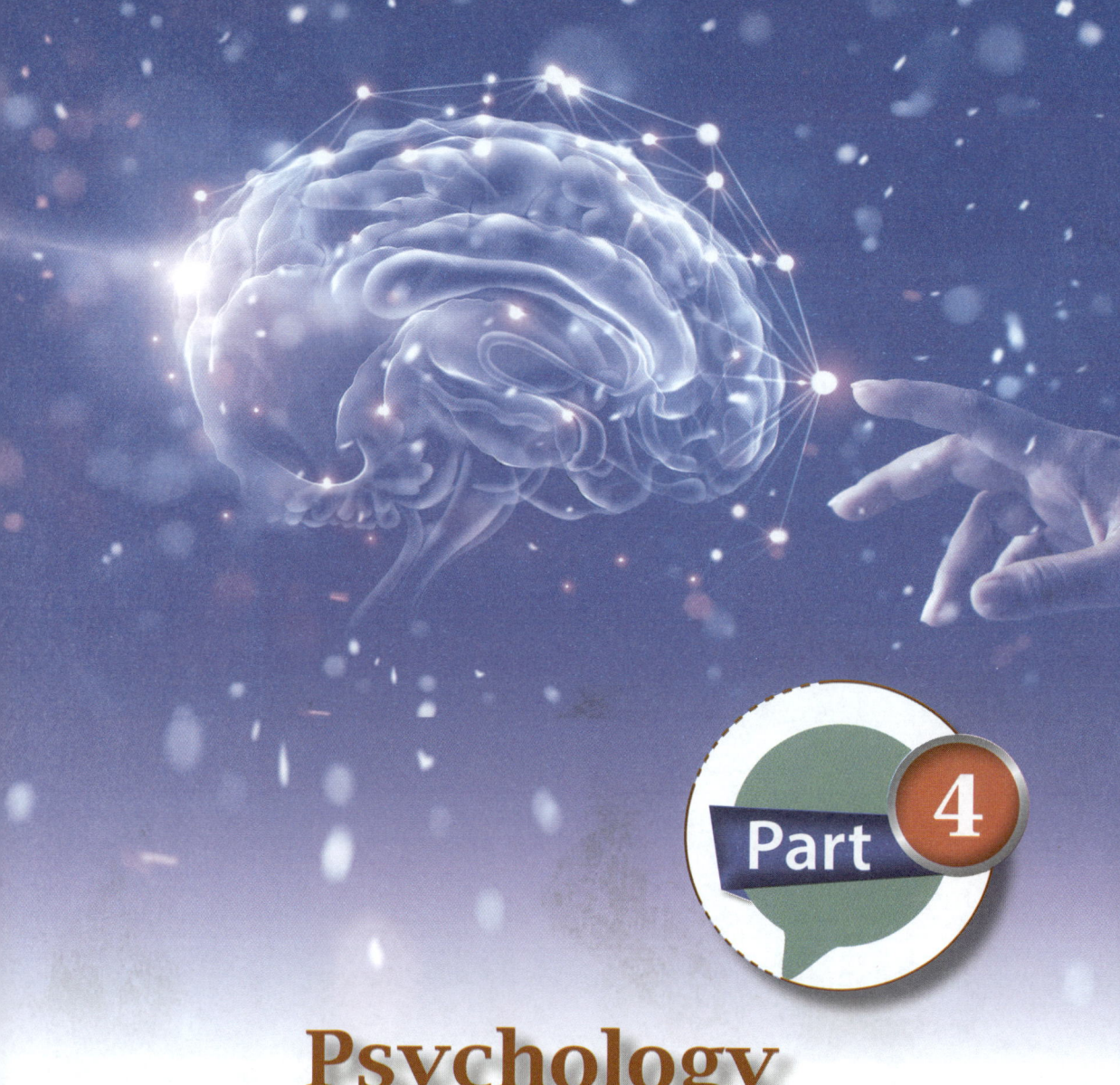

Psychology

Part 4

Part Outline

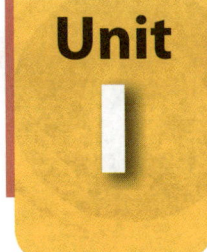

Unit 1

Introduction

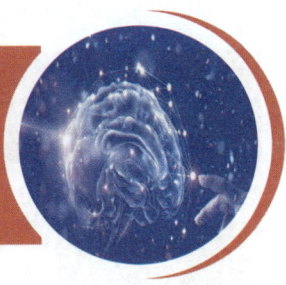

DEFINITION

Psychology is defined as the science that studies the mental processes, especially those affecting behavior of the human beings. The mental processes, which affect human behavior are thinking, feeling, reasoning, desiring, intelligence, motives and emotions. The study of psychology helps to get an insight into human behavior.

PURPOSE OF STUDYING PSYCHOLOGY

Knowledge of psychology is essential for a nurse to know others and herself/himself to differentiate normal and abnormal behavior and to help others and herself/himself to develop normal mental health. Understanding a patient as an individual is the basis of good nursing. A nurse in her daily works meets many people, like patients and their relatives, visitors, families and her own co-workers. Each individual is different in different ways. To deal with different people including patients in a smooth way, the nurse should have some knowledge of psychology.

SCOPE OF PSYCHOLOGY

Psychology has different branches, such as normal psychology, abnormal psychology, educational psychology, children's psychology, medical psychology and so on. Medical psychology deals with patients suffering from disorders of the mind. The persons trained in medicine and psychology are known as psychiatrists. The basic purpose of psychology is to study or investigate human behavior.

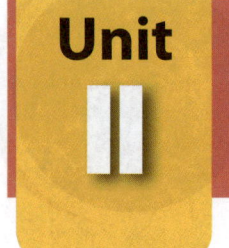

Unit II

Psychology of Human Behavior

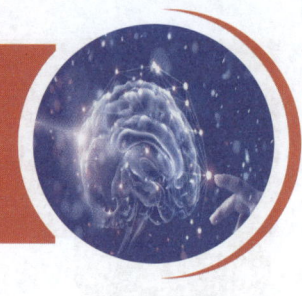

DYNAMICS OF BEHAVIOR

Behavior is the result of physical and mental factors interacting together. The physical basis of behavior is contained in the cerebral cortex, hypothalamus and thalamus, situated in the brain.

Behavior consists of our:

- Physical responses, habits and skills
- Organic responses such as feelings, emotions and tensions of the individual
- Intellectual responses, such as perceiving, thinking and reasoning

BODY-MIND RELATIONSHIP

Any state of mind affects the body and the state of body always affects the mind. Mind and body cannot be separated. Emotions stimulate the nerve centers and cause bodily changes, for example, facial expressions while crying or laughing. Similarly, when one is tired or fatigued he/she is prone to bad emotions, such as anger, fear or anxiety. Emotions also cause internal physiological effects, such as loss of appetite, nausea, vomiting, etc. There are a group of diseases known as 'psychosomatic' diseases, such as essential hypertension, peptic ulcer, etc. They are mostly physical expressions of psychological conditions. These diseases are stated to be due to the mind acting upon the body. All emotions, such as sorrow, joy, anger, etc. have their effects upon the body. A person who is not mentally healthy cannot be physically healthy. The definition of health given by World Health Organization (WHO) is:

"Health is a state of complete physical, mental and social well-being and not merely an absence of disease or infirmity."

This statement also indicates a strong relationship between our body and mind.

MOTIVATION

Motivation is an inner force, which drives an individual to certain action. It also determines the human behavior. Without motivation, learning cannot take place and behavior change cannot be expected. The terms, motives, needs, wants, desires and urges are almost same and these terms are interdependent yet interrelated. An individual is motivated to follow certain behavior to satisfy the basic human needs.

MAIN HUMAN NEEDS

The main human needs can be classified as follows:

- **Biologic needs** such as food for hunger, water for thirst, medicine for sick, etc.
- **Social needs** are love, recognition, education, acceptance, etc.
- **Economic needs** are economic securities, which everyone wants.

UNCONSCIOUS MOTIVES

According to psychologists, the human mind has the following three levels:

1. **Conscious mind:** The conscious experiences are being aware/knowing, feeling, etc. for example, we know that a patient is ill and feels sorry for his/her illness.
2. **Subconscious mind**: The subconscious mind is the second level of the function of mind, for example, we tend to forget things of lesser importance happening around us. Many of our daily actions are performed in this way.
3. **Unconscious mind:** The third level of unconscious mind stores all our forgotten past experiences, such as repressed wishes, desires, fears, etc. Many of these come to the surface during sleep and are responsible for dreams and for abnormal behavior. Many kinds of the abnormal behaviors and mental disorders (e.g., psychoneurosis) are said to be due to the unconscious part of the mind forcing its way into conscious mind.

 Stimulant

Psychoanalysis is a technique used by the psychologists to study the unconscious mind. Dream analysis, hypnosis and word associations are some of the techniques employed in psychoanalysis.

MENTAL HEALTH

Mental health is a part of total health of the body. 'Sound mind is in a sound body' is an old saying. The proverb which is of Greek origin, insists that the mind and body should be both healthy and sound. A healthy person can think normally and act instantly in any given situation. The definition of health given by the World Health Organization (WHO) includes physical, mental and social well-being (Fig. 1).

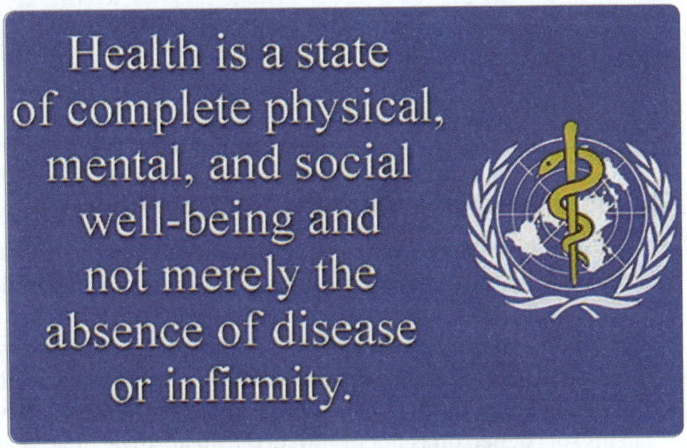

As such, mental health is an important component of health. It is not only concerned with early detection, diagnosis and treatment of mental disorders, but also with the preservation and promotion of good mental health, and prevention of mental illness.

Health is a state of complete physical, mental, and social well-being and not merely the absence of disease or infirmity.

Figure 1: Definition of health by WHO

Foundations and Contributing Factors of Mental Health

The foundation of mental health is laid in early childhood. The contributing factors of mental health are:

- **Good physical health:** Good physical health is the basis and stepping stone of mental health. All the systems of the body are to be in good working conditions so that the body could perform in unison. Those who are having defective functioning of the systems of the body, are easy victims to mental illness.
- **Basic needs:** Mental health cannot be attained unless the basic needs of an individual are satisfied. Mainly one's physical, psychological and social needs must be met for the promotion of his/her mental health.

Unit II ❖ Psychology of Human Behavior

- **Habits:** Certain habits, such as work, study, play, sleep and rest contribute to mental health. Control of emotions both at home and outside, learning to adjust cheerfully to the surroundings, appreciations for others and respecting the rights of others, cultivation of self-confidence, setting reasonable goals for oneself are some of the attitudes, which one should cultivate for developing good mental health (Fig. 2).

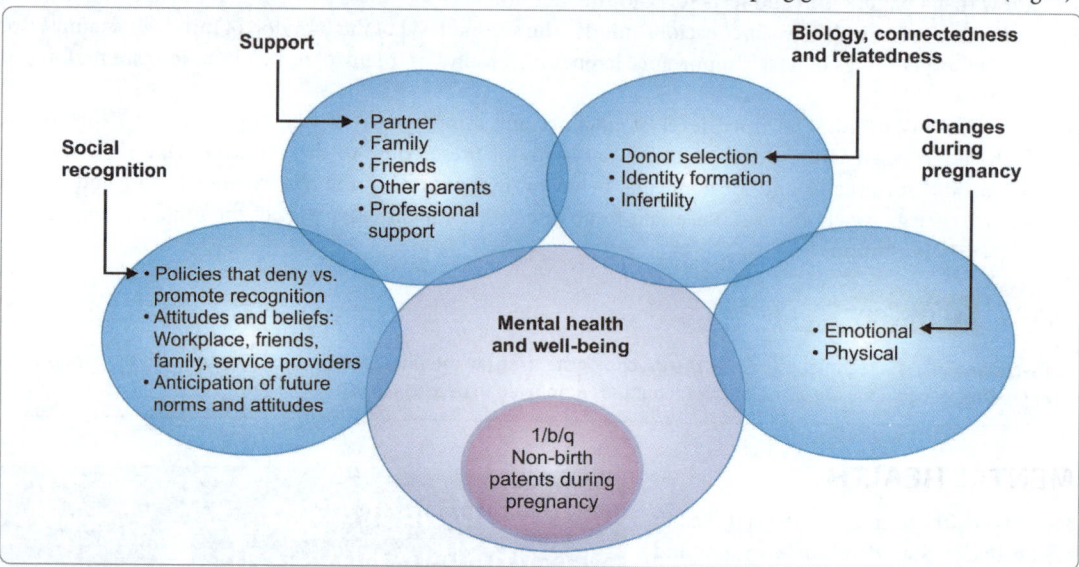

Figure 2: Contributing factors of mental health

Characteristics of a Mentally Healthy Person

- A mentally healthy person is satisfied with himself/herself. He/she feels happy, calm and cheerful and does not feel pity about himself/herself. There are no conflicts and such person is not at 'war' with self.
- A mentally healthy person is well-adjusted. Such person can easily get along with others. He/she accepts criticism and is not easily upset. This kind of person understands the emotional needs of others and tries to be considerate and courteous in his/her dealings with others.
- A mentally healthy person has good emotional control and he/she does not get easily affected by emotions. This sort of person is not dominated by fear, anger, love, jealousy, guilt or worries. He/she faces problems boldly and solves them intelligently.

EMOTIONS

Emotions are strong feelings of an individual. It is an important component of a human personality and it further motivates the behavior. Some of the important emotions are: anger, fear, love, hate, jealousy, moodiness, joy, sorrow, pity, sympathy, etc.

What Characterizes Emotions?

An emotional experience is characterized by both external and internal changes in the human being.

- **External changes:** The external changes or expressions are apparent and easily seen by others such as facial expressions, changes in the voice and changes in the posture, etc. By studying the facial expressions, we can find out if a person is angry, happy or depressed. They accompany an emotional state to communicate reaction and intention of actions.

- **Internal changes:** The internal changes or the physiological components are brought by emotions and these can be observed through bodily symptoms, such as rapid pulse, respiration, increased blood pressure, tension and pain. Usually, these changes are temporary and subside when the individual returns to the normal stage from the state of intense emotion.

Role of Emotions in Health and Sickness

An emotional state determines and represents human behavior. Anger can make a person rude. Disorders of emotions interfere with the efficiency of an individual such as lack of concentration, lack of appetite, increased risk of accidents, lack of sleep, palpitation, etc. Emotional disorders in children may appear in the form of aggressiveness and antisocial behaviors. If the emotional disorders are sustained by a person, they will be harmful to that individual. Due to disturbed emotional states, diseases such as insomnia, hypertension, peptic ulcer, etc. occur. Emotional crisis may even predispose to mental diseases. Some specific emotions are fear, anger, anxiety and love.

Control of Emotions

A well-adjusted mentally healthy person is able to keep his/her emotions under control. Children should be raised with love and appreciation from parents and others so that they will have emotional maturity. For adults, happy family is the basis of emotional adjustment. Anxious parents need reassurance and their fear should be allayed.

Methods of Controlling Emotions

- Cultivate hobbies and good habits of reading and recreation
- Avoid mental conflicts
- Understand own limitations and adjust accordingly
- Develop a sense of humor

The study of psychology helps us to understand the basis of emotions and the need to keep emotions under control.

HABITS

Habits are accustomed way of doing things. Habits accumulated through generation become customs and customs in turn create social behavior. Habits once formed persist and influence human behavior. Habits may be good or bad. Habits build up human personality. An individual should not become a slave to his/her habits, rather should remain a master of habits. Good habits promote health and bad habits may ruin an individual, e.g., smoking, alcoholism, etc. Eating and sleeping at regular time are good habits. It is the job of psychologists and sociologists to find out how good habits can be developed and bad ones are eliminated.

ATTITUDES

Attitudes are acquired characteristics of an individual. They are long-lasting dispositions of the mind. They are not learnt from textbooks but are acquired by social interactions. Attitudes are acquired by oneself and not taught by anyone. Like habits, attitudes are of many kinds, such as attitude to sickness, attitude to life, attitude to family planning, etc. Once an attitude is formed, it is difficult to change. The responsibility to develop good attitude in children from childhood devolves upon parents, teachers, religious leaders and elders. A nurse should cultivate positive attitudes, such as kindness, understanding, consideration and dedicated service. Developing good attitude toward our life is an essential factor for a comfortable and happy life.

Unit II ❖ Psychology of Human Behavior

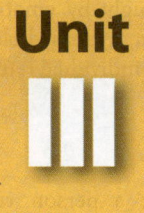

Unit III

Learning, Thinking, Reasoning and Problem Solving

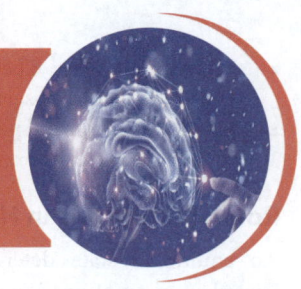

LEARNING

Definition

Learning is necessary for human survival and progress. Leaning means acquiring knowledge, skills, and formation of habits and perception. To a large extent, learning depends on intelligence. Learning is both conscious and unconscious and is a continuous process in human life.

Conditions Affecting Learning

- **Intelligence of the individual:** Learning depends upon the intelligence and mental ability of an individual. The mental faculty is related to heredity, nutrition, and IQ. Children with low IQ are poor learners and sometimes they may not learn at all, even if all the other factors are favorable.
- **Age:** There is an old saying that "you cannot teach an old dog new tricks". The highest curve of learning reaches at the 22–25 years of age. After the age of 30, there is a sharp decline in learning.
- **Learning situation:** Physical facilities for learning, such as institution, teachers, textbooks and audio-visual aids promote learning.
- **Motivation:** In order to learn effectively, there must be adequate motivation. The powerful motives, such as encouragements, praise, rewards and success stimulate the learning of students.
- **Physical health of the individual:** Physically handicapped persons, like deaf, dumb, or chronically sick people cannot learn well although exceptions may be there (Step up).
- **Mental health of the individual:** Worries, anxieties, and fears, interfere with learning.

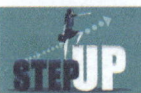

Stephen Hawking
Stephen Hawking was one of the most well-known physicists in the world, and was diagnosed with ALS when he was 21. Hawking spoke with the assistance of a computer in the later years of his life and was a full-time powerchair user since 1980s. His in-depth studies of the universe, specifically the framework of general relativity and quantum mechanics, became a popular introduction to the field for lay persons, and Hawking was a popular figure in pop culture as well—appearing on hugely popular television shows such as *The Simpsons* and *Star Trek: The Next Generation*. His best-selling work, *A Brief History of Time*, stayed on the Sunday Times bestsellers list for an astounding 237 weeks.

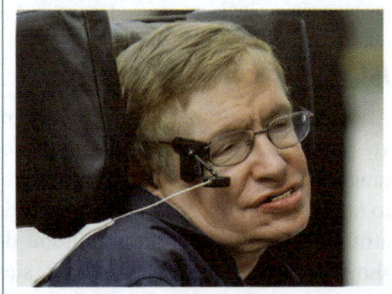

Stephen Hawking

Helen Keller

She was an American author, political activist, and lecturer. Helen Keller was the first deaf and blind person to earn a Bachelor of Arts degree. Her story was famously portrayed in the play and film, *The Miracle Worker,* which documented how her teacher Anne Sullivan was finally able to develop a language that Helen could understand. Helen wrote a total of twelve published books, including her spiritual autobiography, *My Religion,* and was also a member of the Socialist Party in America. She campaigned heavily for women's rights and other labor rights, and was also awarded the Presidential Medal of Freedom by Lyndon Johnson in 1964.

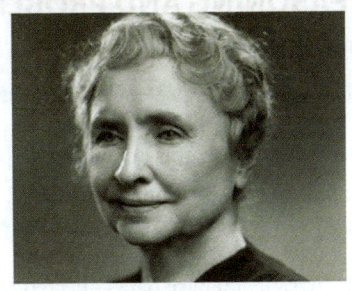
Helen Keller

TYPES OF LEARNING THEORIES

Psychologists have proposed a number of theories about the types of learning, such as:

- **Learning by conditioned reflex:** It is well known that when a dog sees food, it begins to salivate. This is an inborn reflex. Pavlov, the Russian Physiologist linked two stimuli to produce a newly-learned response. He discovered that if a bell was rung when the dog was not fed, the ringing of bell alone could induce salivation naturally. This is called conditioned reflex. The psychologists proposed that learning takes place partly by this mechanism.
- **Trial and error method:** The child 'tries and tries again' repeatedly using a number of approaches until accidentally the ideal approach becomes obvious.
- **Learning by observation and imitation:** We learn a good deal by observation and imitation of others. A child learns language by observation and imitation. A child copies or imitates gestures, facial expressions and movements, such as walking, from others. Observation is most important in healthcare industry. Observation promotes attention, discrimination, recognition and helps to understand patient's condition and make decisions based on these observations.
- **Learning by doing:** In this type, there is co-ordination of muscular responses with sensory impulses. Nursing skills for doing procedures are learnt by doing only for example, learning typing, musical instruments, etc.
- **Learning by remembering:** We learn by memorizing or remembering some dates, events, some faces, etc.
- **Learning by Insight:** We solve a problem by insight or exploration. When a disease is diagnosed some insight is involved. Human beings learn by a combination of methods, which is already in their insight.

THINKING

Definition

Thinking is an active mental process. Man is a thinking animal. Thinking includes perception, memory, imagination and reasoning. The anatomical basis of thinking is cerebral cortex. In fact, the actual purpose of education is to help and teach people to think and not merely to memorize facts and figures to reproduce.

- 'Imaginative thinking' is a mental process, which involves the thinking in the absence of original sensory stimuli. Daydreaming and thinking of our future plans are examples of imaginative thinking.
- The highest form of thinking is said to be 'creative thinking', e.g., an artist painting a picture. Creative thinking is said to be responsible for new inventions and discoveries.

Unit III ❖ Learning, Thinking, Reasoning and Problem Solving

REASONING AND PROBLEM-SOLVING

Definition

The important aspect of thinking is problem-solving, which is considered as the highest stage of human learning. Reasoning can be part of problem-solving. Some of the problems in our life are simple, whereas many other problems are more complex and difficult, and require thinking and reasoning.

Reasoning requires intelligence:

There are several steps in reasoning process, such as:

- Collection of information from the subject
- Arrangement of data collected carefully
- Observation of the implications
- Drawing conclusions
- Testing the conclusions

An intelligent person reasons the matters well. Reasoning is not always fully correct. Fallacies may occur. In difficult or complex problems, repetition of all processes may be required to reach a conclusion.

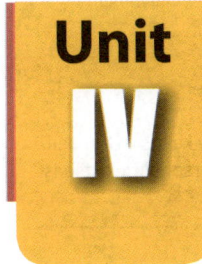

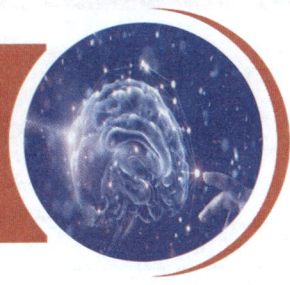

Unit IV
Personality

DEFINITION

Personality is the sum total of a person's heredity and environment. It is a declaration of which type of a person an individual is. Personality is a keyword in psychology because it implies the physical and mental traits or features of an individual. It is important to remember that the personality of the nurse affects the well-being of the patient and the success of her work depends, to a great extent, on her personality.

COMPONENTS OF PERSONALITY

Mainly there are four components of personality mentioned as follows:

1. **Physical traits or features,** such as height, weight, facial expression, physical health, etc. For a lay person personality means an impressive appearance and a healthy body.
2. **Emotional features** are strong feelings, such as fear, anger, love, jealousy, worries, etc. Such feelings affect the makeup of an individual's personality.
3. **Intelligence:** The intellectual ability of a person affects his personality. An intelligent person, who has a good personality and subnormal intelligence, is described as a 'dull' person.
4. **Behavior:** Behavior is a reflection of one's personality. Behavior is described using terms, such as gentle, kind, affectionate, balanced, submissive and aggressive. When we assess a human personality, all these components should be taken into consideration.

TRAITS OF PERSONALITY

A trait is described as an ability to behave in a consistent manner in different situations. Human personality is a bundle of traits. The basic personality traits are established by the age of six years. Some traits such as good manners are cultivated, some may be modified depending on the society in which we are placed, e.g., sense of humor.

Some of the personality traits are cheerfulness, good manners, loyalty, honesty, sportsmanship, reliability, kindness, sense of humor, tactfulness, patience, humbleness, willing to help others, etc.

The public expect some of the personality traits from a nurse, such as kindness, honesty, patience, tolerance, perseverance, consciousness, thoroughness in the subject and initiative. It is possible to cultivate these traits by learning, observing seniors and by practical experiences.

Stimulant

- The Swiss Psychiatrist, Carl Jung (1875–1961) divided personalities into extrovert and introvert.
- **An extrovert** is a person who is practical, active and easily mixes with others.
- **An introvert** is a person who is reserved and shy, he suffers or hides everything and generally keeps to himself/herself and does not mingle freely with others. Most people exhibit characteristics of both personalities at least in particular situations.

PROCESS OF DEVELOPMENT OF PERSONALITY

Human life consists of definite stages of growth mentioned below. Each stage is marked by distinctive psychology.

- **Infancy:** It is the first one year of life. The infant is hardly a social creature. There is rapid physical and mental growth. The infant is totally dependent on the mother. By the end of first year, the infant is able to stand up for short time and try to walk with a little support and enjoys simple tricks and games.
- **Pre-school child:** There is considerable growth of brain at this stage. He feeds himself, speaks, loves his home, fears darkness, loves stories and wants to assume responsibility and begins to mix with other children.
- **School age:** This stage ranges from 5 to 12 years. The child is active all the time. By the age of 8 years his/her mental powers are fully developed. His/her brain is almost the size of an adult. The child begins to reason out matters, gradually detaches himself from family and shows more attachment to his playmates and friends, and begins to form groups. The period of childhood terminates with the onset of puberty which is about 11 years in case of girls and 13 years in case of boys.
- **Adolescence:** This stage is also called 'teenage'. It is a turbulent period in one's life—a period of dreams, adventures, love and romance. The teens strive for independence and dislike parental authority. They are fully aware of social values and norms. There is rapid physical growth.
- **Adults:** The person becomes matured and more balanced. Physical and mental characteristics are fully developed. There are no rigid demarking lines when changing from adolescence to adulthood.
- **Old age:** There is no definite time to start old age in a person. Due to many reasons a person gets his old age even before the expected chronological age. Whatever is the reason, old age is a gradual process marked by decline in physical powers of sense organs marked by psychological changes, such as impaired memory, rigidity of outlook, irritability, bitterness, inner withdrawal and social maladjustments.

FACTORS INFLUENCING GROWTH AND DEVELOPMENT

- **Heredity:** The genetic factors, such as height, weight, mental and social aspects and personality influence the growth and personality development of a person.
- **Constitutional factors:** The constitution of an individual is an effective factor to determine the type of his/her personality. We are always impressed by an individual who has a muscular and a well-proportioned body. Height, weight, physical defects, health and strength affect one's personality. There can be three types of personality based on constitution:
  - Short and stout
  - Tall and thin
  - Muscular and well-proportioned.

- **Biological factors:** The working of the nervous system, glands and blood chemistry determine our characteristics and habitual modes of behavior. These factors form biological basis of personality. Adrenal gland, thyroid gland, pituitary gland and endocrine gland affect personality. Personality defects lead to the development of inferiority complex and the mental mechanism of compensation. This aspect also includes the mental ability of the child.
  - **Age:** The growth rate is maximum during fetal life, infancy and at the time of puberty.
  - **Sex:** At the age of 10–11 years, the female children show sudden increase in weight and height during the onset of puberty and male children grow well between the ages of 13 and 15 years.
  - **Nutrition:** Malnutrition, especially deficiency of protein during early life slows down growth.
  - **Infection:** Chronic illness or recurrent illness slows down growth and development.
- **Intelligence:** Intelligence is mainly hereditary. Persons, who are very intelligent can make better adjustment in home, school and society than those who are less intelligent.
- **Sex differences:** Sex differences play a vital role in the development of personality of an individual. Boys are generally more assertive and vigorous. They prefer adventures. Girls are quieter and get more affected by personal, emotional and social problems.
- **Nervous system:** Development of personality is influenced by the nature of nervous system.
- **Environment:** The sociologists emphasize that the personality of the individual develops in a social environment. It is in the social environment that he comes to have moral ideas, social attitudes and interests. This enables him/her to develop personality. Economic factors and standard of living affect growth and development. Children from well to do families have better height and weight and good personality. The important aspects of the environment are as follows:
  - Physical environment
  - Social environment
  - Family environment
  - Cultural environment
- **Psychological factors:** Tender love, care and proper child-parent relationship affect growth and development favorably. The basic needs of the child must be met such as needs for maternal protection, love and understanding in the home, need for health protection, treatment of sick children, adequate food and shelter, education, need for play and recreation, need for social protection and special needs of the handicapped. When these needs are met, they positively affect the personality of a person.

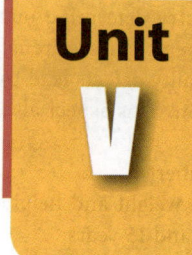

Unit V

Intelligence

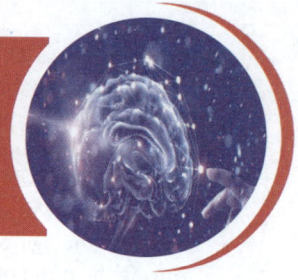

DEFINITION

Intelligence is an important factor of personality. Intelligence is the ability to see meaningful relationships between things. It includes perceiving, knowing, reasoning and remembering. The work of a nurse requires intelligence. The observation of symptoms, understanding and anticipating the needs and complaints of patients and to predict the outcome, etc. require intelligence. Psychologists say that intelligence results from the interplay between heredity and environment.

TYPES OF INTELLIGENCE

Some psychologists describe that intelligence has two aspects, **general intelligence** and **special intelligence**. General intelligence is the ability to solve problems of everyday life and special intelligence is the ability displayed in special fields like mathematics, games, music, painting, etc.

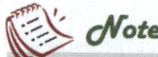 *Note*

Mental Age

Many attempts have been made to measure intelligence. The first test was devised in 1896 by the scientists Benet and Simon. They developed the concept of mental age, that is if a child could do the test devised for 5 years of age, but could not do a test devised for 6 years of age was credited with a mental age of 5 years. By such tests the mental age level is realized, but the brightness or dullness of the child/individual is not indicated. It is a sp-cognitive test.

INTELLIGENCE QUOTIENT (IQ)

It is an improved test to realize mental age. It is obtained by dividing the mental age by chronological age and multiplying by 100.

$$IQ = \frac{\text{Mental age}}{\text{Chronological age}} \times 100$$

When the mental age is the same as chronological age, the IQ is 100. The highest the IQ, the more brilliant the child is. Eighty percent of the people have an IQ of near 100.

Levels of Intelligence

Terms used	IQ range
Idiot	0–24
Imbecile	25–49
Moron	50–69
Borderline	70–79
Low normal	80–89
Normal	90–109
Superior	110–119
Very superior	120–139
Near genius	140 and above

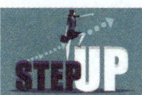

The most common types of IQ tests are:
- Stanford-Binet intelligence scale
- Universal nonverbal intelligence
- Differential ability scales
- Peabody individual achievement test
- Wechsler individual achievement test
- Wechsler adult intelligence scale
- Woodcock Johnson tests of cognitive disabilities

Advantage of IQ Test

Patients with high IQ tax the nurses a good deal. A rapid decline of IQ (dementia) occurs when the brain is damaged by either tumors, injury, drugs, alcohol or infection. Intelligence tests are conducted to recognize the children who need special education, college and professional education and to provide educational guidance.

Disadvantage of IQ Test

Intelligence tests have its own limitations because they cannot measure the intelligence accurately or indicate one's character or emotions.

NOTES

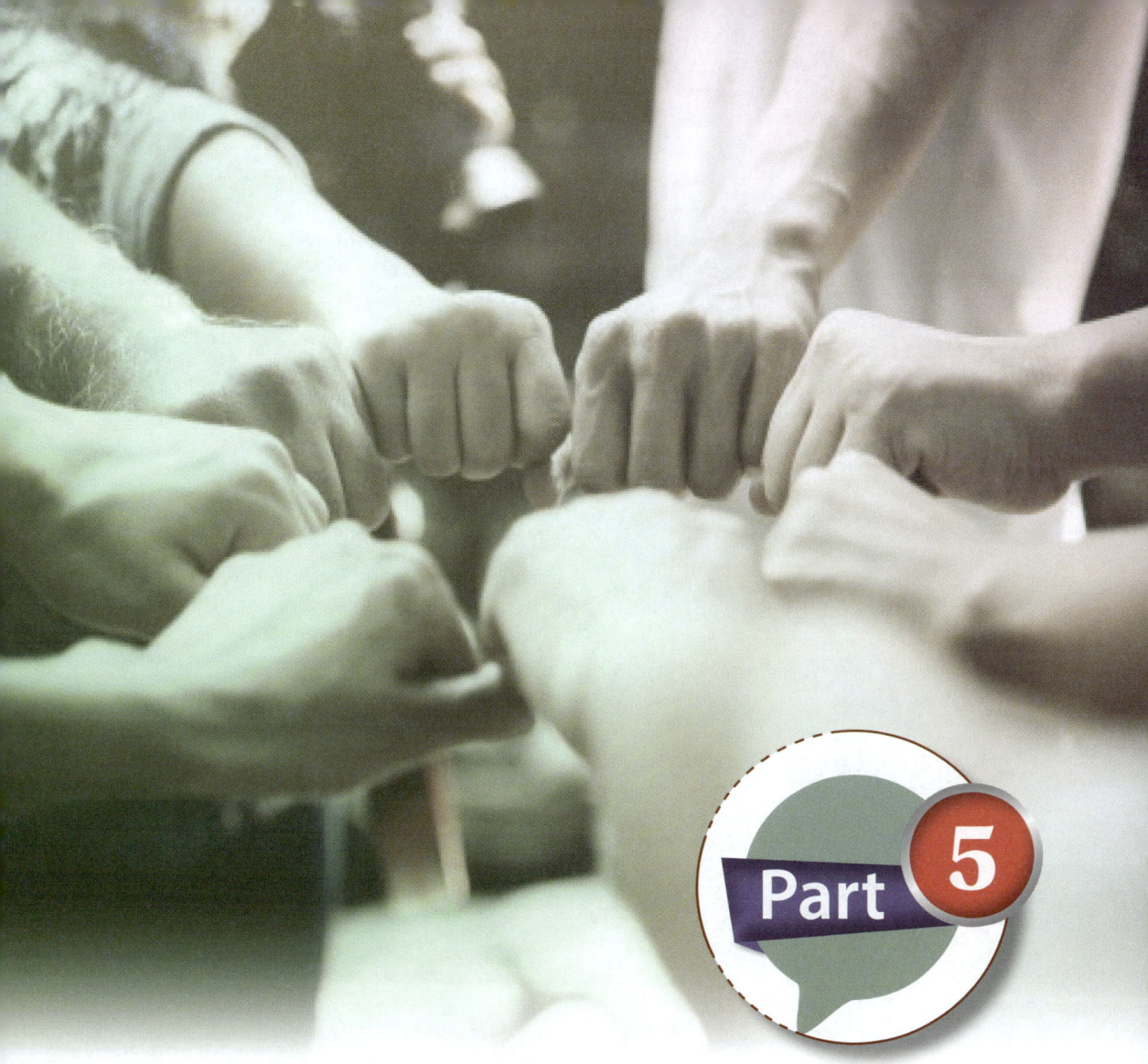

Part 5

Sociology

Part Outline

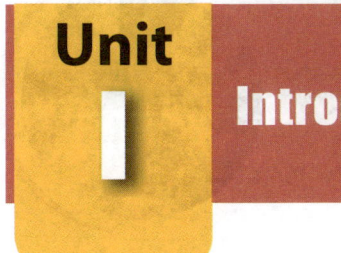

Unit I

Introduction

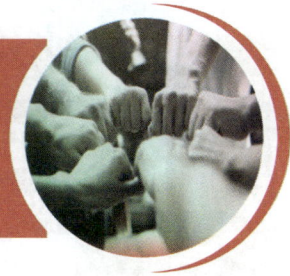

Illness is not only a medical problem but it is also social and psychological problem. The problems presented by a patient are not always purely medical but they are also psychosocial. Diseases such as tuberculosis, leprosy and venereal diseases have etiological causes lying in the social problems. Doctors and nurses should possess the knowledge of biological, behavioral and social sciences for the successful functioning in the field of health care.

DEFINITION OF SOCIOLOGY

In different books, different definitions conveying almost same meanings are given. But a very simple definition of sociology is as follows:

"Sociology is the scientific study of the development of human relationships and organizations." That is, interpersonal and intergroup relationships which are distinct in their behaviors, of an individual.

IMPORTANCE OF SOCIOLOGY IN NURSING

- The study of **sociology** helps **nurses** to identify the psychosocial problems of patients, which inturn helps *to* **improve** the quality of treatment.
- Sociology helps nurses to give a culturally competent and sensitive care.
- It guides nurses to respect the social values and norms of the patient.
- It helps nurses to understand the relationship between disease and the social factors.
- Knowledge on societal customs and superstitions may help the nurse to handle such patients during management of diseases.

Unit
II
Individual

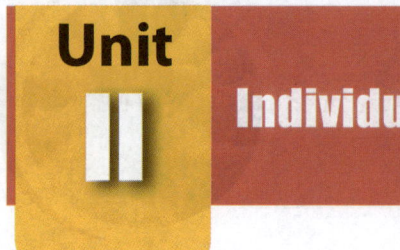
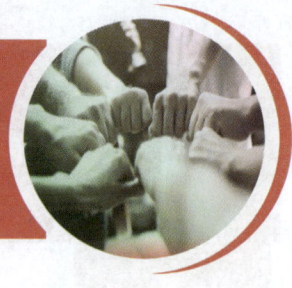

RIGHTS OF AN INDIVIDUAL

The Universal Declaration of Human Rights speaks about the right to health in the following terms:

"Everyone has the right to a standard of living adequate for the health and well-being of himself and of his family, including food, clothing, housing and medical care and necessary social services, and the right to security, in the event of unemployment, sickness, disability, widowhood, old age or other lack of livelihood in circumstances beyond his control. Motherhood and childhood are entitled to special care and assistance. All children, whether born in or out of wedlock, shall enjoy the same social protection."

Constitution of World Health Organization (WHO) expressed the human rights as:

The enjoyment of the highest attainable standard of health is one of the fundamental rights of every human being without distinction of race, religion, political belief, economic or social condition.

Most countries of the world have accepted the idea of the right to health.

The Constitution of India guarantees the following seven broad categories of fundamental rights:

1. The right to equality
2. The right to freedom of speech and expressions
3. The right against exploitation
4. The right to freedom of practice and propagation of religion
5. The right to minorities to conserve their culture
6. The right to property
7. The right to constitutional remedies for the enforcement of fundamental rights.

RESPONSIBILITIES FOR ACHIEVING HEALTH

Although health has been recognized as fundamental right of every human being, it has to be achieved by individual effort. It cannot be given by one person to another person.

The responsibility to attain good health not only rests on the individual but also upon the community or state. Responsibilities regarding personal health, such as diet, care of skin, teeth, recreation, exercise, cultivation of healthful habits, immunization, early reporting when falling sick, optimum utilization of available health services, etc. must be accepted by the individual to achieve maximum health.

POLICIES OF THE GOVERNMENT TO SAFEGUARD THE HEALTH OF THE CITIZENS

In civilized societies, state government assumes responsibility to safeguard or promote the health and welfare of its citizens. State government has the policies toward safeguarding the health of citizens. Its main points are:

- Prevent the abuse of health and strength of workers, such as men, women and children, and check the vocation of entering in unsuited work to their age or strength.
- Children and youth are protected against exploitation and against moral and material abandonment.
- Giving assistance to education, employment, old age, sickness and disablement, etc.
- Securing just and humane conditions for work and maternity relief.
- State shall regard raising the level of nutrition, standard of living conditions of the people and improvement of public health among its primary duties.

Main Policies Implemented by Government of India

Under the National Health Mission, the government has launched several schemes like:

- Reproductive, Maternal, Newborn, Child and Adolescent Health (RMNCH+A) program essentially looks to address the major causes of mortality among women and children.
- Rashtriya Bal Swasthya Karyakram (RBSK) is an important initiative aiming at early identification and early intervention for children from birth to 18 years to cover 4 'D's that is Defects at birth, Deficiencies, Diseases, Development delays including disability.
- The Rashtriya Kishor Swasthya Karyakram: The key principle of this programme is adolescent participation and leadership, Equity and inclusion, Gender Equity and strategic partnerships with other sectors and stakeholders.
- Janani Shishu Suraksha Karyakaram to motivate those who still choose to deliver at their homes to opt for institutional deliveries.
- National AIDS Control Organisation was set up so that every person living with HIV has access to quality care and is treated with dignity.
- Revised National TB Control Program is a state-run tuberculosis control initiative of Government of India with a vision of achieving a TB free India.
- National Leprosy Eradication Programme was initiated by the government for early detection through active surveillance by the trained health workers.
- The Government of India has launched Mission Indradhanush with the aim of improving coverage of immunization in the country.
- Government of India has implemented National Mental Health Program to ensure the availability and accessibility of minimum mental healthcare for all in the foreseeable future.
- Pulse Polio is an immunization campaign established by the government of India to eliminate polio in India by vaccinating all children under the age of five years.
- Pradhan Mantri Swasthya Suraksha Yojana (PMSSY) was announced with objectives of correcting regional imbalances in the availability of affordable/ reliable tertiary healthcare services.
- Rashtriya Arogya Nidhi which provides financial assistance to the patients that are below poverty line and are suffering from life-threatening diseases.
- National Tobacco Control Programme was launched with the objective to bring about greater awareness about the harmful effects of tobacco use and about the Tobacco Control Laws.
- Integrated Child Development Service was launched to improve the nutrition and health status of children in the age group of 0-6 years, lay the foundation for proper psychological, physical and social development of the child.
- Rashtriya Swasthya Bima Yojana is a government-run health insurance program for the Indian poor.

Unit II ❖ Individual

Unit III

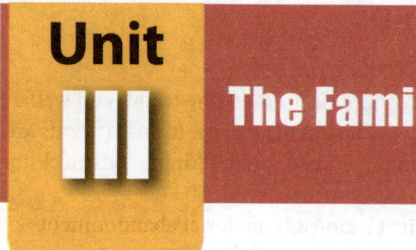

The Family

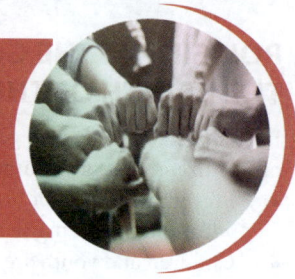

DEFINITION

The family is a basic unit in all societies. A family is defined as a 'Group' of biologically-related individuals living together and eating from a common kitchen.

- **As a biological unit,** the family members share some biological characteristics.
- **As a social unit** the family members share a common dwelling and social environment.
- **As a cultural unit** the family members reflect the culture of wider society and also determine the behavior and attitude of its members.

THE FAMILY CYCLE

The family cycle involves a life cycle of an elementary family and this is given as follows:

- **Stage of formation**: This phase begins with the marriage of a man to a woman to form their family.
- **Stage of growth:** In this phase, children are born and the family size increases.
- **Stage of retraction**: Children are grown up and leave the original family including the parents, to form their own family.
- **Stage of disintegration:** Here the parental family disintegrates due to the death of one parent or both the parents.

This is the common family cycle in our society but not rigid.

TYPES OF FAMILIES

Mainly there are three types of families:

1. **The nuclear family or elementary family:** It is universal in all human societies, consists of married couple and their children. The members of family occupy the same house and generally the husband plays a dominant role in the family.
2. **The joint family or extended family**: This is a family grouping and is very common in India. It consists of a number of married couples and their children living together in the same house. All are blood-related, property is held in common, and senior male member controls the internal and external affairs of the family. This family has the motto that 'Union is Strength'. In India, joint family system is gradually breaking up.
3. **The three-generation family:** In this type of family, there are representatives of three generations—grandfather, father and grandchildren. Such families are formed when young couples continue to live with their parents and have their own children.

BASIC NEEDS OF THE FAMILY

The important basic needs of a family as follows:

- **Physical needs** such as:
  - Food
  - Shelter
  - Clothing
  - Safe physical environment, such as safe water, disposal of wastes, etc.
- **Psychosocial needs** such as:
  - A happy home
  - A safe working environment, freedom from poverty
  - Adequate medical care
  - Care of special groups, such as mothers, children, aged and handicapped
  - Social security
- **Biological needs** such as:

  Freedom from communicable diseases, control of insects and vectors, rodents and planned parenthood.

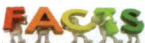

Planned Parenthood

- Planned parenthood or family planning may be defined as 'children by choice not by chance'. A planned family is a happy family. The current slogan in India is 'we are two and we have two'. The Government of India is advocating 'small family norm'—that is every married couple should not have more than two or three children.

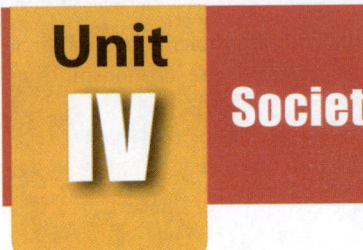

Unit IV — Society

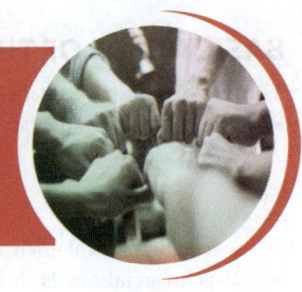

DEFINITIONS

- **Society:** A society is a group of people of common origin, language and history that is living together in an organized community.
- **Socialization:** Socialization is the process of adapting an individual according to the society, customs of the society and by doing this, he or she becomes a useful member of the society.

STRUCTURE OF A SOCIETY

The factors of the structure of a society are caste, income and occupation.

1. **Caste:** Indian society is generally based on caste system. There are four main divisions of castes in India—Brahmins, Kshatriyas, Vaishyas and Shudras. These are further divided into subcastes.
2. **Income:** On the basis of income, people have been grouped into classes as, upper class, middle class and lower class. Upper class people enjoy better standards of life.
3. **Occupation:** In India, there is no satisfactory occupational class system however it can be used for classifying people.

CLASSIFICATION OF SOCIETY

The society is classified into two groups based on the place of living.

1. Rural Societies

India is a land of villages. The villagers are almost self-sufficient as they have almost everything they require. Rural people primarily depend on agriculture. Societies in the villages are the rural societies. Castes, religion, rituals, kinship, marriage and economy are some of the aspects of an Indian village or Rural Society.

2. Urban Societies

Towns and cities comprise the urban society. They are relatively large, dense and permanent settlements of people. It has been said that civilization means city and city means civilization. City represents the way of living of man in modern age. Cities are the melting pots of races, people and cultures. In cities, the occupational pattern of the people is different. Social life is impersonal and less intimate. Traditional patterns of belief and behavior tend to be broken down. New ideas and patterns of behavior originate which further spread to villages. There is diversity of occupation. They depend less on agriculture.

SOCIAL PROBLEMS

In a community, there are both individual and social problems. When individual problems affect a large number of people, it becomes social problems. Some of the present social problems are alcoholism, drug addictions, vagrancy, juvenile delinquency, prostitution, AIDS, etc. Some of the social problems have medical implications, e.g. venereal diseases. Many of the social problems are solved by social and political actions, such as social welfare programs, social assistance and social legislations in the community to curb the social evils.

Here some of the social problems have been discussed:

Prostitution

Prostitution is the business or practice of engaging in sexual activity for money. It is an age-old social evil. It is a social problem in most urban areas however less prevalent in rural areas.

Causes of Prostitution

- Changes in environment
- Break down of family relations (family disorganization)
- Parental quarrels
- Want of affection (Dereliction)
- Illegitimate love
- Source of getting money easily
- Low lQ
- Low moral standards
- Poverty

Government of India has passed an Act in 1956 known as "The Suppression of Immoral Traffic Act" to control prostitution. But it cannot be controlled by legal measures alone. Social welfare measures, such as marriage counselling services, after care and rehabilitation programs are needed to minimize this problem.

Delinquency

A delinquent is one who shows deviation from normal behavior, especially among juveniles. He/she is one who has committed an offence such as theft, sexual offence, murder, burglary, etc. Delinquency is a social problem in many communities. The causes responsible for delinquency are social maladjustments, poverty, disturbed home conditions, alcoholism, drug addiction and modern ways of living.

Handicapped

A person having a condition that markedly restricts his/her ability to function physically, mentally, or socially is known as handicapped. These people in the society are another social problem.

It comprises six main categories:
1. The blind
2. The deaf
3. The orthopedically handicapped
4. The leprosy affected
5. The mentally retarded
6. The emotionally and socially handicapped

Unit IV ❖ Society

The people suffering from above-mentioned categories are increasing in the society. In all civilized countries, the handicapped people are looked after in proper manner. The rehabilitation services available for the handicapped in India are:

- Medical care facilities
- Education for the blind, deaf and orthopedically handicapped
- Vocational training
- Job placement and sheltered work shops
- Pensions, scholarships and allowances for the education and training of the handicapped.

Indian Government included provision for the establishment of four national institutes for the blind, deaf, orthopedically handicapped and mentally retarded in the "Fifth Five-Year Plan."

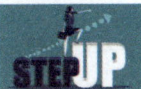

"The Rights of Persons with Disabilities Bill - 2016" was implemented on 27 December 2016. The Bill replaced the existing PwD Act, 1995, which was enacted 21 years back. It fulfills the obligations to the United National Convention on the Rights of Persons with Disabilities (UNCRPD), to which India is a signatory. This law gives equal rights to the disabled persons.

This bill covers the following mentioned disabilities:

The Rights of Persons with Disabilities Bill, 2016 Types of disabilities have been increased from existing 7 to 21	
1. Blindness	12. Muscular dystrophy
2. Low-vision	13. Acid attack victim
3. Leprosy-cured persons	14. Parkinson's disease
4. Locomotor disability	15. Multiple sclerosis
5. Dwarfism	16. Thalassemia
6. Intellectual disability	17. Hemophilia
7. Mental illness	18. Sickle cell disease
8. Cerebral palsy	19. Autism spectrum disorder
9. Specific learning disability	20. Chronic neurological condition
10. Speech and language disability	21. Multiple disabilities including deaf, blindness
11. Hearing impairment (deaf and hard of hearing)	

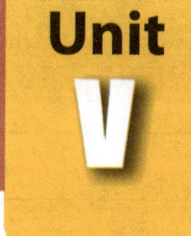

Unit V

The Community

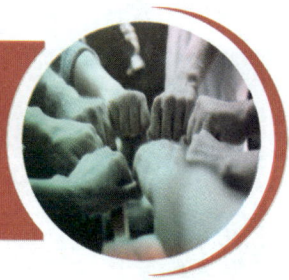

DEFINITION

A community is a network of human relationships. It is a major functioning unit of society. It is the place where our home is located, children are educated, sick people are treated in hospitals and their individual basic needs and desires are met.

From the time of birth to death, all normal human beings are part of a group, family or community. No man can live alone without the help of others.

CHARACTERISTICS OF A COMMUNITY

- The community has a particular geographic area.
- It is composed of people living together.
- People cooperate to satisfy their basic needs.
- There are common organizations, such as markets, schools, stores, banks, hospitals and other offices to deal with the people of the community.

CULTURE AND CULTURAL PATTERNS

The culture and cultural patterns define the way of life. "Culture is defined as the training and refinement of mind, tastes and manners." Culture is the product of human society and man is largely a product of cultural environment. Culture is heritage from one generation to another. In general, culture stands for the mode of living, religion, language, customs, habits, beliefs, etc. In other words, culture is the whole way of life of a person.

A health worker should be aware of the cultural patterns of the people, they are dealing with; because cultural factors are involved in all aspects of community health, nutrition, mother and child health, personal hygiene, environment, etc. There are great differences in the cultural patterns of people about nutrition, care of mother and child health, personal hygiene, environmental sanitation, outlook of health and diseases.

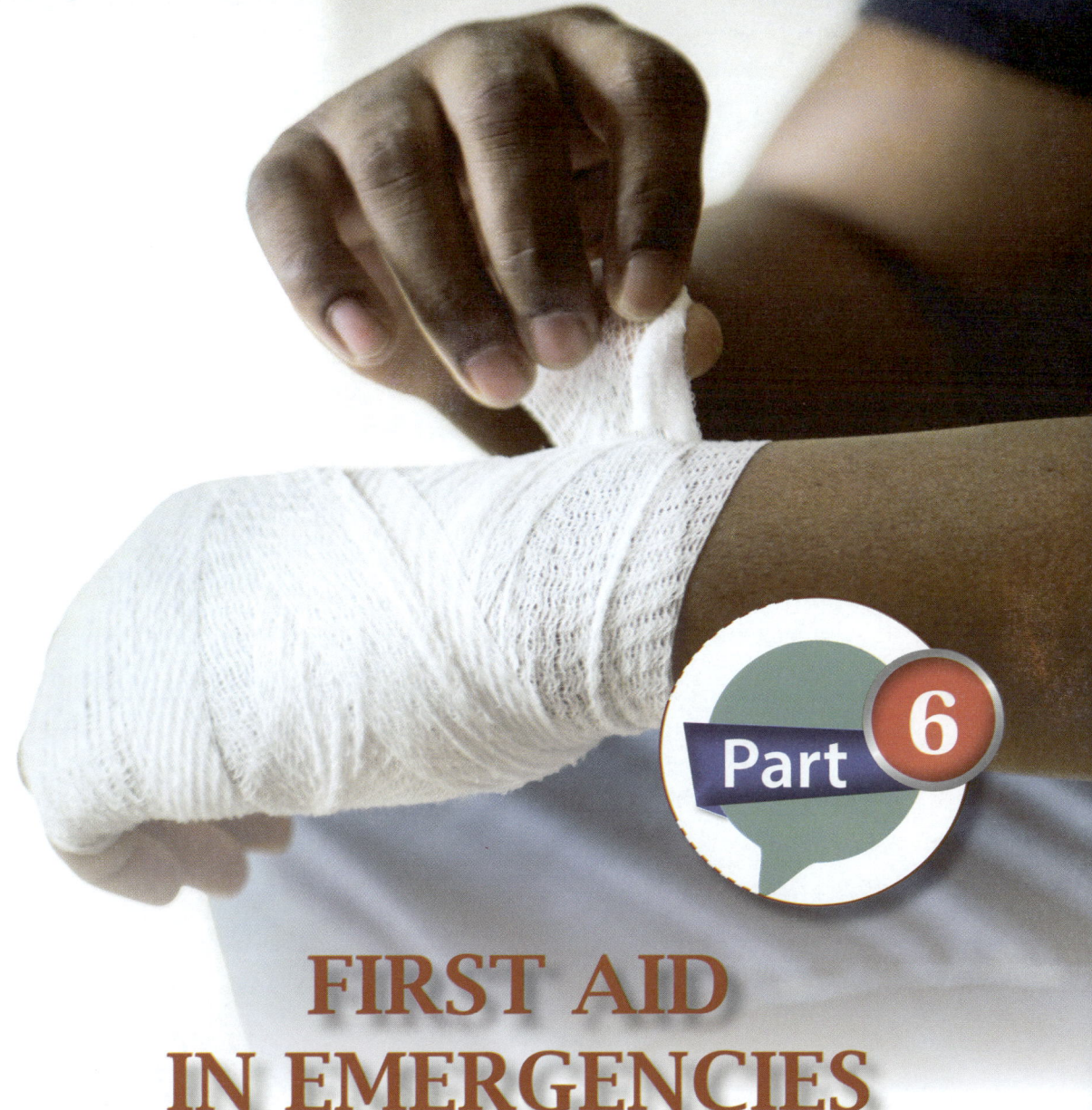

Part 6

FIRST AID IN EMERGENCIES

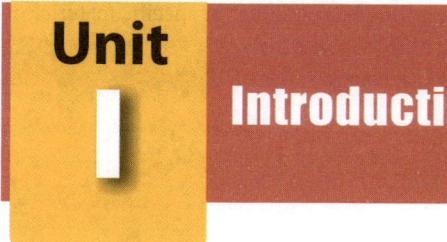

Unit

1

Introduction

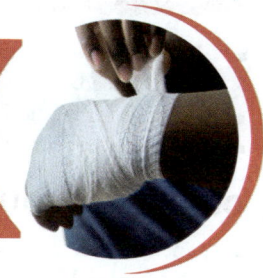

FIRST AID

First aid is the immediate treatment given to the victim of trauma or sudden illness before proper medical aid is available.

Purposes of First Aid

- To save life.
- To prevent further injury, complications or deterioration of the condition of the patient.
- To relieve pain by providing comfortable position, reassurance or by any other suitable measures possible.
- To arrange for available medical attention as early as possible by taking the patient to the hospital by suitable transport.
- To assist doctor by giving the details of accident or injury and the first aid treatment given.

Importance of First Aid

- Prior to medical aid, first aid is given to save life, to prevent deterioration and to help recovery of patient/victim.
- It provides quick medical treatment until professional assistance arrives.
- It helps to ensure that the right medical assistance is provided.
- The knowledge in first aid also benefits the individuals themselves.
- It helps people during various emergency situations.

Principles of First Aid

- Reach the site of accident as early as possible.
- Avoid asking unnecessary questions to the patient or his/her relatives, which may waste time.
- Understand the cause of the casualty.
- Remove the causative agent of accident from the patient or remove the patient from the agent, if possible, e.g., fire, electricity, poisonous insects, etc.
- Make out whether the patient is conscious, unconscious, dead or alive.
- Make sure about the immediate first aid measure to be adopted such as stopping the bleeding, restoration of breathing, etc.
- Keep a record of the patient, details of event and treatment given.
- Keep the patient warm and comfortable as far as possible.

- Improvise the proper arrangement of articles to avoid wasting time by searching for specific materials in time of need.
- Arrange for medical aid as soon as possible.
- Reassure the patient and the relatives.

QUALITIES REQUIRED FOR A FIRST AIDER

- The first aider should be a good observer.
- He/she should be self-confident and calm even under stress.
- Should have leadership ability to control the crowd and to get help from people, like visitors.
- He/she should be able to recognize priority needs.
- First aider must be sympathetic and tactful in handling the anxious relatives.
- He/she should be aware of one's limitations and abilities and avoid assuring the patient and relatives or declaring the patient dead, if so.
- The person must be skilled in administration or application of methods of first aid.

Stimulant

Remember the 3 Ps for first aid as follows:

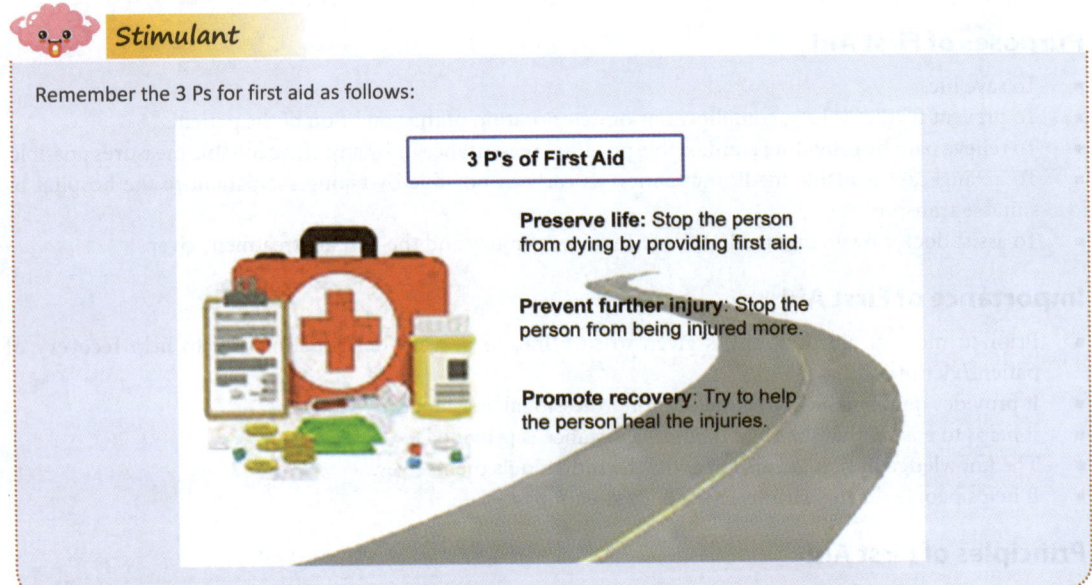

3 P's of First Aid

Preserve life: Stop the person from dying by providing first aid.

Prevent further injury: Stop the person from being injured more.

Promote recovery: Try to help the person heal the injuries.

Stimulant

Remember PRICE when giving first aid to injured

P	R	I	C	E
Protect the injury from further damage	**Rest** your injury for a few days to ease pain	**Ice** the area experiencing the pain	**Compress** the area with a bandage to limit swelling	**Elevate** your injury preferably above the heart

RULES OF FIRST AID

- Be calm, quick and methodical. Find out all the major injuries and wounds and treat them suitably.
- If respiration is stopped, start artificial respiration.
- Try to stop bleeding as early as possible.
- Try to prevent shock to the patient and in case patient is serious, try to move him/her to the nearest hospital instead of waiting to prevent shock on the spot.
- Keep the patient comfortable and warm and do not move him unnecessarily.
- Reassure the relatives by encouraging words and get their cooperation.
- Do not allow crowd around the patient. Let him/her get fresh air.
- Do not cause injury to the patient while moving and removing clothes. Get medical aid as early as possible or shift the patient to the nearest hospital.
- Remember that the aim of first aid is to save life, relieve pain and to prevent further injury or complications.
- The success of first aid depends upon directing the activities according to situation, common sense and experience.

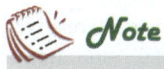 *Note*

Do's and Don'ts of first aid

Do's	Don'ts
Before handling casualty, use	First aider can never
• Mask • Gloves • Head cover	• Prescribe medicine • Declare death

SCOPE OF FIRST AID

- The scope of first aid is very vast. Accidents may occur to any one at any time and at any place because of natural calamities, burns, electric shock, insect bites, snakebite or through any other means. The first aider reaches the site when any accident occurs or is informed about a casualty.
- On reaching the spot, first-hand information must be collected by the first aider himself, from the patient itself, if patient is conscious, or from the nearest relatives or onlookers, so that an idea of the injury sustained could be formed.
- He/she should collect the information such as when the accident occurred, how it happened, the site of particular injury caused and whether the patient became unconscious due to the accident.
- **Then the first aider should examine the patient for:**
  - **Pulse:** Feel the pulse whether normal or not. If not felt, check whether the patient is dead or unconscious.
  - **Respiration:** Absent, low, fast, gasping respiration is serious and needs urgent medical treatment.
  - **Pallor:** The degree of whiteness of the tongue, conjunctiva and nails indicates the severity of bleeding.
  - **Cyanosis:** Blueness of tongue and lips indicates lack of oxygen.
  - **Bleeding:** Watch for bleeding from injured site/sites, ears, nose, mouth, etc.

Unit I ❖ Introduction

- **Fracture:** Check for fracture that may have occurred in any bones of the body.
- **Burns:** If burn has occurred, monitor the extent of area involved.
- **Poisons:** Look for the smell of poison or stain of poison on the skin or cloth.
- After getting the extremely essential information and examining the patient (taking a very limited time), the treatment should be given promptly, according to the priority.
- Any complaints of the patient or relatives or even minute injury should be dealt with seriously.
- After rendering the first aid treatment, the patient should be taken to the doctor or to the hospital for proper and systematic treatment.

APPROACH TO FIRST AID

- When the accident occurs in a house or institution there will be facilities for first aid treatment, which can be planned methodically. However, if it is a road or public place, the treatment has to be altered according to the available facilities. As delay is dangerous, try to transport the patient to the nearest hospital. The approach and method of first aid depends on the circumstances and the place of the accident. A deliberate approach is essential.
- Before starting any first aid treatment, get the permission from the patient or the nearest relatives. Observe and examine the patient and make sure that any life-saving methods as artificial respiration is needed. Try to remove the preventable causes of the accident if seen on observation as fire or electricity or such any other sources.
- Shock is treated according to the severity. Every symptom seen in patient should be considered on its own merit and treatment should be given accordingly.
- If there are large numbers of casualties at the spot, the treatment should be started from the more severe to the lesser one. Stopping of breathing, hemorrhage and weakness of the patient require urgent care. Such patients should be shifted to the hospital immediately.
- If the accident occurred at home or in an institution, doctor may be called to the spot as the shifting may be delayed due to many reasons. The first aider can give the first aid treatment and the relatives or bystanders can go and bring the doctor.
- The bystanders should control crowd and the need of shifting a casualty to the hospital depends on the environment and the condition of the patient. Always remember that you are only a first aider and not a doctor. The use of intelligence and common sense of the first aider is more valuable in such situations.

IMPORTANT POINTS OF ATTENDING A CASUALTY

To attend a casualty, the first aider should consider many details and the methods to be adapted to decide the treatment.

Alarming Conditions Requiring First Aid

Usually, three main conditions call for first aid. They are:

1. **Stopping of breathing:** If **breathing is affected** and patient is cyanosed, artificial breathing is required.
2. **Severe bleeding:** If there is severe bleeding from a wound, it may cause death due to great loss of blood, which needs the application of pressure on pressure points.
3. **Shock:** If there is shock with symptoms, like cold and clammy skin, severe perspiration, pale face, nausea and vomiting, the patient needs treatment for shock immediately and the care for injury.

CONCEPT OF EMERGENCY

Definition

An emergency is a situation that poses an immediate risk to health, life, property, or environment. Most emergencies require urgent intervention to prevent a worsening of the situation. The emergency nursing is care of patients who require prompt medical attention to avoid long-term disability or death.

The most important basic concept in emergency medicine is traditionally remembered by the mnemonic 'ABC' which stands for Airway, Breathing, Circulation. The care provider first makes sure that the patient has an open airway, is breathing appropriately, and has circulation intact (i.e., pulses, normal skin color and no uncontrolled bleeding).

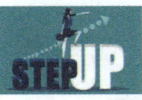

Triage in Nursing
- The term 'triage' comes from French word 'trier', and it was originally applied to a process of sorting, probably around 1792, by Baron Dominique Jean Larrey, Surgeon in Chief to Napoleon's Imperial Guard. Triàge was **developed** by the army surgeon Larrey during the Napoleonic era. 'Nurse Triage' refers to the formal process of early assessment of patients attending an accident and emergency (A&E) department by a trained nurse, to ensure that they receive appropriate attention, in a suitable location, with the required degree of urgency.
- **Simple triage and rapid treatment** (**START**): First aiders use START to evaluate victims and accordingly assign them to one of the following four categories (Fig. 1):
  1. Deceased/expectant (black)
  2. Immediate (red)
  3. Delayed (yellow)
  4. Walking wounded/minor (green)

Contd...

Unit I ❖ Introduction

STEP**UP**

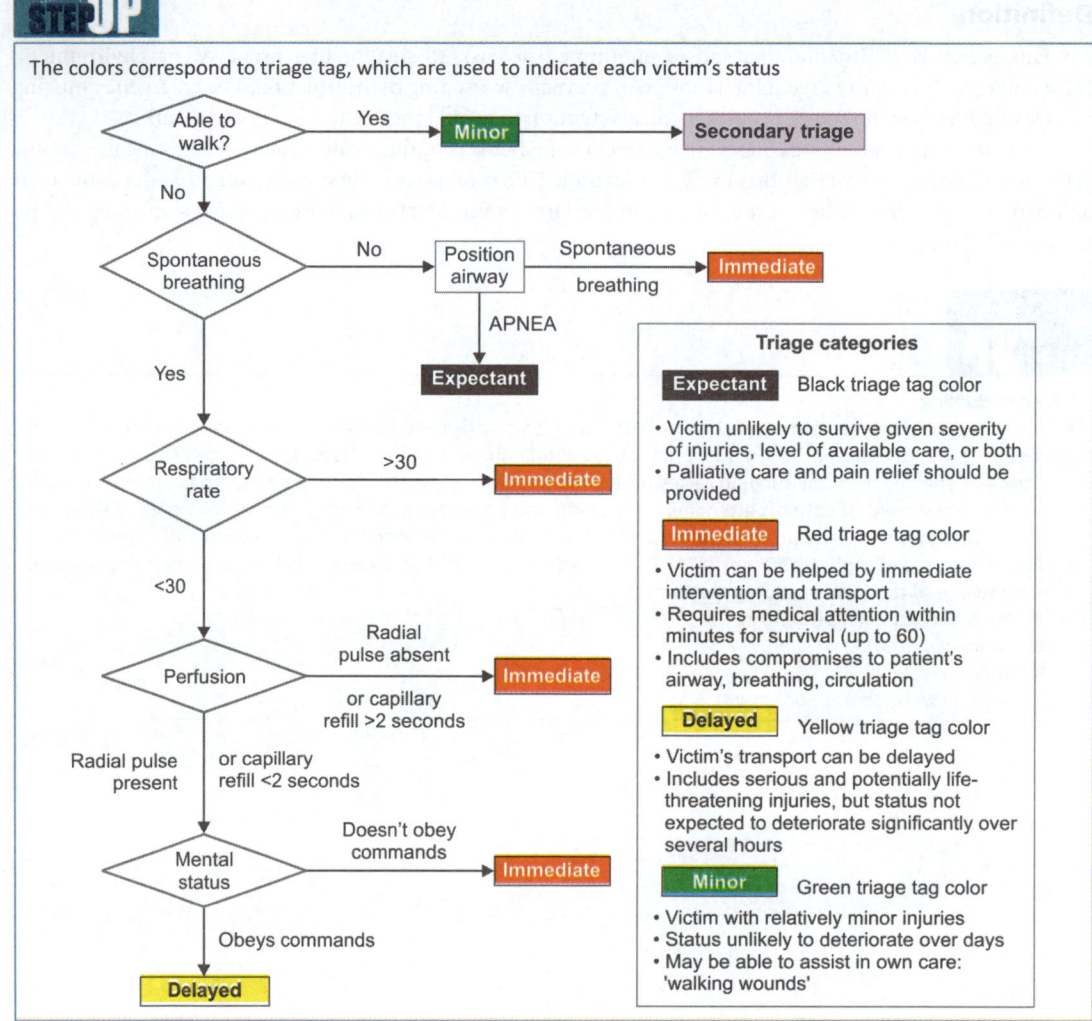

Figure 1: START triage

Introduction

When an emergency strikes, there is no time to start researching how to respond. From natural disasters to traffic accidents, we never know when a situation will arise that will demand quick thinking, cool nerves and a little bit of know-how. In many emergency cases, the best thing we can do is to stay calm and collected. Heightened emotions tend to hamper our critical thinking skills and our ability to think quickly. In addition to staying 'cool under pressure', several concrete skills can make the difference in life-and-death situations. Triage nursing is the support in such emergency situations.

Unit I ❖ Introduction

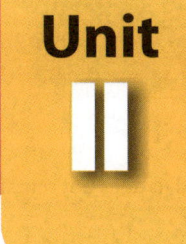
Procedures and Techniques in First Aid

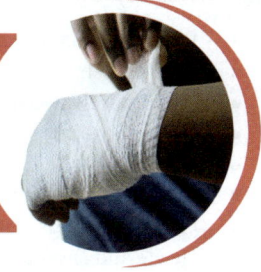

First Aid Kit

DEFINITION

A first aid kit is a collection of supplies and equipment that is used to give medical treatment. A well-stocked first aid kit, kept in easy reach, is a basic necessity.

PREPARATION OF FIRST AID KIT

Different sizes of first aid kits are available at a chemist's shop. Items of individual choice can be bought and kept in the first aid box (Fig. 1). Articles should be arranged in the box properly. Everything should be ready for an immediate use. Even though the kits are of different size, the following items should be included.

Dressing Articles

- Gauze dressings of different sizes in individual sterile packages
- Rolls of gauze bandages 5 and 8 cm wide
- Adhesive bandages in assorted sizes
- Rolls of absorbent cotton
- Adhesive tapes
- Mild antiseptics
- Cotton cutting scissors–1
- Surgical scissors–1
- Artery forceps–1
- Dissecting forceps—toothed and nontoothed–1 each
- Drainage tube
- Safety pins
- Tube of petroleum jelly–1
- Laundered and ironed linen sheet about 1 meter square for making sling or bandages.
- Paper and pen to mark the information and observations about the patient
- Tongue depressor
- Airway
- Splints
- Thermometer
- Syringe and needles

- Rubber catheter and tourniquet
- Mackintosh
- Small towels two or three
- Match box–1
- Candles
- Medium size torch–1
- Gauze dressings, cotton and bandages are available in sterile packets. Once it is opened, it does not remain sterile and should be replaced.
- Other items like soap, salt, potassium permanganate crystals, milk of magnesia, medicine glass, drinking glass and medicine dropper, etc. are to be kept in the bag.
- In an emergency, clean rags or clothing shall be used if sterile dressings are finished.

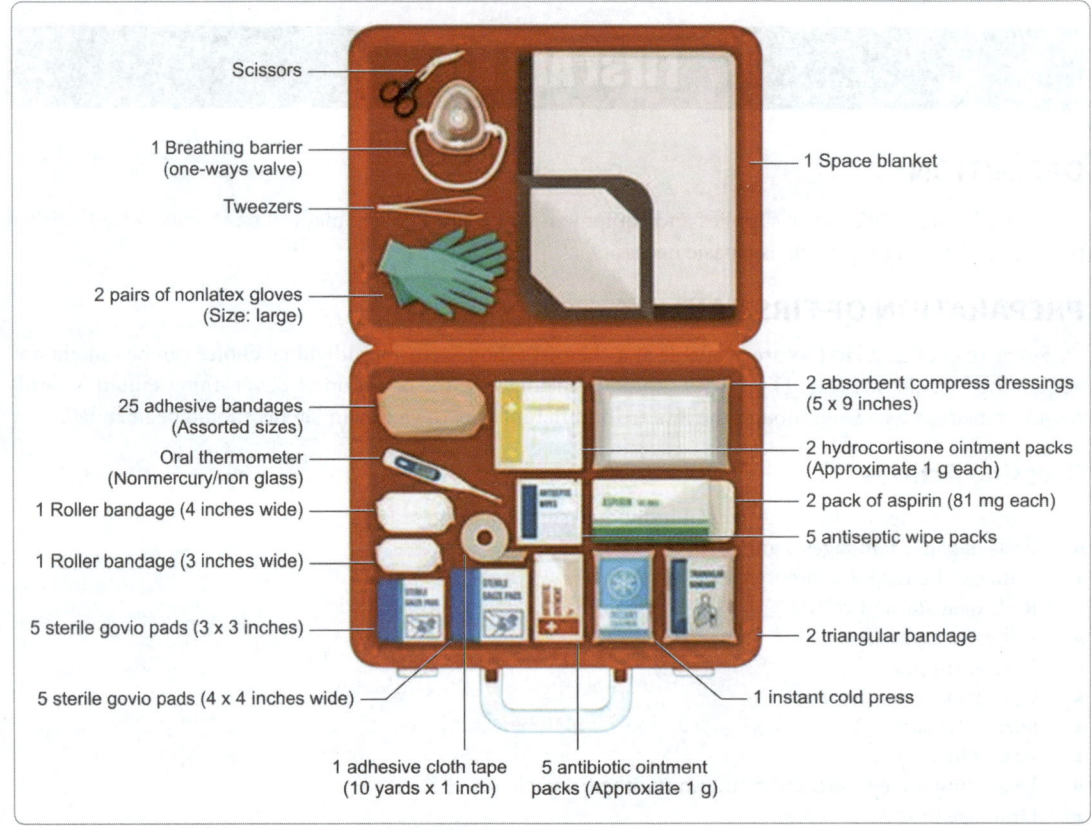

Scissors

1 Breathing barrier
(one-ways valve)

Tweezers

2 pairs of nonlatex gloves
(Size: large)

1 Space blanket

25 adhesive bandages
(Assorted sizes)

Oral thermometer
(Nonmercury/non glass)

1 Roller bandage (4 inches wide)

1 Roller bandage (3 inches wide)

5 sterile govio pads (3 x 3 inches)

5 sterile govio pads (4 x 4 inches wide)

2 absorbent compress dressings
(5 x 9 inches)

2 hydrocortisone ointment packs
(Approximate 1 g each)

2 pack of aspirin (81 mg each)

5 antiseptic wipe packs

2 triangular bandage

1 instant cold press

1 adhesive cloth tape
(10 yards x 1 inch)

5 antibiotic ointment
packs (Approxiate 1 g)

Figure 1: A model of first aid kit

Medicines

When first aid is to be given to a large number of people after a disaster, necessary items like syringes and needles, infusion sets and medicines are required. The drugs to be included are normal saline, glucose saline, dextrose in water in different strengths, distilled water for injection, atropine, adrenaline, aminophylline, calcium gluconate, meperidine, nikethamide, phenobarbitone, diazepam, antitetanus serum, tetanus toxoid, 2% lignocaine, etc.

Disinfectants and Antiseptics

Some of the disinfectants and antiseptics commonly used are:

- **Dettol:** Used to clean wounds and surrounding area of the wound. (2–4 teaspoon full in 500 mL of water). It is also used to sterilize instruments which cannot be sterilized by heat.
- **Savlon:** Used to wash equipment, disinfect soiled linen, spray in patient's room and to clean the wounds (half an ounce to 2 liters of water).
- **Potassium permanganate crystals:** To use as gargles (one crystal to one cup of water), bladder washes (1:60), insect bites and purification of water.
- **Rectified spirit:** Used for disinfection of skin, instruments and ampoules. It should not be used over wounds or raw area as it removes coagulum formed on raw area.
- **Boric acid:** Used for mouthwash, irrigation of urinary bladder, skin, inflammation of mucous membrane and skin, burns, bed sore, etc. (Strength - 5%). It can be used as dusting powder or in ointment form also.
- **Triiodine:** 2% for disinfection of skin and treatment of wounds.
- **Iodoform:** Composed of iodine, potash and alcohol. It relieves pain in raw mucous membrane and prevents putrefaction in wounds with pus.
- **Iodophores:** For example, povidone iodine. Used on boils, furunculosis, burns, ulcers, tinea, surgical scrub, disinfecting surgical instruments, nonspecific vaginitis.
- **Merbromin:** Salt of mercury with weak antiseptic action for dressing wounds.
- **Acriflavine:** An antiseptic 1:1000 for dressing wounds
- **Glycerine acriflavine:** Useful in edematous and infected wounds
- **Hydrogen peroxide:** It is used for cleaning infected wounds. On contact with tissues, it releases necrotic materials. Tissue debris and necrotic material float on the bubbles formed. Some heat is generated in the process.
- **Silver nitrate:** Silver nitrate sticks are used for cauterizations of wounds and hypertrophic granulation tissues. Solutions of 0.01 to 10% are used for local applications. A solution of 1:1000 strength is used for irrigation of urinary bladder.
- **Gentian violet:** 1% solution is used for application in infected wounds, mucous membranes and serous surfaces. It can be used in fungal infections of throat and vagina.
- **Carbolic acid:** It is used to cauterize dog bites, snake bites, etc. It is also used to sterilize sharp instruments, like surgical scissors and scalpels. But the instruments should be washed with sterile water after taking from carbolic acid, before use. (Strength 1:20 for one hour to sterilize instruments).
- **Chlorhexidine:** Nonirritant, more active against gram +ve bacteria. It is used for surgical scrub, neonatal bath, mouthwash and general skin antiseptic. It is most widely used antiseptic in the hospitals.

Dressing, Bandaging and Splinting

DEFINITION

A bandage is a piece of material used either to cover wounds, to keep dressings in place, to apply pressure to control bleeding, to support a medical device such as a splint, or on its own to provide support to the body. It can also be used to restrict a part of the body (Fig. 2).

Bandages are strips of different materials in varying lengths and widths. It is used in the size according to the purpose and part to which it is to be applied. They are commonly made out of linen, flannel, calico, crape or elastic net.

PURPOSES OF BANDAGING

- To secure dressing in position
- To control bleeding
- To immobilize an injured part of the body
- To prevent or reduce swelling
- To relieve pain by supporting an injured limb

Bandage should be applied firm enough to retain dressing and splints in position but should not be too tight to cause injury to the part or to interfere the circulation of blood. Bluish discoloration and loss of sensation of the fingers or nails are dangerous signs, which indicate that the bandaging is too tight. In case of pressure bandage applied to arrest bleeding from a limb, it should be tight enough to stop the bleeding but it is released after a reasonable short period and reapplied if needed again.

Parts of Bandages

The parts of bandages are head, body and free end or tail (Fig. 2).

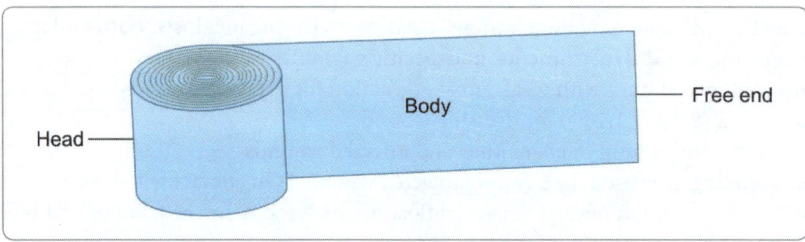

Figure 2: Head, body and tail or free end of the bandage

Usually a single bandage is used to apply. But in places, like head, double-headed roller bandage is required. In this, the free ends of two-roller bandages are sewed together leaving the heads to close together, on the same side of the bandage.

Types of Bandages

- Roller bandages
- Triangular bandages
- Special bandages like 'T' bandage or many tailed bandages.
- Tubular Bandages.

Roller Bandages

Roller bandages are long strips of material.

Purposes of Applying Roller Bandages

- To cover and retain dressings and splints in position
- To prevent or to reduce swelling by pressure bandage
- To give support for a sprained or dislocated joint
- To prevent or control hemorrhage
- To restrict movement
- To correct deformity

Roller bandages are prepared in different lengths and widths depending upon the site to be applied and made out of cotton cloth, calico, crape or elastic net or such other materials. Before use, the bandage should be firmly rolled.

Most roller bandages are 6 yards long except the very narrow bandages, which are short. The width depends on the part of the body to be bandaged. The usual width is as follows:

Part to be bandaged	Usual width
Fingers	1 inch
Arm	2–2.5 inches
Leg	3–3.5 inches
Trunk	4–6 inches
Head	2 inches

Types of Roller Bandages

There are two types of roller bandages:
1. **An elastic roller bandage**: It is used to apply support to a strain or sprain and is wrapped around the joint or limb many times. It should be applied firmly, but not tightly enough to reduce circulation (Fig. 3).
2. **Cotton or linen roller bandages:** These are used to cover gauze dressings. They come in many different widths and are held in place with tapes, clips or pins (Figs 4A and B).

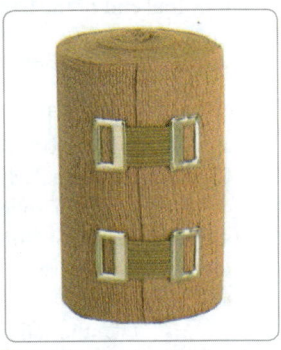

Figure 3: Elastic roller bandage

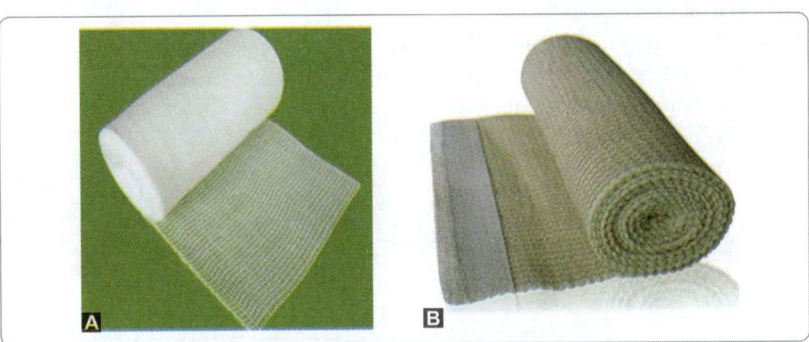

Figures 4A and B: Cotton or linen roller bandages

Rules for the Application of Roller Bandages

- Select the bandage of the proper size and tightly rolled.
- Face the patient while bandaging except applying it to the head.
- Comfort of the patient is of first consideration except for arresting hemorrhage and correcting deformity. Therefore, keep the patient in comfortable position.
- Support the injured area while bandaging.
- Neatness and economy must be considered but bandaging should fulfill the purpose and cover the dressing completely.

Unit II ❖ Procedures and Techniques in First Aid

- Bandages should be firm and applied with even pressure throughout. However, the extremities should be carefully watched for any signs of swelling or cyanosis due to the interference of circulation by too tight bandaging.
- Hold the roller of the bandage in the right hand when applying it to the left hand of the patient and in the left hand when applying bandage to right hand of the patient.
- Place some pads of cotton wool on the part to be bandaged so that the bandages does not slip or cause cutting into the skin underneath.
- Hold the end of the roller bandage over the outer aspect of the injured part and wind it around twice one on the other to fix it.
- Wind the bandage from below upwards and from inside to outwards.
- Cover 2/3 of the previous loop of the bandage by the next one and continue.
- Do not bandage the part too tight or too loose.
- At the completion, fix the end of the bandage with a safety pin, a piece of sticking plaster or dividing the terminal end of the bandage longitudinally and tying the two ends around the bandaged part.

Applying the Roller Bandage

The turns in the application of roller bandages follow a certain path/way. The following are the five basic forms of bandaging that can be used to apply most types of bandages:

- **Circular bandage**: It is used to hold dressings on body parts such as arms, legs, chest or abdomen. Strips of cloth or gauze roller bandage or triangular bandage folded down to form strip of bandage (cravat) are used for application of circular bandage. In this technique the layers of bandage are applied over the top of each other (Figs 5A and B).
  - **Procedure**
    - Take the roll on the inner aspect.
    - Unroll the bandage either toward you or laterally, holding the loose end until it is secured by the first circle of the bandage.
    - Two or three turns may be needed to cover an area adequately.
    - Hold the bandage in place with tape or a clip or a knot.
    - Almost all bandaging techniques start and end with a few circular bandaging turns.

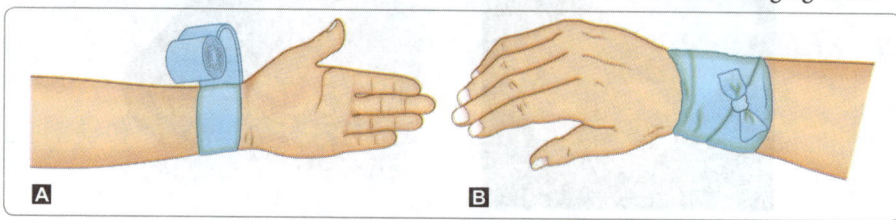

Figures 5A and B: Circular bandage

- **Simple spiral bandage:** Simple spiral bandage is used in spiral form over a limb where there is uniform thickness such as finger, wrists, etc. Bandage is applied obliquely around the part, each turn covering two-third (2/3) of the preceding one and the edges being parallel and at the end, it is fixed with safety pin or bandage pin (Figs 6A to C).

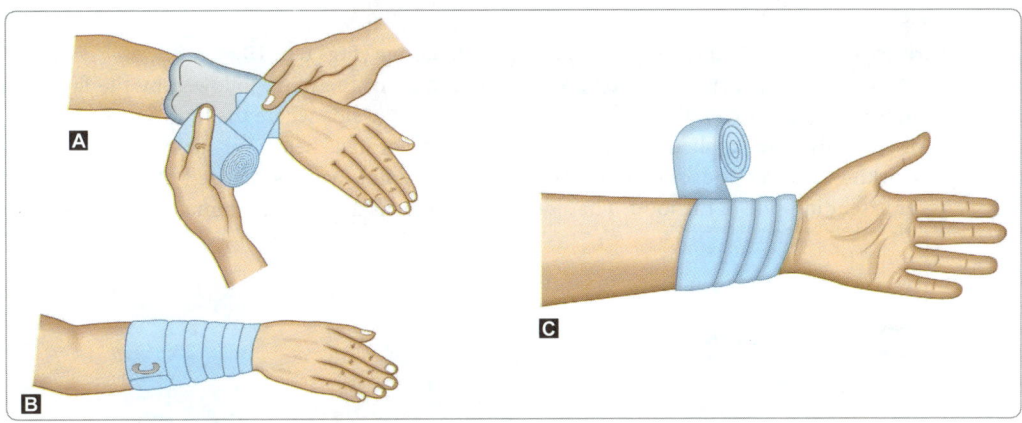

Figures 6A to C: Simple spiral bandage

- **Reverse spiral bandage:** This is a modified spiral in which the roll of the bandage is reversed downwards on itself at each round. It is used in lower and upper arms and on legs. In this, the bandage is folded back on itself by 180° after each turn (Figs 7A to C).

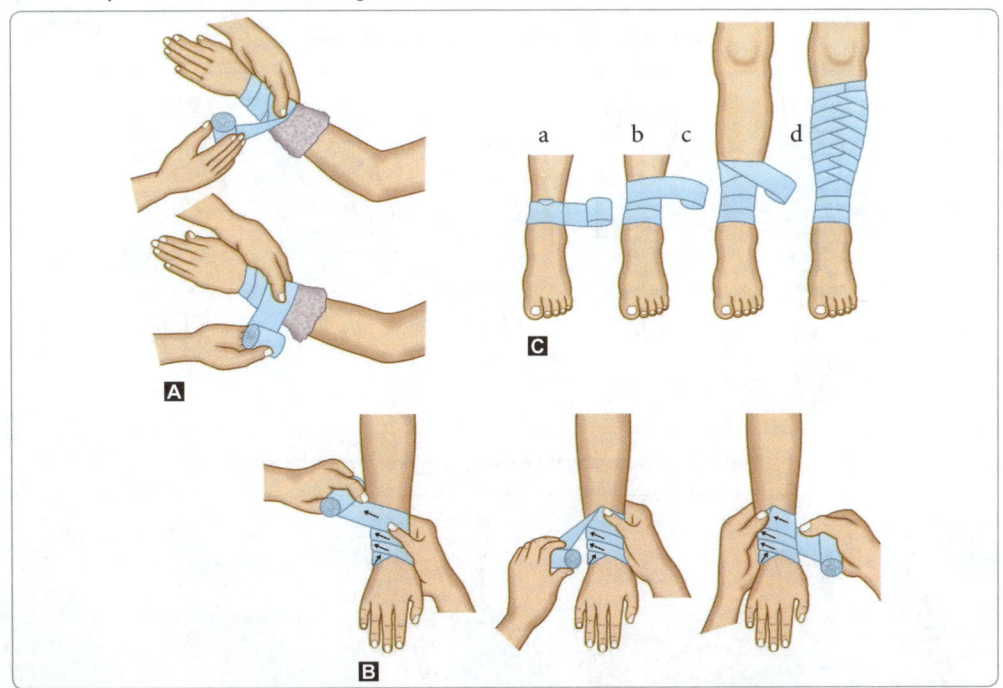

Figures 7A to C: Reverse spiral bandage

- **Figure of eight bandage:** The bandage is applied obliquely up and down alternately, so that the loops appear like a figure of eight. This is done for the forearm, elbow, knee joint and leg. This bandaging technique involves two turns, with the strips of bandage crossing each other at the side where the joint flexes or extends. It is usually used to bind a flexing joint or body part below and above the joint.

Unit II ❖ Procedures and Techniques in First Aid

● **Procedure**
There are two ways of bandaging figure of eight bandage (Figs 8 to 10):

1. Initially a circular turn is made around the middle of the joint, followed by the fanning out upwards and downwards. The turns should cross at the side where the limb flexes.

2. It can also be applied from a starting point located below or above the joint crease, working towards the joint itself. The cross-over points will be located at either the flexing or extending side of the joint. The side where the turns do not cross remains uncovered.

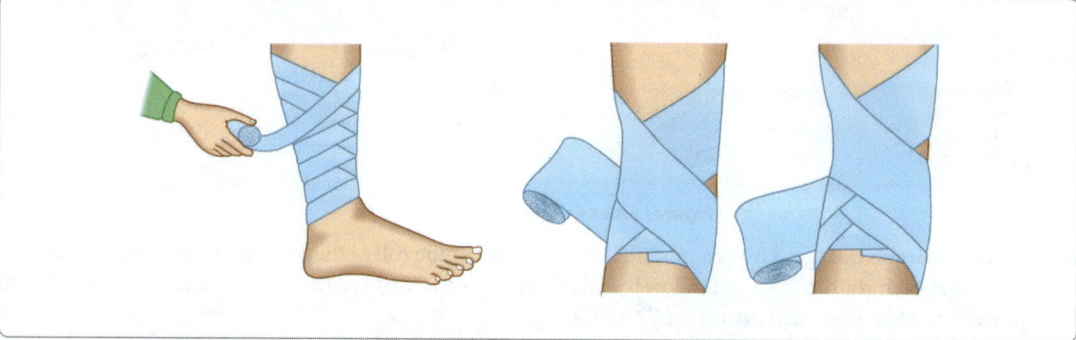

Figure 8: Figure of eight bandage of the leg

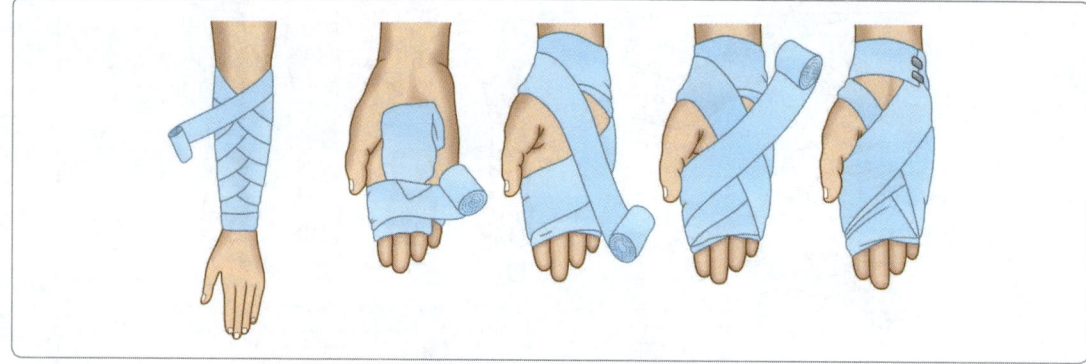

Figure 9: Figure of eight bandage on forearm and hands

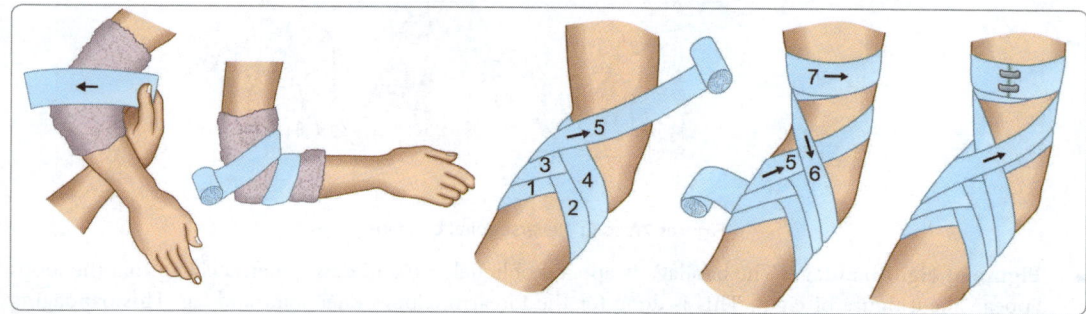

Figure 10: Figure of eight bandage for elbow

■ **Spica bandage:** It is a modified form of figures of eight bandages for bandaging the elbow, knee joint, groin, hip, shoulder, thumb and heels. It is used for bandaging large areas such as the shoulder and hip (Figs 11 to 17).

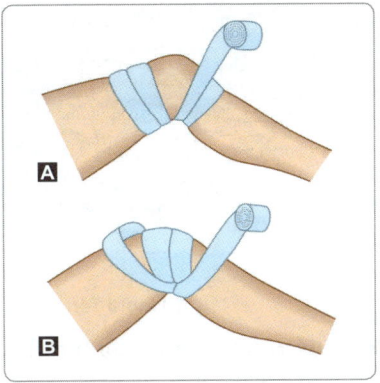

● **Procedure**

a. Anchor the bandage below the joint (around the upper arm or thigh).

b. Wrap the bandage across the joint and around the trunk of the body (chest or abdomen).

c. Return and cross the previous wrap.

d. Wrap the bandage behind the limb, overlapping one-third of the anchor wrap.

e. Continue to wrap (Steps b, c, and d) until the joint is sufficiently supported.

f. Tape, clip, or tie the end of the bandage.

Figure 11A and B: Figure of eight bandage for the knee joint or spica

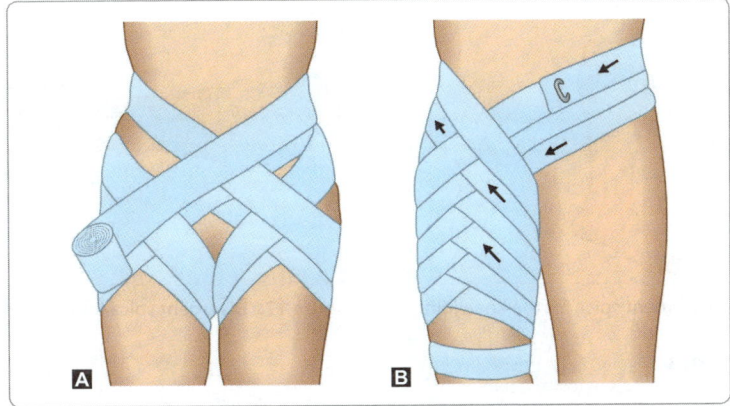

Figures 12A and B: (A) Spica for the hip; (B) Spica for the groin

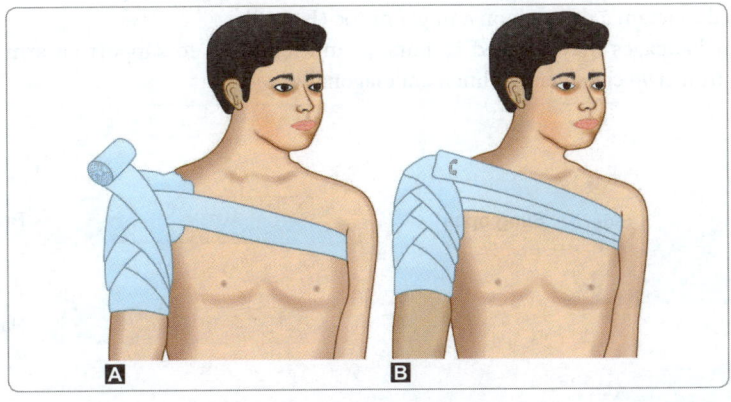

Figures 13A and B: Spica for the shoulder

Unit II ❖ Procedures and Techniques in First Aid

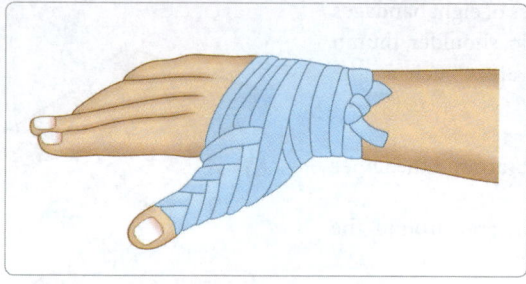

Figure 14: Spica for the thumb

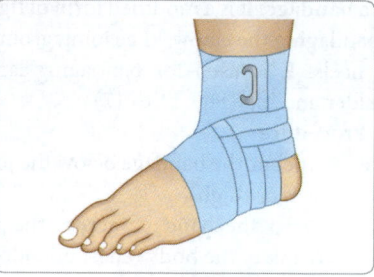

Figure 15: Spica for the heel

- **Divergent spica** is a form of figure of eight in which the turn goes alternately above and below ending above and is used for bent joints as elbow knee or heel.

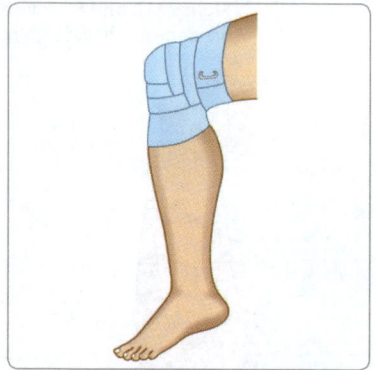

Figure 16: Divergent spica for the knee joint

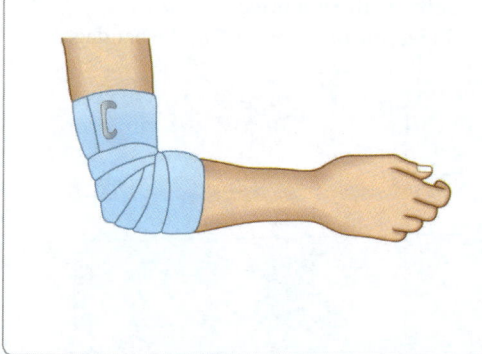

Figure 17: Divergent spica for the elbow

Triangular Bandages

- A triangular bandage is used as an arm sling or as a pad to control bleeding. It may also be used to support or immobilize an injury to a bone or joint or as improvised padding over a painful injury. A tubular gauze bandage is used to retain a dressing on a finger or toe (Fig. 18).
  - Triangular bandages may be used in nursing and for slings to support an arm after injury. It is prepared from a 90 cm square of linen cut diagonally.

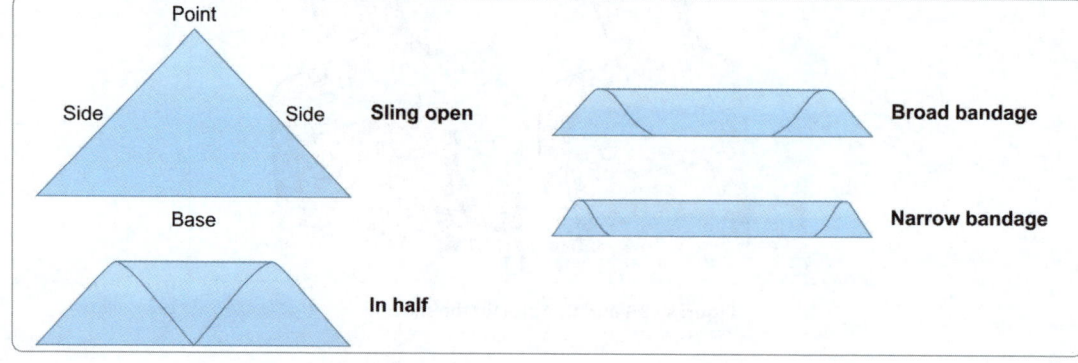

Figure 18: Parts of triangular bandage and foldings

- **Triangular bandage for the head (Figs 19A and B):**
  - ○ Place the base folded bandage on the forehead at the level of the eyebrows.
  - ○ Take the two ends backwards. Cross them over the body of the bandage hanging over the nape of the neck and tie them over the forehead.
  - ○ Bring the free end of the point forward and pin it.

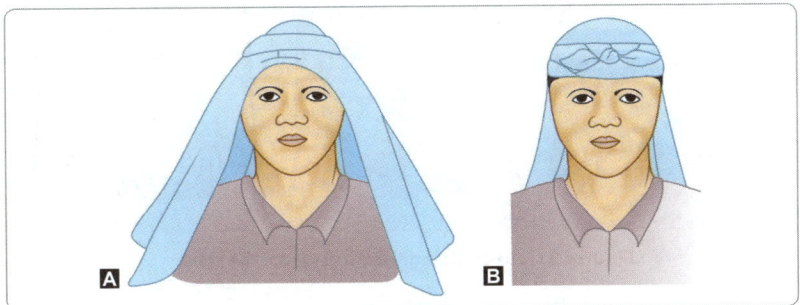

Figures 19A and B: Triangular bandage for the head

- **Triangular bandage to the hand (Figs 20A to E):**
  - ○ Place the bandage on a flat surface and keep the hand on it, fingers directed towards the apex of the triangle.
  - ○ Turn the apex back over the fingers
  - ○ Cross the other two ends backwards and tie them over the apex on the back of the hand near the wrist
  - ○ Pin the point over the knot.

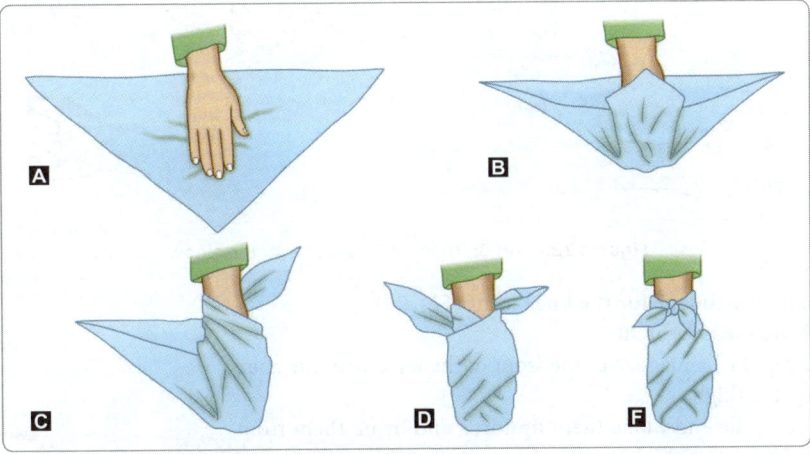

Figures 20A to E: Triangular bandage for the hand

- **Triangular bandage to the chest (Figs 21A to C)**
  - ○ Place the center of the bandage over the chest, its apex over the shoulder on the uninjured side.
  - ○ Carry the other two ends backwards and tie them over the back in such a way that one end remain longer than the other.
  - ○ Tie the longer end to the apex on the shoulder.
  - ○ If the injury is on the back, reverse the procedure.

Unit II ❖ Procedures and Techniques in First Aid

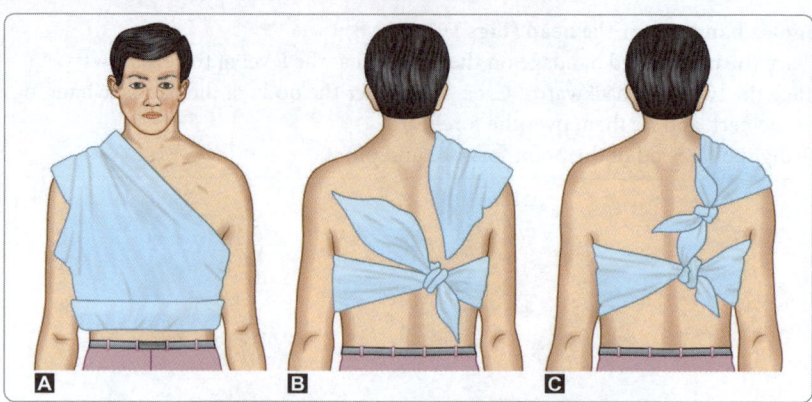

Figures 21A to C: Triangular bandage for the chest

- **Triangular bandage for the elbow (Fig. 22):**
  - Bend the elbow at 90°.
  - Bend right hand to the left side and left hand to the right side.
  - Place the apex of the triangular bandage on the back of the upper arm and the middle of the base on the forearm.
  - Cross the other two ends in front of the elbow and round the arm and tie them above the elbow in one side. Bring the apex downwards and pin over the tie on the side.

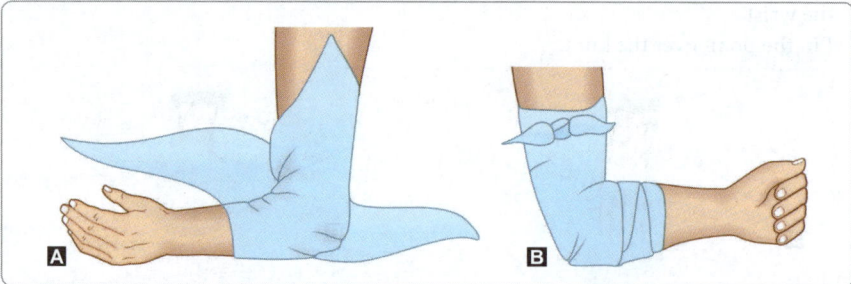

Figures 22A and B: Triangular bandage for the elbow

- **Triangular bandage for the knee joint (Fig. 23):**
  - Bend the knee at 90°.
  - Keep the bandage over the front of the knee with the apex on the thigh.
  - Cross the ends, take them upwards and bring them from back of the thigh to the front of the thigh. Tie them together.
  - Bring the apex downwards and pin over the tie in front.
- **Triangular bandage for the foot (Figs 24A to E):**
  - Place the bandage on the floor
  - Ask the patient to place his foot on the center of the bandage, the toes directed towards the apex.
  - Draw the apex backwards over the ankle.

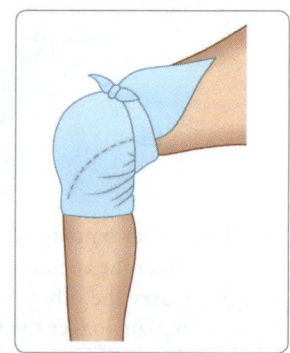

Figure 23: Triangular bandage for the knee joint

- o Draw the ends round the ankle at the back.
- o Bring them forwards and tie them in front of the ankle.
- o Bring the apex down in front of the knot and pin it over the knot.

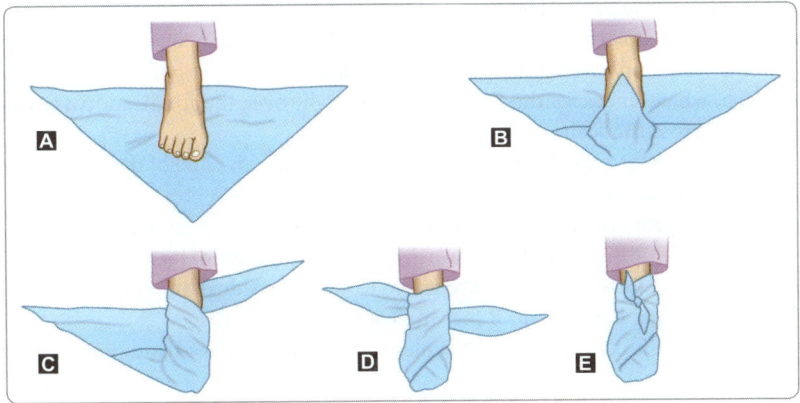

Figures 24A to E: Triangular bandage for the foot

Tubular Bandages

- Tubular gauze is an elastic retention net bandage that holds dressings in place without tape. Stockinette dressing bandage tubular gauze is ideal for fragile skin or simple convenience that a tubular net bandage provides (Fig. 25).

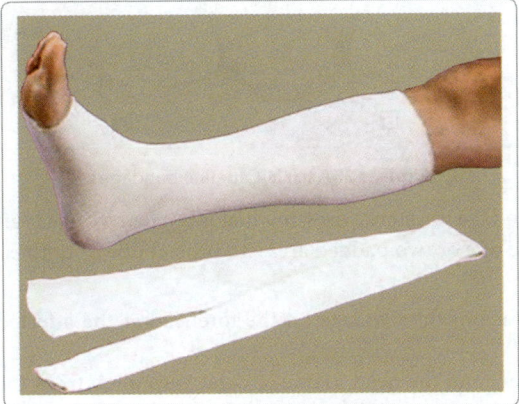

Figure 25: Tubular bandage

Head and Other Bandages

- **Capeline bandage:** Capeline bandage covers the head or an amputation stump like a cap (Figs 26A to C). This is used when the whole head is to be covered. A double-headed roller bandage is needed for this.

  Procedure:
  - Patient is seated comfortably and the nurse stands behind the patient.
  - The center of the outer surface of the bandage is placed in the center of the forehead holding the rolls in each hands of the nurse.

Unit II ❖ Procedures and Techniques in First Aid

- The usual length is 6 yards of each roll in each hand.
- The lower border of the bandage should be just above the eyebrows.
- The head of the bandage is brought around over the temples of the head and above the ears and reaches the nape of the neck. Here the ends are crossed.
- The upper bandage is carried on around the head. The other bandage is brought over the center of the top of the scalp and extends to the root of the nose.
- The bandage, which encircles the head is now brought over the forehead, covering and fixing the bandage could cross the scalp.
- This bandage is then brought back over the scalp slightly to one side of the center, thus covering one margin of the original turn.
- At the back, it is again crossed and fixed by the encircling bandage and is turned back over the scalp to the opposite side of the centerline, covering the other margin of its original turn.
- These backward and forward turns are repeated to alternate side of the center, each one being in turn fixed by the encircling bandage until the whole scalp is covered.
- Finally, the bandage is completed by a circular turn around the head and pinned in the center of the forehead.

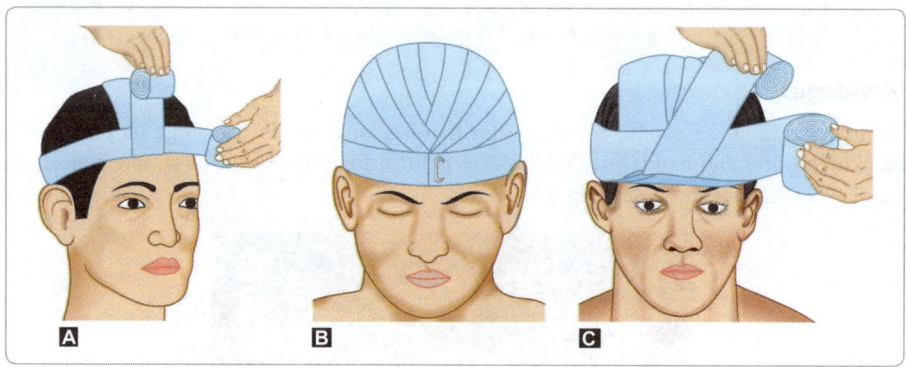

Figures 26A to C: Capeline bandages

- **Ear bandage:** An ear bandage is a sterile dressing that is applied to an ear after the wound has closed up. An ear bandage can have one or two padded areas, to protect one or both ears (Fig. 27).

Procedure:
- Keep the outer surface of the bandage on the forehead at the affected side.
- Carry the bandage around the head in one circular turn away from the injured ear towards the sound side and carry the bandage around the back of the head, low down in the nape of the neck and carry it obliquely to the head again and repeat the same.
- Each turn being slightly higher than the previous one, as it covers the dressing but slightly lower as it covers the hair.
- Continue until the whole dressing is covered and complete the bandage by one straight turn around the forehead, pinning where all the turns cross one another.
- It is better to take the bandage around the forehead between each turn covering the dressing, which will keep it tighter. But this makes a heavy bulk around the head.

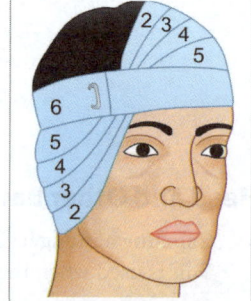

Figure 27: Ear bandage

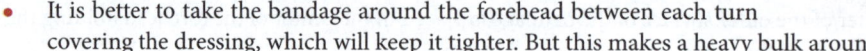

■ **Eye bandage:** Eye care bandages are used for protecting injured eyes and healing lazy eye (Fig. 28).
  ● **Reasons for applying an eye bandage:**
    ○ To maintain gentle pressure over an eye pad
    ○ To arrest hemorrhage
    ○ To reduce swelling after eyelid surgery
    ○ Following eye surgery, e.g., enucleation
    ○ For a child, and ensure that the pad is not disturbed.

Procedure:
● Lay the outer surface of the bandage against the forehead on the affected side and take the circular turn around the head bandaging away from the injured eye.
● Carry the bandage on, around the head until it reaches the ear on the sound side for the second time.

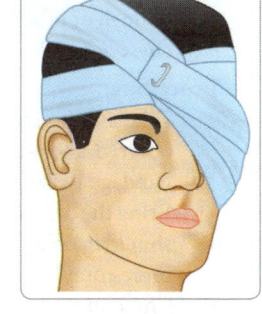

Figure 28: Bandage for the eye

● Take it obliquely to the back of the head, under the prominence, at the back of the skull and from there bring it upwards beneath the ear of the affected side, over the pad of the eye to the circular turn and continue over the head to the starting point.
● Repeat this turn two or three times until the dressing is covered.
● Finish it with a safety pin just above the unaffected eye.
● The pattern resembles that of the ear bandage but there are few turns.
● The bandage should be light in weight and should not obstruct the view of the good eye.

■ **Jaw bandage:** A jaw bandage is used to temporarily stabilize the jaw after a fracture or dislocation (Figs 29A to C). Before applying a bandage to a casualty's jaw, remove all foreign material from the casualty's mouth. If the casualty is unconscious, check for obstructions in the airway.

It serves a twofold purpose:
1. Stops the bleeding and protects the wound
2. It also immobilizes a fractured jaw

Procedure:
● Place the bandage under the chin and carry its ends upward. Adjust the bandage to make one end longer than the other.
● Take the longer end over the top of the head to meet the short end at the temple and cross the ends over.
● Take the ends in opposite directions to the other side of the head and tie them over the part of the bandage that was applied first.

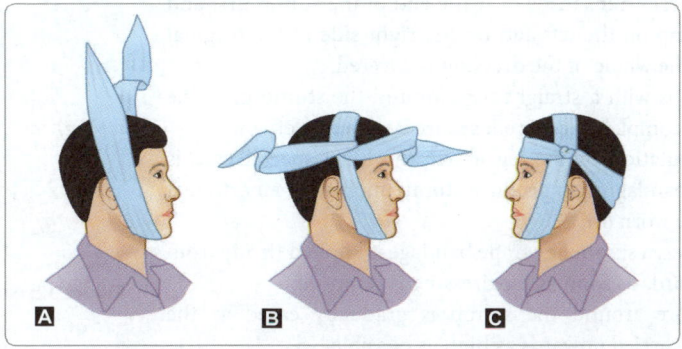

A   B   C

Figures 29A to C: Bandage for the jaw

Unit II ❖ Procedures and Techniques in First Aid

- **Breast bandage to support one breast**
  - The breast is bandaged by using a four-inch roller bandage of gauze, flannel, or other material. It is used as an option for lymphedema of the chest or trunk (Fig. 30).

  Procedure:
  - Take a three-inch bandage and start bandaging below the breast to be covered and working away from it towards the sound side, carry the bandage twice around the waist.
  - Bring the bandage up under the breast to be supported over the opposite shoulder obliquely down across the back or under the arm and once more round the waist on covering two-third of the previous turn.
  - These turns are repeated until the breast is sufficiently covered.
- **Bandaging both breasts (Fig. 31):**
  - Take two circular turns around the waist as for the single breast, starting under the right breast and bring the bandage up, under the right breast over the left shoulder obliquely down across the back, under the right arm and across the front of the waist, horizontally.
  - Carry the bandage under the left arm up, across the back to the right shoulder and down across the chest under the left breast.
  - From here, it is passed under the left arm and is turned horizontally across the back to beneath the right breast again.
  - These turns are repeated until both breasts are covered.
- **Stump bandage:** A stump bandage is an elastic bandage applied to an amputation stump in order to control postoperative edema and to shape the stump (Figs 32 and 33). It helps to protect the healing tissue, holds the wound dressing in place, reduce swelling, and shape the residual limb for a prosthesis.

  Procedure:
  - Place patient in a comfortable position with leg flat.
  - Take a four-inch elastic bandage.
  - Keep the end of the bandage in the center of the upper side of the limb and carry the bandage, over the center of the thumb to the same level behind, holding the turns back and front with the thumb and fingers of the other hand of the nurse.
  - Repeat the recurrent turns over the end of the stump first and on the stump on the left and on the right side of the original turn until the whole of the dressing is covered.
  - Fix the loops with a straight turn around the stump until the dressing is completely covered; secure it with a safety pin.
  - In an amputation of the leg above the knee special care is needed in bandaging to produce stump upon such an artificial limb can be worn on.
  - In such cases, a six-inches crape bandage is applied firmly from below upwards as soon as the dressing is removed.
  - The pressure around the stump is gradually eased as the bandage is carried upwards as high as possible.

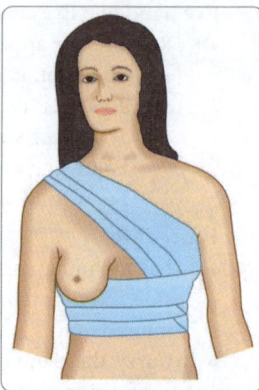

Figure 30: Breast bandage to support one breast

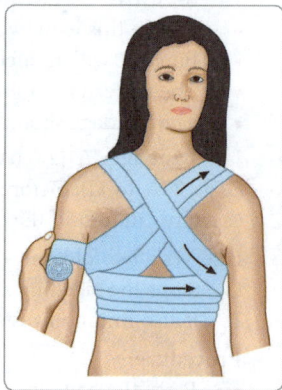

Figure 31: Bandaging both breasts

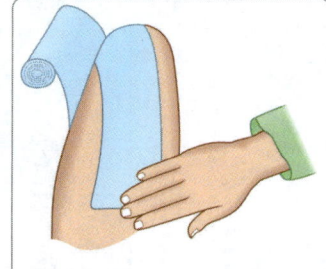

Figure 32: Stump bandage for limb

- The object is to produce a conical stump owing to stretching.
- Such bandage may require reapplication several times daily and the patient should not be allowed to go about on crutches when such a bandage is worn.

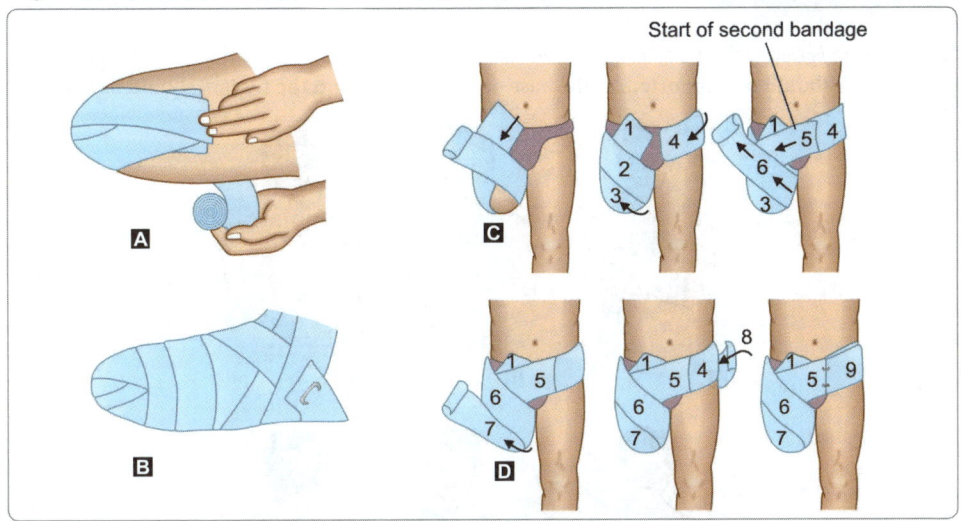

Figures 33A to D: Stump bandage of the leg above the knee

SLINGS

Definition

Slings are supportive materials made out of the same items for making bandages to support fractured ribs or collar bones or fractured, plastered or splinted upper limbs. It is prepared from a 90 cm. square of linen, cut diagonally.

Uses of Slings

- To support injured arms
- To prevent pull by upper arms in injuries to chest, shoulder, collar bones or neck

Types of Slings

Arm Sling

An arm sling is used in cases of fractured ribs, injuries of upper limbs and in cases of fracture in the arm, forearm, wrists and hands after application of splints or plaster casts and bandaging (Figs 34A to F).

Method of Application of Arm Sling

- A triangular bandage is used.
- Take 90 cm of square linen, make it diagonal in two layers or cut diagonally and take one of it.
- Put it on the chest of the patient directing the apex to the injured elbow and the upper end around the back of the neck.
- Place the forearm horizontally across the chest over the spread cloth, elbow at 90° and bring the hanging end up so that the forearm is covered by the bandage.

- Tie the end of the taken up lower end to the upper end around the neck using a reef knot, in the pit above the collar bone of the affected side.
- Bring the point at the elbow to the front and secure it with a safety pin so as to form a pocket to support the elbow.
- When the sling is tied well, the arm should be comfortable, lying just above the belt line. The wrist should not dangle but should be supported by the base of the bandage and the fingers should be visible.

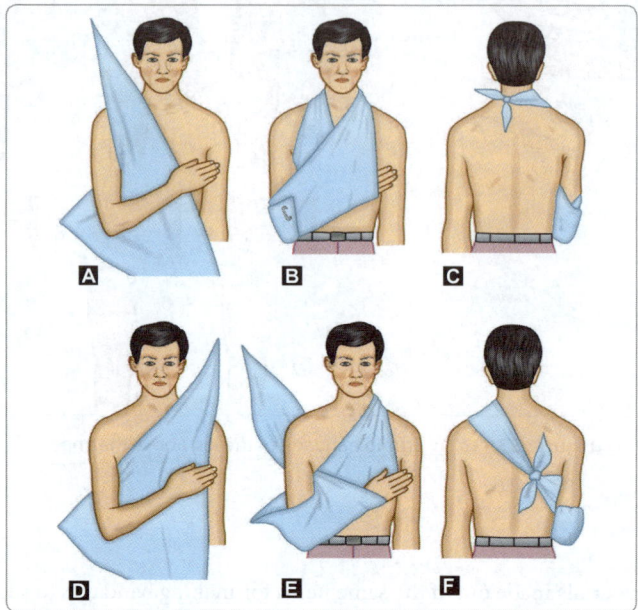

Figures 34A to F: Supporting an arm with a triangular bandage

Collar and Cuff Sling

- This sling is used to support the wrist only (Figs 35A and B).
- The elbow is bent and the forearm is placed across the chest in such a way that the fingers touch the opposite shoulder. In this position the sling is applied.
- A clove-hitch is passed around the wrist and the ends tied in the hollow above the collar bone on the injured side.

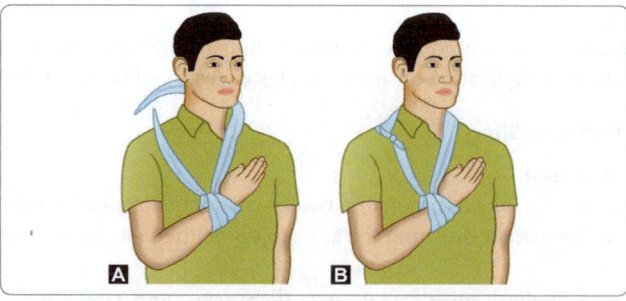

Figures 35A and B: Collar and cuff sling

Triangular Sling (St John Sling)

- A triangular sling is used for the fracture of the collarbone to keep the hand raised up giving relief from pain due to fracture (Figs 36A to C).
- Place the forearm across the chest with the fingers pointing toward the opposite shoulder and the palm over the breast bone.
- Place an open bandage across the chest with one end over the hand and the point below the elbow.
- Tuck the base of the bandage comfortably under the forearm and hand.
- Fold the lower end also round the elbow and take it up and cross the back over the uninjured shoulder and tie it with the other free end into the hollow above the collar bone.
- Tuck the point between forearm and bandage
- Tuck the fold so formed, backwards over the lower half of the arm and fix it with a safety pin.

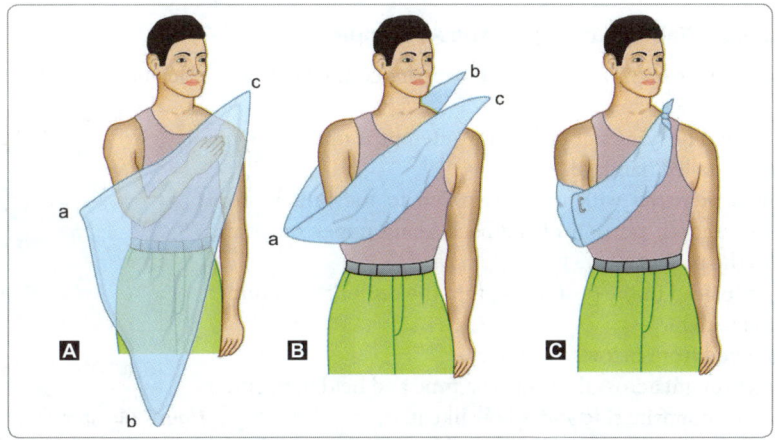

Figures 36A to C: Triangular sling (St John sling) for the fracture of the collar bone

SPECIAL BANDAGES

Types of Special Bandages

The two very common special bandages are shown in Figures 37 and 38.

'T' Bandage

- It consists of two strips of flannel about 4 inches wide, stitched together in a form of a 'T'.
- The horizontal strip is made long enough to pass round the body usually the hip and the vertical strip is passed up between the legs.
- It is then pinned to the horizontal strip to keep rectal or perineal dressings in position.

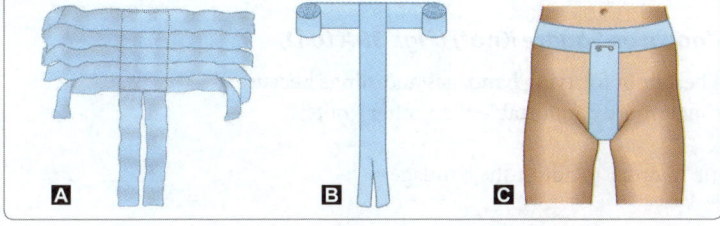

Figures 37A to C: T' bandage

Many Tailed Bandage or Abdominal Binder

It is used for abdominal wound, certain chest dressings and for the part where the use of a roller bandage causes great amount of movement and exertion for the patient to apply it.

- Abdominal binder consists of a number of strips or tails of flannel or cotton material, 4–6 inches wide and of sufficient length to encircle the part and overlap at least 8 inches.
- Each strip overlies the one above by two-thirds of its width and the whole is secured in the center by a piece of the same material.
- There should not be hard ridges to hurt the patient.
- Bandages for the chest are sometimes provided with two tails stitched to the top of the back piece and standing slightly outwards which pass over the shoulder and are pinned to the front of the bandage when the other tails are folded over to keep the bandage from slipping down.

Application of a Many Tailed Bandage to the Abdomen

Two people are required to apply a many-tailed bandage comfortably and efficiently, however in an emergency one can manage it (Fig. 38).

- The patient should be lying flat before any attempt is made to apply or adjust a many-tailed bandage.
- The bandage is prepared with the tails rolled to the center, from either end, the smooth portion of the back being upper most and placed next to the patient.
- The bandage is placed in the position so that the center bands under the back of the patient.
- Bandage is applied from below to upwards.
- One tail being brought across the body at a time and held in position by a tail from the opposite side and follow like it.
- The last tail is brought around the body or obliquely downwards and secured with a safety pin.

Figure 38: Application of an abdominal binder or many-tailed bandage

Many tailed bandages are also applied to maintain the intra-abdominal pressure and to prevent shock and collapse in cases of childbirth and after paracentesis. In such cases, the bandage is applied from above downwards.

The disadvantages of an abdominal binder are respiratory difficulty and hypotension due to compression on the vena cava.

KNOTS

Definition

A good knot holds but is easy to open if necessary (Figs 39A to D)· There are different knots for different purposes and all knots are not good for all purposes. Some of the knots that are useful in bandaging are:

Reef Knot (Also Known as Square Knot) (Figs 39A to D)

The reef knot is the best knot for tying bandages and slings because:

- It lies flat, making it more comfortable than other knots.
- It does not slip.
- It is easy to untie in order to adjust the bandage.

Procedure

- Take one end of a bandage in each hand
- Lay the end from the right hand over the one from the left hand and pass it under to form a half-knot. This will transfer the ends from one hand to the other
- Tighten by pulling one loop against the other or by pulling only on the ends
- Place knots so they do not cause discomfort by pressing on skin or bone, particularly at the site of a fracture or at the neck, when tying a sling.
- If the knot is uncomfortable, place soft material underneath as padding.

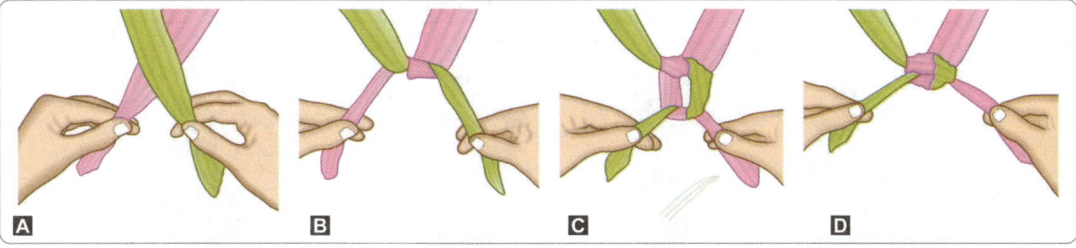

Figures 39A to D: Reef knot

Clove Hitch

Clove-hitch is made with a narrow bandage. Two loops are made and laid one on top of the other. A clove hitch is two successive half-hitches around an object. It is most effectively used as a crossing knot. It is used to tie the colored arm sling. A clove-hitch is passed round the wrist and the ends are tied in the hollow above the collar bone on the injured side (Figs 40A and B).

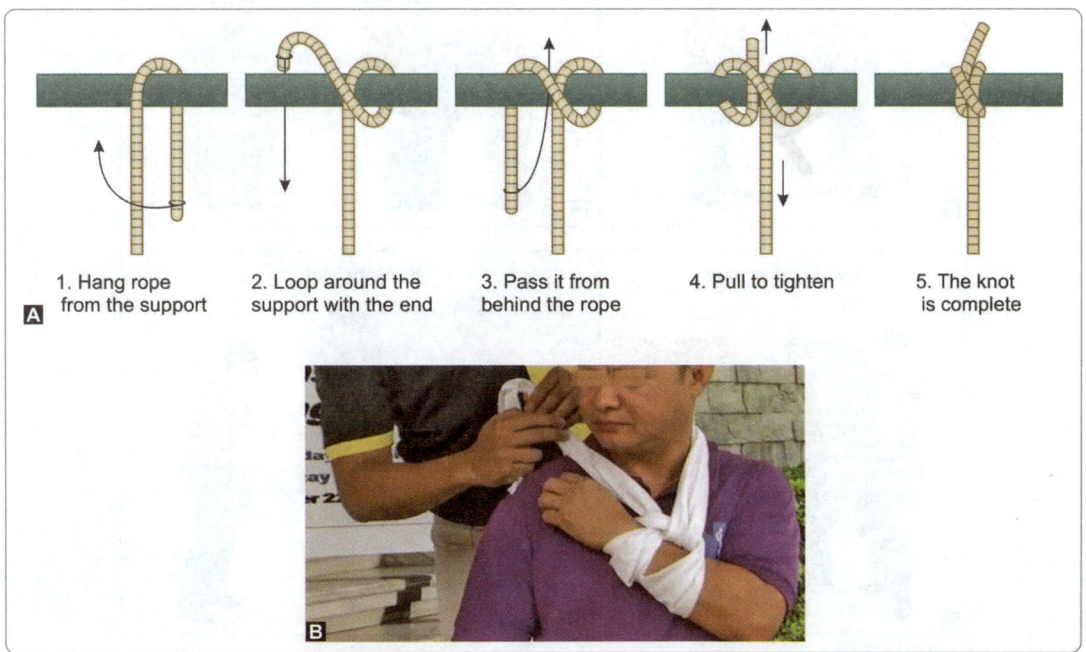

1. Hang rope from the support
2. Loop around the support with the end
3. Pass it from behind the rope
4. Pull to tighten
5. The knot is complete

Figures 40A and B: (A) Method of using clove hitch; (B) Method of putting clove hitch

Unit II ❖ Procedures and Techniques in First Aid

Transportation of the Injured

It is the process of moving an injured person to a hospital or other treatment center. Once you have rescued the casualty from the immediate danger, slow down! Casualties should not be moved before the type and extent of injuries are evaluated and the required emergency medical treatment is given. There are various methods of transporting the injured (Figs 41A to E).

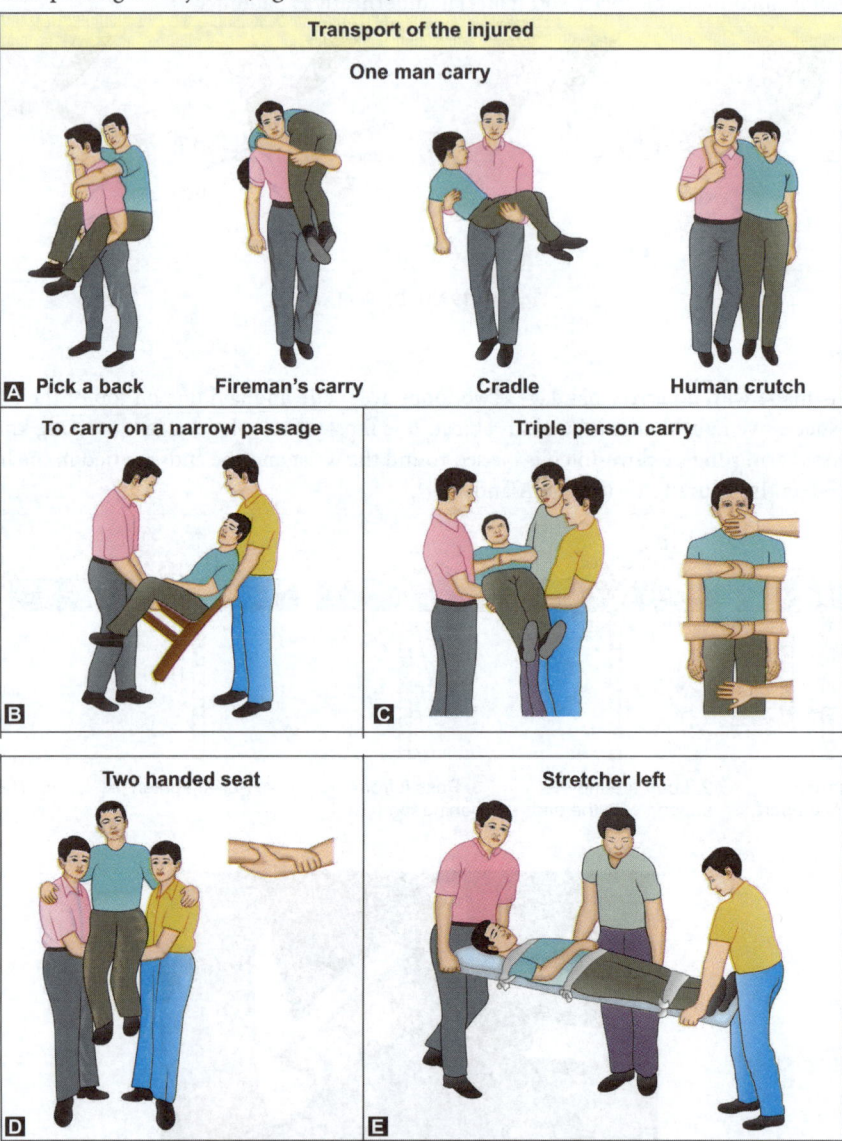

Figures 41A to E: Transporting the victim

Types of Drag and Carry

Drag and carry techniques are required to evacuate a sick or injured person from an emergency scene to a location of safety. Causalities must be carried carefully and should be correctly handled, otherwise their injuries may become more serious or possibly fatal. Situation permitting, evacuation of a causality should be organized and un-hurried. Each movement should be performed as deliberately and gently as possible. Manual carries are tiring for the rescuer and involve the risk of increasing the severity of the casualty's injury. Choose the evacuation techniques that will be least harmful, both to rescuer and the victim. Some of the rescue drag and carry techniques are as follows:

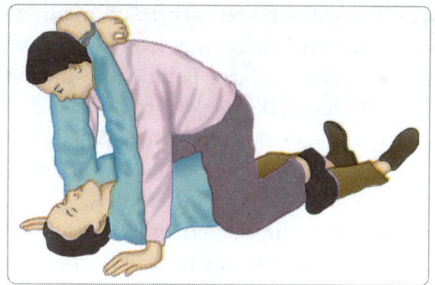

Figure 42: Tied-hands crawl/Fireman's drag

- **Tied-hands crawl/Fireman's drag**: The tied-hands crawl may be used to drag an unconscious casualty for a short distance. It is particularly useful when you must crawl underneath a low structure, but it is the least desirable because the casualty's head is not supported (Fig. 42).
  - Place the casualty face up. Cross the casualty's wrists and tie them together
  - Kneel astride the casualty and lift the arms over your head so that the casualty's wrists are at the back of your neck
  - When you crawl forward, raise your shoulders high enough so that the casualty's head will not bump against the deck
- **Crawling technique:** Use a triangular bandage, a torn shirt, etc. to tie the casualty's hands together and place them around your neck. This way you can move a person much heavier than yourself (Fig. 43).
- **One person arm carry:** Single rescuer to lift a victim safely by arm carry (Fig. 44). Rescuer holding the victim around the victim's back and under the knees
- **Walking assist:** This method requires the injured or ill person to be conscious (Fig. 45).
  - Place the injured or ill person's arm across your shoulders and hold it in place with one hand.
  - Use your other hand and place it around the person's waist to support them.

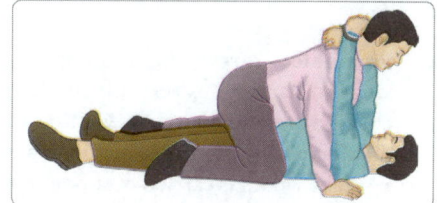

Figure 43: Crawling technique

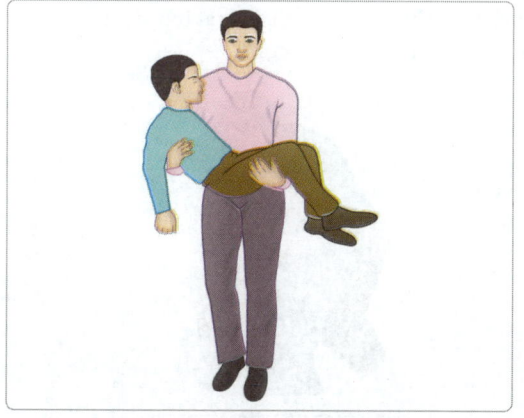

Figure 44: One person arm carry

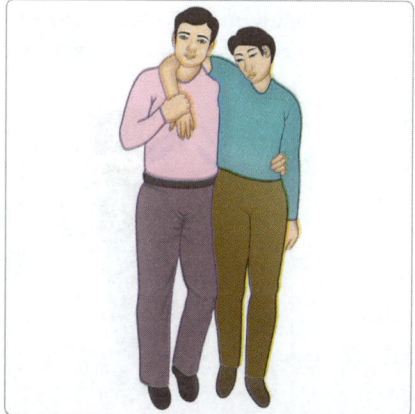

Figure 45: Walking assist

Unit II ❖ Procedures and Techniques in First Aid

- **Two-person seat carry:** This method requires two people to assist the conscious person in need of transport (Fig. 46).
  - Put one arm behind the person's thighs and the other across the person's back.
  - Interlock your arms with those of the second person assisting in the transport so that it goes behind the person's legs and across their back.
  - Lift the injured or ill person that is sitting on the seat created by the arms of the first-aiders.
- **One person carry:** This method can be used for both conscious and unconscious persons. Similar methods include piggyback style, fireman carry, or pack-strap carry (Fig. 47).
  - Kneel in front of the person with your back toward him.
  - Bring your arms around the victim's knees.
  - Grasp his hands over your chest.

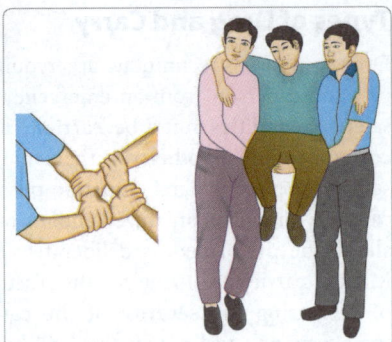

Figure 46: Two-person seat carry

Note

- Avoid injury to your own back by keeping straight and lifting with your legs.

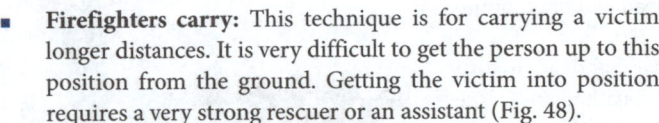

- **Firefighters carry:** This technique is for carrying a victim longer distances. It is very difficult to get the person up to this position from the ground. Getting the victim into position requires a very strong rescuer or an assistant (Fig. 48).
  - The victim is carried over one shoulder
  - The rescuer's arm, on the side that the victim is being carried, is wrapped across the victim's legs and grasps the victim's opposite arm.

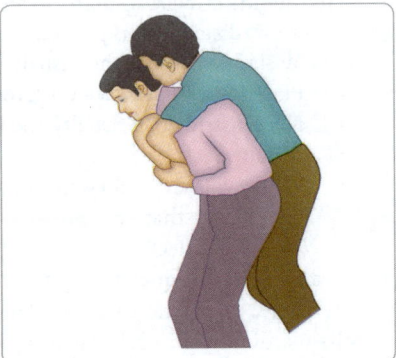

Figure 47: One person carry

- **One person pack-strap carry:** This method is better for longer distances to lift a victim safely (Fig. 49).
  - Place both the victim's arms over your shoulders.
  - Cross the victim's arms, grasping the victim's opposite wrist
  - Pull the arms close to your chest
  - Squat slightly and drive your hips into the victim while bending slightly at the waist
  - Balance the load on your hips and support the victim with your legs.

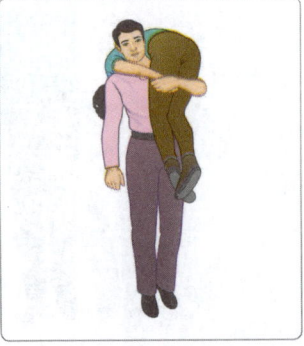

Figure 48: Firefighters carry

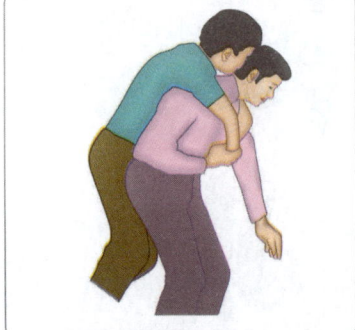

Figure 49: One person pack-strap carry

■ **Drag methods:** This method includes the blanket drag, ankle drag and the clothes drag (Fig. 50).

- **Blanket drag method**
    - With this method, gather half of the blanket and place it against the person's side.
    - Roll the person toward you and reach over to place the blanket so that it is positioned under the person.
    - Roll the person on the blanket and gather the blanket at the head and drag.

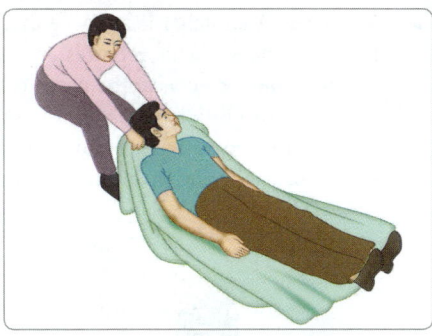

Figure 50: Drag methods

- **Ankle drag method**
    - With the ankle drag method, firmly grasp the person's ankles and move backward in a straight line (Fig. 51).

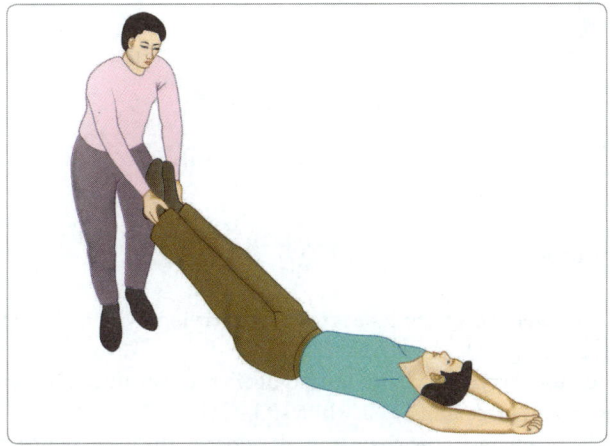

Figure 51: Ankle drag method

- **Clothes drag method**
    - In this method, grasp the person's clothing behind the neck (Fig. 52) (gather enough to secure a firm grip).
    - Use the clothing to pull the person head first.

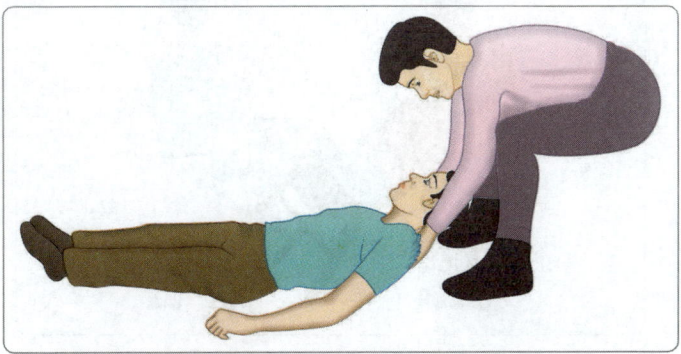

Figure 52: 'Clothes drag' method for moving a victim

Unit II ❖ Procedures and Techniques in First Aid

■ **Stretcher:** A stretcher is a device that is used to transport an ill or injured person by having the person lie on the object. This requires at least two people to help assist in the transport. When a stretcher is not available, objects can be used to create one. There are several ways to make a stretcher. One of the techniques is given here (Figs 53A and B).

● Use two poles that are somewhat longer than the victim's length.
● Take a shirt and push the poles through the sleeves.

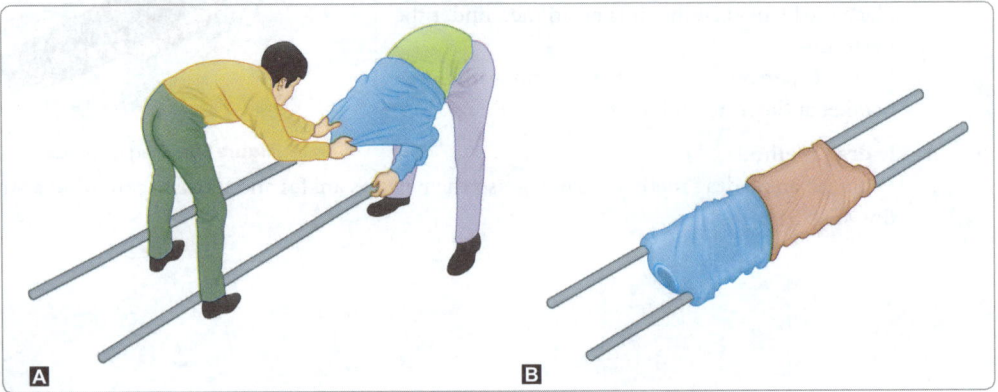

Figures 53A and B: Stretcher

 **Note**

● You can also use a tarp or blanket and wrap the poles in between.

■ **Chair carry, chair stretcher:** This technique is used for carrying a victim for longer distances and is used for unconscious victims (Fig. 54).

This is a good method for carrying a victim up and down stairs or through narrow or uneven areas.

● Pick the victim up and place him or have him sit in a chair
● The rescuer at the head grasps the chair from the sides of the back, palms in
● The rescuer at the head then tilts the chair back onto its rear legs
● For short distances or stairwells, the second rescuer should face in and grasp the chair legs
● For longer distances, the second rescuer should separate the victim's legs, back into the chair and on the command of the rescuer at the head, both rescuers stand using their legs.

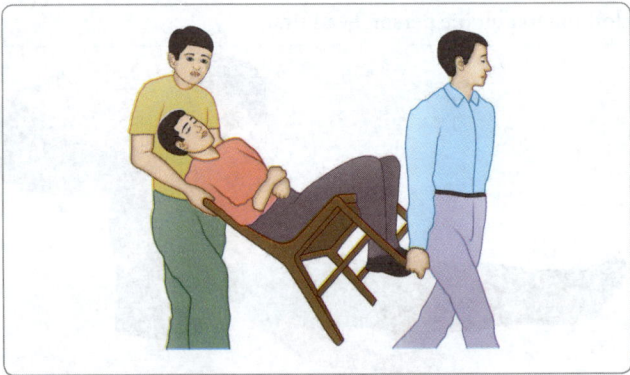

Figure 54: Chair carry/chair stretcher

Unit II ❖ Procedures and Techniques in First Aid

- **Fireman's lift (Figs 55A and B):**
  - The bearer grasps the patient's left wrist with the right hand.
  - The bearer's head is placed under the patient's left armpit, drawing the patient's body over the bearer's left shoulder.
  - The bearer's left arm should encircle both thighs, and then lift the patient.
  - The patient's wrist is transferred to the bearer's left hand, thus leaving one hand free to remove obstacles or to open doors.

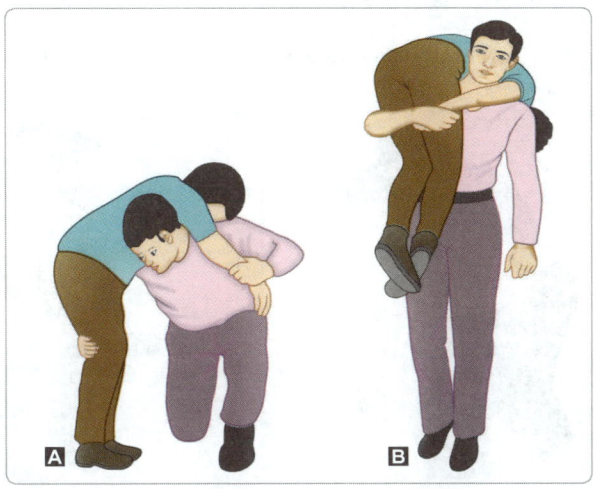

Figures 55A and B: Fireman's lift

- **Four-handed basket seat:** This technique is for carrying conscious and alert victims to moderate distances. The victim must be able to stand unsupported and hold themselves upright during transport (Fig. 56).
  - Position the hands as indicted in the graphic
  - Lower the seat and allow the victim to sit
  - Lower the seat using your legs, not your back
  - When the victim is in place stand using your legs, keeping your back straight

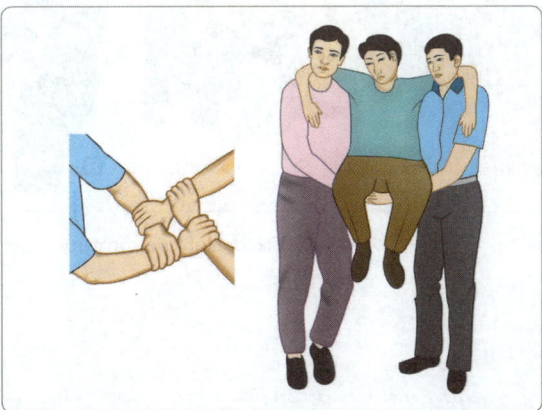

Figure 56: Four-handed basket seat

- **Pack-strap carry (Fig. 57):**
  - The patient is supported along the bearer's back.
  - The patient's right arm is brought over the bearer's right shoulder and held by the bearer's left hand.
  - The patient's left arm is brought over the left shoulder and held by the bearer's right hand.
  - The patient is thus carried on the back, with the arms resembling pack straps.
- **Piggyback carry (Fig. 58):**
  - The patient is supported along the bearer's back with the knees raised to the sides of the bearer's torso.
  - This leaves the patient practically in a sitting position astride the bearer's back, with arms around the bearer's neck or trunk.

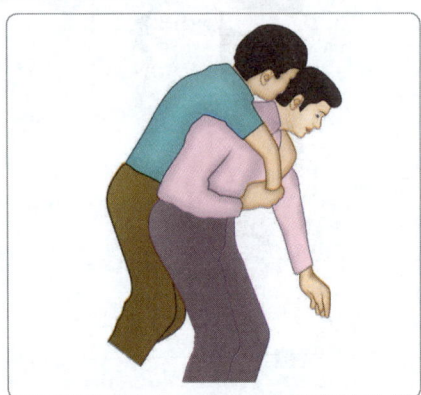 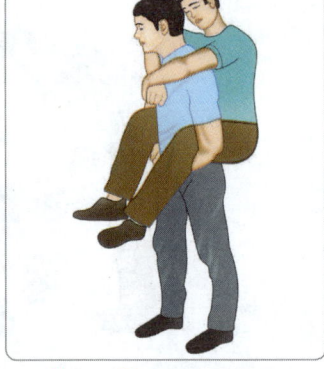

Figure 57: Pack-strap carry   **Figure 58:** Piggyback carry

- **Six- or eight-person carry:** This is done as the three person carry, except three or four bearers are on each side of the patient, thus dividing the patient's weight more uniformly (Figs 59A and B).

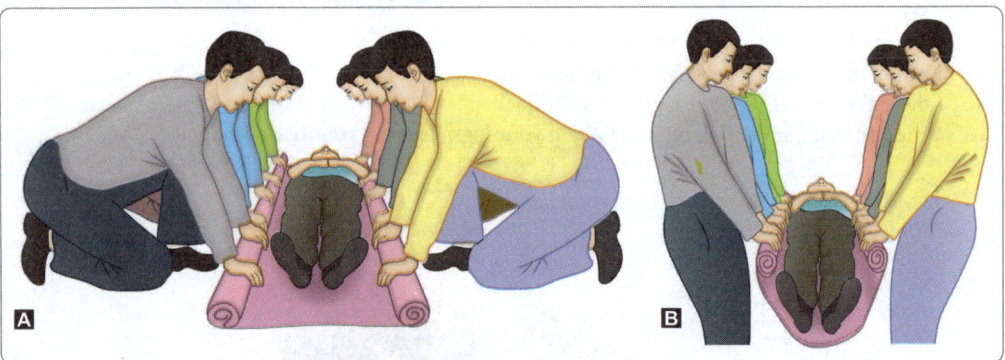

Figures 59A and B: Six- or eight-person carry

■ **Three- or four-person carry (Fig. 60):**

 • This is the litter-type carry used by emergency squads.

 • Three persons kneel on one side of the patient, place their hands under the patient, and lift up.

 • The head bearer supports the patient's head and shoulders, the center bearer lifts the waist and hips and the third bearer lifts both the lower extremities.

 • A fourth person, if available, should help steady the patient while he or she is being lifted.

■ **Vehicles:**

 • If an ambulance is not available, stretchers can be improvised with ropes and chairs, ladders, or poles.

 • The patient should always be tied to the stretcher during transportation.

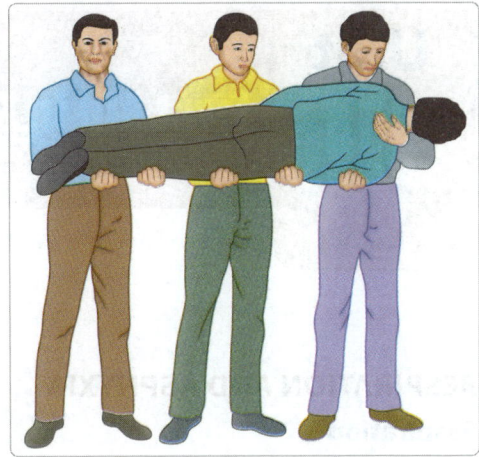

Figure 60: Three- or four-person carry

 • Several bearers will be necessary to assist entering and leaving the vehicle.

   o **Ambulances:**

     ♦ Shift the patient into the ambulance using a stretcher.

     ♦ Two of the most widely used rescue stretchers are the canvas and bamboo 'Neil-Robertson' and the tubular metal and plastic 'Paraguard' stretchers. The latter has the particular virtue of folding to half-size for ease of storage.

   o **Special transport systems:**

     ♦ In addition to the rescue stretcher, special transport systems may be involved in bridging the gap between the accident site and the ambulance. Helicopters, hovercraft, land rovers or lifeboats may be needed.

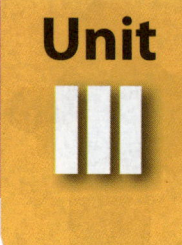

Unit III

First Aid in Emergencies

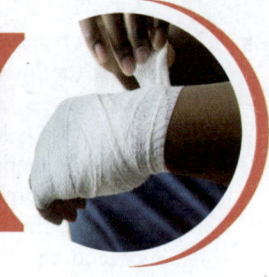

RESPIRATION AND ASPHYXIA

Respiration

It is the process of taking in or inhaling (when air enters the lungs), and exhaling or expiration (when air leaves the lungs). During inspiration, lungs expand and air is drawn in and when the thoracic cavity contracts, the air is drawn out of the lungs. This cycle of inspiration and expiration occurs 16–20 times in a minute.

Asphyxia or Suffocation

It is a condition in which the lungs do not get sufficient air or sufficient oxygen for the oxygenation of deoxygenated blood.

Signs and Symptoms of Asphyxia

- Patient with asphyxia experiences weakness, dizziness and breathlessness.
- Bluish discoloration of the face, lips, nails, tip of the nose and fingers.
- Neck veins are swollen.
- If the asphyxia is due to lack of oxygen in the air or an airway obstruction, the patient makes great efforts to breathe.
- If the asphyxia is due to depression of respiratory center, respiration is slow and fluttering. The patient becomes unconscious. In acute and severe asphyxia there might be involuntary relaxation of sphincter muscles and passage of urine and stools.

 *Note*

The most important and first step in the management of asphyxia is to clear the airway

Causes of Asphyxia

It is a fatal condition, which occurs if there is not enough oxygen available for the tissues of the body. Such lack of oxygen may be due to an insufficient amount of oxygen in the air breathed in or any interference with or injury to the respiratory system. The following are the conditions that result in asphyxia:

- Low oxygen levels in the air, like high altitude, sewers, coal mines, etc.
- Gas poisoning
- Consumption of atmospheric oxygen and smoke, e.g., burning buildings
- Obstruction of air passages, like foreign body or food, external compression by hanging, strangulation, etc.

- It could be due to *drowning* where water enters the respiratory tract causing bronchospasm and lack of access of air
- Depression of respiratory center by morphine or barbiturate poisoning
- Compression of thoracic cavity due to fall of earth, sand or mines or collapse of house, etc.
- Respiratory diseases, like bronchial asthma or pulmonary tuberculosis, etc.

Drowning

- Turn the face of the patient downwards, head on one side, arms stretched beyond the head
- Infants and children may be held upside down for some time
- Raise the middle part of the body with the help of hands so that the water may drain out of the lungs
- Remove wet clothes and keep the patient warm
- When patient is recovered give him/her sweet warm drinks
- Do not let the patient to sit up
- When the water is drained out completely, treat for the shock according to the condition of the patient (Fig. 1).

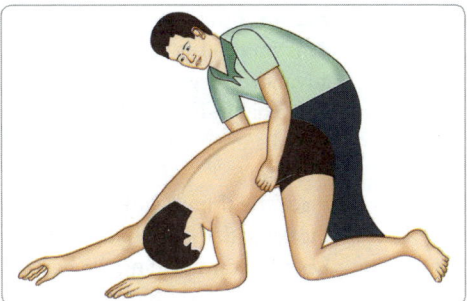

Figure 1: Removal of water from the lungs in drowning

In Hanging or Strangulation

Cut the ligature or string around the neck and treat for the asphyxia and shock.

Choking

Partial or complete obstruction of internal air passage due to obstruction by food, fluid or foreign bodies is known as choking (Figs 2A and B).

- **Choking due to foreign body in the airway:**

  As first aid, different methods can be adopted to remove foreign body from the airway.
  - **Back blows:**
    - Stand on one side and slightly behind the patient.
    - Place the left hand over the sternum of the patient to support, the head being at a lower level than the chest.
    - Give four sharp blows rapidly over the spine between the shoulder blades.

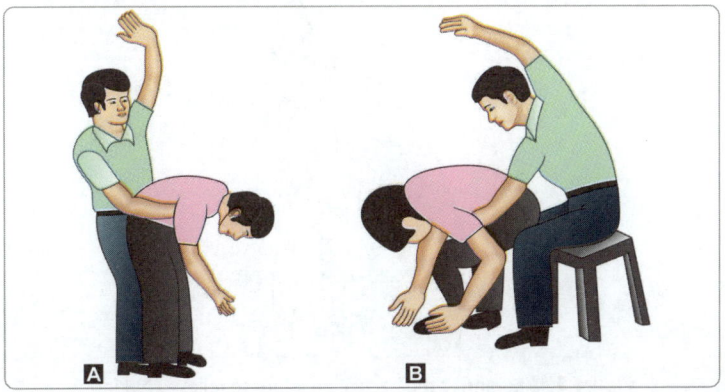

Figures 2A and B: Slapping the back to relieve choking

Unit III ❖ First Aid in Emergencies

- **Heimlich's maneuver or manual abdominal thrust:**
  - Stand behind the patient with arms around the patient's waist.
  - Grasp one wrist with the other and place the thumb side of the fist against the patient's abdomen between the umbilicus and rib cage.
  - Then quickly press the fist inwards and upwards four times (Fig. 3).
- **Manual chest thrusts:**
  - This method is to be used for obese patients and in case of advanced pregnancy.
  - Stand behind the patient with arms directly under the patient's armpits encircling the chest at the level of the middle of the sternum.
  - Place the thumb side of the right fist over the sternum, grasp the fist with the left hand and exert four rapid backward thrusts.
  - Lean forward placing the head of the patient below the level of the chest, if possible (Fig. 4).
- **Flapping the back of an infant to relieve choking:**
  - To remove the foreign body from the airway of an infant or a child, abdominal thrusts cannot be used because of the risk of injury to abdominal viscera (Fig. 5).
  - In such condition, hold the infant upside down with head lower than the chest.
  - Holding the infant by his/her legs in the left hand upside down, smack his back hard three or four times, rapidly on the spine between the shoulder blades with the heel of the right hand.
  - If it is not successful, lay the child in prone position with the head hanging downwards over your left thigh supporting the head on the left arm and give sharp smacks between the shoulders.
  - If it is not successful, induce vomiting by passing two fingers right to the back of the throat.
  - Take the child immediately to the hospital and get the medical aid.
  - Once the airway is clear, the patient may start breathing on his/her own. Ensure that child gets the fresh air. If the patient cannot breath, give artificial respiration.

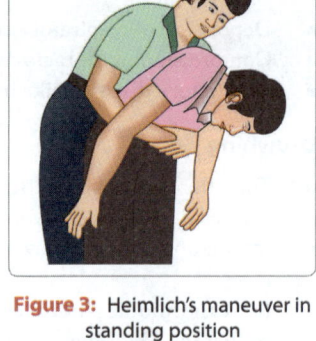

Figure 3: Heimlich's maneuver in standing position

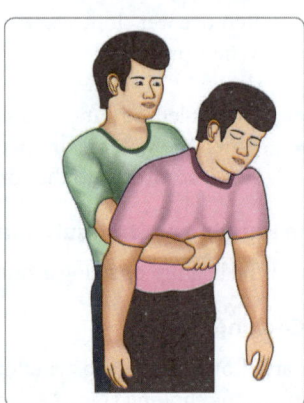

Figure 4: Manual chest thrusts

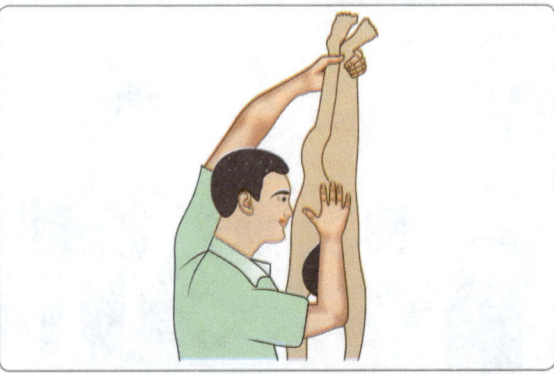

Figure 5: Slapping at the back of an infant to relieve choking

ARTIFICIAL RESPIRATION (EXTERNAL RESPIRATORY RESUSCITATION)

Artificial respiration or ventilation is means of assisting or stimulating respiration. It is a metabolic process referring to the overall exchange of gases in the body by pulmonary ventilation, external respiration, and internal respiration. There are several methods of giving artificial respiration practiced as first aid.

Methods of Artificial Respiration

The most successful and commonly used methods are:

- **Mouth-to-mouth method:** It was discovered during the Second World War and was found to be best and easiest method to be used in conditions of respiratory distress.
- Silvester's method (Armlift chest pressure method)
- Schafer's method (Prone pressure method)

Asphyxia of severe degree may be found along with unconsciousness. The general causes are:

- The tongue has fallen back into the throat.
- Vomitus has collected in the throat.
- Some foreign materials have collected in the air passages.
- When a casualty is unconscious, make sure that he/she is breathing freely. Begin to work immediately as every minute is critical and do not make delay.

Preparation of the Patient for Starting Artificial Respiration

- Loosen the clothing at the waist, chest and neck.
- Tilt the head backwards while supporting the neck with palm. This will lift the tongue to its normal position so that the air passages are cleared and the casualty may begin to breathe after a gasp.
- If the breathing does not start by the above treatment, help in the movement of chest and lungs four or five times, which will be enough to start breathing. If breathing has not started even now, mouth-to-mouth breathing is started (Fig. 6).

  - **Mouth-to-mouth respiration:**
    - o Place the patient on his back.
    - o Loosen the clothing on his neck, chest and waist.
    - o Remove any dentures if present.
    - o Clear the patient's mouth with a handkerchief twisted on your fingers.
    - o Place the right hand under the neck and the left hand on forehead and tilt the head backwards.
    - o Using the hand under the neck, lift the chin of the patient upwards.
    - o If the patient starts breathing on his own, maintain the chin in that position itself.

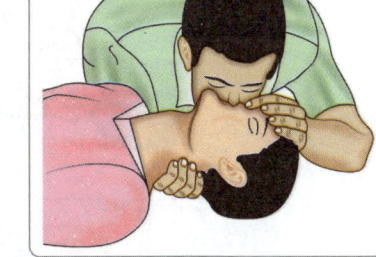

Figure 6: Mouth-to-mouth respiration

    - o If breathing has not started, pinch the patient's nostrils together, take a deep breath, cover the patient's mouth firmly with your own mouth and breathe into his/her lungs.
    - o See through the angle of your eye that his chest rises.
    - o Remove your mouth from the patient's mouth and turn your head away.
    - o The air in the patient's lungs escapes.
    - o Repeat this procedure rapidly three or four times to saturate the patient's blood with oxygen.
    - o Repeat this procedure about 12 times per minute and continue until the patient starts breathing on his/her own.

Unit III ❖ First Aid in Emergencies

- Take the patient to the hospital in ambulance.
- This routine is similar for infants and children except that the mouth and nose of the child is to be covered by your mouth and less force has to be used than for an adult.
- In certain situations, mouth-to-mouth respiration cannot be given when the face is damaged, or the lower jaw is fractured or if the lips and mouth have been burnt by a poison. In such cases, other manual methods are used.

- **Silvester's method (arm-lift chest pressure):**
  - Place the patient, face upwards (Figs 7A and B).
  - Place a folded blanket under the shoulders of the patient to raise them so that the head falls backwards.
  - Kneel near the head.
  - Grasp the patient's forearms near the wrist, cross them over the lower part of the chest and lean forward to press the crossed arms for two seconds.
  - Then pull the arms upwards and outwards with a sweeping movement and place them on the ground nearby your own knees for three seconds. Again bring the hands back and give pressure on the chest as before.
  - Repeat the cycle for 12 times per minute.
  - This method is useful when the patient cannot be placed with face down.
  - It is more effective than the prone pressure method.
  - Take the patient to the hospital in ambulance as early as possible.

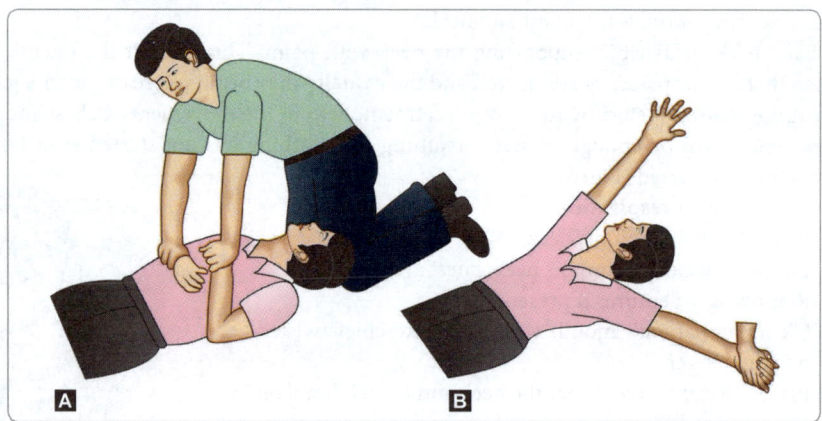

Figures 7A and B: Sylvester's method

- **Schafer's method (prone pressure method):**
  - Place the patient in prone position, head turned to one side, hands resting on the floor on both sides of the head.
  - Kneel by the side of the patient at the level of the hips.
  - Place the hands over the lower part of the back, wrists almost touching, thumbs forward and fingers opposed.
  - Keep your upper limbs straight as you lean forward so as to apply pressure by the weight of the body.
  - Then rock backwards to release pressure.
  - Repeat the cycle twelve times per minute until respiration starts normally, if the heart is working.
  - Arrange for the ambulance and take the patient to the hospital (Figs 8A and B).

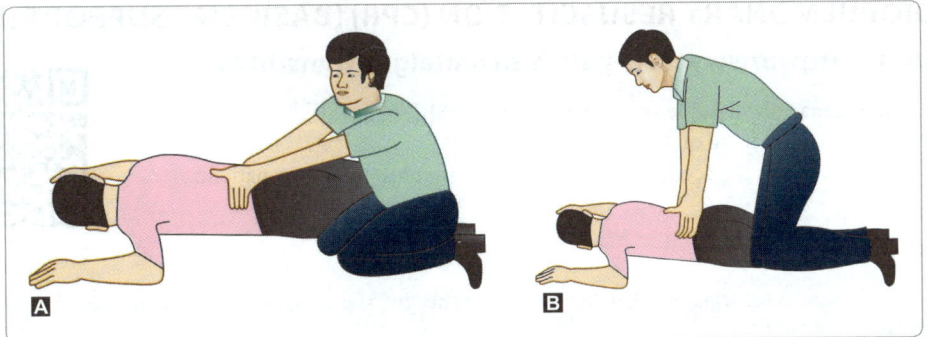

Figures 8A and B: Schafer's method

EXTERNAL CARDIAC MASSAGE (EXTERNAL CARDIAC RESUSCITATION)

The heart may stop functioning (cardiac arrest) due to some diseases of the heart or it may be secondary to respiratory failure. In both the conditions, there is deficiency of oxygenated blood in circulation in the rest of the body and irreversible damage may occur to the vital organs resulting in death of the patient, unless the heart is made to function immediately.

A sharp striking is given to the sternum with a closed fist from a height of 20–25 cm. If the heart does not start beating with this method, external cardiac massage is to be started.

Signs and Symptoms of Cardiac Arrest

- Loss of consciousness
- Cyanosis
- Failure to feel the pulse in the wrist or neck
- Heart sounds cannot be heard from the chest if ear is kept close to the patient's chest
- Pupils dilated

External cardiac massage achieves rhythmic compression of the heart between the sternum and the vertebral column so that blood is pumped into the pulmonary and systemic circulation. Mechanical stimulation of the heart induces it to contract on its own, so that on cessation of the massage, the heart continues to beat by itself (Figs 9A to C).

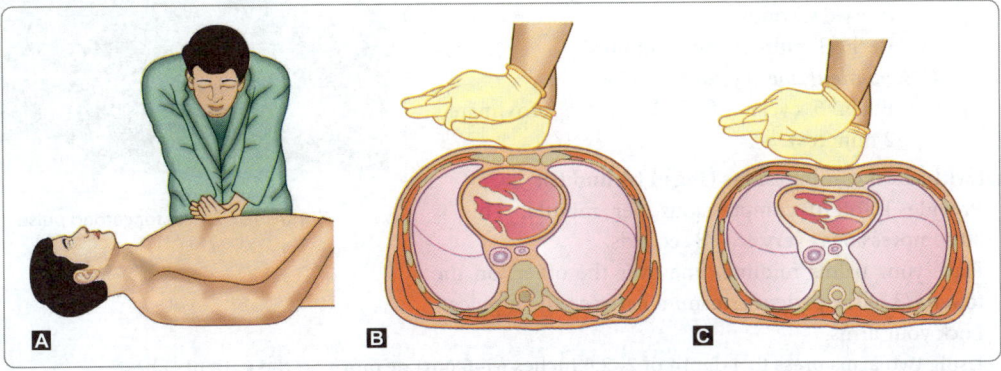

Figures 9A to C: External cardiac massage

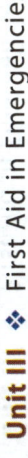

Unit III ❖ First Aid in Emergencies

CARDIOPULMONARY RESUSCITATION (CPR) [BASIC LIFE SUPPORT (BLS)]

For Adults (https://www.acls-pals-bls.com/algorithms/bls/)

The following scenario will guide you in performing CABD.

■ You found an adult lying on the ground.

■ Assess to make sure the scene is safe for you to respond to the down patient.

Mnemonic

A common acronym in BLS used to guide CPR providers about the appropriate steps to assess and treat patients in respiratory and cardiac distress is:
CABD (Circulation, Airway, Breathing, Defibrillate).

■ **Assess responsiveness**: Stimulate and speak to the adult asking if he/she is ok. Look at the chest and torso for movement and normal breathing.

If unresponsive:

● One provider—first call the emergency response team and bring an AED to the patient.

● Two providers—have someone near, call the emergency response team and bring the AED.

● Place patient supine on a hard flat surface.

🧠 **Stimulant**

AED: An automated external defibrillator (AED) is an emergency life-saving device that is used in the event of sudden cardiac arrest. It is a portable device that analyses the heart rhythm and administers an electrical charge to the heart, if needed to establish a regular heartbeat in the event of a cardiac arrest.

■ Circulation

● Check the patient for a carotid pulse (Fig. 10) for 5–10 seconds. (Do not check for more than 10 seconds.)

If the patient has a pulse:

○ Move to the airway and rescue-breathing portion of the algorithm.

○ Provide 10 rescue breaths per minute (1 breath every 6 seconds).

○ Recheck pulse every 2 minutes.

If the patient doesn't have a pulse:

○ Begin 5 cycles of CPR (lasts approximately 2 minutes).

Start with chest compressions (Figs 11A and B):

■ Provide 100–120 compressions per minute. This is 30 compressions every 15–18 seconds.

■ Place your palms midline, one over the other, on the lower 1/3 of the patient's sternum between the nipples.

■ Lock your arms.

■ Using two arms press to a depth of 2–2.4 inches (5–6 cm) or more on the patient's chest.

■ Press hard and fast.

■ Allow for full chest recoil with each compression.

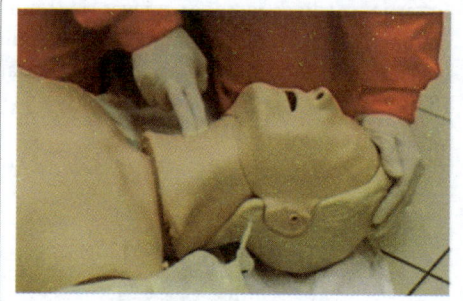

Figure 10: Assess for carotid pulse

- 1 cycle of adult CPR is 30 chest compressions to 2 rescue breaths.
- If two providers are present, switch rolls between compressor and rescue breather every 5 cycles.

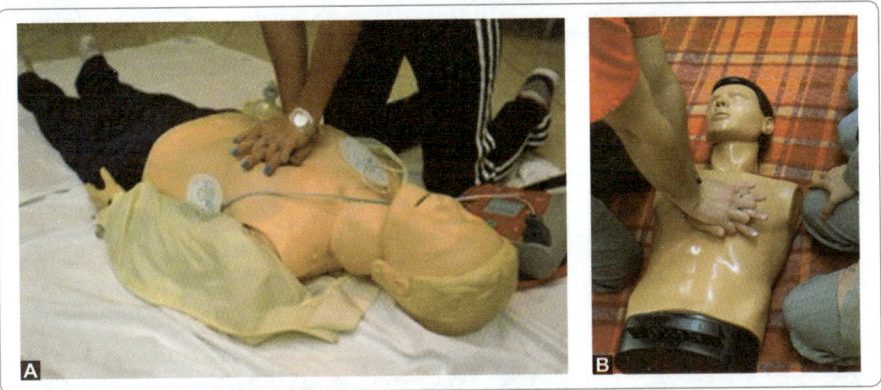

Figures 11A and B: Chest compressions

Airway

In the event of an unwitnessed collapse, drowning, or trauma:
- Use the jaw thrust maneuver. (This maneuver is used when a cervical spine injury cannot be ruled out.):
- Place your fingers on the lower rami of the jaw.
- Provide anterior pressure to advance the jaw forward.

In the event of a witnessed collapse with no reason to assume a C-spine injury: **Use the head tilt-chin lift maneuver:**
- Place your palm on the patient's forehead and apply pressure to tilt the head backward.
- Place the fingers of your other hands under the mental protuberance of the chin and pull the chin forward and cephalic (Fig. 12).

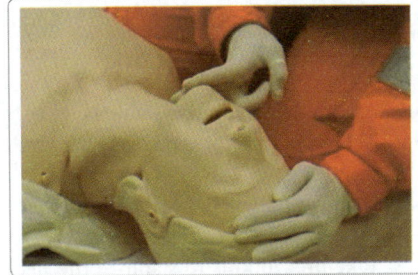

Figure 12: Head tilt-chin lift maneuver

Breathing:
- Scan the patient's chest and torso for possible movement during the 'assess unresponsiveness' portion of the algorithm.
- Watch for abnormal breathing or gasping.

If the patient is breathing adequately:
- Continue to assess and maintain a patent airway and place the patient in the recovery position. (Only use the recovery position if it is unlikely to worsen patient injury.)

If the patient is not breathing or is breathing inadequately (Figs 13A and B).

If the patient has a pulse:
- Commence rescue breaths immediately.

If the patient has no pulse:
- Begin CPR.
- Use a barrier device if available.
- Pinch the patient's nose closed.
- Make a seal using your mouth over the mouth of the patient or use a pocket mask or bag mask.

- Each rescue breath should last for approximately 1 second.
- Watch for chest rise.
- Allow time for the air to expel from the patient.

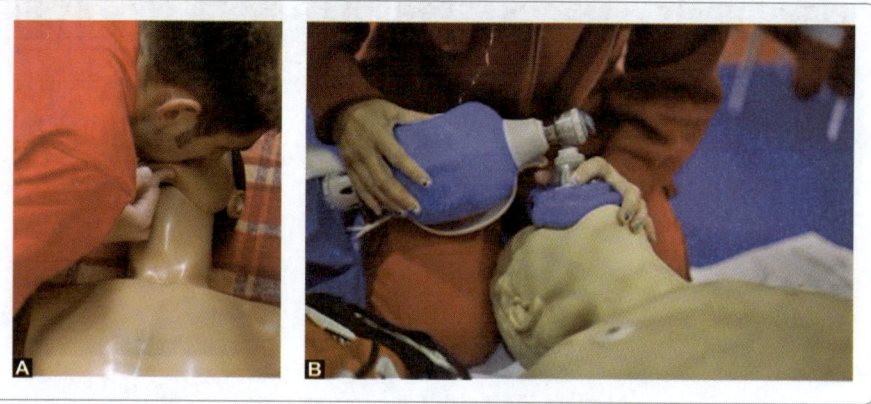

Figures 13A and B: Cardiopulmonary resuscitation

Recovery Position (Lateral Recumbent or 3/4 Prone Position)

- This position is used to maintain a patent airway in the unconscious person.
- Place the patient close to a true lateral position with the head dependent to allow fluid to drain.
- Assure the position is stable (Fig. 14).
- Avoid pressure of the chest that could impair breathing.
- Position patient in such a way that it allows turning onto her back easily.
- Take precautions to stabilize the neck in case of cervical spine injury.
- Continue to assess and maintain access of airway.
- Avoid the recovery position if it will sustain injury to the patient.

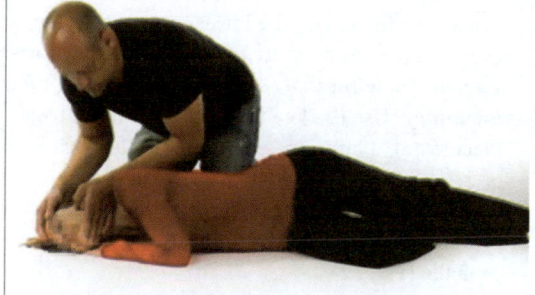

Figure 14: Recovery position

Defibrillate

Arrival of the automated external defibrillator (AED) (Fig. 15)

- Turn AED on now! (early defibrillation is the single most important therapy for survival of cardiac arrest and should be done as soon as it arrives).
- Follow verbal AED prompts.
- Firmly place appropriate pads (adult/pediatric) to patient's skin to the indicated locations (pad image).
- A short pause in CPR is required to allow the AED to analyze the rhythm.

If the rhythm is not shockable:

- Initiate 5 cycles of CPR.
- Recheck the rhythm at the end of the 5 cycles of CPR.

If the shock is indicated:

- Assure no one is touching the patient or is in mutual contact of a good conductor of electricity by yelling "Clear, I'm Clear, you're Clear!" prior to delivering a shock.
- Press the shock button when the providers are clear of the patient.
- Resume 5 cycles of CPR.

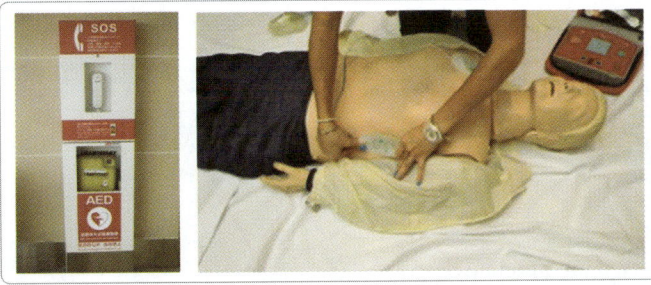

Figure 15: Automated external defibrillator for survival of cardiac arrest

For an Infant (Fig. 16)

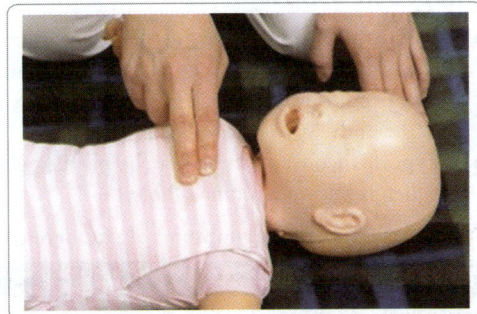

- Provide 100–120 compressions per minute. This is 30 compressions every 15–18 seconds.
- **One provider:** Place two fingers on the sternum of the lower chest. One between the nipple line and the other 1 cm below.
- **Two providers**: Encircle the infant's torso with both hands with both thumbs pointing cephalic positioned 1 cm below the nipples over the sternum.
- Chest compressions should be at least 1.5 inches or 1/3 the depth of infant's chest.
- Press hard and fast.
- Allow for full chest recoil.
- Only allow minimal interruptions to the chest compressions.

Figure 16: Cardiopulmonary resuscitation in infants

(One provider: 1 cycle is 30 chest compressions to 2 rescue breaths and two providers: 1 cycle is 15 chest compressions to 2 rescue breaths)

For a Child Older than 1 Year of Age to Puberty (Fig. 17)

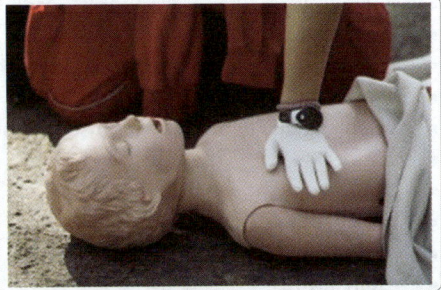

- Provide 100–120 compressions per minute. This is 30 compressions every 15–18 seconds.
- Use one or two arms.
- Place one or both of your palms midline, one over the other, on the lower sternum, between the nipples.
- Press at least to 1/3 the depth of patient's chest or 2 inches.
- Press hard and fast.
- Allow for full chest recoil with each compression.
- Allow for only minimal interruptions to chest compressions.

Figure 17: Cardiopulmonary resuscitation in older child

Unit III ❖ First Aid in Emergencies

- **One provider:** 1 cycle is 30 chest compressions to 2 rescue breaths.
- **Two providers:** 1 cycle is 15 chest compressions to 2 rescue breaths.

COMMON CASUALTIES AND MANAGEMENT

The common casualties, which need immediate attention, are as follows:

- Unconsciousness
- Convulsions
- Hemorrhage
- Shock
- Poisoning
- Bites and stings
- Burns and scalds
- Foreign bodies
- Injuries to the bones, joints and muscles

A few of the casualties have been discussed here along with their cause and management:

Unconsciousness

- **Definition:** Unconsciousness is a condition in which the patient does not respond to external stimuli. Any interferences with the normal functioning of the brain and nerves bring about loss of sensitivity. It may occur due to some disease of the brain or due to some serious injury and diseases in any other parts of the body.
- **Types:** Unconsciousness may be partial, which is called stupor or it may be complete unconsciousness, which is known as coma (Table 1).

Table 1: Differences in symptoms of stupor and coma

Stupor	Coma
• Do not respond on calling name or talking to the patient, but can be aroused with difficulty	• No response at all in coma
• Patient will resist to open the eyes while attempting by others.	• Lids can be opened by others without resistance
• Pupils of the eyes contract when light is allowed to fall on it	• There is no response to light. Pupil is widely dilated in deep coma

Common causes of unconsciousness:

- Common fainting
- Brain injuries like cerebral injury, cerebral hemorrhage or cerebral tension
- Apoplexy
- Epilepsy
- Poisoning by narcotic drugs, alcohol or sedative drugs
- Asphyxia due to drowning, poisons or strangulation
- Shock
- Heat strokes or exhaustion
- Heart attacks
- Electric shocks
- Convulsions
- Medical diseases like insulin coma, hepatic coma, cerebrovascular accidents, acute fever, meningitis, etc.

- Hemorrhage
- Hysteria

Management of unconscious patients or patient who has fainted:
- Keep the patient flat on the floor with head turned to one side. If not possible keep the patient in prone position with face resting and turned to one side.
- In both these positions no pillow is kept under head and the face is turned to one side to allow the secretions, if any, to flow out.
- Prevent the tongue from falling back by placing two fingers behind the angle of the jaw on each side and pressing the jaw together. If that fails, open the mouth, clear it and pull the tongue forward holding it with a handkerchief gently.
- Remove false teeth, if any.
- Avoid crowd around and let the fresh air come in. If in a room, open the windows and doors to get fresh air.
- Loosen the clothes from around the neck, chest and waist.
- Keep the patient warm.
- Watch for vomiting.
- Watch pulse rate and respiration.
- Arrange for medical aid.
- Do not give anything orally as it may enter in wind pipe and choke the patient.
- Do not apply heat.
- Sprinkle cold water on the face or wipe the face with a towel dipped in cold water.
- Do not leave the patient alone or unattended.
- If breathing is stopped or about to stop, turn the patient into the required posture and start artificial respiration.
- It is better to remove the patient to a sheltered place on a stretcher.
- On return to the consciousness, wet the lips with water.
- Once the patient recovers fully, tea or coffee can be given.

Common fainting is due to the reduction of blood supply to the brain. The pulse and respiration rates are rapid and patient appears pale. Better to raise the foot end of the patient slightly to allow more blood to the brain. Besides the measures mentioned above, some smelling salt is used or slashed onion is given to smell.

Sunstroke

- **Sunstroke** occurs due to prolonged exposure to the sun. It starts with headache, sometimes vomiting, dizziness, cramps and dryness of throat. Temperature rises to 38°C. Pulse becomes rapid and goes weak, respiration is shallow and irregular and the patient becomes weak.
- **Management:** Move the patient to a cool place in a shade. Adopt measures to lower body temperature like, starting fans, applying ice bags, giving tepid sponging, etc.
  Try other measurers as mentioned in the management of unconscious patient.

Convulsions

Hysterical Fits

Hysteria is a psychiatric disorder, which can be expressed in a number of ways. Hysteria is one of the physiological manifestations of psychological expressions. Patient is not really unconscious but pretends to be so. Usually, no physical injury occurs as the patient falls with care. The patient may have convulsive limb movements. Limbs may be rigid; eyes are tightly closed, or fluttering, open or closed. There may be frothing at the angle of mouth. Incontinence of urine and feces does not occur. Fits never occur when the patient is left alone. Patient responds soon to rest, sprinkling of cold water on the face and inhalation of smelling salt or slashed onion.

Persons exhibit these signs when he/she needs help from others therefore, the problem should be investigated. The solving of a problem is not within the scope of a first aider. So the patient should be sent to a doctor to get the condition treated.

Convulsions in Children

Convulsions can occur in children (under 3 years) due to high fever. Other causes of convulsions are low blood sugar level, fall or rise in the sodium level in the blood, low level of magnesium or calcium in the blood, cerebral palsy, worries, etc. The child rolls up his/her eyes, and body becomes stiff. A number of convulsions occur, body becomes blue, froth comes from the mouth and child passes into unconsciousness state.

Management:
- Keep the child on his back on a flat surface with face turned to one side.
- Keep a spoon or folded cloth between teeth to prevent tongue bite.
- Prevent the child from falling down from the cot.
- Do not try to stop the convulsions forcefully. Trying to stop the convulsions by holding him will not stop it in spite, it may aggravate the convulsions by stimulation.
- After convulsion has stopped, keep the child in recovery position. That is, prone position turned to left side, right upper and lower limbs flexed, left upper arm kept at ease behind the body, head tilted backwards and upwards to keep the airway clean.
- Loosen clothes around neck, chest and waist.
- Do not give anything orally.
- If the convulsion is due to fever, try to reduce fever by application of ice bag, putting fan and tepid sponging.
- Call medical aid or transfer the patient to the hospital.

Convulsions in Adults

Usually convulsions in adults occur due to epilepsy.

Stages:
- There will be a period of *aura*—with signs of premonitory symptoms, like blurring of vision, flashes in front of eyes and ringing in the ears.
- In the next stage patient cries out aloud (cry).
- The next stage is *tonic phase* characterized by rigidness of the body in which limbs are held stiff, extended and breathing is arrested for 0.5 minutes.
- This is followed by **clonic phase** characterized by convulsions of 0.5–1 minute. Tongue may be bitten and lips and tongue become blue.
- Patient may pass urine involuntary and becomes unconscious after the clonic phase, which is called *postictal phase* for a variable interval.

Management:
- When the premonitory symptoms are seen, put the patient in a safe place.
- Allow plenty of fresh air to the patient and don't allow crowd to gather around him.
- Remove dentures, hair pin, etc. if any.
- Loosen the clothes around neck, chest and waist.
- Put the patient in recovery position during unconsciousness.

- Keep mouth gag, spoon or a folded handkerchief between the teeth to prevent biting the tongue.
- Nothing should be given orally.
- Arrange for medical aid to prevent further convulsions.
- Follow the general rules for treatment of an unconscious patient.
- When child recovers, give a warm sweet drink.
- Advise him to follow the treatment for epilepsy to control the condition.

When the patient becomes normal, instruct the patient and relatives to:
- Carry a card with the patient stating his/her address and the diagnosis, so that if a fit occurs on the road, aid may be available easily.
- Avoid driving and swimming.
- Avoid contact with fire, bathing alone in river or tanks, electricity, machines, etc.

Hemorrhage

Hemorrhage or bleeding is the loss of blood from the body through an injury or ulceration or through an orifice because of break in the continuity of blood vessels.

Classification of Hemorrhage

- **According to the site of hemorrhage:** Bleeding is of two types:
  1. **External or revealed hemorrhage** is bleeding from an injury in the skin with or without damage in the underlying tissues.
  2. **Internal or concealed hemorrhage** is bleeding in the organs or body cavities, which are not visible outside the skin.
- **According to the type of vessel involved:**
  - **Arterial bleeding:** Bleeding may be from arteries called arterial bleeding. Blood is bright red in color, flows in spurts and can be arrested by compression over the artery between the heart and the site of injury.
  - **Venous bleeding:** Bleeding from veins is venous bleeding. Blood is bluish red in color, flows continuously without spurts and cannot be arrested by compression above the site.
  - **Capillary bleeding:** Bleeding from capillaries is called capillary bleeding. Blood is bright red in color, amount is much less than arterial and venous bleeding and blood flows (as oozing), in the total space of injury.
- **Depending upon the time of occurrence of bleeding:**
  It may be termed *as primary hemorrhage, reactionary hemorrhage and secondary hemorrhage.*
  - **Primary hemorrhage** occurs at the time of injury.
  - **Reactionary hemorrhage** occurs within 36 hours after injury, usually between 4 and 6 hours due to recovery from shock, establishment of collateral circulation, slipping of ligatures, and dislodgement of clot, sealing the injured vessel.
  - **Secondary hemorrhage** occurs within 3–10 days after injury due to infection at the site of injury, which causes softening of tissues, ulceration, sloughing, etc.
- **According to size of hemorrhage:**
  - **Patechial hemorrhage:** Minute pin size hemorrhage in the skin and/or mucous membrane.
  - **Purpura:** Small areas of hemorrhage (up to 1 cm) into skin and mucous membrane.
  - **Ecchymosis:** A large (over 1–2 cm in diameter) extravasation of blood into the skin and mucous membrane.
  - **Hematoma:** Extravasation of large amount of blood into tissue with resultant swelling is known as hematoma (mostly acute)

Unit III ❖ First Aid in Emergencies

Causes of Hemorrhage

Predisposing causes of hemorrhage are:

- Bleeding disorders like hemophilia
- Purpura
- Jaundice
- High blood pressure
- Deficient coagulation of blood due to the administration of anticoagulant drugs like heparin

External Hemorrhage

It is the bleeding, which is visible.

Signs and symptoms of severe external bleeding:

Patient complains of blood loss, feeling of cold, thirst and dyspnea. He/she is pale, cold and clammy extremities, weak, restless, rapid breathing, rapid thready pulse, low blood pressure. Usually the bleeding will be combined from arteries, veins and capillaries.

Management or arresting bleeding:

- Keep the patient on his/her back comfortably.
- Lift the affected part above the level of the heart, if not contraindicated.
- If there is any foreign body in the wound, do not try to remove it while giving the first aid, as it may increase bleeding.
- Apply direct pressure over the bleeding area with sterile pad of gauze or several thickness of rag pieces. Maintain pressure for 5-15 minutes. If bleeding has stopped on removal of pad, apply an antiseptic cream over the wound and keep dressings of tight sterile material.

In order to stop bleeding one of the following methods are applied:

- **Pressure points:** Pressure point is a point at which an artery can be compressed between the compressing finger and an underlying bone to cut off blood supply to the site of bleeding. If a direct method fails to control bleeding, we can apply pressure over a pressure point between the site of injury and the heart.

The important pressure points are shown in Figure 18.

The most important pressure points are described here and are marked in the figure.

- **Temporal pressure points:** Thumb is kept on the upper margin of the ear and the rest of the palm over the back of the head. Pressure is applied above an inch in front of the upper part of the ear and backwards against the temporal bone. The temporal artery runs at this place before it gives of branches.
- **Occipital pressure points:** It is four fingers behind the ears in both sides. Pressure is applied just below the occipital bone on the side with the thumb.
- **Facial pressure points:** Thumb is kept on the lower position of the lower jaw and the fingers on the back of the head and neck. Pressure is applied on the artery at a point at the junction between the middle third and posterior line of the lower jaw.

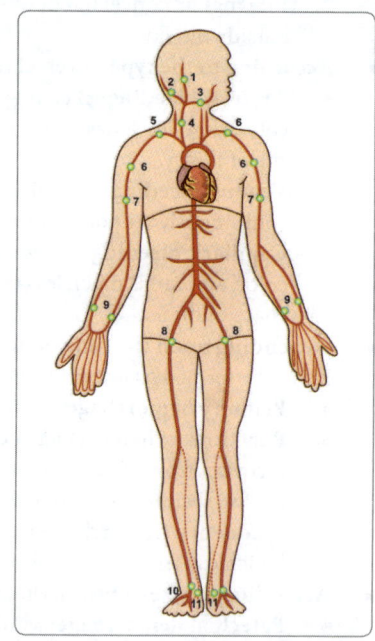

Figure 18: Diagram of the pressure points
Abbreviations: 1. Temporal, 2. Occipital, 3. Facial, 4. Carotid, 5. Subclavian, 6. Axillary, 7. Brachial, 8. Femoral, 9. Radial or Ulnar 10. Anterior Tibial, 11. Posterior Tibial

- **Carotid pressure points:** Two in number, one on either side of the neck. Pressure is applied by the thumb, and is placed on the side of the neck; up above in the side of the trachea and is pressed against the vertebral column behind, with the other fingers of the same hand to stop the bleeding in head area.
- **Subclavian pressure points:** These are two in number, on either side behind the inner end of the clavicle, blood vessel going to the armpit. Pressure is applied by pressing one thumb on top of the other in the hollow above and behind the middle of the collar bone so that the artery is pressed against the first rib.
- **Axillary pressure points:** These are two in number, right and left, it can be pressed by the thumb against the head of the humerus in the armpit.
- **Brachial pressure points:** These points are situated on each side on both hands. It can be pressed against the humerus, with the thumb placing at the inner side of the upper arm.
- **Femoral pressure points:** Femoral pressure points are present on both sides of groin. Femoral arteries are present in the thighs and these supply blood to the lower extremities. To apply pressure on femoral artery, compress at about the center of the groin with the thumb against the horizontal portion of the pelvic bone. Use the left thumb for the right groin and the right thumb for the left depending on the side of the thigh. Knees is slightly bent (Fig. 19).

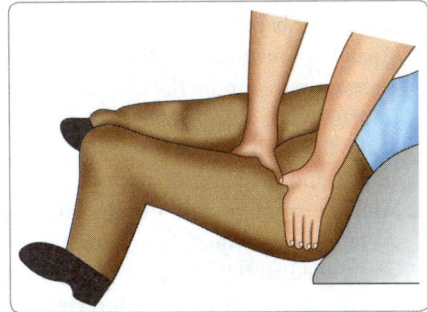

Figure 19: Femoral pressure points

- **Radial or ulnar pressure points:** These are present on both hands. Each of them can be compressed by pressing the thumb against the respective bones just above the wrist, when bleeding occurs in the palm.
- **Anterior and posterior pressure points** are situated just above the ankle joint of the leg.

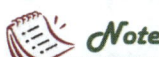 **Note**

Finger pressure over a pressure point can be used only until a tourniquet can be applied because it cannot be maintained for long time.

- **Tourniquet:** A tourniquet is a constrictive band made with a piece of bandage material or split rubber tube and is applied to a limb, to arrest arterial hemorrhage. Tourniquet is no longer used in first aid since its use may cause permanent damage to muscles or nerve supply.

  A tourniquet can be applied around a limb only over a **single bone** that is in the arm or thigh. It causes circular compression of the limb including its blood vessels.

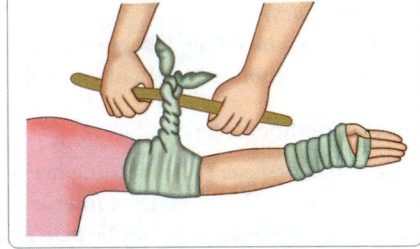

Figure 20: Arrest of bleeding by twist

Tourniquet must be applied between the bleeding site and the heart. The three types of tourniquets in use are:
  - (i) **Fabric tourniquet:** It is a linen tourniquet, which is not elastic. Therefore, it has to be tightened by twisting (Fig. 20).

(ii) **Esmarch's tourniquet:** It is a strong rubber tube of 1.5 meters long with a metal chain at one end and a metal hook at the other. After winding the tube tightly around the limb, compression is maintained by fixing the hook in the chain (Fig. 21).

(iii) **Band tourniquet:** Flat rubber band or tube or a belt can be used as a band tourniquet. It is more elastic (Fig. 22).

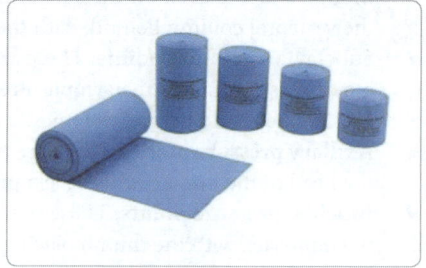

Figure 21: Esmarch's tourniquet

Principles of applying the tourniquets:
- Tourniquet should be applied as close to the affected area as possible and should be tied over a layer of clothing or soft pad to reduce pain and avoid pinching of the skin; never apply over bare skin.
- A rubber tourniquet is stretched with both hands, wrapped several times around the limb and tied.
- Tourniquet should be tightened enough to stop bleeding and make the limb pale. If not tight enough, the limb becomes bluish and bleeding increases as venous return is cut off while arterial blood flow to the limb continues.
- A fabric tourniquet is wrapped around the limb twice and pulled as tight as possible and then tightened further by twisting it with a stick inserted into the knot until the bleeding stops.

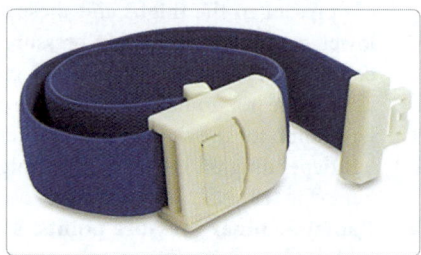

Figure 22: Band tourniquet

- A tourniquet should not be left tied for more than 20 minutes in the upper limbs and in the lower limbs because tissues can die because of prolonged lack of oxygen.
- If transporting the patient to hospital takes longer time than the mentioned period, the tourniquet should be released for a few minutes and then tied tight again, if needed.
  (The time of keeping a tourniquet tight on the limbs may vary slightly in different books)
- Pin a note to the patient's clothing on which the time of application and time of the last released tourniquet should be recorded. Make sure that the tourniquet is always visible. Do not cover it with cloth.

Dangers of tourniquet:
Tourniquets may save life but they must be used with caution.
- **Gangrene:** Application of a tourniquet can result in gangrene and loss of a limb if not loosened every 20 minutes.
- **Increased bleeding:** If a tourniquet is not applied tight enough, the flow of blood will not stop but it will stop the venous return of blood to the heart and increase the bleeding instead of controlling.

Internal Hemorrhage

Internal hemorrhage is the bleeding in the organs or body cavities which cannot be seen from outside.

The signs and symptoms of internal bleeding are same as external bleeding except revealed bleeding. In abdominal bleeding, there may be pain in abdomen and tenderness on touch.

Management and first aid:
The principles of management in internal bleeding are:
- Complete bed rest in a head low position.
- Allow no movements.
- Keep him/her warm with blankets.

- Nothing is given orally as it is likely that patient is to be given anesthesia and to undergo operation, when taken to hospital.
- Shift the patient to hospital as early as possible.

Bleeding from Special Cavities and Regions

- **Bleeding from the nose (epistaxis):** Bleeding from the nose may be due to breaking of small blood vessels in the nose or due to insertion of sharp objects like pencil or by direct injury to the nose or by high blood pressure.

    Management and first aid for epistaxis
    - Make the patient to sit with head slightly tilted forward.
    - Ask him/her to breathe through mouth.
    - Allow blood to drip from the nose to a bowl.
    - Pinch the soft part of the nose (Fig. 23).
    - Apply ice to the forehead and root of the nose.
    - If these measures fail, put a gauze roll in the nose.
    - If available keep a swab soaked in adrenaline in saline.
    - Seek medical aid as soon as possible.

- **Ruptured varicose veins:** A patient may have bleeding from limbs by rupturing of varicose veins.

    Management:
    - Keep the patient flat comfortably.
    - Reassure the patient.
    - Elevate the limb with bleeding.
    - Keep the wound covered and put bandage firmly. Apply pressure to pressure points, if needed.
    - Send for medical aid.
    - Observe and treat for shock.

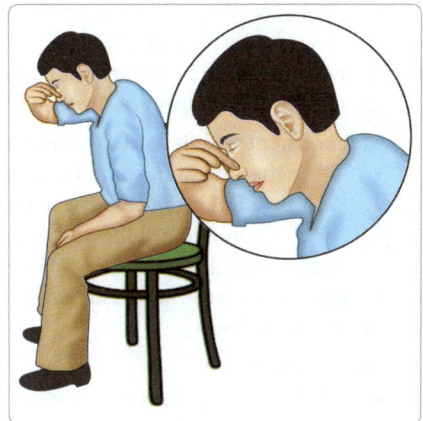

Figure 23: First aid for epistaxis

- **Hemoptysis:** Coughing of blood is called hemoptysis. A patient may cough out blood due to a deep chest injury or due to diseases of the lungs such as tuberculosis or cancer.

    Signs and symptoms of hemoptysis:
    - History of coughing out blood
    - Blood will be frothy due to air bubbles from lungs
    - Blood is bright red in color
    - No food particles in the vomitus
    - Reaction of blood is alkaline
    - Features of respiratory diseases are present

    Management and first aid of hemoptysis:
    - Keep the patient flat with head and shoulders slightly raised and the face turned to one side; or allow him to sit up right.
    - Reassure the patient and remain with him.
    - Nothing orally is given.
    - Keep him reasonably warm by blanket but no hot water bag or too much covering should be applied.
    - Arrange ambulance and take him/her to hospital as soon as possible.

- **Hematemesis:** Vomiting of blood is known as hematemesis due to peptic ulcer, acute gastritis, cancer of the stomach, bleeding esophageal varices or deep injury caused in the stomach.

Unit III ❖ First Aid in Emergencies

Signs and symptoms of hematemesis:

- History of vomiting blood.
- No froth present in vomitus.
- Vomitus is mixed with food particles.
- Blood in the vomitus is seen brown or coffee ground color.
- Reaction of blood in vomitus is acidic due to the presence of hydrochloric acid in the stomach.
- Other features of stomach disorders are seen.

Management and first aid of hematemesis:

- Keep the patient flat with face turned to one side. Left or right lateral positions also can be used.
- Do not give anything orally.
- Reassure the patient and do not leave him alone.
- Seek medical aid urgently.

- **Hematuria:** Blood in the urine is called hematuria. It may be due to injury to the kidneys or urinary tract, urinary stones or cancer of the urinary bladder.

  Management and first aid of hematuria:

  - Keep the patient in comfortable position.
  - Plenty of fluids orally is given, if not contraindicated.
  - Keep the urine until the doctor sees it.
  - Seek medical aid.

- **Bleeding from a tooth socket:** After teeth extraction, bleeding from teeth socket may occur immediately or after a few hours.

  Management:

  - Push a small plug of cotton wool into the bleeding socket.
  - Place the larger pad of cotton wool over the cotton plug and ask the patient to clench the teeth to compress the bleeding site.
  - Avoid spitting, gargling, etc.
  - Do not remove the plug for about 15–20 minutes after stopping the bleeding.

- **Bleeding from the anus:** Bleeding from the anus may be from upper gastrointestinal tract in which the blood may be black due to the alteration of blood (oxidation) during its passage down to the bowel. If the bleeding is from colon or rectum, blood is bright red in color, often due to bleeding piles or due to some other serious conditions such as ulcerative colitis or cancer of the colon. Usually, such bleeding does not need any first aid. If it needs urgent treatment, the management includes:

  - Put the patient in bed with head end in low position.
  - For bleeding piles, apply ice pack locally.
  - Do not apply any hot application to the abdomen.
  - Seek medical aid as soon as possible.

Shock

Shock is a general depression of the vital functions of the body. Shock occurs immediately or soon after emotional or physical trauma, due to loss of circulating blood. This loss may actually manifest as hemorrhage or due to an impaired circulation, without bleeding. Both reasons cause a lowered blood pressure resulting in a diminished supply of blood to the vital centers of the brain. When there is no external bleeding, blood pools in the abdominal or peripheral vessels that have been dilated. So, there is disproportion of the circulating blood in the cardiovascular system and the central cerebral blood vessels. All casualties should be treated for shock.

Causes of Shock

- Strong emotions
- Pain
- Electrical shock
- Foreign proteins given in transfusion
- Snake bite
- Severe injury
- Hemorrhage
- Burns causing loss of fluids and pain
- Dehydration
- Exposure to sunstroke

Signs and Symptoms of Shock

Signs:

- **Appearance:**
  - Patient is pale
  - Skin is cold and clammy
  - Sunken eyes
- **Physical signs:**
  - Subnormal temperature
  - Rapid and thready pulse
  - Fast, shallow and irregular respiration may become gasping
  - Low blood pressure
  - Limbs are flaccid
  - Patient becomes unconscious
- **Mental state:**
  The patient is usually anxious but may become apathetic.

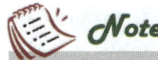 *Note*

Signs are observations which can be noted by others. **Symptoms** are subjective feelings that the patient complains.

Symptoms:
- Nausea
- Vertigo
- Thirst

Management and treatment:
- Keep the patient at rest, lying down if possible and reassure him.
- Loosen the tight clothing.
- If the patient stops breathing, resuscitation methods are used.
- Treat the injury if there is any.
- Keep the patient warm by the use of blankets to a temperature as near to normal body temperature.
- Warm sweet drinks may combat shock, but administer only when the patient is conscious.
- Get medical aid as quickly as possible.
- Do not remove clothing unnecessarily as this may cause further injury or loss of body heat.

Unit III ❖ First Aid in Emergencies

- Always check surroundings to ensure safety of patient as fallen electrical wires, etc.
- Never try to treat the casualty beyond the limits of first aid.
- Do not allow crowd around the casualty. The help of onlookers should be used for telephoning for medical aid, obtaining blankets, bandages, splints, warm drinks, etc.
- Inform the relatives or friends which may relieve their worries.

The person who telephones for medical aid should give the following information:
- The exact location of the patient
- Condition of the patient
- The number of casualties requiring attention

 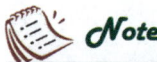 *Note*

Treatment for shock should always be given to all casualties.
The treatment of shock can be summarized as:
- Rest and assurance
- Treatment of injury
- Maintenance of temperature
- Warm glucose fluids if not contraindicated
- Seeking medical aid

Fluids should not be given to patients who are:
- Semiconscious patients
- Unconscious patients
- Patient who is unable to swallow
- Patient who is likely to require anesthesia
- Poisoning, bites and stings

Poisoning

A poison is a substance that causes death, injury or harm to organisms, when taken into the body in enough quantity. It can harm or destroy life. Poison can be consumed accidentally or deliberately for suicidal purpose or may be administered for homicidal purpose. Poison may enter the body by any of the following routes:

- **Oral route,** e.g., insecticides, alcohol, drugs, acids, alkalies contaminated or decomposed foods.
- **Inhalation,** e.g., carbon monoxide, carbon dioxide, anesthetic gases or any other poisonous gases.
- **Injections**, e.g., narcotics, sedatives.
- **Bites**, e.g., snake bite, scorpion sting, dog bite, bites of other wild animals.
- **Skin**, e.g., pesticides.

Types of Poisons

- **Corrosive poisons, which can burn tissues:**
  - Acids, e.g., Sulfuric acid.
  - Alkalies, e.g., caustic soda.
  - Disinfectants, e.g., Lysol, dettol .
  - Bleaching agents, e.g., chlorine.

- **Signs and symptoms of corrosive poisoning:**
  - Burns to lips and mouth.
  - Severe abdominal pain if the patient is conscious.
  - Severe shock.

Management and treatment for corrosive poisoning:

- Send for medical aid.
- Do not induce vomiting.
- Give water to dilute the poison.
- Give egg white or milk to soothe the burnt tissues.
- Dilute acids can be used to neutralize alkaline poisoning. For example, equal parts of lemon juice and water or one part of vinegar to three parts of water.
- Treat the patient for shock.
- Collect any bottles or containers, which have held the poison, if any, for further investigation and treatment.
- Save any vomitus for pathological analysis.

- **Noncorrosive poisons:**
  - Sedations
  - Aspirin
  - Iron
  - Other medicines

Management for the poisoning by the ingestion of medications or noncorrosive poisoning:

- If the patient is semiconscious or unconscious, do not induce vomiting and do not give anything by mouth.
- Keep the patient's airway clear.
- Start resuscitation methods if respiration ceases.
- Take the patient to the hospital or send for a doctor.
- If the patient is conscious, induce vomiting.

- **Kerosene or substances containing kerosene poisoning:**
  - Kerosene
  - Insecticides
  - Furniture polish
  - Shoe polish

Management of poisoning by kerosene or substances containing kerosene:

- Do not induce vomiting.
- Give the patient a glass of milk.
- Take the patient to the hospital.

General Management of any Type of Poisoning

- Remove the poison by the use of an emetic.
- Neutralize the poison if vomiting is not advised.
- Dilute the poison if vomiting is not advisable and an antidote cannot be given.
- Send for medical aid.
- Collect the bottles which may have contained the poison and a sample of any vomitus and take them to the hospital for analysis.
- If the first aider is not sure about the treatment to be given, contact the casualty department of a hospital and be prepared to state the name of the substance and the approximate amount ingested.
- If the patient is conscious, try to find out what has been swallowed, in what quantity and at what time.
- After vomiting has stopped, give milk or egg albumin to the patient, and tea or coffee for drinking.
- In case of gaseous poisoning, take the patient out of the room, avoid crowd around, let the fresh air, loosen the clothing and give artificial respiration, if needed.

Unit III ❖ First Aid in Emergencies

- Take the patient to a doctor as early as possible.
- For poisoning through skin, wash the contaminated area with plenty of cold water. Remove any contaminated clothing, but be careful and avoid touching the chemical yourself.
- Encourage the patient to drink as much water as he/she can. Watch for development of twitching and fits.
- If the poison has been ingested, administer universal antidote, which is composed of 2 parts of activated charcoal (burnt toast), one part of magnesium oxide (milk of magnesia) and one part of tannic acid (strong tea).
- Administer a specific antidote, e.g., weak acid for strong alkali, weak alkali for strong acid, starch for iodine.
- Inform the police.

Method of inducing vomiting:
- With your index finger, tickle the back of the patient's throat.
- Give two glasses of tepid water.
- Give 60 gm of common salt in 300 mL of water.
- Give syrup of ipecac—oral dose of 15 mL followed by a large amount of water; repeated after half an hour, if necessary.

Precaution: Do not induce vomiting if the patient is unconscious or suspected to have ingested strong acid or alkali.

Contraindications for inducing vomiting
- Patients who have swallowed a corrosive poison.
- When substances containing kerosene have been ingested, vomiting is contraindicated as pneumonia may result.
- If the patient is semiconscious or unconscious.
- If the patient is convulsing, inducing vomiting is contraindicated. Manage as an unconscious patient.

 *Note*

Poisoning is best avoided rather than treated. There is an old saying that *'prevention is better and easy than cure"*. It is a valuable proverb in this regard and is completely applicable to prevent poisoning.

Precautions to Prevent Poisoning

The following precautions will be helpful in preventing certain poisoning:
- Do not store medicines for longer period than needed.
- Keep away medicines from the reach of children.
- Do not take medicines in the dark.
- Always read the label before taking medicines.
- Do not pour harmful liquids in the bottles of lemonade or other drinks. Children may mistake the contents for their favorite drink.
- Do not keep the detergents, domestic cleaners and acids under the sink where children can find them.
- Do not take medicines without medical advice.
- Avoid the production of carbon monoxide by burning the coal in closed room.
- Use household cooking gas with care.
- Avoid contact with dogs, which are not immunized for rabies.
- Avoid possible contact with snakes, scorpions and wild animals.

Food Poisoning

Food poisoning occurs due to ingestion of contaminated or decomposing food, due to the presence of bacteria or virus in the food. Onset is rapid and within a few hours after ingestion of contaminated food, patient will have abdominal pain, blood and mucus in stool, fever and vomiting, which may precede diarrhea. More than one person may be affected at times and suffer from this condition.

Management

- Take the patient to the hospital
- Investigate the type of organisms affected
- Analysis of food particles taken from vomitus or aspirated from stomach
- Keep the patient warm
- Provide facilities for defecation and hand washing
- Avoid dehydration
- Treat to prevent shock

Acute Alcoholic Intoxication

In mild cases of alcoholic intoxication, there will be smell of alcohol, rowdiness, disorientation, irrelevant talk and incoordination.

In moderate intoxication, there will be unconsciousness, hypotonia and normal or slightly dilated pupils. In severe intoxication, the patient is in deep coma, irregular breathing and dilated pupils. Head injury may be associated due to falling in the semiconscious or unconscious stage.

Management

- Take the patient to the hospital.
- Restrain him/her by chemical or physical method until he/she is conscious. Keep under sedation, if required.

Bites and Stings

Bites and stings should always be taken seriously because their effects can be fatal.

Snake Bite

In most of the cases snakes bite only when provoked. All snakes are not poisonous. Even the bite of a poisonous snake is not always dangerous because when a snake bites in its defense, little or no venom is injected. The snake must be identified because no antivenom is needed if it is nonpoisonous. If it is poisonous, the species of snake must be identified so that specific antivenom shall be given. If the snake cannot be found or identified, general antivenom should be given.

Signs and symptoms:
- The patient shows history of snake bite.
- There are two fang marks at a finger's breadth (½ an inch) apart.
- Intense pain is experienced by the patient at the site of bite of a viper.
- The area is swollen and blackened.
- Bleeding may be seen at the site of bite and in different parts of the body.
- Patient vomits, collapses and coma follows.

Stimulant

- From 15 minutes to two hours after the bite of a **cobra** or similar snakes, neurotoxic effects like giddiness, lethargy, muscular weakness and spreading paralysis are seen.
- Breathing becomes slow and labored.
- After two hours, if treatment is not given, respiration ceases with or without convulsions and heart stops functioning.
- A bite by a **sea snake** is felt as a sharp initial prick, which gradually becomes painless. After one to two hours, generalized muscular pain and stiffness develop starting in the neck, shoulders and lips. Urine turns brown in color. Respiratory failure may occur.

Management and first aid (Fig. 24):

- Make the patient lie down and let him/her rest. Reassure the patient as he/she will be frightened even though his/her life is not in danger. Explain the treatment being given.
- **If the bite is on a limb:**
  - Apply a constrictive bandage at a site between the site of bite and the heart, to diminish the circulation of venom.
  - If the bite is on the lower limb, apply the bandage around the thigh.
  - If the bite is on the upper limb, apply the bandage around the arm.
  - Immobilize the injured part to minimize the circulation.
  - Send for medical aid or take the patient to the hospital.
  - Wash the area with cold water and soap. Cold pack or ice pack over the area will help to reduce the flow of blood to and from the part.
- **If the site of bite is in a place where constriction bandage cannot be applied**:
  - Wash the bitten area with cold water and soap and make a 3 mm deep cuts through each fang mark with sterile razor blade to cause bleeding and drainage of the venom.
  - Apply suction to the wound with a pump.
  - Keep the patient at rest to reduce circulation and spread of venom.
  - Shift the patient to the hospital as soon as possible.
  - Cauterization or application of potassium permanganate crystals locally are controversial because it will inhibit bleeding and drainage of poison.
  - Observe for any signs of respiratory distress or cardiac failure. The first aider must be ready to commence artificial respiration and cardiac massage.
  - If possible, kill the snake and take it with the patient to the hospital for identification. This step will help in the administration of specific antivenom.

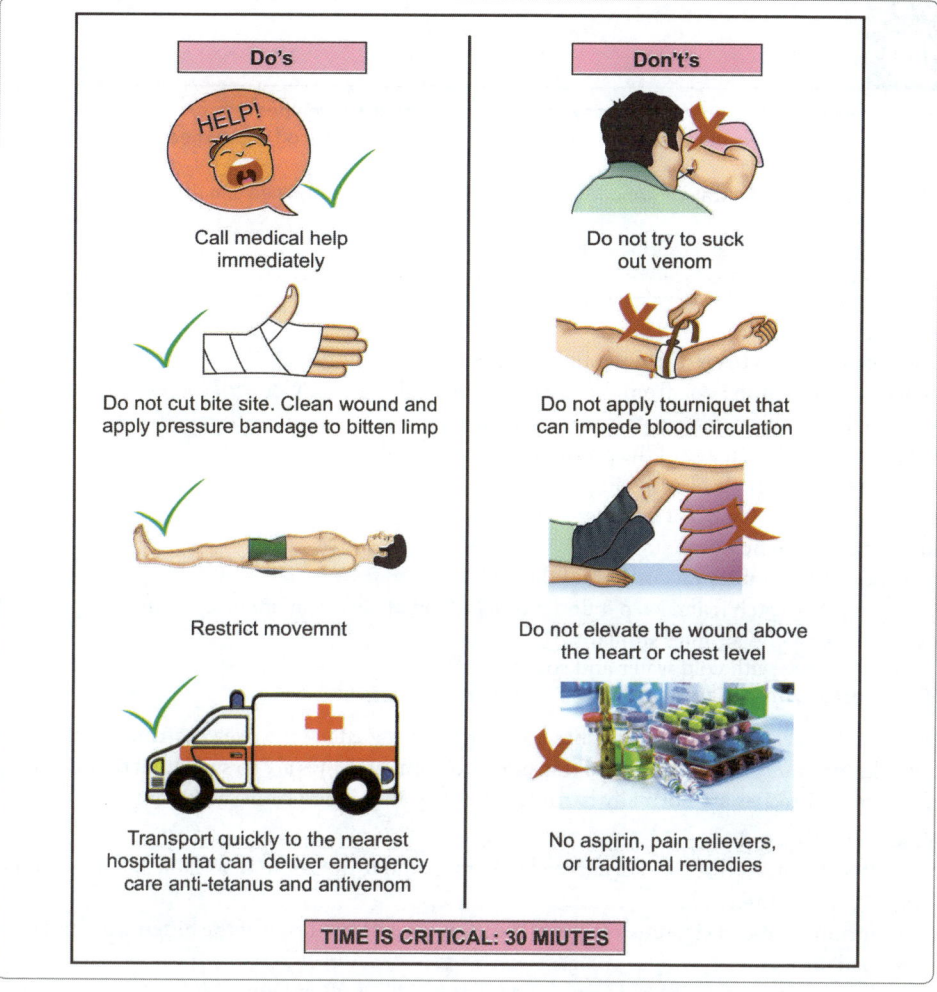

Figure 24: Do's and don'ts in first aid for snake bite

Dog Bite

Dog bite is sometimes very serious as it may cause infection. If the dog is suffering from rabies, it will be transmitted to victims. This condition is known as hydrophobia (fear of water). The dog should not be killed but it should be chained and kept under observation for ten days. If the dog is healthy after this period, there is no danger of rabies.

Aim of first aid in dog bite:
- To prevent rabies or other infections
- To get medical aid

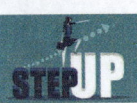

- The limbs of the dog become paralyzed and the dog crawls, refusal of food and a special shape in the nose are early features.
- Dog becomes restless and wanders about anxiously, the eyebrows are wrinkled and there is a hunted look on the face.
- Hind limbs get paralyzed early causing staggering gait.
- The tone of the dog's bark gets altered due to the spasm of the muscles of the throat.

Management:
- All dog bites must be treated as potentially as bite by a rabid dog.
- Remove the saliva of the dog from the site of bite by washing with plenty of soap and running water.
- Do not apply carbolic acid or potassium permanganate on the wound within half an hour of the bite and allow bleeding and drainage of the poison from the wound.
- Dry the site and apply sterile dressing.
- If bleeding is severe, control it by other measures.
- Take the patient to the hospital.
- Check the status of rabies vaccination of the dog.
- If it is a stray dog, catch it and keep it under observation of development of signs and symptoms of rabies.
- Treat the bites of wild animals similarly.

Insect Bite and Stings—Stings of Mites, Ticks and Leeches

Mites, ticks and leeches are found in marshes and jungles. They attach themselves firmly to the skin of man. Mites and ticks may carry typhus fever and transmit it to humans. Mites are so small that they cannot be easily seen and removed. Leeches are normally harmless, but they suck blood from the victim.

Management and first aid:
- Do not try to remove the insects manually as their mouth parts may remain in the skin and cause inflammation and infection.
- Put the burning end of a cigarette or a small burning stick to the body of the bitten ticks and leeches and they will fall off.
- Application of salt or juice of betel leaves and tobacco will result in falling off leeches from the skin.
- Clean the area with methylated spirit after removing the insect.
- Apply weak ammonia or soda bicarbonate or antihistamine content or pressed garlics, which relieve irritation.

Scorpion Sting

The toxicity of the venom of a scorpion is worse than that of snakes but the luck is that only a small quantity of venom is injected in one bite. There is severe local irritation and burning pain radiating from the site. There may be headache, giddiness, nausea, profuse perspiration and muscular cramps. In some severe bites, unconsciousness may develop. Children may die due to lung edema.

Management and first aid:
- Tie a tourniquet or rubber tube above the site of the sting, if it is on the leg or forearm.
- Incise the site if necessary to drain of the venom through bleeding.

- Wash the site with plain water, dilute solution of potassium permanganate, ammonia or borax.
- Apply ice pack locally to diminish the absorption of the venom.
- Arrange for immediate medical aid.

Bee Sting

Usually, the bees attack a person in groups and not by a single one. While biting, the bee leaves the sting with poison sac at the site of sting. Locally, there is intense pain. The area becomes swollen, red and tender.

Management and first aid:
- The sting should be removed with a mosquito forceps or with the tip of a needle or pin sterilized by flaming or boiling.
- Do not attempt to remove the sting with fingers as it causes the risk of injection of more venom into the tissues.
- Wash the site with soap and water.
- Apply tincture iodine, washing soda, ammonia or pressed garlic locally.

A bee or wasp sting on the tongue is dangerous because the tongue may swell up and block the throat, interfering with respiration.

Management and first aid when sting is on tongue:
- Give ice to the patient to suck
- If the tongue swells up and obstruct respiration, hold it with a handkerchief and pull it well forward until the doctor comes.
- If the patient becomes unconscious, put him in recovery position, maintain the airway patent and give the care as mentioned under the care of unconscious patient.

Burns and Scalds

- Burns are injuries caused by heat, like fire, contact with hot metals, radiation, electricity or chemicals.
- Scalds are caused by moist heat due to boiling water, steam or hot oil and hot tar.

Classification of Burns

- **Superficial burns:**
  First degree   -   Reddening of skin
  Second degree   -   Blistering of the skin
- **Third degree:**
  Deep burns   -   Subcutaneous tissue and muscle destruction.

The two important factors, which determine the condition of the patient, are the size of the burnt area and his/her age. A small third degree burn is less serious than a large second degree. All patients who have suffered burns are in shocked stage, especially children and elderly patients. Therefore, a more accurate assessment of the condition of the patient is made on admission by applying the 'Wallace's Rule of Nine' and Lund and Browder chart (Fig. 25).

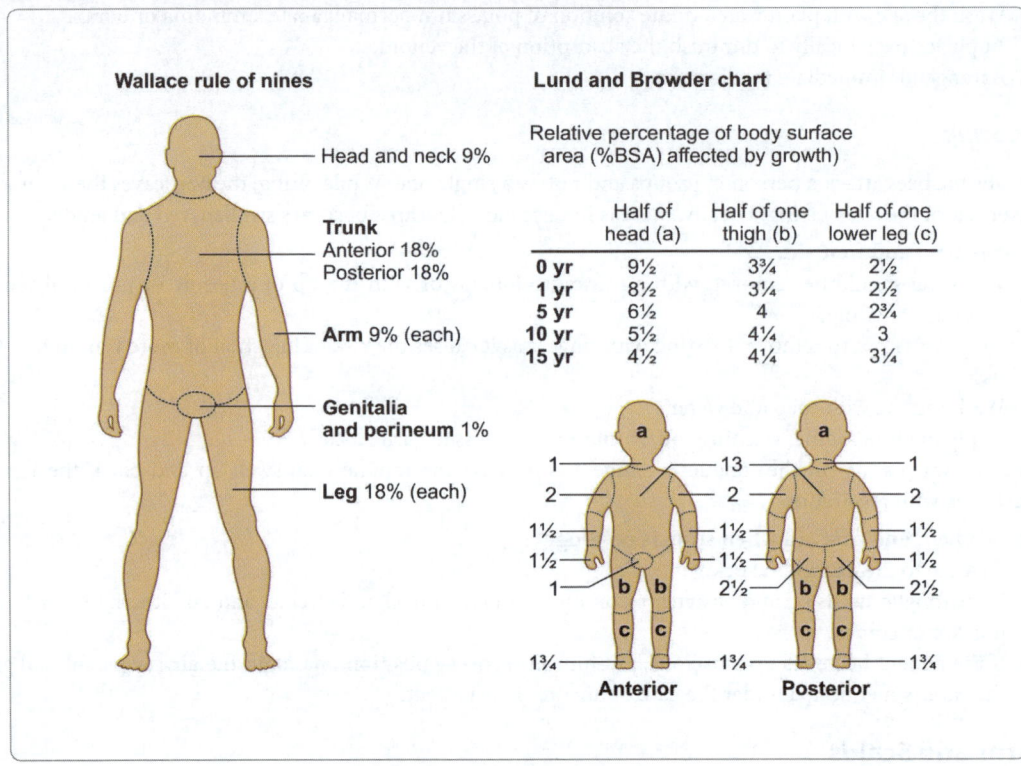

Figure 25: Wallace's rule of nines

Management and treatment of burns:

- If the clothing of the patient catches fire, extinguish the flame quickly by wrapping a blanket or other similar material around him/her to smother the flames.
- Send for medical aid.
- Ask the patient to lie down soon instead of running with flames. Rolling in the ground will help to extinguish the flames.
- Cover the patient with a clean sheet. It is important to separate the adjacent surfaces like groin, axilla and in between fingers, when covering the burnt area.
- Bandage loosely to keep the dressing in position.
- As all burn-patients are liable to develop shock, cover the patient with a blanket. However, the blanket should not come in direct contact with the burnt area as it may cause infection as well as stick on to the raw surface.
- Reinforce the dressings and check the bandage, if necessary.
- Particular care must be taken when dealing with burns to treat shock and to prevent infection. The following rules must be observed:
  - Do not break blisters.
  - Do not apply creams, lotions or oils on blisters.
  - Do not cover burns directly with fluffy materials, cotton wool or blankets.
  - Do not remove burnt clothing adherent to the skin.
  - Encourage the patient to take rest as increased movement will cause more pain, therefore will increase shock. Sometimes, sedatives may be ordered by the doctor.

Complications:
1. **Early complications:** Shock and infection.
2. **Late complications:** Scarring and contractures leading to loss or limitation of movements.

Treatment of superficial burns to small areas:
- Immerse the part in cold water.
- Cover the area with clean non-fluffy material.
- Keep the patient warm and reassure him.
- Take the patient to a doctor or to the casualty department of a hospital.

Chemical Burns

A chemical burn occurs when skin or eyes or any part of body comes in contact with an irritant, like an acid or a base. Chemical burns are also called caustic burns. They may cause a reaction on skin or within body. These burns can affect internal organs, if swallowed.

Types of chemicals:
1. **Acids,** e.g., sulfuric acid, carbolic acid, etc.
2. **Alkalis,** e.g., caustic soda
3. **Disinfectants,** e.g., Lysol, mercury compounds, etc.

Chemical Burns to Eyes

A chemical burn may occur when a chemical comes in contact with the eyes. Alkalis are particularly dangerous to the eyes.

Management:
- Wash the eyes thoroughly with water. To wash the eye, hold open the eyelids gently and allow a stream of cold water over the eye. As a quickest method, hold the head of the patient under a tap with the affected eye turned to the flow.
- After washing thoroughly, take the patient to an ophthalmologist for consultation.

First aid for burns has been depicted through the following Figure 26.

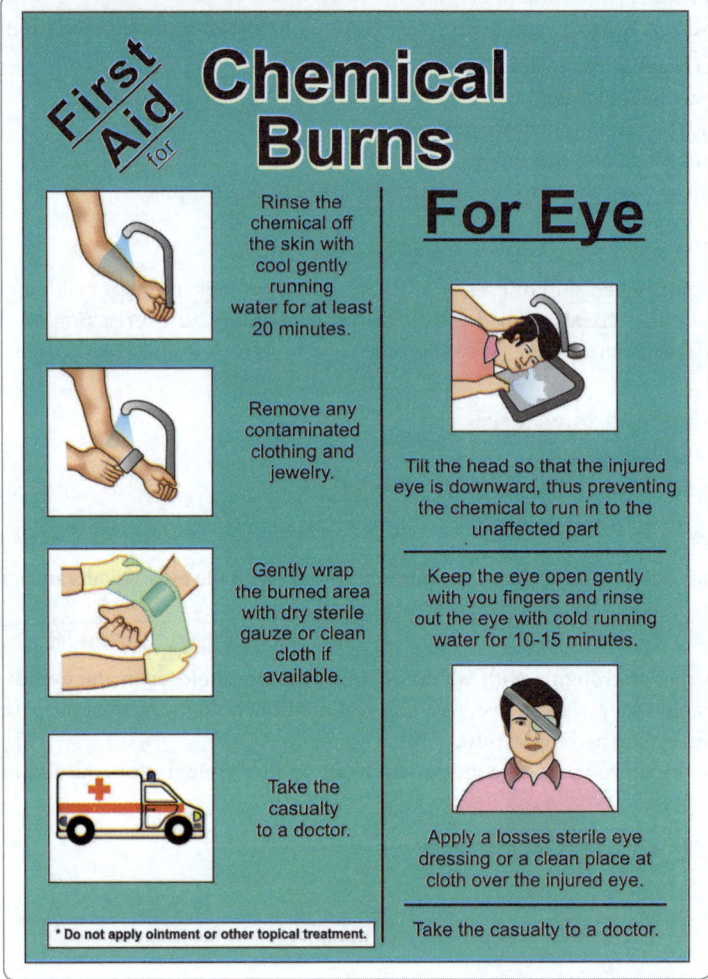

Figure 26: First aid for chemical burns

Lime Burns to the Eye

Lime or quicklime is a chemical irritant. It may adhere to the conjunctiva, and result in opacification of the cornea with marked reduction of vision. It may cause in loss of the eyeball.

Management:

- To prevent further complications, remove all particles of lime before the eye is irrigated.
- Evert the eyelids and remove the lime particles using a clean handkerchief or tissue paper.
- Wash the eye with cold water.
- Take the patient to an ophthalmologist or casualty of the hospital for consultation.
- Patients who had burns of the eye will be more comfortable if the affected eye is covered with a pad of soft material, and kept in position by a tape.

Foreign Bodies

- **Foreign bodies in the eye:** Many foreign objects enter the conjunctiva of the eye as a result of mishaps that occur during everyday activities. Dirt and sand fragments typically enter the eyes because of debris that may come with blowing wind. Sharp materials like metal or glass can get into the eye as a result of explosions or accidents with tools such as hammers, drills, or lawnmowers. The most common types of foreign objects that may enter in the eyes are:
  - Eyelashes' hair
  - Dried mucus
  - Sawdust
  - Dirt
  - Sand
  - Cosmetics
  - Contact lenses
  - Metal particles
  - Glass shards

  Management and first aid:
  - Don't rub eyes.
  - Lift the upper eyelid up and out over the lower lid, and then roll your eyes around.
  - Flush eyes generously with water, and keep eyes open during flushing.
  - Repeat the previous steps until the object is eliminated.
  - If there is an object embedded in the eye, do not remove it, as this may cause further damage. Instead, cover the eye with an eye shield or gauze and seek prompt medical attention.

- **Foreign bodies in the ear, nose and throat:** Foreign bodies in the ear, nose, and breathing tract (airway) sometimes occur in children.

- **Foreign bodies in the ear:** Foreign bodies can either be in the ear lobe or in the ear canal. Some of the items that are commonly found in the ear canal include the following:
  - Food
  - Insects
  - Toys
  - Buttons
  - Pieces of crayon
  - Small batteries

  Management and first aid:
  - Don't try to remove the object yourself. Seek the help of a healthcare professional as soon as possible.
  - Reassure the victim and try to keep them calm.
  - Remove the object if possible. If the object is clearly visible, pliable and can be grasped easily with tweezers, then gently remove it.
  - Don't probe the ear with a tool such as a cotton swab or matchstick.
  - Try using gravity. Tilt the head to the affected side to dislodge the object.
  - Try using oil for an insect. If the foreign object is an insect, tilt the person's head so that the ear with the insect is upward. Try to float the insect out by pouring mineral oil, olive oil or baby oil into the ear. The oil should be warm, but not hot. Don't use oil to remove an object other than an insect. If an insect has found its way into the ear, in case of a child, support baby's head with the affected ear facing up. Gently flood the ear with slightly warm water; the insect should float out. If this doesn't work, take the baby to a healthcare professional.

Unit III ❖ **First Aid in Emergencies**

- Try washing the object out. Use a rubber-bulb ear syringe and warm water to irrigate the object out of the canal, (again provided no ear tubes are in place and you don't suspect the eardrum is perforated).
- **Foreign bodies in the nose:** Objects that are put into the nose are usually soft things. These will include, but are not limited to, tissue, clay, and pieces of toys, or erasers.

  Management and first aid:
  - Don't probe at the object with a cotton swab or other tool.
  - Don't try to inhale the object by forcefully breathing in. Instead, breathe through mouth until the object is removed.
  - Blow your nose gently to try to free the object, but don't blow hard or repeatedly. If only one nostril is affected, close the opposite nostril by applying gentle pressure and then blow out gently through the affected nostril.
  - If the object is visible and it can be easily grasped, then gently remove it with tweezers. Don't try to remove an object that isn't visible or easily grasped.
  - Seek emergency medical assistance.
- **Foreign bodies in the throat:** A foreign body in the throat can cause choking and it will be a medical emergency that needs immediate attention. The foreign body can get stuck in many different places within the airway. The child may then inhale deeply and the object may become lodged in the 'airway' tube (trachea) instead of the 'eating' tube (esophagus).

  Management:
  - Management is similar to management of choking.

Injuries to the Bones, Joints and Muscles

Causes of Injuries to Bones and Joints

- Falling, tripping
- Motor vehicle accidents
- Running, walking, exercise
- Sports, physical activity
- Sudden impact

Types of injuries to bones and joints:
- **Fractures:** A fracture is a break or crack in the bone and needs to be treated by a doctor.
- **Dislocation:** A dislocation is the movement of a bone at a joint from its normal position. When the bone is moved out of place, the joint no longer functions.
- **Sprain:** A sprain is tearing of the ligaments of a joint. Sprains mostly occur at the ankle, knee, wrist and fingers.
- **Strain:** A strain is the stretching and tearing of a muscle. They usually occur in the neck, back, thigh, or the back of the lower leg.

Management and first aid:
- Protect the fractured area with a sling made of a triangular piece of cloth.
- Use padded boards, pillows, or newspapers to splint the fracture.
- Protect the neck from any turning or bending. Do not move until a neck brace or spine board has been applied.
- Use **RICE** method when dealing with a sprain or strain.

The RICE method is a simple self-care technique that helps reduce swelling, ease pain, and speed up healing (Fig. 27).

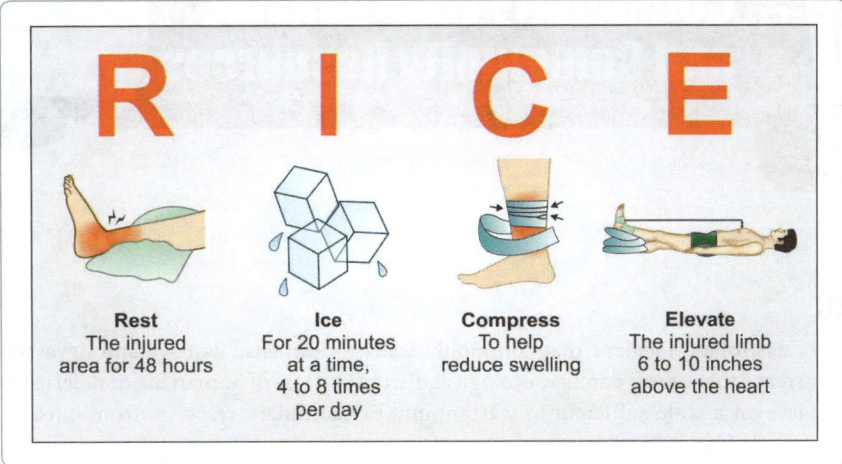

Figure 27: Self-care in sprain and strain

- **Rest:** Do not move or straighten the injury.
- **Immobilize:** Try to stabilize the person in the position he/she was found. Splint or sling the injured part only and use caution if moving the person.
- **Cold:** Indirectly cool the part using ice for up to 20 minutes.
- **Elevate:** Only elevate the part if it does not cause more pain.
  ■ Seek medical assistance.

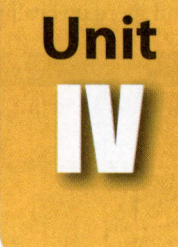

Unit IV

Community Emergencies and Community Resources

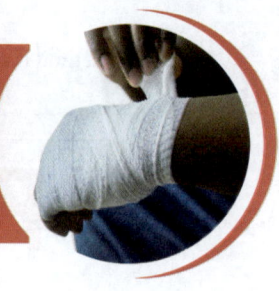

DISASTER

A disaster is a catastrophic incident that commonly leads to immense damage and devastation. Disaster means any occurrence that causes damage, ecological disruption, loss of human life or deterioration of health and health services on a scale sufficient to warrant and extraordinary response from outside the affected community or area (WHO, 1995).

Types

Following two types of disasters can be seen:
1. Natural disasters
2. Man-made disasters

Various types of disasters are enumerated as table here:

Major natural disasters	Minor natural disasters
• Food • Cyclone • Drought • Earthquake	• Cold wave • Thunderstorms • Heat waves • Mud slides • Storm
Major man-made disasters	**Minor man-made disasters**
• Setting of fires • Epidemic • Deforestation • Pollution due to prawn cultivation • Chemical pollution • Wars	• Road/train accidents, riots • Food/poisoning • Industrial disaster/crisis • Environmental pollution

1. **Natural disasters:** These include droughts, earthquakes, tsunamis, forest fires, landslides and mudslides, blizzards, hurricanes, tornadoes, floods and volcanic disruptions.
2. **Man-made disasters:** These include hazardous substance accidents (e.g., chemicals, toxic gases), radiologic accidents, dam failures, resource shortage (e.g., food, electricity and water), structural fire and explosions and domestic disturbances (e.g., terrorism, bombing and riots), bioterrorism, explosions, fires, toxic materials, pollution, civil unrest (e.g., riots, demonstrations), terrorist attacks, etc.

Differences between man-made and natural disaster are explained here:

Natural disasters	Man-made disasters
When disasters occur due to natural forces they are called natural disasters	Man-made disasters are influenced by humans and they are often a result of negligence and human error among other factors
Natural disasters include things such as floods, volcanic eruptions, earthquakes, floods, tornadoes, landslides and hurricanes.	Human-made disaster involves an element of human intent, negligence, or error or involving a failure of a man-made system
Natural disaster occurs due to forces of nature	Human-made disasters occur as a result of human action
Natural disasters are disasters that take place regardless of human action	Human action can increase the likelihood and impact of natural disasters

Phases of a Disaster

Figure 1 shows different phases of disasters:

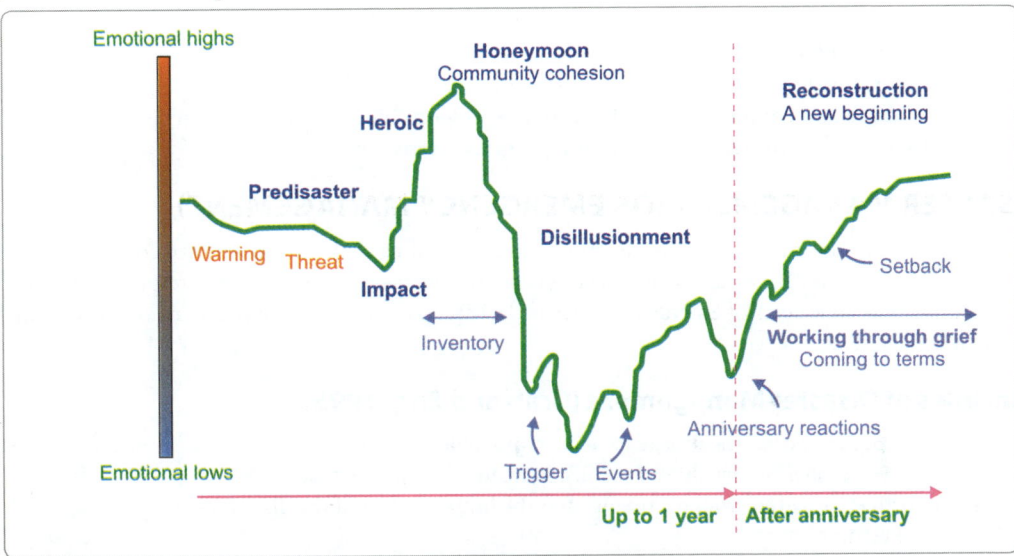

Figure 1: Phases of disaster

The following are three phases of disaster:

1. **Preimpact phase:**
   - It is the initial phase of the disaster.
   - Warning is given prior to the actual occurrence.
   - Emergency centers are opened.
   - Communication through radio, television and community must be given.

2. **Impact phase:**
   - This occurs at the time of disaster.
   - The impact phase continues until the threat of further destructions has passed and the emergency plan is in effect.
   - Emergency operation center (EOC) are established.
   - Physical and psychological support to the victims is provided in this phase.

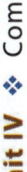

Unit IV ❖ Community Emergencies and Community Resources

3. **Postimpact phase:** Recovery begins during the emergency phase and ends with the return of normal community order and functioning. This phase may last for a lifetime for persons in the impact area (e.g., victims of the atomic bombing of Hiroshima).

This phase can be divided into:

Heroic phase:
- It is characterized by a high level of activity with a low level of productivity.
- There is a sense of altruism, and many community members exhibit adrenaline-induced rescue behavior. Risk assessment may be impaired.

Honeymoon phase:
- It is characterized by a dramatic shift in emotions.
- Disaster assistance is readily available. Community bonding occurs. Optimism exists that everything will return to normal quickly.

Disillusionment phase:
- It is in contrast to the honeymoon phase.
- Communities and individuals realize the limits of disaster assistance.

Reconstruction phase:
- It is characterized by an overall feeling of recovery.
- Individuals and communities begin to assume responsibility for rebuilding their lives, and people adjust to a new 'normal' while continuing to grieve losses.

DISASTER MANAGEMENT (OR EMERGENCY MANAGEMENT)

It is the creation of plans through which communities reduce vulnerability to hazards and cope with disasters. Disaster management is defined as the organization and management of resources and responsibilities to deal with all humanitarian aspects of emergencies, particularly preparedness, response and recovery to minimize the impact of disasters.

Principles of Disaster Management (Grab and Eng, 1995)

- Prevent the occurrence of the disaster whenever possible.
- Minimize the number of casualties if the disaster cannot be prevented.
- Prevent further casualties from occurring after the initial impact of the disaster.
- Rescue the victims.
- Provide first aid to the injured.
- Evacuate the injured to medical facilities.
- Provide definitive medical care.
- Promote reconstruction of lives.

Phases of Disaster Management

The phases of disaster management are (Fig. 2):
- Response
- Recovery
- Mitigation
- Preparedness

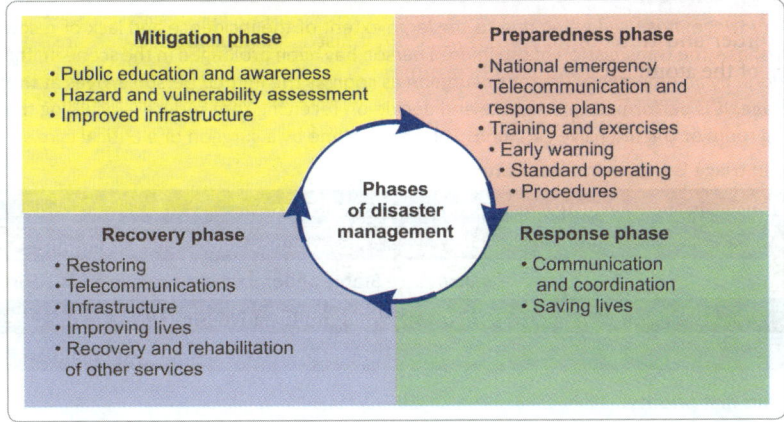

Figure 2: Phases of disaster management

Role of Nurse in Disaster

Figure 3 shows the roles of a nurse in a disaster.

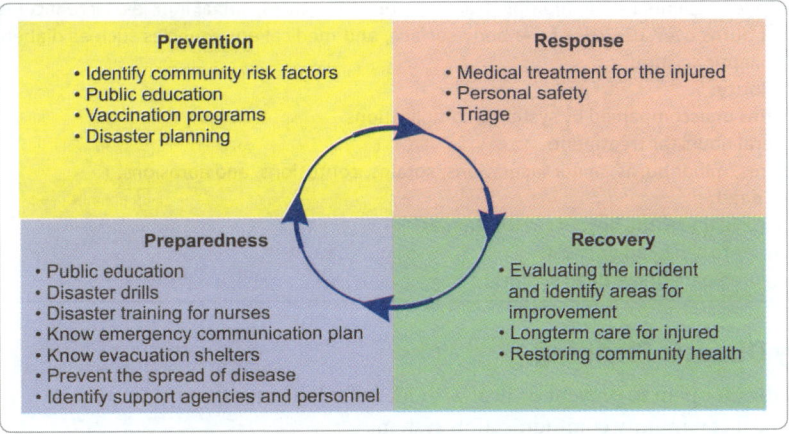

Figure 3: Role of a nurse in disaster

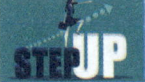

Triage
- **Triage (categorizing):** One of the most important roles of the nurse is assessing the clients and categorizing them. This process is called Triage.
- **Meaning:** Triage is derived from the French word 'trier', which means separating, categorizing or classifying, and refers to the categorization, classification, and prioritization of patients and injured people, based on their urgent need for treatment.
- **Stages of triaging:** Triage is usually performed at three stages:
  (i) **Primary triage:** It is carried out at the scene of the incident by an emergency technician aims at the prompt assessment of the injured person and rapid transfer to the treatment center.

Contd...

(ii) **Secondary triage:** It is used when due to the large extent of the incidence and lack of resources in the pre-hospital phase, the transmission of the injured person has been prolonged in the scene. In these cases, triage will be done by an emergency doctor or surgeon as soon as the injured person arrives at the hospital.

(iii) **Third triage:** It is performed to prioritize and decide on receiving care services, including transferring to the operating room or the intensive care unit. This step is done by a surgeon or a critical care specialist.

Color coding in triage is shown in table here:

Triage category	Priority	Color	Conditions
Immediate	1	Red	Chest wounds, shock, open fractures, 2–3 burns
Delayed	2	Yellow	Stable abdominal wound, eye and CNS injuries
Minimal	3	Green	Minor burns, minor fractures, minor bleeding
Expectant	4	Black	Unresponsive, high spinal cord injury

Red—most urgent, first priority:
- Life-threatening injuries, shock, chest wounds, internal hemorrhage, head injuries producing increased loss of consciousness, partial -or full-thickness burns over 20–60% of the body surface, chest pain.
- Poor chance of survival.

Yellow—urgent, second priority:
- Injuries with systemic effects and complications but yet not in shock, withstand 30–60 minutes.
- Category includes patients having multiple fractures, open fractures, spinal injuries, large lacerations; partial-or full- thickness burns over 10–20% of the body surface, and medical emergencies such as diabetic coma, insulin shock; and epileptic seizure.

Green—third priority:
- Minimal injuries unaccompanied by systemic complications.
- Can wait several hours for treatment.
- Closed fractures, minor burns, minor lacerations, sprains, contusions, and abrasions.

Black—dying or dead:
- Would not survive under the best of circumstances.
- Crushing injuries to the head or chest.
- Hopelessly injured patients or dead victims.

Community Disaster Planning

- Develop a disaster plan to prevent or deal with identified disaster threats.
- Identify a local community communication system.
- Identify disaster personnel, including private and professional volunteers, local emergency personnel, agencies, and resources.
- Identify regional backup agencies or personnel.
- Identify specific responsibilities for various personnel involved in disaster coping and establish a disaster chain of command.

Role of Police Force in Disaster Management

Police organization has to see itself as a major player in disaster management. It will continue to have the first responder role, given its proximity to the incidence site and relationship with the people. The police is among the first responders in any crisis because:
- Local police arrive first.
- Possess well developed communication system
- Familiar with local terrain

- Wider reach, every village covered
- Better knowledge of local people feelings and mindset
- People recognize police as first responder uniformed and disciplined

Role of Police before Disaster—Prevention and Preparedness Phase

- Emergency traffic plan
- Detail communication plan
- Identification of building
- Security plan
- Resource mapping
- Training

Role of Police during Disaster—Emergency Response Phase

- Search and rescue (SAR).
- **Deployment of resources**—Restoration of communication system/liaisoning with rescue team
- Prevention of commission of cognizable offences including all offences against property, human body and public tranquility
- Security during relief distributions/relief management
- Isolate disaster sites and control site access for safety of victims, general public and efficiency of incident operation
- Camp management
- Emergency transportation and traffic regulation
- Coordination with various agencies
- Casualty information/disposal of dead
- Family liaison officers
- Media management
- VIP security
- Crowd management

Role of Emergency Medical Services

Ambulance services provide a critical link between health care and disaster management systems.
- They provide prehospital care for patients experiencing medical emergencies in disasters; and medical transport to tertiary health care facilities by road, air and water.
- They may also be involved in ensuring that people at risk are moved out of problematic situation particularly those with health concerns.

Role of Voluntary Agencies

Nongovernmental Organizations (NGOs) are playing very important role in different stages of disaster reduction.
- The NGOs have some important skills for rescue, coordination and for relief activities.
- They have the flexibility to respond quickly and efficiently at the local level and are often the first organizer's groups to reach the disaster site.
- The role of NGOs in the predisaster phase should include awareness generation, education, training, and formation of village level task force, disaster management committees and teams, development of disaster management plans, conduct of mock drills, vulnerability assessment and coordination with government and non-government agencies.

Unit IV ❖ Community Emergencies and Community Resources

- In the immediate phase, the NGO response is focused on emergency food relief, temporary shelter, emergency medical aid, debris removal and habitat restoration, trauma counseling, and raising families.
- Some NGOs also distribute temporary shelter materials among disaster-affected people soon after the disaster.
- Rejuvenating people's spirits and raising awareness about reconstruction challenges is also an important part of NGOs intervention.
- The NGOs can play a key role in the immediate aftermath of disasters by extending assistance in rescue and first aid, sanitation and hygiene, damage assessment and assistance to external agencies bringing relief materials.
- During the postdisaster phase, the NGOs can take a lead by providing technical and material support for safe construction, revival of educational institutions and restoration of means of livelihood. They assist the government in monitoring the pace of implementation for various reconstruction and recovery programs.

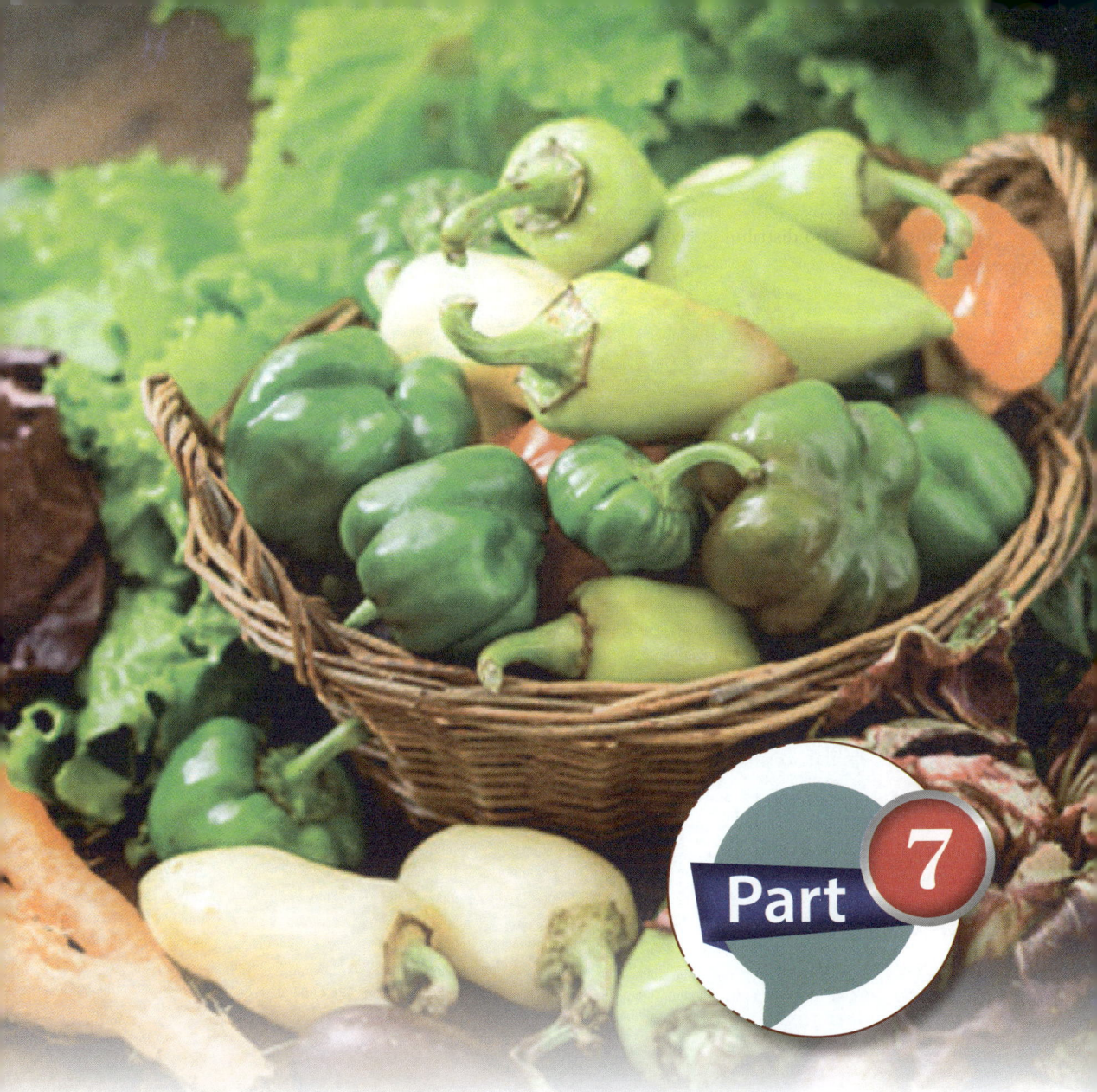

Nutrition

Unit 1

Introduction

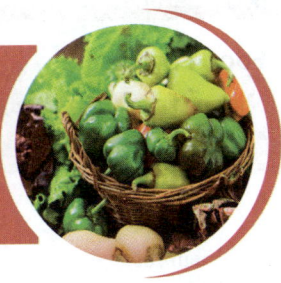

DEFINITIONS

- **Nutrition:** Nutrition is a science that deals with the food consumed by human beings or simply the study of daily diet. Nutrition consists of all the processes or activities by which the human body receives the food and further uses it for growth, development, regulation of body functions and repairs.
- **Dietetics:** It is the science dealing with the planning of nutrition and preparation of food.
- **Food:** It is any substance, which can be used by the body for its growth, development, regulation of body functions and repairs.

NUTRIENTS OR NUTRIMENTS (FOOD)

These are food substances that nourish, promote and strengthen the body with proteins, carbohydrates, fats, minerals, vitamins and water.

Food is one of the basic factors of the health. Man takes food to satisfy hunger. Hunger is one of the natural experiences and basic needs of man. Everyone fetches food and take it daily. Animals find their own food without being taught by anyone and they eat it according to their need and keep themselves healthy. Human beings study about the required food factors and try to take the most suitable food for the health.

Nurses are concerned about nutrition more than just keeping themselves alive. They want to be healthy and need to have energy to do the strenuous work and they have to be living examples for their patients. In order to fulfil this need, they have to learn themselves and teach others what to eat so that the body may be properly built up and supplied with energy and remain protected. This knowledge about food is necessary to prevent and overcome diseases. Therefore it is mandatory and important that every nurse should study and understand the principles of nutrition.

Nutrition deals with the way in which the human body receives and uses food materials necessary for its growth and development and keeping it in good condition. This starts with eating food. The food is swallowed, and digested as it passes through stomach and small intestine. During digestion, food is broken into simple substances. These substances are absorbed in liquid form in the blood stream and carried to the liver where they are either stored or changed further, or sent out to the other parts of the body for use, as required. Some of the absorbed substances are used to supply heat and energy to the body, some are used to build and repair the tissues, some of these absorbed substances are utilized to control the chemical changes taking place in the body or to protect the body from disease. Finally, the waste products which are not useful to the body are excreted as feces.

Therefore, the food we take should contain all the required food factors needed to perform all the above mentioned functions in the body. When the food satisfies all the required food factors, it is a proper diet or nutrition.

Food Factors

The important food factors are:

- Carbohydrates
- Proteins
- Fats
- Minerals
- Vitamins
- Water

The food we take contains almost all of these food factors to a certain extent. The main food factors, namely protein, fat and carbohydrate along with water, satisfy the immediate need of body when we eat food.

 Stimulant

Composition of human body
Human body is composed of components of food factors. An average composition of body is given as follows:

Water	63%
Proteins	17%
Fats	12%
Minerals	7%
Carbohydrates	1%

Types of Food

- **Food factors are grouped on the basis of their functions.**
- **Energy-yielding foods,** which are rich in carbohydrate and fat, e.g., cereals, sugar, roots and tubers.
- **Body-building foods,** which are rich in proteins, e.g. meat, fish, milk and pulses.
- **Protective foods,** which are rich in proteins; vitamins and minerals, e.g., milk, eggs, green leafy vegetables and fruits.

Functions of Food

Main functions of the food are:

- **Supply of heat and energy for work and play:** As a source of energy, food for the human body may be compared to petrol or gas for a car and steam or current for an engine. Without petrol or gas the car will not run; without steam or current the engine will not move. When a man starves for one or two days, he feels weak, lacks energy and is unable to work. Energy needed for work and play is supplied mainly by carbohydrate and fat although protein may also be used.
- **Body building and repair:** To build a new car, entirely new parts should be put together. If one part wears out, it must be replaced by a new part. In the human body, the food elements are essential for the building of new parts for the growth and repair or renewal of tissues, which are worn out. Proteins and mineral elements are the main essential food constituents for growth, repair and maintenance of the body.
- **Maintenance and regulation of tissue functions**: All machinery needs lubrication in order to run smoothly and to prevent friction. The basic food constituents adequate for growth, repair and energy are not sufficient for the body. It still needs other nutrients to regulate the various body processes; some are required for growth, others for producing energy and still others for preventing the body from diseases. Protein and mineral salts along with vitamins help for the third function of food.

Unit I ❖ Introduction

- **Control of body processes and protection of the body** are similarly carried out by proteins, minerals, vitamins.

INTERRELATION OF NUTRIENTS

When considering and comparing with a machine, it seems obvious that human body is a wonderful machine.

The various functions of nutrients are related to each other which are as follows:

- Food for heat and energy—carbohydrates, fats and proteins
- Food for growth and repair—proteins and mineral elements
- Food for regulation and protection—proteins, mineral elements and vitamins.

There are very few foods which contain only one nutrient. Most foods contain several nutrients, but there is no single food found in nature, which contains all the nutrients essential for body. Each nutrient has separate function (as well as it is related to all other nutrients, especially to the three main functions of the body). In many cases deficiency or excess of one nutrient influences the requirement for others. Also excessive intakes of one nutrient may interfere with the metabolism of another.

The interrelationship of nutrients is clear from the Figure 1 given here.

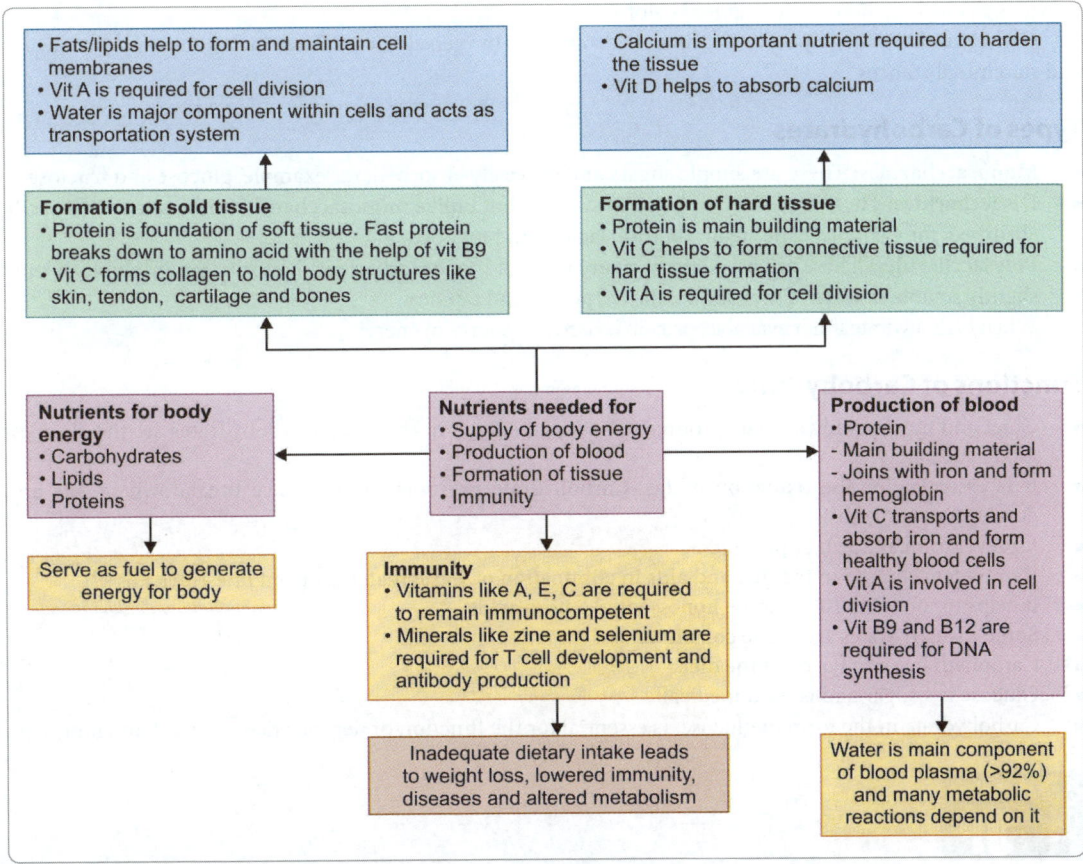

Figure 1: Interrelationship of nutrients

Unit I ❖ Introduction

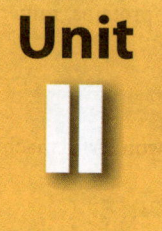

Unit II

Food Factors—Functions and Sources

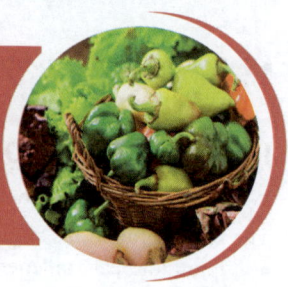

CARBOHYDRATES

Carbohydrate is a simple sugar or a compound formed by the combination of two or more simple sugars. Carbohydrates are the chief and main source of energy and warmth and form the bulk in the diet, and are stored in the form of glycogen in the liver and muscles. Indian food is composed of more carbohydrates and provides as much as 90% of the required calories.

Carbohydrates are composed of carbon, hydrogen and oxygen elements. They include a number of sugary and starchy substances.

Types of Carbohydrates

- **Monosaccharides:** These are simple sugars and get easily absorbed, for example, glucose and fructose.
- **Disaccharides:** These are less complex than starches but unlike monosaccharides they cannot be directly absorbed, for example, cane sugar, sucrose, lactose and maltose.
- **Polysaccharides:** These are made up of many units of monosaccharides. Majority are insoluble or only slightly soluble in water, for example, starch, potato and tapioca.
- When carbohydrate is not available, protein is used as a source of energy.

Functions of Carbohydrate

- Chief and most readily available source of heat and energy in the body. Carbohydrates are the cheapest food available.
- It is essential for the oxidation of fat. Carbohydrate prevents the excessive breakdown of fats and development of ketosis.
- It prevents breakdown of protein.
- It provides cellulose in the diet and aids in elimination of waste materials from intestines.
- It helps in the synthesis of some nonessential amino acids.
- Some carbohydrates are tissue constituents.
- Carbohydrates add flavor to the diet.
- Glucose is a sugar and is used medically.
- Carbohydrate in the form of glucose, is essential for the function of nervous tissues, heart and lungs.

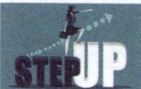

This medicine works by quickly increasing the amount of glucose in blood. Glucose is also used to provide calories (in the form of carbohydrates), to a person who cannot eat because of illness, trauma, or other medical condition.

Sources

- Chief sources of carbohydrate in foods are sugars and starches.
- Cane sugar and jaggery are a good source of disaccharide sugar.
- Fruits are rich source of carbohydrates.
- Starch is present in cereals, dhals, roots and tubers.
- Nuts contain some amount of carbohydrates.
- Cellulose or roughage are complex carbohydrates. They are not digested by intestinal enzymes. They have no nutritive value. These are present in tough fibers of vegetables, cereals, fruits and roots. Roughage helps to prevent constipation and intestinal cancer.

RDA Recommendations

Recommended Dietary Allowance (RDA)/Daily requirement: RDA for carbohydrate is 130 g/day for adults and children. It provides 50–60% of the total caloric requirement of the body.

PROTEIN

Proteins are the main organic constituents of the animal body which form the basis of muscular tissue, the protective structure of body as bones, cartilage, skin, hair, nails and provide a large part of the total solids of the body.

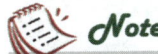

Note

One-fourth of the body solids are proteins.

These are required for the growth and repair of tissues. Although many nutrients are needed for growth and repair, chiefly protein and minerals are required. Protein forms the basic structure of all cells of the body and the minerals are often associated with protein for special function, for example, calcium and phosphorus in bone, iron in hemoglobin of blood.

Amino Acids

The principal constituents of proteins are amino acids. There are 21 significant amino acids in the body. Out of 21 amino acids, **8 are essential amino acids** that are provided in the diet and the remaining **13 are nonessential amino acids,** manufactured in the body. Food items which provide all essential amino acids are **called complete proteins or first class proteins**, for example, animal proteins derived from milk, eggs, liver, meat, etc.

Foods that lack one or more essential amino acids are called *incomplete protein* or second-class protein, for example, vegetable protein from cereals, pulses, etc.

Functions of Proteins

- Protein is necessary for the growth and repair of tissues in the body.
- Protein is a necessary constituent of normal secretions of the body, such as enzymes and hormones and for antibodies and hemoglobin.
- Protein is essential for maintaining the correct osmotic pressure in the body. Hypoproteinemia or deficiency of protein in the blood upsets the osmotic pressure and is one of the causes of edema.

Unit II ❖ Food Factors—Functions and Sources

- Protein has a stimulating effect upon metabolism which is known as the specific dynamic action of protein.
- Protein may be used as a source of energy, but since it has more important functions as given above, the greater part of the daily requirement of calories should come from carbohydrate and fat and not from protein.

RDA Recommendations

RDA/daily requirements of protein: Although the recommendation of protein by ICMR is 1 g/kg or 0.8 grams of protein per kilogram of body weight, the requirement for growing children and pregnancy and lactation is higher.

Sources

Table 1 exhibits different sources of protein.

Table 1: Sources of protein

Complete or first class protein	Incomplete or second class proteins
• Milk (Cow's milk) ⎱ • Curds ⎰ • Mutton ⎱ Animal • Beef ⎰ sources • Liver • Fish • Eggs (Hen's) • Ground nuts • Soybeans ⎱ Plant sources • Green gram ⎰	• Wheat ⎱ • Ragi ⎰ • Rice (Parboiled) ⎱ Plant • Red gram ⎰ sources • Dhal • Bengal gram

Most of the animal proteins are complete proteins.

Effect of Protein Deficiency

During infancy and for children under five years, it results in Kwashiorkor, marasmus, mental retardation, stunted growth and development. In adults, lack of proteins causes anemia, poor development of muscles, underweight, susceptibility to infection, etc. In pregnancy, deficiency of proteins causes premature babies, underweight babies, still births and other abnormalities.

FATS

Fats are composed of carbon, hydrogen and oxygen elements, like carbohydrate and it is an important source of energy, characterized by their insolubility in water and greasy feel. The basic units of lipids/fats are the fatty acids.

Functions of Fat

- One gram of fat provides 9 calories of energy and it is a concentrated form of energy.
- They act as transport media for fat-soluble vitamins, like A, D, E and K.
- They act as cushion to protect organs like liver, spleen, intestines, etc. against friction.
- The subcutaneous fat helps in temperature regulation.

- Dietary fats provide essential fatty acids like linoleic acid, which cannot be synthesized by the body. It prevents the skin from drying and scaling.
- Fatty foods give a feeling of fullness, satisfaction and make the food tastier.
- Normal amount of fat deposit in the body maintains a shapely figure.

RDA Recommendations

RDA/daily requirements of fat: Indian food gives 15–20% of energy from dietary fats. Western diet provides about 40% of calories from dietary fats. Minimum adult—20 g/day, pregnancy—30 g/day, lactating mothers—45 g/day. Children—22–25 g/day requirements of fats are unknown. 50% of the fat should be from animal sources.

Sources of Fat

- Vegetable sources of fats are derived from oily seeds, like groundnuts, coconut, mustard, cotton seeds, sunflower seeds and custard seeds.
- Animal sources of fats are derived from animal products, like milk, meat, fish oil, etc.

VITAMINS

Vitamins are organic compounds required in small quantities for the growth and metabolism of the body. These substances are not manufactured in the body. Therefore, these have to be provided in the diet. A well-balanced diet contains vitamin in sufficient amount.

The daily requirement of Vitamins varies considerably and changes during different stages of health and disease.

Factors Affecting the Requirements of Vitamins

- **Age:** Growing children need greater amount than others do, especially vitamin D.
- **Size:** Larger a person, greater the requirement of vitamin
- **Febrile period:** Disease state and antibiotic therapy demands increased amount of vitamins.
- Vitamin demands are more to individuals who perform exercises .
- Increased intake of carbohydrate increases the need of vitamin, especially vitamin B group.
- During pregnancy and lactation larger quantities of vitamin are required, especially vitamin D.

Types of Vitamin

Vitamins are classified into two main groups:
- Fat-soluble vitamins, like A, D, E and K.
- Water-soluble vitamins, like vitamin B complex group and vitamin C (Ascorbic Acid).

Fat-soluble Vitamins

Vitamin A

Vitamin A is fat-soluble. It is available as *retinal* in animal source and has *carotene* in plant sources.

Functions:
- It is required for the formation of retinal pigments of the eyes.
- Vitamin A helps to form and maintain healthy teeth, skeletal and soft tissue, mucus membranes, and skin.
- Vitamin A promotes good eyesight, especially in low light

Sources of vitamin A:

- Animal sources, like ghee, butter, liver, fish.
- Plant sources, like drumstick leaves, yellow fruits like papaya mango, apricots, oranges, etc. carrots and other vegetables.

Deficiency of vitamin A causes:

- Scaliness of the skin and sometimes acne
- Failure of growth
- Diseases of the eyes
- Night blindness due to lack of formation of retinal pigments
- Lowered resistance in children. Vitamin A is also called **'anti-infection' vitamin**.

RDA Recommendations

- **RDA/requirements of vitamin A:** For men and women the requirement is 5000 IU/day

Pregnant woman	6000	IU
Lactating woman	8000	IU
Infants	1000	IU
Toddlers	2000	IU
School children	5500	IU

Vitamin D

Functions:

- Vitamin D improves absorption of calcium and phosphorus and keeps normal blood level of these elements.
- Vitamin D is required for development of bones and teeth and it also prevents rickets. It has anti-rickety properties.

RDA Recommendations

RDA/requirements of vitamin D: Infants, children, women during pregnancy and lactation need 400 IU of vitamin D per day. Adults need no vitamin D in diet as it is prepared by the skin in the presence of sunlight.

Sources:

It is present in less quantity in plant sources. In the body, it is synthesized by the action of ultraviolet rays from the sun. Human milk is very poor in vitamin D and cannot meet the dietary requirements.

Deficiency of vitamin D causes:

- Rickets in children between the age of 6 months and 2 years
- Osteomalacia in adults—softening of the bones

Vitamin E

It is also known as **antisterility vitamin**. Other name is '**tocopherol' or alpha-tocopherol**.

Functions:

- Vitamin E functions mainly as an antioxidant, which means it helps protect cells from damage caused by unstable molecules called free radicals.
- It protects cells from damage and it might aid in lowering the risk of a variety of health problems, from heart disease to cancer and possibly even dementia.
- Vitamin E is required for functioning of the immune system. As a powerful antioxidant, it helps cells fight off infection.
- This vitamin also helps to protect eyesight.
- Vitamin E plays an important role in the production of hormone-like substances called prostaglandins, which are responsible for regulating a variety of body processes, such as blood pressure and muscle contraction.

RDA Recommendations

- **RDA/requirements of vitamin:** The recommended dietary allowance (RDA) for vitamin E is 15 milligrams (or 22.4 IU).
- RDA for lactating women is 19 mg (28.4 IU).

Sources:

- Nuts, such as almonds, peanuts and hazelnuts.
- Rich in vegetable oils such as sunflower, wheat germ, safflower, corn and soybean oils.
- Sunflower seeds and green leafy vegetables such as spinach and broccoli contain vitamin E.

Deficiency causes:

- Sterility in males due to degeneration of testis and habitual abortion in females.
- Degeneration of renal tubules and myocardium has also been reported.

Vitamin K

Functions:

- It is necessary for the production of clotting factors in the liver of adults and newborns.
- Vitamin K is used by body in the treatment of bleeding and also in defects of absorption due to lack of bile salts in the intestines.

Sources:

- **Animal source:** Liver is a rich source of vitamin K.
- **Plant sources:** Cabbage, tomato, soybeans, beans, fruits, etc.

RDA Recommendations

- **RDA/requirements:** Adults get enough of vitamin K from the daily food.
- Newborn infants are usually given 1 mg of Vitamin K intramuscularly on the first day of life to prevent hemorrhagic diseases.

Unit II ❖ Food Factors—Functions and Sources

Water-soluble Vitamins

Vitamin B Complex Group

These are water-soluble vitamins.
- Vitamin B_1 (thiamine)
  - **Functions:**
    - o Essential for metabolism of carbohydrates.
    - o Essential for the nutrition and functions of nervous system.
  - **Sources:**
    - o Yeasts, legumes, liver, cereals, milk, egg yolks.
  - **Deficiency causes:**
    - o Beriberi
    - o Wernicke's encephalopathy.

RDA Recommendations

- **RDA/dietary requirements of vitamin B_1:** 0.4–0.7 mg/day. The RDA for adults is 1.2 mg/day for men and 1.1 mg/day for women. During pregnancy and lactation, a woman needs 1.5 mg/day.

- Vitamin B_2 (riboflavin)
  - **Functions:**
    - o Required for carbohydrate metabolism.
    - o Necessary for healthy skin and eyes.
  - **Sources:**
    - o Egg yolk, wheat germ, meat, cereals except rice, liver, soybeans, pulses and milk.
  - **Deficiency causes:**
    - o Beriberi
    - o Pellagra
    - o Kwashiorkor
    - o Many diseases of the mouth, eyes, nose, ears and dermatitis.

RDA Recommendations

- **RDA/daily requirements of Vitamin B_2:** The normal recommended daily allowance (RDA) of riboflavin is dependent on age, gender and reproductive status. RDA of vitamin B_2 is 1.3 milligrams daily for men and 1.1 mg for women. A higher dose of 3 mg/day can help to prevent cataracts.

- Vitamin B_3 (nicotinic acid or niacin)
  - **Functions:**
    - o Required for carbohydrate metabolism.
    - o Required for central nervous system, alimentary system and skin.
  - **Sources:**
    - o Cereals, milk, cheese, yeast, eggs, meat, liver and pork.
  - **Deficiency causes:**
    - o **Pellagra** which is marked by dermatitis along with diarrhea and dementia, known as three Ds.
    - o Diseases of the mouth, like sore mouth, glossitis, etc.

- ○ Loss of appetite, abdominal pain and diarrhea.
- ○ Diseases of nervous system, like depression, apathy, sleeplessness, disorientation, confusion and other nervous disorders.
- ○ It may cause anemia.

RDA Recommendations

RDA/daily requirements of vitamin B$_3$ (nicotinic acid or niacin): The recommended daily amount of niacin for adult males is 16 mg a day and for adult women who are not pregnant, 14 mg a day. Children need between 2 and 16 mg daily, depending on age.

- ■ Vitamin B$_6$ (pyridoxine)
  - ● **Functions:**
    - ○ Essential for metabolism of fat and protein
    - ○ Essential for functioning of nervous system
    - ○ Needed for the formation and maturation of white bood cells (neutrophils).
  - ● **Sources:**
    - ○ Egg yolk, pulses, meat, yeast, cereals, liver and peas.
  - ● **Deficiency causes:**
    - ○ Dermatitis
    - ○ Peripheral neuropathy
    - ○ Muscular weakness
    - ○ Seizures
    - ○ Growth Retardation
    - ○ Anemia

RDA Recommendations

RDA/daily requirements of Vitamin B$_6$ (pyridoxine): The current recommended daily amount (RDA) for B$_6$ is 1.3–1.7 mg for adults over 19 years of age.

Note

- • Patients who are taking isonicotinylhydrazide (INH) for tuberculosis treatment develop deficiency of pyridoxine that requires additional supplement.

- ■ Vitamin B$_5$ (pantothenic acid)
  - ● **Function:**
    - ○ Required for carbohydrate and fat metabolism.
  - ● **Sources:**
    - ○ Widely distributed in animal and plant sources.
  - ● **Deficiency causes:**
    - ○ No definite deficiency state is proved.

RDA Recommendations

RDA/daily requirements of vitamin B$_5$ (pantothenic acid): Infants require 1.7 mg; children need 2–4 mg; men and women 14 years and older need 5 mg; pregnant and breastfeeding women need 6–7 mg.

- Vitamin B$_9$ (folic acid)
  - **Functions:**
    - Helps the body to produce and maintain new cells, and prevents changes to DNA that may lead to cancer. It maintains basic unit of genes (DNA) and thus promotes growth.
    - Essential for the maturation of red blood cells.
  - **Sources:**
    - Yeast, liver, kidney, milk and green leafy vegetables.

RDA Recommendations

RDA/daily requirements of vitamin B$_9$ (folic acid)
- **Normal adults:** 100 mg/day.
- **Pregnant woman:** 300–400 mg/day.
- **Children:** 100 mg/day.
- Requirements increase during pregnancy, infancy, in the use of anticancer and convalescent and antituberculosis drugs.

  - **Deficiency causes:**
    - Megaloblastic anemia
- Vitamin B$_{12}$ (cyanocobalamin)
  - **Functions:**
    - Promotes growth
    - Essential for the maturation of RBC
    - Needed for fat and carbohydrate metabolism
    - Helps to prevent diarrhea mainly due to antibiotic therapy.
  - **Sources:**
    - It is present in liver, meat, kidneys and milk.
    - It is absent in foods of plant origin therefore pure vegetarians suffer from vitamin B$_{12}$ deficiency diseases.
  - **Deficiency causes:**
    - Pernicious anemia, which makes it hard for body to absorb vitamin B$_{12}$.
    - Affects the major nerves of the spinal cord and functions of the nervous system.
    - Atrophic gastritis, in which stomach lining thins down.
    - Immune system disorders such as Grave's disease or lupus.

RDA Recommendations

RDA/daily requirements of vitamin B$_{12}$ (cyanocobalamin): The typical general supplemental dose of vitamin B$_{12}$ is 1–25 mcg/day. The recommended dietary allowances (RDAs) of vitamin B$_{12}$ are: 1.8 mg; older children and adults, 2.4 mcg; pregnant women, 2.6 mg; and breastfeeding women, 2.8 mg 1–2 mcg/day.

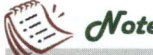 **Note**

Vitamin B$_{12}$ is provided by a well-balanced diet and produced in the large intestines by intestinal bacteria.

Ascorbic Acid (Vitamin C)

Ascorbic acid is also known as vitamin C. It is a water-soluble vitamin, which is destroyed by heat and is hardly left in cooked food.

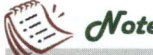 **Note**

Copper vessels destroy vitamin C.

Functions:
- It is essential for the formation of connective tissue.
- It aids in iron absorption.
- It is required to prevent bleeding disorders.
- It improves resistance of the body.

Sources:
- Fruits like oranges, lemon, sweet lime, amla and guava.
- Vegetables like tomatoes, drumstick leaves, cabbage, cauliflower and potatoes.

Deficiency causes:
- **Scurvy:** It occurs due to the failure of wounds to heal because of vitamin C deficiency. Deficiency affects growth of bone and fractured bones do not heal well.
- Breaking the blood vessels due to lack of ascorbic acid.

 RDA Recommendations

RDA/daily requirements of Vitamin C: Infants need 20–30 mg daily from second month: 1–2 teaspoons of orange juice daily or double the amount of tomato juice per day can meet the requirement.
- Adults and pregnant woman require 40 mg of vitamin C per day.
- Lactating women need liberal amount of ascorbic acid although the requirements are only 80 mg/day.

MINERALS

Minerals are inorganic substances found in nature having a definite chemical composition. These are widely distributed in vegetables and animal kingdom. Usually enough amount of minerals are provided by a well-balanced diet.

Types of Minerals

Depending upon the requirement, minerals are divided into two groups:
1. **Major minerals:** These are minerals required in macro quantities, such as calcium, phosphorus, sodium, potassium and chlorine.
2. **Trace elements:** Elements like iron, iodine and zinc required in micro quantities.

Unit II ❖ Food Factors—Functions and Sources

Major Minerals

Calcium

Ninety-nine percent of body calcium is in the blood and bones. Calcium contributes 1.5–2% of total body weight.

Functions:

- Calcium is required for the growth of teeth and bones.
- Required for the adequate functioning of heart muscles.
- Calcium activates a number of enzymes.
- Calcium is required for metabolic functions and clotting of blood.

Sources:

- Milk and milk products are best dietary sources of calcium.
- Ragi, wheat and tapioca provide a large quantity of calcium.
- Vegetables are usually poor sources of calcium except green leafy vegetables.

Deficiency of calcium causes:

- Rickets
- Osteomalacia
- Tetany
- Dental caries
- Growth retardation

RDA Recommendations

RDA/daily requirements of calcium:
- Children below 10 years need 500–1000 mg of calcium per day.
- Children above 10 years require 1000–1500 mg of calcium per day.
- Adults require 500 mg of calcium per day.
- Pregnant and lactating women require 1000 mg of calcium per day.

Phosphorus

Functions:

- It is required for the metabolism of cells.
- It is an important constituent of bone and teeth.
- It helps to maintain the acid base balance of the body.

Sources:

If the dietary contents of calcium and proteins are adequate, phosphorus requirements are met easily. Other sources of potassium are meat, wheat, legumes and fish products.

Deficiency causes:

No clear-cut deficiency disease has been reported.

RDA Recommendations

- **RDA/daily requirements of phosphorus:** 1–2 g that is readily obtained from ordinary meals. The Linus Pauling Institute supports the RDA for phosphorus as 700 mg/day for adults.

Sodium, Potassium and Chlorine

- These are present in foods and are required for normal functioning of the body. These three elements are related to one another.
- Potassium is present mainly inside the blood cells and soft tissues while sodium is present mainly in the fluids bathing the cells, like blood plasma and tissue fluids.

Functions:

These three elements are necessary for the carriage of carbon dioxide by blood and is further transported from the cells to the lungs to be excreted.

- **Sodium** is important for regulating the movement and use of water within the body because it helps to maintain osmotic pressure.
- **Chlorine** is necessary for the production of hydrochloric acid in the stomach. Sodium, potassium and **calcium** help in for the correct functioning of the body.
- **Potassium** is present in almost all foods, and is sufficient to meet the daily requirements. It is difficult to remove potassium from the food.

Sources:

- Sodium chloride is available to body when we eat cooked foods.
- **Sodium, potassium and chlorine** are present in adequate quantities in normal nutrition and deficiency is not usual.

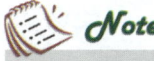 *Note*

- In diet therapy, sometimes it is necessary to restrict sodium intake.

Trace Elements

Iron

The major amount of iron in body is in the form of hemoglobin, but smaller amount is present in the liver and bone marrow. The total amount of iron present in the body is average 3.5 g.

- **Functions:**
  - Iron is essential for the formation of hemoglobin.
  - The chief function of iron is to transport oxygen to tissues.
  - Iron present in the nucleus of cells is very necessary for the oxidation in the tissues.
- **Sources:**
  - Liver, egg yolk, meat, green leafy vegetables, jaggery, etc. Iron from animal source is better absorbed than vegetable source.

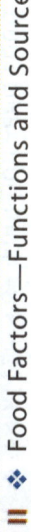

Unit II ❖ Food Factors—Functions and Sources

RDA Recommendations

RDA/daily requirements of iron: These vary according to the age, sex and physiological changes like pregnancy and lactation.

- Infants
- Children   1 mg/kg/daily
- 1–10 years   8–12 mg/kg/daily
- 10–12 years   15 mg/kg/daily
- Adolescents   15 mg/kg/daily
- Adults
- Men   10 mg/kg/daily
- Women   20 mg/kg/daily
- Pregnant women   40–50 mg/kg/daily
- Lactating women   30–40 mg/kg/daily

- **Deficiency causes:**
  - **Anemia:** Iron deficiency leads to anemia.

Iodine

It is the best-known trace element.

- **Functions:**
  - It is essential for the formation of thyroxine, which is required for the maintenance of normal cell metabolism.
- **Sources:**
  - Best source is common salt, which is extracted from seawater.
  - It is also available in cod liver oil and seafish.
- **Deficiency causes:**
  - Swelling of the thyroid gland in front of the neck which is known as goiter.

RDA Recommendations

RDA/daily requirements of iodine: 0.2 mg of iodine is recommended daily. 'Iodized salt' is marketed by the Government of India to prevent goiter.

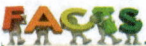

Potassium iodide is mixed with common salt, known as iodized salt.

Other Inorganic (Trace) Elements

There are other inorganic elements, which are essential for human nutrition but are needed in the body only in very small amounts.

- **Copper** functions with iron in the formation of hemoglobin.
- **Cobalt** is present in vitamin B_{12} that is also necessary for the formation of hemoglobin.
- **Zinc** is found mainly in pancreatic tissue and has an important part in the formation and storage of insulin in the gland.

Unit II   Food Factors—Functions and Sources

These elements are needed in small amounts and an adequate diet can meet the requirements of all trace elements. So, it is not necessary to consider any special source of these elements in the diet.

WATER

Water is an extremely essential need for the human body. One may live without food for a few days but cannot live without water. Therefore, water is more important than food for human body.

Water Content in Human Body

- Body consists of an average 60–70% of water or fluids which is distributed in different parts of the body.
- About seven liters of water/fluid is produced in the alimentary tract and most of it is absorbed.
- Even though the exact amount is not recorded, a certain amount of water in cerebrospinal water/fluid is produced by the brain, which flows to the spinal canal and is absorbed there itself.
- A small amount of water/fluid is produced in the eyes and it keeps the eyes wet and controls the movement.
- Urinary system secretes a large amount of water/fluid and a good amount of it is excreted as urine through bladder and urethra.
- According to the physical exertion, atmospheric condition and the intake of water, a particular amount of water is lost from the skin through perspiration.

Retention of fluid in the tissues causes edema and excessive loss of water/fluid from the body produces dehydration.

Functions of Water in the Body

- Water is essential for the formation of blood and other fluids in the body, and for the excretion of waste products from the body.
- For the digestion and absorption of food materials in the body, water is needed.
- For the regulation of body temperature, water is needed.
- Water is essential to produce the serous fluids in the joints and in between the layers of serous membranes covering the organs of the body.
- Water is extremely essential for the proper functioning of all the organs in the body.

The body gets water through drinking as water and as other fluids, through foods and fruits. Water is lost from the body through urinary system as urine, through gastrointestinal system with stools; as perspiration through skin; and through respiratory system as moisture. To keep balance between the intake and loss of fluid in the body, the intake should tally according to the output. An average adult should take a minimum of two liters of water daily. Depending upon the condition of the disease, the intake of fluids in a patient should be regulated by oral administration or through any other routes.

Because of strenuous physical exertion and in hot climate, increased amount of water is needed by the body and a large amount of water is lost from the body. Comparatively, the body of children consists of part that is more fluid. Therefore, if fluid is lost from the body of children due to any reason, the condition deteriorates rapidly and dehydration occurs. Depending upon the weight of the child, the fluid requirement can be calculated. 165 mL of water per kilogram of body weight is a reasonable requirement and that amount should be administered as different forms of fluids to the child per day.

Unit II ❖ Food Factors—Functions and Sources

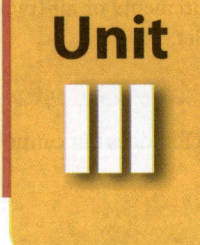

Unit III

Normal Dietary Requirements

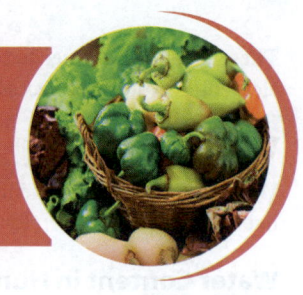

METABOLISM

Metabolism is the changes that take place in nutrients from the time of their absorption to their reaching as the end products of the various processes through which they pass and release energy.

When food is eaten it is digested in the gastrointestinal tract so that it is broken down into substances simple enough to be absorbed into the blood stream. These substances are then carried to the various parts of the body where they are used for building up and repairing tissues, this process is called *anabolism* or they are broken down further to produce energy, and this process is called *catabolism*. Anabolism and catabolism together are called *metabolism*.

BASAL METABOLIC RATE

It is the amount of energy required by a person who is awake while at complete physical and mental rest and has not consumed food for 12–14 hours. Basal metabolic rate (BMR) never goes to zero during life because of the energy required for respiration and circulation.

Every activity of the body requires energy, even maintaining the vital processes, such as respiration and circulation. We need energy to do activities, like moving about and doing any physical work. The harder the physical work done, the greater is the amount of energy required by the body; and the less physical work done, the smaller is the amount of energy required. When the body is at complete rest, the energy requirement is at its lowest.

Measurement of energy and calorie: All forms of energy can be converted into heat. It is often convenient to measure energy as heat. The unit for the measurement of heat is called calorie. The calorie is the (usually capital 'C' is used for Calorie) amount of heat required to raise the temperature of one kilogram (1000 g) of water through one degree centigrade.

Unit of calorie is called 'Joule'.
1 Calorie = 4.184 Kilojoule.
It is calculated approximately as 4 Kilojoule.
A Joule is a very small unit, so the term Kilojoule (1000 Joules) is used.

Factors Affecting Basal Metabolic Rate

- **Surface area of the body:** The larger the surface area of the body the greater is the exchange of heat.
- **Sex:** Males need more calories than females.
  - 40 calories per square meter of body per hour for man.
  - 37 calories per square meter of body per hour for woman.
- **Age:** Growing children and adolescents need higher calories.

- **Diseases:** Some diseases, especially diseases of the thyroid may raise or lower BMR.
- **Undernutrition:** Prolonged or chronic undernutrition may reduce BMR.
- **Mental status:** Psychological tension caused by worry or stress will increase BMR.
- **Body size**: Metabolic rate increases as weight, height and surface area increases.
- **Climate and body temperature:**
  - The BMR of people in tropical climates is generally 5–20% higher than their counterparts living in more temperate areas because it takes energy to keep the body cool.
  - Exercise performed in hot weather also imposes an additional metabolic load.
  - Body-fat content and effectiveness of clothing determine the magnitude of increase in energy metabolism in cold environments.
- **Hormonal levels**: Thyroxine (T_4), the key hormone released by the thyroid glands has a significant effect upon metabolic rate.
- **Health**: Fever, illness, or injury may increase resting metabolic rate two-fold.

ENERGY METABOLISM

Definition: The expenditure or using up of the energy in the body is known as energy metabolism.

Factors Affecting Total Energy Requirements

- Weight of the person
- Specific dynamic action of the food
- Age of the person
- Temperature
  - Amount of work done
  - External temperature
- Muscular activities increase calorie requirement
- **Pregnancy:** In pregnancy calorie requirements increase due to growth of fetus, placenta, etc.

Food Items Which Supply Energy

As mentioned previously, the functions of nutrients are related to each other. Any food may contain one or more nutrients. However, carbohydrates, fats and proteins are the nutrients, which give calories to the body.

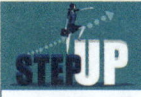

- The calorific value of these nutrients and many common foods has been determined by burning a known weight of the nutrient or food in an atmosphere of oxygen in an instrument known as **Bomb Calorimeter**.
- The values for carbohydrates, proteins and fats as obtained in the Bomb Calorimeter are given as follows:

Carbohydrate	1 g	gives	4 calories (4 Cal)
Protein	1 g	gives	4 calories (4 Cal)
Fat	1 g	gives	9 calories (9 Cal)

BALANCED DIET

Balanced diet is an adequate diet containing all the essential nutrients in the right amount and correct proportion. A balanced diet is one that has correct amount of body-building protein, energy-giving carbohydrate or fat as well as protective food that contain vitamins and minerals. It is important that, to have a balanced diet, the foods items are mixed with different items and are eaten together.

Unit III ❖ Normal Dietary Requirements

Effect of Nutrition on Health

The essence of nutrition is providing sufficient quantity of food required to supply adequate calories, proteins, carbohydrates, fats, vitamins and minerals.

Good nutrition helps in:
- Physical growth of the body
- Building defense mechanism in the body
- Prevention of nutritional deficiency diseases
- Reduction of mortality and morbidity rates.

MENU PLANNING

Factors to be Considered in Planning Food

A good meal should be nutritious, well-cooked with careful combination of foods and flavors. In the planning of meals, the following factors should be considered:

General Factors
- The number of members in the house.
- Occupation and income of the family.
- Food requirement of each member in the house.
- Consider that the children, old people, pregnant and lactating women are vulnerable groups and need particular foods.
- Changes in food according to the caste and religion of people.
- Consideration to the racial discrimination of the people in the house.
- Nutritional adequacy or the provision of palatable foods that are rich in essential nutrients.
- The food budget, which is influenced by the family income, knowledge of the shopper, family's likes and dislikes of food and their goals and values.

Social Factors

Ignorance and poverty of people are the most important causes of malnourishment and deficiency diseases in our country. Therefore, the knowledge of the people about the need of good nutrition for health, along with social development and economic situation, determines the standard of quality and quantity of food and the health status of the individuals and family.

Cultural Factors
- **Customs and habits:** Customs and habits are passed from generations to generation, e.g., millions of people prefer white polished rice.
- **Religion:** It has a powerful influence on the type of food consumed, e.g. vegetarians and nonvegetarians.
- **Food fads:** Food fads are personal likes and dislikes about certain food.
- **Poverty:** Protective food items, such as meat, fish and eggs are costly therefore, these are not part of the diet of poor people.
- **Ignorance:** Ignorance is the root cause of most health problems and faulty dietary habits in India. Malnutrition and undernutrition are always due to shortage of food, especially because of poverty and ignorance.

SPECIAL DIETS

Diet in Pregnancy

Pregnancy and lactation are natural phenomena, which create greater demands upon the body. A woman receiving an adequate diet during pregnancy is more likely to have a safe delivery of a healthy child. Therefore, a pregnant woman needs an adequate diet during that period. The needed nutrients for the child growing in the uterus are obtained from the blood of the mother. Inadequate and improper diet of the mother may lead to complications in developing fetus, such as prematurity, congenital defects and still birth. Toxemia of pregnancy may also occur.

The weight of an infant at birth is a reflection of the weight gained by the woman during pregnancy and this weight gain depends upon the food taken by the mother. The weight gain during pregnancy is usually 8–10 kg. Most of this should occur during the last trimester when the growth of the fetus is most rapid. During the second half of the pregnancy, calorie intake should be increased by 300 calories and protein by 14 g/day. Not only proteins, but vitamins and especially iron, calcium and phosphorous are also important in the diet of pregnant women. All these food factors are especially essential for the development of bones, teeth and hair and the general growth of the fetus in the uterus and these should be included in the diet of the mother. Milk is a good source of most of these nutrients.

During the first three months of normal pregnancy, the diet need not be different from an average normal diet of a woman. After the third month, all essential nutrients are supplied to the fetus in proper amount. Food items like meat, fish, pulses, vegetables and green leafy vegetables, fruits, nuts, sugar or jaggery and an increased amount of milk and cereals, like rice and wheat are given in adequate quantity during pregnancy to meet the increased calorie requirement, and for the proper growth of the fetus. As far as possible, first class proteins should be selected.

Diet in Lactation

Postnatal period is the time when the mother needs complete rest to regain health and she is in lactation stage too. A lactating woman experiences increased hunger and thirst and she needs careful feeding. For the first 12 hours after delivery, easily digestible soft food should be given. After 12 hours, the mother will have a normal appetite and a regular diet should be continued. This will help to increase the secretion of milk. The nutritional demands of the lactating woman are greater than that of in pregnancy. The requirements of calories, proteins, iron, calcium and vitamins are also increased. The Indian Council of Medical Research (ICMR) laboratories recommend 2700 calories per day with 110 grams of protein for a lactating woman. Three-fourths of the protein must be from first class protein. Calcium requirement must be increased to 2 g/day. A lactating woman should take plenty of fluids as water, milk and other drinks for the production of more milk and proper functioning of body and keeping fluid balance of the body. At least four glasses of milk and one egg per day should be taken regularly. Food should include cereals, pulses, fruits, meat, fish, green leafy vegetables, other vegetables and green gram in an increased amount. Since cow's milk is highly nutritious, the amount shall be increased to at least 500 mL/day.

Unit III ❖ Normal Dietary Requirements

Unit IV
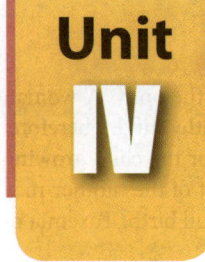

Cooking
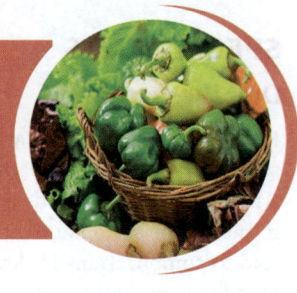

WHY DO WE NEED COOKING?

Meeting the nutritional requirement is a basic need for everyone. An increasing emphasis is being placed today on the importance of adequate food for maintaining good health. Besides medications and appropriate treatments, adequate nourishment has to be provided to the patient and it must be recognized as a part of care while giving patient care, if he/she has to gain full benefit for treatment. It is a fact that a large number of people are suffering from malnutrition and deficiency diseases in varying degrees. One nurse may not be sufficient in this matter. Although, when a nurse is giving care to one or few patients, she is responsible for giving proper attention while providing adequate nutrition to them. In fulfilling this responsibility of meeting the nutritional needs of the patients effectively, the nurse must have a good knowledge of the science of nutrition, an intelligent understanding of the principles of diet therapy and skill in the preparation and serving of foods to patients. On the basis of this view, the required food factors and the need of food in healthy state and disease in humans are already discussed in detail in **previous chapters** of this book.

Practical knowledge of cookery and skills in cooking are important for every nurse. In well-established hospitals, there are special departments and specially-trained and qualified persons to deal with the aspect of diet for the patients. But in small hospitals, this responsibility rests on the nurses itself. A nurse has to recognize the needs of food according to the disease, preparation of food items and to make the alterations in food for his/her patients. Not only that, the nurse is the most suitable person to impart necessary knowledge about food and feeding to the patients and their relatives during health and disease. Every nurse should have at least a basic knowledge about food that it is one of the essential factors of health; and cooking of the food is necessary; and the ability of feeding a patient is a requirement for the successful functioning.

PURPOSES OF COOKING

The purposes of cooking and the effects of different methods of cooking are important factors to be considered while preparing food for sick people and for those who need to restrict one or more of nutrients to cure themselves. Different methods of cooking are used in different types of diets. Food is cooked for the following purposes:

- To make the food more digestible
- To develop new flavor and taste in food
- To make the food more safe by destroying harmful bacteria and parasites in it.

METHODS OF COOKING

- **Boiling:** Cooking by boiling in water or other liquids.
- **Simmering**: It is a modification of boiling using water or other liquid (just under boiling point).
- **Pouching:** It is similar to simmering using water or other liquids in an open pan.

- **Steaming**: Food is cooked with the help of steam (water vapors), which come out from boiling water.
- **Stewing:** It is to simmer food very slowly with only very little water or liquid in a covered pan on top of the stove.
- **Frying:** Cooking the food in very hot fat or oil. It is one of the quickest methods and is done in an open pan.
- **Baking:** Cooking food in oven or closed container, with hot air all around like bread, biscuits and cakes.
- **Roasting:** It is similar to baking but food is placed in hot fat in a baking tin in the oven so that it cooks partly in hot fat and partly in hot air, e.g., meat and root vegetables. It is one of the quickest methods.
- **Grilling:** It is a method of cooking food by exposing it directly to high heat in bright, hot fire or with the help of a special grilling plate fitted to stove, which is heated by gas or electricity.

KITCHEN EQUIPMENT REQUIRED FOR COOKING FOOD

There should be a convenient room with needed tables and proper water supply and the following equipment:

Kitchen scale	For weighing the items
Measuring cups and liter measures	To measure the liquid forms
Mixing bowls	To mix the items
Strainers (metal and wire)	To filter the fluid mixtures (a clean piece of cloth or muslin can also be used)
Knives of various sizes	For cutting like vegetable knife, chopping knife, kitchen knife and bread knife
Spoons of various sizes	To take, or measure or mix the items such as table spoons, desert spoons, tea spoons, set of standard measuring spoons, and wooden spoons of different sizes.
Forks	To pick up items
Egg whisk or beater	To beat the eggs
Lemon squeezer	To squeeze the lemon or citrus fruits
Grinder	To grind the items
Wooden board	For chopping and rolling items
Rolling pin	To roll the mixed items
Meat mincer or grinder	To cut the meat in very small pieces
Saucepans of various sizes	To keep various items or mixing the items
Equipment and cleaning aid	To clean the vessels and other items
Handling equipment like tongs	To hold and take the hot vessels from stove or heater
Thick-padded cloth	To handle the hot vessels and pan
Towels	To dry the vessels and spoons
Tray cloths and covers	To use in trays and to cover the items in tray
Mop cloths	To clean the floor
Dusters	To clean and dry the tables
Scrubbing brush or coconut fiber	To clean the vessels by rubbing
Cleaning powders	To clean soiled vessels
Soap in soap dish and towels	To wash hands and dry
Mixer with different jars	To mix or powder the items
Refuse bin or dustbin with cover	To keep the waste materials (covered)

All the above-mentioned articles should always be kept clean, neatly arranged and ready for use at any time.

RECIPES

Majority of cookery books have a section of recipes to cater for the taste of various people. The following may be taken as basic recipes for the preparation of light and easily digestible foods. Recipes are divided into the following groups:

- **Clear fluid food items are:** Clear tea, black coffee, clear soups, fruit juice, raw tomato juice, whey, lime juice with or without salt or sugar, barley water with or without salt and albumen water.
- **Full fluid food items are:**
  - Milk and coffee with or without sugar
  - Milk and tea with or without sugar
  - Cocoa and milk with or without sugar
  - Beaten egg (egg flip) with or without sugar
  - Fortified milk drinks with or without sugar
  - Dhal soup
  - Vegetable soup
  - Butter milk with or without salt.
- **Light cereal preparations are:**
  - Different kinds of congees like,
  - **Broken double-boiled rice congee** with milk, with or without salt or sugar
  - **Ragi congee** with or without milk or sugar
  - **Arrowroot congee** with or without milk or sugar or salt
  - **Sago congee** with or without milk or sugar or salt
  - **Barley congee** with or without milk or sugar or salt
  - **Toast** as prepared in home
  - **Rusk** prepared in bakery
- **Vegetable preparations**: Vegetables boiled in water and strained with or without salt
- **Egg preparations:** Soft-cooked eggs, hard-boiled eggs, poached eggs, scrambled egg or buttered egg, omelette.
- **Fish and meat preparations:** Steamed fish, creamed fish, creamed chicken, minced liver.
- **Light puddings like:**
  - Fruit jelly
  - Milk jelly
  - Baked custard
  - Corn flour pudding
  - Ice cream, etc.

RECIPES OF LIGHT PUDDINGS

Preparation method of few light puddings has been given here as:
- **Fruit jelly**

  Ingredients:
  - 500 mL fruit juice
  - 100 g sugar
  - 20 g powdered gelatin

  Method: Put all ingredients into a pan and warm gently, stirring all the time. Turn into a rinsed mould and allow it to set, preferably in a refrigerator. Keep cold until served.

- **Milk jelly**
  Ingredients:
  - 500 mL milk
  - 50 g sugar
  - Strip of lime or orange peel
  - 15 g powdered gelatin

  Method: Put the lime or orange peel in the milk. Bring to boiling point and strain the milk in a pan having gelatin and sugar. Keep stirring until all ingredients are dissolved. Keep on cooking for some more time, stirring from time to time until the mixture has consistency of thick cream. Pour into rinsed moulds and allow it to set, preferably in a refrigerator. Keep cold until served.

- **Baked custard**
  Ingredients:
  - 1 egg
  - 180 mL milk
  - Sugar to taste

  Method: Beat the egg lightly, heat the milk and pour over the beaten egg, stirring all the time. Add sugar to taste and stir well. Pour the mixture into a greased dish and sprinkle a little grated nutmeg on top if desired. Stand the dish in a baking tin with hot water halfway up its sides. Bake in a moderate oven until set.

  If steamed custard is required, pour the mixture into individual greased moulds, place in a steamer and simmer until set.

- **Corn flour pudding**
  Ingredients:
  - 500 mL milk
  - Thin strips of lime or orange peel or other flavoring agent
  - 30 g sugar
  - 15 g custard powder
  - 30 g corn flour

  Method: Pour about three-quarters of the milk into a saucepan, add the orange rind or other flavoring, sugar and a pinch of salt and bring it to boil slowly. Mix the corn flour and custard powder together with the remaining cold milk. Pour the boiling milk into the mixed custard and corn flour, stirring well. Add it to the pan and boil for a few minutes until it thickens. Pour into individual moulds and allow to set until cold, preferably in a refrigerator. Keep cold until served.

- **Ice cream:**
  - Milk 25 mL
  - 1 egg
  - Sugar 20 g
  - Flavoring agent

  Method: Beat the egg lightly and mix in the milk and sugar. Heat over a low flame or in a double boiler until the mixture begins to thicken. Remove from the heat and cool quickly. Add flavor as desired and freeze. Keep cold until served.

Unit IV ❖ Cooking

NOTES

APPENDICES

 TRACHEAL SUCTIONING

Tracheal suctioning is the removal of secretions from tracheobronchial tree through an endotracheal tube or tracheostomy tube with the help of mechanical suction device.

Goal

To maximize the amount of secretions removed with minimal adverse effects associated with the procedure

Purposes

- To stimulate coughing
- To prevent infection and atelectasis
- To provide effective ventilation
- To prevent aspiration of food, blood and gastric fluid
- To prevent lower respiratory tract infection from retained secretions
- To maintain a patent airway by removing retained tracheobronchial secretions
- To improve oxygenation and to improve the work of breathing
- To collect secretions for diagnostic testing

Types of Tracheal Suctioning

- Open suction
- Closed suction

Preliminary Assessment

- Assess the rate, depth and rhythm of respirations
- Auscultate breath sounds
- Note noisy, wet, or gurgling respirations
- Note signs and symptoms of hypoxemia and hypercapnia (restlessness, confusion, etc.)
- Assess patient's ability to cough and the amount and character of sputum
- Assess vital signs and signs and symptoms of infection
- Note any drainage from mouth
- Assess accidental extubation. Keep extra tracheostomy tube and obturator at bedside

Articles Required

Articles	Purpose
Wall suction or portable suction unit	For performing suctioning
Connecting tubing and collecting bottle	For attaching to the suction unit
An oxygen source, Ambu bag or ventilator connections	For hyperoxygenation
Sterile normal saline solution or sterile water	Solutions used for irrigation
Sterile suction catheter	For performing suctioning
Sterile container or basin	For pouring solution for clearing the suction tubings
Disposable sterile gloves and clean gloves	For preventing contact with secretions
Required PPE including goggles, mask apron etc.	For preventing contact with secretions
Tracheostomy care kit with tracheal dilator	For Emergency resuscitation if required
Overbed table	For positioning the patient
Mackintosh and towel	For protecting the linen
Clean tissues	For wiping during and after suctioning
Stethoscope	For respiratory assessment
Monitoring device, e.g., pulse oximetry	For assessing hypoxia
Kidney tray or paper bag	For disposing soiled waste
Oral care tray	For performing oral hygiene

Procedure

Steps	Procedure	Rationale
1.	Assess patient need for suctioning (respiratory assessment using stethoscope for signs of hypoxia), risk for aspiration and inability to protect own airway or clear secretions adequately. Place pulse oximetry probe on the patient's finger. 	Physical signs and symptoms indicate the need for suctioning.
2.	Explain the procedure to the patient.	Allays anxiety and wins confidence and cooperation.
3.	Ensure the patient's privacy by screening the patient.	Helps to promote dignity

Contd...

Steps	Procedure	Rationale
4.	Position the patient in semi-Fowler's or high Fowler's position with head turned to the side or sitting upright. Unconscious patients should be placed in the lateral position. 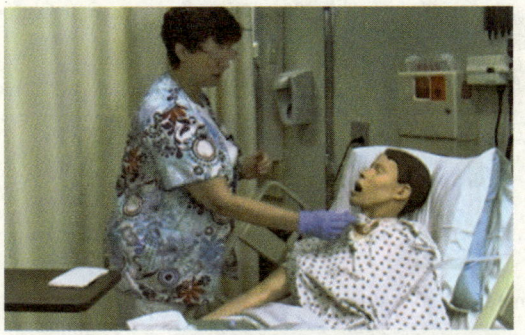	This facilitates ease of suctioning and prevents aspiration. It also promotes lung expansion and effective coughing. Side placement promotes forward drainage of secretions.
5.	Increase supplemental oxygen therapy to 100% or as ordered by physician. 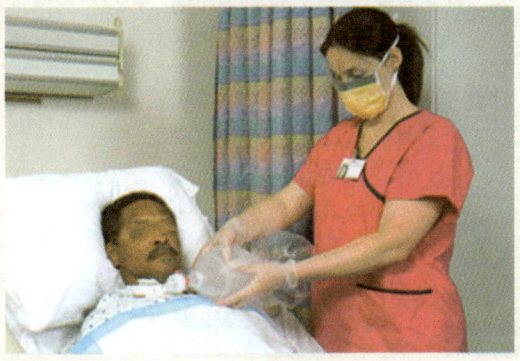	This is in preparation for the hypoxia that is precipitated by suctioning, both from mechanical interruption and cessation of oxygen flow briefly. Deep breathing helps to reduce suction-induced hypoxemia.
6.	Gather articles at the bedside.	Organization promotes skilled performance.
7.	Place mackintosh and towel on patient's chest. 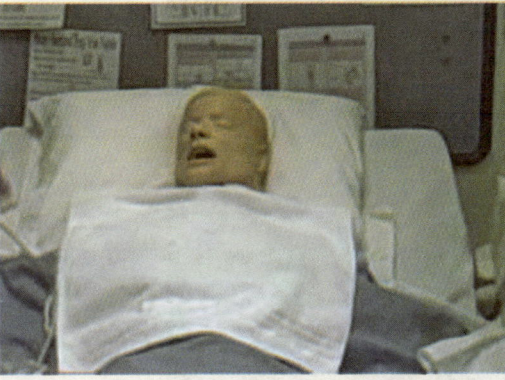	Prevents patient from coming in contact with secretions.

Contd...

Appendix 1: Tracheal Suctioning

Steps	Procedure	Rationale
8.	Wash hands and wear appropriate personal protective equipment (PPE). 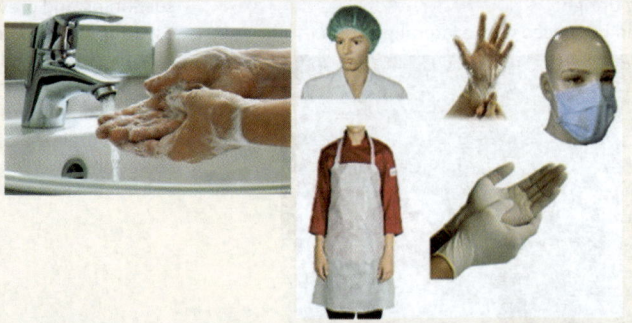	Prevents the transmission of microorganisms. Protective equipment protects you from contact with secretions.
9.	Date and open the bottle of normal saline solution or sterile water. 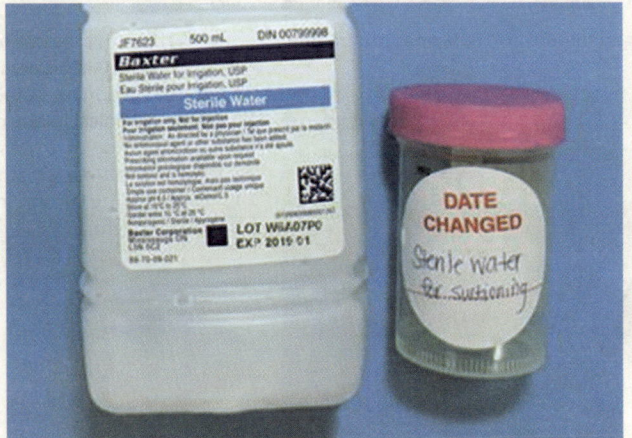	Prevents use of contaminated solution.
10.	Using strict aseptic technique, open the suction catheter kit or the packages containing the sterile catheter, container and sterile gloves. 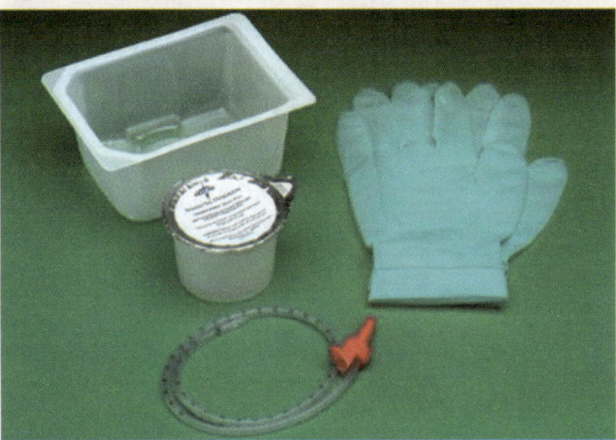	Ensures sterility of the procedure.

Contd...

Steps	Procedure	Rationale

Don the sterile gloves.

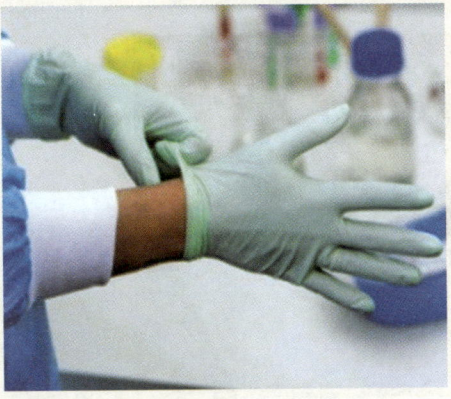

Water is used to clear connection tubing in between suctions. (at least three times)

Consider your dominant hand sterile and your nondominant hand nonsterile. Using your nondominant hand, pour the saline solution into the sterile container.

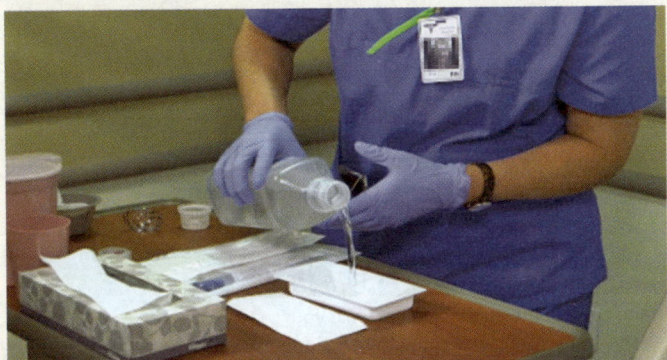

Fill sterile container with approximately 100 mL of sterile normal saline solution or sterile water.

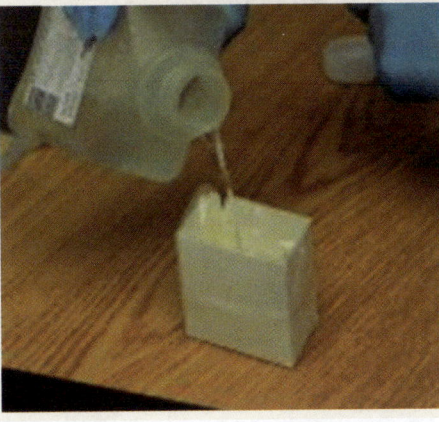

Contd...

Steps	Procedure	Rationale
11.	Attach one end of connection tubing to the suction machine and the other end to the suction catheter.	This prepares equipment to function effectively.

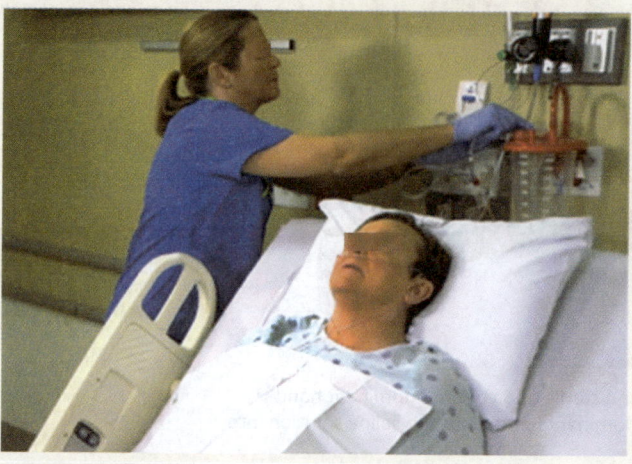

Pick up the catheter with your dominant (sterile) hand and attach it to the connecting tubing.

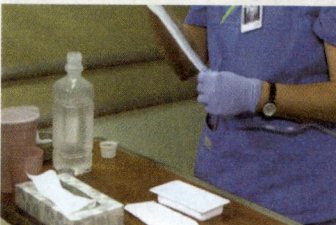 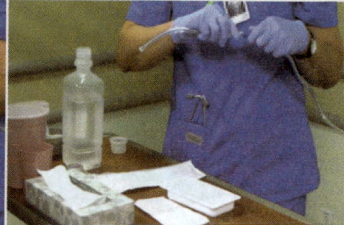

Use your nondominant hand to control the suction valve while your dominant hand manipulates the catheter. Do not allow the suction catheter to touch any unsterile surface.

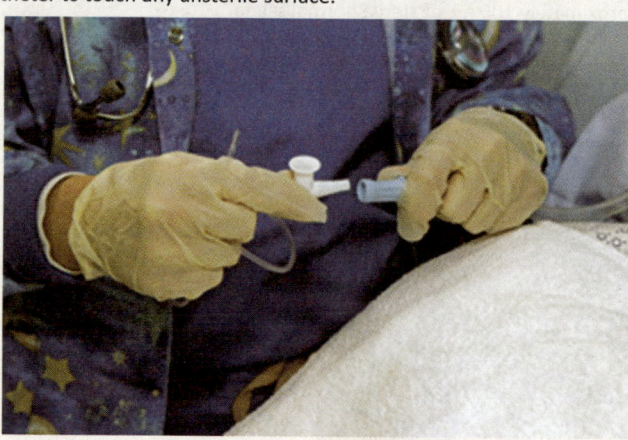

Contd...

Steps	Procedure	Rationale
12.	Turn on suction from the wall or portable unit to the required level and set the pressure according to your facility's policy.	Elevated pressure settings increase risk of trauma to mucosa and can induce greater hypoxia.

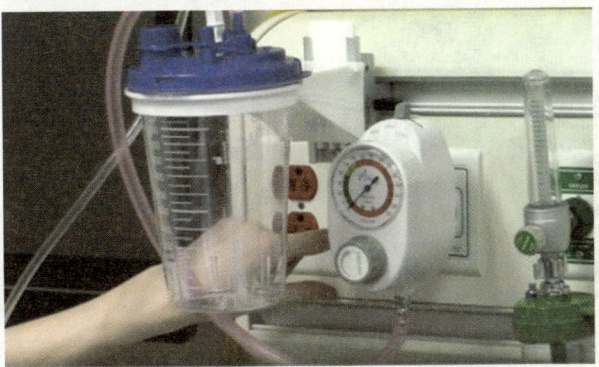

| | Test function by covering hole on the suction catheter with your thumb and suctioning up a small amount of water. | Tube occlusion tests suction apparatus |

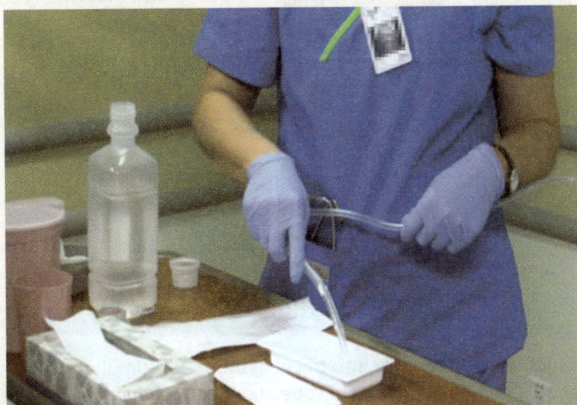

Turn on suction apparatus to appropriate negative pressure for: adults—100–120 mm Hg children—50–100 mm Hg infants—40–60 mm Hg.

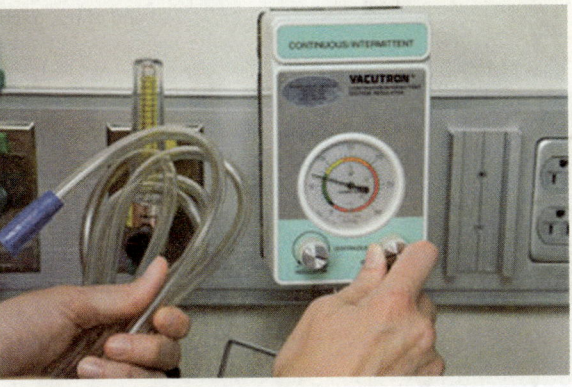

Contd...

Appendix 1: Tracheal Suctioning

Steps	Procedure	Rationale
13.	Preoxygenate the patient with the Ambu bag or through the ventilator with 100% oxygen. 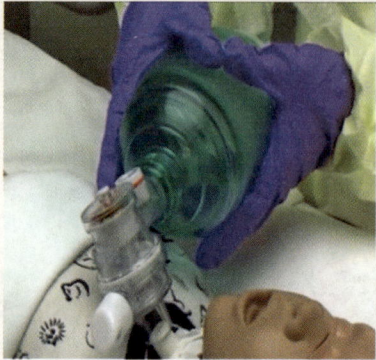	This helps to reduce suction-induced hypoxia.
14.	Dampen catheter in the sterile water to lubricate. 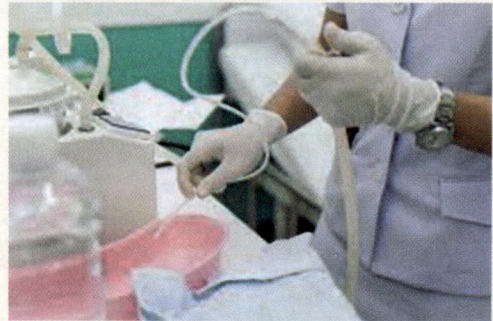 Disconnect tube from oxygen source with unsterile hand.	Lubrication prevents mucosal trauma when catheter is inserted.
15.	Using sterile hand, gently insert suction catheter fully into tracheal tube. The tip of the suction catheter should be below the end of tube. 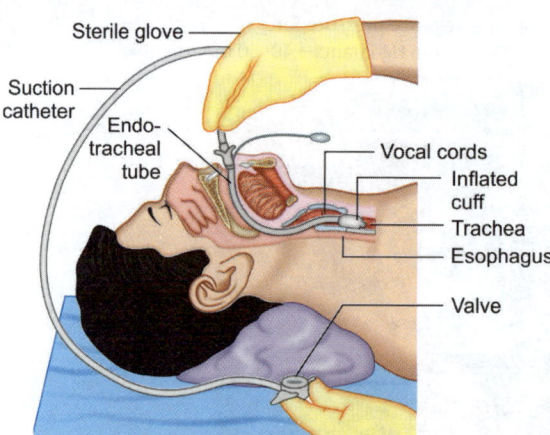	Stimulation of coughing generally indicates catheter is below end of the tube. This helps to reduce chance of a mucous plug forming in the end of the tracheal tube.

Contd...

Steps	Procedure	Rationale

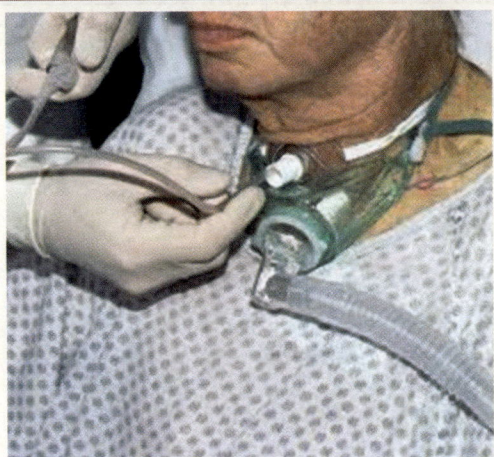

| 16. | Apply intermittent suction by quickly opening and closing suction port with unsterile hand, and withdraw catheter using a rotating motion. The entire suctioning process should not exceed 10—15 seconds in duration. Ensure that the emergency resuscitation equipment is kept ready for use, if required. | Intermittent suction minimizes tracheal tissue damage. Suction is applied only as catheter is being removed to minimize hypoxia. |

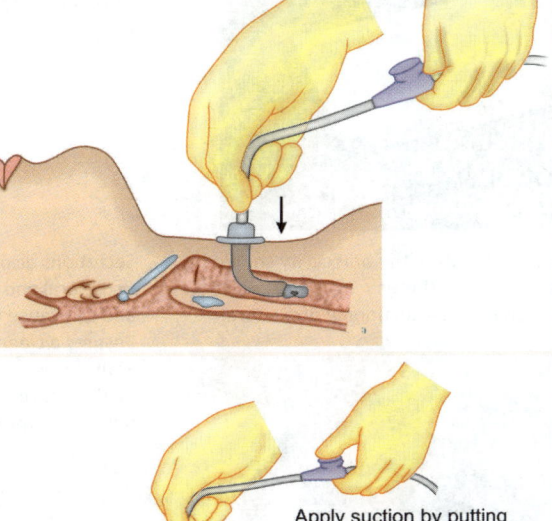

Apply suction by putting your thumb over the hole in the catheter while you gently pull the catheter back out. Gently roll the catheter between your thumb and forefinger as you pull the catheter out

Contd...

Appendix 1: Tracheal Suctioning

Steps	Procedure	Rationale
17.	Oxygenate, reoxygenate and hyperinflate patient's lungs with ambu bag and 100% oxygen after each suctioning attempt. 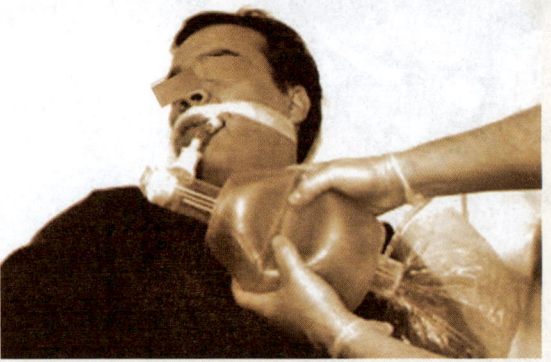	Prevents hypoxia.
18.	Flush the catheter with sterile water. 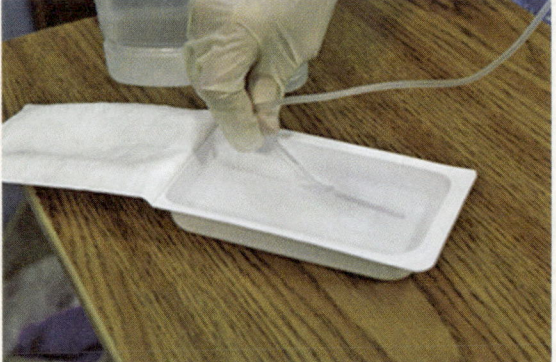	Clearing secretions before they dry reduces probability of transmission of microorganisms and enhances delivery of preset suction pressures. It also prevents the connection tubing from plugging.
19.	Once tracheal suctioning has been completed, the oral cavity should be cleansed and suctioned using the suction catheter. Oral hygiene should follow any tracheostomy suctioning procedure. 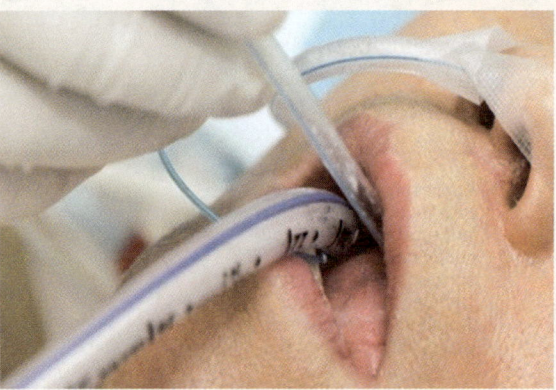	Secretions also accumulate in the oral and nasopharynx and can cause tissue damage. Ensures a clean, moist oral cavity. Replace oxygen to prevent or minimize hypoxia.

Contd...

Appendix 1: Tracheal Suctioning

Steps	Procedure	Rationale
20.	After completing suctioning, pull your glove off over the coiled catheter and discard it. If the catheter has to be reused, place catheter in a clean dry area for reuse with suction turned off.	Ensures safe disposal of catheter and gloves without contamination.
21.	Reassess respiratory status and O_2 saturation for improvements. 	Facilitates comparison of respiratory status with the baseline assessment.
22.	Ensure patient is in a comfortable position and call bell is within reach.	This promotes patient comfort.
23.	Clean up supplies, discard the used items and replace with new supplies so they will be ready for the next suctioning.	Having the supplies at the bedside facilitates a quick response.
24.	Remove gloves and wash hands. 	Prevents the transmission of microorganisms.
25.	Document procedure with the date, time including: • Reason for suctioning • Technique used • Amount, color, consistency and odor (if any) of the secretions • The client's respiratory status before and after the procedure • Any complications and the nursing action taken • The client's tolerance for the procedure. • Any significant events along with signature of the nurse.	Documentation fosters quality care.

Appendix 1: Tracheal Suctioning

ORAL SUCTIONING

Suctioning

Suctioning is the mechanical aspiration of pulmonary secretion from a patient with an artificial airway in place, in order to clear and maintain a patent airway.

Types of Suctioning

The type of suctioning depends on the anatomy of the region that is being suctioned.

- **Oral suctioning:** Insertion of catheter into the mouth of the patient.
- **Nasopharyngeal suctioning:** Insertion of the catheter on a downward slant through the nostril into the floor of the nasopharynx.
- **Endotracheal suctioning:** Insertion of the catheter into the ET tube to the appropriate depth.
- **Airway stoma:** Insertion of the catheter into the stoma, e.g., tracheostomy suctioning.

Oral Suctioning

Oral suctioning is a method used to clear secretions from the mouth and oropharynx through the application of negative pressure via a suction catheter or bulb syringe.

- It is the use of an oral suction catheter or a rigid plastic suction catheter, known as a Yankauer in order to remove pharyngeal secretions through the mouth.
- Oral suctioning involves the mouth.
- Oropharyngeal involves the mouth and the pharynx and sometimes the trachea.

Purposes

- The purpose of oral suctioning is to maintain a patent airway and improve oxygenation by removing mucous secretions and foreign material (vomit or gastric secretions) from the mouth and throat (oropharynx).
- Oral suctioning is useful to clear secretions from the mouth in the event when a patient is unable to remove secretions or foreign matter by effective coughing.

Indications

Patients who benefit the most include those with CVAs, drooling, impaired cough reflex related to age or condition, or impaired swallowing.

Contraindications

Oral suction should not be performed in patients with:

- Loose teeth
- Facial fractures
- Clotting disorders
- Laryngeal or oral carcinoma
- Recent head and neck surgeries
- Severe bronchospasm
- Stridor
- Restlessness/anxiety

Suctioning Devices

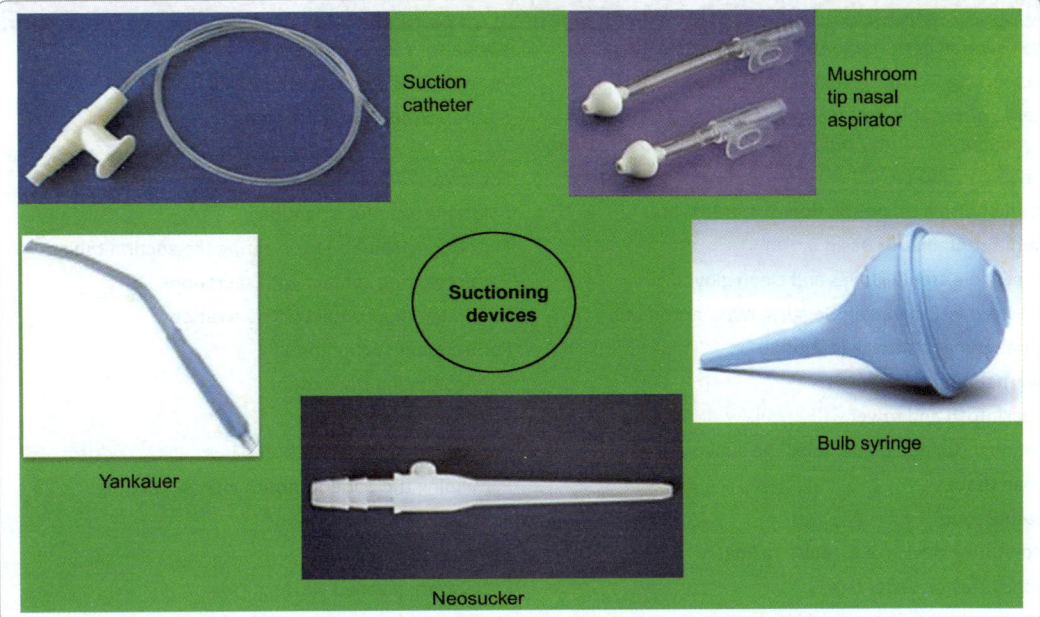

Suction catheter

Mushroom tip nasal aspirator

Suctioning devices

Bulb syringe

Yankauer

Neosucker

General Instructions

- A verbal or written consent should be obtained depending on the patient's condition.
- Know which patients are at risk for aspiration and are unable to clear secretions because of an impaired cough reflex.
- Keep all the necessary supplies readily available at the bedside and ensure suction is functioning.
- Preparation for suctioning depends on an emergent versus a non-emergent need for suctioning. In cases of acute respiratory distress, where obstruction of the airway or the airway adjunct is suspected, suctioning must be performed emergently with even minimal preparation.
- Care should be taken to maintain sterility while suctioning the endotracheal/tracheostomy tubes. Suctioning of the oropharynx or the nasopharynx does not require complete sterility.
- Avoid mouth sutures, sensitive tissues and any tubes located in the mouth or nares.
- Avoid stimulating the gag reflex.
- Know appropriate suctioning limits and the risks of applying excessive pressure or inadequate pressure.
- Always perform a pre- and postrespiratory assessment to monitor patient for improvement.
- If an abnormal side effect occurs (e.g., increased difficulty in breathing, hypoxia, discomfort, worsening vital signs, or bloody sputum), notify appropriate health care provider.
- Do not perform suctioning in the mouth for longer than 10 seconds at a time.
- Empty the canister as required
- The suction unit battery should be charged regularly as per instructions.
- Ensure that the suction catheter has a large hole for the thumb to cover to initiate suction, along with smaller holes along the end, through which mucous enters when suction is applied.
- The oral suctioning catheter is not used for tracheotomies due to its large size.

Appendix 2: Oral Suctioning

Articles Required

Articles	Purpose
Wall suction or portable suction unit	For performing suctioning
Connecting tubing and collecting bottle	For attaching to the suction unit
Sterile disposable oral suction catheters (#10 to #16 French for an adult) / bulb syringe/ or Yankauer catheter	For performing oral suctioning
An oxygen source	For oxygen administration
Sterile normal saline solution or sterile water	Solutions used for irrigation
Sterile container or basin	For pouring solution for clearing the suction tubings
Disposable sterile gloves and clean gloves	For preventing contact with secretions
Required PPE including Goggles, mask apron etc.	For preventing contact with secretions
Oropharyngeal airway (optional)	For frequent suctioning
Overbed table	For positioning the patient
Mackintosh and towel	For protecting the linen
Optional: Tongue blade, tonsil tip suction device	For depressing tongue
Clean tissues	For wiping the patient mouth after suctioning
Stethoscope	For respiratory assessment
Monitoring device, e.g., pulse oximetry	For assessing hypoxia
Kidney tray or paper bag	For disposing soiled waste
Mouth care tray if required	For performing oral care after oral suctioning

Procedure

Steps	Procedure	Rationale
1.	Assess patient need for suctioning (respiratory assessment using stethoscope for signs of hypoxia), risk for aspiration, and inability to protect own airway or clear secretions adequately. Place pulse oximetry probe on the patient's finger.	Physical signs and symptoms indicate the need for suctioning.
2.	Explain the procedure to the patient	Allays anxiety and wins confidence and cooperation.
3.	Ensure the patient's privacy by screening the patient.	Helps to promote dignity
4.	Position the patient in semi-Fowler's or high Fowler's position with head turned to the side or sitting upright. Unconscious patients should be placed in the lateral position.	This facilitates ease of suctioning and prevents aspiration. It also promotes lung expansion and effective coughing. Side placement promotes forward drainage of secretions.
5.	Preoxygenation with 100% oxygen should be initiated prior to suctioning.	This is in preparation for the hypoxia that is precipitated by suctioning, both from mechanical interruption and cessation of oxygen flow briefly.

Contd...

Steps	Procedure	Rationale
6.	Gather articles at the bedside.	Organization promotes skilled performance.
7.	Place Mackintosh and towel on patient's chest.	Prevents patient from coming in contact with secretions.
8.	Wash hands and wear appropriate PPE.	Prevents the transmission of microorganisms. Protective equipment protects you from contact with secretions.
9.	Check date and open the bottle of normal saline solution or sterile water.	Prevents use of contaminated solution.
10.	Using strict aseptic technique, open the suction catheter kit or the packages containing the sterile catheter, container and sterile gloves. Don the gloves.	Ensures sterility of the procedure. Water is used to clear connection tubing in between suctions (at least three times)
	Consider your dominant hand sterile and your nondominant hand nonsterile. Using your nondominant hand, pour the saline solution into the sterile container.	
	Fill sterile container with approximately 100 mL of sterile normal saline solution or sterile water.	
11.	Attach one end of connection tubing to the suction machine and the other end to the Yankauer.	This prepares equipment to function effectively.
	Pick up the catheter with your dominant (sterile) hand and attach it to the connecting tubing.	
	Use your nondominant hand to control the suction valve while your dominant hand manipulates the catheter. Do not allow the suction catheter to touch any unsterile surface.	
12.	Turn on suction from the wall or portable unit to the required level and set the pressure according to your facility's policy.	Elevated pressure settings increase risk of trauma to mucosa and can induce greater hypoxia.
	Test function by covering hole on the suction catheter with your thumb and suctioning up a small amount of water.	Tube occlusion tests suction apparatus
	Set regulator to appropriate negative pressure: Wall suction, 80–150 mm Hg; portable suction, 7–15 mm Hg for adults. (For detail refers Appendix 1)	

Contd...

Appendix 2: Oral Suctioning

Steps	Procedure	Rationale
13.	Remove patient's oxygen mask if present. Nasal prongs may be left in place. 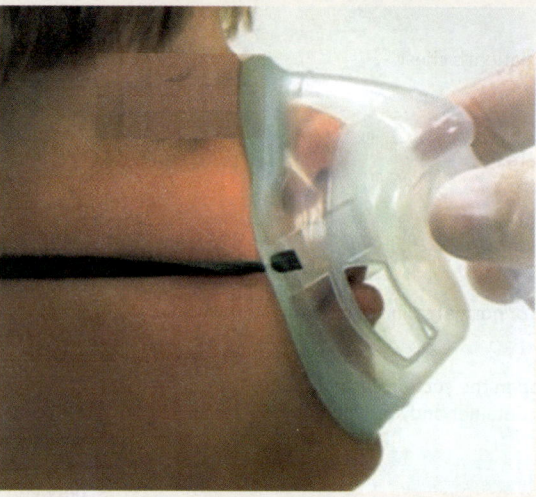 Instruct the client to cough and breathe slowly and deeply several times before beginning suction. 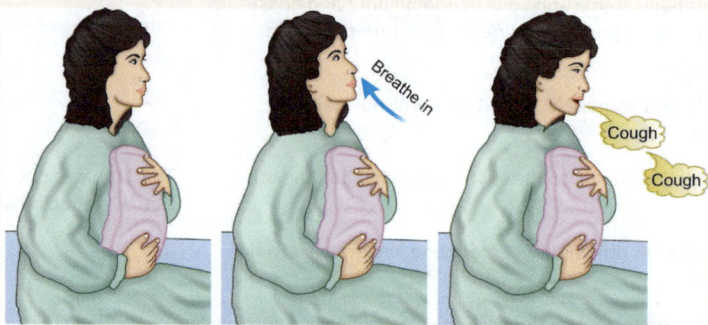	Coughing helps loosen secretions and may decrease amount of suction necessary, while deep breathing helps minimize or prevent hypoxia.
14.	Insert suction catheter into client's mouth and apply suction by covering the thumb hole. Leave the vent open when introducing the catheter. 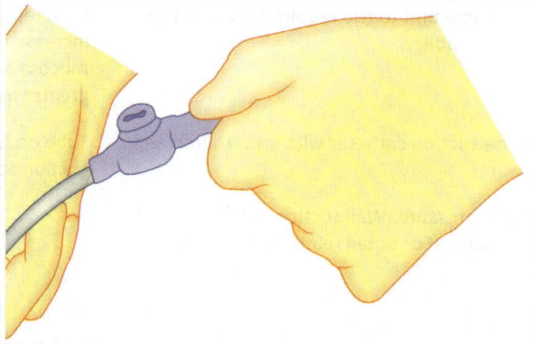	Rolling the tube back and forth ensures suctioning in all areas Coughing helps move secretions from the lower airways to the upper airways.

Contd...

Steps	Procedure	Rationale
	Apply suction by placing the thumb over vent and withdraw the catheter with a rotating motion.	

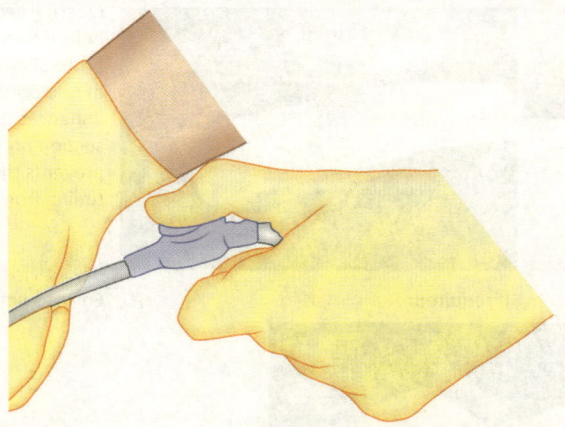

Run catheter along gum line to the pharynx in a circular motion, keeping Yankauer moving.

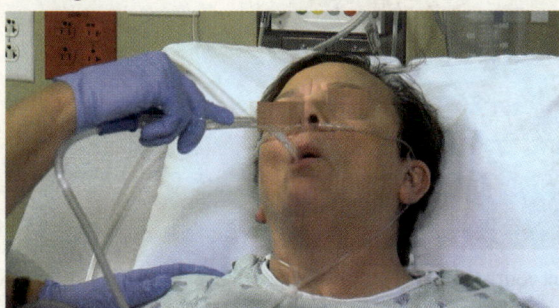

Apply intermittent suction, take care not to allow suction tip to invaginate oral mucosal surfaces with continuous suction. Encourage patient to cough.

| 15. | Apply suction for a maximum of 10–15 seconds. Allow patient to rest in between suction for 30 seconds to 1 minute. | |

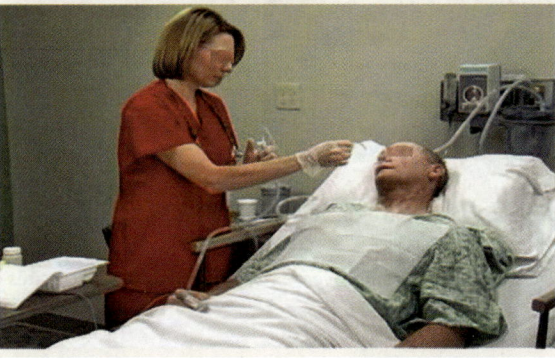

Contd...

Steps	Procedure	Rationale
16.	If required, replace oxygen on patient and clear out suction catheter by placing yankauer in the basin of water. 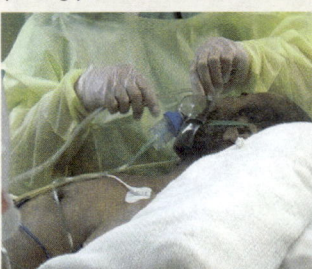 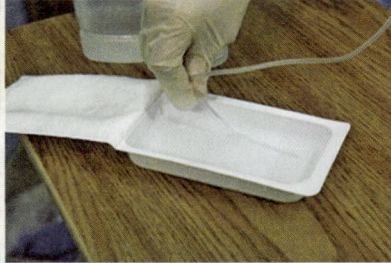	Replace oxygen to prevent or minimize hypoxia. Clearing secretions before they dry reduces probability of transmission of microorganisms and enhances delivery of preset suction pressures. It also prevents the connection tubing from plugging.
17.	Reassess and repeat oral suctioning if required. 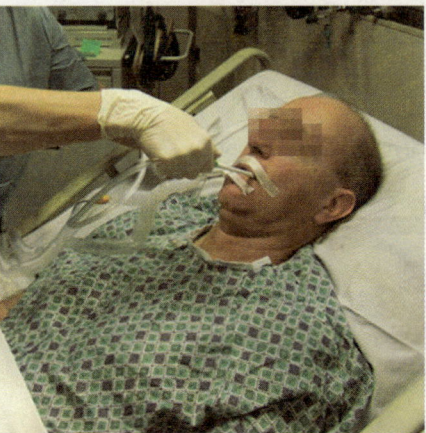	Ensures patency of airway
18.	After completing suctioning, pull your sterile glove off over the coiled catheter and discard it. 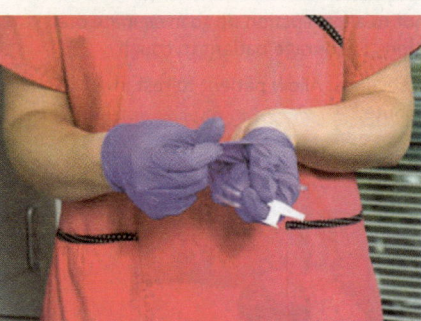 If the catheter has to be reused, place catheter in a clean dry area for reuse with suction turned off.	Ensures safe disposal of catheter and gloves without contamination.
19.	Reassess respiratory status and O_2 saturation for improvements.	Facilitates comparison of respiratory status with the baseline assessment.

Contd...

Appendix 2: Oral Suctioning

Steps	Procedure	Rationale
20.	Ensure patient is in a comfortable position and call bell is within reach. Provide oral hygiene if required.	This promotes patient comfort.
21.	Clean up supplies, Discard the used items and replace with new supplies so they will be ready for the next suctioning.	Having the supplies at the bedside facilitates a quick response.
22.	Remove clean gloves and wash hands.	Prevents the transmission of microorganisms.
23.	Document procedure with the date, time including • Reason for suctioning • Technique used • Amount, color, consistency and odor (if any) of the secretions • The client's respiratory status before and after the procedure • Any complications and the nursing action taken • The client's tolerance for the procedure along with signature of the nurse	Documentation fosters quality care.

3 NASOPHARYNGEAL SUCTIONING

Nasopharyngeal suctioning is a technique used to clear secretions from the nasopharynx through the application of negative pressure via a suction catheter or bulb syringe.

Purpose

- To remove secretions from the pharynx by a suction catheter inserted through the nostril.

Indications

- Nasopharyngeal suction is indicated when there is evidence of retained secretions but the patient is not able to clear the secretions independently
- If the secretions are too deep in the airway for nasal suction.

Contraindications

- Unexplained hemoptysis (the coughing up of blood from the lungs or bronchi) or known clotting disorder
- Laryngospasm (stridor)
- Bronchospasm
- Basal skull fractures and other causes of cerebrospinal fluid leakage via the ear
- Pneumothorax
- Recent esophageal or tracheal anastomoses and other forms of tracheobronchial trauma
- Occluded nasal passages
- Unexplained nasal bleeding
- Severe hypoxemia/hypoxia
- Raised intracranial pressure
- Acute hypo or hypertension

Preliminary Assessment

- Assess the institution policy to determine whether a physician's order is required for nasopharyngeal suctioning.

- Assess the client's blood gas or oxygen saturation values and check vital signs.
- Assess the client's ability to cough and deep breathe to determine the ability to move secretions up the tracheobronchial tree.
- Assess the client's history for a deviated septum, nasal polyps, nasal obstruction, traumatic injury, epistaxis, or mucosal swelling.

Articles Required

Articles	Purpose
Wall suction or portable suction unit	For performing suctioning
Connecting tubing and collecting bottle	For attaching to the suction unit
An oxygen source	For oxygen administration
Sterile normal saline solution or sterile water	Solutions used for irrigation
Sterile nasopharyngeal suction catheter (#10 to #16 French for an adult)	For performing nasopharyngeal suctioning
Sterile container or basin	For pouring solution for clearing the suction tubings
Disposable sterile gloves and clean gloves	For preventing contact with secretions
Required PPE including goggles, mask, apron etc.	For preventing contact with secretions
Nasopharyngeal airway (optional)	For frequent suctioning
Overbed table	For positioning the patient
Mackintosh and Towel	For protecting the linen
Clean tissues	For wiping the patient nose during and after suctioning
Stethoscope	For respiratory assessment
Monitoring device, e.g., pulse oximetry	For assessing hypoxia
Kidney tray or paper bag	For disposing soiled waste
Sterile lubricant	For preventing mucosal damage by lubricating the suction tip.

Procedure

Steps	Procedure	Rationale
1.	Assess patient need for suctioning (respiratory assessment using stethoscope for signs of hypoxia), risk for aspiration, and inability to protect own airway or clear secretions adequately. Place pulse oximetry probe on the patient's finger.	Physical signs and symptoms indicate the need for suctioning.
2.	Explain the procedure to the patient.	Allays anxiety and wins confidence and cooperation.
3.	Ensure the patient's privacy by screening the patient.	Helps to promote dignity.
4.	Position the patient in semi-Fowler's or high Fowler's position with head turned to the side or sitting upright. Unconscious patients should be placed in the lateral position.	This facilitates ease of suctioning and prevents aspiration. It also promotes lung expansion and effective coughing. Side placement promotes forward drainage of secretions.

Contd...

Steps	Procedure	Rationale
5.	Increase supplemental oxygen therapy to 100% or as ordered by physician. Encourage the client for deep breathing.	This is in preparation for the hypoxia that is precipitated by suctioning, both from mechanical interruption and cessation of oxygen flow briefly. Deep breathing helps to reduce suction-induced hypoxemia.
6.	Gather articles at the bedside.	Organization promotes skilled performance.
7.	Place Mackintosh and towel on patient's chest.	Prevents patient from coming in contact with secretions.
8.	Wash hands and wear appropriate PPE	Prevents the transmission of microorganisms. Protective equipment protects you from contact with secretions.
9.	Check date and open the bottle of normal saline solution or sterile water.	Prevents use of contaminated solution.
10.	Using strict aseptic technique, open the suction catheter kit or the packages containing the sterile catheter, container and sterile gloves. Don the sterile gloves.	Ensures sterility of the procedure. Water is used to clear connection tubing in between suctions (at least three times)
	Consider your dominant hand sterile and your nondominant hand nonsterile. Using your nondominant hand, pour the saline solution into the sterile container. Fill sterile container with approximately 100 mL of sterile normal saline solution or sterile water.	
11.	Attach one end of connection tubing to the suction machine and the other end to the suction catheter.	This prepares equipment to function effectively.
	Pick up the catheter with your dominant (sterile) hand and attach it to the connecting tubing. Use your nondominant hand to control the suction valve while your dominant hand manipulates the catheter. Do not allow the suction catheter to touch any unsterile surface.	
12.	Turn on suction from the wall or portable unit to the required level and set the pressure according to your facility's policy.	Elevated pressure settings increase risk of trauma to mucosa and can induce greater hypoxia.
	Test function by covering hole on the suction catheter with your thumb and suctioning up a small amount of water.	Tube occlusion tests suction apparatus.
	Set regulator to appropriate negative pressure: wall suction, 80–150 mm Hg; portable suction, 7–15 mm Hg for adults.	
13.	Remove patient's oxygen mask or nasal prongs if present.	This may hinder the procedure. Coughing helps loosen secretions and may decrease amount of suction necessary, while deep breathing helps minimize or prevent hypoxia.

Contd...

Appendix 3: Nasopharyngeal Suctioning

Steps	Procedure	Rationale
	Instruct the client to cough and breathe slowly and deeply several times before beginning suction.	

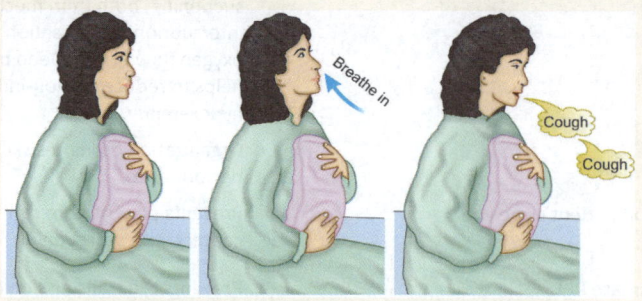

| 14. | Open lubricant. Squeeze small amount onto open sterile catheter package without touching package. Lubricate 3" to 4" of the catheter tip with irrigating solution. Water soluble lubricant is used to avoid lipoid aspiration pneumonia. | Lubrication prevents mucosal trauma when catheter is inserted. Excessive lubricant can occlude catheter. |

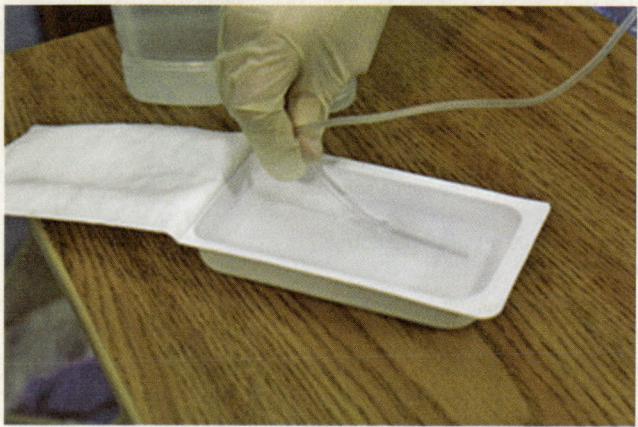

| 15. | Measure catheter from the tip of the nose to the tip of the earlobe. It is approximately 16 cm in adults; 8–12 cm in older children; 4–8 cm in young children and infants. | Proper placement ensures removal of pharyngeal secretions. |

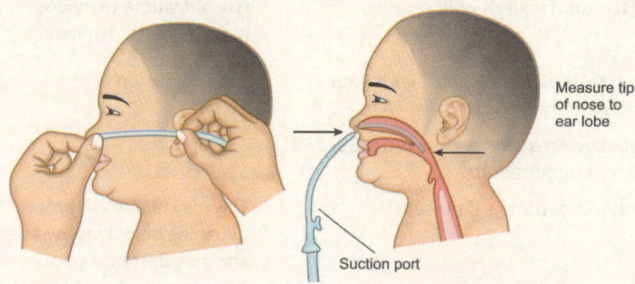

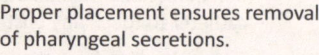

Contd...

Appendix 3: Nasopharyngeal Suctioning

Steps	Procedure	Rationale
16.	Raise the tip of the client's nose with your nondominant hand to straighten the passageway and facilitate insertion of the catheter. Follow natural course of nares slightly slant catheter downward and advance to back of pharynx. Advance the catheter as far as possible to the measured length. Without applying suction, gently insert the suction catheter into the client's nares.	Rolling the tube back and forth ensures suctioning in all areas.

Leave the vent open when introducing the catheter.

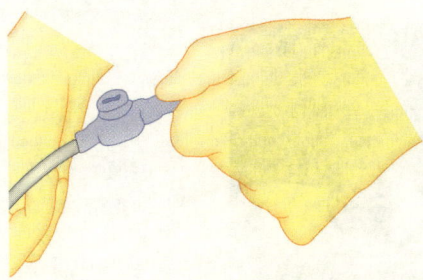

Roll the catheter between your fingers to help it advance through the turbinates. Continue to advance the catheter, approximately 5"–6" (12.7–15 cm), until you reach the pool of secretions or the client begins to cough.

Using intermittent suction, withdraw the catheter from the nose with a continuous rotating motion to minimize invagination of the mucosa into the catheter's tip and side ports.

Apply suction for only 10–15 seconds at a time to minimize tissue trauma.

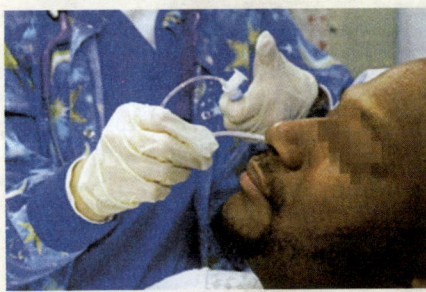

Apply suction by placing the thumb over vent and withdraw the catheter with a rotating motion.

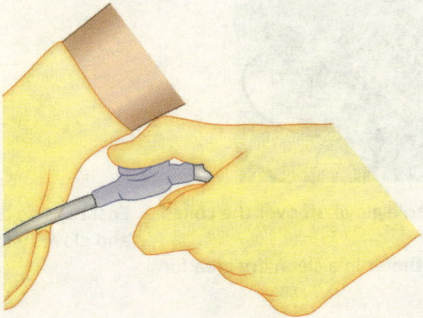

Contd...

Appendix 3: Nasopharyngeal Suctioning

Steps	Procedure	Rationale
17.	Repeat the procedure, up to 3 times, until gurgling or bubbling sounds stop and respirations are quiet. Allow 30 seconds to 1 minute to allow reoxygenation and reventilation. If the client has no history of nasal problems, perform alternate suctioning between nostrils. If repeated nasopharyngeal suctioning is required, the use of a nasopharyngeal or oropharyngeal airway will help with catheter insertion, reduce traumatic injury and promote a patent airway. 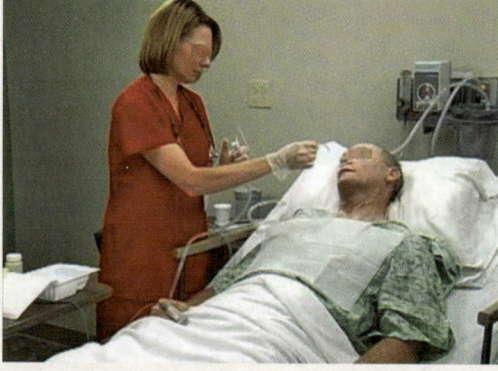	Alternate suctioning in nostrils minimize traumatic injury.
18.	If required, replace oxygen on patient and clear out suction catheter by placing it in the basin of water. 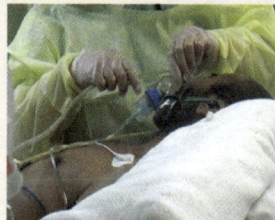 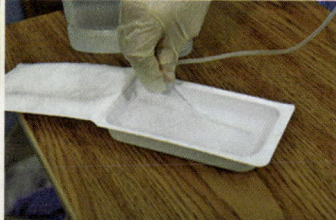	Replace oxygen to prevent or minimize hypoxia. Clearing secretions before they dry reduces probability of transmission of microorganisms and enhances delivery of preset suction pressures. It also prevents the connection tubing from plugging.
19.	Reassess and repeat suctioning if required. 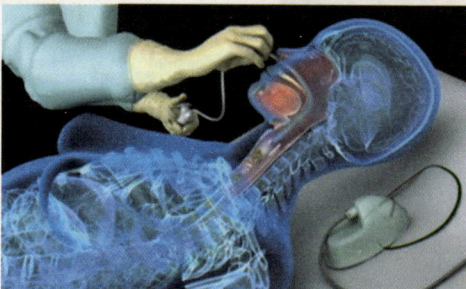	Ensures patency of airway
20.	After completing suctioning, pull your sterile glove off over the coiled catheter and discard it. If the catheter has to be reused, place catheter in a clean dry area for reuse with suction turned off.	Ensures safe disposal of catheter and gloves without contamination.

Contd...

Steps	Procedure	Rationale
21.	Reassess respiratory status and O_2 saturation for improvements.	Facilitates comparison of respiratory status with the baseline assessment.
22.	Ensure that patient is in a comfortable position and call bell is within reach.	This promotes patient comfort.
23.	Clean up supplies, Discard the used items and replace with new supplies so they will be ready for the next suctioning.	Having the supplies at the bedside facilitates a quick response.
24.	Remove gloves and wash hands.	Prevents the transmission of microorganisms.
25.	Document procedure with the date, time including • Reason for suctioning • Technique used • Amount, color, consistency and odor (if any) of the secretions • The client's respiratory status before and after the procedure • Any complications and the nursing action taken • The client's tolerance for the procedure along with signature of the nurse.	Documentation fosters quality care.

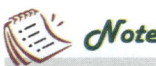 *Note*

Preoxygenation should be used with caution in oxygen sensitive clients such as those with chronic heart and lung conditions and those with pneumonia.

 4 MAINTAINING INTAKE OUTPUT CHART

Fluid Balance Chart

It is known as the **Fluid-Balance Chart.** It is the measurement and recording of all intake of fluids and all outputs during 24 hours period with the purpose of assessing the fluid and electrolyte balance and early detection of any abnormalities.

Purposes of Intake and Output

- The intake and output chart is a tool used for the purpose of documenting and sharing information.
- It ensures accurate record keeping.
- It prevents circulatory overload.
- It prevents dehydration.
- It aids in analyzing trends in fluid status.
- It contributes to accurate assessment record.
- It helps us to ensure that whatever is taken by the patient especially fluids either via the gastrointestinal tract (enterally) or through the intravenous route (parenterally) is excreted or removed from the patient.

Indications of Intake and Output Chart

- In case of dehydration
- Congestive heart failure
- Taking diuretics or corticosteroids
- Severe vomiting or diarrhea
- Patients with kidney impairment
- Fluid and electrolyte imbalance
- Dark concentrated urine
- Excessive perspiration

Appendix 4: Maintaining Intake Output Chart

- Recent surgical procedure
- Client's with burns
- Dialysis patients
- Any bleeding
- Dry mucous membrane
- Decreased or little urine output

Importance of Maintaining I/O Chart

It helps us determine the patient's fluid status especially:

- Hydration status
- Status of dehydration
- Fluid overload
- Rule out any obstruction

Normal Fluid Balance

Intake		Output	
Ingested liquid	1500 mL	Urine	1500 mL
Ingested food	800 mL	Skin loss	600 mL
Metabolism	200 mL	GI loss	100 mL
		Loss through lungs	300 mL
Total	2500 mL/day	Total	2500 mL/Day

Structure of Intake Output Chart

- The intake-output chart is so named because on one side is the intake and on the other side is the output.
- I/O charts are usually single sheets of standard A4 paper and are often separated from the main medical record e.g., placed on a clip board.
- The chart is a table where the rows divide the chart into time intervals.
- The columns indicate the type and amount of the fluid that has been given and the mode and site of administration, the fluid output including urine, discharges or drainage.
- Normally the empty chart is pre-printed and the data is entered in ink.
- Measurements of volume are in mL.
- The chart is for a 24 hours period but, for practical reasons, it does not follow the calendar day (i.e., from 12 midnight to 12 midnight of the next day). Rather, it follows the nursing shift, i.e., usually from 7 a.m. on the starting day to 7 a.m. the next day.
- While the order or plan may extend into the nursing morning shift of the next day, the intake and output measurements end with the night shift. Charting is then started on a new form.

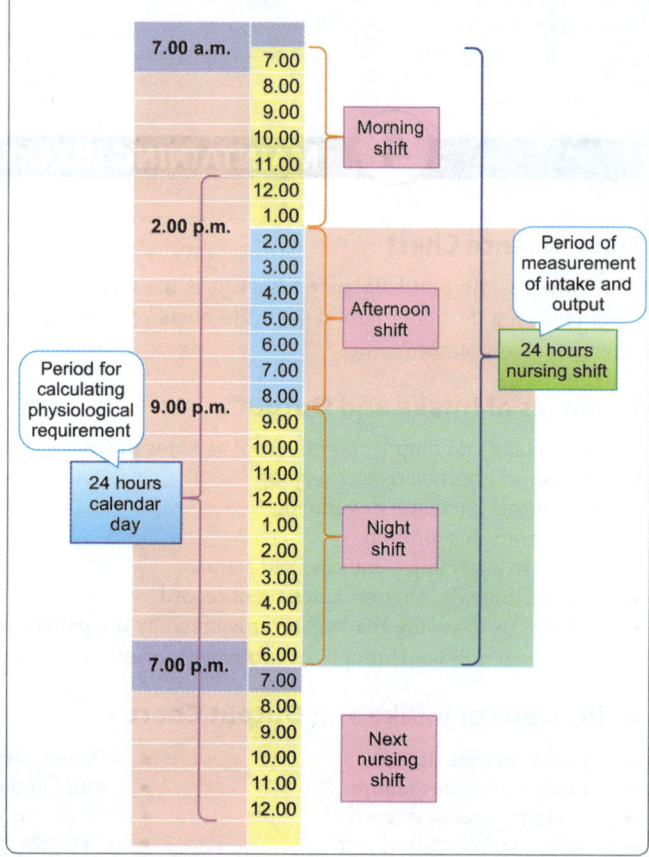

Appendix 4: Maintaining Intake Output Chart

- It is important to document the name of the patient, the registration number/medical record number and the (starting) date for which the chart is used.
- At the end of the patient's stay, the charts should be reincorporated as part of the medical record.
- All relevant particulars of the input and output data are charted in the appropriate time-interval (period) on the chart under the relevant chart headings (column and row titles).
- The amount of both, the input and the output is totaled for every shift (sub-total) and for the 24 hours period (grand total) starting at 7.00 a.m. and ending at 6.59 a.m. the next day.

INTAKE-OUTPUT CHART

Name					Registration number			
Date								

TIME	INTAKE (ml)				OUTPUT (ml)			
MORNING SHIFT	Method		Site		Urine	N/G Aspirate	Drains Stoma etc.	Stool B.O.
07.00 a.m.	Type of Fluid	Addition	Amount					
			Put up	Gone in				
02.00 p.m.		Remainder						
		Total at end of shift						

TIME	INTAKE (ml)				OUTPUT (ml)			
AFTERNOON SYIFT	Method		Site		Urine	N/G Aspirate	Drains Stoma etc.	Stool B.O.
02.00 p.m.	Type of Fluid	Addition	Amount					
			Put up	Gone in				
09.00 p.m.		Remainder						
		Total at end of shift						

TIME	INTAKE				OUTPUT			
NIGHT SHIFT	Method		Site		Urine	N/G Aspirate	Drains Stoma etc.	Stool B.O.
09.00 p.m.	Type of Fluid	Addition	Amount					
			Put up	Gone in				
07.00 a.m.		Remainder						
		Total at end of shift						

Contd...

Appendix 4: Maintaining Intake Output Chart

	NOTES		SHIFT TOTAL (ml)		24 HOUR BALANCE (ml)			
Morning			Intake		**From**		**To**	
Shift			Output		**Date**		**Date**	
					Time		**Time**	
Afternoon			Intake		**Total Intake**			
Shift			Output					
Night			Intake		**Total Output**			
Shift			Output		**Difference**			

Data Entered for the Input

- Water
- Juice
- Milk/coffee/tea
- Yogurt
- Ice

- IV fluids
- Enteral/Tube feedings
- Any liquid
- Blood transfusion

Documenting IV Infusion

- At the beginning of putting up an IV infusion
- At the beginning of a shift
- Whenever a pack is finished and another is put up
- Whenever the regime is changed
- The nurse enters the actual time that he/she starts the infusion rather than the time planned
- The nurse on duty calculates the cumulative total at the end of the shift
- The remainder or amount left-over of any IV fluid or enteral fluid in the container is noted to be carried forward to the next shift in the 'remainder' column

TIME	INTAKE					OUTPUT			
	Method		**Site**			Urine	N/G Aspirate	Drains Stoma etc.	Stool B.O.
NIGHT SHIFT	*Intravenous Infusion*		*Peripheral vein left hand*						
		Type of Fluid	**Additions**	**Amount**					
09.00 p.m.				**Put up**	**Gone in**				
Carry forward	*Dextrose 5 %*		*Nil*	100					
					100				
10.00 p.m.	*Normal saline in Dextrose 5 %*		*1 gm KCl*	500					
					500				
03.00 a.m.	*Dextrose 5 %*		*Nil*	500					
04.00 a.m.						300			
					400				
7.00 a.m.			**Remainder**	100					
			Total at end of shift	1000		300			

Cumulative Total (Each Shift)

Data Entered for the Output

The type of fluid that is excreted or drained out is indicated by the headings on separate columns. These include:

- Urine
- Nasogastric aspirate
- Drainage from drainage tubes, stomas etc.
- Stool/feces (only the occurrence of passage of stool is recorded. In children with diarrhea the loss may be measured)
- Vomiting
- Blood
- NG drainage
- For children—weigh the diapers. 1 g of diaper weight = 1 mL of urine

Measuring Urine Output

- In a patient, who is alert and not on a urinary drainage catheter, the patient or care giver collects the urine in a urinal or bottle each time urine is passed.
- The amount is usually measured by a nurse or nursing aid using a measuring jug and recorded on the chart.
- Dependable patients may also be allowed to measure the urine and record them on a slip of paper before recording them. The nurse copies the amount onto the I/O chart.
- Urine output may need to be measured at the end of a shift or more often (e.g., hourly).
- As the urinary catheter is attached through into a collapsible plastic with markings, the amount can be read from these markings or by emptying the entire content of the bag into a measuring jug when it is full or at the end of the shift or day.

Measuring Losses from Drainage Tubes

- To measure the loss, one method is to read from markings on drainage bags/bottles.
- After reading the loss for the current period, she may use an ink marker or tape to indicate on the bag or bottle the level when it was last read.
- The amount at the end of a shift is calculated by subtracting the amount of the previous reading from the accumulated amount.
- In the second method, reading is done and then the whole bag or bottle is emptied.
- Other forms of fluid or semi-fluid may be discharged by the body. These include:
  - Intestinal contents
  - Gastric juice from a nasogastric tube
  - Urine from a nephrostomy tube
  - If the patient has a fistula originating from the jejunum or ileum, the intestinal contents are collected into a jejunostomy or ileostomy bags.

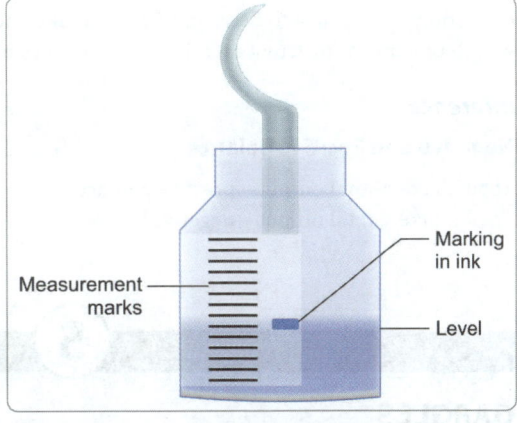

Appendix 4: Maintaining Intake Output Chart

- Measurement of the output is made by transferring the content into a measuring–container or aspirated with a syringe.
- The time of measurement for each output is written on a separate row unless it coincides with the time when the input was recorded. There should be enough rows on the chart to record the time of intake as well as output.

Articles Required

Articles	Purpose
Intake and output chart	For documentation
Calibrated drinking glass	For measuring the intake
Bedside commode/male and female urinal	For excretion of urine
Calibrated container	For measuring urine output or other outputs
Gloves	For preventing contact with body secretions
Weighting scale	For measuring the diapers

Procedure

- Explain the purpose and procedure for measuring I/O to the client.
- Record the volume for all fluids consumed.
- Make sure that all IV fluids or tube feedings are being administered at the prescribed rate. Ensure that the nurse who adds additional IV fluid containers also records the volume.
- Keep track of fluid volumes used to irrigate drainage tubes or flush feeding tubes.
- Wear gloves.
- Measure and record the volume of voided urine, urine collected in a catheter drainage bag, liquid stool or other.
- Wash hands.
- Check the volume remaining in currently infusing IV fluids.
- Record the total amount of all fluid intake and output volumes.
- Compare the data to determine if the intake and output are approximately the same.
- Report major differences in I/O to the client's physician.

Inference

Negative and Positive Balance

Total intake > total output—positive balance
Total intake < total output—negative balance

GARGLING

GARGLES

In order to gargle, concentrated, clear aqueous solution is used in the posterior region of mouth to prevent the throat infection.

Gargling is the act of bubbling liquid in the mouth. In this, air is forced through liquid and it is held at the back of the mouth causing it to bubble and flurry.

It is also described as washing of one's mouth and throat with a liquid that is kept in motion by breathing through it with a gurgling sound.

Purposes

- Gargling can moisten a sore throat and bring temporary relief.
- Gargling with salt water can alleviate symptoms and even help to prevent upper respiratory infections.
- It also helps to remove the mucus build-up in the respiratory tract and nasal cavity.
- It may help relieve the symptoms of the common cold.

Uses

- Astringent
- Antiseptic/antibacterial
- Antisoreness

SALT WATER GARGLE

Salt water gargles are an easy and natural home remedy that helps to soothe the inflammation of the throat.

Mechanism of Action

- The addition of salt to a glass of warm water is used as a gargle.
- This creates an osmosis effect where the concentration of salt draws fluids from the mouth and throat tissues to relieve a painful infection.
- It also breaks up thick mucus, which can remove irritants like allergens, bacteria and fungi from the throat.

Benefits of Gargling with Salt Water

- Soothes inflammation and prevents recurrence of infection.
- It can help to alleviate throat inflammation caused by seasonal allergies, colds, and sinus infections.
- Pain caused by bleeding gums and canker sores can also be lessened by a periodic salt water gargle.
- Salt water neutralizes acids caused by invading bacteria. This, in turn, helps keep a balanced pH level in your mouth (the bacteria would much prefer a steamy, acidic home), which can help prevent gingivitis.
- Salt water can also guard against the spread of fungal infections such as the yeast Candidiasis.
- A salt water gargle can thin the sore-throat-causing mucus build-up in the respiratory tract and nasal cavity.

Side Effects of a Salt Water Gargle

Too much salt can dehydrate the mouth and throat tissues.

Articles Required

A tray containing:

Articles	Purpose
A cup of warm water	For gargling
Table salt	For gargling
Spoon	For stirring the salt in warm water
Kidney tray	For collecting the waste and spit out water
Tissue paper or a wash cloth	For wiping the mouth
Towel	For spreading under the neck in order to protect the clothing

Appendix 5: Gargling

Procedure

Steps	Procedure	Rationale
1.	Explain the procedure to the patient	Allays anxiety and wins confidence and cooperation.
2.	**Preparation of a salt water gargle:** • Wash hands • Take a glass full of warm pure water and not tap water.	Hot water may burn the mouth. Use pure water because tap water often includes chlorine, which could irritate the throat and weaken the immune system.

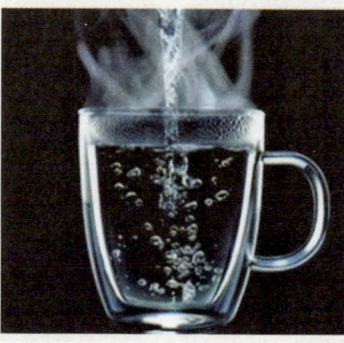

• Add a pinch of salt or quarter to half a spoon of table salt to it.

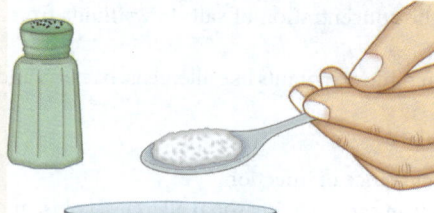

• Simply stir until it is completely dissolved.

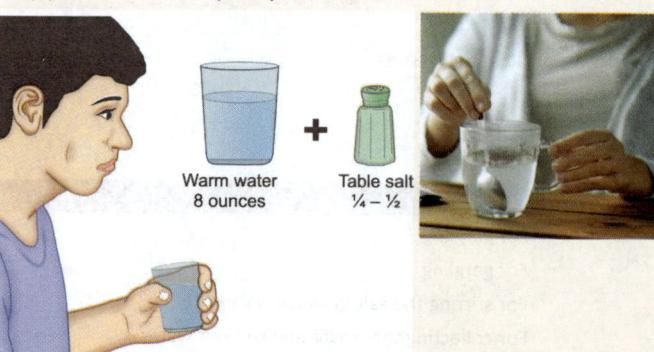

Warm water 8 ounces + Table salt ¼ – ½

Contd...

Steps	Procedure	Rationale
3.	Arrange the articles near to the patient	Organization promotes skilled performance.
4.	Wash hands 	Prevents transmission of microorganisms
5.	Place a towel down the neck of the patient 	Prevents soiling of clothes
6.	Take a large sip of the warm salt water solution 	Ensures entry of adequate water into the back of the throat.

Ask the patient to tilt head back, and gargle the solution holding it into the back of the throat for 15–30 seconds

Contd...

Steps	Procedure	Rationale
7.	Swish the water around the teeth and gums before spitting it out into the wash basin or kidney tray.	Washes out debris present in the mouth.

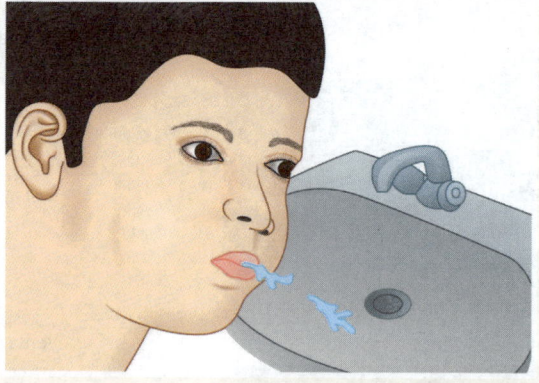

Steps	Procedure	Rationale
8.	Repeat this method until the cup of salt water is finished. And the procedure has to be repeated every four hours until sore throat subsides.	Soothes the throat.

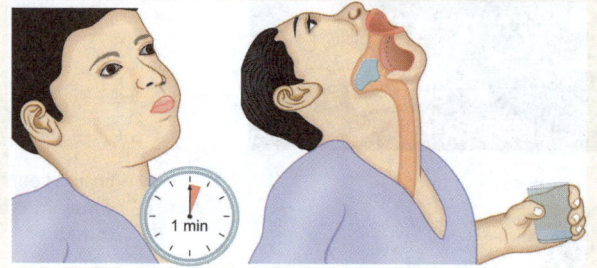

Steps	Procedure	Rationale
9.	Replace the articles and wash hands.	Prevents transmission of microorganisms.

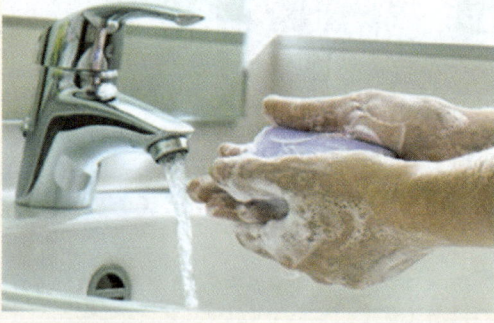

Steps	Procedure	Rationale
10.	Document the procedure, with date and time, the response of the patient along with the signature of the nurse.	Documentation fosters quality care.

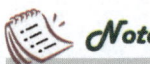 **Note**

Readymade solutions are available as gargles, e.g., betadine, hydrogen peroxide, hexidine, phenol

Appendix 5: Gargling

6 INSTILLATION OF EAR DROPS

Ear Drops

Ear drops are medications that are instilled into the auditory canal to produce the local effects, solutions ordered to treat the ear are often referred to as otic **(pertaining to the ear) drops.**

Purposes

- To combat infection
- To soften the ear wax
- To produce local anesthesia and to reduce pain in the ear
- To kill an insect lodged in the auditory canal
- To facilitate removal of a foreign body
- To treat infection or inflammation

Pre Requisites

- Check the physician's order for installation of ear drops and any specified instructions with regard to the side of instillation that is right ear/left ear etc.
- Check the ten rights of medication administration.
- Certain medications are contraindicated for certain ear disorders. Hence, know the diagnosis of the patient and the therapeutic effect of the medication.
- The auditory canal should be thoroughly cleaned before instilling the ear drops.
- Drops must be warm when they are instilled into the ear, otherwise it may cause vertigo. In order to warm the ear drops, place the container in a bowl of warm water or rinse the dropper 3 or 4 times in hot water and then take the medications.
- Place the patient in a side-lying position or in the dorsal recumbent position with the head turned to one side with the affected ear uppermost.
- Before instilling a solution into the ear, the nurse should inspect the ear for signs of drainage, an indication of a perforated tympanic membrane. Eardrops are usually contraindicated when the tympanic membrane is perforated.

Articles Required

A clean tray containing:

Article	Purpose
Hand washing solution or hand rub	For hand washing
Medication bottle with sterile dropper	For ear instillation
Small bowl—2 One bowl to place cotton balls or cotton tipped applicator One bowl to keep hot water.	To plug the ear after application and to clean the ear To warm the solution if it is cool

Contd...

Article	Purpose
Small cotton balls or cotton tipped applicator	For cleaning the ear and to plug the ear

Disposable gloves (optional) as per Institution policy	For preventing cross infection
Kidney tray	For collecting soiled waste
Tissue paper	For wiping the ears
Mackintosh and towel	For protecting the linen

Preparation of Patient

- Explain the procedure to the patient.
- Position the patient comfortably.
- Ensure that the patient is not allergic to any of the ear drops ingredients.
- Examine the ear for any discharge.

Position of Patient

- Sitting (on a comfortable chair) and tilting the head to the side with the ear to be treated facing up; or
- Side lying down with the affected ear up.

Preparation of Unit

- An area of good lighting
- Arrange all the necessary articles near to the bedside

Procedure

Steps	Procedure	Rationale
1.	Explain the procedure to the patient. Provide privacy.	Allays anxiety and helps to win the confidence and cooperation of the patient.
2.	Arrange the articles at the bedside.	Organization facilitates skilled procedure.

Contd...

Steps	Procedure	Rationale
3.	Position the patient comfortably, either in a chair with or in a side lying position with the affected ear facing upwards. Place the mackintosh and towel under the head. 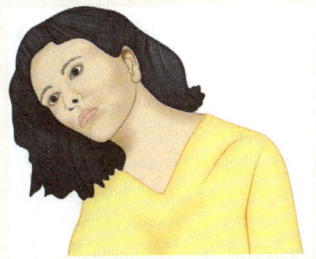 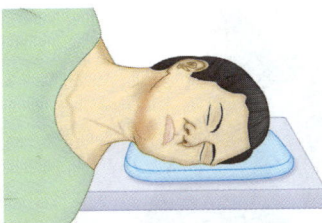	Facilitates comfortable administration of ear drops. Prevents soiling of linen and clothes.
4.	Wash hands and don gloves 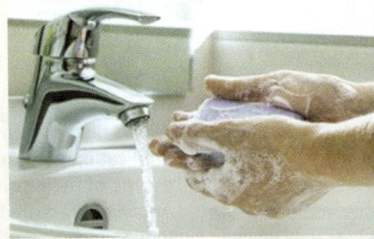 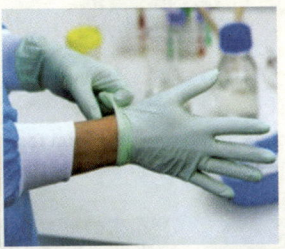	Prevents cross infection.
5.	With your non dominant hand straighten the ear canal by pulling the pinna • Down and back for children • Upward and outward for adults 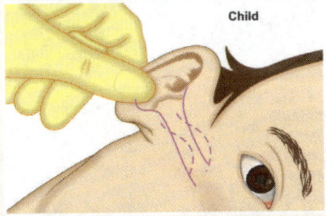 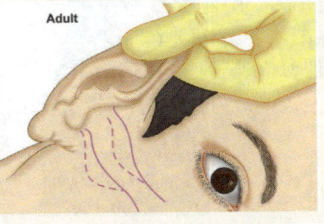	Pulling the pinna straightens ear canal.
6.	With your dominant hand, draw up medication into ear dropper, ensuring correct dosage. Hold dropper tip just above ear canal. 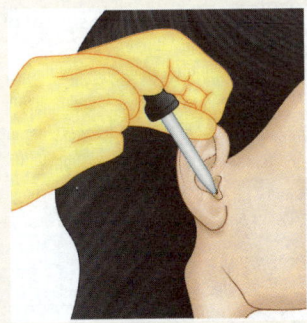 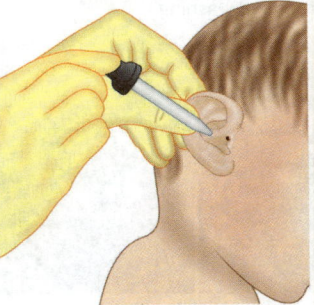	Touching the ear with the dropper tip may contaminate the medication. Allows the air to escape from the auditory canal.

Contd...

Appendix 6: Instillation of Ear Drops

Steps	Procedure	Rationale
	Do not touch the ear with the dropper tip. Instil the drops into the side wall of the auditory canal by holding the dropper at least ½ inch above the ear canal. 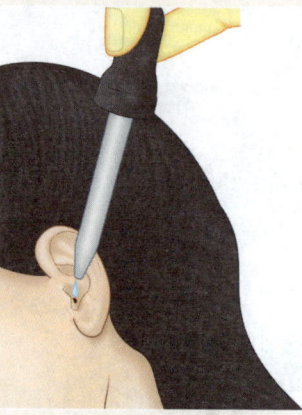	
7.	Instruct the patient to remain in the same position for at least few minutes. Apply gentle pressure to tragus several times. Plug the ear with a cotton or gauze piece, if indicated. 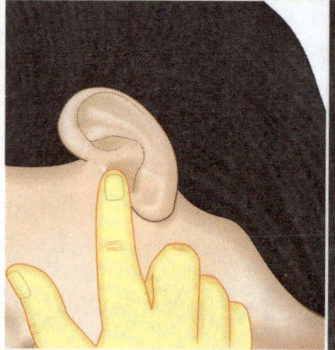 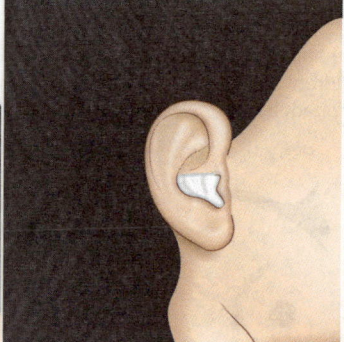	Allows distribution of medication and prevents escape of medication. Applying pressure helps to move medication toward tympanic membrane.
8.	Replace articles and assist patient to a comfortable and safe position.	Ensures patient safety and comfort.
9.	Remove gloves and perform hand washing 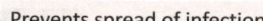 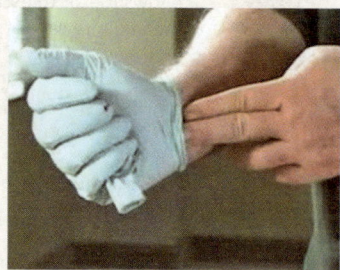 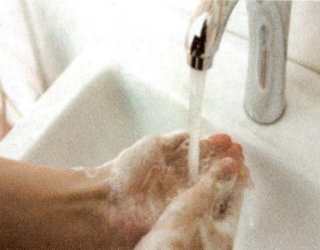	Prevents spread of infection

Contd...

Steps	Procedure	Rationale
10.	Document date, time, name of the drug, dose, route, the side of the ear the medication was instilled into, number of drops and patient's response to procedure with signature.	Documentation fosters quality care

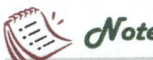 *Note*

- Allow 3 or 4 drops to trickle down on one side of the canal so that the drops may reach up to the ear drum.
- Ask the patient to remain in the same position for a few minutes following instillation.
- Any complaint made by the patient should not be ignored.
- Medication should never be forced into the ear canal especially if it is occluded (as by wax). Forcing medication into an occluded eardrum can injure the eardrum.

7   INSTILLATION OF EYE DROPS

Eye Drops

Medications are administered or instilled in mucous membranes of eye for various therapeutic purposes. Instillation of eye drop is the dispensation of a sterile ophthalmic medication into a patient's eye.

Purposes

- To combat infection
- To relieve inflammation
- To relieve pain and discomfort
- To dilate or constrict the pupil
- To treat eye disorders such as glaucoma
- To diagnose foreign bodies and corneal abrasions

Indications

- Routine—eye examination
- Healing—vitamin C eye drops for severe chemical injury
- Lubrication—paraffin for comfort and to prevent recurrent corneal erosions
- Emergency use—eye irrigation for chemical burns
- Diagnostic procedures—dilating drops and fluorescein dye
- Analgesic and anesthetic—local anesthetic for eye examination
- Mydriasis—pupil dilation for visualization of fundus
- Procedural—anesthetic eye drops before eye wash
- Prophylaxis—seasonal conjunctivitis
- Therapeutic glaucoma

Contraindications

- Allergies to the medications

Prerequisites

- Check the physicians order for instillation of eye drops or ointment and any specified instructions with regard to the site of instillation, right eye/left eye/both eyes etc.
- Check the ten rights of medication administration.
- Certain medications are contraindicated for certain eye disorders. Hence, know the diagnosis of the patient and the therapeutic effect of the medication.
- **Inspect the eye drops**: Look at the liquid inside the container closely.
  - Check for anything floating in the solution (unless there are supposed to be particles in the drops). Don't use the drops if they have small bits floating in them.
  - Be sure the product says 'ophthalmic' somewhere on the label. It is easy to confuse ear drops that say 'otic' on the label, with those that are to be administered in the eye.
  - Check the medication for any discoloration, cloudiness and precipitation. Do not use, if present.
  - Inspect the container to be sure it has not been damaged. Check the tip of the container, without touching it, to be sure there is no visible damage or discoloration.
- When separate bottles are used for each eye, label it as left eye and right eye.
- Eye drops and ointment should be administered:
  - At the correct time
  - In the correct strength
  - Via the correct route
  - To the right person
  - Into the correct eye
- To improve flow of ointment, hold tube in hand for several minutes to warm it before use.
- Do not allow medication in an eye dropper to flow back into the bulb of the dropper.
- Do not return the remaining medication of the eye dropper back into the bottle after instillation.
- To prevent wastage, take only the required amount of solution in the dropper.
- Read specific instructions given on the leaflets supplied with the medications.
- Never use any solution or ointment which is unlabeled to instill in the eye.
- Instruct a contact lens wearer to avoid drops with preservatives as these increase corneal contact time and may lead to corneal toxicity.
- Do not share eye drops

 Note

- When both eye drops and eye ointment are prescribed, always instill the eye drops first and then eye ointment.
- Eye drops are sterile products. Don't try to open it using safety pins. Use only pointed tip inside the cap to pierce the bottle.

Articles Required

Article	Purpose
Hand washing solution or hand rub	For hand washing
A clean tray containing: Medication bottle with sterile dropper or ointment tube	For eye instillation
Small bowl–2 One bowl to place cotton balls or gauze pledgets One bowl to keep cooled boiled water/normal saline	For removing the dried crust or left over ointment or dust and wiping the eye

Contd...

Appendix 7: Instillation of Eye Drops

Article	Purpose
Small cotton squares or gauze pledgets 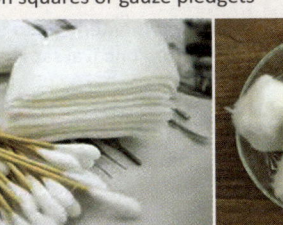 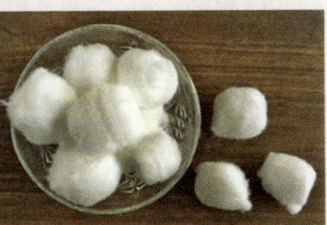	For removing the dried crust and wiping the eye
Normal saline solution or cooled boiled water	For softening the dried crust and removing
Disposable gloves (optional) as per institution policy	For preventing cross infection
Drops dispenser or ointment applicator (Optional)	For comfortable instillation of medication
Tissue paper	For wiping the eye
Kidney tray	For collecting the soiled waste
Mackintosh and towel	To protect linen

Preparation of Patient

- Explain the procedure to the patient
- Position the patient comfortably
- Inform the patient that Eye medications may cause burning or blurring for a few minutes.
- Ensure that the patient is not allergic to any of the eye drops or ointment ingredients
- Examine the eyes and eyelids for signs of improvement or deterioration everytime before application

Position of Patient

- Sitting (on a comfortable chair) or
- Lying down (semi-prone or recumbent) with the head supported with a pillow.

Preparation of Unit

- Administer eye drops in an area of good lighting
- Arrange all the necessary articles near to the bedside

Procedure

Steps	Procedure	Rationale
1.	Explain the procedure to the patient. Explain the need and reason for instilling drops or ointment.	Helps to win the confidence and cooperation of the patient.
2.	Screen the patient	Provides privacy.
3.	Position the patient comfortably, either in a chair with the head well supported or place the head over a pillow if patient is lying down. Place the mackintosh and towel under the head.	Helps to prevent solution or tears flowing towards the other eye. Facilitates easy view of the eye to apply drops

Contd...

Appendix 7: Instillation of Eye Drops

Steps	Procedure	Rationale
4.	Wash hands and apply gloves	Prevents cross infection
5.	Cleanse the eyelids and lashes with cotton balls or gauze pledgets moistened with cooled boiled water or sterile normal saline when there are crusty or purulent deposits on the eyelids.	Prevent debris entering into the eye when the conjunctival sac is exposed.
6.	Dip cotton ball in boiling water/normal saline. Squeeze out excess liquid and use the moist cotton ball to wipe and clean crusts around the eyelids.	Helps to prevent solution or tears flowing toward the other eye.
7.	Use one cotton ball or pledget for only one stroke, moving from the inner to the outer canthus of the eye.	Prevents carrying of debris to the lacrimal duct.
8.	Wash hands again before proceeding with instilling the eye drops.	Prevents cross infection
9.	Unscrew the bottle and keep the cap on a clean tissue paper. Do not touch the tip of the dropper.	Prevents entry of Microorganisms

Contd...

Appendix 7: Instillation of Eye Drops

Steps	Procedure	Rationale
10.	Gently agitate the bottle around gently for 30–40 seconds before inserting drops	Ensures the drug is properly mixed
11.	Ask the patient to look up at the ceiling or behind.	Helps to ensure the eye drop does not land directly onto the sensitive cornea.

Steps	Procedure	Rationale
12.	Gently pull the lower eye lid and the dropper is held perpendicular to the eye. This can be done by **Method I:** Pulling downward with one finger	The pocket so formed can hold one drop of medicine

Method II: Pinching the lower lid. This creates a pocket into which a drop may be inserted.

Contd...

Appendix 7: Instillation of Eye Drops

Steps	Procedure	Rationale
13.	Squeeze the upturned dropper bottle and Instil the eye drop into the space (fornix) or the pocket by holding the bottle approximately 1–2 cm (1/2–3/4 in) above conjunctival sac. Make sure the drop goes in, if in doubt apply one more drop. Alternatively, an eye drop applicator can be used. 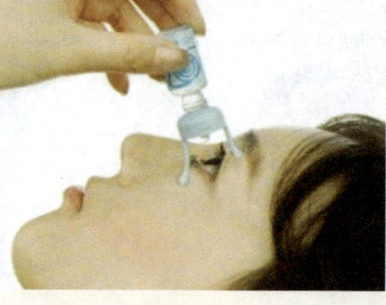	Squeezing helps free flow of medication. Instillation from a distance prevents • Contamination of the dropper • Accidental injury to cornea and other structures
14.	Release the eyelid and ask the patient to gently close the eyes for one minute. 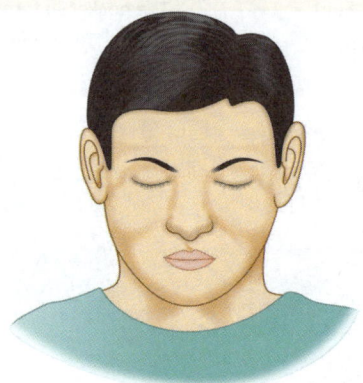	Ensures absorption of drug and avoids spillage of medicine out of the eye.
15.	Apply gentle pressure over the area of lacrimal sac between the root of the nose and junction of upper and lower eye lids. Hold the pressure for 1–3 minutes. 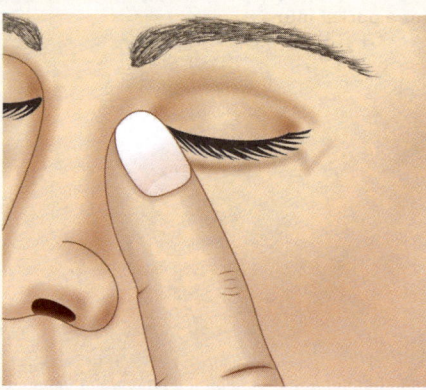	Prevents the eye drops from draining down these ducts to the nose. 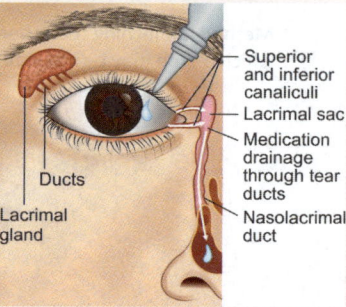

Labels on image 4:
Superior and inferior canaliculi
Lacrimal sac
Medication drainage through tear ducts
Nasolacrimal duct
Ducts
Lacrimal gland

Contd...

Steps	Procedure	Rationale
16.	Ask him/her to blink the eye	Blinking helps to distribute the medication.
17.	Wipe any extra drops and tears from the closed lids or cheek with a tissue paper or gauze pledgets.	Promotes comfort

Steps	Procedure	Rationale
18.	If more than one eye drop has to be applied, wait at least five minutes before applying the second eye drop.	Immediate administration makes the first drop from being washed out by the second before it has had time to work.

Steps	Procedure	Rationale
19.	If drops land on outer lid margins, repeat procedure	Accidental spillage may hamper exact delivery of dosage.
20.	Replace the bottle cap immediately after use.	Keeps the medication clean.
21.	Replace all articles	Helps to keep the unit clean
22.	Remove gloves and wash hands	Prevents cross infection
23.	Position the patient comfortably	Ensures patient comfort

Appendix 7: Instillation of Eye Drops

Procedure for Applying Eye Ointment

Steps	Procedure	Rationale
1.	Explain the procedure to the patient	Helps to win the confidence and cooperation of the patient
2.	Position the patient comfortably, either in a chair with the head well supported or place the head over a pillow, if he/she is lying down.	Helps to prevent solution or tears flowing towards the other eye. Facilitates easy view of the eye to apply drops
3.	Wash hands	Prevents cross infection
4.	Cleanse the eyelids and lashes with cotton balls or gauze pledgets moistened with cooled boiled water or sterile normal saline when there are crusty or purulent deposits on the eyelids.	Prevent debris entering into the eye when the conjunctival sac is exposed
5.	Dip cotton ball in boiling water/normal saline. Squeeze out excess liquid and use the moist cotton ball to wipe and clean crusts around the eyelids.	Helps to prevent solution or tears flowing towards the other eye.
6.	Use one cotton ball or pledget for only one stroke, moving from the inner to the outer canthus of the eye.	Prevents carrying of debris to the lacrimal duct.
7.	Wash hands	Prevents cross infection
8.	Read the prescription thoroughly to establish the site in the eye where ointment has to be applied. For example, may be for structures other than the eye, such as an eyelid wound.	Ensures correct dosage of medicine at appropriate site to hasten quick recovery
9.	Ask the patient to look up at the ceiling or behind.	This helps to ensure the eye drop does not land directly onto the sensitive cornea.
10.	**Two methods:** • Instil a thin ribbon of the ointment squeezed directly into the lower fornix from the inner canthus to the outer canthus • A small line of ointment can be squeezed onto the appropriate applicator. Gently place the applicator in the lower fornix without touching the cornea.	Helps to make sure your eye gets the correct amount of medication

Contd...

Steps	Procedure	Rationale
11.	Ask the patient to gently close the eyes.	The ointment may take a few moments to melt and spread over the eye.
12.	The applicator is withdrawn at the outer canthus with the eyes still closed.	Avoids spillage of ointment
13.	Wipe the excess ointment from the eyelids using a tissue paper or gauze pledget.	Promotes comfort
14.	Ask the patient roll his/her eye behind closed lids.	Helps to distribute the medication
15.	Discard a small amount of ointment on a sterile cotton ball and wipe the top of the tube. Replace the cap.	Facilitates comfortable usage of medication next time. Dried crusts of ointment if present may block the passage.
16.	Replace all articles	Helps to keep the unit clean
17.	Wash hands	Prevents cross infection
18.	Position the patient comfortably	Ensures patient comfort

 Stimulant

Closed eye technique: Recommended for patients who find it difficult to have drops instilled directly into the eye, for example, children or older people. Use this technique as a last resort.
- Ask the patient to lie flat or with his/her head tilted back
- Administer a drop of the medication onto the closed eyelid in the nasal corner
- Ask the patient to open the eye and close it gently once the drug has entered it

Postprocedure Care

- Do not try to push tears that overflow back into the eye.
- Do not rub eyes.
- Do not massage the eyeball after the instillation of medications.
- Observe for possible side effects.
- If drops are for reuse they should be labelled and returned to the fridge or storage area.
- Eye medications may cause burning for a few minutes. However, if the medications cause redness, or swelling of the eye lids, or severe itching inform your eye doctor immediately.
- Store at correct temperature.
- Avoid contaminating eye dispenser from contact with eye, eyelid, eyelashes, or finger.
- When administering drugs such as Beta blocker drops, the punctum (tear duct) should be occluded by applying the forefinger for approximately three to five minutes to limit systemic absorption through the nasal passages. Beta blockers can cause bronchoconstriction, hypotension, bradycardia, nausea, diarrhea, anxiety, depression, hallucinations and fatigue.

Appendix 7: Instillation of Eye Drops

Safety Considerations

- After administration of eye drops or ointments, patients must be advised against driving or operating machinery until their vision has cleared and/or their eyes have stopped stinging.
- It is important to read the instructions carefully regarding storage of eye medications. Correct medication storage is essential.
- Some eye drops, such as chloramphenicol, must be stored in a refrigerator before and after opening while others are stored in the refrigerator after opening only.
- In hospital settings, eye drops should be discarded after seven days and replaced if the treatment continues.
- In non-hospital settings, drop bottles should be replaced every 28 days.
- Write down the first date of opening on the bottle to remember when to stop its use.

Documentation Record

- Time on which the medication was instilled
- The eye onto which the medication was instilled
- Type, strength and amount (dosage) of the medication
- Any adverse effects noticed
- Patient response

INSTILLATION OF NASAL DROPS OR SPRAY

Nasal Instillation

Nasal instillation is delivering medicine directly into the nose and onto the nasal membranes.

Purposes

- To combat infection of the nasal cavity or sinuses
- To provide astringent effect
- To relieve inflammation and congestion in case of rhinitis
- To give local anesthesia
- To shrink swollen mucous membranes
- To loosen secretions and facilitate drainage

Prerequisites

- Check the physician's order for instillation of nasal drops and any specified instructions with regard to the side of instillation, right nose/left nose/both etc.
- Check the ten rights of medication administration.
- Avoid oil based solutions as nasal drops, since it interferes with the normal ciliary action and may cause aspiration pneumonia if aspirated into the lungs because oily solutions will not be absorbed and will act as a foreign body.
- See that the anterior nares are clean and free from discharges.

Articles Required

Article	Purpose
Hand washing solution or Hand rub	For hand washing
A Clean tray containing: Medication bottle with sterile dropper	For nasal instillation
Small bowl	To place cotton balls or cotton tipped applicator
Small cotton balls or cotton tipped applicator	For cleaning the nose
Disposable gloves (optional) as per Institution policy	For preventing cross infection
Kidney tray	For collecting soiled waste
Tissue paper/rag pieces	For wiping the nose
Mackintosh and towel	For protecting the linen
Sputum mug	For spitting medication that enters the throat.

Preparation of Patient

- Explain the procedure to the patient.
- Position the patient comfortably.
- Ensure that the patient is not allergic to any of the nasal drops or spray.
- Examine the nose for any discharge, swelling etc.

Preparation of Unit

- Administer in an area of good lighting
- Arrange all the necessary articles near to the bedside

Procedure for Instilling Nasal Drops

Steps	Procedure	Rationale
1.	Explain the procedure to the patient. Explain that the patient may feel a burning sensation or choking sensation or both as the drop trickles down the throat.	Allays anxiety and helps to win the confidence and cooperation of the patient.
2.	Screen the patient.	Provides privacy.
3.	Arrange the articles at the bedside.	Organization facilitates skilled procedure.

Contd...

Appendix 8: Instillation of Nasal Drops or Spray

Steps	Procedure	Rationale
4.	Position the patient comfortably, in supine position with hyperextending the neck. Place the mackintosh and towel under the head. 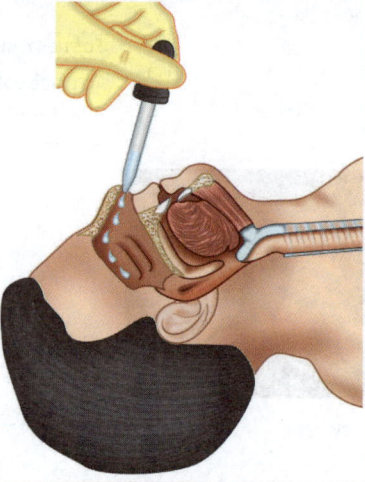	Facilitates comfortable administration of nasal drops Prevents soiling of linen and clothes
5.	Provide patient with tissues and Instruct the client to blow the nose unless contraindicated 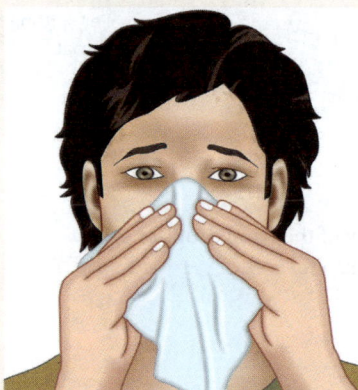	Removes mucous and secretions that might hinder absorption of medication
6.	Wash hands and don gloves 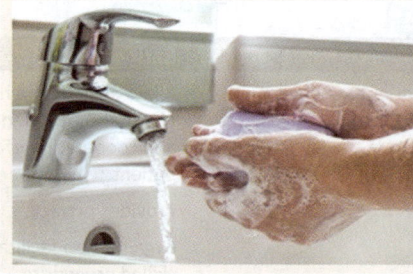 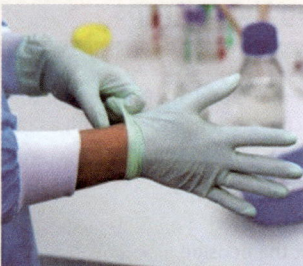	Prevents cross infection

Contd...

Steps	Procedure	Rationale
7.	Draw fluid into medication dropper with enough for both nares. Ask patient to breathe through the mouth. 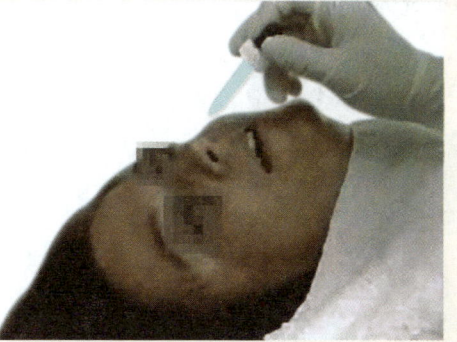	Breathing through the mouth will help prevent aspiration of the medication

Hold dropper about 1 cm above nares and drop 2–3 drops of medication into one nare and then the other.

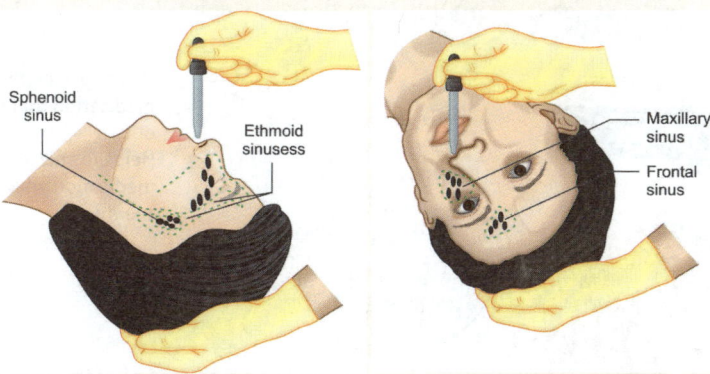

If it is nasal spray, instruct the patient to close one nostril and breathe gently through the other as the spray is being administered. Repeat in another nostril.

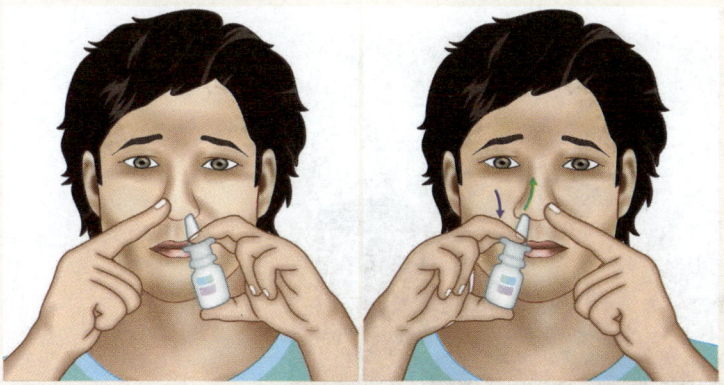

Care should be taken not to touch the nares with the dropper/spray bottle.

Contd...

Appendix 8: Instillation of Nasal Drops or Spray

Steps	Procedure	Rationale
8.	Position patient with head back for few minutes. And make the patient lower his/her head to eye level and gently move it left and right to allow the medication to flow to the lower part of the nose. 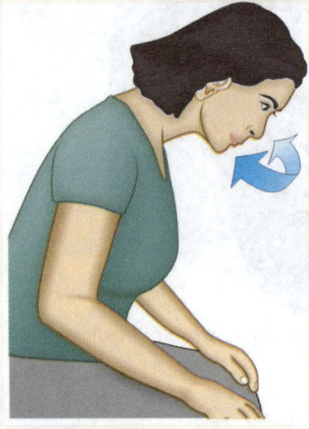	This position prevents escape of the medication
9.	Provide tissue paper or rag pieces. 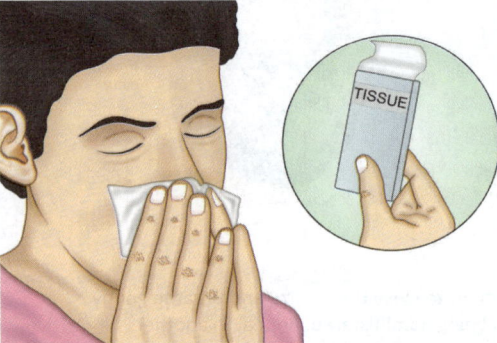	Helps to wipe the medication that escapes out Helps to spit the medication which enters the throat
	Provide sputum mug. 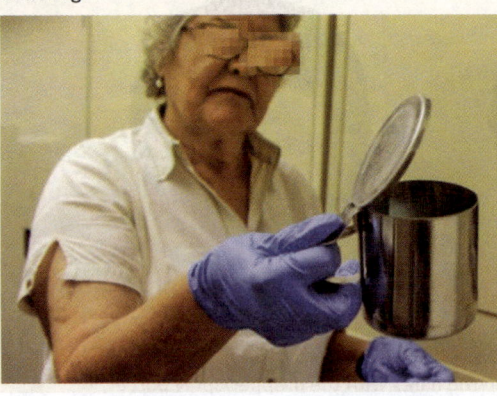	

Contd...

Steps	Procedure	Rationale
10.	Replace articles and assist patient to have a comfortable and safe position.	Ensures patient safety and comfort
11.	Remove gloves and perform hand washing	Prevents spread of infection
12.	Document date, time, name of the drug, dose, route, the side of the nose the medication was instilled into, number of drops and patient's response to procedure with signature.	Documentation fosters quality care

 *Note*

- Ask the patient to remain in the same position for sometime after the instillation of the drug. This allows the solution to flow into the posterior nares. It gives time for the medication to act on the mucus membranes of the anterior portion and then it can drain into the posterior nares.
- Be careful not to infect the dropper by touching it on the tip of the nose. Contamination of the dropper will cause contamination of the medicine in the container.

 9 NASAL SPRAYS

These are liquid medicines that are sprayed into the nose.
Both solution and suspension formulations can be formulated as nasal sprays.

Purposes

- Used to relieve the symptoms of sinusitis, hay fever, allergic rhinitis and non-allergic (perennial) rhinitis.
- Reduces inflammation and histamine production in the nasal passages.
- Relieves nasal congestion, runny nose, itchy nose and sneezing.

Types

Nasal spray comes in many forms:
- A regular spray, e.g., Otrivin spray (Xylometazoline)

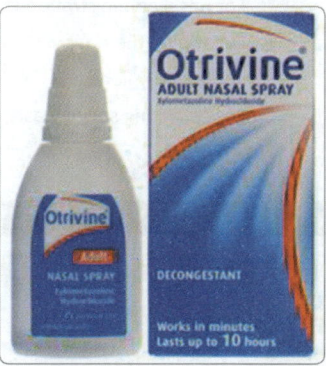

- Metered-dose spray pumps or a pump spray, e.g., Afrin pump mist (oxymetazoline)

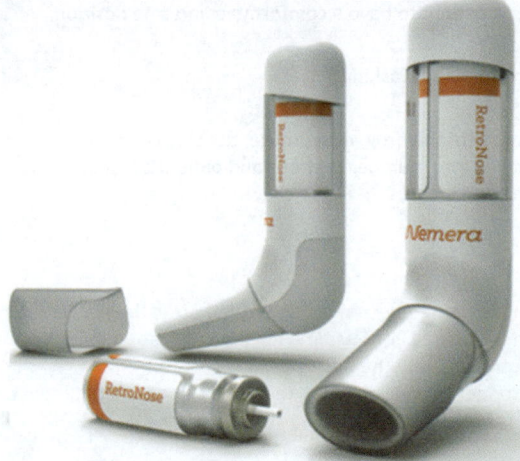

- Mucosal atomization device (MAD—commonly used in emergency, e.g., teleflex (naloxone)

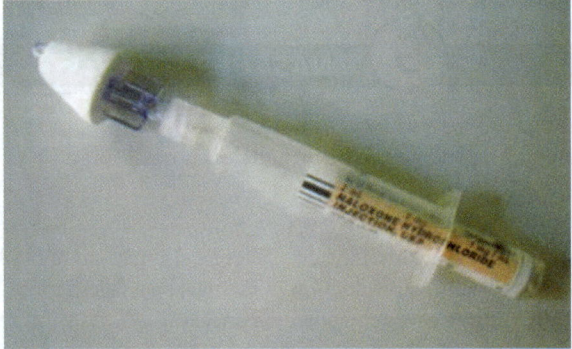

Articles Required

Articles	Purpose
Nasal spray	For nasal administration
Tissue paper	For wiping the nose
Handrub	For hand hygiene
Kidney tray	For collecting soiled waste

Procedure

Steps	Procedure	Rationale
1.	Explain the procedure to the patient	Allays anxiety and wins confidence and cooperation
2.	Arrange the articles at the bedside	Organization promotes skilled performance

Contd...

Steps	Procedure	Rationale
3.	Ask the patient to gently blow the nose (or use a saline spray or rinse, then wait 10 minutes before using the spray medication).	Helps to clear the nasal passages

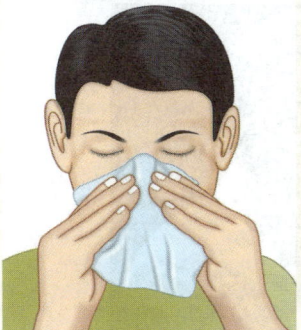

Steps	Procedure	Rationale
4.	Perform hand hygiene. Wear PPE as per Institution policy.	Prevents transmission of microorganisms
5.	Shake the nasal spray bottle gently. Prime the bottle by spraying the product one or more times into the air or into a tissue paper until a mist form. Care should be taken not to spray on face.	Helps in mixing up of medication

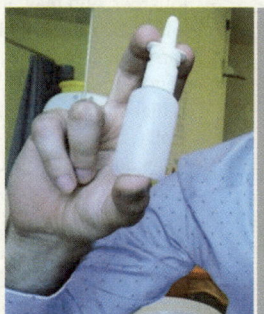 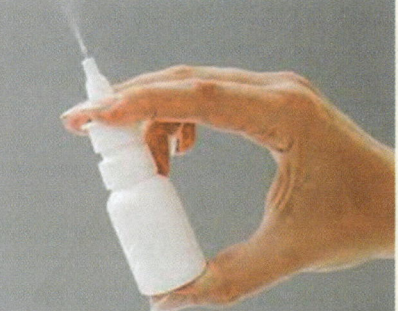

Steps	Procedure	Rationale
6.	Tilt the head forward for about 45 degrees. Support the head with one hand.	Tilting the head back allows the medicine to flow through the nose to the throat and may be swallowed and absorbed into the gastrointestinal tract. Supporting the head prevents neck strain

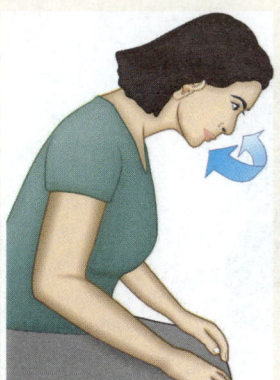 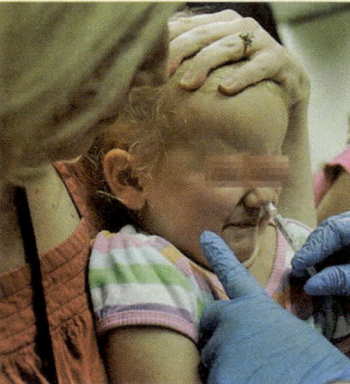

Contd...

Appendix 9: Nasal Sprays

Steps	Procedure	Rationale
7.	Close the nostril that is not receiving the medication. Do this by gently pressing on that side of nose. 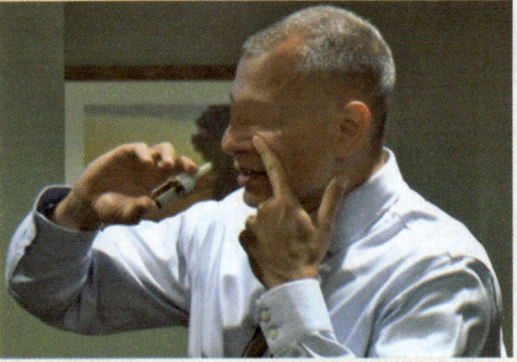	Breathing through the mouth will help prevent aspiration of the medication
8.	Gently put the nozzle into one nostril using the opposite hand—right hand for left nostril and vice versa. Avoid pushing it in hard. Direct the nozzle slightly away from the midline to avoid contact with the septum. 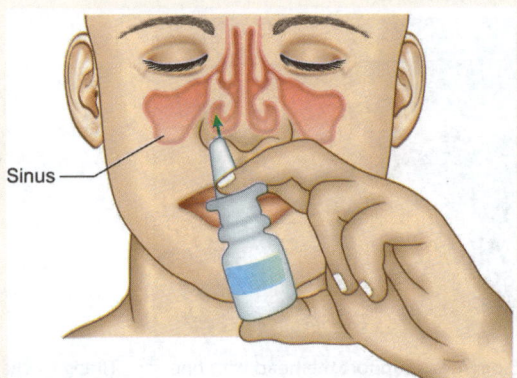 Sinus	Pushing hard avoids damaging the septum. It may result in a higher concentration on the areas likely to be most inflamed and may promote wider distribution within the nose, because the concentration of ciliated cells is higher in the lateral nasal wall • Avoiding the septum might reduce the risk of nosebleed
	Aim the nozzle toward the hole inside the nose: • Slightly to the outside, not towards the septum • Inwards towards the middle of the head (parallel to the roof of the mouth), not towards the top of the nose. If it is a pump spray, hold the bottle with the index and middle fingers on each side of the bottle and the thumb on the bottom of the bottle. 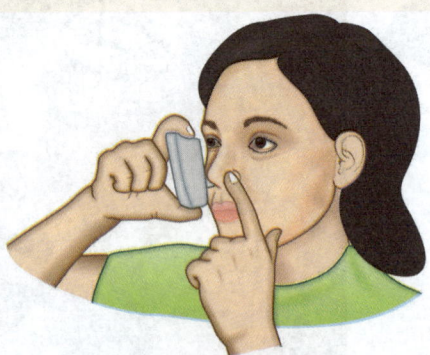	

Contd...

Steps	Procedure	Rationale
9.	Breathe in deeply through that nostril as you squeeze the bottle or by pressing down the pump with the index and middle fingers. Breathe in gently and deeply through that nostril and press to spray at the same time. Squirt once or twice (2 different directions). Remove the bottle and sniff once or twice. Avoid sniffing hard during or after spraying. 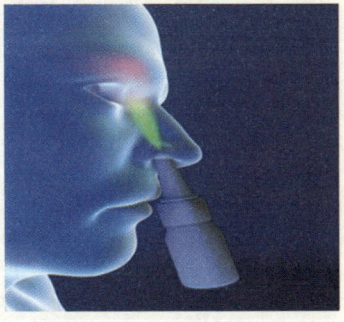	This improves the distribution of the spray. Vigorously inhaling while spraying does not improve distribution and could increase oropharyngeal deposition. Sniffing could force the spray into the back of the throat instead of inside the nose where it needs to work.
10.	Repeat if directed. Wait at least 10 seconds between sprays. Repeat steps for the other nostril. If you have been advised to use two different nasal sprays, use one, wait 10 minutes, then use the other 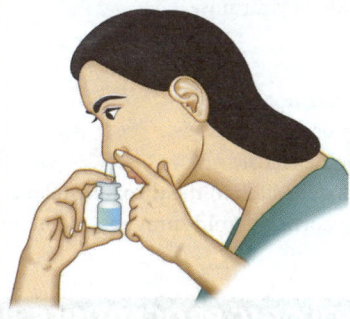	Helps in drug absorption and prevents untoward effects
11.	Instruct the patient to keep the head tilted back for several minutes and to breathe slowly through nose. Instruct the patient not to blow the nose for several minutes 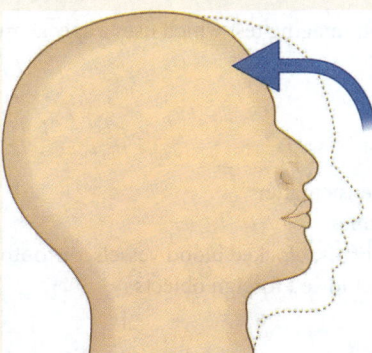	Facilitates drug absorption and prevents escape of the medication

Contd...

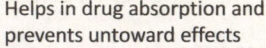

Appendix 9: Nasal Sprays

Steps	Procedure	Rationale
12.	Wipe the tip of the spray device with a tissue paper. Put the cap back on the bottle. Wait a few minutes to blow the nose after using the nasal spray.	Prevents contamination of the bottle
13.	Wash your hands	Prevents transmission of microorganisms
14.	Document the procedure with date and time, medicines used, patient response, any adverse events along with the signature of the nurse.	Documentation fosters quality care

Errors to Avoid

- Spray tip touching anything besides the inside of your nose.
- Forgetting to prime the spray device
- Skipping doses
- Wrong head position (should be tilted forward, not back)
- Pushing the nozzle too hard or far into the nose
- Blowing nose hard after spraying (the medicine is lost)
- Sniffing hard after spraying (the medicine is deposited in the throat instead of the nose)
- Using saline sprays or irrigations after using corticosteroid spray instead of before

(10) RADIOLOGIC PROCEDURES

X-RAY

An X-ray (also called radiography) is a common imaging test which uses a special method for taking pictures of areas inside the body.

Purposes

- To see inside the body
- To differentiate between soft tissues and dense matter
- To locate fractures and infections in the bones
- To detect benign or cancerous tumors, arthritis, blocked blood vessels, or tooth decay
- To diagnose digestive tract problems or swallowed foreign objects

General Instructions

- Collect history specifically related to child bearing age/pregnant, if they are breastfeeding
- Informed consent in certain radiologic procedures

- Provide privacy
- Collect the previous film and note review if any
- Through explanation regarding the procedure. It is essential to inform before taking an X-ray, that small amounts of radiation will be exposed that can be dangerous for the developing fetus.
- **Need for fasting:**
  - This is required depending on the type of X-ray test
  - Usually required only for certain X-rays of digestive tract
  - Medicines can be taken only with a small sip of water
- **Attire:**
  - Dress comfortably for an X-ray
  - Wear loose clothing that can easily be removed
  - If undergoing a chest X-ray, patient has to normally undress from the waist up and wear a hospital gown during the test.
- Remove all jewelry, glasses and metal objects.
- Empty bladder prior to the procedure for an abdominal X-ray
- Do not drink excessively on the morning of the procedure.
- Some X-ray tests use a contrast medium - barium or iodine or a pill or an injection that helps to outline a specific area of body on the X-ray image.

Nurse's Responsibility

During the Procedure

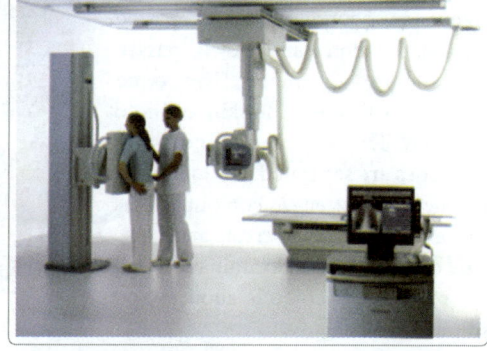

- The patient is asked to stand or lie in front of the film plates.
- The X-ray technician will align the X-ray machine to take images of the specified body parts.
- Electromagnetic radiation is passed through the body and captured on film in the form of a radiograph to make X-ray images.
- Patient may be asked to hold breath to show up more clearly chest and lung on the x-ray image. Or he may be asked to hold still and/or move to different positions like front and side views.
- The duration of the exam will vary, but the average is about 15 minutes.

ULTRASONOGRAPHY

Ultrasound imaging is also called ultrasound scanning or sonography or sonogram.

Ultrasound imaging is a diagnostic procedure that involves exposing part of the body to high-frequency sound waves to produce images of soft tissues within the body.

Preparation

- The steps you will take to prepare for an ultrasound will depend on the area or organ that is being examined.
- Fasting for eight to 12 hours before abdominal ultrasound.
- Ultrasound of the gallbladder, liver, pancreas, or spleen, requires a fat-free meal the evening before the test and then to fast until the procedure.
- For other examinations, patient is asked to drink lot of water and hold urine for better visualization of bladder.

Appendix 10: Radiologic Procedures

Patient Preparation

Type of Exam	Patient Preparation of Exam
Abdominal ultrasound	• Nothing to eat or drink 8 hours prior to exam
Pelvic ultrasound or transvaginal ultrasound	• Arrive at exam with a full bladder (drink 32–40 oz or water 45 minutes prior to exam time)
Lower extremity venous Doppler ultrasound	• No preparation required
Thyroid ultrasound	• No preparation required
Carotid ultrasound Doppler	• No preparation required
Bilateral renal artery ultrasound	• Nothing to eat or drink 8 hours prior to exam
Renal ultrasound	• Arrive at exam with a full bladder (drink 32–40 oz of water 45 minutes prior to exam time)
Soft tissues ultrasound	• No preparation required

Procedure

A special lubricating jelly is applied to the patient's skin. A hand-held transducer emitting silent, high-frequency sound waves is placed against the body and slowly passed over the area of interest. The sound waves pass through the skin and into the body. The returning sound waves or echoes are separated and identified by the transducer. A computer uses those sound waves to create an image. The duration of the examination will vary, but the average is about 30-60 minutes.

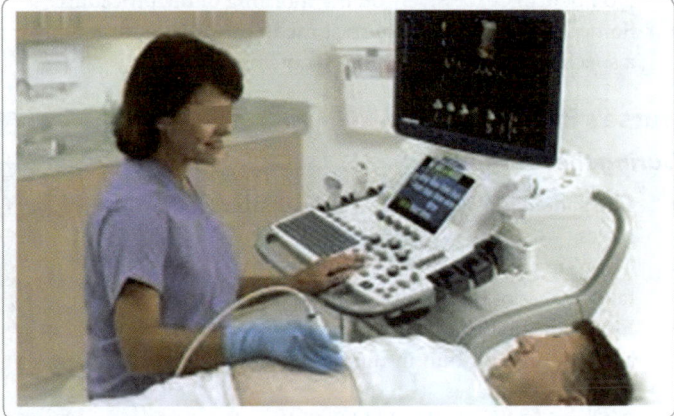

CT SCAN

A computerized tomography (CT) scan or computerized axial tomography (CAT) scans are special X-ray tests that produce cross-sectional images of the body using X-rays and a computer.

Purposes

CT examination helps to:
- Quickly identify injuries to the lungs, heart and vessels, liver, spleen, kidneys, bowel or other internal organs in cases of trauma.
- Guide biopsies and other procedures such as abscess drainages and minimally invasive tumor treatments.
- Plan for and assess the results of surgery, such as organ transplants or gastric bypass.
- Stage, plan and properly administer radiation treatments for tumors as well as monitor response to chemotherapy.
- Measure bone mineral density for the detection of osteoporosis.

Preparation for Procedure

Depending on part of the body to be scanned, instruct the patient to:

- Wear a hospital gown
- Remove metal objects such as a belt, jewelry, dentures and eyeglasses, which might interfere with image results
- Refrain from eating or drinking for a few hours.
- A special dye called contrast material may be needed for some CT scans
- Uncooperative patients and children may require a sedative.

Procedure

- CT scanners are shaped like a large doughnut standing on its side.
- Patient is instructed to lie on a narrow, motorized table that slides through the opening into a tunnel.
- Straps and pillows may be used to help to stay in position.
- The table moves the patient into the scanner.
- Detectors and the X-ray tube rotate around the patient. Each rotation yields several images of thin slices of the body.

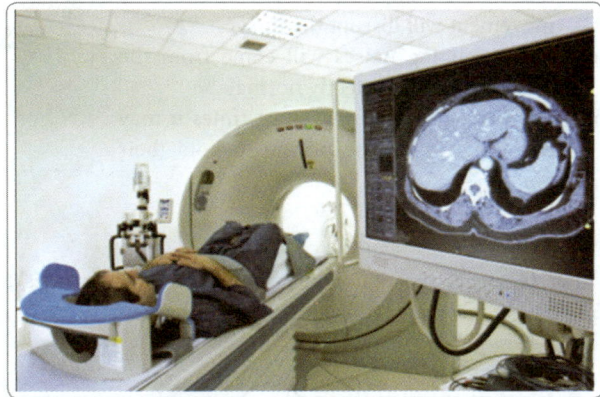

- Buzzing and whirring noises may be heard during the procedure.
- Patient should avoid coughing, wriggling or producing other large motion during the scans.
- A technologist in a separate room sees and hears the patient.
- Technologist may ask the patient to hold the breath at certain points to avoid blurring of images.
- Bones appear white on the X-ray. Soft tissue, such as the heart or liver, shows up in shades of gray. Air appears black.

Postprocedure Care

Drink lots of fluids to help remove the contrast material from the body.

MAGNETIC RESONANCE IMAGING (MRI)

MRI uses a strong magnetic field and radio waves to create detailed images of the organs and tissues within the body.

Patient Preparation

- Ask the patient to change into a gown.
- As magnets are used, it is critical that no metal objects are present in the scanner.
- The doctor will ask the patient to remove any metal jewelry or accessories that might interfere with the machine.
- A person will probably be unable to have an MRI if they have any metal inside their body, such as bullets, shrapnel, or other metallic foreign bodies. This can also include medical devices, such as cochlear implants, aneurysm clips, and pacemakers.
- Earplugs or headphones will be provided to block out the loud noises of the scanner.

Appendix 10: Radiologic Procedures

Procedure

- MRIs employ powerful magnets which produce a strong magnetic field that forces protons in the body to align with that field.
- The MRI technician will communicate with the patient via the intercom to make sure that they are comfortable. They will not start the scan until the patient is ready.
- During the scan, it is vital to stay still. Any movement will disrupt the images.
- Loud clanging noises will come from the scanner. This is perfectly normal.
- Depending on the images, at times it may be necessary for the person to hold their breath.

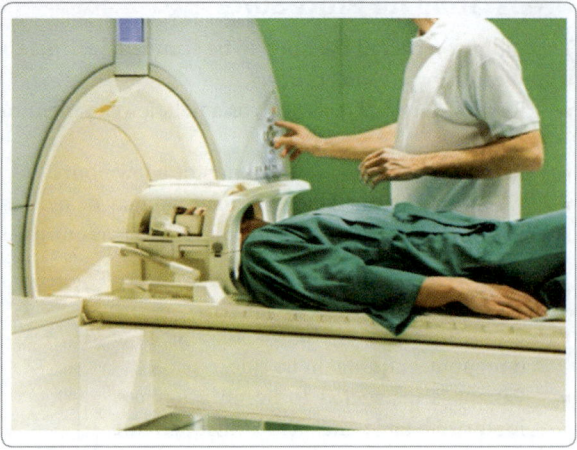

Postprocedure Care

After the scan, the radiologist will examine the images to check whether any more are required. If the radiologist is satisfied, the patient can go home.

 ENDOSCOPIC PROCEDURES

Endoscopy is a **nonsurgical diagnostic and therapeutic procedure** where specialized equipment called endoscope is used to examine a person's internal parts of the body.

Purposes

- To determine the cause of any abnormal symptoms
- To remove a small sample of tissue
- To visualize inside the body during a surgical procedure, such as repairing a stomach ulcer, or removing gallstones or tumors

Types of Procedures

There are many endoscopic procedures. Some of the common procedures are:
- GI endoscopy
  - Upper GI endoscopy—gastroscopy and duodenoscopy
  - Lower GI endoscopy—sigmoidoscopy and colonoscopy
- Cystourethroscopy
- Laryngoscopy
- Bronchoscopy
- Arthroscopy

Upper GI Endoscopy

An upper gastrointestinal (GI) endoscopy or esophagogastroduodenoscopy (EGD) is a procedure used to visualize the upper GI (gastrointestinal) tract including esophagus, stomach and duodenum.

Indications

The most common indications for diagnostic EGD include:

- Dyspepsia unresponsive to medical therapy or associated with systemic signs
- Dysphagia or odynophagia
- Persistent gastroesophageal reflux symptoms
- Occult gastrointestinal bleeding
- Surveillance for malignancy

Pre-procedural Care

- Endoscopic procedures require a formal, informed signed consent form.
- Explain the procedure to the patient, the significance of any preparation and any postprocedural sequelae.
- Instruct the patient to fast and restrict fluids for 6–8 hours prior to the procedure to reduce the risk of aspiration related to nausea and vomiting. The patient may be required to be NPO after midnight.
- Sedatives are administered prior to the procedure to relax the patient and facilitate passage of the scope.
- If the patient wears dentures, removal of the dentures prior to oral insertion of the scope.

Nurse's Responsibility

During Procedure

- The procedure typically takes between 10 and 20 minutes to complete.
- The patient is placed by placing the patient on the left side. A plastic mouth guard is placed between the teeth to prevent damage to the teeth and endoscope.
- A thin, flexible tube called an endoscope which has a lens and light source and projects images on a video monitor is introduced into the patient's mouth.
- Air or carbon dioxide gas is gently introduced through the endoscope to open the esophagus, stomach and intestine, allowing the endoscope to be passed through these areas to see completely.

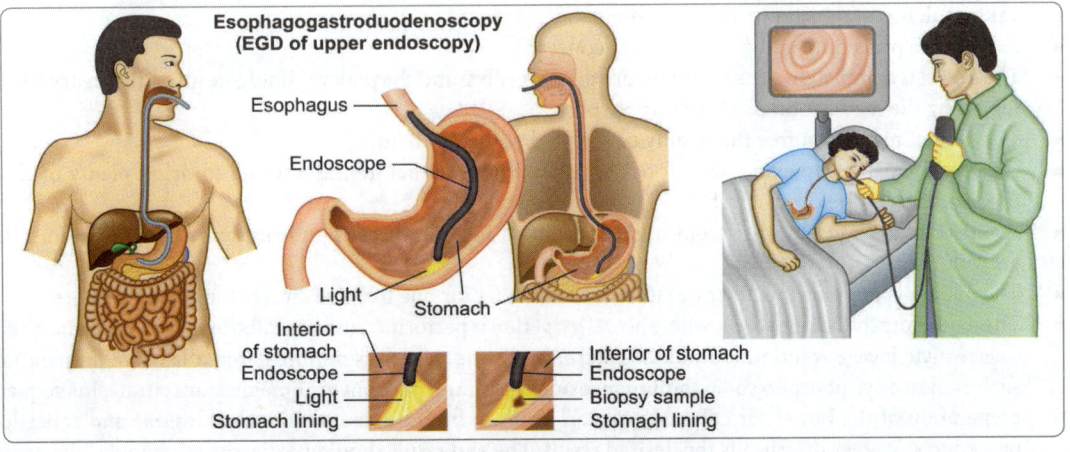

Fig: Esophagogastroduodenoscopy

Appendix 11: Endoscopic Procedures

After Procedure

- Withhold foods, fluids and oral medications until the patient is fully alert and gag reflex has returned.
- Monitor vital signs.
- Patient may have a sore throat for 1–2 days, but this should resolve.
- There are no dietary restrictions after endoscopy. The patient may resume regular diet. Most patients are able to eat immediately after endoscopy without problems.
- Ask the patient to drink plenty of fluids (>2 L/day), including juices, water, broth and sports drinks after the procedure.
- Advice the patient to take rest for the remainder of the day after the procedure. Patient can resume normal activities as he can tolerate.
- No driving for 24 hours after the procedure due to the effects of the sedating medications.

Lower GI Endoscopy or Colonoscopy

Colonoscopy is the endoscopic examination of the large colon and the distal part of the small intestine with a CCD camera or a fiber optic camera on a flexible tube passed through the anus to visualize the colon.

Purposes

- To screen for colon polyps or colorectal cancer
- To diagnose a change in bowel habits, like persistent diarrhea
- To find out the reason for Iron deficiency anemia
- To screen a family history of colon cancer
- To monitor for a personal history of colon polyps or colon cancer
- To rule out chronic, unexplained abdominal or rectal pain
- As a diagnostic tool for patients with symptoms such as lower gastrointestinal bleeding, change in bowel habit or abdominal pain
- To evaluate or follow up inflammatory bowel disease
- For interventions such as removal of foreign bodies, polypectomy, stricture dilatation and stenting (for example of a malignancy).

Patient's Preparation

- Take a full medical history from the patient.
- Explain the procedure and gain informed consent.
- The bowel is completely cleaned out before the procedure and the patient should be given full instructions regarding the medication used for this purpose.
- The patient may be on free fluids only or a light diet the day before.
- Instruct the patient to avoid solid food for at least one day before the test and to drink plenty of clear fluids on the day before the test.
- Avoid drinking red liquids. Avoid high fiber foods including seeds and nuts for the week before the procedure.
- The patient is put on a low fiber or clear-fluid only diet for one to three days before the procedure.
- The day before the colonoscopy, whole bowel irrigation is performed using a solution of polyethylene glycol - electrolyte lavage solution (PEG-ES). Alternatively, the patient is administered a laxative preparation such as bisacodyl, phospho soda, sodium picosulfate, sodium phosphate or magnesium citrate. Inadequate preparation of the bowel for colonoscopy can result in both missed pathological lesions and cancelled procedures. Watery diarrhea is the desired result. The end result should be diarrhea that looks like urine.

- It is better to avoid aspirin and ibuprofen combinations at least ten days prior to the procedure to avoid the risk of bleeding if a polypectomy is to be performed.
- Adequate hydration is important before, during and after bowel preparation regardless of the bowel preparation administered.

Nurse's Responsibility

During the Procedure

- Observe the patient's tolerance of the procedure. Provide reassurance, commentary and support.
- Although colonoscopy can be performed in unsedated state, intravenous sedation with midazolam or fentanyl and pethidine is recommended during the procedure.
- The patient is positioned in the left lateral position.
- After an initial rectal examination to assess the sphincter tone, the endoscope is lubricated and passed via the anus towards the rectum, colon and the terminal ileum.
- Air or carbon dioxide and sterile water or saline will be gently pumped through the scope into the colon to inflate it. Instruct the patient that he/she may feel bloating or gas cramps as the air opens the colon.
- Once the whole colon has been viewed, the endoscope is removed slowly, allowing full visualization again on withdrawal. Biopsies may be taken during removal.
- Assess and document patient's status on completing the procedure.

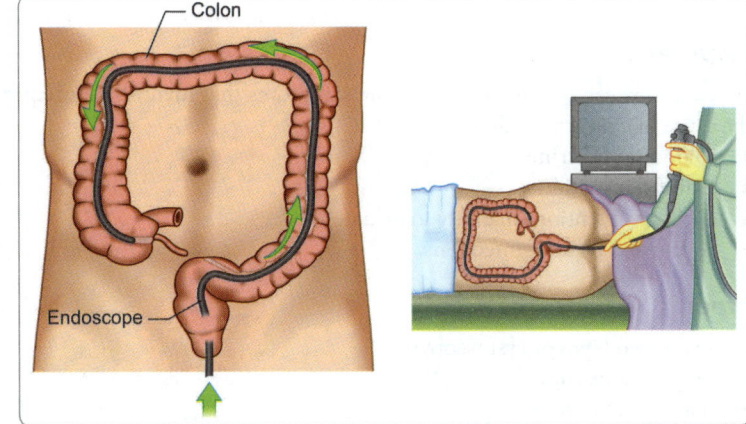

Fig: Colonoscopy

After the Procedure

- Assess and monitor the patient until complete recovery.
- Document all care given and any unusual events that occurred.
- Provide written instructions regarding diet, medications, activity restrictions, follow-up and complications.

Potential Complications

- **Major complications:**
  - Colonic perforation
  - Hemorrhage
  - Over-sedation
  - Cardiorespiratory events
  - Septicemia
- **Minor complications:**
  - Incomplete procedure due to abdominal discomfort
  - Rectal bleeding

Cystoscopy or Cystourethroscopy

It is otherwise called as bladder scope or cystourethrography or prostatography. A cystoscopy is an invasive diagnostic and interventional procedure that allows for direct visualization of the urethra, urethral sphincter, prostate, bladder and ureteral orifices through the transurethral insertion of a cystoscope into the bladder.

Purposes

A cystoscopy can be used to investigate symptoms that involve the urethra or the bladder and to determine the cause of concerns such as:
- Blood in the urine
- Painful urination
- Urinary retention (inability to urinate)
- Recurrent bladder infections

Types

There are two types of cystoscopy:
1. Rigid cystoscopy
2. Flexible cystoscopy

Nurse's Responsibility

Before Cystoscopy

- Assess patient's understanding of the procedure and answer any queries.
- Obtain informed consent.
- Withhold blood thinning medications.
- Provide instruction for fasting and non-fasting preparation.
- Establish an IV line.
- Instruct patient to empty the bladder prior to the procedure and to change into the hospital gown provided.
- Administer sedation and other medications as ordered.
- Antimicrobial prophylaxis in high risk groups.
- Skin preparation.

During Cystoscopy

- Place patient in a lithotomy position.
- The cystoscope or a ureteroscope is inserted to examine the urethra
- The scope will need to be directed anteriorly as it is advanced into the bladder.
- In men, the penis should be angled 45°–60° relative to the abdominal wall as the scope passes through the anterior urethra. Once beyond the membranous urethra, the scope is directed anteriorly to enter the bladder.
- The lower urinary tract is systematically evaluated as the scope is advanced into the bladder.
- Upon entering the bladder, the mucosa should be carefully inspected. Prior to removing the scope, the bladder should be drained.
- Other procedures—diagnostic or therapeutic may be performed as per the indications.
- Upon completion of the examination and related procedures, the cystoscope is withdrawn.
- Specimen is sent to the laboratory.

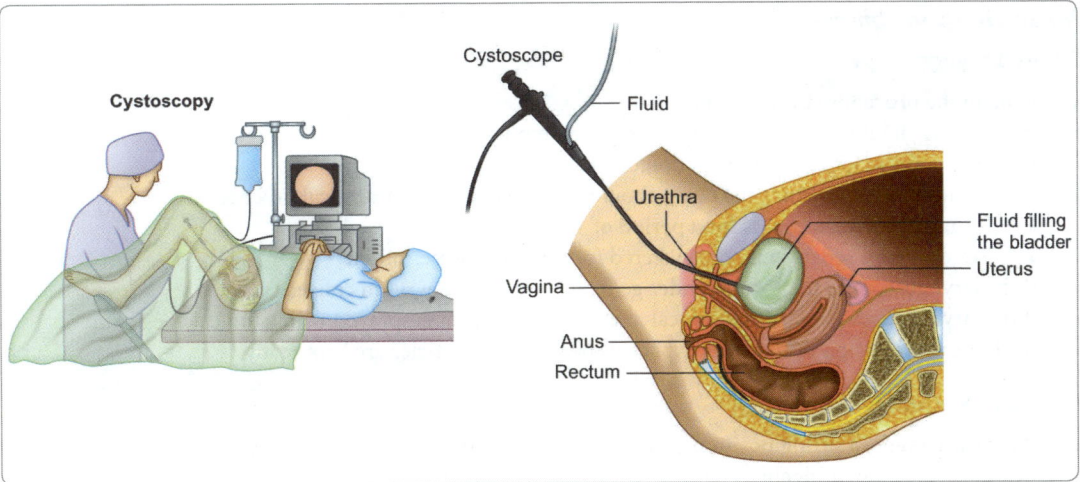

After Cystoscopy

- Monitor and record vital signs.
- Assess the patient's ability to void at least 24 hours after the procedure.
- Observe the color which may be Pink-tinged urine.
- Encourage increased fluid intake as indicated.
- Encourage deep breathing exercises.
- Provide warm sitz baths and administer mild analgesics as ordered.
- Watch out for signs of serious complications like sepsis, bladder perforation, hematuria.

Laryngoscopy

Laryngoscopy is the visualization of the interior of the larynx through introduction of the laryngoscope through the mouth.

Indications

A laryngoscope can be recommended for patients with:
- Problems with voice, including uncharacteristic breathing or hoarseness, weak voice, or complete loss of voice
- Unexplained pain in the throat or ear
- Difficulties in swallowing
- A palpable lump in the throat
- Coughing up bloody mucus
- Injuries to the throat
- Narrowing of the throat
- Obstructions in the airway
- Signs and symptoms of cancer in the voice box (larynx)

Appendix 11: Endoscopic Procedures

Nurse's Responsibility

Before Laryngoscopy

- Explain the procedure to the client.
- Instruct the client to breathe quietly through the mouth.
- Darken the room for clear visualization of structures.
- For the direct laryngoscopy, the client should be prepared as for a surgical procedure.
  - Withheld food and fluids for a period of 4 to 6 hours.
  - Pre-operative sedation is administered for the client as per order.
- If the laryngoscopy is to be done under general anesthesia, a written consent is taken.
- If the laryngoscopy is done under local anesthesia the throat is sprayed with a topical anesthetic.
- If a biopsy or excision of tissues is expected the necessary articles are kept ready.

During Procedure

- Place the patient in sitting position or supine position with neck hyperextended.
- Administer anesthetic agent as per the type of laryngoscope used.

Direct Flexible Laryngoscopy

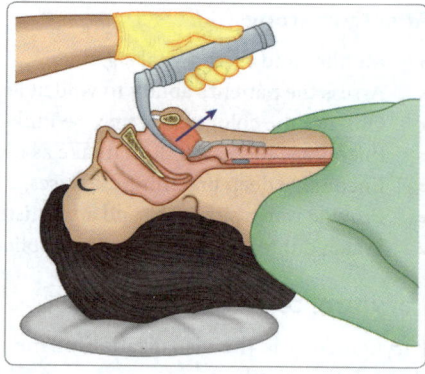

- Patients are often numbed using local anesthetic in spray form. This prevents pain and dulls the gag reflex.
- A flexible laryngoscope is inserted via the nasal cavity and pushed down into the throat.

Indirect Laryngoscopy

- This approach involves the use of special mirror with a light source is provided via headgear.
- This is placed toward the back of a patient's throat to get a closer look at the affected area.

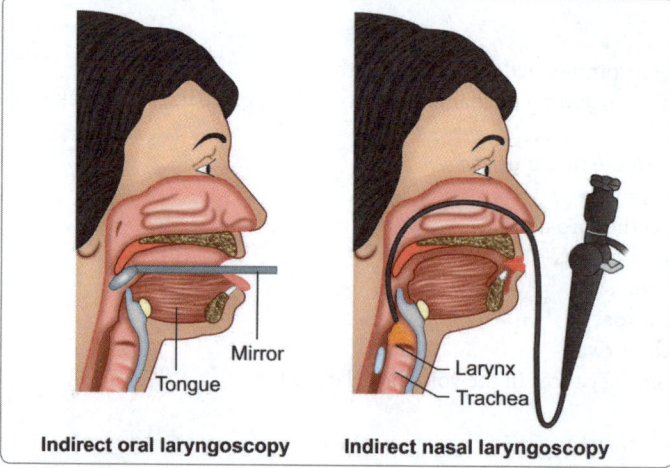

Indirect oral laryngoscopy   Indirect nasal laryngoscopy

After Care of the Patient

- Following laryngoscopy the client who had general anesthesia is kept flat in bed without a pillow under the head.
- If it is done under local anesthesia the swallowing reflexes are absent in the client; therefore the client is kept in a side-lying position to drain the saliva.
- The client is given nothing to eat or drink until the gag reflex returns.
- Before oral feeds are started, provide sips of water to check the client's ability to swallow.
- Watch for the signs of complications like:
  - Coughing and spitting of blood
  - Pain or swelling in the throat and neck
  - Restlessness and breathing difficulty
- Record the procedure in the nurse's record with date

Arthroscopy

Arthroscopy is an endoscopic procedure that allows direct visualization of a joint through a small incision.

Indications

- Arthritis—helpful in diagnosis and treatment of inflammatory, non-inflammatory and infectious types of arthritis and non-inflammatory degenerative arthritis or osteoarthritis.
- Various joint injury such as cartilage tears or meniscus tears, ligament strains and tears, cartilage deterioration underneath the patella or kneecap
- Evaluation of knees and shoulders
- Examine and treat conditions of the wrist, ankles and elbows
- Removing loose tissues, chips of bone or cartilage or foreign objects (plant thorns) that are lodged in the joint

Nurse's Responsibility

Before the Procedure

- Patients who are on anticoagulants (blood thinners) should have these medications carefully adjusted prior to surgery.
- Physical examination, blood tests, urinalysis are done prior to the procedure.
- ECG and chest X-ray for patients who have a history of heart or lung problems and generally anyone over the age of 50
- Signs of ongoing infection in the body usually postpone arthroscopy, unless it is being done for possible infection of the joint in question.

During Procedure

- The procedure is carried out in the operating room or as a day-care procedure under sterile conditions.
- An injection of a local anesthetic into the joint or general anesthesia is used.
- A large bore needle is then inserted and the joint is distended with saline.
- The arthroscope, a small tube that contains optical fibers and lenses, is introduced through the tiny incision in the skin into the joint to be examined.
- Joint structures, synovium and articular surfaces are visualized because the arthroscope is connected to a video camera and the interior of the joint is seen on a television monitor.

Appendix 11: Endoscopic Procedures

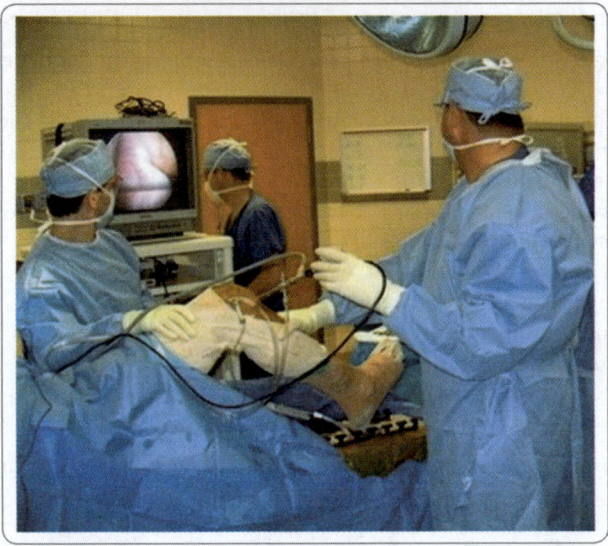

After the Procedure

- Wrap the joints with a compression dressing to control swelling
- Apply ice over the area to control edema and discomfort
- Keep the joint extended and elevated to reduce swelling
- Advice the patient to limit activity following procedure
- Monitor neurovascular function
- Administer analgesics per doctor's prescription to control discomfort

Complications

- Infection
- Hemarthrosis
- Thrombophlebitis
- Stiffness
- Delayed wound healing

Bronchoscopy

Bronchoscopy is an invasive procedure that permits the direct examination of the larynx, trachea, and bronchi using either a flexible fiberoptic bronchoscope or a rigid metal bronchoscope.

Indications

Bronchoscopy may be performed in patients for diagnostic and/or therapeutic purposes:

Diagnostic Bronchoscopy

- Direct visualization of the tracheobronchial tree for any abnormalities such as inflammatory process, tumors, or strictures
- Direct visualization of the larynx to determine the presence of a vocal cord paralysis
- Aspiration of a specimen for culture and sensitivity and for cytological examination

- Biopsy of tissue from suspected lesions
- Cough
- Wheeze/stridor
- Abnormal chest X-ray
- Persistent pneumothorax

Therapeutic Bronchoscopy

- Removal of excessive secretions, mucus plugs, benign or malignant tumors to clear airways
- Removal of foreign objects or other obstructions
- Control of bleeding in the bronchi
- Palliative laser therapy or radiation therapy for bronchial tumors
- Stent placement, Brachytherapy, Laser therapy, Photodynamic therapy, Balloon dilatation, electrocautery, Cryotherapy.

Nurse's Responsibility

Before the Procedure

- A signed consent form is obtained from the patient.
- Obtain medical history. Ask for any history of allergies to anesthetic agents and list of medicines the patient is taking.
- Check for NPO status. Withhold food and fluids for 612 hours prior to the examination to decrease the risk of aspiration.
- Obtain baseline vital signs and monitor vital signs.
- Instruct the patient to do oral care and remove any dentures if appropriate.
- Administer preoperative medications as ordered. Explain to the patient that an IV sedative such as propofol may be given as an anesthetic agent.
- Prepare for local anesthesia. If the bronchoscopy is not conducted under general anesthesia, inform the patient that a topical anesthetic (e.g., lidocaine) will be sprayed on the pharynx to prevent coughing and gagging as the scope is passed down through the throat. Explain that the spray may have a bitter taste to it.
- Relieve anxiety. Reassure the patient that airway blockage won't occur.
- Prepare emergency resuscitation equipment at the bedside. Laryngospasm and respiratory distress may occur following the procedure.

During the Procedure

- Position the client. Place patient in a sitting or supine position and provide supplemental oxygen as ordered.
- A local anesthetic is flushed into the patient's throat.
- A bronchoscope is inserted through the patient's mouth or nose.
- When the bronchoscope reaches above the vocal cords, about 3 to 4 mL of 2% to 4% lidocaine is sprayed through the scope's inner channel to the vocal cords to anesthetize distant areas.
- The practitioner examines the anatomic structure of the trachea and bronchi, notes the color of the mucosal lining and inspects for tumors or inflamed areas.
- Tissue samples may be collected from a suspect area. A bronchial brush is needed to collect sample cells from the surface of a lesion and a suction apparatus to remove foreign materials or mucus plugs may be used. Bronchoalveolar lavage may be performed to diagnose the infectious causes of infiltrates in an immunocompromised patient or to remove copious secretions.
- Secure specimen. Send the properly labeled specimen to the laboratory immediately.

Appendix 11: Endoscopic Procedures

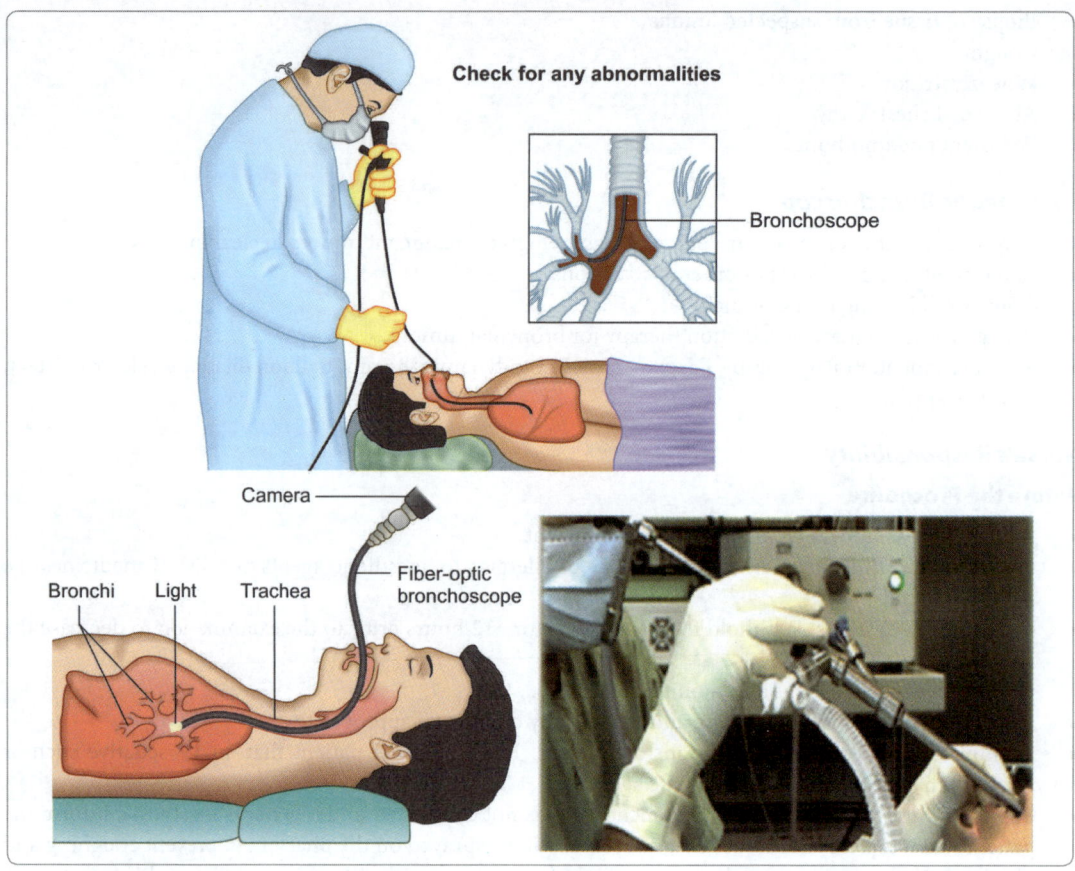

Check for any abnormalities

Bronchoscope

Camera

Bronchi   Light   Trachea   Fiber-optic bronchoscope

After the Procedure

- Assess bleeding episodes. Observe the patient's sputum and report for any excessive bleeding. Explain that a minimal amount of blood streak is expected and normal for few hours after the procedure.
- Assess respiratory status. Watch out for signs of bronchial spasm or bronchial perforation such as facial crepitus, hypoxemia, hemorrhage, and chest tightness.
- Monitor vital signs. Changes in the vital signs or any discomforts felt by the patient may indicate a possible complication.
- Position the patient. Place the conscious patient in a semi-Fowler's position while for an unconscious patient, place on one side with the head of the bed slightly raised.
- Reinforce diet. Maintain NPO status until the anesthesia has worn off and the gag reflex has returned. The patient may resume his normal diet, starting with sips of water or ice chips.
- Prevent aspiration. Provide an emesis basin, and instruct the patient to spit out saliva rather than swallow it.
- Relieve anxiety and provide comfort measures. Reassure the patient that hoarseness, loss of voice and sore throat may occur temporarily. Offer lozenges or a soothing liquid gargle to relieve discomfort until gag reflex returns.

Complications

- Bleeding from the site of the biopsy
- Fever
- Hypoxemia
- Laryngospasm
- Pneumothorax or a collapsed lung

BLOOD TRANSFUSION

The transfusion of blood or blood products is the administration of whole blood, its components, or plasma-derived products.

The transfusion of blood or blood products is the administration of whole blood, its components, or plasma-derived products. Blood transfusion is a therapeutic measure where the whole blood or components of the blood, e.g., plasma or erythrocytes are administered into the venous circulation for restoration of **blood** or plasma volume.

Purposes

- To restore blood volume after hemorrhage
- To maintain hemoglobin levels in severe anemia
- To replace specific blood component
- To restore oxygen-carrying capacity of blood
- To provide platelets and clotting factors

Indications

The primary indication for a blood transfusion is to improve the oxygen-carrying capacity of the blood. Other indications for different blood products and their components are:

- **Packed red blood cells:** PRBC's are used when the client is in need of increased oxygen transporting red blood cells as may occur with:
  - Postoperative patients
  - An acute hemorrhage.
- **Platelets:** Platelets are administered to clients who are adversely affected with:
  - A platelet deficiency
  - A serious bleeding disorder, such as thrombocytopenia
  - Platelet dysfunction that requires the clotting factors that are in platelets.
- **Fresh frozen plasma:** Fresh frozen plasma is administered to clients who are in need of clotting factors or are in need of increased blood volume as occurs in:
  - Hypovolemia
  - Hypovolemic shock.

  Fresh frozen plasma does not have to be typed and cross matched to the client's blood type because plasma does not contain antigen carrying red blood cells.
- **Albumin:** Albumin is administered to clients who need expanded blood volume and/or plasma proteins.
- **Clotting factors and cryoprecipitate:** Clotting factors and cryoprecipitate are administered to clients affected with a clotting disorder including the lack of fibrinogen.
- **Whole blood:** Whole blood is typically reserved for only cases of severe hemorrhage. Whole blood contains clotting factors, red blood cells, white blood cells, plasma, platelets and plasma proteins.

Appendix 12: Blood Transfusion

Common Abbreviations used in Blood Transfusion

- RBC – Red Blood Cells
- PRBC – Packed Red Blood Cells
- LR-RBC – Leukoreduced Red Blood Cells
- RDP – Random Donor Platelets
- SDP – Single Donor Platelets
- LR-Pooled Platelets – Leuko Reduced Pooled Platelets

Types of Blood Transfusion

The most common types of blood transfusion are:
- **Allogenic blood transfusion:** Blood that is donated by another person.
- **Autologous transfusion:** It is the transfusion of one's own blood.

Blood type compatibility has been presented in table as follows:

Blood Type	Gives	Receives
A+	A+, AB+	A+, A-, O+, O-
O+	O+, A+, B+, AB+	O+, O-
B+	B+, AB+	B+, B-, O+, O-
AB+	AB+	Everyone
A-	A+, A-, AB+, AB-	A-, O-
O-	Everyone	O-
B-	B+, B-, AB+, AB-	B-, O-
AB-	AB+, AB-	AB-, A-, B-, O-

Guidelines for use of blood and blood products:

Component	Average volume	Storage temperature	Shelf life	Compatibility
Whole blood	450 mL	1–6°C	35 days	
PRBC'S	180–350 mL	1–6°C	21–35 days	ABO, Rh, cross matched
FFP (Fresh frozen plasma)	100–150 mL/unit 250 ML/unit	<–20°C	1 year	ABO
Platelets whole blood derived	50 mL/bag pooled to usual dose of 4–6 bags	20–24°C	5 days	Preferably ABO
Cryoprecipitate	10–15 mL/Unit Pooled to usual dose of 4–6 bags	<–20°C	1 year	Any group
Leucocyte depleted RBC's	200–250 mL	1–6°C	1 day	

Contd...

Component	Volume per unit	Dose	Number of donors	Storage	Need to defrost	Storage after defrosting	Time to transfusion	Filter required
Packed red cells	180–350 mL (mean 28 mL)	4 mL/kg equivalent to 1 unit will raise Hb by 1 g/dL	1	Designated temperature-controlled refrigerator at 4 + 2°C for 35 days	No	N/A	4 hours after removal from storage	Blood transfusion set with 170–200 micron filter
Fresh frozen plasma	240–300 mL (mean 273 mL)	10-15 mL/kg or 1:1 with RBC in major hemor-rhage	Multiple	Designated temperature controlled freezer at -30° for 24 months	Yes - takes 15–30 minutes	Can be stored in blood fridge for 24 hours	4 hours after removal from storage	As above
Platelets	200–300 mL	1 adult therapeutic dose increases platelet count by 20–40 × 10°/liter	Multiple	Temperature controlled at 22 + 2°C with continuous agitation for 5 days	No	N/A	As soon as possible over 30–60 minutes they should not be put in the fridge	As above but not through giving set which has been used for other blood products
Cryoprecip-itate	100–250 mL (mean 152 mL)	2 × 5 donor pools (equivalent to 10 single donor units) raise plasma fibrinogen by 1 g/L	Multiple	Designated temperature-controlled freezer at -30°C for 24 months	Yes–takes 15–30 minutes	Must be kept at ambient tempera-ture for up to 4 hours	As soon as possible it should not be put in the fridge	As above

Articles Required

Articles	Purpose
Unit of blood or blood components	For blood transfusion
Blood administration set either a straight line or a Y set (Y set is preferred)	For administration of blood products
Normal saline solution	For priming
IV dressing	For securing the site
Venipuncture set containing a 16G or 18G needle.	For starting IV line in patients who do not have venous access.
Alcohol swab	For wiping the IV port
Disposable gloves (sterile), apron, mask	For performing safe procedure
Hand rub	For hand hygiene

Contd...

Appendix 12: Blood Transfusion

Articles	Purpose
Mackintosh and towel	For securing the linen
Vital signs tray and pulse oximetry	For checking TPR, BP and Oxygen Saturation
Kidney tray	For discarding soiled waste materials
BMW waste bins	For safe disposal of bio hazard articles

Preparation of Patient

- Verify the physician's order for the specific blood or blood product. This includes:
  - Type of blood product
  - Amount to be infused
  - Date, time, rate and duration of infusion
  - Any modifications to be done on a blood component (e.g., irradiation)
  - Specific transfusion requirements
  - Possible sequence in which multiple components are to be transfused
  - Any pre or post transfusion medications
- Obtain the patient's past transfusion history and note any known allergies and previous transfusion reactions.
- Verify patency of IV site. The patient's IV cannula must be patent and without complications, such as infiltration or phlebitis.
- Verify that blood typing and cross-matching (also known as a G & S) have been completed within the past 96 hours.
- Assess laboratory values such as hematocrit, coagulation values and platelet count.
- Check that the patient has properly completed and signed the transfusion consent form. Consent is mandatory for all blood and blood product transfusions.
- Know the indications for the transfusion and explain the same to the patient.
- All blood products taken from the blood bank must be started within 30 minutes and administered within 4 hours due to the risk of bacterial proliferation in the blood component at room temperature.
- Obtain patient's base line data before the transfusion. This includes temperature, pulse, respiration and blood pressure, oxygen saturation.
- Obtain the correct blood component for the patient.
- Check the requisition form and the blood bag label for the following details by two nurses:
  - Patient name
  - Identification number
  - Blood type and Rh group
  - The blood donor number
  - Expiry date of blood
  - Check blood for any abnormalities like gas bubbles, change in color, cloudiness, presence of clots and excess air.
  - Make sure that the blood is left at room temperature for no more than 30 minutes before starting the transfusion. RBCs deteriorate and lose their effectiveness after 2 hours at room temperature. Adhere to the Institution's policy for returning the blood if it has not been started. As blood components warm, the risk of bacterial growth also increases.
- Ensure that the duty doctor counter checks and signs before starting the transfusion.

Procedure

Steps	Procedure	Rationale
1.	Identify the patient and explain the procedure and its purpose to the patient such as blood product to be transfused, approximate length of time and desired outcome of transfusion	Allays anxiety and wins confidence and cooperation
2.	Close the doors and windows. Screen the patient 	Provides privacy and prevents drought
3.	Arrange the articles at the bedside	Organization promotes skilled performance
4.	Obtain and record the patient's pretransfusion baseline vital signs, including temperature, pulse, respiration, blood pressure and oxygen saturation level. If the patient is febrile (temperature >37.8°C or 100°F), notify the health care provider before initiating the transfusion 	Baseline data facilitates for easy comparison before, during and after the procedure
5.	Have emergency equipment available at the bedside like oxygen, suction apparatus, etc. 	Facilitates immediate attention to tackle potential complications, as prompt intervention may be required to prevent serious complications

Contd...

Steps	Procedure	Rationale
6.	Wash hands and wear appropriate PPE 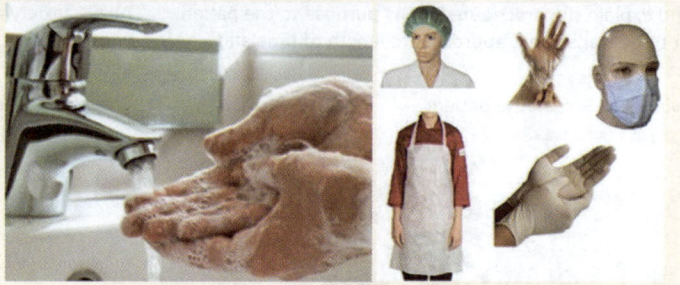	Prevents transmission of micro organisms
7.	Place the patient in a comfortable position 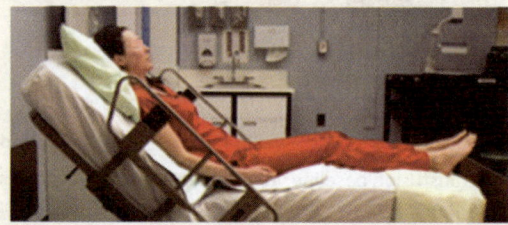	Proper positioning promotes comfort and aids relaxation
8.	Place Mackintosh and towel under the IV access site. Assess the patency of IV line or initiate venous access 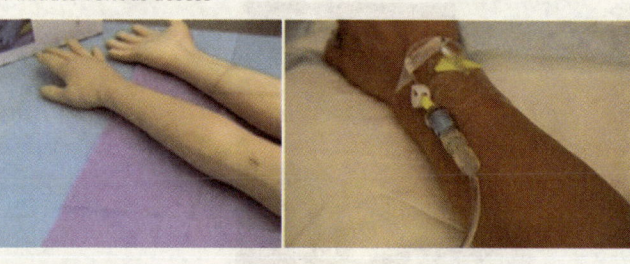	Protects the linen from soiling
	If patient does not have an intravenous access, perform venipuncture on a suitable vein. Select a large vein 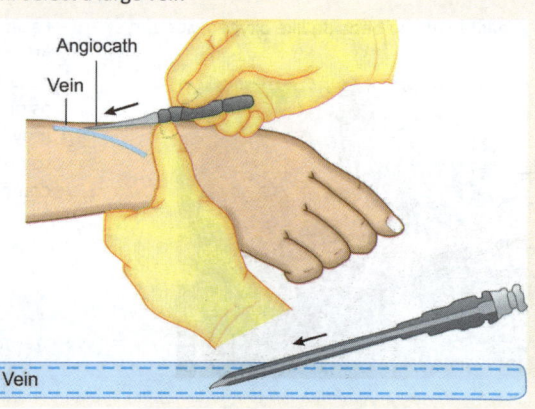	Large vein and large needle prevents destruction of RBC's during transfusing

Contd...

Appendix 12: Blood Transfusion

Steps	Procedure	Rationale
	Appropriate needle gauge is based on clinical status of patient, urgency of transfusion and venous access: • 18G for trauma/surgery • 20–22G for elective medical/geriatric Patient Transfusion set must be Luer-locked to a 2.0 mL maximum extension tubing, either directly to cannula 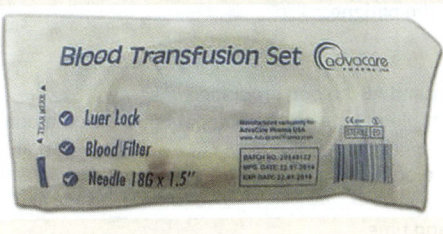	
9.	Prime the IV line with 0.9% NS 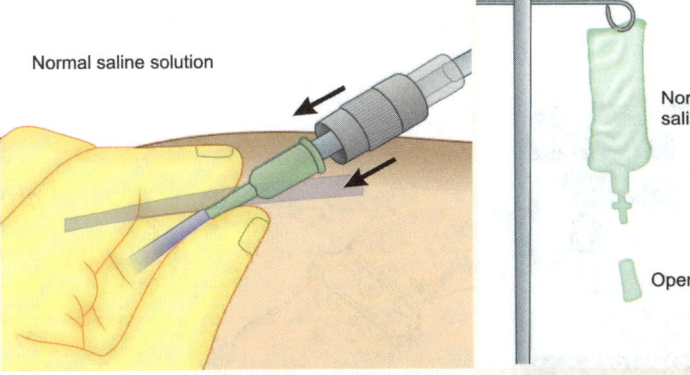	Dextrose causes lysis of RBCs, Ringer's Solution, medication and other additives and hyper alimentation solution are incompatible
10.	Obtain blood products from the blood bank within 30 minutes of planned transfusion Assess blood bag for any signs of leaks or contamination, such as clumping, clots, gas bubbles, or a purplish discoloration. Return to blood bank if blood bag contains any of the above signs 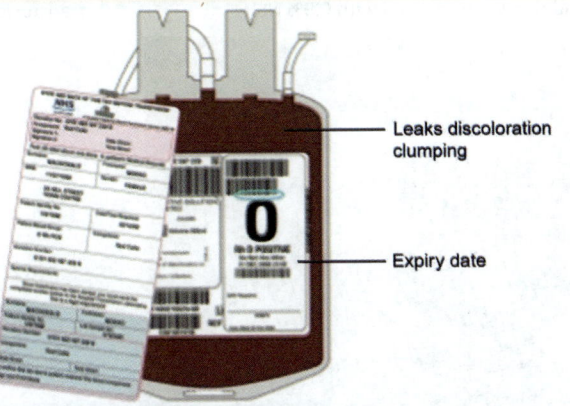	Complete visual inspection of product prevents untoward complications

Contd...

Appendix 12: Blood Transfusion

Steps	Procedure	Rationale
11.	Initial verification must be completed by two trained staff competent in blood transfusion administration process which includes • Identification data of the patient • Physician order • Consent • Type of blood product and ABO blood grouping • Confirming the patient blood type and Rh compatibility with the donor blood type and Rh • Serial number on the blood bag • Date of collection • Product expiry date and time • Special requirements (e.g., irradiated) • G & S expiry date • Compatibility tag and label attached to blood product	Proper verification ensures safe administration of blood

Steps	Procedure	Rationale
12.	Administer pre-medications as ordered. Medications must be administered through an IV infusion set and the IV site cleared with 0.9% NS	Ensures priming of transfusion set

Contd...

Steps	Procedure	Rationale
13.	Final verification must be completed by the same two staff members. In addition to the above verification, recipient identification and product check is confirmed. Invert product 5–10 times gently	Helps to mix the cell within the plasma

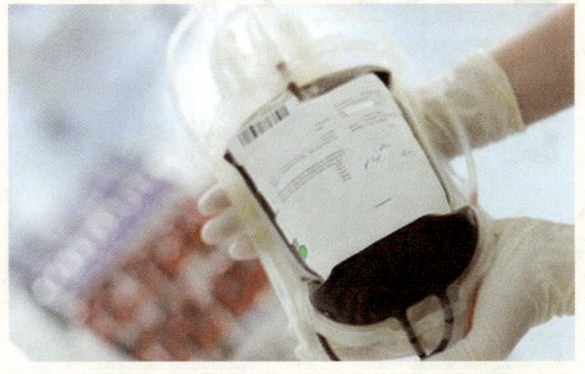

14.	Prime the blood product administration set using aseptic technique: Take a straight blood transfusion set	Aseptic technique ensures safe transfusion of blood

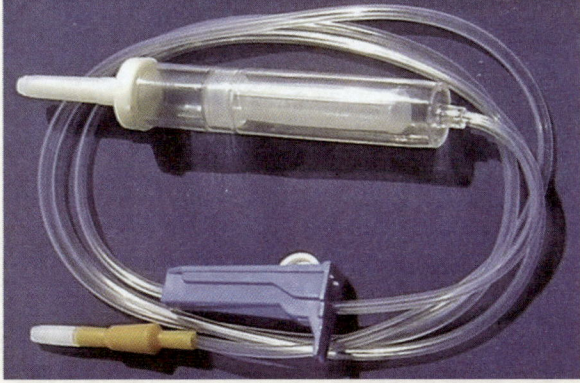

Insert spike of the blood administration set into the blood product container

Prevents entry of air thus preventing air embolism

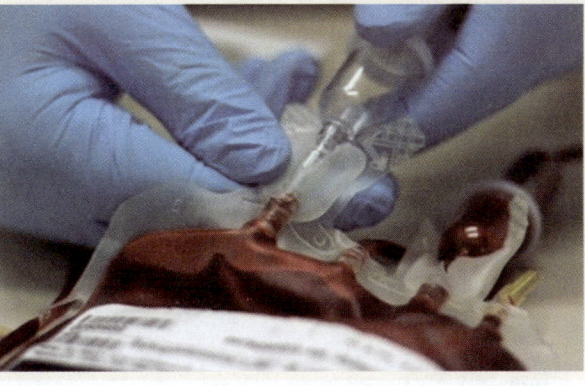

Contd...

Appendix 12: Blood Transfusion

Steps	Procedure	Rationale
	Close clamp. Completely cover the filter with product 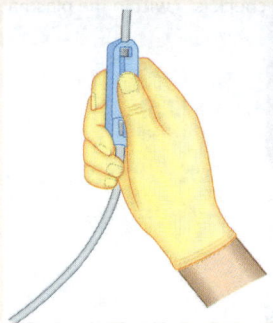 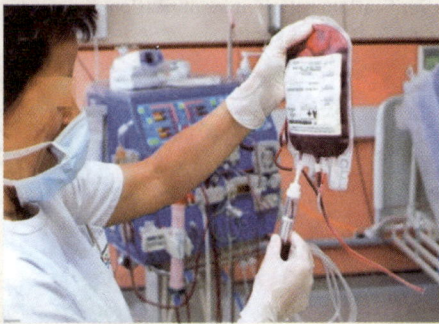 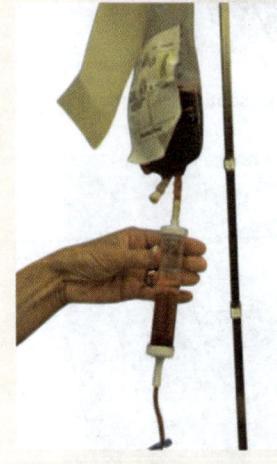	
15.	Obtain vital signs immediately prior to transfusion, then 15 minutes after initiation, then every hour until transfusion is complete 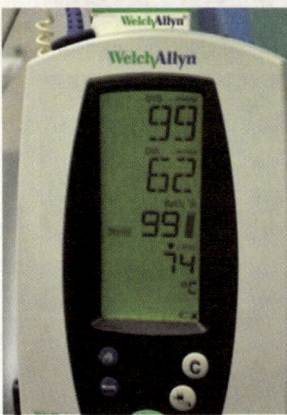	Monitoring vital signs facilitates early recognition of untoward effects

Contd...

Steps	Procedure	Rationale
16.	Disconnect the NS infusion and connect blood administration set and start transfusion with due care to maintain asepsis 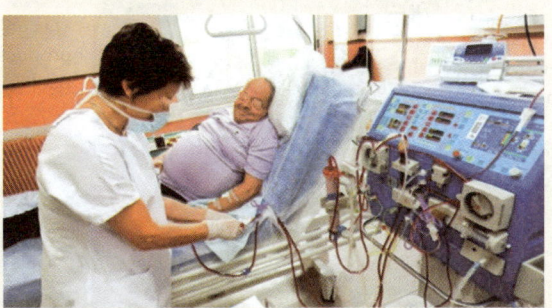 Advise patient on the signs and symptoms of transfusion reaction and what and when to report	Ensures safe administration This helps the patient to easily identify any side effects immediately to the care giver
17.	Start infusion slowly at 2 mL/min. Initiate red cells slowly (25 mL in the first 15 minutes). For all other blood transfusions, refer to the blood and product sheet. The infusion rate may be increased if there are no signs of circulatory overload 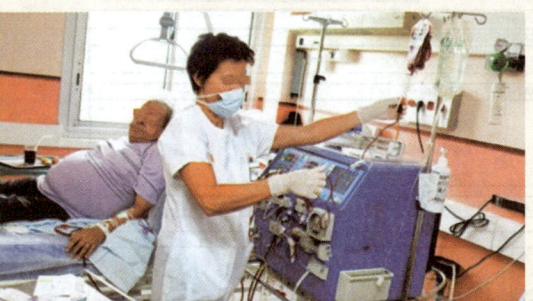	Infusing small amounts of blood component initially minimizes volume of blood to which patient is exposed, thereby minimizing severity of reaction and also prevents circulatory overload
18.	For each and every unit of blood transfusion remain with the patient for the first 5 minutes and assess for clinical signs of transfusion reaction Complete transfusion within 4 hours of receipt of the product from the blood bank 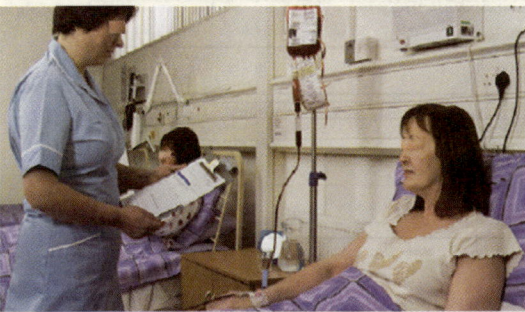	Most transfusion reactions occur within first 15 minutes of a transfusion

Contd...

Appendix 12: Blood Transfusion

Steps	Procedure	Rationale
19.	Assess and observe for clinical signs and symptoms of reactions up to 24 hours post-transfusion In the event of a transfusion reaction, stop the infusion. Manage transfusion reactions as per protocol Complete required transfusion reaction form Return remaining blood to blood bank for further investigation 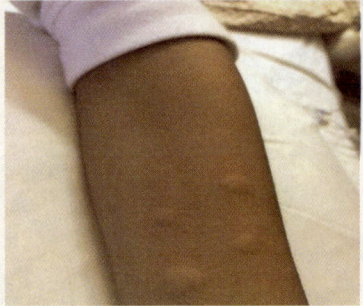	Helps to prevent life threatening complications This helps to analyze the products in the blood bank

---

Baptist Hospital of Miami   Baptist Children's Hospital

TRANSFUSION REACTION INVESTIGATION REPORT

INSTRUCTIONS TO NURSES: (Protocol GPL-13)
1. Immediately stop transfusion. Keep vein open with slow saline drip.
2. Verify that patient identification and Transfusion Slip data are the same.
3. Immediately notify attending and ordering physicians and Transfusion Service.
4. Order a Transfusion Reaction Evaluation Workup, upon physician request.
5. Send **STAT** to Transfusion Service:
   • a properly labeled post transfusion specimen, including control number,
   • Transfusion Reaction Investigation Report form, with Section I & II completed
   • blood component with tubing and Transfusion Slip attached.
6. Send urine specimen labeled "Blood Reaction", when available.

SECTION I - (This section to be completed by R.N.)
TRANSFUSION DATA

Date of Transfusion	Time Started	Time Stopped	Approximate Volume Given	Type of Component	Unit Number

PATIENT HISTORY

Diagnosis: _____   Previous Reactions: ☐ YES ☐ NO

Prior Transfusions: ☐ YES ☐ NO   Type, if known: _____

If YES, when: ___   Previous Pregnancies: ☐ YES ☐ NO

SECTION II - CLINICAL FINDINGS - (This section to be completed by R.N.)

SYMPTOMS - Check as appropriate	Immediate	Delayed
Chills	☐	☐
Fever	☐	☐
Dyspnea	☐	☐
Nausea	☐	☐
Vomiting	☐	☐
Bleeding	☐	☐
Shock	☐	☐
Pain	☐	☐
B/P changes	☐	☐
Itching	☐	☐
Rash/Hives	☐	☐
Chest Pain	☐	☐
Dark Urine	☐	☐
Headache	☐	☐
Other / Specify		

VITAL SIGNS	Pre-Transfusion	Post-Transfusion
Temperature		
Blood Pressure		
Pulse		

Patient Bedside Clerical Check	Errors Detected	
Patient's Name	☐ YES	☐ NO
Patient's Date of Birth	☐ YES	☐ NO
Medical Record Number	☐ YES	☐ NO
Control Number	☐ YES	☐ NO
Unit/Patient ABO/Rh	☐ YES	☐ NO

Name of attending / ordering physician:

Name & Signature of R.N.:   Date / Time:

SECTION III - CONCLUSIONS - (This section to be completed by Pathologist)

☐ Not Classified	☐ Mild Allergic	☐ Hemolytic
☐ Febrile, Non-hemolytic	☐ Anaphylactic	☐ Delayed Hemolytic
☐ Sepsis	☐ Circulatory Overload ☑	☐ TRALI

Comments: _____

Pathologist's Name (print)   Signature   Date / Time

03400B1670   Form #1670 (Rev. 8/09)

Contd...

Steps	Procedure	Rationale
20.	After completing the transfusion, flush administration set with maximum of 50 mL of normal saline and re-establish IV as per physician orders	Facilitates patency of transfusion set by preventing stasis of blood products and its clotting
21.	Obtain vital sign and compare with base line assessment	Helps to detect post transfusion complications
22.	Discard waste in biohazard waste container **Blood and body fluid bags** **Dispose in yellow bag**	This prevents the spread of infection through biohazard waste
23.	Replace articles, discard PPE and wash hands	Prevents transmission of microorganisms
24.	Document procedure which may include: • Transfusion record form • All vital signs and reactions • Initiation and termination of transfusion • Any significant findings • The name of the second nurse who did the two person verification process • The name and amount of the specific type of transfusion such as 1 unit of packed red cells • The number of the blood product • IV site • Size of the angiocath that was used • Duration of the transfusion • Patient reaction • Along with the signature of the staff	Documentation fosters quality care

Appendix 12: Blood Transfusion

■ 0.9% sodium chloride is the only solution that should be infused through the administration set immediately before or after blood. Normal saline is compatible with blood; ringer's lactate, dextrose, hyperalimentation and other intravenous solutions with incompatible medications are not compatible with blood and blood products.
■ When required, red blood cells should only be warmed using a specifically designed commercial device and following the manufacturer's instructions.
■ Drugs must not be added to blood.
■ Red cells should be collected from the blood refrigerator immediately prior to transfusion.
■ Commence the transfusion within 30 minutes and complete within 4 hours of removal from the controlled temperature storage facility. If the infusion is not commenced within 30 minutes, the pack must be returned to the laboratory and labelled.
■ A new administration set should be used if the patient has multiple transfusions over more than 12 hours to prevent bacterial growth.
■ Administration set should also be changed between different types of blood component and if ABO group of blood being transfused is changed.
■ Specific blood administration tubing is required for all blood transfusions. Blood tubing is changed every 4 hours or 4 units, whichever comes first.

Transfusion Reactions

Transfusion reactions are defined as adverse events associated with the transfusion of whole blood or one of its components.

Complications	Signs/Symptoms	Treatment	Extraneous
Febrile transfusion reaction	1 degree rise in temperature May have chills, malaise	Supportive -acetaminophen	Most Common
Hemolytic transfusion reaction	Fever, chills, pain at the site of reaction, nausea/vomiting, shock, dark urine	STOP the transfusion Lots of IV fluids +/− diuretics	Worst reaction. Often a clerical issue - ABO incompatibility
Allergic reaction	Urticaria, pruritus, hives. Anaphylaxis is rare	Symptomatic -antihistamines. Do NOT need to stop transfusion	**Note:** They are not actually allergic to blood but secondary to antibodies in the blood
Transfusion related acute lung injury (TRALI)	Dyspnea, hypoxemia, bilateral chest Dy infiltrates (think ARDS)	STOP the transfusion -airway control, supportive care	Most common cause of death associated with transfusions but...better prognosis than most ARDS
Transfusion associated circulatory overload (TACO)	Dyspnea, edema	Give blood slowly (over 3–4 hours) Diuretics with transfusion	Often occurs in the elderly and chronically anemic

    CHEST PHYSIOTHERAPY

Chest physiotherapy (CPT) is a group of therapies where a spectrum of mechanical techniques is used for the noninvasive clearance of pulmonary secretions from the airways.

Appendix 13: Chest Physiotherapy

Purposes of CPT

- To help patients breathe more freely and to get more oxygen into the body
- To prevent the accumulation of secretions
- To improve respiratory efficiency
- To improve the mobilization of secretions
- To regain the most efficient breathing pattern
- To improve the distribution of ventilation
- To improve the cardiopulmonary exercise tolerance
- To promote expansion of the lungs
- To strengthen respiratory muscles

Precautions

Chest physiotherapy should not be performed on patients with the following conditions:
- Bleeding in the lungs
- Head or neck injuries
- Fractured ribs
- Collapsed lungs
- Acute asthma
- Pulmonary embolism
- Active hemorrhage
- Some spinal injuries
- Open wounds or burns

Risks

The risks and complications associated with chest physiotherapy are:
- Oxygen deficiency if the head is kept lowered for drainage
- Increased intracranial pressure
- Temporary lowering of blood pressure
- Bleeding in the lungs
- Pain or injury to the ribs, muscles, or spine
- Vomiting
- Inhalation of secretions into the lungs
- Heart irregularities

Components of CPT

Chest physiotherapy includes
- Postural drainage or mean gravity-assisted bronchial drainage
- Chest percussion
- Chest vibration
- Turning
- Deep breathing exercises and coughing
- Incentive spirometry

Bronchial Drainage/Postural Drainage

It is a therapeutic modality that uses gravity-assisted positioning designed to improve pulmonary hygiene.

Appendix 13: Chest Physiotherapy

Definition

Postural drainage is the positioning of a patient with an involved lung segment to facilitate the drainage of bronchopulmonary secretions from the tracheobronchial tree with the help of gravity. It involves placing the patient's body in various positions that are intended to drain secretions from the patient's lung segments into the central airways using gravity.

Goal

The fundamental goal of postural drainage is to move loosened secretions toward the proximal airway for eventual removal.

The applied anatomy of lungs helps a nurse to administer postural drainage appropriately.

The nurse must understand the location of the involved lung segments and the proper position to optimize drainage into the proximal airway.

- **Lung lobes and segments:** The lungs are divided into lobes, segments and subsegments and fluid drainage is directed centrally to the hilum.
  - The right lung is composed of three lobes: the upper lobe, the middle lobs and the lower lobe.
  - The left lung is made up of only two lobes: the upper lobe and the lower lobe.
  - The lobes are divided into smaller divisions called segments.
    - The upper lobes on the left and right sides are each made up of three segments: apical, posterior and anterior.
    - The left upper lobe includes the lingual, which corresponds to the middle lobe on the right.
    - The lower lobes each include four segments: superior, anterior, basal, lateral basal and posterior basal.

Right Side	Left Side
Upper Lobe	**Upper Lobe**
• Apical	• Apical-posterior
• Posterior	• Anterior
• Anterior	
Middle Lobe	**Lingula**
• Lateral	• Superior
• Medial	• Inferior
Lower Lobe	**Lower Lobe**
• Superior	• Superior
• Medial basal	• Anteromedial basal
• Anterior basal	• Lateral basal
• Lateral basal	• Posterior basal
• Posterior basal	

Best Time to Perform Postural Drainage

- Postural drainage should be done several times each day.
- Postural drainage should precede meals by 30–60 minutes.
- The duration of treatment continues as long as the patient tolerates the therapy.
- This may last up to 1 hour in certain patients (e.g., CF patients).

Appendix 13: Chest Physiotherapy

Articles Required

A tray containing:

Articles	Purposes
Hand rub	For washing hands
Gloves, gown and mask as indicated	For caregiver protection
Suction equipment	For patients who are unable to clear secretion
Sputum cup or kidney basin	For collecting expectorated sputum
Light towel	For covering area of chest during percussion.
Pillows	For supporting patient and for comfort
Bed or table that can be adjusted or a tilt table	For placing in a range of positions
Tissue papers	For wiping the secretions
Incentive spirometer	For spirometry
Vibrators/massagers approved for physiotherapy	For performing vibrations

Preparation

- Ensure that several hours have passed since the patient has eaten
- Perform a baseline respiratory assessment
- Place the patient on a pulse oximetry
- Place the patient in the position to permit gravity drainage of secretion
- Administer bronchodilators, if needed, to relax the airway muscles

Procedure

Steps	Procedure		Rationale
1.	Explain the procedure to the patient		Proper explanation reduces anxiety and promotes cooperation.
2.	Perform hand hygiene and wear required PPE		Prevents the spread of microorganisms.

Contd...

Appendix 13: Chest Physiotherapy

Steps	Procedure	Rationale
3.	Loosen any tight clothing	Facilitates performance of chest physiotherapy easily.
4.	Place sputum container and tissues within the reach of the client.	Helps to spit the expectorant
5.	Lower head of bed slowly so that client's head is positioned in no greater than 25 downward angle. Right Left Raise 12 inches **Right middle lobe**	Gravity helps to mobilize secretion
6.	Instruct client to remain in position for 3–15 minutes and to inform if any discomfort is felt.	Facilitates proper drainage of secretions

Contd...

Steps	Procedure	Rationale
7.	Instruct client to turn to other side, then to supine position, then the procedure is repeated. The positions are changed to drain different segments of the lungs.	Helps to drain all the segments of lungs

Anterior

Right   Left

Anterior segments (upper lobes)

Steps	Procedure	Rationale
8.	Instruct the client to take deep breathe between position changes.	Facilitates lung expansion and helps in comfort

Breath in   **Breath out**

Steps	Procedure	Rationale
9.	Instruct client to expectorate secretions. If the client is unable to expectorate, perform suctioning. Note the color and characters of sputum.	This helps to clear the chest and airways

Appendix 13: Chest Physiotherapy

Contd...

Steps	Procedure	Rationale
10.	Auscultate chest areas for improved breath sounds. Compare patient respiratory assessment pre and post postural drainage. 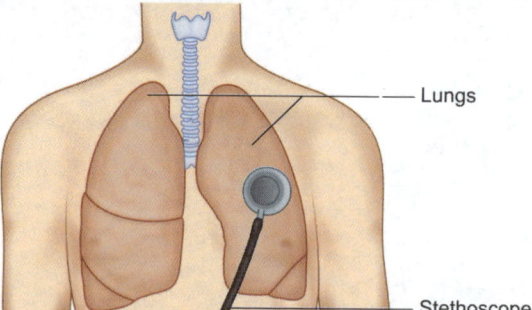	Helps to identify the effect of postural drainage
11.	Remove gloves and wash hands. 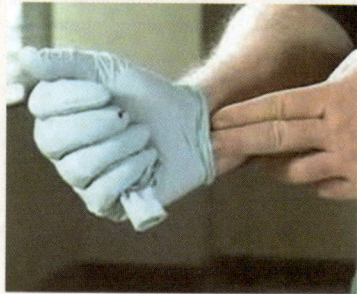 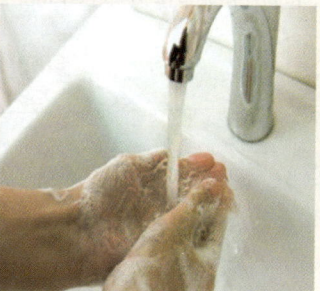	Prevents transfer of microorganisms
12.	Perform oral hygiene following secretion expectoration. 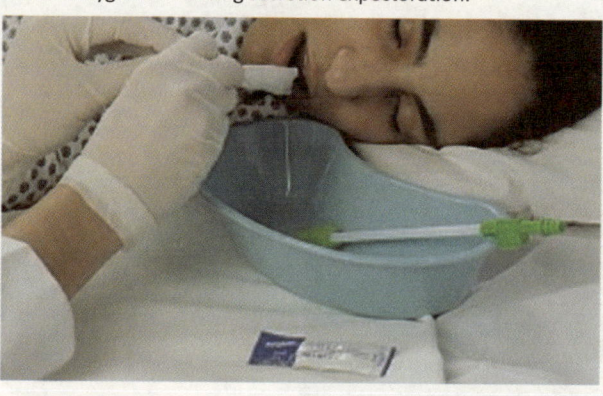	Helps to prevent discomfort produced by the odor of the sputum
13.	Document the procedure with date, time, quantity of sputum, color and other characters with signature.	Documentation fosters quality care

Lungs

Stethoscope

Postural Drainage Positions for CPT

Lung segment	Position	CPT	Representation
Upper Lobes			
Posterior segment	Patient leans forward 30° over the back of a chair (or in bed).	Vibration and percussion can be performed over the upper portion of the back on either side, if ordered.	Right posterior segment Left posterior segment
Apical segment	Patient leans backward 30°.	Vibration and percussion can be performed between the clavicle and the top of the scapula on either side, if ordered.	Upper lobes, apical segment

Contd...

Appendix 13: Chest Physiotherapy

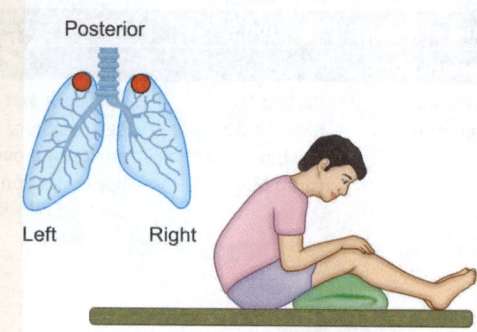

Posterior apical segment

| Anterior segment | Patient lies supine with a pillow under the knees, which enables the abdominal muscles to relax and makes breathing easier. | Vibration and percussion can be performed between the clavicle and nipple of a male patient on either side, if ordered. It may not be possible in a female patient. | 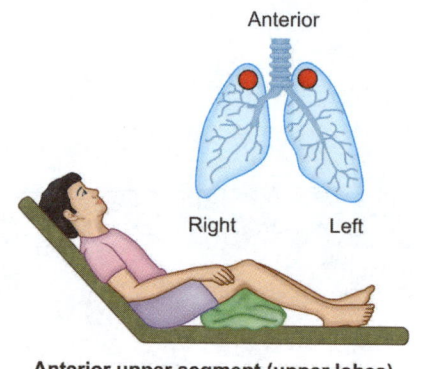 |

Anterior upper segment (upper lobes)

Right Middle and Left Lingual

| Right lateral and medial segments | • Same position is used to drain both lobes.
• Patient lies one-fourth turn up from the back-down position and a pillow may be placed between flexed knees.
• The foot of the bed is elevated 15° (14 inches). | Vibration and percussion can be performed below the right nipple area in a male patient, if ordered. It may not be possible in a female patient. | 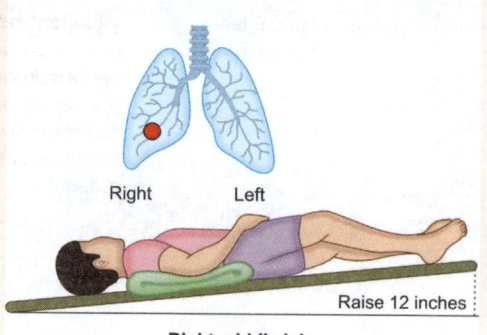 |

Raise 12 inches

Right middle lobe

Contd...

Appendix 13: Chest Physiotherapy

| Left superior and inferior lingual segments | • Same position is used to drain both lobes.
• Patient lies one-fourth turn up from the back-down position and a pillow may be placed between flexed knees.
• The foot of the bed is elevated 15° (14 inches). | Vibration and percussion can be performed below the left nipple area in a male patient, if ordered. It may not be possible in a female patient. | 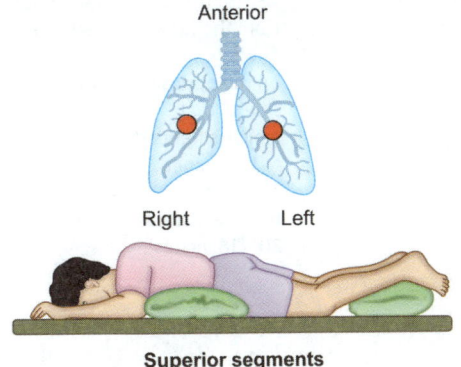
Superior segments

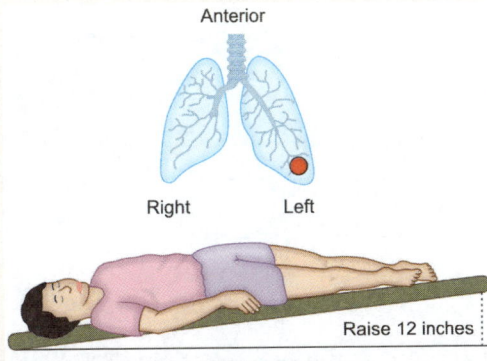
Left lingular |

Lower Lobes

| Posterior basal segment | • Patient lies face down on the bed with the pillow between hips.
• The foot of the bed is elevated 30° (18 inches). | Vibration and percussion can be performed over the appropriate lobe, if ordered. | 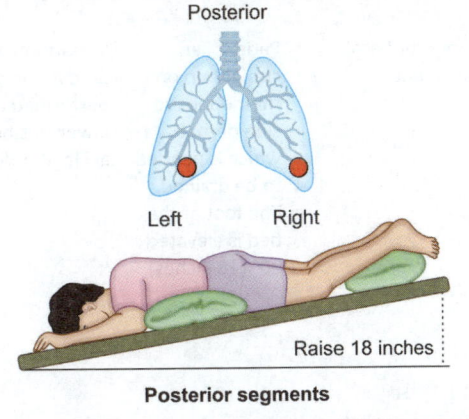
Posterior segments |

Contd...

Appendix 13: Chest Physiotherapy

Lateral basal segment	• Patient lies one-fourth turn up from the face-down position on the opposite side of that which is needed to be drained. • The foot of the bed is elevated 30° (18 inches).	Vibration and percussion can be performed over the posterolateral areas of the lower ribs, if ordered.	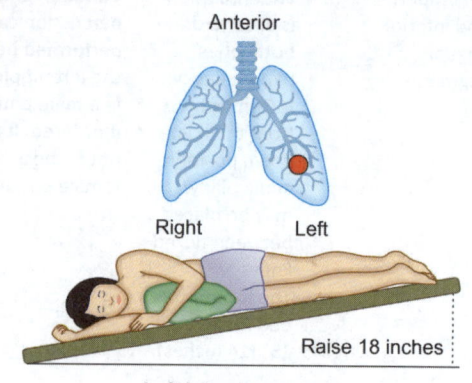 **Left lateral segments**
			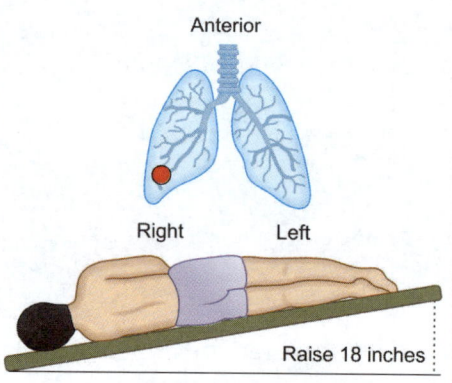 **Right lateral segments**
Anterior basal segment	• Patient lies straight up on their opposite side of that which is needed to be drained. • The foot of the bed is elevated 30° (18 inches).	Vibration and percussion can be performed over the lower ribs below the axilla, if ordered.	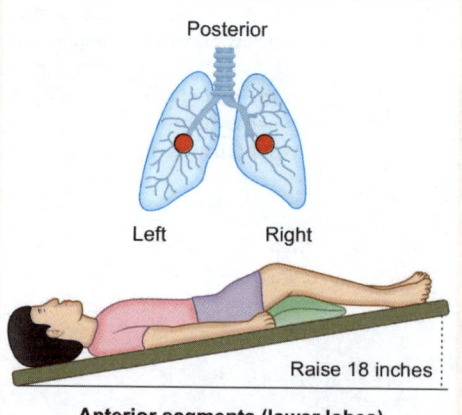 **Anterior segments (lower lobes)**

Contd...

Superior segment	• Patient lies face down on the bed with a pillow beneath the hips. • The bed is in the flat position.	Vibration and percussion can be performed in the middle of the back below the scapula on whichever side is needed, if ordered.	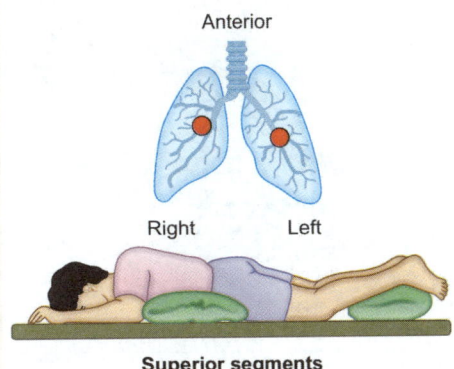

Chest Percussion

Percussion aids in the removal of secretions from the tracheobronchial tree. Percussion is done by cupping the hand so as to allow a cushion of air to come between the percussor hand and the patient. Mechanical energy is produced by compression of the air between the cupped hand and the chest wall. If this is done properly, a popping sound (similar to striking the bottom of a ketchup bottle) will be heard when the patient is percussed. There should be a towel between the patient and the percussor hand in order to prevent irritation of the skin. Proper force and rhythm can be accomplished by placing the hands not farther than 5 inches from the chest and then alternating flexing and extending of the wrists (similar to a waving motion). The procedure should last 5–7 minutes per affected area.

Percussion is applied over the surface landmarks of the bronchial segments that are being drained. The hands rhythmically and alternately strike the chest wall. Incisions, skin grafts, and bony prominences should be avoided during percussion.

Procedure

1. Wash hands and don gloves.
2. Cover area to be percussed with gown or cloth towel.
3. Holding arms with elbows slightly flexed, cup your hands with thumbs and fingers closed, keeping wrists loose and relaxed.
4. Rhythmically flex and extend wrists to clap over area.
5. This motion produces vibrations that loosen secretions for easier removal with coughing or suctioning.
6. Percuss by alternating hands.
7. Slowly and rhythmically percuss each area for 3–5 minutes.
8. Do not percuss over bone, breasts, or other tender area. Vibrations are not transmitted to the chest wall through bone or breast tissue and percussion in these areas can cause discomfort.
9. Encourage client to cough after percussion of lung areas.
10. Auscultate all lung areas for changes in breath sounds.

Appendix 13: Chest Physiotherapy

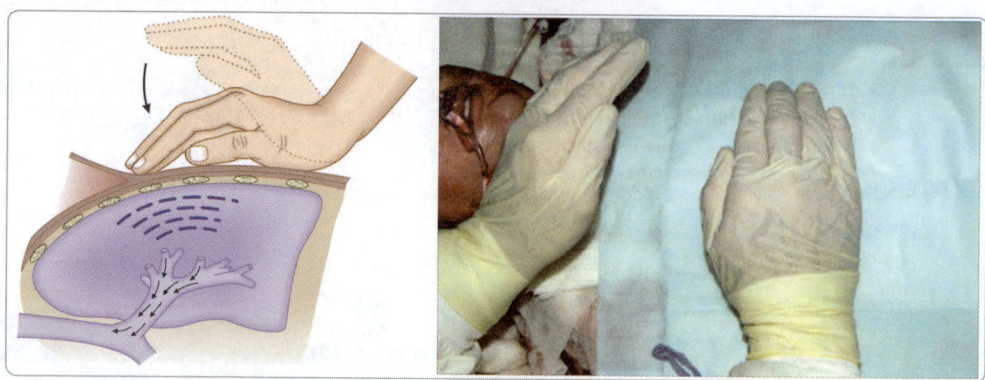

Vibration/Shaking

Vibration/shaking is a shaking movement used to move loosened secretions to larger airways so that they can be coughed up or removed by suctioning. Vibration involves rapid shaking of the chest wall during exhalation. The nurse vibrates the thoracic cage by placing both hands over the percussed areas and vibrating into the patient, isometrically contracting or tensing the muscles of their arms and shoulders.

Vibration frequencies in excess of 200/min can be achieved if the procedure is done correctly. Vibration has mechanical effect in moving secretions towards the main bronchi and also stimulates cough reflex.

Procedure

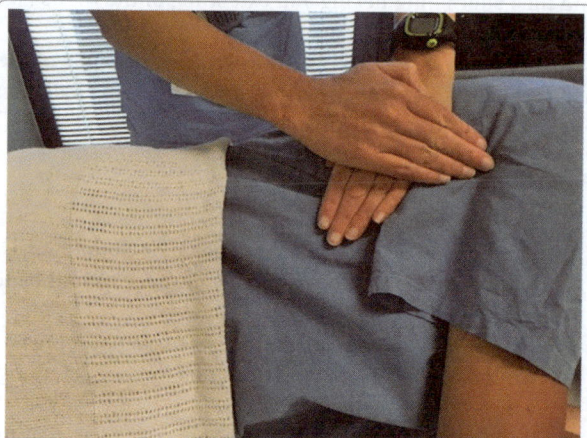

1. It should ideally be performed during expiratory phase.
2. Vibration is applied either by placing both hands directly on the ribcage and over the chest wall or cupping with some facemask like device/single hand and gently compressing and rapidly vibrating the chest wall as patient exhales.
3. After every three or four vibrations, patient should be motivated for deep coughing using diaphragm and abdominal muscles.
4. Patient must be adequately rested in phases.
5. After each cycle of vibration, chest should be auscultated with stethoscope for any new change/improvement in breath sounds.
6. Each cycle of vibration should be decided according to the patient's tolerance and clinical response: usually 10–15 minutes.
7. Vibration is to be avoided over the patient's breasts, spine, sternum, and rib cage to prevent any discomfort to the patient.
8. During shaking patient is placed in supine position with the hands placed on the anterior aspect of chest or one hand anteriorly or posteriorly. In side lying position, the hands may be placed together on the lateral aspect of the thorax anteriorly or posteriorly.

Appendix 13: Chest Physiotherapy

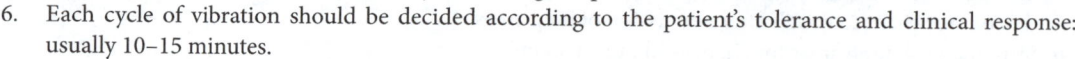

Turning

Turning from side to side permits lung expansion. The patient may turn on his or her own, or be assisted by a caregiver. Turning should be done at a minimum of every two hours if the patient is bedridden. The head of the bed can also be elevated in order to promote drainage.

Breathing Exercises

Breathing exercises play an important role in overall pulmonary rehabilitation program of acute and chronic pulmonary disorders.

Purposes

- To retrain respiratory muscles
- To improve ventilation
- To decrease work of breathing

Types of Breathing Exercises

- Deep breathing exercises
  - Diaphragmatic breathing
  - Purse lip breathing
- Respiratory muscle training
- Segmental breathing or local basal expansion exercises
  - Apical expansion exercises
  - Upper lateral costal expansion exercises
  - Lower lateral costal expansion exercises
  - Posterior basal expansion exercises
- Glossopharyngeal breathing

Deep Breathing Exercises

- Deep breathing helps to expand the lungs and forces an improved distribution of the air into all sections of the lungs. There are two types of deep breathing exercises.

Diaphragmatic Breathing Exercise

Diaphragmatic breathing strengthens the diaphragm, decreases the use of accessory muscles and allows for better emptying of the lungs. It helps the patient breathe in a controlled manner during activities that produce dyspnea. Advise the patient to stop exercise if shortness of breath occur.

Procedure

1. Explain the procedure to the patient.
2. Ask the patient to clear the nasal passages.
3. The patient should stand firmly or sit in semi-Fowler's position.
4. The patient's back should kept straight. This helps to promote full expansion of the lungs.
5. Place one hand on stomach just below the ribs and the other hand at mid chest.
6. The knees should be flexed.

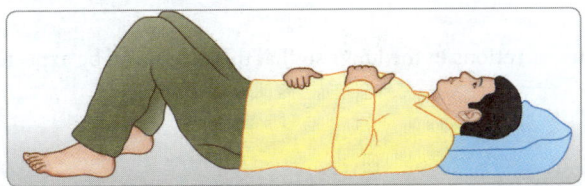

Appendix 13: Chest Physiotherapy

- Instruct the patient to inhale slowly and deeply through the nose letting the abdomen protrudes as far as it will.

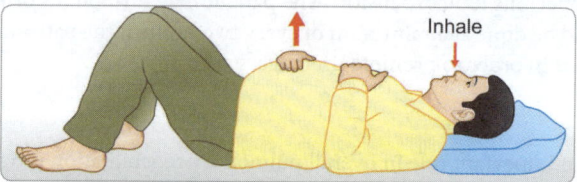

- Instruct the patient to hold his breath for at least 3 seconds.
- Instruct the patient to exhale slowly through pursed lips while tightening the abdominal muscles.
- Press firmly inward and upward on the abdomen while breathing out. This facilitates slower and complete emptying of the lungs.

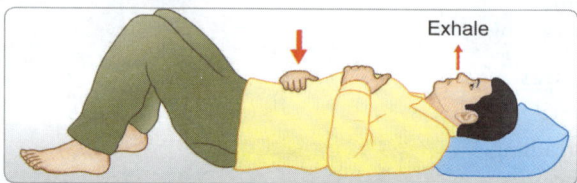

- This procedure should be done for 1 minute followed by a rest period of 2min.
- Work up to 2 minutes four times daily in different positions like supine, sitting, standing and walking.

Pursed-lip Breathing

Pursed lip breathing slows the respiratory rate, decreases the dynamic compression of the airways and thus keeps the airways open longer.

Procedure

1. Explain the procedure to the patient.
2. Ask the patient to clear the nasal passages.
3. The patient should stand firmly or sit in semi-Fowler's position
4. The patient's back should kept straight. This helps to promote full expansion of the lungs.
5. Have the patient inhale slowly through the nose to the count of 2.
6. Instruct the patient to exhale slowly and evenly against pursed lips to the count of 4 while contacting (tightening) the abdominal muscles.
7. Avoid exhaling forcefully.
8. Pursing the lips increases the intrabronchial, intra-alveolar pressure (helps maintain them open)

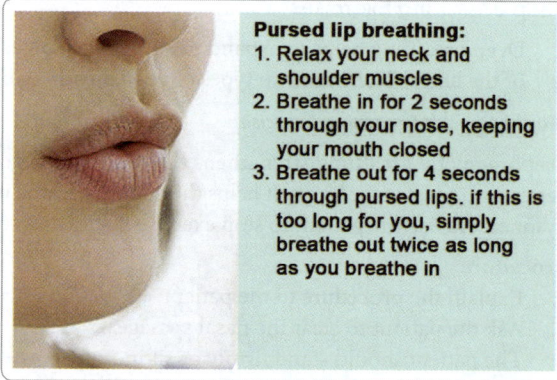

Pursed lip breathing:
1. Relax your neck and shoulder muscles
2. Breathe in for 2 seconds through your nose, keeping your mouth closed
3. Breathe out for 4 seconds through pursed lips. if this is too long for you, simply breathe out twice as long as you breathe in

Coughing

Coughing helps to break up secretions in the lungs so that the mucus can be expectorated or suctioned out if necessary.

Appendix 13: Chest Physiotherapy

Procedure

1. Ask the patient to sit upright or semi-Flower's position. This facilitates deep inhalation.
2. Instruct the patient to place one hand on stomach just below the ribs and the other hand at mid chest with the knees flexed.
3. Instruct the patient to take slow inspiration deeply through the nose and watch for chest movement.
4. Instruct him to hold breath to count of 5.
5. Ask the patient to exhale forcefully and then release air while flexing forward and simultaneously having short puffs or coughs.
6. Repeat for 3 deep coughs or until mucus is expectorated.
7. This procedure is repeated several times a day.

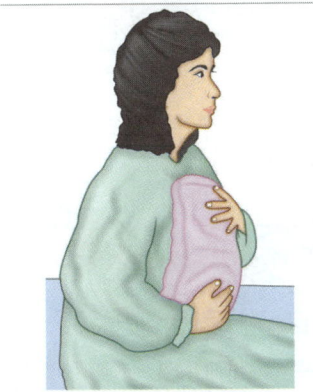

Step 1
- Sit on the edge of a bed or a chair. Or lie on your back with your knees slightly bent
- Lean forward slightly. Hold a pillow firmly against your incision with both hands
- Breathe out normally

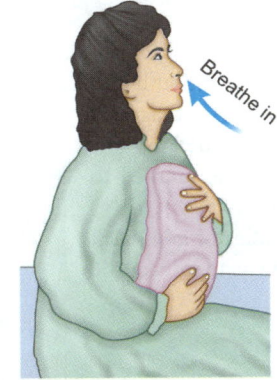

Step 2
- Breathe in slowly and deeply through your nose
- Then breathe out fully through your mouth. Repeat
- Take a third deep breath. Fill your lungs as much as you can

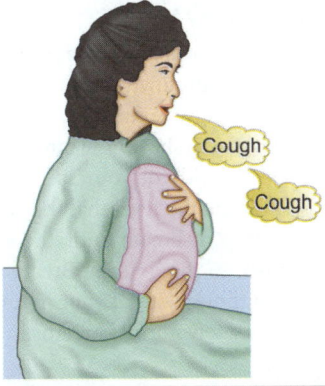

Step 3
- Cough 2 or 3 times in a row
- Try to push all of the air out of your lungs as you cough
- Then relax and breathe normally
- Repeat as directed

Incentive Spirometry (IS)

- Incentive Spirometry helps to achieve sustained maximal inspiration (SMI).
- The physiologic principle of SMI is to produce a maximal transpulmonary pressure gradient by generating a more negative intrapleural pressure. This pressure gradient produces alveolar hyperinflation with maximal airflow during the inspiratory phase.

Goals

- To optimize lung inflation
- To prevent atelectasis
- To optimize the cough mechanism by providing larger lung volumes
- To assess the effectiveness of therapy or detect the onset of acute pulmonary disease.

Appendix 13: Chest Physiotherapy

Procedure

Using your incentive spirometer

Your incentive spirometer will show how well you are breathing. Using it will help you get back to breathing your best. And it can help you avoid complications by keeping your lungs clear and active after surgery or an illness.

Get ready

1. Sit upright, or as far upright as you can.
2. If you have an incision, apply light pressure to it with a pillow.
3. Breathe normally a few times.

A deep, steady breath

4. Exhale normally. Close your lips around the mouthpiece.
5. Breathe in slowly and steadily through your mouth until your lungs are full. The volume indicator (see diagram) will rise to show how much air you've breathed in.
6. On the side of your spirometer, move the marked to show the top level that the volume incdicator got to.
7. Hold your breath until the volume indicator goes back down to the bottom. Breathe out slowly, then take the mouthpiece out of your mouth.
8. Take a few normal breaths.

Repeat

9. Repeat steps 4 to 8 numbers of times. Each time you take a breath, try to move the indicator higher than the time before.
10. After you've done a set of 10 breaths, cough. This will help clear the mucus out of your lungs.
11. Between exercises, put the mouthpiece in a plastic storage bag.

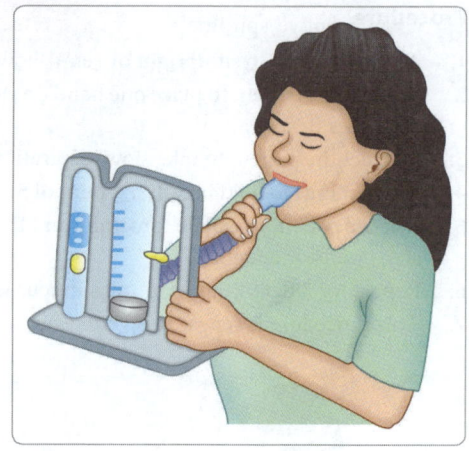

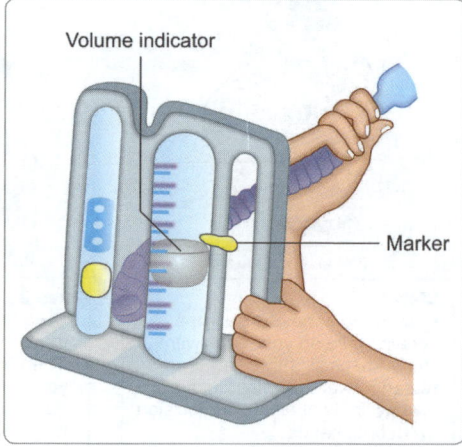

Volume indicator

Marker

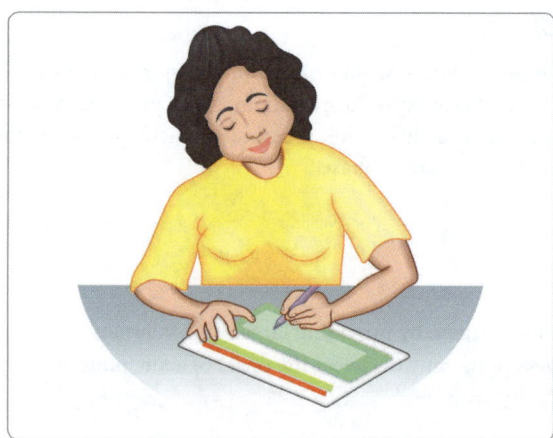

Use your incentive spirometer to times a day. After each set of 10 breaths, record your top score on the incentive spirometer chart on the back of the page. Follow your progress each day.

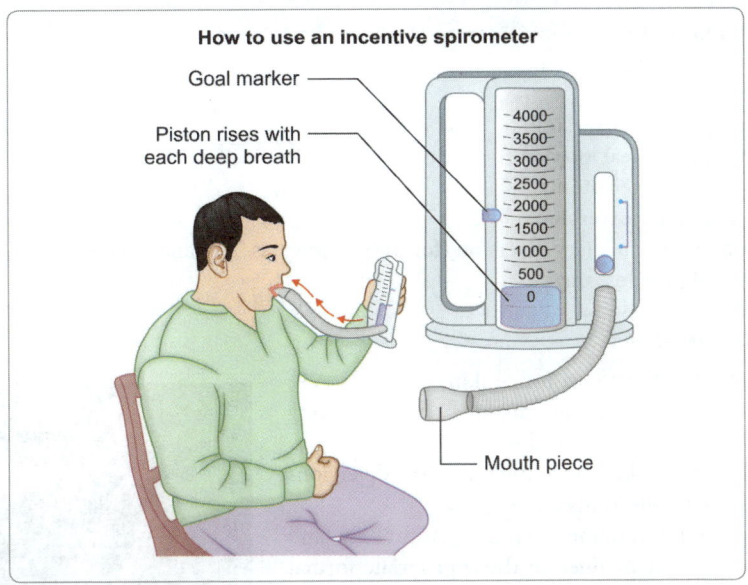

How to use an incentive spirometer

Goal marker

Piston rises with each deep breath

Mouth piece

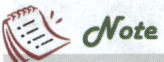 **Note**

Respiratory or pulmonary care nurse plays an important role in performing chest physiotherapy. They have an important role in educating the patient regarding these techniques. In addition to these, they also incorporate many other techniques such as early mobilization, ventilator hyperinflation, etc. especially in the management of critically ill patients.

14 URINARY DIVERSION PROCEDURE

A urinary diversion is required when the bladder can no longer function normally as a reservoir for storing urine. Urinary diversion procedures are performed to divert urine from the bladder to a new exit site.

Definition: Urinary diversion is a surgical procedure that reroutes the normal flow of urine out of the body when urine flow is blocked usually through a surgically created opening in the skin.

Indications

- Cancer of the urinary bladder
- Management of pelvic malignancy
- Birth defects
- Strictures
- Trauma to the ureters and urethra
- Neurogenic bladder
- Chronic inflammatory conditions causing severe ureteral and renal damage

Appendix 14: Urinary Diversion Procedure

Types of Urinary Diversion

- **Based on duration:**
  - Temporary urinary diversion
  - Permanent urinary diversion
- **Based on parts involved:**
  - **Cutaneous urinary diversion:**
    - Ileal conduit (ileal loop)
    - Cutaneous ureterostomy
  - **Continent urinary diversion:**
    - Continent ileal urinary diversion (formerly known as "Indiana pouch")
    - Ureterosigmoidostomy

Nurse's Responsibility

- Assess, monitor stoma and peristomal skin.
- Maintenance and care of stoma/stoma site including changing the accessories like pouches.
- Assessment of neo bladder and other urinary diversions and escalate any complications found.
- Records all care information concisely, accurately and completely, in a timely manner, in the appropriate format and on the appropriate forms.
- Maintains aseptic technique while handling stoma.

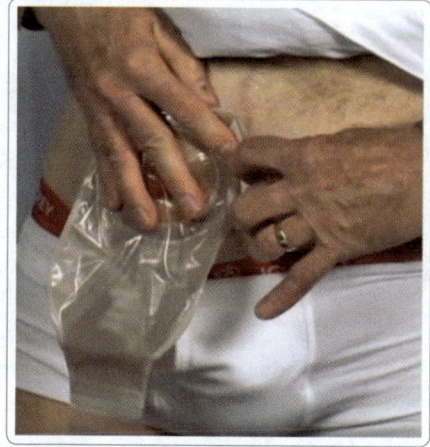

Changing a Pouch

- Drainable pouches need to be changed every 3–5 days.
- Change pouches if there are any leaks or irritation.
- Change the pouch if there is any itching around the stoma
- Urostomy pouches can be changed anytime.

Articles Required

A tray containing:

Articles	Purposes
New pouch	For changing
Damp wash clothes or wipes	For cleaning the stoma
Sizing template	For measuring the stoma and size the opening
Pen	For tracing the size of the stoma
Scissors	For cutting the stomal opening
Kidney tray/paper bag/disposable garbage bag	For discarding the soiled waste
Urine collection container/commode/access to toilet	For safe discarding the urine

Procedure

1. Explain the procedure to the patient
2. Provide privacy
3. Gather supplies

4. Wash hands
5. Remove the old pouch gently and slowly by peeling away one corner of the barrier
6. Discard the used pouch
7. Inspect the stoma and the skin surrounding it
8. Clean skin with water and dry it
9. Apply the new pouch by centering the cut opening over the stoma
10. Emptying a pouch:
    i. Check the pouch level. Empty or change the pouch when it is one third to one half full. Emptying a pouch:
    ii. Check the pouch level. Empty or change the pouch when it is one third to one half full.
11. Empty the pouch on a regular schedule
12. Help the patient to Put on garments and change the linen if needed
13. Replace the articles after washing
14. Wash hands
15. Document the procedure including the date, time, nature of stoma.

Six Easy Steps to Change Ostomy Pouch

Step 1: Wash hands properly under the running water

Step 2: Gently and slowly, remove the pouch while giving support to the skin. Adhesive remover wipes can ease the process

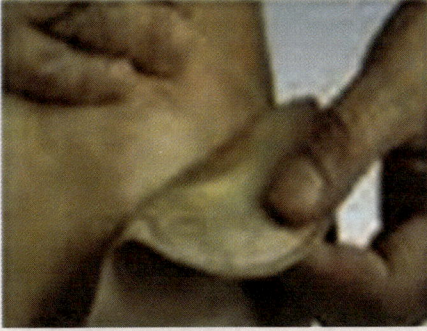

Step 3: Wrap it in a newspaper and put it in an ordinary plastic bag then to the domestic refuse or whichever way is convenient.

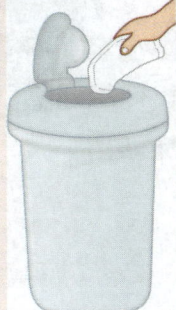

Contd...

Appendix 14: Urinary Diversion Procedure

Six Easy Steps to Change Ostomy Pouch

Step 4: Gently clean around the stoma using lukewarm water and dry wipe taking care not to rub. Do not use soap or any other solvent as it may irritate the skin

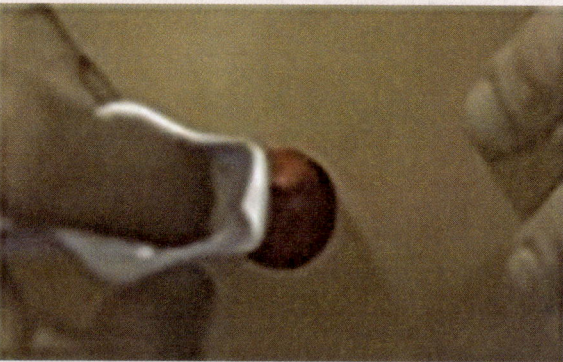

Step 5: Hole in the stoma pouch flange may need to be cut to the correct size.

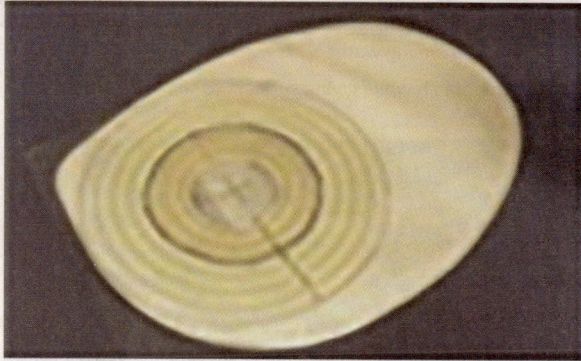

Step 6: After removing the protective cover from the adhesive flange. Fit the pouch over the stoma making sure there are not creases which might cause leakage

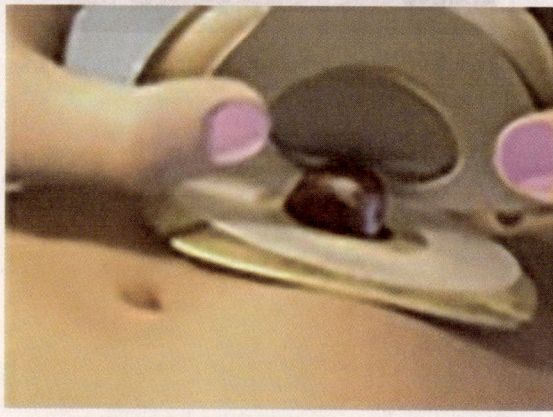

Note: Hold it for 20-30 seconds, for proper adhesion to your skin.

Appendix 14: Urinary Diversion Procedure

VAGINAL IRRIGATION

The vaginal irrigation is also known as vaginal douching. The word "douche" comes from the French word, which means to wash or soak. Douching is the practice of washing or flushing the vagina with water or other fluids at a very low pressure.

Vaginal irrigation or a vaginal douche, is the injection of fluid either plain or medicated solution into the vaginal canal under low pressure in order to cleanse the vaginal tract prior to a surgical procedure or examination or due to vaginal drainage.

Purposes

- Aids in mechanical cleansing of the vaginal tract and the cervix as in leukorrhea.
- Helps to remove any foul odor that may be present.
- Helps to cleanse and irrigate the cervix after cauterization.
- Reduces swelling and promote healing after cauterization.
- As a preoperative procedure on most patients having gynecologic surgery
- For cleansing the vaginal canal, removing an irritating discharge.
- To relieve inflammation and congestion of the genital tract.
- To apply an antiseptic solution to prevent the growth of microorganisms as in preparation of surgery.
- To arrest hemorrhage.
- To stimulate circulation of pelvic organs and promote absorption of exudates.

Solutions Used

- Sterile water
- Normal saline
- Sodium bicarbonate 2%
- Vinegar (acetic acid) 1%
- Savlon 1 in 1000
- Potassium permanganate 1 in 4000
- Boric acid 2%
- Acriflavine 1 in 4000
- Dettol 2%
- Bichloride of mercury 1 in 4000

General Instructions

- Douches are given only on the doctor's orders.
- Never give during pregnancy or menstruation and puerperium as it may carry infection to the uterus.
- Clean the perineum thoroughly before the douches are given. Clean the perineum from above downwards towards the rectum to prevent colon bacilli entering the urethral meatus.
- Usually a 'clean technique' is enough for all patients. However, 'sterile technique' is used in all cases when indicated, e.g., vaginal operations.
- Use solution of correct strength to prevent chemical irritation.
- Adjust the height of the reservoir to regulate the pressure of the solution flowing into the vagina. Therefore, the height of the irrigating can should be not more than 24 inches from the level of the patient's hips.
- Regulate the temperature of the solution according to the purpose of irrigation. For most of the irrigation, a temperature of 40.5ºC is tolerated by the patient. To relieve inflammation and to check bleeding, a higher temperature is used.

- Gravity will aid to the inflow of solution, if the hips are elevated and the head is low. Gravity also aids the outflow of solution if the patient is raised to the sitting position on the completion of the treatment.
- The treatment should not be done hastily if the therapeutic effects are to be achieved. It should take at least 20–30 minutes to give two pints of solution.
- Do the procedure in an adequate light.

Articles Required

A tray containing:

Articles	Purpose
Irrigating can with tubing and a clamp	For using as a reservoir for irrigation
Irrigating solution	For irrigating the vagina
A sterile douche tray with douche and Douche nozzle	For directing the fluid into the vaginal canal
Bath blanket	For providing privacy for the patient
Jug with extra fluid	For complete irrigation of vagina
Bedpan or douche pan with cover	For receiving the return flow
IV pole	For adjusting the height of the irrigating can
Sponge holding forceps	For cleaning the perineum
A small bowl with wet cotton swabs	For cleaning the perineum
A small bowl with dry cotton balls or gauze pieces	For drying the perineum
Cotton applicators	For applying the medication, if ordered
Mackintosh and towel	For protecting the bedding and the garments
Vaginal speculum, If required	For examining the vagina and to apply the medication
Kidney tray and paper bag	For discarding the soiled wastes
Extra sheets and garments	For changing after the procedure
Screen	For providing privacy

Procedure

Steps	Procedure	Rationale
1.	Explain the procedure to the patient including the sequence of the procedure and the level of cooperation expected.	Allays anxiety and wins confidence and cooperation.
2.	Provide privacy with screens. Close the doors and windows as needed.	Maintains client's self esteem

Contd...

Steps	Procedure	Rationale
3.	Ask the patient to void.	Reduces the discomfort of a full bladder.
4.	Assist the patient to a dorsal recumbent position with knees flexed and hips rotated laterally on the bed pan. Or place the patient on a sims' position. The hips should be higher than the shoulders to aid in the gravity flow. A pillow under the back will make the patient more comfortable. Remove the back rest and extra pillow if any. Bring the patient to the edge of the bed to avoid over reaching. Adjust the height of the bed to the comfortable working of the nurse.	Facilitates comfort and ensures ease of access to the vagina. Proper positioning prevents back strain to the nurse
5.	Place the mackintosh and towel under the patient.	Prevents soiling of linen and clothing.
6.	Cover the patient with a bath blanket or a sheet and fanfold the top covers to the foot end of the bed. Drape the patient as for any gynecological examinations and expose only the perineum. Remove the bottom garments or raise it above the waist level.	Minimum exposure lessens embarrassment and helps to provide warmth.
7.	Keep all the articles arranged at the bedside.	Organization facilitates accurate skill performance.

Appendix 15: Vaginal Irrigation

Contd...

Steps	Procedure	Rationale
8.	Wash hands. Wear appropriate PPE	Prevents transfer of microorganisms.
9.	Pour the solution into the can and allow little solution to run through the tubing. 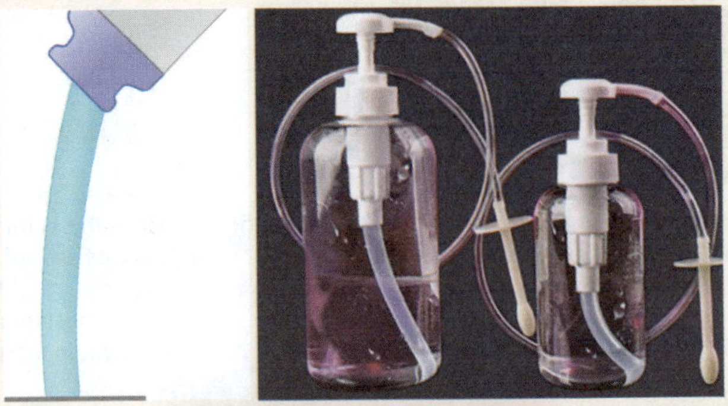 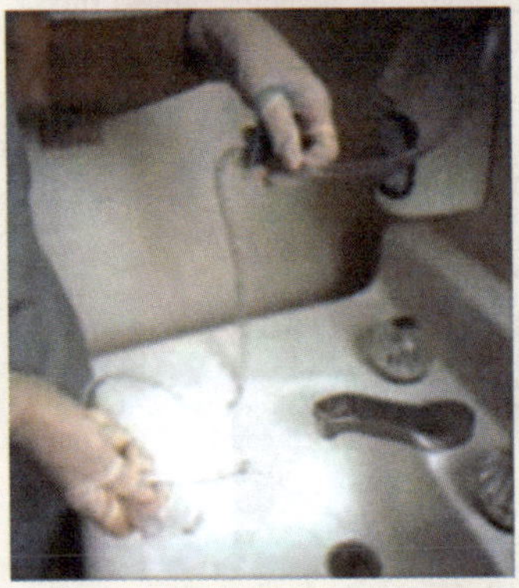	Height of can determines the force of fluid.

Tighten the clamp.

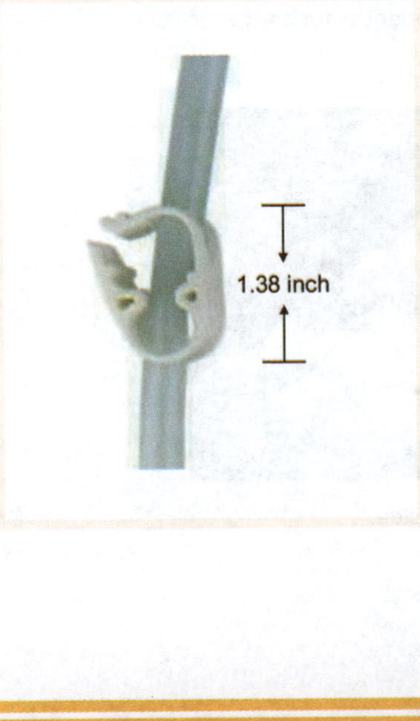

1.38 inch

Contd...

Steps	Procedure	Rationale
	Hang the can on the IV pole not more than 24 inches/30 cm/2 feet from the level of the patient's hip. 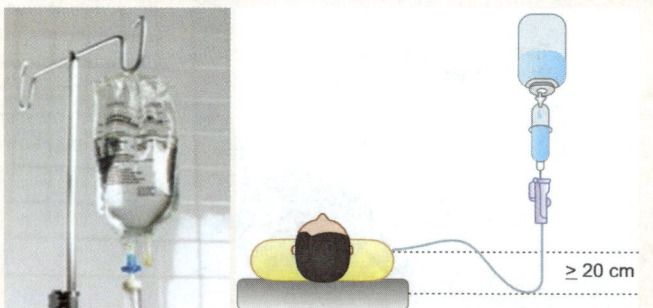	
10.	Clean the perineum with wet swabs using the sponge holding forceps. 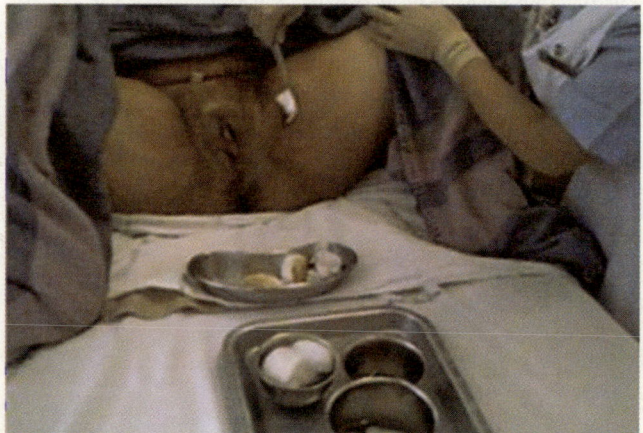	This prevents the infection carried to the vaginal canal.
11.	Examine the douche nozzle for any cracks and connect it to the tubing attached to the can. Wet and lubricate the douche nozzle. 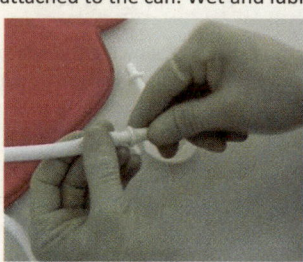 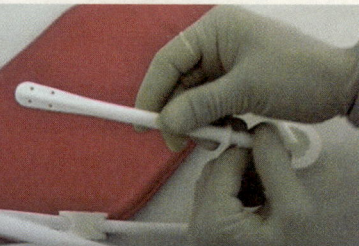	Cracks in the douche nozzle may cause injury of the vaginal wall. Lubrication helps to prevent friction and tissue trauma.

Contd...

Appendix 15: Vaginal Irrigation

Steps	Procedure	Rationale
12.	Assess the temperature of water by pouring a little amount on the wrist. 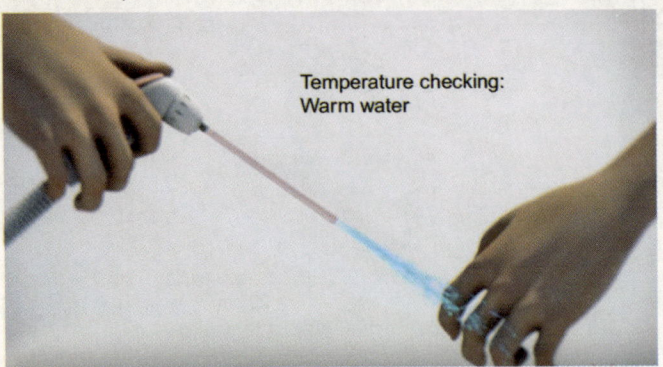 Temperature checking: Warm water Allow small amount of solution to flow over the vulva. Regulate the flow of fluid by adjusting the screw clamp. 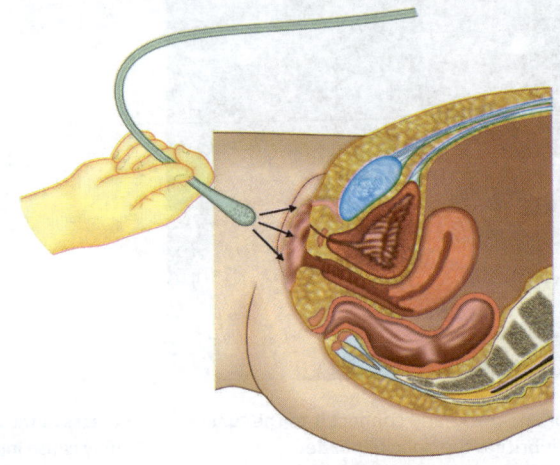	Pouring solution over the vulva removes any gross discharge. It also helps to determine the tolerance of the patient to the temperature of the solution. Too much pressure in a vaginal irrigation may force infections into the cervical canal.
13.	Separate the labia with the thumb and forefinger of the left hand and gently insert the nozzle into the vagina about 2–3 inches or about 7 cm. 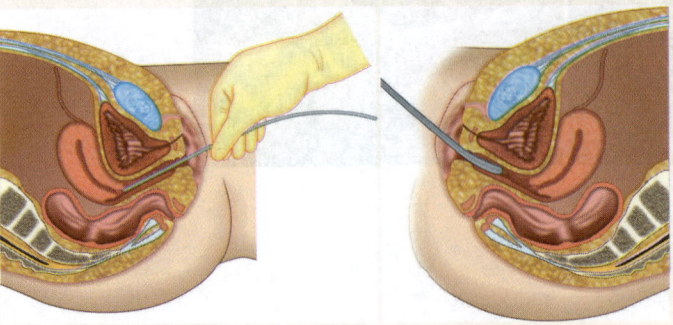	Following the anatomical curve will prevent injury to the vaginal mucosa.

Contd...

Steps	Procedure	Rationale

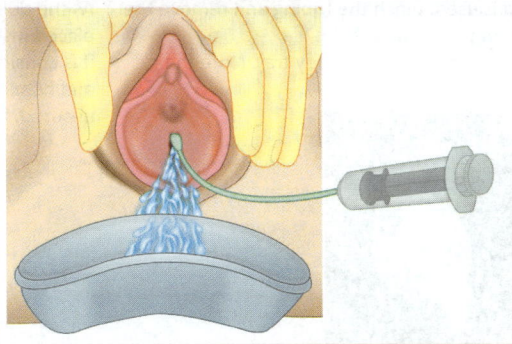

Direct the nozzle downward and backwards along the curve of the vaginal canal.

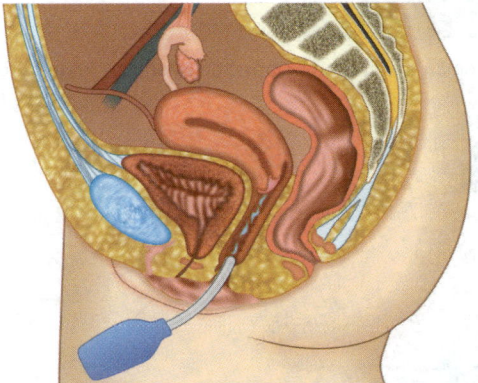

| 14. | Allow the fluid to run in a steady stream. Rotate the nozzle. As the solution runs in, it flows out again into the bedpan. | Rotating the nozzle ensures thorough cleansing of the vaginal walls including the anterior, posterior and lateral fornices (pouches). |

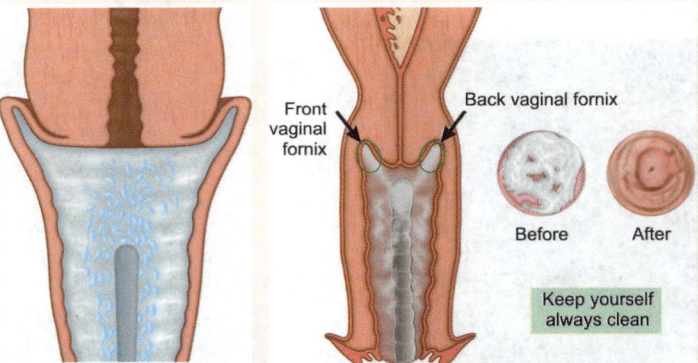

Front vaginal fornix

Back vaginal fornix

Before   After

Keep yourself always clean

Contd...

Appendix 15: Vaginal Irrigation

Steps	Procedure	Rationale
15.	When a required amount of fluid is used, pinch the tubing and remove the nozzle from the vaginal canal. Clamp the tubing. Disconnect the douche nozzle and place it in the kidney tray. Note the character of the return flow. 	As the douche nozzle is placed inside the vagina, it is considered as infected and hence safe disposal is ensured.
16.	Help the patient to a sitting position on the bedpan to drain the solution from the vaginal canal. Remove the bedpan, turn the patient to one side and dry the perineum and buttocks. 	Helps to drain the solution by gravity after cleansing. Promotes comfort.

Contd...

Steps	Procedure	Rationale
17.	If any medication is to be applied, insert the speculum into the vagina to visualize the cervix and apply the medications using the cotton applicators. Apply a perineal pad.	Perineal pad prevents staining of the garments by the medications.
18.	Remove the mackintosh and towel and re-arrange the bed. Change the garments and bed linen as necessary. Adjust the position of the patient in bed and make her comfortable.	Promotes warmth and comfort.
19.	Take all the articles to the utility room. Note the character of the fluid in the bedpan. Empty the bedpan and clean it as usual. Rinse the douche nozzle in cold running water first and then with warm soapy water. Rinse it thoroughly under the running water again and put it for boiling, or disinfect it in an appropriate disinfectant. Clean all the articles and dry them and store them in their proper place.	Ensures use for another patient. Safe disposal protects from contamination.
20.	Remove PPE and perform hand hygiene	Prevents transfer of microorganisms.
21.	Document the procedure on the nurse's record with date and time, type and the amount of solution used, amount and type of vaginal discharge present (if any) and the patient's reaction to the douche along with the signature of the nurse.	Documentation fosters quality care.

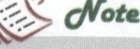

Note

- If the woman is menstruating give a douche as per doctor's prescription.
- Remember the pressure of an aqueous solution in a container has been established as ½ pound for every one foot of elevation. The pressure of the irrigating fluid used for vaginal irrigation should not exceed one pound.
- In performing vaginal irrigation to patients with gonorrhea, wear gown and use gloves and goggles.
- Use smaller nozzles for virgins.
- If a glass nozzle is used, it must be carefully examined for cracks before and after the insertion to prevent injury to the vaginal wall.

Appendix 15: Vaginal Irrigation